SPARKS & TAYLOR'S

Nursing Diagnosis Reference Manual

Tenth Edition

Linda Lee Phelps, DNP, RN
Clinical Assistant Professor
College of Nursing and Health Innovation
Arizona State University
Phoenix, Arizona

Wolters Kluwer

Philadelphia • Baltimore • New York • London
Buenos Aires • Hong Kong • Sydney • Tokyo

Acquisitions Editor: Natasha McIntyre
Director of Product Development: Jennifer Forestieri
Development Editor: Annette Ferran
Editorial Coordinator: Emily Buccieri
Production Project Manager: Marian Bellus
Editorial Assistant: Dan Reilly
Design Coordinator: Terry Mallon
Manufacturing Coordinator: Karin Duffield
Prepress Vendor: S4Carlisle Publishing Services

10th edition

Credits

Nursing diagnoses, definitions, and characteristics from Herdman, T. H., and Kamitsuru, S. (Eds.). Nursing Diagnoses: Definitions and Classification 2015–2017. Copyright © 2014, 1994–2014 by NANDA International. Used by arrangement with John Wiley & Sons Limited.

Suggested NOC labels: Moorhead, S., Johnson, M., & Maas, M. L., & Swanson, E. (2013). *Nursing Outcomes Classification (NOC)* (5th ed.). St. Louis: Mosby.

Suggested NIC labels: Bulechek, G. M., Butcher, H. K., Dochterman, J. M., & Wagner, C. (2013). *Nursing Interventions Classification (NIC)* (6th ed.). St. Louis: Mosby

The clinical treatments described and recommended in this publication are based on research and consultation with nursing, medical, and legal authorities. To the best of our knowledge, these procedures reflect currently accepted practice. Nevertheless, they can't be considered absolute and universal recommendations. For individual applications, all recommendations must be considered in light of the patient's clinical condition and, before administration of new or infrequently used drugs, in light of the latest package-insert information. The authors and publisher disclaim any responsibility for any adverse effects resulting from the suggested procedures, from any undetected errors, or from the reader's misunderstanding of the text.

9 8 7 6 5 4 3 2 1

Printed in China

Library of Congress Cataloging-in-Publication Data

Names: Phelps, Linda Lee, author. | Ralph, Sheila Sparks, author. | Taylor, Cynthia M., author.
Title: Sparks & Taylor's nursing diagnosis reference manual / Linda Lee Phelps, DNP, RN, Clinical Assistant Professor, College of Nursing and Health Innovation, Arizona State University, Phoenix, Arizona.
Other titles: Nursing diagnosis reference manual
Description: Tenth edition. | Philadelphia : Wolters Kluwer Health, 2017. | Revision of: Sparks & Taylor's nursing diagnosis reference manual / Sheila Sparks Ralph, Cynthia M. Taylor. 2014. 9th ed. | Includes bibliographical references and index.
Identifiers: LCCN 2016051171 | ISBN 9781496347817 (paperback)
Subjects: LCSH: Nursing diagnosis—Handbooks, manuals, etc. | BISAC: MEDICAL / Nursing / Assessment & Diagnosis.
Classification: LCC RT48.6 .S66 2017 | DDC 616.07/5—dc23 LC record available at https://lccn.loc.gov/2016051171

Care has been taken to confirm the accuracy of the information presented and to describe generally accepted practices. However, the author(s), editors, and publisher are not responsible for errors or omissions or for any consequences from application of the information in this book and make no warranty, expressed or implied, with respect to the currency, completeness, or accuracy of the contents of the publication. Application of this information in a particular situation remains the professional responsibility of the practitioner; the clinical treatments described and recommended may not be considered absolute and universal recommendations.

The author(s), editors, and publisher have exerted every effort to ensure that drug selection and dosage set forth in this text are in accordance with the current recommendations and practice at the time of publication. However, in view of ongoing research, changes in government regulations, and the constant flow of information relating to drug therapy and drug reactions, the reader is urged to check the package insert for each drug for any change in indications and dosage and for added warnings and precautions. This is particularly important when the recommended agent is a new or infrequently employed drug.

Some drugs and medical devices presented in this publication have Food and Drug Administration (FDA) clearance for limited use in restricted research settings. It is the responsibility of the health care provider to ascertain the FDA status of each drug or device planned for use in his or her clinical practice.

CCS1216

LWW.com

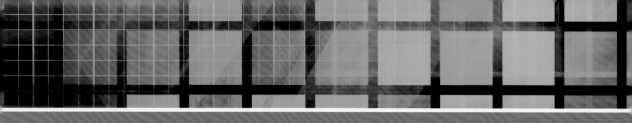

CONTRIBUTORS AND REVIEWERS

CONTRIBUTORS

Elizabeth Braun, MSN, RN, CPN, CNE
Adjunct Clinical Lecturer
Indiana University Health
Indiana University School of Nursing
Indianapolis, Indiana

Maria Holmes, MSN-Ed, RN
Assistant Professor
Clinical Site Coordinator
School of Nursing
Hampton University
Hampton, Virginia

Kelly Holt, MScN, RN, CPMHN(C)
Assistant Clinical Professor
School of Nursing
McMaster University
Hamilton, Ontario
Clinical Nurse Specialist
Mood Disorders Program
St. Joseph's Healthcare Hamilton
Hamilton, Ontario

Carel Mountain, DNP, RN, CNE
Associate Degree Nursing Program
Shasta College
Redding, California

Christine Ullom, DNP, RNC-NIC, CNE, CHSE
Director of Nursing Education
Danville Area Community College
Danville, Illinois

REVIEWERS

Staci Boruff, PhD, RN
Professor of Nursing
Department of Nursing
Walters State Community College
Morristown, Tennessee

Sheila Holland, RN, MSN
Associate Professor of Nursing
Nelms School of Nursing
Jackson State Community College
Jackson, Tennessee

Laly Joseph, DVM, DNP, RN, C, MSN, ARNP, ANP, BC
Assistant Professor of Clinical
School of Nursing and Health Studies
University of Miami
Coral Gables, Florida

Cathleen Kunkler, MSN, RN, ONC, CNE
Director of Nurse Education, Associate Professor
Corning Community College
Corning, New York

Beatriz C. Nieto, PhD, RN
Associate Professor
School of Nursing
The University of Texas -Pan American
Edinburg, Texas

Janette Petro
Community College of Allegheny County
Monroeville, Pennsylvania

Dwayne Pettyjohn, RN-BSN
Program Leader
Nursing Department
Camosun College
Victoria, British Columbia, Canada

L. Jane Rosati, EdD, MSN, RN
Professor
School of Nursing
Daytona State College
Daytona Beach, Florida

Laurie Singel, PhD, MSN, RN-BC
Ila Faye Miller School of Nursing & Health Professions
University of the Incarnate Word
San Antonio, Texas

Susan K. Tucker, RN, DNP, CNE
Program Director
Nursing Education
Gadsden State Community College
Gadsden, Alabama

PREFACE

Sparks and Taylor's Nursing Diagnosis Reference Manual, tenth edition, offers clearly written, authoritative care plans to meet the health care needs of patients throughout the life span. This edition contains care plans for 25 new nursing diagnoses, updated information for 14 nursing diagnoses, and updated definitions and content to meet the 2015–2017 NANDA-I standards. The Applying Evidence-Based Practice feature at the beginning of each section provides evidence-based scenarios for each stage of the life cycle. A new feature in this edition highlights interventions that meet the Quality and Safety Education for Nurses (QSEN) criteria for patient-centered care or safe practice. Look for the icons throughout the book: EBP I PCC QI S T&C

The nursing process is the foundation for all nursing actions. Each care plan included in *Sparks and Taylor's Nursing Diagnosis Reference Manual*, tenth edition, has been constructed utilizing the nursing process. More than 340 comprehensive plans of care for NANDA-I approved nursing diagnoses are distributed throughout eight sections of the book. The care plans were written and reviewed by leading nursing clinicians, educators, and researchers. Each care plan is complete and can be used independently, thereby eliminating the need to search for material in different places.

Sparks and Taylor's Nursing Diagnosis Pocket Guide, third edition, is a pocket-sized companion to this manual. The pocket guide contains one care plan for each diagnosis and is organized using the NNN Taxonomy of Nursing Practice and the ICNP intervention terminology. The pocket guide's compact two-page care plan design is functional in any setting. Both the pocket guide and the reference manual include the linkages between NANDA International and the Nursing Interventions Classification (NIC) and Nursing Outcomes Classification (NOC) labels. You'll find the care plans invaluable in every health care setting you encounter throughout your career.

STUDENT AND INSTRUCTOR RESOURCES

Visit thePoint to find additional resources for students and instructors. Available resources include journal articles, case studies, assignments, evidence-based practice research articles, a QSEN map, a concepts-base curriculum map, and more!

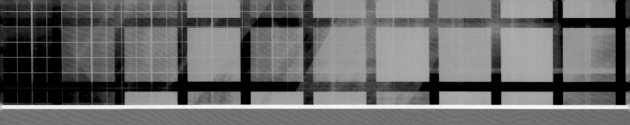

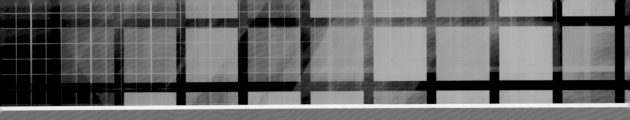

ACKNOWLEDGMENTS

I wish to express my appreciation to the nurses who contributed to the *Nursing Diagnosis Reference Manual*, tenth edition. Their expertise and commitment to quality patient care made this work possible. I am also grateful to Annette Ferran and Natasha McIntyre from Wolters Kluwer for their assistance, patience, and support.

I dedicate this book to all nurses, students to expert clinicians, who are dedicated to providing quality patient care.

CONTENTS

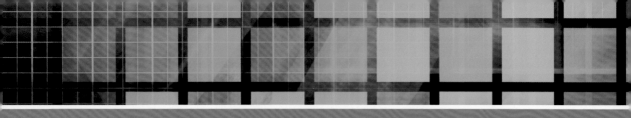

OVERVIEW OF THE NURSING PROCESS

The nursing process provides a framework for independent nursing action, promotes a consistent structure for professional practice, and helps bring focus more precisely on each patient's health care needs. The nursing process is a systematic method for making decisions and implementing care. Steps in the nursing process include

- assessing the patient's problems
- forming a diagnostic statement
- identifying expected outcomes
- creating a plan to achieve expected outcomes and solve the patient's problems
- implementing the plan or assigning others to implement it
- evaluating the plan's effectiveness.

These phases of the nursing process—assessment, nursing diagnosis formation, outcome identification, care planning, implementation, and evaluation—are dynamic, flexible, and frequently overlap. The American Nurses Association has established these phases to meet professional Standards of Practice (American Nurses Association, 2015).

Becoming familiar with the nursing process has many benefits. It will allow you to apply your knowledge and skills in an organized, goal-oriented manner. It will also enable you to communicate about professional topics with colleagues from all clinical specialties and practice settings. Using the nursing process is essential to documenting nursing's role in the provision of comprehensive, quality patient care.

The recognition of the nursing process is an important development in the struggle for greater professional autonomy. By clearly defining those problems a nurse may treat independently, the nursing process has helped to dispel the notion that nursing practice is based solely on carrying out the physician's orders.

Nursing remains in a state of professional evolution. Nurse researchers and expert practitioners continue to develop a body of knowledge specific to the field. Nursing literature is gradually providing direction to students and seasoned practitioners for evidence-based practice. A strong foundation in the nursing process will enable you to better assimilate emerging concepts and to incorporate these concepts into your practice. (See Table 1, *Nursing's Approach to Problem Solving*.)

ASSESSMENT

The first and most critical phase in the nursing process—assessment—consists of the patient history, the physical examination, and pertinent diagnostic studies. Nurses also collect information about patient strengths and areas where potential problems exist. The other nursing process phases—nursing diagnosis formation, outcome identification, planning care, implementation, and evaluation—depend on the quality of the assessment data for their effectiveness.

TABLE 1. NURSING'S APPROACH TO PROBLEM SOLVING

Dynamic and flexible, the phases of the nursing process resemble the steps that many other professions rely on to identify and correct problems. Here's how the nursing process phases correspond to the standard problem-solving method.

NURSING PROCESS	PROBLEM-SOLVING METHOD
Assessment	
• Collect and analyze subjective and objective data about the patient's health problem	• Recognize the problem • Learn about the problem by obtaining facts
Diagnosis	
• State the health problem	• State the nature of the problem
Outcome identification	
• Identify expected outcomes	• Establish goals and a time frame for achieving them
Planning	
• Write a care plan that includes the nursing interventions designed to achieve expected outcomes	• Think of and select ways to achieve goals and solve the problem
Implementation	
• Put the care plan into action • Document the actions taken and their results	• Act on ways to solve the problem
Evaluation	
• Critically examine the results achieved • Review and revise the care plan as needed	• Decide if the actions taken have effectively solved the problem

A properly recorded initial assessment provides

- a way to communicate patient information to other caregivers
- a method of documenting initial baseline data
- a foundation on which to build an effective care plan

Your initial patient assessment begins with the collection of data (patient history, physical examination findings, and diagnostic study data) and ends with a statement of the patient's deficiency in, risk for, or readiness for enhancement of a specific problem that is written as the nursing diagnosis.

Building a Database

The information you collect when taking the patient's history, performing a physical examination, and analyzing test results serves as your assessment database. Your goal is to gather and record information that will be most helpful in assessing your patient. You can't realistically collect—or use—*all* the information that exists about the patient. To limit your database appropriately, ask yourself these questions:

- What data do I want to collect?
- How should I collect the data?
- How should I organize the data to make care planning decisions?

Your answers will help you to be selective in collecting meaningful data during patient assessment.

The well-defined database for a patient may begin with admission signs and symptoms, chief complaint, or medical diagnosis. It may also center on the type of patient care given in a specific setting, such as the intensive care unit (ICU), the emergency department (ED), or an outpatient care center. For example, you wouldn't ask a trauma patient in the ED about a family history of breast cancer, nor would you perform a routine breast examination. You would, however, do these types of assessment during a comprehensive health checkup in an outpatient care setting.

If you work in a setting where patients with similar diagnoses are treated, choose your database from information pertinent to this specific patient population. Even when addressing patients with similar diagnoses, complete a thorough assessment to make sure unanticipated problems don't go unnoticed.

Collecting Subjective and Objective Data

The assessment data you collect and analyze fall into two important categories: subjective and objective. The patient's *history*, embodying a *personal perspective* of problems and strengths, provides *subjective data*. It's your most important assessment data source. Because it's also the most subjective source of patient information, it must be interpreted carefully.

In the *physical examination* of a patient—involving inspection, palpation, percussion, and auscultation—you collect *objective data* about the patient's health status or about the pathologic processes that may be related to illness or injury. In addition to adding to the patient's database, this information helps you interpret the patient's history more accurately by providing a basis for comparison. Use it to validate and amplify the historical data. However, don't allow the physical examination to assume undue importance—formulate your nursing diagnosis by considering *all* the elements of your assessment, not just the examination.

Laboratory test results are another objective form of assessment data and the third essential element in developing your assessment. Laboratory values will help you to interpret—and, usually, clarify—your history and physical examination findings. The advanced technology used in laboratory tests enables you to assess anatomic, physiologic, and chemical processes that can't be assessed subjectively or by physical examination alone. For example, if the patient complains of fatigue (history) and you observe conjunctival pallor (physical examination), check the patient's hemoglobin level and hematocrit (laboratory data).

Both subjective (history) and objective (physical examination and laboratory test results) data are essential for comprehensive patient assessment. They validate each other and together provide more data than either can provide alone. By considering history, physical examination, and laboratory data in their appropriate relationships to one another, you'll be able to develop a nursing diagnosis on which to formulate an effective care plan.

Taking a Complete Health History

This portion of the assessment consists of the subjective data you collect from the patient. A complete health history provides the following information about a patient:

- Biographical data, including ethnic, cultural, health seeking, and spiritual factors
- Chief complaint (or concern)
- History of present illness (or current health status)
- Health promotion behaviors, motivation
- Past health history
- Family medical history
- Psychosocial history
- Activities of daily living (ADLs)
- Review of systems

Follow this orderly format in taking the patient's history, but allow for modifications based on the patient's chief complaint or concern. For example, the health history of a patient with a localized allergic reaction will be much shorter than that of a patient who complains vaguely of mental confusion and severe headaches.

If the patient has a chief complaint, use information from the health history to decide whether problems stem from physiologic causes or psychophysiologic maladaptation and how nursing interventions may help. The depth of such a history depends on the patient's cooperation and your skill in asking insightful questions.

A patient may request a complete physical checkup as part of a periodic (perhaps annual) health maintenance routine. Such a patient may not have a chief complaint. Therefore, this patient's health history should be comprehensive with detailed information about lifestyle, self-image, family and other interpersonal relationships, and degree of satisfaction with current health status.

BOX 1. USING AN ASSESSMENT CHECKLIST

Use an assessment checklist such as this to ensure that you cover all key points during your health history interview. Although the format may vary from one facility to another, all assessment checklist guides include the same key elements.

- ***Reason for hospitalization or chief complaint:*** As patient sees it
- ***Duration of this problem:*** As patient recalls it (Has it affected the patient's lifestyle?)
- ***Other illnesses and previous experience with hospitalization(s):*** Reason, date(s), results, impressions of previous hospitalizations, problems encountered, effect of this hospitalization on education, family, child care, employment, finances
- ***Observation of patient's condition:*** Level of consciousness, well-nourished, healthy, color, skin turgor, senses, headaches, cough, syncope, nausea, seizures, edema, lumps, bruises or bleeding, inflammation, integrity of skin, pressure areas, temperature, range of motion, unusual sensations, paralysis, odors, discharges, pain
- ***Mental and emotional status:*** Cooperative, understanding, anxious, language, expectations, feelings about illness, state of consciousness, mood, self-image, reaction to stress, rapport with interviewer and staff, compatibility with roommate
- ***Review of systems:*** Neurologic, EENT (eye, ear, nose, throat), pulmonary, cardiovascular, GI (gastrointestinal), GU (genitourinary), skin, reproductive, musculoskeletal, and so forth
- ***Allergies:*** Food, drugs, other allergens, type of reaction
- ***Medication:*** Dosage, why taken, when taken, last dose, does the patient have it, any others taken occasionally, recently, why, use of over-the-counter drugs or cough preparations, use of alcohol or recreational drugs
- ***Prostheses:*** Pacemaker, intermittent positive-pressure breathing unit, tracheostomy tube, drainage tubes, feeding tube, catheter, ostomy appliance, breast form, hearing aid, glasses or contact lenses, dentures, false eye, prosthetic limb, cane, brace, walker, does the patient have the device, need anything
- ***Hygiene patterns:*** Dentures, gums, teeth, bath or shower, when taken
- ***Rest and sleep patterns:*** Usual times, aids, difficulties
- ***Activity status:*** Self-care, ambulatory, aids, daily exercise
- ***Bladder and bowel patterns:*** Continence, frequency, nocturia, characteristics of stools and urine, discharge, pain, ostomy, appliances, who cares for these, laxatives, medications
- ***Meals and diet:*** Feeds self, diet restrictions (therapeutic and cultural or preferential), frequency, snacks, allergies, dislikes, fad diets, usual dietary intake
- ***Health practices:*** Breast self-examination, physical examination, Papanicolaou test, testicular self-examination, digital rectal examination, smoking, electrocardiogram, annual chest X-ray, practices related to other conditions, such as glaucoma testing, urine testing, weight control
- ***Lifestyle:*** Parent, family, number of children, residence, occupation, recreation, diversion, interests, financial status, religion, sexuality, education, ethnic background, living environment
- ***Typical day profile:*** As patient describes it
- ***Informant:*** From whom did you obtain this information, patient, family, old records, ambulance driver

Be sure to record health history data in an organized fashion to ensure the information will be meaningful to everyone involved in the patient's care. Some health care facilities provide patient questionnaires or computerized checklists. (See Box 1, *Using an Assessment Checklist*.) These forms make history-taking easier, but they aren't always available. Therefore, you must know how to take a comprehensive health history without them. This is easy to do if you develop an orderly and systematic method of interviewing. Ask the history questions in the same order every time. With experience, you'll know which types of questions to ask in specific patient situations.

REVIEW OF SYSTEMS

When interviewing the patient, use this review of systems as a guide.

- *General*: Overall state of health, ability to carry out ADLs, weight changes, fatigue, exercise tolerance, fever, night sweats, repeated infections
- *Skin:* Changes in color, pigmentation, temperature, moisture, or hair distribution; eruptions; pruritus; scaling; bruising; bleeding; dryness; excessive oiliness; growths; moles; scars; rashes; scalp lesions; brittle, soft, or abnormally formed nails; cyanotic nail beds; pressure ulcers
- *Head*: Trauma, lumps, alopecia, headaches
- *Eyes*: Nearsightedness, farsightedness, glaucoma, cataracts, blurred vision, double vision, tearing, burning, itching, photophobia, pain, inflammation, swelling, color blindness, injuries (also ask about use of glasses or contact lenses, date of last eye examination, and past surgery to correct vision problems)
- *Ears*: Deafness, tinnitus, vertigo, discharge, pain, and tenderness behind the ears, mastoiditis, otitis or other ear infections, earaches, ear surgery
- *Nose*: Sinusitis, discharge, colds, or coryza more than four times per year; rhinitis; trauma; sneezing; loss of sense of smell; obstruction; breathing problems; epistaxis
- *Mouth and throat*: Changes in color or sores on tongue, dental caries, loss of teeth, toothaches, bleeding gums, lesions, loss of taste, hoarseness, sore throats (streptococcal), tonsillitis, voice changes, dysphagia, date of last dental checkup, use of dentures, bridges, or other dental appliances
- *Neck*: Pain, stiffness, swelling, limited movement, or injuries
- *Breasts:* Change in development or lactation pattern, trauma, lumps, pain, discharge from nipples, gynecomastia, changes in contour or in nipples, history of breast cancer (also ask whether the patient knows how to perform breast self-examination)
- *Cardiovascular*: Palpitations, tachycardia, or other rhythm irregularities; pain in chest; dyspnea on exertion; orthopnea; cyanosis; edema; ascites; intermittent claudication; cold extremities; phlebitis; orthostatic hypotension; hypertension; rheumatic fever (also ask whether an electrocardiogram has been performed recently)
- *Respiratory*: Dyspnea, shortness of breath, pain, wheezing, paroxysmal nocturnal dyspnea, orthopnea (number of pillows used), cough, sputum, hemoptysis, night sweats, emphysema, pleurisy, bronchitis, tuberculosis (contacts), pneumonia, asthma, upper respiratory tract infections (also ask about results of chest X-ray and tuberculin skin test)
- *Gastrointestinal*: Changes in appetite or weight, dysphagia, nausea, vomiting, heartburn, eructation, flatulence, abdominal pain, colic, hematemesis, jaundice (pain, fever, intensity, duration, color of urine), stools (color, frequency, consistency, odor, use of laxatives), hemorrhoids, rectal bleeding, changes in bowel habits
- *Renal and genitourinary*: Color of urine, polyuria, oliguria, nocturia (number of times per night), dysuria, frequency, urgency, problem with stream, dribbling, pyuria, retention,

passage of calculi or gravel, sexually transmitted disease (discharge), infections, perineal rashes and irritations, incontinence (stress, functional, total, reflex, urge), protein or sugar ever found in urine

- *Reproductive*: Male—lesions, impotence, prostate problems (also ask about use of contraceptives and whether the patient knows how to perform a testicular self-examination); female—irregular bleeding, discharge, pruritus, pain on intercourse, protrusions, dysmenorrhea, vaginal infections (also ask about number of pregnancies; delivery dates; complications; abortions; onset, regularity, and amount of flow during menarche; last normal menses; use of contraceptives; date of menopause; last Papanicolaou test)
- *Neurologic*: Headaches, seizures, fainting spells, dizziness, tremors, twitches, aphasia, loss of sensation, weakness, paralysis, numbness, tingling, balance problems
- *Psychiatric*: Changes in mood, anxiety, depression, inability to concentrate, phobias, suicidal or homicidal thoughts, hallucinations, delusions
- *Musculoskeletal*: Muscle pain, swelling, redness, pain in joints, back problems, injuries (such as fractured bones, pulled tendons), gait problems, weakness, paralysis, deformities, range of motion, contractures
- *Hematopoietic*: Anemia (type, degree, treatment, response), bleeding, fatigue, bruising (also ask whether patient is receiving anticoagulant therapy)
- *Endocrine* and *metabolic*: Polyuria, polydipsia, polyphagia, thyroid problem, heat or cold intolerance, excessive sweating, changes in hair distribution and amount, nervousness, swollen neck (goiter), moon face, buffalo hump

ENSURING A THOROUGH HISTORY

When documenting the health history, be sure to record both negative and positive findings; that is, note the absence of symptoms that other history data indicate might be present. For example, if a patient reports abdominal pain and burning, ask about experiencing nausea and vomiting or noticing blood in stools. Record the presence or absence of these symptoms.

Remember that the information you record will be used by others who will be caring for the patient. Recorded information can be used as a legal document in a liability case, a malpractice suit, or an insurance disability claim. With these considerations in mind, record history data thoroughly and precisely. Continue your questioning until you're satisfied that you've recorded sufficient detail. Don't be satisfied with inadequate answers, such as "a lot" or "a little"; such subjective terms must be explained within the patient's context to be meaningful. If taking notes seems to make the patient anxious, explain the importance of keeping a written record. To facilitate accurate recording of the patient's answers, familiarize yourself with standard history data abbreviations.

When you complete the patient's health history, it becomes part of the permanent written record. It will serve as a subjective database with which you and other health care professionals can monitor the patient's progress. Remember that history data must be specific and precise. Avoid generalities. Instead, provide pertinent, concise, detailed information that will help determine the direction and sequence of the physical examination—the next phase in your patient assessment.

Physical Examination

After taking the patient's health history, the next step in the assessment process is the *physical examination*. During this assessment phase, you obtain objective data that usually confirm or rule out suspicions raised during the health history interview.

Use four basic techniques to perform a physical examination: *inspection, palpation, percussion,* and *auscultation* (IPPA). These skills require you to use your senses of sight, hearing, touch, and smell to formulate an accurate appraisal of the structures and functions of body systems. Using IPPA skills effectively lessens the chances that you'll overlook something important during the physical examination. In addition, each examination technique collects data that validate and amplify data collected through other IPPA techniques.

Accurate and complete physical assessments depend on two interrelated elements. One is the critical act of sensory perception, by which you receive and perceive external stimuli. The other element is the conceptual, or cognitive, process by which you relate these stimuli to your knowledge base. This two-step process gives meaning to your assessment data.

Develop a system for assessing patients that identifies problem areas in priority order. By performing physical assessments systematically and efficiently instead of in a random or indiscriminate manner, you'll save time and identify priority problems quickly. First, choose an *examination method.* The most commonly used methods for completing a total systematic physical assessment are *head-to-toe* and *major body systems.*

The head-to-toe method is performed by systematically assessing the patient by—as the name suggests—beginning at the head and working toward the toes. Examine all parts of one body region before progressing to the next region to save time and to avoid tiring the patient or yourself. Proceed from left to right within each region so you can make symmetrical comparisons; that is, when examining the head, proceed from the left side of the head to the right side. After completing both sides of one body region, proceed to the next.

The major body systems method of examination involves systematically assessing the patient by examining each body system in priority order or in an established sequence.

Both the head-to-toe and the major body systems methods are systematic and provide a logical, organized framework for collecting physical assessment data. They also provide the same information; therefore, neither is more correct than the other. Choose the method (or a variation of it) that works well for you and is appropriate for your patient population. Follow this routine whenever you assess a patient, and try not to deviate from it.

To decide which method to use, first determine whether the patient's condition is life-threatening. Identifying the *priority* problems of a patient suffering from a life-threatening illness or injury—for example, severe trauma, a heart attack, or GI hemorrhage—is essential to preserve the patient's life and function and prevent additional damage.

Next, identify the *patient population* to which the patient belongs, and take the common characteristics of that population into account in choosing an examination method. For example, elderly or debilitated patients tire easily; for these patients, you should select a method that requires minimal position changes. You may also defer parts of the examination to avoid tiring the patient.

Try to view the patient as an integrated whole rather than as a collection of parts, regardless of the examination method you use. Remember, the integrity of a body *region* may reflect adequate functioning of many body *systems*, both inside and outside the region in question. For example, the integrity of the chest region may provide important clues about the functioning of the cardiovascular and respiratory systems. Similarly, the integrity of a body *system* may reflect adequate functioning of many body *regions* and of the various systems within these regions.

You may want to plan your physical examination around the patient's *chief complaint* or *concern*. To do this, begin by examining the body system or region that corresponds to the chief complaint. This allows you to identify priority problems promptly and reassures the patient that you're paying attention to his chief complaint.

Physical examination findings are crucial to arriving at a nursing diagnosis and, ultimately, to developing a sound nursing care plan. Record your examination results thoroughly, accurately,

BOX 2. DOCUMENTATION TIPS

Remember these rules about documenting your initial assessment:

- Always document your findings as soon as possible after you take the health history and perform the physical examination.
- Complete documentation of your assessment away from the patient's bedside. Jot down only key points while you're with the patient.
- If you're using an assessment form, answer every question. If a question doesn't apply to your patient, write "N/A" or "not applicable" in the space. (Unanswered questions give the appearance that the question was not assessed.)
- Focus your questions on areas that relate to the patient's chief complaint. Record information that has significance and will help you build a care plan.
- If you delegate the job of filling out the first section of the form to another nurse or an ancillary nursing person, remember—you must review the information gathered and validate it if you aren't sure it's correct.
- Always accept accountability for your assessment by signing your name to the areas you've completed.
- Always directly quote the patient or family member who gave you the information if you fear that summarizing will lose some of its meaning.
- Always write or print legibly, in ink.
- Be concise, specific, and exact when you describe your physical findings.
- Always go back to the patient's bedside to clarify or validate information that seems incomplete.

and clearly. Although some examiners don't like to use a printed form to record physical assessment findings, preferring to work with a blank paper, others believe that standardized data collection forms can make recording physical examination results easier. These forms simplify comprehensive data collection and documentation by providing a concise format for outlining and recording pertinent information. They also remind you to include all essential assessment data.

When documenting, describe exactly what you've inspected, palpated, percussed, or auscultated. Don't use general terms, such as *normal*, *abnormal*, *good*, or *poor*. Instead, be specific. Include positive and negative findings. Try to document as soon as possible after completing your assessment. Remember that abbreviations aid conciseness. (See Box 2, *Documentation Tips*.)

NURSING DIAGNOSIS

According to NANDA International, the nursing diagnosis is a "clinical judgment concerning a human response to health conditions/life processes, or vulnerability for that response, by an individual, family, group, or community. A nursing diagnosis provides the basis for selection of nursing interventions to achieve outcomes for which the nurse has accountability" (Herdman & Kamitsuru, 2014, p. 464). The nursing diagnosis must be supported by clinical information obtained during patient assessment. (See Box 3, *Nursing Diagnoses and the Nursing Process*.)

Each nursing diagnosis describes a patient problem that a nurse can legally manage. Becoming familiar with nursing diagnoses will enable you to better understand how nursing practice is distinct from medical practice. Although the identification of problems commonly overlaps in nursing and medicine, the approach to treatment clearly differs. Medicine focuses on curing disease; nursing focuses on holistic care that includes care and comfort. Nurses can independently diagnose and treat the patient's response to illness, certain health problems and risk for health problems, readiness to improve health behaviors, and the need to learn new health

BOX 3. NURSING DIAGNOSES AND THE NURSING PROCESS

When first described, the nursing process included only assessment, planning, implementation, and evaluation. However, during the past three decades, several important events have helped to establish diagnosis as a distinct part of the nursing process.

- The American Nurses Association (ANA), in its 1973 publication *Standards of Nursing Practice*, mentioned nursing diagnosis as a separate and definable act performed by the registered nurse. In 1991, the ANA published its revised standards of clinical practice, which continued to list nursing diagnosis as a distinct step of the nursing process.
- Individual states passed nurse practice acts that listed diagnosis as part of the nurse's legal responsibility.
- In 1973, the North American Nursing Diagnosis Association, now NANDA International, began a formal effort to classify nursing diagnoses. NANDA International continues to meet biennially to review proposed new nursing diagnoses and examine applications of nursing diagnoses in clinical practice, education, and research. Their most recent meeting was held in May 2012 in Houston, Texas. NANDA International also publishes *Nursing Diagnoses: Definitions and Classification 2015–2017*, a complete list of nursing diagnoses, definitions, and defining characteristics. Currently, members of NANDA-I are working in cooperation with the ANA and the International Council of Nurses to develop an International Classification of Nursing Practice.
- The emergence of the computer-based patient record has underscored the need for a standardized nomenclature for nursing.

information. Nurses comfort, counsel, and care for patients and their families until they're physically, emotionally, and spiritually ready to provide self-care.

Developing Your Diagnosis

The nursing diagnosis expresses your professional judgment of the patient's clinical status, responses to treatment, and nursing care needs. In effect, the nursing diagnosis *defines* the practice of nursing. Translating the patient's history, physical examination, and laboratory data into a nursing diagnosis involves organizing the data into clusters and interpreting what the clusters reveal about the patient's ability to meet the basic needs. In addition to identifying the patient's needs in coping with the effects of illness, consider what assistance the patient requires to grow and develop to the fullest extent possible.

Your nursing diagnosis describes the cluster of signs and symptoms indicating an actual or potential health problem that you can identify—and that your care can resolve. Nursing diagnoses that indicate potential health problems can be identified by the words "risk for," which appear in the diagnostic label. There are also nursing diagnoses that focus on prevention of health problems and enhanced wellness.

Creating your nursing diagnosis is a logical extension of collecting assessment data. In your patient assessment, you asked each history question, performed each physical examination technique, and considered each laboratory test result because it provided evidence of how the patient could be helped by your care or because the data could affect nursing care.

To develop the nursing diagnosis, use the assessment data you've collected to develop a problem list. Less formal in structure than a fully developed nursing diagnosis, this list describes the patient's problems or needs. It's easy to generate such a list if you use a conceptual model or an accepted set of criterion norms. Examples of such norms include normal physical and psychological development and Gordon's functional health patterns.

You can identify the patient's problems and needs with simple phrases, such as *poor circulation, high fever,* or *poor hydration*. Next, prioritize the problems on the list, and then develop the working nursing diagnosis.

Writing a Nursing Diagnosis

Some nurses are confused about how to document a nursing diagnosis because they think the language is too complex. However, by remembering the following basic guidelines, you can ensure that your diagnostic statement is correct:

- Use proper terminology that reflects the patient's *nursing* needs.
- Make your statement concise so it's easily understood by other health care team members.
- Use the most precise words possible.
- Use a problem and cause format, stating the problem and its related cause.

Whenever possible, use the terminology recommended by NANDA-I.

NANDA-I diagnostic headings, when combined with suspected etiology and supported by defining characteristics or risk factors (Herdman & Kamitsuru, 2014, p. 26), provide a clear picture of the patient's needs. Thus, for clarity in charting, start with one of the NANDA-I categories as a heading for the diagnostic statement. The category can reflect an actual or potential problem. Consider this sample diagnosis:

- *Heading:* Impaired physical mobility
- *Etiology:* Related to pain and discomfort following surgery
- *Signs and symptoms (these are the defining characteristics or risk factors)*: "I can't walk without help." Patient hasn't ambulated since surgery on ____ (give date and time). Range of motion limited to 10 degrees flexion in the right hip. Patient can't walk 3 feet from the bed to the chair without the help of two nurses.
- This format links the patient's problem to the etiology without stating a direct cause-and-effect relationship (which may be hard to prove). Remember to state only the patient's problems and the probable origin. Omit references to possible solutions. (Your solutions will derive from your nursing diagnosis, but they aren't part of it.)

Avoiding Common Errors

One major pitfall in developing a nursing diagnosis is writing one that nursing interventions can't treat. Errors can also occur when nurses take shortcuts in the nursing process, either by omitting or hurrying through assessment or by basing the diagnosis on inaccurate assessment data.

Keep in mind that a nursing diagnosis is a statement of a health problem that a nurse is licensed to treat—a problem for which you'll assume responsibility for therapeutic decisions and accountability for the outcomes. A nursing diagnosis is *not* a

- diagnostic test ("schedule for cardiac angiography")
- piece of equipment ("set up intermittent suction apparatus")
- problem with equipment ("the patient has trouble using a commode")
- nurse's problem with a patient ("Mr. Jones is a difficult patient; he's rude and won't take his medication.")
- nursing goal ("encourage fluids up to 2,000 mL/day")
- nursing need ("I have to get through to the family that they must accept the fact that their father is dying.")
- medical diagnosis ("cervical cancer")
- treatment ("catheterize after each voiding for residual urine").

At first, these distinctions may not be clear. The following examples should help clarify what a nursing diagnosis is:

- Don't state a need instead of a problem.
  - Incorrect: Fluid replacement related to fever
  - Correct: Deficient fluid volume related to fever

- Don't reverse the two parts of the statement.
  - Incorrect: Lack of understanding related to noncompliance with diabetic diet
  - Correct: Noncompliance with diabetic diet related to lack of understanding
- Don't identify an untreatable condition instead of the problem it indicates (which can be treated).
  - Incorrect: Inability to speak related to laryngectomy
  - Correct: Social isolation related to inability to speak because of laryngectomy
- Don't write a legally inadvisable statement.
  - Incorrect: Skin integrity impairment related to improper positioning
  - Correct: Impaired skin integrity related to immobility
- Don't identify as unhealthful a response that would be appropriate, allowed for, or culturally acceptable.
  - Incorrect: Anger related to terminal illness
  - Correct: Ineffective therapeutic regimen management related to anger over terminal illness
- Don't make a tautological statement (one in which both parts of the statement say the same thing).
  - Incorrect: Pain related to alteration in comfort
  - Correct: Acute pain related to postoperative abdominal distention and anxiety
- Don't identify a nursing problem instead of a patient problem.
  - Incorrect: Difficulty suctioning related to thick secretions
  - Correct: Ineffective airway clearance related to thick tracheal secretions

How Nursing and Medical Diagnoses Differ

You assess your patient to obtain data in order to make a nursing diagnosis, just as the physician examines a patient to establish a medical diagnosis. It is important to understand the differences between the two and remember that they sometimes overlap. You perform a complete assessment to identify patient problems that nursing interventions can help resolve; your nursing diagnoses state these problems. (Some problems may be secondary to medical treatment.) If you plan your care of a patient around only the medical aspects of an illness, you'll probably overlook significant problems.

For example, suppose the patient's medical diagnosis is a fractured femur. In your assessment, take a careful history. Include questions to determine whether the patient has adequate financial resources to cope with prolonged disability. To assess the patient's capacity to adjust to the physical restrictions caused by the disability, gather data about his or her previous lifestyle.

Suppose your physical examination of this patient—in addition to uncovering signs and symptoms pertaining to the medical diagnosis—reveals actual or potential skin breakdown secondary to immobility. Your nursing diagnoses, in that case, may include home maintenance management impairment, diversional activity deficit (related to prolonged immobility), and risk for skin integrity impairment.

The care plan you prepare for this patient should include the nursing interventions suggested by your nursing diagnoses as well as the nursing actions necessary to fulfill the patient's medical treatment plan. When integrated into a care plan, the nursing and medical diagnoses describe the complete nursing care the patient needs. See Box 4 for examples of differences between medical and nursing diagnoses.

BOX 4. EXAMPLES OF MEDICAL AND NURSING DIAGNOSES

Study the following examples here to better understand the difference between medical and nursing diagnoses:

- Frank Smith, age 67, complains of "stubborn, old muscles." He has difficulty walking, as you can see by his shuffling gait. During the interview, Mr. Smith speaks in a monotone and seems very depressed. Physical examination shows a pill-rolling hand tremor. Laboratory tests reveal a decreased dopamine level.
  - *Medical diagnosis:* Parkinson's disease
  - *Nursing diagnoses:* Impaired physical mobility related to decreased muscle control; disturbed body image related to physical alterations; deficient knowledge related to lack of information about progressive nature of illness
- For 5 consecutive days, Judy Wilson, age 26, has had sporadic abdominal cramps of increasing intensity. Most recently, the pain has been accompanied by vomiting and a slight fever. Your examination reveals rebound tenderness and muscle guarding.
  - *Medical diagnosis:* Appendicitis
  - *Nursing diagnoses:* Acute pain related to biologic agents; deficient fluid volume related to vomiting
- During an extensive bout with respiratory tract infections, Tom Bradley, age 7, complains of throbbing ear pain. Tom's mother notes his hearing difficulty and his fear of the pain and possible hearing loss. On inspection, his tympanic membrane appears red and bulging.
  - *Medical diagnosis:* Acute suppurative otitis media
  - *Nursing diagnoses:* Acute pain related to swollen tympanic membrane; fear related to progressive hearing loss.

OUTCOME IDENTIFICATION

During this phase of the nursing process, you will identify expected outcomes for the patient. Derived from the patient's nursing diagnoses, expected outcomes are goals that are measurable, patient focused, realistic, clear, concise, and time limited. These goals may be short- or long-term. Short-term goals include those of immediate concern that can be achieved quickly. Long-term goals take more time to achieve and usually involve prevention, patient teaching, and rehabilitation.

In many cases, you can identify expected outcomes by converting the nursing diagnosis into a positive statement. For instance, for the nursing diagnosis "impaired physical mobility related to a fracture of the right hip," the expected outcome might be "The patient will ambulate independently before discharge."

When writing the care plan, state expected outcomes in terms of the patient's behavior—for example, "the patient correctly demonstrates turning, coughing, and deep breathing." Also, identify a target time or date by which the expected outcomes should be accomplished. The expected outcomes will serve as the basis for evaluating your nursing interventions.

If possible, consult with the patient and the patient's family when establishing expected outcomes. As the patient progresses, expected outcomes should be increasingly directed toward planning for discharge and follow-up care.

Outcome statements should be tailored to your practice setting. For example, on the ICU, you may focus on maintaining hemodynamic stability, whereas on a rehabilitation unit, you would focus on maximizing the patient's independence and preventing complications. (See Box 5, *Understanding NOC.*)

BOX 5. UNDERSTANDING NOC

The Nursing Outcomes Classification (NOC) is a standardized language of patient or client outcomes that was developed by a nursing research team at the University of Iowa. It contains 385 outcomes organized into 33 classes and 7 domains. Each outcome has a definition, list of measurable indicators, and references. The outcomes are research based, and studies are ongoing to evaluate their reliability, validity, and sensitivity. More information about NOC can be found at the Center for Nursing Classification and Clinical Effectiveness (*www.nursing.uiowa.edu/cnc*).

Writing Expected Outcome Statements

Expected outcomes must be stated in measurable terms. Measurable terms describe observable results and provide the criteria for success; they clearly describe the expected result after interventions are implemented. Avoid ambiguous language such as *better, improve,* or *decrease* because such terms are difficult to quantify. When writing expected outcomes in your care plan, always start with a specific action verb that focuses on the patient's behavior. By telling your reader how the patient should *look, walk, eat, drink, turn, cough, speak*, or *stand*, for example, you give a clear picture of how to evaluate progress.

Avoid starting expected outcome statements with *allow, let, enable*, or similar verbs. Such words focus attention on your own and other health care team members' behavior—not on the patient's.

With many documentation formats, you won't need to include the phrase "The patient will..." with each expected outcome statement. You will, however, have to specify which person the goals refer to when family, friends, or others are directly concerned.

Make sure target dates are realistic. Be flexible enough to adjust the date if the patient needs more time to respond to your interventions.

PLANNING

The nursing care plan refers to a written plan of action designed to help you deliver quality patient care. It includes relevant nursing diagnoses, expected outcomes, and nursing interventions. Keep in mind that the care plan usually forms a permanent part of the patient's health record and will be used by other members of the nursing team. The care plan may be integrated into an interdisciplinary plan for the patient. In this instance, clear guidelines should outline the role of each member of the health care team in providing care.

Benefits of a Care Plan

To provide quality care for each patient, you must plan and direct that care. Writing a care plan allows you to document the scientific method used throughout the nursing process. In the care plan, you summarize the patient's problems and needs (as nursing diagnoses) and identify appropriate nursing interventions and expected outcomes. A care plan that's well conceived and properly written helps decrease the risk of incomplete or incorrect care by

- *Giving direction*: A written care plan gives direction by showing colleagues the goals you have set for the patient and gives clear instructions for assisting in goal achievement. The care plan also makes clear exactly what to document on the patient's progress notes. For instance, the plan should list what observations to make and how often, what nursing measures to take and how to implement them, and what to teach the patient and the patient's family before discharge.

- *Providing continuity of care*: A written care plan identifies the patient's needs to each caregiver and tells what must be done to meet those needs. With this information, nurses caring for the patient at different times can adjust their routines to meet the patient's care demands. A care plan also provides caregivers with specific instructions on patient care, eliminating the confusion that can exist. If the patient is discharged from your health care facility to another, your care plan can help ease this transition.
- *Establishing communication between you and other nurses who will care for the patient, between you and health care team members in other departments, and between you and the patient*: Soliciting the patient's input as you develop the care plan demonstrates that you value the patient's opinions and feelings. By reviewing the care plan with other health care team members, and with other nurses, you can regularly evaluate the patient's response or lack of response to the nursing care and medical regimen.
- *Serving as a key for patient care assignments*: If you're a team leader, you may want to delegate some specific routines or duties described in each nursing intervention—not all of them need your professional attention.

Reviewing the Planning Stages

Formulating the care plan involves three stages:

- *Assigning* priorities to the nursing diagnoses: Any time you develop more than one nursing diagnosis for the patient, you must assign priorities to them and begin your care plan with those having the highest priority. High-priority nursing diagnoses involve the patient's most urgent needs (such as emergency or immediate physical needs). Intermediate-priority diagnoses involve nonemergency needs, and low-priority diagnoses involve needs that don't directly relate to the patient's specific illness or prognosis.
- *Selecting* appropriate nursing actions (interventions): Next, you'll select one or more nursing interventions to achieve each of the expected outcomes identified for the patient. For example, if one expected outcome statement reads, "The patient will transfer to chair with assistance," the appropriate nursing interventions include placing the wheelchair facing the foot of the bed and assisting the patient to stand and pivot to the chair. If another expected outcome statement reads, "The patient will express feelings related to recent injury," appropriate interventions might include spending time with the patient each shift, conveying an open and nonjudgmental attitude, and asking open-ended questions.
- *Documenting* the nursing diagnoses, expected outcomes, nursing interventions, and evaluations on the care plan: Reviewing the second part of the nursing diagnosis statement (the part describing etiologic factors) may help guide your choice of nursing interventions. For example, for the nursing diagnosis "Risk for injury related to inadequate blood glucose levels," you would determine the best nursing interventions for maintaining an adequate blood glucose level. Typical interventions for this goal include observing the patient for evidence of hypoglycemia and providing an appropriate diet. Try to think creatively during this step in the nursing process. It's an opportunity to describe exactly what you and your patient would like to have happen and to establish the criteria against which you'll judge further nursing actions.

The planning phase culminates when you write the care plan and document the nursing diagnoses, expected outcomes, nursing interventions, and evaluations for expected outcomes. Write your care plan in concise, specific terms so that other health care team members can follow it. Keep in mind that because the patient's problems and needs will change, you'll have to review your care plan frequently and modify it when necessary.

Elements of the Care Plan

Care planning formats vary from one health care facility to another. For example, you may write your care plan on a form supplied by the hospital, or you can use software that's approved by your facility. Nearly all care planning formats include space in which to document the nursing diagnoses, expected outcomes, and nursing interventions. In many health care facilities, you may also document assessment data and discharge planning on the care plan.

No matter which format you use, be sure to write the care plan in ink (and sign it), even though you may have to make revisions if your nursing interventions don't work. Remember—the patient's care plan becomes part of the permanent record and shouldn't be erased or destroyed. The information must remain intact, enabling you and other health care team members to readily refer to nursing interventions used in the past. (See Box 6, *Guidelines for Writing a Care Plan.*)

Be specific when writing your care plan. By discussing specific problems, expected outcomes, nursing interventions, and evaluations for expected outcomes, you leave no doubt as to what needs to be done by other health care team members. For example, when listing nursing interventions, be sure to include *when* the action should be implemented, *who* should be involved in each aspect of implementation, and the *frequency, quantity*, and *method* to be used. Specify dates and times when appropriate. List target dates for each expected outcome.

If your nursing interventions have resolved the problem on which you've based the nursing diagnosis, write "discontinued" next to the diagnostic statement on the care plan, and list the date you discontinued the interventions. If your nursing interventions haven't resolved the problem by the target date, reevaluate your plan and do one of the following:

- Extend the target date, and continue the intervention until the patient responds as expected.
- Discontinue the intervention, and select a new one that will achieve the expected outcome.

BOX 6. GUIDELINES FOR WRITING A CARE PLAN

Keeping these tips in mind will help you write an accurate and useful care plan.

- Write your patient's care plan in ink—it's part of the permanent record. Sign your name.
- Be specific; don't use vague terms or generalities on the care plan.
- Never use abbreviations that may be confused or misinterpreted. In general, it's better to use only established abbreviations and acronyms.
- Take time to review all your assessment data *before* you select an approach for each problem. (*Note:* If you can't complete the initial assessment, immediately note "insufficient database" on your records.)
- Write down a specific expected outcome for each problem you identify, and record a target date for its completion.
- Avoid setting an initial goal that's too high to be achieved. For example, the outcome for a newly admitted patient with stroke stating, "Patient will ambulate with assistance," is an unrealistic initial goal because several patient outcomes will need to be achieved before this goal can be addressed.
- Consider the following three phases of patient care when writing nursing interventions: What observations to make and how often, what nursing measures to do and how to do them, and what to teach the patient and family before discharge.
- Make each nursing intervention specific.
- Make sure nursing interventions match the resources and capabilities of the staff. Combine what's necessary to correct or modify the problem with what's reasonably possible in your setting.
- Be creative when you write your patient's care plan; include a drawing or an innovative procedure if either will make your directions more specific.
- Don't overlook any of the patient's problems or concerns. Include them on the care plan so they won't be forgotten.
- Make sure your care plan is implemented correctly.
- Evaluate the results of your care plan, and discontinue any nursing diagnoses that have been resolved. Select new approaches, if necessary, for problems that haven't been resolved.

You'll need to update and modify a patient's care plan as problems (or priorities) change and resolve, new assessment information becomes available, and you evaluate the patient's responses to nursing interventions.

IMPLEMENTATION

During this phase, you put your care plan into action. Implementation encompasses all nursing interventions directed toward solving the patient's nursing problems and meeting health care needs. While you coordinate implementation, you also seek help from other caregivers, the patient, and the patient's family. (See Box 7, *Understanding NIC.*)

Implementation requires some (or all) of the following interventions:

- Assessing and monitoring (e.g., recording vital signs)
- Therapeutic interventions (e.g., giving medications)
- Making the patient more comfortable and helping him with ADLs
- Supporting the patient's respiratory and elimination functions
- Providing skin care
- Managing the environment (e.g., controlling noise to ensure a good night's sleep)
- Providing food and fluids
- Giving emotional support
- Teaching and counseling
- Referring the patient to appropriate agencies or services.

Incorporate these elements into the implementation stage:

- *Reassessing:* Although it may be brief or narrowly focused, reassessment should confirm that the planned interventions remain appropriate.
- *Reviewing and modifying the care plan*: Never static, an appropriate care plan changes with the patient's condition. As necessary, update the assessment, nursing diagnoses, implementation, and evaluation sections. (Entering the new data in a different color of ink alerts other staff members to the revisions.) Date the revisions.
- *Seeking assistance*: Determine, for example, whether you need help from other staff members or additional information before you can intervene.

Documentation

Implementation isn't complete until you've documented each intervention, the time it occurred, the patient's response, and any other pertinent information. Make sure each entry relates to a nursing diagnosis. Remember that any action not documented may be overlooked during quality assurance monitoring or evaluation of care. Thorough documentation offers a way for you to take rightful credit for your contribution in helping a patient achieve the highest possible level

BOX 7. UNDERSTANDING NIC

The Nursing Interventions Classification (NIC) is a research-based clinical tool that standardizes and defines the knowledge base for nursing practice; it was developed by a nursing research team at the University of Iowa. It contains 554 interventions organized into 30 classes and 7 domains. Each intervention has a definition, list of indicators, publication facts line, and references (Bulechek, Butcher, Dochterman, & Wagner, 2013). The interventions are research based, and studies are ongoing to evaluate the effectiveness and cost of nursing treatments. More information about NIC can be found at the Center for Nursing Classification and Clinical Effectiveness (www.nursing.uiowa.edu/cnc).

BOX 8. NURSING INTERVENTIONS: THREE TYPES

Knowing the three types of nursing interventions will help you document implementation appropriately.

- *Independent interventions.* These interventions fall within the purview of nursing practice and don't require a physician's direction or supervision. Most nursing actions required by the patient's care plan are independent interventions. Examples include patient teaching, health promotion, counseling, and helping the patient with activities of daily living.
- *Dependent interventions.* Based on written or oral instructions from another professional—usually a physician—dependent interventions include administering medication, inserting indwelling urinary catheters, and obtaining specimens for laboratory tests.
- *Interdependent interventions.* Performed in collaboration with other professionals, interdependent interventions include following a protocol and carrying out standing orders.

of wellness. After all, nurses use a unique and worthwhile combination of interpersonal, intellectual, and technical skills when providing care. (See Box 8, *Nursing Interventions: Three Types.*)

Evaluation

In this phase of the nursing process, you assess the effectiveness of the care plan by answering such questions as:

- How has the patient progressed in terms of the plan's projected outcomes?
- Does the patient have new needs?
- Does the care plan need to be revised?

Evaluation also helps you determine whether the patient received high-quality care from the nursing staff and the health care facility.

Steps in the Evaluation Process

Include the patient, family members, and other health care professionals in the evaluation. Then follow these steps:

- *Select evaluation criteria:* The care plan projected outcomes—the desired effects of nursing interventions—form the basis for evaluation.
- *Compare the patient's response with the evaluation criteria*: Did the patient respond as expected? If not, the care plan may need revision.
- *Analyze your findings*: If your plan wasn't effective, determine why. You may conclude, for example, that several nursing diagnoses were inaccurate.
- *Modify the care plan*: Make revisions (e.g., change inaccurate nursing diagnoses) and implement the new plan.
- *Reevaluate*: Like all steps in the nursing process, evaluation is ongoing. Continue to assess, plan, implement, and evaluate for as long as you care for the patient.

Questions to Answer

When evaluating and documenting the patient's care, collect information from all available sources—for example, the patient's medical record, family members, other caregivers, and the patient. Include your own observations.

During the evaluation process, ask yourself these questions:

- Has the patient's condition improved, deteriorated, or remained the same?
- Were the nursing diagnoses accurate?
- Have the patient's nursing needs been met?

- Did the patient meet the outcome criteria documented in the care plan?
- Which nursing interventions should I revise or discontinue?
- Why did the patient fail to meet some goals (if applicable)?
- Should I reorder priorities? Revise expected outcomes.

NURSING DIAGNOSES AND CRITICAL PATHWAYS

In a growing number of health care settings—inpatient and outpatient, acute and long-term care—critical pathways are being used to guide the process of care for a patient. Critical pathways describe the course of a specific health-related condition. A critical pathway may be used along with or instead of a nursing care plan, depending on the standards set by the individual health care facility. These tools may also be referred to as clinical pathways, care maps, collaborative care plans, or multidisciplinary action plans. (See Box 9, *Developing a Critical Pathway*.)

The concept of the critical pathway evolved out of the growth of managed care and the development of the case management model in the early 1990s. Pressure from managed care organizations to control costs led to the evolution of case management.

In case management, one professional—usually a nurse or a social worker—assumes responsibility for coordinating care so that patients move through the health care system in the shortest time and at the lowest cost possible.

Early on, case managers used the nursing process and based their plans on nursing diagnoses. Over time, however, it became evident that a multidisciplinary approach was needed to adequately monitor the length of stay and reduce overall costs. This led to the development of the critical pathway concept.

In critical pathways, a time line is defined for each condition and for the achievement of expected outcomes. By reading the critical pathway, caregivers can determine on any given day where the patient should be in his or her progress toward optimal health.

BOX 9. DEVELOPING A CRITICAL PATHWAY

The critical pathway is an interdisciplinary tool that requires the collaborative efforts of all disciplines involved in patient care. The interdisciplinary team must decide on a diagnosis, select a set of achievable outcomes, and agree on a plausible time line for achieving the desired outcomes. Note that when establishing standard practices for treatment of a given condition, it has usually proved difficult for physicians to achieve consensus.

ESTABLISHING A TIME LINE

Time intervals allocated on a critical pathway vary according to the patient's condition and its acuity. For a hip replacement, the time line extends over days; for a cardiac catheterization procedure, time intervals are expressed in hours. In the postanesthesia period, a critical pathway can be defined in minutes.

Average length of stay is an important concept in developing a critical pathway. If agency data indicate that the average length of stay for an inpatient who has had a modified radical mastectomy with reconstruction is 4 days, then the team begins planning around a 4-day stay.

BUILDING THE PATHWAY

The interdisciplinary team must choose a framework for developing outcomes and interventions. Some agencies build pathways around nursing diagnoses. If interdisciplinary collaboration is strong, an agency may build pathways around general aspects of care; for example, pain, activity, nutrition, assessment, medications, psychosocial status, treatments, teaching, and discharge planning.

In an acute care setting, outcomes and interventions for each aspect of care are determined for each day of an expected length of stay. In long-term care and other community-based settings, progress may be measured in longer intervals.

The critical pathway provides a method for physicians and nurses to standardize and organize care for routine conditions. These pathways also make it easier for case managers to track data needed to

- streamline utilization of material resources and labor
- ensure that patients receive quality care
- improve the coordination of care
- reduce the cost of providing care

The most successful critical pathways have been developed for medical diagnoses with predictable outcomes, such as hip replacement, mastectomy, myocardial infarction, and cardiac catheterization. Critical pathways work best with high-volume, high-risk, high-cost conditions or procedures for which there are predictable outcomes.

Care Planning for Students

Developing a care plan helps the nursing student improve problem-solving technique, learn the nursing process, improve written and verbal communication, and develop organizational skills. More important, it shows how to apply classroom and textbook knowledge to practice.

Because the purpose is to teach the care planning process, the student care plan is longer than the standard plan used in most health care facilities. In a step-by-step manner, student care plans progress from assessment to evaluation. However, some teaching institutions model the student care plan on the plan used by the affiliated health care institution, adding a space for the scientific rationale for each nursing intervention selected.

Writing out all of your planned actions enables you to review planned nursing activities with your clinical instructor. This is an opportunity to consider whether you have complete assessment data to support your diagnoses and interventions and whether you've taken into consideration all the problems that a more experienced nurse is likely to identify. See Box 10 for an explanation of each section of a care plan.

The Importance of Nursing Diagnoses

Using a critical pathway can be helpful, especially for nursing students and new graduates. You may be assigned to provide care to a particular patient for only 1 or 2 days. Seeing the entire pathway and examining the outcomes the patient is expected to achieve will help you obtain a broader clinical perspective on care.

Using a critical pathway as a guide for delivering care does not negate the need to formulate and utilize nursing diagnoses. Nursing diagnoses continue to define the primary responsibility of nursing—to diagnose and treat human responses to actual or potential health problems. The full nursing care needs of any patient are unlikely to be documented in a critical pathway. When using a pathway, always keep in mind that the patient may require nursing intervention beyond what's specified in the critical pathway.

For example, a patient enters a hospital for a hip replacement and can't communicate verbally because of a recent stroke. The critical pathway wouldn't include measures to assist the patient to disclose personal needs. Therefore, you would develop a nursing care plan around the diagnosis "Impaired verbal communication related to decreased circulation to the brain."

Even if you practice in a clinical setting that relies on critical pathways to fill documentation requirements, the *Nursing Diagnosis Reference Manual*, tenth edition, will prove to be a valuable resource for identifying and treating each patient's unique nursing needs. Creating a care plan based on carefully selected nursing diagnoses and using it along with a critical pathway will enable you to provide your patients with high-quality collaborative care that includes a strong nursing component.

BOX 10. CARE PLANS

All care plans contain the following sections:

- *Diagnostic statement.* Each diagnostic statement includes a NANDA-I–approved diagnosis and, in most cases, a related etiology. This edition of the *Nursing Diagnosis Reference Manual* contains all the diagnoses approved by NANDA-I to date.
- *Definition.* This section offers a brief explanation of the diagnosis.
- *Assessment.* This section suggests parameters to use when collecting data to ensure an accurate diagnosis. Data may include health history, physical findings, psychosocial status, laboratory studies, patient statements, and other subjective and objective information.
- *Defining characteristics.* This section lists clinical findings that confirm the diagnosis. For diagnoses expressing the possibility of a problem, such as "Risk for injury," this section is labeled *Risk factors.*
- *Expected outcomes.* Here you'll find realistic goals for resolving or ameliorating the patient's health problem, written in measurable behavioral terms. You should select outcomes that are appropriate to the condition of your patient. Outcomes are arranged to flow logically from admission to discharge of the patient. Outcomes identified by NOC research have been added to correlate with the NANDA-I expected outcomes.
- *Interventions and rationales.* This section provides specific activities you carry out to help attain expected outcomes. Each intervention contains a rationale, highlighted in italic type. Rationales receive typographic emphasis because they form the premise for every nursing action. You'll find it helpful to consider rationales before intervening. Understanding the why of your actions can help you see that carrying out repetitive or difficult interventions is an essential element of your nursing practice. More importantly, it can improve critical thinking and help you to avoid mistakes. Interventions from NIC research have been added to correlate with the interventions.
- *Evaluations for expected outcomes.* Here you'll find evaluation criteria for the expected outcomes. These criteria will help you determine whether expected outcomes have been attained or provide support for revising outcomes or interventions to meet changing patient conditions.
- *Documentation.* This section lists critical topics to include in your documentation—for example, patient perceptions, status, and response to treatment as well as nursing observations and interventions. Using the information provided in this section will enable you to write the careful, concise documentation required to meet professional nursing standards.

REFERENCES

American Nurses Association. (2015). *Nursing: Scope and standards of practice* (3rd ed.). Silver Spring, MD: Author.

Herdman, T. H. & Kamitsuru, S. (Eds.). (2014). *NANDA International, Inc. nursing diagnoses: Definitions and classification, 2015–2017* (10th ed.). Oxford: Wiley-Blackwell.

PART I

Adult Health

APPLYING EVIDENCE-BASED PRACTICE

The Question

Does weight cycling (yo-yo dieting) have any long-term adverse health effects?

Evidence-Based Resources

Bosy-Westphal, A., Kahlhöfer, J., Lagerpusch, M., Skurk, T., & Müller, M. J. (2015). Deep body composition phenotyping during weight cycling: Relevance to metabolic efficiency and metabolic risk. *Obesity Reviews*, *16*, 36–44. doi:10.1111/obr.12254

Bosy-Westphal, A., & Müller, M. J. (2014). Measuring the impact of weight cycling on body composition: A methodological challenge. *Current Opinion in Clinical Nutrition & Metabolic Care*, *17*(5), 396–400. doi:10.1097/MCO.0000000000000092

Delahanty, L. M., Pan, Q., Jablonski, K. A., Aroda, V. R., Watson, K. E., Bray, G. A., ... Franks, P. W. (2014). Effects of weight loss, weight cycling, and weight loss maintenance on diabetes incidence and change in cardiometabolic traits in the diabetes prevention program. *Diabetes Care*, *37*(10), 2738–2745. doi:10.2337/dc14-0018

Guth, E. (2014). JAMA patient page. Healthy weight loss. *JAMA*, *312*(9), 974. doi:10.1001/jama.2014.10929

Messier, L., Elisha, B., Schmitz, N., Gariepy, G., Malla, A., Lesage, A., ... Strychar, I. (2014). Weight cycling and depressive symptoms in diabetes: A community-based study of adults with type 2 diabetes mellitus in Quebec. *Canadian Journal of Diabetes*, *38*(6), 456–460. doi:10.1016/j.jcjd.2014.01.005

Montani, J. P., Schutz, Y., & Dulloo, A. G. (2015). Dieting and weight cycling as risk factors for cardiometabolic diseases: who is really at risk? *Obesity Reviews*, *16*, 7-18. doi: 10.1111/obr.12251

Murphy, R. A., Patel, K. V., Kritchevsky, S. B., Houston, D. K., Newman, A. B., Koster, A., ... Harris, T. B. (2014). Weight change, body composition, and risk of mobility disability and mortality in older adults: A population-based cohort study. *Journal of the American Geriatrics Society*, *62*(8), 1476–1483. doi:10.1111/jgs.12954

Stevens, V. L., Jacobs, E. J., Patel, A. V., Juzhong, S., McCullough, M. L., Campbell, P. T., & Gapstur, S. M. (2015). Weight cycling and cancer incidence in a large prospective U.S. cohort. *American Journal of Epidemiology, 182*(5), 394–404. doi:10.1093/aje/kwv073

Evaluating the Evidence

Almost half of all adults in the United States have attempted to lose weight. Many of these individuals try diet after diet to lose extra pounds only to gain them back, creating a vicious cycle of weight loss and gain. This type of dieting is called yo-yo dieting or cycling (Stevens et al., 2015). Because many individuals try to lose weight, it is important to investigate whether this method of dieting has any long-term adverse effects.

Multiple studies (Bosy-Westphal, Kahlhöfer, Lagerpusch, Skurk, & Müller, 2015; Bosy-Westphal & Muller, 2014; Delahanty et al., 2014; Messier et al., 2014; Montani, Schutz, & Dulloo, 2015; Stevens et al., 2015) have explored the relationship between weight cycling and increased risk for adverse health effects. Unfortunately, there isn't a clear or unanimous conclusion on whether weight fluctuation is related to development of disease or illness. Although most studies conclude there is no overall increased risk of adverse health effects, specifically from weight cycling, there may be increased risks for certain individuals and conditions.

Two diseases in which obesity is a risk factor are diabetes and cancer. Overweight individuals considered at risk for either of these diseases are often told to lose weight. A study by Delahanty et al. (2014) examined the relationship between weight cycling and incidence of diabetes. The study's results indicated an association with increased risk of hypertension and diabetes. Messier et al. (2014) examined the effects of weight cycling by patients already diagnosed with type 2 diabetes. The results concluded there are no increased associated risks in diabetic patients. In turn, Stevens et al. (2015) investigated whether weight cycling increased cancer risk and found no evidence to indicate any overall increased risks.

Another concern associated with weight cycling is that the body may gain too much fat in comparison with lean muscle mass or there will be a negative impact on body fat distribution. Two studies (Bosy-Westphal et al., 2015; Bosy-Westphal & Müller, 2014) investigated the effects of weight cycling on body mass. Although both studies indicate there is no evidence of overall adverse effects on body composition when weight cycling, Bosy-Westphal & Müller (2014) warn that dieters with a starting weight within normal limits may experience adverse effects. Evidence indicates that severe weight loss in individuals who are considered within normal weight range may regain a higher amount of abdominal fat mass.

Although some studies in the past have associated weight cycling with mortality, many didn't differentiate weight cycling that is initiated by intentional weight loss from that initiated by illness. One recent study explored the differences. Murphy et al. (2014) found that in older adults (aged 70 to 79), there is a possible relationship between unintentional weight change and a higher risk of mortality. However, results from this study indicated that there is no relationship between intentional weight change and the risk of mortality.

In conclusion, although study results are divided on the risks, there is evidence that suggests weight cycling does not have overall negative effects on health. These findings may be significant because estimates indicate that nearly half of Americans have yo-yo dieted while attempting to lose weight.

Applying the Results and Making a Decision

Maintaining a stable weight over time is definitely the best practice. However, overweight people should not stop exercising and trying to lose weight just because they have a history of cycling. Studies have shown that cycling can be beneficial when attempting to lose weight.

Because there is no associated overall increased risk for adverse health effects, overweight and obese individuals should be encouraged to attempt weight loss even if the weight will eventually be regained (Stevens et al., 2015).

Reevaluating Process and Identifying Areas for Improvement

A history of unsuccessful weight loss should not dissuade an individual from future attempts to shed pounds, nor should it diminish the role of a healthy diet and regular physical activity. Eating healthy foods and participating in routine physical activity has shown the best results for maintaining a stable weight (Guth, 2014). Those who practice yo-yo dieting should not give up, and if they gain back the weight, there is evidence that losing it again will not be detrimental to their health.

INTRODUCTION

This section includes approximately 200 alphabetically organized diagnostic labels and associated care plans that identify adult health problems responsive to independent nursing action. Many focus on meeting the patient's actual physiologic needs. For example, you'll find care plans that will assist you to plan the care of a patient with decreased cardiac output, help an injured patient maintain joint range of motion, and teach an immunosuppressed patient measures to prevent infection. In addition, you'll find plans for warding off potential health problems, such as risk for infection or injury.

Other care plans focus on the psychological and psychosocial problems of adulthood. For example, if a patient with a chronic illness experiences related emotional difficulties, such diagnostic labels as *hopelessness, ineffective role performance*, and *disturbed body image* may help pinpoint the patient's needs. If a patient lacks adequate financial, social, or spiritual resources, appropriate care plans provide instructions for documenting such hardships and interventions for ameliorating them.

Still other care plans focus on more specialized patient problems. For example, you'll find plans for patients undergoing surgery.

In summary, the diagnostic labels and associated care plans covered in this section encompass the full range of nursing responsibilities. To make full use of this broad database, you'll need to perform a complete and careful nursing assessment. When appropriate, include questions about the patient's cultural background. Ask about self-concept, stressors, daily living habits, and coping mechanisms. Discuss the patient's health goals. How well does the patient understand his or her condition? Will family members or friends take an active role in patient care? Your assessment should also include information derived from your own observations.

Use information gathered during assessment to select an accurate diagnostic statement and an appropriate care plan. That way, you can ensure your adult patient comprehensive, individualized, and consistent nursing care.

ACTIVITY INTOLERANCE

related to imbalance between oxygen supply and demand

Definition

Insufficient physiologic or psychological energy to endure or complete required or desired daily activities

Assessment

- History of circulatory disease, respiratory disease, or both
- Patient's perception of tolerance for activity
- Current medications, effectiveness
- Respiratory status, including pulse oximetry; pulmonary function studies; and respiratory rate, depth, and pattern at rest and with activity
- Cardiovascular status, including blood pressure, complete blood count, stress electrocardiogram (ECG) results, and heart rate and rhythm at rest and with activity
- Knowledge, including understanding of present condition; perception of need to maintain or restore an activity level consistent with capabilities; and physical, mental, and emotional readiness to learn

Defining Characteristics

- Abnormal blood pressure response to activity
- Abnormal heart rate response to activity
- ECG change (e.g., arrhythmia, conduction abnormality, ischemia)
- Exertional discomfort
- Exertional dyspnea
- Fatigue
- Generalized weakness

Expected Outcomes

- Patient will state desire to increase activity level.
- Patient will state understanding of the need to increase activity level gradually.
- Patient will identify controllable factors that cause fatigue.
- Patient's blood pressure and pulse and respiratory rates will remain within prescribed limits during activity.
- Patient will state a sense of satisfaction with each new level of activity attained.
- Patient will demonstrate skill in conserving energy while carrying out daily activities to tolerance level.
- Patient will explain illness and connect symptoms of activity intolerance with deficit in oxygen supply or use.

Suggested NOC Outcomes

Activity Tolerance; Discharge Readiness; Endurance; Energy Conservation; Psychomotor Energy; Self-Care: Activities of Daily Living (ADLs); Self-Care: Instrumental Activities of Daily Living (IADLs)

Interventions and Rationales

- Discuss with patient the need for activity. *Lack of activity causes physical deconditioning and may also have a negative impact on psychological well-being.*
- PCC Identify activities the patient considers desirable and meaningful. *Engaging patient in activities that have personal meaning gives the patient a greater sense of independence and may motivate patient to continue developing tolerance.*
- Encourage patient to help plan activity progression, being sure to include activities the patient considers essential. *Participation in planning may encourage patient compliance with the plan.*
- Instruct and help patient to alternate periods of rest and activity. *Providing rest periods prevents fatigue and encourages patient to continue improving activity tolerance.*
- Remove barriers that prevent patient from achieving goals that have been established *to minimize factors that may decrease patient's exercise tolerance.*
- S Monitor physiologic responses to increased activity (including respirations, pulse oximetry, heart rate and rhythm, and blood pressure). Document the time after each period of exercise. Wait 5 minutes and measure physiologic responses. *Values should return to normal within 5 minutes or less.*
- PCC Teach patient how to conserve energy while performing ADLs—for example, sitting in a chair while dressing, wearing lightweight clothing that fastens with Velcro or a few large buttons, and wearing slip-on shoes. *These measures reduce cellular metabolism and oxygen demand.*

PCC

- Teach patient exercises for increasing strength and endurance *to improve breathing and promote general physical reconditioning.*
- Support and encourage activity to patient's level of tolerance *to help foster patient's independence.*
- Before discharge, formulate a plan with patient and caregivers that will enable the patient either to continue functioning at maximum activity tolerance or to gradually increase tolerance. For example, teach patient and caregivers to monitor patient's pulse during activities, to recognize the need for oxygen (if prescribed), and to use oxygen equipment properly. *Participation in discharge planning encourages patient satisfaction and compliance.*

Suggested NIC Interventions

Body Mechanics Promotion; Energy Management; Environmental Management; Exercise Promotion; Exercise Therapy: Muscle Control; Mutual Goal Setting; Oxygen Therapy; Progressive Muscle Relaxation

Evaluations for Expected Outcomes

- Patient states a desire to increase activity level.
- Patient identifies a plan to increase activity level.
- Patient lists factors that cause fatigue.
- Patient's blood pressure and pulse and respiratory rates remain within normal parameters.
- Patient expresses satisfaction with increase in activity level.
- Patient is proficient in conserving energy while performing ADLs.
- Patient demonstrates an understanding of the relationship between signs and symptoms of activity intolerance and deficit in oxygen supply or use.

Documentation

- Patient's perception of need for activity
- Patient's priorities in performing selected activities
- Patient's description of physical effects of various activities
- Observations made while patient performs activities
- Skills demonstrated by patient in conserving energy during activity
- New activities patient was able to perform
- Evaluations for expected outcomes

REFERENCES

Bogunovic, L., Hunt, D., Prather, H., Schoenecker, P. L., & Clohisy, J. C. (2014). Activity tolerance after periacetabular osteotomy. *American Journal of Sports Medicine*, *42*(8), 1791–1795. doi:10.1177/0363546514535906

Durheim, M. T., Smith, P. J., Babyak, M. A., Mabe, S. K., Martinu, T., Welty-Wolf, K. E., … Blumenthal, J. A. (2015). Six-minute-walk distance and accelerometry predict outcomes in chronic obstructive pulmonary disease independent of Global Initiative for Chronic Obstructive Lung Disease 2011 Group. *Annals of the American Thoracic Society*, *12*(3), 349–356. doi:10.1513/AnnalsATS.201408-365OC

Inah, K., & Haejung, L. (2014). Effects of a progressive walking program on physical activity, exercise tolerance, recovery, and post-operative complications in patients with a lung resection. *Journal of Korean Academy of Nursing*, *44*(4), 381–390. doi:10.4040/jkan.2014.44.4.381

The pernicious complications of resident immobility and inactivity. (2014). *Canadian Nursing Home*, *25*(4), 19–20.

ACTIVITY INTOLEVRANCE

related to immobility

Definition

Insufficient physiologic or psychological energy to endure or complete required or desired daily activities

Assessment

- History of present illness
- Past experience with prolonged bed rest
- Neurologic status, including level of consciousness, orientation, and motor and sensory status
- Respiratory status, including arterial blood gas analysis; incentive spirometry; breath sounds; and rate, depth, and pattern of respiration at rest and with activity
- Cardiovascular status, including blood pressure, skin color, hemoglobin level and hematocrit, and heart rate and rhythm at rest and with activity
- Musculoskeletal status, including range of motion (ROM) and muscle size, strength, and tone

Defining Characteristics

- Abnormal blood pressure response to activity
- Abnormal heart rate response to activity
- Electrocardiogram change (e.g., arrhythmia, conduction abnormality, ischemia)
- Exertional discomfort
- Exertional dyspnea
- Fatigue
- Generalized weakness

Expected Outcomes

- Patient will regain and maintain muscle mass and strength.
- Patient will maintain maximum joint ROM.
- Patient will perform isometric exercises.
- Patient will help perform self-care activities.
- Heart rate and rhythm and blood pressure will remain within expected range during periods of activity.
- Patient will state understanding of and willingness to cooperate in maximizing activity level.
- Patient will perform self-care activities to tolerance level.

Suggested NOC Outcomes

Activity Tolerance; Endurance; Energy Conservation; Self-Care: Activities of Daily Living (ADLs); Self-Care: Instrumental Activities of Daily Living (IADLs)

Interventions and Rationales

- Perform active or passive ROM exercises to all extremities every 2 to 4 hours. *These exercises foster muscle strength and tone, maintain joint mobility, and prevent contractures.*
- Turn and reposition patient at least every 2 hours. Establish a turning schedule for the dependent patient. Post schedule at bedside and monitor frequency. *Turning and repositioning prevents skin breakdown and atelectasis, and improves lung expansion.*
- Maintain proper body alignment at all times *to avoid contractures and to maintain optimal musculoskeletal balance and physiologic function.*
- Encourage active exercise:
  - Provide a trapeze or other assistive device whenever possible. *Such devices simplify moving and turning for many patients and help them to strengthen upper-body muscles.*
  - PCC Teach isometric exercises *to help patient maintain or increase muscle tone and joint mobility.*
  - Have patient perform self-care activities, assist with turning and transfer. Begin slowly and increase daily, as tolerated. *Performing self-care activities helps patient regain independence and enhances self-esteem.*
- PCC Provide emotional support and encouragement *to improve patient's self-concept, and motivate patient to perform ADLs.*
- PCC Involve patient in planning and decision making *to encourage greater compliance with activity plan.*
- S Monitor physiologic responses to increased activity level, including respirations, heart rate and rhythm, and blood pressure *to ensure they return to normal within 2 to 5 minutes after stopping exercise.*
- PCC Teach caregivers to assist patient with self-care activities in a way that maximizes patient's potential. *This enables caregivers to participate in patient's care and encourages them to support patient's independence.*
- S Make sure that a case manager or social worker has assessed patient's home and made the appropriate modifications to accommodate patient's level of mobility. *Making adjustments in the home allows patient a greater degree of independence in performing ADLs, thus better conserving energy.*

Suggested NIC Interventions

Activity Therapy; Body Mechanics Promotion; Energy Management; Exercise Promotion: Strength Training; Exercise Therapy: Ambulation; Exercise Therapy: Balance; Exercise Therapy: Joint Mobility; Exercise Therapy: Muscle Control

Evaluations for Expected Outcomes

- Patient regains and maintains preillness muscle mass and strength, as demonstrated by increased activity level.
- Patient demonstrates maximum joint ROM.
- Patient performs isometric exercise _____ times per day.
- Patient assists caregiver in performing self-care activities.
- Patient's blood pressure and heart rate and rhythm remain within normal parameters.
- Patient verbalizes understanding of the need to maximize activity level.
- Patient performs self-care activities at optimal level within restrictions imposed by illness.

Documentation

- Patient's perceptions about the importance of maintaining optimal levels of activity within restrictions imposed by the illness
- Activities performed by patient
- Observations of physical findings in response to activity
- Teaching activities performed with patient or caregivers

REFERENCES

Bogunovic, L., Hunt, D., Prather, H., Schoenecker, P. L., & Clohisy, J. C. (2014). Activity tolerance after periacetabular osteotomy. *American Journal of Sports Medicine*, *42*(8), 1791–1795. doi:10.1177/0363546514535906

Durheim, M. T., Smith, P. J., Babyak, M. A., Mabe, S. K., Martinu, T., Welty-Wolf, K. E., ... Blumenthal, J. A. (2015). Six-minute-walk distance and accelerometry predict outcomes in chronic obstructive pulmonary disease independent of Global Initiative for Chronic Obstructive Lung Disease 2011 Group. *Annals of the American Thoracic Society*, *12*(3), 349–356. doi:10.1513/AnnalsATS.201408-365OC

Inah, K., & Haejung, L. (2014). Effects of a progressive walking program on physical activity, exercise tolerance, recovery, and post-operative complications in patients with a lung resection. *Journal of Korean Academy of Nursing*, *44*(4), 381–390. doi:10.4040/jkan.2014.44.4.381

The pernicious complications of resident immobility and inactivity. (2014). *Canadian Nursing Home*, *25*(4), 19–20.

RISK FOR ACTIVITY INTOLERANCE

related to presence of circulatory or respiratory problems

Definition

Vulnerable to experiencing insufficient physiological or psychological energy to endure or complete required or desired daily activities, which may compromise health

Assessment

- History of present illness
- Past experience with immobility or prescribed bed rest
- Cardiovascular status, including blood pressure, heart rate and rhythm at rest and with activity, complete blood count, skin temperature and color, edema, and chest pain or discomfort
- Respiratory status, pulse oximetry, auscultation of breath sounds, pain or discomfort associated with respiration, and rate, rhythm, depth, and pattern of respirations at rest and with activity
- Neurologic status, including level of consciousness; orientation; and mental, sensory, and motor status
- Musculoskeletal status, including range of motion (ROM), muscle size, strength, and tone, and functional mobility as follows:
  0 = completely independent
  1 = requires use of equipment or device
  2 = requires help, supervision, or teaching from another person
  3 = requires help from another person and equipment or device
  4 = dependent; doesn't participate in activity

Risk Factors

- Circulatory problems
- History of previous intolerance
- Inexperience with an activity
- Physical deconditioning
- Respiratory condition

Expected Outcomes

- Patient will maintain muscle strength and joint ROM.
- Patient will carry out isometric exercise regimen.
- Patient will communicate understanding of the rationale for maintaining activity level.
- Patient will avoid risk factors that may lead to activity intolerance.
- Patient will perform self-care activities to tolerance level.
- Patient's blood pressure, pulse, and respiratory rate will remain within prescribed range during periods of activity (specify).

Suggested NOC Outcomes

Activity Tolerance; Endurance; Energy Conservation; Self-Care: Activities of Daily Living (ADLs); Self-Care: Instrumental Activities of Daily Living (IADLs)

Interventions and Rationales

- Position patient to maintain proper body alignment. Use assistive devices as needed *to maintain joint function and prevent musculoskeletal deformities.*
- Turn and position patient at least every 2 hours. Establish turning schedule for the dependent patient. Post at bedside and monitor frequency. *Turning helps prevent skin breakdown by relieving pressure, and reduces the risk of atelectasis and pneumonia.*
- Assess patient's level of functioning using the functional mobility scale *to determine patient's capabilities.*
- Communicate patient's level of functioning to all staff. *Communication among staff members ensures continuity of care and enables patient to preserve identified level of independence.*
- Unless contraindicated, perform ROM exercises every 2 to 4 hours. Progress from passive to active, according to patient tolerance. *ROM exercises prevent joint contractures and muscular atrophy.*
- Encourage active movement by helping patient use trapeze or other assistive devices *to improve muscle tone and enhance self-esteem.*
- PCC Teach patient how to perform isometric exercises *to maintain and improve muscle tone and joint mobility.*
- Assist patient in carrying out self-care activities, turning, and transfer. Increase patient's participation in self-care, as tolerated, *to foster independence and improve mobility.*
- PCC Encourage patient to become involved in planning care and making decisions related to treatment. *Participation in planning enhances patient compliance and self-esteem.*
- PCC Teach patient, family member, or other caregiver methods to maximize patient's participation in self-care. *Informed caregivers can encourage patient to become more independent.*

S
- Assess patient's physiologic response to increased activity (blood pressure, respirations, heart rate, and rhythm). *Monitoring vital signs help to assess tolerance for increased exertion and activity.*

S PCC
- Teach patient symptoms of overexertion, such as dizziness, chest pain, and dyspnea, *to help patient take responsibility for monitoring activity level.*
- Explain rationale for maintaining or improving activity level. Discuss factors that increase risk of activity intolerance. *Education helps patient avoid activity intolerance.*
- Encourage patient to carry out ADLs. Provide emotional support, and offer positive feedback when patient displays initiative. *Offering emotional support enhances patient's self-esteem and motivation.*

Suggested NIC Interventions

Energy Management; Exercise Promotion: Strength Training; Exercise Therapy: Joint Mobility; Hope Instillation; Self-Care Assistance; Teaching: Prescribed Activity/Exercise; Body Mechanics Promotion

Evaluations for Expected Outcomes

- Functional mobility scale indicates that muscle strength and joint ROM remain stable.
- Patient demonstrates isometric exercises.
- Patient explains rationale for maintaining activity level.
- Patient states at least five risk factors for activity intolerance.
- Patient performs self-care activities in preparation for discharge.
- Patient doesn't exhibit evidence of cardiovascular or respiratory complications during or after activity.

Documentation

- Patient's expressions of motivation to maintain maximum activity level within restrictions imposed by illness
- Activities performed by patient
- Teaching instructions provided to patient and family member or other caregivers
- Patient's physiologic response to increased activity
- Evaluations for expected outcomes

REFERENCES

Casaburi, R., & Duvall, K. (2014). Improving early-stage diagnosis and management of COPD in primary care. *Postgraduate Medicine*, *126*(4), 141–154. doi:10.3810/pgm.2014.07.2792

Elbehairy, A. F., Ciavaglia, C. E., Webb, K. A., Guenette, J. A., Jensen, D., Mourad, S. M., ... O'Donnell, D. E. (2015). Pulmonary gas exchange abnormalities in mild chronic obstructive pulmonary disease. Implications for dyspnea and exercise intolerance. *American Journal of Respiratory & Critical Care Medicine*, *191*(12), 1384–1394. doi:10.1164/rccm.201501-0157OC

Kongoji, K., Yoneyama, K., Koyama, K., Mitarai, T., Kamijima, R., Kida, K., ... Akashi, Y. J. (2014). Early defects identified by computed tomography angiography are associated with left ventricular dysfunction and exercise intolerance following acute myocardial infarction. *Japanese Journal of Radiology*, *32*(10), 585–591. doi:10.1007/s11604-014-0344-7

Yates, B. C., Norman, J., Meza, J., Stanek Krogstrand, K., Harrington, S., Shurmur, S., ... Schumacher, K. (2015). Effects of partners together in health intervention on physical activity and healthy eating behaviors. *Journal of Cardiovascular Nursing*, *30*(2), 109–120. doi:10.1097/JCN.0000000000000127

INEFFECTIVE ACTIVITY PLANNING

related to unrealistic perception of personal competence

Definition

Inability to prepare for a set of actions fixed in time and under certain conditions

Assessment

- Patient's perception of problem, coping mechanisms, problem-solving ability, decision-making competencies
- Neurologic status, including level of consciousness; orientation; and mental, sensory, and motor status
- Cultural status, including affiliation with racial, ethnic, or religious groups

Defining Characteristics

- Excessive anxieties toward a task to be undertaken
- Failed pattern of behavior
- Lack of plan or resources
- Lack of sequential organization
- Procrastination
- Unmet goals for chosen activity
- Verbalization of fear or worries regarding a task to be undertaken

Expected Outcomes

- Patient will demonstrate improved self-confidence to accomplish tasks.
- Patient will demonstrate improved concentration in task planning and execution.
- Patient will minimize procrastination.
- Patient will articulate personal goals for activity planning and completion.
- Patient will verbalize diminished fear and anxiety concerning task planning and execution.

Suggested NOC Outcomes

Cognition; Cognition Orientation; Concentration; Decision-Making; Information Processing; Memory

Interventions and Rationales

- PCC Assess patient's concerns related to activity planning and execution *to be able to suggest strategies to overcome challenges.*
- Model effective techniques for planning and executing activities. *Patients who are challenged by planning and executing activities often find it helpful to observe practical approaches instead of solely hearing theoretical information.*
- PCC Teach behavior management strategies *to help patient minimize fears of failure.*
- Praise successes in any steps of planning or executing activities. *Positive reinforcement enhances self-confidence.*

- Refer or collaborate with physical and/or occupational therapists in managing the patient's activity. *Colleagues in related disciplines bring valuable additional perspectives to complex clinical situations.*

Suggested NIC Interventions

Anxiety Reduction; Behavior Management; Calming Technique; Memory Training; Planning Assistance; Sequence Guidance

Evaluations for Expected Outcomes

- Patient demonstrated improved self-confidence and concentration with task accomplishment.
- Patient was able to minimize procrastination.
- Patient stated personal goals for activity planning and execution.
- Patient verbalized diminished fear and anxiety concerning task planning and execution.

Documentation

- Patient's statements of improved self-confidence in task accomplishment
- Patient's stated goals for activity planning and execution
- Evaluations for expected outcomes

REFERENCES

Barz, M., Parschau, L., Warner, L. M., Lange, D., Fleig, L., Knoll, N., & Schwarzer, R. (2014). Planning and preparatory actions facilitate physical activity maintenance. *Psychology of Sport & Exercise, 15*(5), 516–520. doi:10.1016/j.psychsport.2014.05.002

Caudroit, J., Boiché, J., & Stephan, Y. (2014). The role of action and coping planning in the relationship between intention and physical activity: A moderated mediation analysis. *Psychology & Health, 29*(7), 768–780. doi:10.1080/08870446.2014.884223

Lovell, G. P., & Butler, F. R. (2015). Physical activity behavior and role overload in mothers. *Health Care for Women International, 36*(3), 342–355. doi:10.1080/07399332.2014.942901

Norberg, E., Boman, K., Löfgren, B., & Brännström, M. (2014). Occupational performance and strategies for managing daily life among the elderly with heart failure. *Scandinavian Journal of Occupational Therapy, 21*(5), 392–399. doi:10.3109/11038128.2014.911955

RISK FOR INEFFECTIVE ACTIVITY PLANNING

Definition

Vulnerable to an inability to prepare for a set of actions fixed in time and under certain conditions, which may compromise health

Assessment

- History of experience with illness, hospitalization, and surgery
- Health history, including accidents, exposure to pollutants, falls, hyperthermia, hypothermia, poisoning, sensory or perceptual changes (auditory, gustatory, kinesthetic, olfactory, tactile, and visual), and trauma
- Behavioral status, understanding of health problem and treatment plan, past history with health care providers, participation in health care planning and decision making; recognition and realization of potential growth, health, and autonomy

- Mobility status, including range of motion; presence of prosthesis; and limb abnormality, impairment, or injury

Risk Factors

- Flight behavior when faced with proposed solution
- Hedonism
- Insufficient information processing ability
- Insufficient social support
- Pattern of procrastination
- Unrealistic perception of events
- Unrealistic perception of personal abilities

Expected Outcomes

- Patient will express an interest in activity planning.
- Patient will minimize procrastination.
- Patient will set attainable realistic goals for activity planning and completion.
- Patient will demonstrate ability to make decisions and resolve problems.

Suggested NOC Outcomes

Information Processing; Decision-Making; Concentration; Motivation

Interventions and Rationales

- Assess patient's support system. *Family involvement can help patient to feel more in control.*
- PCC Assess patient's feelings related to decision making and activity planning *to help identify underlying fears.*
- Assist the patient to set simple, achievable short-term goals *to promote feeling of achievement.*
- PCC Educate patient regarding recognition of early symptoms of anxiety related to decision making. *This will keep the anxiety from escalating.*
- Explore possible behavior management strategies *that will minimize fears of failure.*
- PCC Listen to patient's concerns *to validate their feeling and your willingness to help.*
- Provide positive reinforcement for independent behaviors. *This will promote confidence and feeling of achievement.*
- Explore the use of alternative methods to minimize concerns regarding activity planning, for example, therapeutic breathing techniques or temporary avoidance technique, *which will allow the buildup of confidence before taking action.*
- PCC Provide community resources for follow-up support *to ensure continuation of care.*
- S Refer to behavioral specialist as needed *to provide care for more complex issues.*

Suggested NIC Interventions

Anxiety Reduction; Behavior Management; Behavior Modification

Evaluations for Expected Outcomes

- Patient plans activities.
- Patient minimizes procrastination.

- Patient has reasonable goals.
- Patient has good decision-making skills.

Documentation

- Patient's expressions of concern about lack of activity planning
- Observations of physiologic and behavioral manifestations of lack of activity
- Interventions performed to promote activity planning
- Patient's response to interventions
- Evaluations for expected outcomes

REFERENCES

Barz, M., Parschau, L., Warner, L. M., Lange, D., Fleig, L., Knoll, N., & Schwarzer, R. (2014). Planning and preparatory actions facilitate physical activity maintenance. *Psychology of Sport & Exercise, 15*(5), 516–520. doi:10.1016/j.psychsport.2014.05.002

Caudroit, J., Boiché, J., & Stephan, Y. (2014). The role of action and coping planning in the relationship between intention and physical activity: A moderated mediation analysis. *Psychology & Health, 29*(7), 768–780. doi:10.1080/08870446.2014.884223

Lovell, G. P., & Butler, F. R. (2015). Physical activity behavior and role overload in mothers. *Health Care for Women International, 36*(3), 342–355. doi:10.1080/07399332.2014.942901

Norberg, E., Boman, K., Löfgren, B., & Brännström, M. (2014). Occupational performance and strategies for managing daily life among the elderly with heart failure. *Scandinavian Journal of Occupational Therapy, 21*(5), 392–399. doi:10.3109/11038128.2014.911955

DECREASED INTRACRANIAL ADAPTIVE CAPACITY

Definition

Intracranial fluid dynamic mechanisms that normally compensate for increases in intracranial volumes are compromised, resulting in repeated disproportionate increases in intracranial pressure (ICP) in response to a variety of noxious and nonnoxious stimuli

Assessment

- Reason for hospitalization
- History of recent head trauma
- Cardiovascular status, including vital signs, skin color and temperature, carotid and apical pulses, heart sounds, jugular vein distention, electrocardiography, and history of hypertension
- Gastrointestinal status, including bowel elimination patterns, dietary intake, and abdominal inspection, palpation, and auscultation
- Musculoskeletal status, including range of motion (ROM); joint and muscle symmetry; muscle size, strength, and tone; functional mobility; contractures, subluxation, dislocation, and atrophy; previous trauma; and degenerative joint diseases
- Neurologic status, including mental status; cranial nerve function; cerebellar function; reflexes (deep tendon, superficial, and pathologic [Babinski's reflex]); peripheral sensory system (pain, position, and vibration); pupillary size and reactivity; use of anticonvulsant, neuroleptic, antidepressant, antimanic, analgesic, or illicit drugs; history of head injury; alcohol abuse; history of lethargy, restlessness, stupor, headaches, seizures, tremors, paresthesia, paresis, incoordination, ticks, fasciculation, pain, psychiatric disorders, or abnormal posturing (decorticate or decerebrate); and tests such as computed tomography scan,

magnetic resonance imaging, cerebral arteriography, electroencephalography, evoked potential studies, and Glasgow Coma Scale
- Respiratory status, including chest expansion; rate, depth, and pattern of respirations; tracheal position; fremitus; auscultation of lung fields; arterial blood gas (ABG) analysis, pulse oximetry, and mixed venous oxygen saturation; history of lung disease; tobacco use; and use of bronchodilators, antibiotics, or diuretics
- Sensory status, including visual and auditory acuity, use of hearing aid or eye glasses, tactile sensitivity eye disorders, and hearing loss

Defining Characteristics

- Baseline ICP equal to or greater than 10 mm Hg
- Disproportionate increase in ICP following stimuli
- Elevated P2 ICP waveform
- Repeated increase in ICP equal to or greater than 10 mm Hg for equal to or more than 5 minutes following external stimuli
- Volume–pressure response test variation (volume: pressure ratio 2, pressure–volume index less than 10)
- Wide-amplitude ICP waveform

Expected Outcomes

- Patient will maintain patent airway, effective breathing patterns, and normal ABG levels.
- Patient will show no evidence of fever.
- Patient's position will promote venous drainage from brain.
- Patient won't experience sustained rise in ICP in response to stimulation.
- Patient's environment will be modified to reduce noxious stimuli.
- Patient will maintain regular bowel function.
- Patient will maintain skin integrity.
- Patient will remain free from signs and symptoms of infection.
- Patient won't show evidence of neurologic compromise.
- Patient and family members will express feelings about treatment and recovery.

Suggested NOC Outcomes

Electrolyte & Acid–Base Balance; Fluid Balance; Neurologic Status; Neurologic Status: Consciousness; Wound Healing: Primary Intention

Interventions and Rationales

- Perform thorough nursing history and head-to-toe assessment and document *to establish baseline of patient's condition for future comparison and to ensure continuity and consistency of care among nursing staff.*
- S Monitor neurologic status, including level of consciousness, pupillary size and reactivity, eye movement, selected reflexes, and motor and sensory function *to identify changes that indicate increased ICP.*
- S Monitor vital signs and hemodynamic parameters (mean arterial blood pressure and pulmonary artery pressure) *to assess hemodynamic stability and to note trends.*
- Maintain ICP monitoring systems, if used. Use sterile technique for dressing changes. Maintain closed system. *Sterile technique prevents contamination of equipment and subsequent infections.*

- Monitor ICP waveforms for trends over time (A waves, B waves, C waves). Assess intracranial pulse waves (P1 percussion waves, P2 tidal waves, P3 dicrotic waves). Monitor for damped waveforms, absent waveforms, or abnormally high or low readings. *Waveforms provide information about cerebral compliance. Cerebral compliance is the body's attempt to cope with changes in intracranial content (brain tissue, blood volume, and cerebral spinal fluid). Compliance is expressed as a mathematical ratio between volume and pressure changes within the skull.*
- Assess cerebral perfusion pressure. *Adequate cerebral perfusion pressure is critical to prevent cerebral ischemia.* Cerebral perfusion pressure is calculated by taking mean arterial pressure and subtracting ICP.
- Assess temperature every 2 hours. *Fever increases cerebral metabolic demands, cerebral blood flow, and ICP.*
- S Maintain patent airway. Assess rate, depth, and rhythm of respirations *to monitor lung expansion and presence of abnormal sounds.*
- Suction patient only if needed. Limit suctioning to 10 to 15 seconds/pass of catheter. *Suctioning stimulates coughing and Valsalva maneuver; Valsalva maneuver increases intrathoracic pressure, decreases cerebral venous drainage, and increases cerebral blood volume, resulting in increased ICP.*
- Administer 100% oxygen for 1 minute before and after suctioning. Hypercapnia results in cerebral vasodilation, increased cerebral blood volume, and increased ICP. *Giving supplemental oxygen helps avoid hypoxemia and tissue ischemia.*
- Administer lidocaine, if prescribed, IV or into endotracheal (ET) tube before suctioning. *Lidocaine suppresses cough reflex, thereby preventing increases in ICP.*
- Monitor ABG levels. Observe for signs and symptoms of respiratory distress. *Hypercapnia results in vasodilation, increased cerebral blood volume, and increased ICP. Hypoxia may contribute to tissue ischemia.*
- Elevate head of bed 15° to 30° or as ordered. Keep patient's head and neck straight. Use sandbags, rolled towels, or small pillows to keep head in neutral position. Avoid hip flexion of 90° or more. *Neutral head position promotes venous drainage from head. Some positions cause increased intra-abdominal and intrathoracic pressure that can interfere with venous drainage from head.*
- When performing neurologic assessment, use minimal amount of stimuli required to obtain a response. *Unpleasant or painful stimuli increase ICP.*
- Limit environmental noise as much as possible. *Auditory stimuli can contribute to increased ICP.*
- Monitor for seizure activity. Maintain seizure precautions. Administer anticonvulsant drugs, as prescribed. *Tonic–clonic seizures increase intrathoracic pressure, decrease cerebral venous outflow, and increase cerebral blood volume, thereby raising ICP.*
- Maintain intake and output. Maintain fluid restriction, if ordered. *Fluid restriction helps decrease extracellular fluid, thereby decreasing ICP.*
- Administer osmotic diuretics, if prescribed. Monitor for signs and symptoms of dehydration (increased sodium, serum osmolality, and decreased urine output). *Osmotic diuretics pull fluid from nonedematous areas of brain, thereby decreasing ICP.*
- Administer loop diuretics, if prescribed, *to decrease water in injured brain tissue and to decrease overall body water, thereby reducing cerebral edema and lowering ICP.* Monitor for signs of dehydration and hypokalemia, which are adverse effects of diuretics.
- Turn and reposition patient every 2 hours and as needed *to prevent pressure ulcer formation.*
- While turning, keep patient's head in neutral position *to promote venous drainage from head.*
- Use a draw sheet to reposition patient. Instruct patient to exhale, if conscious, when turning or moving in bed *to avoid Valsalva maneuver, which can increase ICP by increasing intrathoracic and intra-abdominal pressures.*

- Monitor and record bowel movements. Administer stool softeners, as prescribed. Instruct patient not to hold breath or strain on defecation. *Straining associated with constipation can cause Valsalva maneuver, thereby increasing ICP.*
- PCC Instruct patient, if able to follow simple commands, to avoid pushing against footboard or digging heels into mattress when moving up in bed. Remove footboard if possible, especially if patient has decerebrate or abnormal posturing. *Isometric muscle contraction can increase ICP.*
- Perform passive ROM exercises *to maintain muscle tone and prevent atrophy and contractures.*
- Maintain normothermia. Administer antipyretics if ordered. Apply hypothermia blanket. Assess rectal temperature every 30 minutes while patient is on blanket. Control shivering. Administer chlorpromazine, if prescribed. *Shivering causes isometric muscle contraction, which can increase ICP.*
- Continue frequent neurologic assessment. Compare results with previous findings. *Frequent assessment allows detection of subtle changes in neurologic signs that indicate improvement or deterioration in patient's status.*
- PCC Try to limit painful procedures, if possible. Avoid unnecessary tension or pulling on tubes (such as ET tube or indwelling urinary catheter). *Unpleasant or painful stimuli increase ICP.*
- Involve family members in gentle stroking of patient's face, hand, or arm. *Touch provided by family members may lower ICP in some patients.*
- Speak in a low, soft voice. Provide nursing care in calm, reassuring manner. Explain all procedures before touching patient. *Explanations can help prevent emotional upsets that may increase ICP.*
- Avoid discussion of upsetting topics near patient's bedside. Patient may be upset by discussion of prognosis, treatment procedures, or patient's level of pain. Instruct patient's family members not to discuss upsetting topics within patient's hearing range. *Emotional upsets may increase ICP.*
- Ask family members to bring in audiotapes of familiar voices and patient's favorite music. Play audiotapes through earphones if appropriate. *Family members' voices and preferred music have been shown to decrease ICP in some patients.*
- Provide uninterrupted rest periods as much as possible. Avoid awakening patient during rapid eye movement (REM) sleep. *Cerebral blood flow increases during REM sleep.* Don't carry out nursing activities known to increase ICP during that time. *Nursing procedures performed during REM sleep may cause additional elevations in patient's ICP.*
- Schedule sufficient time, at least 10 minutes, between nursing care activities (such as bathing, turning, and suctioning) *to allow patient to rest and to avoid cumulative effects of continuous activity on ICP. Close spacing of activities has been known to cause sustained increases of ICP.*
- PCC Encourage patient and family to express feelings associated with diagnosis, treatment, and recovery. *Expression of feelings helps patient and family cope with treatment.*
- PCC Refer patient and family to appropriate support groups *to assist them in dealing with the injury, diagnosis, or recovery.*

Suggested NIC Interventions

Acid–Base Management; Cerebral Edema Management; Fluid–Electrolyte Management; Intracranial Pressure (ICP) Monitoring; Respiratory Monitoring; Neurologic Monitoring; Cerebral Perfusion Monitoring

Evaluations for Expected Outcomes

- Patient maintains effective breathing patterns, patent airway, and normal ABG levels.
- Patient shows no evidence of fever.
- Patient maintains proper positioning to promote venous drainage from brain.
- Patient shows no evidence of sustained increase in ICP in response to stimulation.
- Patient's environment contains fewer noxious stimuli as a result of modifications.
- Patient is free from constipation.
- Patient has intact skin.
- Patient has no signs or symptoms of infection.
- Patient shows no evidence of neurologic compromise.
- Patient and family members openly express fear, anxiety, anger, and other feelings associated with treatment and recovery.

Documentation

- Results of initial nursing assessment
- Monitoring procedures and results
- Nursing interventions and patient's response
- Instructions to patient, family, or caregiver and their demonstrated understanding of those instructions
- Evaluations for expected outcomes

REFERENCES

Kukreti, V., Mohseni-Bod, H., & Drake, J. (2014). Management of raised intracranial pressure in children with traumatic brain injury. *Journal of Pediatric Neurosciences*, *9*(3), 207–215. doi:10.4103/1817-1745.147572

Lazaridis, C., Yang, M., DeSantis, S. M., Luo, S. T., & Robertson, C. S. (2015). Predictors of intensive care unit length of stay and intracranial pressure in severe traumatic brain injury. *Journal of Critical Care*, *30*(6), 1258–1262. doi:10.1016/j.jcrc.2015.08.003

Roth, C., Ferbert, A., Deinsberger, W., Kleffmann, J., Kästner, S., Godau, J., ... Gehling, M. (2014). Does prone positioning increase intracranial pressure? A retrospective analysis of patients with acute brain injury and acute respiratory failure. *Neurocritical Care*, *21*(2), 186–191. doi:10.1007/s12028-014-0004-x

INEFFECTIVE AIRWAY CLEARANCE

related to retained secretions

Definition

Inability to clear secretions or obstructions from the respiratory tract to maintain a clear airway

Assessment

- History of present illness
- Patient's perception of ability to clear airway
- Knowledge of physical condition
- Neurologic status, including level of consciousness, orientation, and sensory and motor status

- Respiratory status, including symmetry of chest expansion; use of accessory muscles; cough (productive or nonproductive); respiratory rate, depth, and pattern; sputum characteristics; palpation for fremitus; percussion of lung fields; auscultation for breath sounds; pulse oximetry; chest X-ray; arterial blood gas (ABG) values; and hemoglobin level and hematocrit; pulmonary function studies
- Psychosocial status, including interest, motivation, and knowledge

Defining Characteristics

- Absence of cough
- Adventitious breath sounds
- Alteration in respiratory pattern
- Alteration in respiratory rate
- Cyanosis
- Difficulty verbalizing
- Diminished breath sounds
- Dyspnea
- Excessive sputum
- Ineffective cough
- Orthopnea
- Restlessness
- Wide-eyed look

Expected Outcomes

- Airway will remain patent.
- Adventitious breath sounds (crackles, rhonchi, wheezes, or stridor) will be absent.
- Chest X-ray will show no abnormality.
- Oxygen level will be in normal range.
- Patient will breathe deeply and cough to remove secretions.
- Patient will expectorate sputum.
- Patient will demonstrate controlled coughing techniques.
- Ventilation will be adequate.
- Patient will demonstrate skill in conserving energy while attempting to clear airway.
- Patient will state understanding of changes needed to diminish oxygen demands.

Suggested NOC Outcomes

Anxiety Level; Anxiety Self-Control; Aspiration Prevention; Respiratory Status: Airway Patency; Respiratory Status: Ventilation

Interventions and Rationales

- Assess respiratory status at least every 4 hours or according to established standards. *Obstruction in the airway leads to atelectasis, pneumonia, or respiratory failure.*
- Turn patient every 2 hours. Always position for maximal aeration of lung fields and mobilization of secretions. *This prevents pooling and stasis of respiratory secretions.*
- Mobilize patient to full capabilities *to facilitate chest expansion and ventilation.*
- Avoid placing patient in supine position for extended periods. Encourage lateral, sitting, prone, and upright positions as much as possible *to enhance lung expansion and ventilation.*
- When helping patient cough and deep breathe, use whatever position best ensures cooperation and minimizes energy expenditure, such as raising the head of the bed or sitting on side of bed. *Such positions promote chest expansion and ventilation of basilar lung fields.*
- Suction, as ordered, to stimulate cough and clear airways. Be alert for progression of airway compromise. Maintaining a patent airway will *prevent respiratory distress.*

- Perform postural drainage, percussion, and vibration to facilitate secretion movement. Monitor sputum, noting amount, odor, and consistency. *Sputum amount and consistency are indicators of hydration status and effectiveness of therapy. Foul-smelling sputum may indicate respiratory infection.*
- PCC Teach patient an easily performed cough technique *to clear airway without fatigue.*
- Provide adequate humidification *to loosen secretions.*
- Encourage adequate water intake (3 to 4 L [3 to 4 L/day]) *to ensure optimal hydration and loosening of secretions, unless contraindicated.*
- Encourage sputum expectoration *to remove pathogens and prevent spread of infection.* Provide tissues and paper bags for hygienic disposal *to prevent spreading infection.*
- Give expectorants, bronchodilators, and other drugs, as ordered, and monitor effectiveness. *These measures enhance clearance of secretions from airways.*
- Provide bronchodilator treatments before chest physical therapy *to optimize results of the treatment.*
- Administer oxygen, as ordered, *to promote oxygenation of cells throughout the body.*
- Monitor ABG values and hemoglobin levels *to assess oxygenation and ventilatory status.* Report deviations from baseline levels; oxygen saturation should be higher than 90%.
- If conservative measures fail to maintain partial pressure of arterial oxygen ($Pa{O_2}$) within an acceptable range, prepare for endotracheal intubation, as ordered, *to maintain artificial airway and optimize* $Pa{O_2}$ *level.*
- PCC Assess patient's learning needs, and provide appropriate information *to help prevent recurrence of obstruction and promote change in daily activities to reduce oxygen demands.*

Suggested NIC Interventions

Airway Management; Aspiration Precautions; Cough Enhancement; Infection Protection; Oxygen Therapy; Positioning; Respiratory Monitoring; Ventilation Assistance

Evaluations for Expected Outcomes

- Patient's airway remains clear and allows for adequate ventilation.
- Auscultation of patient's lung fields reveals no adventitious breath sounds.
- Patient's chest X-ray is normal.
- Patient's oxygen level remains within normal range.
- Patient coughs and deep breathes to expectorate secretions.
- Patient expectorates sputum.
- Patient performs controlled coughing techniques.
- Patient doesn't experience dyspnea or change in respiratory pattern.
- Patient performs energy conservation techniques.
- Patient demonstrates understanding of changes needed to diminish oxygen demands.

Documentation

- Patient's perceptions of ability to cough
- Observations of physical findings
- Effectiveness of medications
- Patient's attempts to clear airway
- Maneuvers performed to clear airway
- Evaluations for expected outcomes

REFERENCES

Hanlon, P. (2015). Secretion and airway clearance: Techniques and devices offer a range of treatment options. *RT: The Journal for Respiratory Care Practitioners*, *28*(8), 11–14.

Hanlon, V. D., White, F., Hustosky, A. E., McCormick, C. A., Hayes, E. J., & Wilson, A. (2014). Benefits of standardizing additional airway clearance in the trauma patient population. *Journal of Trauma Nursing*, *21*(3), 127–132. doi:10.1097/JTN.0000000000000045

Jarvis, K., Pirvu, D., Barbee, K., Berg, N., Meyer, M., Gaulke, L., ... Roberts, C. (2014). Change to a standardized airway clearance protocol for children with bronchiolitis leads to improved care. *Journal of Pediatric Nursing*, *29*(3), 252–257. doi:10.1016/j.pedn.2013.11.007

Sole, M. L., & Bennett, M. (2014). Comparison of airway management practices between registered nurses and respiratory care practitioners. *American Journal of Critical Care*, *23*(3), 191–200. doi:10.4037/ajcc2014424

Strickland, S. L. (2015). Year in review 2014: Airway clearance. *Respiratory Care*, *60*(4), 603–605. doi:10.4187/respcare.04095

RISK FOR ALLERGY RESPONSE

Definition

Vulnerable to an exaggerated immune response or reaction to substances, which may compromise health

Assessment

- Risk management
- Pharmacological function
- Physical regulation
- Knowledge level, including patient's current understanding of physical condition and physical, mental, and emotional readiness to learn

Risk Factors

- Allergy to insect sting
- Exposure to allergen (e.g., pharmaceutical agent)
- Exposure to environmental allergen (e.g., dander, dust, mold, pollen)
- Exposure to toxic chemical
- Food allergy (e.g., avocado, banana, chestnut, kiwi, peanut, shellfish, mushroom, tropical fruit)
- Repeated exposure to allergen-producing environmental substances

Expected Outcomes

- Patient will not experience an adverse reaction to allergen.
- Patient will recognize personal risk factors for allergic reaction.
- Patient will express awareness of personal allergy.
- Patient will ask questions if new information requires clarification.

Suggested NOC Outcomes

Risk Control; Risk Detection; Knowledge: Medication; Knowledge: Diet; Immune Hypersensitivity Response; Allergy Response: Localized

Interventions and Rationales

- Determine whether patient has had any previous allergic reaction to substances, and explore related details of the reaction. *Thorough history will provide a more effective prevention plan.*
- Suggest that patient keep a diary noting when symptoms occur. *This will help in the development of a risk reduction plan.*
- Assess for presence of any other conditions that may indicate an altered immune response, for example, multiple food intolerances, sensitivity to flowers or perfumes. *This will help to identify those at risk and promote early interventions for risk reduction.*
- Remove any known allergens from patient environment if possible *to reduce risk of reaction in patient.*
- Assist with any allergy testing and any prescribed treatment interventions such as long-term prophylaxis, *and reinforce treatment plan as needed.*
- S Review signs and symptoms of allergic reaction and emergency interventions *to ensure rapid response to critical situations.*
- PCC Instruct patient and family to inform health care providers of allergy to medications, and consider wearing a warning bracelet *to further protect patient from unnecessary harm.*
- Assist patient to modify environment *to minimize exposure to allergens.*
- For food allergens: Encourage patient to read all food labels *to minimize exposure.* Suggest development of a food allergen card to use when dining out. *This will help chefs prepare a safe meal.*
- For airborne allergens: Encourage frequent washing of bed linens, and using vacuum with special filter *to minimize exposure.*
- S Refer patient to primary provider to discuss possible need for emergency medication, for example, EpiPen. *This will ensure immediate treatment for severe allergic reaction.*

Suggested NIC Interventions

Allergy Management; Risk Identification; Teaching: Individual

Evaluations for Expected Outcomes

- Patient has no episodes of reaction to allergens.
- Patient recognizes possibility of adverse reaction allergen and the response needed.
- Patient asks questions regarding the use of EpiPen or other measures to reduce allergic response.

Documentation

- Patient's expressions of concern about adverse reaction and symptoms of previous episodes of allergic reactions
- Observations of physiologic and behavioral manifestations of adverse reaction to allergens
- Interventions performed to allay adverse reaction
- Patient's response to interventions
- Evaluations for expected outcomes

REFERENCES

Conkin, C., & Mathen, G. (2015). Food allergy management: Improving patient safety. *Journal of the Academy of Nutrition & Dietetics*, *115*, A35. doi:10.1016/j.jand.2015.06.121

Dinakar, C., & Lang, D. M. (2015). Quality measures in allergy, asthma, and immunology. *Annals of Allergy, Asthma & Immunology*, *114*(6), 435–439. doi:10.1016/j.anai.2015.03.012

Harvey, A. R., Basavaraju, S. V., Chung, K. W., & Kuehnert, M. J. (2015). Transfusion-related adverse reactions reported to the National Healthcare Safety Network Hemovigilance Module, United States, 2010 to 2012. *Transfusion*, *55*(4), 709–718. doi:10.1111/trf.12918

Hohler, S. E. (2015). Latex allergies. *OR Nurse*, *9*(1), 12–19. doi:10.1097/01.ORN.0000457107.47873.aa

Schmiedl, S., Rottenkolber, M., Hasford, J., Rottenkolber, D., Farker, K., Drewelow, B., ... Thürmann, P. (2014). Self-medication with over-the-counter and prescribed drugs causing adverse drug reaction-related hospital admissions: Results of a prospective, long-term multi-center study. *Drug Safety*, *37*(4), 225–235. doi:10.1007/s40264-014-0141-3

ANXIETY

related to situational crisis

Definition

Vague uneasy feeling of discomfort or dread accompanied by an autonomic response (the source is often nonspecific or unknown to the individual); a feeling of apprehension caused by anticipation of danger. It is an alerting signal that warns of impending danger and enables the individual to take measures to deal with that threat

Assessment

- Current health status
- Patient's perception of problem, onset of problem, recent stressors, life changes, and other precipitants
- Mental status, including orientation to time, place, and person; insight regarding current situation; judgment; abstract thinking; general information; mood; affect; recent and remote memory; thought processes; and thought content
- Coping and problem-solving ability
- Ability to perform activities of daily living
- Sleep habits
- Dietary and nutritional status
- Available support systems, including family members, friends, clergy, and health care agencies

Defining Characteristics

Behavioral

- Decrease in productivity
- Extraneous movement
- Fidgeting
- Glancing about
- Hypervigilance
- Insomnia
- Poor eye contact
- Restlessness
- Scanning behavior
- Worried about change in life event

Affective

- Anguish
- Apprehensiveness
- Distress
- Fear
- Feeling of inadequacy
- Helplessness
- Increase in wariness
- Irritability
- Jitteriness
- Overexcitement
- Rattled
- Regretful
- Self-focused
- Uncertainty
- Worried

Physiologic

- Facial tension
- Hand tremors
- Increase in perspiration
- Increase in tension
- Shakiness
- Trembling
- Voice quivering

Sympathetic

- Alteration in respiratory pattern
- Anorexia
- Brisk reflexes
- Cardiovascular excitation
- Diarrhea
- Dry mouth
- Facial flushing
- Heart palpitations
- Increase in blood pressure
- Increase in heart rate
- Increase in respiratory rate
- Pupil dilation
- Superficial vasoconstriction
- Twitching
- Weakness

Parasympathetic

- Abdominal pain
- Alteration in sleep pattern
- Decrease in heart rate
- Decreased blood pressure
- Diarrhea
- Faintness
- Fatigue
- Nausea
- Tingling in extremities
- Urinary frequency
- Urinary hesitancy
- Urinary urgency

Cognitive

- Alteration in attention
- Alteration in concentration
- Awareness of physiologic symptoms
- Blocking of thoughts
- Confusion
- Decrease in perceptual field
- Diminished ability to learn
- Diminished ability to problem-solve
- Fear
- Forgetfulness
- Preoccupation
- Rumination
- Tendency to blame others

Expected Outcomes

- Patient will identify factors that elicit anxious behaviors.
- Patient will discuss activities that tend to decrease anxious behaviors.
- Patient will practice progressive relaxation techniques a specified number of times per day.
- Patient will cope with current medical situation without demonstrating severe signs of anxiety.

Suggested NOC Outcomes

Anxiety Level; Anxiety Self-control; Concentration; Coping; Hyperactivity Level; Impulse Self-Control; Psychosocial Adjustment: Life Change; Social Interaction Skills; Stress Level; Symptom Control

Interventions and Rationales

- Spend 10 minutes with patient twice per shift. Convey a willingness to listen. Offer understanding and empathy; for example, "I know you're frightened. I'll stay with you." *Specific amount of uninterrupted, non–care-related time spent with anxious patient builds trust and reduces tension. Active listening helps patient ventilate feelings.*
- Give patient clear, concise explanations of anything that's about to occur. Avoid information overload: An anxious patient can't assimilate many details. *Anxiety may impair patient's cognitive abilities.*
- PCC Listen attentively; allow patient to express feelings verbally. *This may allow patient to identify anxious behaviors and discover the source of anxiety.*
- Make no demands on patient. *Anxious patient may respond to excessive demands with hostility and abuse.*
- Identify and reduce as many environmental stressors (including people) as possible. *Anxiety commonly results from lack of trust in the environment.*
- PCC Have patient state what kinds of activities promote feelings of comfort, and encourage patient to perform them. *This gives patient a sense of control.*
- Remain with patient during severe anxiety. *Anxiety is usually related to fear of being left alone.*
- PCC Include patient in decisions related to care, when feasible. *Anxious patient may mistrust own abilities; involvement in decision making may reduce anxious behaviors.*
- PCC Support family members in coping with patient's anxious behavior. *Involving family members in process of reassurance and explanation allays patient's anxiety as well as their own.*
- Allow extra visiting periods with family if this seems to allay patient's anxiety. *This allows anxious patient and family to support each other according to their abilities and at their own pace.*
- PCC Teach patient relaxation techniques to be performed at least every 4 hours, such as guided imagery, progressive muscle relaxation, and meditation. *These measures restore psychological and physical equilibrium by decreasing autonomic response to anxiety.*
- Offer relaxing types of music to patient for quiet listening periods. *Listening to relaxing music may provide distraction and have a calming effect on patient.*
- PCC Refer patient to community or professional mental health resources to provide ongoing mental health assistance. *Encouraging the use of community resources reinforces the notion that anxiety reduction is a long-term process.*

Suggested NIC Interventions

Active Listening; Anger Control Assistance; Anticipatory Guidance; Anxiety Reduction; Behavior Modification: Social Skills; Calming Technique; Coping Enhancement; Simple Guided Imagery; Support Group

Evaluations for Expected Outcomes

- Patient describes at least two situations that increase anxious behaviors.
- Patient states at least two ways to eliminate or minimize anxious behaviors.
- Patient demonstrates progressive relaxation exercises and practices them a specified number of times per day.
- Patient reports being able to cope with current situation without experiencing severe anxiety.

Documentation

- Patient's statement of anxiety and feelings of relief
- Statements about observable signs of patient's anxiety
- Interventions to reduce patient's anxiety
- Effectiveness of nursing interventions that can be observed
- Evaluations for expected outcomes

REFERENCES

Bayrampour, H., McDonald, S., & Tough, S. (2015). Risk factors of transient and persistent anxiety during pregnancy. (2015). *Midwifery*, *31*(6), 582–589. doi:10.1016/j.midw.2015.02.009

Effects of a psycho-cognitive nursing intervention on critical care patients: Pain and anxiety levels. (2015). *CONNECT: The World of Critical Care Nursing*, *9*(4), 158.

Lopes, J. D. L., Barbosa, D. A., Nogueira-Martins, L. A., & Barros, A. L. B. L. D. (2015). Nursing guidance on bed baths to reduce anxiety. *Revista Brasileira de Enfermagem*, *68*(3), 437–443. doi:10.1590/0034-7167.2015680317i

Nursing care for patients developing marked anxiety on being diagnosed with cancer progression after surgery. (2015). *Cancer Nursing*, *38*, S70.

RISK FOR ASPIRATION

Definition

Vulnerable to entry of gastrointestinal secretions, oropharyngeal secretions, solids, or fluids to the tracheobronchial passages, which may compromise health

Assessment

- Neurologic status, including level of consciousness (LOC), orientation, and mental status
- Gastrointestinal (GI) status, including gag and swallow reflexes, inspection of abdomen, abdominal girth, auscultation of bowel sounds, palpation for masses and tenderness, percussion of abdomen, and medications
- Nutritional status, including continuous and intermittent tube feeding
- Respiratory status, including skin color, rate and depth of respiration, cough (productive or nonproductive), auscultation of breath sounds, palpation for fremitus, sputum characteristics (color, consistency, amount, and odor), arterial blood gas values, and chest X-ray
- Vital signs
- Laboratory studies, such as white blood cell (WBC) count and sputum culture

Risk Factors

- Barrier to upper body
- Decrease in GI motility
- Decrease in LOC
- Delayed gastric emptying
- Decreased gag reflex
- Enteral feedings
- Facial surgery
- Facial trauma
- Impaired ability to swallow
- Incompetent lower esophageal sphincter
- Increase in gastric residual
- Increase in intragastric pressure
- Ineffective cough
- Neck surgery
- Neck trauma
- Oral surgery
- Oral trauma
- Presence of oral/nasal tube (e.g., tracheal, feeding)
- Treatment regimen
- Wired jaws

Expected Outcomes

- Patient will tolerate ___ mL of tube feeding.
- Patient's temperature and WBC count will remain normal.
- No pathogens will appear in cultures.
- Respiratory secretions will be clear and odorless.
- Auscultation will reveal no adventitious breath sounds.
- Auscultation will reveal normal bowel sounds.
- Patient and caregiver will discuss measures to prevent aspiration.

Suggested NOC Outcomes

Aspiration Prevention; Mechanical Ventilation Response: Adult; Respiratory Status: Airway Patency; Respiratory Status: Ventilation; Risk Control; Swallowing Status

Interventions and Rationales

- S Assess respiratory status at least every 4 hours *for signs of possible aspiration (increased respiratory rate, cough, sputum production, or diminished breath sounds), which should be treated as early as possible.*
- Monitor and record neurologic status *to detect altered LOC, which could affect ability to swallow food or saliva.*
- S Monitor and record vital signs *to detect signs of aspiration or impaired gas exchange due to aspiration.*
- S Keep suction equipment available at all times, especially when feeding the patient, *to ensure ability to keep airway clear.*
- S Assess patient for gag and swallow reflexes. *Decreased gag or swallow reflex may cause aspiration.*
- Encourage patient to cough and expectorate sputum *to mobilize secretions.* Provide tissues and paper bags for hygienic sputum disposal *to prevent spreading infection.*
- Auscultate for bowel sounds every shift, and report changes. *Delayed gastric emptying and elevated intragastric pressure may promote regurgitation of stomach contents.*
- If patient is receiving tube feedings:
  - Assess cuff inflation for patient with artificial airway, and adjust appropriately *to protect lower airways from oropharyngeal secretions.*
  - Add food coloring to tube feeding if patient has altered state of consciousness, diminished gag reflex, or history of aspiration *to help monitor gastric secretions for aspiration.*
  - Begin regimen with a small, diluted amount, as tolerated and ordered, *to allow adjustment to formula osmolality and avoid nausea, vomiting, and diarrhea.*
  - Elevate head of bed during and after feedings unless contraindicated *to prevent aspiration.*
  - Check for residual tube feeding every shift, and record amount. If more than 50 mL remains, withhold feeding *to prevent vomiting and aspiration. Report findings to physician.*
  - Place tube properly before feeding or giving medication *to protect airway.*
  - Stop feeding immediately if you suspect aspiration; then apply suction, as needed, and turn patient on side *to avoid further aspiration.*
- Assess need for antiemetic drug *to reduce nausea and vomiting.* Administer, if ordered, and monitor for effectiveness.
- Review test results *to identify signs of infection*; report abnormalities.
- PCC Explain treatment to patient and caregivers *to encourage compliance.*

Suggested NIC Interventions

Airway Suctioning; Artificial Airway Management; Aspiration Precautions; Enteral Tube Feeding; Positioning; Vomiting Management

Evaluations for Expected Outcomes

- Patient tolerates ____ mL of tube feeding.
- Patient's temperature and WBC count remain within normal parameters.
- No pathogens appear in patient's cultures.
- Patient's respiratory secretions remain clear and odorless.
- Auscultation of lungs reveals no adventitious breath sounds.
- Auscultation of abdomen reveals normal bowel sounds.
- Patient and caregiver discuss measures necessary to prevent aspiration.

Documentation

- Verification of tube placement
- Tolerance of tube feedings
- Residuals of tube feedings
- Vomiting or aspiration
- Breath sounds
- Patient's indication of situations that may lead to aspiration
- Observations of physical findings
- Interventions performed to prevent aspiration
- Evaluations for expected outcomes

REFERENCES

American Association of Critical Care Nurses. (2016). Prevention of aspiration in adults. *Critical Care Nurse*, *36*(1), e20–e24. doi:10.4037/ccn2016831

DiLibero, J., Lavieri, M., O'Donoghue, S., & DeSanto-Madeya, S. (2015). Withholding or continuing enteral feedings during repositioning and the incidence of aspiration. *American Journal of Critical Care*, *24*(3), 258–262. doi:10.4037/ajcc2015482

Sakai, K., Hirano, H., Watanabe, Y., Tohara, H., Sato, E., Sato, K., & Katakura, A. (2016) An examination of factors related to aspiration and silent aspiration in older adults requiring long-term care in rural Japan. *Journal of Oral Rehabilitation*, *43*(2), 103–110. doi:10.1111/joor.12349

AUTONOMIC DYSREFLEXIA

Definition

Life-threatening, uninhibited sympathetic response of nervous system to a noxious stimulus after a spinal cord injury at T7 or above

Assessment

- History of spinal cord trauma, including level of injury or lesion, and previous episodes of dysreflexia
- Patient's description of symptoms, including headache, nasal congestion, blurred vision, chest pain, diaphoresis and flushing above level of lesion, chilling, paresthesia, cutis anserina ("goose flesh") above level of lesion, metallic taste, and nausea

- Neurologic status, including level of consciousness, orientation, pupillary response, sensory status, and motor status
- Cardiovascular status, including blood pressure, heart rate and rhythm, and skin temperature and color
- Genitourinary status, including urine output, palpation of bladder, signs of urinary tract infection (UTI), and examination of urinary assistive devices such as catheter
- Gastrointestinal (GI) status, including nausea and vomiting, usual bowel elimination pattern, last bowel movement, inspection of abdomen, auscultation of bowel sounds, palpation for masses, and percussion for areas of dullness
- Environmental conditions, including changes in temperature (e.g., cold draft) and objects putting pressure on skin

Defining Characteristics

- Blurred vision
- Bradycardia
- Chest pain
- Chilling
- Conjunctival congestion
- Diaphoresis (above the injury)
- Headache (diffuse pain in different areas of the head and not confined to any nerve distribution area)
- Horner's syndrome
- Metallic taste in mouth
- Nasal congestion
- Pallor (below injury)
- Paresthesia
- Paroxysmal hypertension
- Pilomotor reflex
- Red blotches on skin (above the injury)
- Tachycardia

Expected Outcomes

- Cause of dysreflexia will be identified and corrected.
- Patient will experience cardiovascular stability as evidenced by ____ systolic range, ____ diastolic range, and _____ heart rate range.
- Patient will avoid bladder distention and UTI.
- Patient will have no fecal impaction.
- Patient's environment will have no noxious stimuli.
- Patient will state relief from symptoms of dysreflexia.
- Patient will have few, if any, complications.
- Patient's bladder elimination pattern will remain normal.
- Patient's bowel elimination pattern will remain normal.
- Patient, family members, or caregiver will demonstrate knowledge and understanding of dysreflexia and will describe care measures.
- Patient will experience few or no dysreflexic episodes.

Suggested NOC Outcomes

Knowledge: Disease Process; Neurologic Status; Neurologic Status: Autonomic; Sensory Function Status; Vital Signs Status

Interventions and Rationales

- S Assess for signs of dysreflexia (especially severe hypertension) *to detect condition so that prompt treatment may be initiated.*
- Place patient in sitting position or elevate head of bed to *aid venous drainage from brain, lower intracranial pressure, and temporarily reduce blood pressure.*
- Ascertain and correct probable cause of dysreflexia:
  - Check for bladder distention and patency of catheter. If necessary, irrigate catheter with small amount of solution or insert a new catheter immediately. *A blocked urinary catheter can trigger dysreflexia.*
  - Check for fecal mass in rectum. Apply dibucaine ointment (Nupercainal) or another product, as ordered, to anus and 19 (2.5 cm) into rectum 10 to 15 minutes before removing impaction. *Failure to use ointment may aggravate autonomic response.*
  - Check environment for cold drafts and objects putting pressure on patient's skin, *which could act as dysreflexia stimuli.*
  - Send urine for culture if no other cause becomes apparent *to detect possible UTI.*
- If hypertension persists despite other measures, administer ganglionic blocking agent, vasodilator, or other medication as ordered. *Drugs may be required if hypertension persists or if noxious stimuli can't be removed.*
- Take vital signs frequently *to monitor effectiveness of prescribed medications.*
- PCC Instruct patient, family members, or caregiver about dysreflexia, including its causes, signs and symptoms, and care measures *to prepare them to handle possible emergencies related to condition.* Suggest patient carry an autonomic dysreflexia emergency card such as the one from www.sci-info-pages.com *to provide information quickly for responders unfamiliar with autonomic dysreflexia.*
- Implement and maintain bowel and bladder elimination programs *to avoid stimuli that could trigger dysreflexia.*

Suggested NIC Interventions

Airway Management; Bowel Management; Dysreflexia Management; Fluid Management; Neurologic Monitoring; Surveillance; Temperature Management; Vital Signs Monitoring

Evaluations for Expected Outcomes

- Cause of dysreflexia is identified and corrected.
- Patient experiences cardiovascular stability as evidenced by ___ systolic range, _____ diastolic range, and ___ heart rate range.
- Palpation doesn't reveal a distended bladder or signs of UTI.
- Patient's bowel elimination program is successfully implemented and maintained. Fecal impaction is absent.
- Patient's environment remains free from noxious stimuli.
- Patient expresses relief from signs and symptoms of dysreflexia.
- Patient doesn't experience complications of dysreflexia, including contractures, venous stasis, thrombus formation, skin breakdown, and hypostatic pneumonia.
- Patient's bladder elimination program is successfully implemented and maintained, urinary catheter is patent and without kinking or blockage, and urine output remains within specified volume.
- Patient's bowel elimination pattern remains normal.
- Patient, family member, or caregiver expresses understanding of causes, signs and symptoms, and treatment of autonomic dysreflexia, and demonstrates measures to implement if dysreflexia occurs.

- Because of successful maintenance of bladder and bowel elimination programs, preventive skin care measures, and patient and family teaching, patient experiences few or no dysreflexic episodes.

Documentation

- Objective assessment of dysreflexic episode
- Patient's description of dysreflexic episode
- Interventions to identify and eliminate causes of dysreflexia and patient's response to these
- Instructions given to patient, family, and caregiver
- Patient's expressions of understanding and demonstrated ability to prevent or manage dysreflexic episode
- Implementation, alteration, or continuation of bladder and bowel programs
- Evaluations for expected outcomes

REFERENCES

Colangelo, J. (2014). Care considerations for patients with spinal cord injuries. *Radiologic Technology*, *86*(1), 33–58

Putz, C., Helbig, L., Gerner, H., Zimmermann-Stenzel, M., & Akbar, M. (2014). Autonomic dysreflexia: A possible trigger for the development of heterotopic ossifications after traumatic spinal cord injury? *European Journal of Trauma & Emergency Surgery*, *40*(6), 721–726. doi:10.1007/s00068-013-0353-8

Wyndaele, J. J. (2015). Iatrogenic urological triggers of autonomic dysreflexia: A systematic review. *Spinal Cord*, *53*(7), 499. doi:10.1038/sc.2015.109

RISK FOR AUTONOMIC DYSREFLEXIA

Definition

Vulnerable to life-threatening, uninhibited response of the sympathetic nervous system post-spinal shock, in an individual with spinal cord injury or lesion at T6 or above (has been demonstrated in patients with injuries at T7 and T8), which may compromise health

Assessment

- History of spinal cord trauma or spinal cord tumor, including level of injury or lesion, and previous episodes of dysreflexia
- Neurologic status, including level of consciousness, orientation, pupillary response, sensory status, and motor status
- Cardiovascular status, including blood pressure, heart rate and rhythm, and skin temperature and color
- Genitourinary status, including urine output, palpation of bladder, signs of urinary tract infection (UTI), and urinary assistive devices such as catheter
- Gastrointestinal (GI) status, including nausea and vomiting, usual bowel pattern, bowel habits, last bowel movement, inspection of abdomen, auscultation of bowel sounds, palpation for masses and tenderness, and percussion for areas of tympany and dullness
- Environmental conditions, including changes in temperature (e.g., cold drafts) and objects putting pressure on skin

Risk Factors

Cardiopulmonary Stimuli

- Deep vein thrombosis
- Pulmonary emboli

Gastrointestinal Stimuli

- Bowel distention
- Constipation
- Difficult passage of feces
- Digital stimulation
- Enemas
- Esophageal reflux disease
- Fecal impaction
- Gallstones
- Gastric ulcer
- GI system pathology
- Hemorrhoids
- Suppositories

Musculoskeletal–Integumentary Stimuli

- Cutaneous stimulation (e.g., pressure ulcer, ingrown toenail, dressings, burns, rash)
- Fracture
- Heterotopic bone
- Pressure over bony prominence
- Pressure over genitalia
- Range of motion exercises
- Spasm
- Sunburn
- Wound

Neurologic Stimuli

- Irritating stimuli below level of injury
- Painful stimuli below level of injury

Regulatory Stimuli

- Extremes of environmental temperature
- Temperature fluctuations

Reproductive Stimuli

- Ejaculation
- Labor and delivery period
- Menstruation
- Ovarian cyst
- Pregnancy
- Sexual intercourse

Situational Stimuli

- Constrictive clothing (e.g., straps, stockings, shoes)
- Pharmaceutical agent
- Positioning
- Substance withdrawal (e.g., narcotic, opiate)

Urologic Stimuli

- Bladder distention
- Bladder spasm
- Cystitis
- Detrusor sphincter dyssynergia
- Epididymitis
- Instrumentation
- Renal calculi
- Surgical procedure
- Urethritis
- Urinary catheterization
- UTI

Expected Outcomes

- Risk factors for dysreflexia will be identified and reduced.
- Patient will avoid bladder distention.
- Patient won't experience UTI.
- Patient will maintain normal urinary and bowel elimination patterns.
- Patient will be free from fecal impaction.
- Patient's environment will be free from noxious stimuli that may cause dysreflexia.
- Patient, family member, or caregiver will express understanding of causes of dysreflexia.
- Patient, family member, or caregiver will demonstrate understanding of measures to prevent dysreflexia.

Suggested NOC Outcomes

Neurologic Status: Autonomic; Symptom Severity; Vital Signs Status

Interventions and Rationales

- Assess for risk factors of dysreflexia, such as constipation, fecal impaction, distended bladder, and presence of noxious stimuli. *Identifying risk factors can prevent or minimize dysreflexic episodes.*
- Monitor and record intake and output accurately *to ensure adequate fluid replacement, thereby helping to prevent constipation.*
- Check for bladder distention and patency of catheter. *A blocked catheter can trigger dysreflexia.*
- Check for abdominal distention and assess bowel sounds. Monitor and record characteristics and frequency of stools. *Fecal impaction may lead to dysreflexia.*
- Encourage fluid intake of 3 L daily, unless contraindicated. *Adequate fluid intake helps maintain patency of catheter and aids bowel elimination.*
- Administer laxative, enema, or suppositories, as prescribed, *to promote elimination of solids and gases from GI tract.* Monitor effectiveness.
- PCC Consult with dietitian about increasing fiber and bulk in diet to maximum prescribed by physician *to improve intestinal muscle tone and promote comfortable elimination.*
- Implement and maintain bowel and bladder programs *to avoid stimuli that could trigger dysreflexia.*
- S Monitor vital signs frequently *to ensure effectiveness of preventive measures.* Severe hypertension may indicate dysreflexia.
- PCC Instruct patient, family member, or caregiver about risk factors, signs and symptoms, and care measures for dysreflexia *to help prevent a possible dysreflexic episode and help patient respond appropriately should dysreflexia occur.* Suggest patient carry an autonomic dysreflexia emergency card such as the one from www.sci-info-pages.com *to provide information quickly for responders unfamiliar with autonomic dysreflexia.*

Suggested NIC Interventions

Dysreflexia Management; Neurologic Monitoring; Vital Signs Monitoring

Evaluations for Expected Outcomes

- Risk factors for dysreflexia are identified and reduced.
- Patient avoids bladder distention.
- Patient doesn't experience UTI.
- Patient maintains normal urinary and bowel elimination patterns.
- Patient remains free from fecal impaction.
- Patient's environment is free from noxious stimuli that may cause dysreflexia.
- Patient, family member, or caregiver expresses understanding of causes of dysreflexia.
- Patient, family member, or caregiver demonstrates understanding of measures to prevent dysreflexia.

Documentation

- Presence of risk factors for dysreflexia
- Interventions to minimize risk of dysreflexia and patient's response
- Patient's, family members', or caregiver's expressions of concern about risk of dysreflexia

- Instructions given to patient, family member, or caregiver regarding prevention of dysreflexic episodes
- Implementation or alteration of bowel and bladder program
- Evaluations for expected outcomes

REFERENCES

Colangelo, J. (2014). Care considerations for patients with spinal cord injuries. *Radiologic Technology, 86*(1), 33–58.

Putz, C., Helbig, L., Gerner, H., Zimmermann-Stenzel, M., & Akbar, M. (2014). Autonomic dysreflexia: A possible trigger for the development of heterotopic ossifications after traumatic spinal cord injury? *European Journal of Trauma & Emergency Surgery, 40*(6), 721–726. doi:10.1007/s00068-013-0353-8

Wyndaele, J. J. (2015). Iatrogenic urological triggers of autonomic dysreflexia: A systematic review. *Spinal Cord, 53*(7), 499. doi:10.1038/sc.2015.109

RISK FOR BLEEDING

Definition

Vulnerable to a decrease in blood volume, which may compromise health

Assessment

- Cardiovascular status, including blood pressure, cardiac output, patient and family history of cardiovascular disease, peripheral pulses, and smoking history
- Nutritional status, including dietary patterns, laboratory tests, and serum protein level
- Neurologic status, including level of consciousness (LOC), mental status, motor function, and sensory pattern
- Reproductive status, including number of pregnancies and complications of pregnancy
- Respiratory status, including breath sounds, respiratory rate, and pattern
- Presence of health condition that may interfere with bleeding, such as coagulopathies
- Gastrointestinal (GI) status, including nausea and vomiting, bowel habits, stool characteristics, history of GI problems, disease, or surgery; bowel sounds
- Laboratory studies, including complete blood count, liver profile, serum electrolyte levels, platelet count, and blood coagulation studies

Risk Factors

- Aneurysm
- Circumcision
- Disseminated intravascular coagulopathy
- GI condition (e.g., ulcer, polyps, varices)
- History of falls
- Impaired liver function (e.g., cirrhosis, hepatitis)
- Inherent coagulopathy (thrombocytopenia)
- Insufficient knowledge of bleeding precautions
- Postpartum complications (e.g., uterine atony, retained placenta)
- Pregnancy-related complications (e.g., premature rupture of membranes, placenta previa/abruption, multiple gestation)
- Trauma
- Treatment regimen

Expected Outcomes

- Patient will receive adequate screening/monitoring to alert clinicians of existing risk factors for bleeding.
- Patient will receive appropriate follow-through and evidence-based interventions by clinicians to protect the patient from a bleeding episode.
- Patient will receive appropriate clinician staffing and surveillance for a rapid response to rescue client before bleeding occurs (i.e., avoid a failure to rescue occurrence).
- Patient heart rate, rhythm, blood pressure, and tissue perfusion will remain within expected ranges during episodes of risk.
- Patient will exhibit coping mechanism and functional behavior during episodes of risk.
- Patient and clinicians will identify and avoid risk situations with the potential for trauma injury and falls in the environment.
- Patient will perform self-care activities and functions.
- Patient will experience no bleeding episodes.

Suggested NOC Outcomes

Maternal Status: Antepartum; Maternal Status: Postpartum; Blood Coagulation; Treatment-Related Side Effects: Surgery, Circumcision, Medications, Administration of Blood Products; Circulation Status; Tissue Perfusion: Vital Organs and Cellular; Wound Healing; Blood Loss Severity; Trauma

Interventions and Rationales

- Interview/screen each individual for risk factors for bleeding; *some individuals know their risks for bleeding, others do not, and clinical tests and evaluation by expert clinicians allow for preventive or corrective intervention measures.*
- Anticipate conditions and episodes of care that may precipitate bleeding. *The clinicians in high-risk areas (trauma, emergency departments, ante/intra/postpartum, surgery) must be prepared and aware of patient conditions and changes that could precede a bleeding event.*
- Monitor physiologic responses (vital signs, O_2 level, LOC [behavior]) for values that remain in expected or normal ranges; *early bleeding compensatory mechanisms alter respirations, pulse, and blood pressure, and subtle changes can be detected by a perceptive clinician.*
- Monitor for frank bleeding and for occult bleeding in urine and feces through assessment of wounds, dressings, and eliminated body fluids either by visual inspection or with the aid of easy chemical testing (guaiac hemoccult).
- Correlate interview findings, risk factors, and current episode of care and patient condition *to determine the imminent level of risk for bleeding.*
- Perform vital signs and basic physical assessments according to evidence-based protocols for the in-hospital patient who is at risk for bleeding *until it is assured the patient is no longer at risk for bleeding.*
- Obtain clinical laboratory tests (hemoglobin, hematocrit, CBC, TT, PT, APTT, others) and point-of-care tests (guaiac, urine dip test, gastroccult) *to monitor for trend changes in values that would indicate a risk for bleeding or that a bleeding episode is in process.*
- Examine surgical and wound dressings; *drainage tubes and collection canisters to measure the amount of bleeding and seepage the patient experiences, and compare this with the expected blood loss for similar conditions.*

- PCC Teach about intended effects of medications (heparin, enoxaparin, warfarin, clopidogrel, aspirin) that increase the risk for bleeding or prolong clotting. *This enables the patient to avoid situations that could cause bleeding (shaving, sports, vigorous tooth brushing) and to observe self for bleeding.*
- PCC Teach about unintended or adverse effects of medications (corticosteroids, aspirin, NSAIDs) that increase the risk for bleeding or prolong clotting. *This enables the patient to avoid situations that could cause bleeding (shaving, sports, vigorous tooth brushing) and to observe self for bleeding.*
- PCC Teach the patient gentle alternatives in activities of daily living (ADLs) *to avoid trivial trauma that may cause injury and bleeding.*
- PCC Teach the patient about inherent conditions (thrombocytopenia, hemophilia), and devise an approach to lifestyle *that protects the patient from injury and yet is satisfying and has a positive quality of life.*
- PCC Teach the patient patterns of risk management and promotion of a lifestyle that focuses on health promotion and injury avoidance because this will diminish the possibility of injury. *Having the knowledge to participate safely will increase independence and enhance self-esteem.*
- Provide care that protects the individual with a risk for bleeding from injury *to prevent bleeding.*
- Implement evidence-based interventions that reverse or remove the risk for bleeding or the bleeding condition. *These interventions will prevent the patient from bleeding or will stabilize the patient's physiologic condition and assist in recovery.*
- Provide emotional support to the patient who is experiencing an episode of bleeding and also physiologic compensatory responses such as anxiety, fear, and a sense of dread. *This support provides assurance and is calming.*
- PCC Support the patient to participate in decisions about the treatment regime that places the patient at risk for bleeding. *This active participation encourages greater understanding of the rationale and compliance by the patient with the treatment regime (for medications, see above).*
- PCC Refer the patient at risk for bleeding secondary to treatment goals (i.e., warfarin, INR level) to a case manager or advanced practice nurse *for clinical monitoring and reinforcement of teaching and lifestyle adjustments.*
- Manage and monitor the recovery progress of the patient who experienced a bleeding episode *because the patient may be weak and at safety risk for falls or injury.*
- PCC Refer to a case manager the patient with inherent conditions that require long-term monitoring and management *so that the patient can maintain independence safely.*

Suggested NIC Interventions

Hemodynamic Regulation; Intravenous (IV) Therapy; Circulatory Care; Hypovolemic Management; Vital Signs Monitoring; Fluid Management; Laboratory Data Interpretation; Shock Management

Evaluations for Expected Outcomes

- Patient receives careful monitoring of existing risk factors.
- Patient receives appropriate intervention to protect from bleeding episodes.
- Patient's vital signs remain in the ranges expected during risk for bleeding period.
- Patient exhibits adequate coping mechanisms.
- Patient is able to articulate an understanding of ways to avoid risk situations.
- Patient experiences no incidence of active bleeding.

Documentation

- Recording of assessments for bleeding
- Lab values and vital signs
- Signs of any active bleeding episodes
- Intake and output
- Patient's concern about the risk for bleeding
- Patient's understanding of practical ways in which to avoid risk

REFERENCES

Forslund, T., Wettermark, B., Wändell, P., Euler, M., Hasselström, J., & Hjemdahl, P. (2014). Risks for stroke and bleeding with warfarin or aspirin treatment in patients with atrial fibrillation at different CHADSVASc scores: Experience from the Stockholm region. *European Journal of Clinical Pharmacology*, *70*(12), 1477–1485. doi:10.1007/s00228-014-1739-1

Kärkkäinen, J. M., Koskela, J. M., & Jyrkkä, J. (2015). Alcohol abuse increases rebleeding risk and mortality in patients with non-variceal upper gastrointestinal bleeding. *Digestive Diseases & Sciences*, *60*(12), 3707–3715. doi:10.1007/s10620-015-3806-6

Mounce, M., Essel, C., Kim, T., & Harris, C. M. (2015). Risk factors for bleeding in hospitalized patients with elevated INR: No vitamin K therapy received versus vitamin K received. *Hospital Pharmacy*, *50*(10), 894–899. doi:10.1310/hpj5010-894

RISK FOR UNSTABLE BLOOD GLUCOSE LEVEL

Definition

Vulnerable to variation in blood glucose/sugar levels from the normal range, which may compromise health

Assessment

- Health status, educational level, cultural status, requests for information; demonstrated understanding of material
- Integumentary status, color, elasticity, hygiene, lesions, moisture, sensation, complete blood cell count, hemoglobin/hematocrit, serum albumin, blood coagulation studies, serum electrolytes, mobility status, urinary or bowel incontinence
- Nutritional status, including dietary patterns, laboratory tests, and serum protein level
- Neurologic status, including level of consciousness, mental status, motor function, and sensory pattern
- Behavioral status, understanding of health problem and treatment plan, past history with health care providers, participation in health care planning and decision making; recognition and realization of potential growth, health, and autonomy
- Gastrointestinal (GI) status, including nausea and vomiting; bowel habits; stool characteristics; history of GI problems, disease, or surgery; and bowel sounds
- Laboratory studies, including serum albumin, and glucose

Risk Factors

- Alteration in mental status
- Average daily physical activity is less than recommended for gender and age
- Compromised physical health status
- Delay in cognitive development

- Does not accept diagnosis
- Excessive stress
- Excessive weight gain
- Excessive weight loss
- Inadequate blood glucose monitoring
- Ineffective medication management
- Insufficient diabetes management
- Insufficient dietary intake
- Insufficient knowledge of disease management
- Nonadherence to diabetes management plan
- Pregnancy
- Rapid growth period

Expected Outcomes

- Patient will be free from symptoms of hypoglycemia/hyperglycemia.
- Patient will have serum glucose values in the prescribed desired range.
- Patient will verbalize understanding of how to control blood glucose level.

Suggested NOC Outcomes

Blood Glucose Level; Diabetes Self-Management; Knowledge: Diabetes Management, Weight Control

Interventions and Rationales

- Assess patient for symptoms of low serum glucose level, and maintain a patient airway if indicated. *A low serum glucose may not be detected in some patients until moderate to severe central nervous system impairment occurs, which can lead to a compromised airway and cardiac arrest.*
- Assess for the underlying cause of changes in glucose (e.g., inadequate dietary intake; illness such as nausea, vomiting, or diarrhea; and too much insulin) *to help patient prevent future episodes and adapt treatment strategies and lifestyle changes.*
- PCC Monitor or instruct patient to monitor glucose levels with a glucometer at regular intervals *to identify and respond early to fluctuations in glucose levels that occur outside normal parameters.*
- Assess family understanding of prescribed treatment regimen. *The family plays an important role in supporting the patient.*
- PCC Assess patient's knowledge of hypo/hyperglycemia *to ensure adequate management and prevent future episodes.*
- Monitor for signs and symptoms of hyperglycemia (polyuria, polydipsia, polyphagia, lethargy, malaise, blurred vision, and headache). *Early detection ensures prompt intervention and management.*
- Assess for the underlying cause of elevated serum glucose level, including inadequate dietary intake, illness, and poor medication management *to prevent future episodes and develop treatment strategies such as changes in lifestyle.*
- Perform immediate finger stick with a glucometer *to determine glucose level, which will guide treatment strategies.* Administer insulin, as prescribed, *to treat elevated blood glucose levels.*

- Provide patient with glucose tablets or gel if he or she is conscious and has ability to swallow. Administer intravenous glucose if patient is unconscious or cannot swallow. *Immediate treatment in the form of oral or intravenous glucose must be administered to reverse the low serum glucose level. If patient becomes nauseated, turn patient on side to prevent aspiration.*
- S Protect patient from injuries, such as falls. *Symptoms of low serum glucose place patient at risk for injury, especially when driving and performing other potentially dangerous activities.*
- Evaluate serum electrolyte levels. Administer potassium, as prescribed. *With elevated blood glucose levels, potassium and sodium levels may be low, normal, or high, depending on the amount of water loss. Consider performing serum testing for $HgbA_{1c}$ (glycosylated hemoglobin A_{3C} level) to evaluate average blood glucose levels over a period of approximately 2 to 3 months and to assess the adherence and effectiveness of the treatment regimen.*
- PCC Teach patient and family self-management of hypoglycemia and hyperglycemia including glucose monitoring at regular intervals *to treat abnormal glucose levels early* and medication management, nutritional intake, exercise, and regular follow-up visits with the physician *to ensure adequate understanding and management of the treatment regimen to prevent future hyperglycemic events. Patient and family teaching may include referrals to a diabetic educator, diabetic education classes, and a dietitian.*
- PCC Consult physician if signs and symptoms persist. *Changes in prescribed medications may be needed, such as with oral hypoglycemic agents or insulin dosing.* Call for emergency medical services if patient is unstable outside the hospital.

Suggested NIC Interventions

Bedside Laboratory Testing; Health Education; Health Screening; Nutritional Counseling; Teaching: Disease Process; Teaching: Prescribed Medications

Evaluations for Expected Outcomes

- Patient has no episodes of hypoglycemia or hyperglycemia.
- Patient has glucose readings within prescribed range.
- Patient verbalizes glucose management plan.

Documentation

- Patient's expressions of concern about symptoms of previous episodes of hypoglycemia or hyperglycemia
- Observations of physiologic and behavioral manifestations of poor glucose control
- Interventions performed to allay symptoms of hypoglycemia or hyperglycemia
- Patient's response to interventions
- Evaluations for expected outcomes

REFERENCES

Cheng, A. Y. (2014). Achieving glycemic control in special populations in hospital: Perspectives in practice. *Canadian Journal of Diabetes*, *38*(2), 134–138. doi:10.1016/j.jcjd.2014.02.021

Daly, B., Arroll, B., Kenealy, T., Sheridan, N., & Scragg, R. (2015). Management of diabetes by primary health care nurses in Auckland, New Zealand. *Journal of Primary Health Care*, *7*(1), 42–49.

Kubacka, B. (2014). A balancing act. *Nursing*, *44*(1), 30–38. doi:10.1097/01.NURSE.0000438706.66979.52

DISTURBED BODY IMAGE

related to biophysical changes

Definition

Confusion in mental picture of one's physical self

Assessment

- Physiologic changes
- Behavioral changes
- Patient's and family's perception of patient's present health problem
- Patient's usual pattern of coping with stress
- Marital status
- Patient's role in family
- Patient's past experiences with health problems
- Sleep pattern
- Appetite
- Hobbies and interests
- Occupational history
- Ethnic background and cultural perceptions

Defining Characteristics

- Absence of body part
- Alteration in body function
- Alteration in body structure
- Alteration in view of one's body (e.g., appearance, structure, function)
- Avoids looking at one's body
- Behavior of acknowledging one's body
- Behavior of monitoring one's body
- Change in ability to estimate spatial relationship of body to environment
- Change in lifestyle
- Change in social involvement
- Depersonalization of body part by use of impersonal pronouns
- Emphasis on remaining strengths
- Extension of body boundary (e.g., includes external object)
- Fear of reaction by others
- Focus on past appearance
- Focus on past function
- Focus on previous strength
- Heightened achievement
- Hiding body part
- Negative feeling about body
- Nonverbal response to perceived change in body (e.g., appearance, structure, function)
- Overexposure of body part
- Perceptions that reflect an altered view of one's body appearance
- Personalization of body part by name
- Personalization of loss by name
- Preoccupation with change
- Preoccupation with loss
- Refusal to acknowledge change
- Trauma to nonfunctioning body part
- Alteration in body function (due to anomaly, disease, medication, pregnancy, radiation, surgery, trauma, etc.)
- Alteration in cognitive functioning
- Alteration in self-perception
- Cultural incongruence
- Developmental transition
- Illness
- Impaired psychosocial functioning
- Injury
- Spiritual incongruence
- Surgical procedure
- Trauma
- Treatment regimen

Expected Outcomes

- Patient will acknowledge change in body image.
- Patient will participate in decision making about his or her care (specify).

- Patient will communicate feelings about change in body image.
- Patient will express positive feelings about self.
- Patient will talk with someone who has experienced the same problem.
- Patient will demonstrate ability to practice two new coping behaviors.

Suggested NOC Outcomes

Adaptation to Physical Disability; Body Image; Coping; Grief Resolution; Adaptive Psychosocial Adjustment: Life Change; Self-Esteem

Interventions and Rationales

- PCC While assisting with self-care measures, involve patient in discussions that will provide further insights into patient's coping patterns and self-esteem. *Patient's usual coping patterns and self-perception provide baseline data for assessing potential threat of current situation.*
- PCC Accept patient's perception of self. *The nurse's acceptance validates patient's self-perception and provides reassurance of successfully overcoming crisis.*
- PCC Assess patient's readiness for decision making; then involve patient in making choices and decisions related to care and treatment. *This gives patient a sense of control over environment.*
- PCC Encourage patient to participate actively in performing care. *This gives patient a sense of independence and increases self-esteem.*
- PCC Give patient opportunities to voice feelings. *This helps patient ventilate doubts and resolve concerns.*
- Provide positive reinforcement to patient's efforts to adapt *to increase probability that healthy adaptation will continue.*
- Arrange for patient to interact with others who have similar problems. *A support group allows patient to share mutual support and caring with others who can fully understand. This kind of support will help the patient to respond in social situations without undue embarrassment.*
- PCC Refer patient to a mental health professional for further counseling. *Referral is indicated when patient is adapting poorly to situation.*
- PCC Teach patient coping strategies (specify) *to help overcome maladaptive coping behaviors.*
- PCC Have patient provide feedback about coping behaviors that seem to work. Reinforce the practice of these behaviors. *This allows you to evaluate patient's adaptive abilities.* Positive feedback reinforces adaptability and encourages similar behaviors in future.

Suggested NIC Interventions

Active Listening; Anticipatory Guidance; Body Image Enhancement; Coping Enhancement; Counseling; Grief Work Facilitation; Presence; Self-Care Assistance; Spiritual Support; Support System Enhancement

Evaluations for Expected Outcomes

- Patient acknowledges change in body image.
- Patient takes an active role in planning aspects of care (specify).
- Patient expresses emotions associated with change in body image.
- Patient expresses at least one positive feeling about self daily.

- Patient participates in discussions with support group composed of individuals with a similar change in body image (specify).
- Patient uses at least two healthy coping skills to deal with change in body image.

Documentation

- Words patient uses to describe self, prostheses, adaptive equipment, and limitations
- Body parts that patient focuses on or ignores
- Observations related to change in structure or function of body part
- Observed responses of patient to change in body part, such as touching or not touching
- Health education or counseling provided to help patient cope with altered body image
- Patient's response to nursing interventions
- Evaluations for expected outcomes

REFERENCES

Aguilar Cordero, M. J., Mur Villar, N., Neri Sánchez, M., Pimentel-Ramírez, M. L., García-Rillo, A., & Gómez Valverde, E. (2015). Breast cancer and body image as a prognostic factor of depression: A case study in México City. *Nutricion Hospitalaria*, *31*(1), 371–379. doi:10.3305/nh.2015.31.1.7863

Lewis-Smith, H., Diedrichs, P. C., Rumsey, N., & Harcourt, D. (2016). A systematic review of interventions on body image and disordered eating outcomes among women in midlife. *International Journal of Eating Disorders*, *49*(1), 5–18. doi:10.1002/eat.22480

Rhoten, B. A., Deng, J., Dietrich, M. S., Murphy, B., & Ridner, S. H. (2014). Body image and depressive symptoms in patients with head and neck cancer: An important relationship. *Supportive Care in Cancer*, *22*(11), 3053–3060. doi:10.1007/s00520-014-2312-2

Taylor, C. (2015). Body image concerns after colorectal cancer surgery. *British Journal of Nursing*, *24*, S8–S14.

INEFFECTIVE BREATHING PATTERN

related to respiratory muscle fatigue

Definition

Inspiration and/or expiration that does not provide adequate ventilation

Assessment

- History of respiratory disorder
- Respiratory status, including rate and depth of respiration, symmetry of chest expansion, use of accessory muscles, presence of cough, anterior–posterior chest diameter, palpation for fremitus, percussion of lung fields, auscultation of breath sounds, and pulmonary function studies
- Cardiovascular status, including heart rate and rhythm, blood pressure, and skin color, temperature, and turgor
- Neurologic and mental status, including level of consciousness and emotional level
- Knowledge, including current understanding of physical condition and physical, mental, and emotional readiness to learn

Defining Characteristics

- Abnormal breathing pattern (e.g., rate, rhythm, depth)
- Altered chest excursion
- Bradypnea

- Decrease in expiratory pressure
- Decrease in inspiratory pressure
- Decrease in minute ventilation
- Decrease in vital capacity
- Dyspnea
- Increase in anterior–posterior chest diameter
- Nasal flaring
- Orthopnea
- Prolonged expiration phase
- Pursed-lip breathing
- Tachypnea
- Use of accessory muscles to breathe
- Use of three-point position

Expected Outcomes

- Patient's respiratory rate will stay within 5 breaths/minute of baseline.
- Arterial blood gas (ABG) levels will return to baseline.
- Patient will report feeling comfortable when breathing.
- Patient will report feeling rested each day.
- Patient will demonstrate diaphragmatic pursed-lip breathing.
- Patient will achieve maximum lung expansion with adequate ventilation.
- Patient will demonstrate skill in conserving energy while carrying out activities of daily living (ADLs).

Suggested NOC Outcomes

Mechanical Ventilation Response: Adult; Respiratory Status: Airway Patency; Respiratory Status: Gas Exchange; Respiratory Status: Ventilation; Vital Signs

Interventions and Rationales

- S Assess and record respiratory rate and depth at least every 4 hours *to detect early signs of respiratory compromise.* Also assess ABG levels, according to facility policy, *to monitor oxygenation and ventilation status.*
- S Auscultate breath sounds at least every 4 hours *to detect decreased or adventitious breath sounds;* report changes.
- Assist patient to a comfortable position, for example, by supporting the upper extremities with pillows, providing an overbed table with a pillow to lean on, and elevating head of bed. *These measures promote comfort, chest expansion, and ventilation of basilar lung fields.*
- Perform chest physiotherapy *to aid mobilization and secretion removal* if ordered. Percussion, vibration, and postural drainage enhance airway clearance and respiratory leffort.
- Provide rest periods between breathing enhancement measures *to avoid fatigue.*
- Help patient with ADLs as needed, *to conserve energy and avoid overexertion and fatigue.*
- Administer oxygen as ordered. *Supplemental oxygen helps reduce hypoxemia and relieve respiratory distress.*
- Suction airway as needed. *Retained secretions alter the ventilatory response, thus reducing oxygen, leading to hypoxemia.*
- Schedule necessary activities to provide periods of rest. *This prevents fatigue and reduces oxygen demands.*
- PCC Teach patient about:
  - pursed-lip breathing
  - abdominal breathing
  - performing relaxation techniques
  - taking prescribed medications (ensuring accuracy of dose and frequency and monitoring adverse effects)

- scheduling activities to avoid fatigue and provide for rest periods
  These measures allow patient to participate in maintaining health status and improve ventilation.

PCC
- Refer patient for evaluation of exercise potential and development of individualized exercise program. *Exercise promotes conditioning of respiratory muscles and patient's sense of well-being.*

Suggested NIC Interventions

Acid–Base Monitoring; Airway Management; Airway Suctioning; Anxiety Reduction; Exercise Promotion; Oxygen Therapy; Progressive Muscle Relaxation; Respiratory Monitoring; Ventilation Assistance

Evaluations for Expected Outcomes

- Patient's respiratory rate remains within established limits.
- Patient's ABG levels return to and remain within established limits.
- Patient indicates, either verbally or through behavior, feeling comfortable when breathing.
- Patient reports feeling rested each day.
- Patient performs diaphragmatic pursed-lip breathing.
- Patient demonstrates maximum lung expansion with adequate ventilation.
- When patient carries out ADLs, breathing pattern remains normal.

Documentation

- Patient's expressions of comfort in breathing, emotional state, understanding of medical diagnosis, and readiness to learn
- Physical findings from pulmonary assessment
- Interventions carried out and patient's responses to them
- Evaluations for expected outcomes

REFERENCES

Bradley, H., & Esformes, J. (2014). Breathing pattern disorders and functional movement. *International Journal of Sports Physical Therapy*, *9*(1), 28–39.

Jones, M., Troup, F., Nugus, J., Roughton, M., Hodson, M., Rayner, C., ... Pryor, J. (2015). Does manual therapy provide additional benefit to breathing retraining in the management of dysfunctional breathing? A randomized-controlled trial. *Disability & Rehabilitation*, *37*(9), 763–770. doi:10.3109/09638288.2014.941020

Sulemanji, D. S., Fangping, B., Yandong, J., & Kacmarek, R. M. (2014). A unidirectional breathing pattern improves breathing efficiency in subjects with severe COPD. *Respiratory Care*, *59*(10), 1487–1493. doi:10.4187/respcare.02899

DECREASED CARDIAC OUTPUT

related to altered contractility

Definition

Inadequate blood pumped by the heart to meet the metabolic demands of the body

Assessment

- Mental status, including orientation and level of consciousness (LOC)
- Cardiovascular status, including history of valvular disorder, capillary heart disease, or myopathy; skin color, temperature, turgor, and capillary refill time; jugular vein distention; hepatojugular reflux; heart rate and rhythm; heart sounds; blood pressure; peripheral pulses; electrocardiogram (ECG); exercise ECG; echocardiogram; and phonocardiogram
- Respiratory status, including respiratory rate and depth, breath sounds, chest X-ray, and arterial blood gas values
- Renal status, including weight, intake and output, and urine specific gravity

Defining Characteristics

Altered Heart Rate/Rhythm

- Bradycardia
- ECG change (e.g., arrhythmia, conduction abnormality, ischemia)
- Heart palpitations
- Tachycardia

Altered Preload

- Decreased central venous pressure (CVP)
- Decrease in pulmonary artery wedge pressure (PAWP)
- Edema
- Fatigue
- Heart murmur
- Increase in CVP
- Increase in PAWP
- Jugular vein distention
- Weight gain

Altered Afterload

- Abnormal skin color (e.g., pale, dusky, cyanosis)
- Alteration in blood pressure
- Clammy skin
- Decrease in peripheral pulses
- Decrease in pulmonary vascular resistance (PVR)
- Decrease in systemic vascular resistance (SVR)
- Dyspnea
- Increase in PVR
- Increase in SVR
- Oliguria
- Prolonged capillary refill

Altered Contractility

- Adventitious breath sounds
- Coughing
- Decreased cardiac index
- Decrease in ejection fraction
- Decrease in left ventricular stroke work index
- Decrease in stroke volume index
- Orthopnea
- Paroxysmal nocturnal dyspnea
- Presence of S3 heart sound
- Presence of S4 heart sound

Behavioral/Emotional

- Anxiety
- Restlessness

Expected Outcomes

- Patient's pulse will be greater than ____ but not less than ____.
- Patient's blood pressure will be greater than ____but not greater than ____.
- Patient will exhibit no arrhythmias.
- Skin will remain warm and dry.
- Patient will exhibit no pedal edema.
- Patient will perform activity within limits of prescribed heart rate.
- Patient will express sense of physical comfort after activity.

- Patient will maintain adequate cardiac output.
- Patient will perform stress-reduction techniques every 4 hours while awake.
- Patient will verbalize understanding of reportable signs and symptoms.
- Patient will understand diet, medication regimen, and prescribed activity level.

Suggested NOC Outcomes

Cardiac Pump Effectiveness; Circulation Status; Tissue Perfusion: Abdominal Organs; Tissue Perfusion: Peripheral; Fluid Overload Severity; Vital Signs

Interventions and Rationales

- S Monitor and record LOC, heart rate and rhythm, and blood pressure at least every 4 hours, or more often if necessary, *to detect cerebral hypoxia possibly resulting from decreased cardiac output.*
- Auscultate for heart and breath sounds at least every 4 hours. Report abnormal sounds as soon as they develop. *Extra heart sounds may indicate early cardiac decompensation; adventitious breath sounds may indicate pulmonary congestion and diminished cardiac output.*
- Measure and record intake and output accurately. *Decreased urine output without lowered fluid intake might indicate decreased renal perfusion, possibly from decreased cardiac output.*
- S Promptly treat life-threatening arrhythmias, as ordered, *to avoid crisis.*
- Weigh patient daily before breakfast *to detect fluid retention.*
- Inspect for pedal or sacral edema to *detect venous stasis and reduced cardiac output.*
- Provide skin care every 4 hours *to enhance skin perfusion and venous flow.*
- Gradually increase patient's activities within limits of prescribed heart rate *to allow heart to adjust to increased oxygen demand.* Monitor pulse rate before and after activity *to compare rates and gauge tolerance.*
- Plan patient's activities *to avoid fatigue and increased myocardial workload.*
- Maintain dietary restrictions, as ordered, *to reduce risk of cardiac disease.*
- PCC Teach patient stress-reduction techniques *to reduce patient's anxiety and provide a sense of control.*
- PCC Explain all procedures and tests to *enhance understanding and reduce anxiety.*
- PCC Teach patient and family about chest pain and other reportable symptoms, prescribed diet, medications (name, dosage, frequency, and therapeutic and adverse effects), prescribed activity level, simple methods for lifting and bending, and stress-reduction techniques. *These measures involve patient and family in care.*
- Administer oxygen, as prescribed, *to increase supply to myocardium.*

Suggested NIC Interventions

Cardiac Precautions; Circulatory Precautions; Fluid Management; Hemodynamic Regulation; Vital Signs Monitoring

Evaluations for Expected Outcomes

- Patient's pulse rate remains within set limits.
- Patient's blood pressure remains within set limits.

- Patient doesn't exhibit arrhythmias during monitoring or physical examination.
- Patient's skin remains warm and dry to touch.
- Inspection and palpation don't reveal pedal edema.
- Patient carries out activities of daily living (ADLs) without heart rate exceeding or dropping below set limits.
- Patient doesn't indicate, either verbally or through behavior, chest pain, dyspnea, fatigue, or other forms of discomfort after activity.
- Patient performs stress-reduction techniques every 4 hours.
- Patient describes signs and symptoms of decreased cardiac output, such as dizziness, syncope, clammy skin, fatigue, and dyspnea.
- Patient understands importance of following prescribed diet, taking medications as ordered, and maintaining activity level.

Documentation

- Patient's needs and perception of problem
- Observations of physical findings
- Patient's response to activity
- Development of skills related to diet, medication, activity, and stress management
- Evaluations for expected outcomes

REFERENCES

Caitlin, B. J., Lewis, K. B., Nichols, N., & Parsons, L. M. (2015). Advance care planning and the role of the cardiovascular nurse. *Canadian Journal of Cardiovascular Nursing*, *25*(3), 5–9.

McLaughlin, D., Hoy, L., & Glackin, M. (2015). Heart failure nurse specialist crisis interventions and avoided hospital admissions. *British Journal of Cardiac Nursing*, *10*(7), 326–333.

Unverzagt, S., Oemler, M., Braun, K., & Klement, A. (2014). Strategies for guideline implementation in primary care focusing on patients with cardiovascular disease: A systematic review. *Family Practice*, *31*(3), 247–266. doi:10.1093/fampra/cmt080

DECREASED CARDIAC OUTPUT

related to altered stroke volume

Definition

Inadequate blood pumped by the heart to meet metabolic demands of the body

Assessment

- History of cardiac disorder
- Mental status, including orientation and level of consciousness
- Cardiovascular status, including history of arrhythmias and syncope, jugular vein distention, hepatojugular reflux, heart rate and rhythm, heart sounds, blood pressure, peripheral pulses, electrocardiogram (ECG), exercise ECG, echocardiogram, serum digoxin levels, and skin color, temperature, turgor, and capillary refill time
- Respiratory status, including respiratory rate and depth, breath sounds, chest X-ray, and arterial blood gas values
- Renal status, including weight, intake and output, urine specific gravity, and serum electrolytes

Defining Characteristics

Altered Heart Rate/Rhythm

- Bradycardia
- ECG change (e.g., arrhythmia, conduction abnormality, ischemia)
- Heart palpitations
- Tachycardia

Altered Preload

- Decreased central venous pressure (CVP)
- Decrease in pulmonary artery wedge pressure (PAWP)
- Edema
- Fatigue
- Heart murmur
- Increase in CVP
- Increase in PAWP
- Jugular vein distention
- Weight gain

Altered Afterload

- Abnormal skin color (e.g., pale, dusky, cyanosis)
- Alteration in blood pressure
- Clammy skin
- Decrease in peripheral pulses
- Decrease in pulmonary vascular resistance (PVR)
- Decrease in systemic vascular resistance (SVR)
- Dyspnea
- Increase in PVR
- Increase in SVR
- Oliguria
- Prolonged capillary refill

Altered Contractility

- Adventitious breath sounds
- Coughing
- Decreased cardiac index
- Decrease in ejection fraction
- Decrease in left ventricular stroke work index
- Decrease in stroke volume index
- Orthopnea
- Paroxysmal nocturnal dyspnea
- Presence of S3 heart sound
- Presence of S4 heart sound

Behavioral/Emotional

- Anxiety
- Restlessness

Expected Outcomes

- Patient's pulse will be greater than ____ but not greater than ____.
- Patient's blood pressure will be greater than ___ but not greater than ____.
- Patient's skin will remain warm and dry.
- Patient will experience few or no dyspneic episodes.
- Patient will show no signs of dizziness or syncope.
- Patient will experience no chest pain.
- Patient will practice stress-reduction techniques every 2 hours.
- Patient's cardiac output will remain adequate.
- Patient will have no arrhythmias.
- Patient will verbalize knowledge of reportable signs and symptoms.
- Patient will understand diet, medication regimen, and prescribed activity level.

Suggested NOC Outcomes

Cardiac Disease Self-Management; Cardiac Pump Effectiveness; Circulation Status; Tissue Perfusion: Abdominal Organs; Tissue Perfusion: Cardiac; Tissue Perfusion: Peripheral; Tissue Perfusion: Pulmonary; Vital Signs

Interventions and Rationales

- S • Monitor patient at least every 4 hours for irregularities in cardiac rate or rhythm, dyspnea, fatigue, crackles in lungs, jugular venous distention, or chest pain. *Any or all of these may indicate impending cardiac failure or other complications.* Report them immediately.
- Assess skin temperature every 4 hours. *Cool, clammy skin may indicate decreased cardiac output.*
- Assess respiratory status at least every 4 hours. Report complaints of dyspnea or restlessness. *Adventitious breath sounds or dyspnea may indicate fluid buildup in lungs and pulmonary capillary bed (as in heart failure).*
- Administer oxygen, as ordered, *to increase supply to myocardium.*
- S • Report complaints of dizziness or syncope promptly; *these may indicate cerebral hypoxia resulting from a cardiac rhythm disturbance.*
- Tell patient to report chest pain right away *because it may signal myocardial hypoxia or injury.*
- Plan patient's care to avoid overexertion, *which increases myocardial oxygen demand.*
- Change patient's position frequently *to promote comfort and avoid tachycardia and other sympathetic responses.*
- PCC • Teach patient how to perform stress-reduction techniques, such as deep breathing and meditation, *to allay anxiety, avoid cardiac complications, and promote cardiac healing.*
- Remind patient to practice stress-reduction techniques every 2 hours while awake *to help internalize learned techniques.*
- Give antiarrhythmic drugs as prescribed *to reduce or eliminate arrhythmias.* Monitor for adverse effects.
- Instruct patient to avoid straining during bowel movements, *which may cause stimulation of the vagus nerve, resulting in bradycardia and decreased cardiac output.*
- Administer stool softeners, as prescribed, *to reduce straining during bowel elimination.*
- PCC • Teach patient about reportable symptoms (chest pain, palpitations, weakness, dizziness, and syncope), prescribed diet, medications (name, dosage, frequency, and therapeutic and adverse effects), and activity level. *These measures let patient and caregivers participate in patient's care and help patient make informed decisions about health status.*

Suggested NIC Interventions

Cardiac Care; Energy Management; Fluid Monitoring; Hemodynamic Regulation; Laboratory Data Interpretation; Shock Prevention; Vital Signs Monitoring

Evaluations for Expected Outcomes

- Patient's pulse rate remains within set limits.
- Patient's blood pressure remains within set limits.
- Patient's skin remains warm and dry.
- Patient experiences fewer dyspneic episodes.
- Patient doesn't experience dizziness or syncope.
- Patient doesn't experience chest pain.
- Patient practices stress-reduction techniques every 2 hours.
- Patient's cardiac output remains adequate.
- No arrhythmias are noted during monitoring or physical examination of patient.
- Patient lists signs and symptoms of decreased cardiac output (dizziness, syncope, cool or clammy skin, fatigue, and dyspnea).

- Patient expresses understanding of importance of following prescribed diet, taking medications, and maintaining activity level.

Documentation

- Patient's symptoms
- Observation of physical findings
- Incidents of chest pain, including location, character, duration, and treatment
- Patient's tolerance for activity
- Interventions to control or monitor symptoms and patient's response
- Patient teaching
- Evaluations for expected outcomes

REFERENCES

Caitlin, B. J., Lewis, K. B., Nichols, N., & Parsons, L. M. (2015). Advance care planning and the role of the cardiovascular nurse. *Canadian Journal of Cardiovascular Nursing*, *25*(3), 5–9.
McLaughlin, D., Hoy, L., & Glackin, M. (2015). Heart failure nurse specialist crisis interventions and avoided hospital admissions. *British Journal of Cardiac Nursing*, *10*(7), 326–333.
Unverzagt, S., Oemler, M., Braun, K., & Klement, A. (2014). Strategies for guideline implementation in primary care focusing on patients with cardiovascular disease: A systematic review. *Family Practice*, *31*(3), 247–266. doi:10.1093/fampra/cmt080

RISK FOR DECREASED CARDIAC OUTPUT

Definition

Vulnerable to inadequate blood pumped by the heart to meet metabolic demands of the body, which may compromise health

Assessment

- History of cardiac disorder
- Mental status, including orientation and level of consciousness (LOC)
- Cardiovascular status, including history of arrhythmias and syncope, valvular disorder, capillary heart disease, or myopathy; skin color, temperature, turgor, and capillary refill time; serum digoxin levels; jugular vein distention; hepatojugular reflux; heart rate and rhythm; heart sounds; blood pressure; peripheral pulses; electrocardiogram (ECG); exercise ECG; echocardiogram; and phonocardiogram
- Respiratory status, including respiratory rate and depth, breath sounds, chest X-ray, and arterial blood gas values
- Renal status, including weight, intake and output, urine specific gravity, and serum electrolytes

Risk Factors

- Alteration in heart rate
- Alteration in heart rhythm
- Altered afterload
- Altered contractility
- Altered preload
- Altered stroke volume

Expected Outcomes

- Patient's pulse will be within normal limits.
- Patient's blood pressure will be within normal limits.
- Patient will exhibit no arrhythmias.
- Patient's skin will remain warm and dry.
- Patient will exhibit no pedal edema.
- Patient will show no signs of dizziness or syncope.
- Patient will experience few or no dyspneic episodes.
- Patient will experience no chest pain.
- Patient will express sense of physical comfort after activity.
- Patient will maintain adequate cardiac output.
- Patient will perform stress-reduction techniques.
- Patient will verbalize understanding of reportable signs and symptoms.
- Patient will verbalize understanding of diet, medication, and activity level on cardiac health.

Suggested NOC Outcomes

Cardiac Pump Effectiveness; Circulation Status; Tissue Perfusion: Peripheral; Vital Signs

Interventions and Rationales

- S Monitor and record LOC, heart rate and rhythm, and blood pressure, and report any abnormal results. *Changes from normal limits may indicate decreased cardiac output.*
- S Monitor patient for dyspnea, fatigue, crackles in lungs, jugular venous distention, or chest pain. *Any or all of these may indicate impending cardiac failure or other complications. Report them immediately.*
- Auscultate for heart and breath sounds. Report abnormal sounds as soon as they develop. *Extra heart sounds may indicate early cardiac decompensation; adventitious breath sounds may indicate pulmonary congestion and diminished cardiac output.*
- Measure and record intake and output accurately. *Decreased urine output without lowered fluid intake might indicate decreased renal perfusion, possibly from decreased cardiac output.*
- S Promptly treat life-threatening arrhythmias, as ordered, *to avoid crisis.*
- Weigh patient daily before breakfast *to detect fluid retention.*
- Inspect for pedal or sacral edema to *detect venous stasis and reduced cardiac output.*
- Provide skin care as needed *to enhance skin perfusion and venous flow.*
- Maintain dietary restrictions, as ordered, *to reduce risk of cardiac disease.*
- Report complaints of dizziness or syncope promptly; *these may indicate cerebral hypoxia resulting from a cardiac rhythm disturbance.*
- Tell patient to report chest pain right away *because it may signal myocardial hypoxia or injury.*
- PCC Teach patient stress-reduction techniques *to reduce patient's anxiety and provide a sense of control.*
- Explain all procedures and tests to *enhance understanding and reduce anxiety.*
- PCC Teach patient and family about chest pain and other reportable symptoms, prescribed diet, medications (name, dosage, frequency, and therapeutic and adverse effects), prescribed activity level, simple methods for lifting and bending, and stress-reduction techniques. *These measures involve patient and family in care.*
- Administer oxygen, as prescribed, *to increase supply to myocardium.*

Suggested NIC Interventions

Cardiac Precautions; Circulatory Precautions; Fluid Management; Homodynamic Regulation; Vital Signs Monitoring

Evaluations for Expected Outcomes

- Patient's pulse rate remains within set limits.
- Patient's blood pressure remains within set limits.
- Patient's cardiac output remains adequate.
- Patient doesn't exhibit arrhythmias during monitoring or physical examination.
- Patient's skin remains warm and dry to touch.
- Patient experiences fewer dyspneic episodes.
- Patient doesn't experience dizziness or syncope.
- Patient doesn't experience chest pain.
- Patient will not exhibit pedal edema.
- Patient doesn't indicate, either verbally or through behavior, chest pain, dyspnea, fatigue, or other forms of discomfort after activity.
- Patient performs stress-reduction techniques as needed.
- Patient describes signs and symptoms of decreased cardiac output, such as dizziness, syncope, clammy skin, fatigue, and dyspnea.
- Patient understands importance of diet, medications, and activity on cardiac health.

Documentation

- Patient's needs and perception of problem
- Observations of physical findings
- Patient's response to activity
- Development of skills related to diet, medication, activity, and stress management
- Incidents of chest pain, including location, character, duration, and treatment
- Interventions to control or monitor symptoms and patient's response
- Patient teaching
- Evaluations for expected outcomes

REFERENCES

Caitlin, B. J., Lewis, K. B., Nichols, N., & Parsons, L. M. (2015). Advance care planning and the role of the cardiovascular nurse. *Canadian Journal of Cardiovascular Nursing, 25*(3), 5–9.

Kholdani, C. A., Oudiz, R. J., & Fares, W. H. (2015). The assessment of the right heart failure syndrome. *Seminars in Respiratory & Critical Care Medicine, 36*(6), 934–942. doi:10.1055/s-0035-1564925

McLaughlin, D., Hoy, L., & Glackin, M. (2015). Heart failure nurse specialist crisis interventions and avoided hospital admissions. *British Journal of Cardiac Nursing, 10*(7), 326–333.

Zhu, J., Zhang, X., Shi, G., Yi, K., & Tan, X. (2015). Atrial fibrillation is an independent risk factor for hospital-acquired pneumonia. *PLoS One, 10*(7). doi:10.1371/journal.pone.0131782

IMPAIRED COMFORT

related to illness-related symptoms; insufficient environmental control

Definition

Perceived lack of ease, relief, and transcendence in physical, psychospiritual, environmental, cultural, and/or social dimensions

Assessment

- Patient's understanding of health problem and treatment plan
- Coping mechanisms, problem-solving ability, decision-making competencies
- Quality of relationships, support systems
- Changes in sleep patterns, appetite, and activity level

Defining Characteristics

- Alteration in sleep pattern
- Anxiety
- Crying
- Discontent with situation
- Distressing symptoms
- Fear
- Feeling cold
- Feeling hot
- Feeling of discomfort
- Feeling of hunger
- Inability to relax
- Irritability
- Itching
- Moaning
- Restlessness
- Sighing
- Uneasy in situation

Expected Outcomes

- Patient's heart rate, rhythm, and respiration rate will remain within expected range during rest and activity.
- Patient will maintain muscle mass and strength.
- Patient will report pain using pain scale.
- Patient will report periods of restful sleep.

Suggested NOC Outcomes

Comfort Status; Coping; Knowledge: Health Promotion; Pain Control

Interventions and Rationales

- Monitor pain level using scale 1 to 10. Assess vital signs during times of discomfort, including blood pressure, heart rate and rhythm, and respirations.
- Assess sleeping patterns in response to discomfort.
- Provide a quiet and relaxing atmosphere. Encourage active exercise *to increase a feeling of well-being.*
- Provide pain medications as ordered.
- PCC Teach relaxation exercises and techniques *to promote reduced pain levels, sleep, and reduce anxiety.*
- PCC Include patient in plan of action *to promote self-care.*
- PCC Teach medication administration and schedule *to facilitate pain relief.*
- PCC Teach massage therapy to caregiver *to promote comfort.*
- PCC Refer to pain management clinic if pain cannot be controlled through relaxation and exercise. Refer to physical therapist *to accommodate patient's level of activity.* Refer to massage therapist *to promote relaxation.*

Suggested NIC Interventions

Active Listening; Aroma Therapy; Calming Technique; Coping Enhancement

Evaluations for Expected Outcomes

- Patient's vital signs remained within expected range for rest and activity.
- Patient maintained muscle mass and strength.
- Patient used pain scale when reporting episodes of pain.
- Patient reported period of restful sleep.

Documentation

- Patient record of vital signs
- Patient reports of pain on scale of 1 to 10
- Patient reports of restful sleep
- Evaluations for expected outcomes

REFERENCES

Krinsky, R., Murillo, I., & Johnson, J. (2014). A practical application of Katharine Kolcaba's comfort theory to cardiac patients. *Applied Nursing Research*, *27*(2), 147–150. doi:10.1016/j.apnr.2014.02.004

Slatyer, S., Williams, A. M., & Michael, R. (2015). Seeking empowerment to comfort patients in severe pain: A grounded theory study of the nurse's perspective. *International Journal of Nursing Studies*, *52*(1), 229–239. doi:10.1016/j.ijnurstu.2014.06.010

van Soest-Poortvliet, M. C., van der Steen, J. T., de Vet, H. C., Hertogh, C. M., Onwuteaka-Philipsen, B. D., & Deliens, L. H. (2014). Factors related to establishing a comfort care goal in nursing home patients with dementia: A cohort study among family and professional caregivers. *Journal of Palliative Medicine*, *17*(12), 1317–1327. doi:10.1089/jpm.2014.0205

ACUTE CONFUSION

Definition

Abrupt onset of reversible disturbances of consciousness, attention, cognition, and perception that develop over a short period of time

Assessment

- Age, gender, level of education, occupation, and recent immigration status
- Health history, including use of medications, recent surgery, allergies, history of alcoholism, drug abuse, and depression
- Neurologic status, including level of consciousness (LOC); orientation; thought and speech; mood; affect; memory; visual and spatial ability; judgment and insight; psychomotor activity; perceptions; delusions, illusions, and hallucinations; pain level; recent behavioral changes; and history of transient ischemic attacks, head injury, early dementia, AIDS, or schizophrenia
- Cardiovascular status, including vital signs, skin color, auscultation of carotid artery and heart sounds, and history of coronary artery disease or hypertension
- Respiratory status, including rate, depth, and pattern of respirations; auscultation for breath sounds; smoking history; shortness of breath; and history of chronic obstructive pulmonary disease, cancer, or tuberculosis
- Sensory status, including results of vision and hearing examination, use of corrective lenses or hearing aid, and history of eye or ear disorders
- Nutritional status, including typical daily food intake and weight loss
- Sleep status, including recent change in sleep pattern or environment (recent hospitalization)

Defining Characteristics

- Agitation
- Alteration in cognitive functioning
- Alteration in LOC
- Alteration in psychomotor functioning
- Hallucinations
- Inability to initiate goal-directed behavior
- Inability to initiate purposeful behavior
- Insufficient follow-through with goal-directed behavior
- Insufficient follow-through with purposeful behavior
- Misperception
- Restlessness

Expected Outcomes

- Patient will experience no injury.
- Patient's neurologic status will remain stable.
- Family members will report an improved ability to cope with the patient's confused state.
- Patient will start to participate in activities of daily living (ADLs).
- Patient will report feeling increasingly calm.
- Patient and family members will state the causes of acute confusion.
- Patient and family members will express an understanding of the importance of informing other health care providers about episodes of acute confusion.

Suggested NOC Outcomes

Anxiety Level; Cognition; Cognitive Orientation; Distorted Thought Self-Control; Information Processing; Neurologic Status: Consciousness; Safe Home Environment; Sleep

Interventions and Rationales

- S Assess patient's LOC and changes in behavior *to provide baseline for comparison with ongoing assessment findings.*
- Have a staff member stay at patient's bedside, if necessary, *to protect patient from harm as long as he is confused.*
- Enlist the aid of family member *to help calm patient.*
- Limit noise and environmental stimulation *to prevent patient from becoming more confused. Environmental stimulation tends to exacerbate confused states.*
- S Monitor neurologic status on a regular basis *to detect any improvement or decline in patient's neurologic function.*
- Use appropriate safety measures *to protect patient from injury.* Avoid physical restraints *to prevent agitating patient.*
- PCC Address patient by name and tell your name *to foster patient's awareness of self and environment.*
- Give patient short, simple explanations each time you perform a procedure or task *to decrease confusion.*
- Schedule nursing care to provide quiet times for patient *to help avoid sensory overload.*
- Mention time, place, and date frequently throughout day. Have a clock and a calendar where patient can easily see them. Refer to these aids frequently when orienting patient *to foster awareness of self and environment.*

- Keep patient's possessions in the same place as much as possible. *A consistent, stable environment reduces confusion and frustration and aids completion of ADLs.*
- Ask family members to bring labeled family photos and other favorite articles *to create a more secure environment for patient.*
- Plan patient's routine, and be as consistent as possible in following it. *A consistent routine aids task completion and reduces confusion.*
- Speak slowly and clearly, and allow patient ample time to respond *to reduce frustration and promote task completion.*
- PCC Encourage patient to perform ADLs, dividing tasks into small, critical units. Be patient and specific in providing instructions. Allow time for patient to perform each task. *These measures enhance self-esteem as well as help prevent complications related to inactivity.*
- PCC Encourage family members to share stories and discuss familiar people and events with patient. *Sharing stories and familiar subjects promotes a sense of continuity, aids memory, and creates a sense of security and comfort.* Note that even if patient's short-term memory is impaired, remote memory still may be intact.
- PCC Support family members' attempts to interact with patient *to provide positive reinforcement.*
- Allow time before and after visits for family members to express feelings. *Listening to family members in an open and nonjudgmental manner helps them cope with patient's illness. Listening to their opinions may also help you assess and monitor patient's condition.*
- Reassure patient and family that confusion will be temporary *to help relieve their anxiety.* Always include patient in discussions.
- PCC Confer with physician about diagnostic test results, patient's progress in behavior, and patient's LOC. *A collaborative approach to treatment helps ensure high-quality care and continuity of care.*
- Discuss episodes of acute confusion with patient and family members *to make sure they understand the cause of confusion.*
- Review supportive measures family members can take at home if patient begins to exhibit signs of confusion. Tell them to give patient short explanations of activities; repeat time, place, and date frequently; speak slowly and clearly and allow patient time to respond; and provide patient with a consistent routine. *Teaching empowers patient and family members to take greater responsibility for their health care needs.*
- Stress to patient and family that, in the future, they should inform health care providers about episodes of acute confusion *to help ensure continuity of care.*

Suggested NIC Interventions

Behavior Management: Overactivity/Inattention; Cognitive Stimulation; Delirium Management; Fall Prevention; Hallucination Management; Medication Management; Reality Orientation; Sleep Enhancement

Evaluations for Expected Outcomes

- Patient doesn't experience injury during episodes of acute confusion.
- Patient exhibits a mental status within his or her normal range.
- Family members report an increased ability to cope with patient's confused state.
- Patient performs ADLs to the extent possible.
- Patient reports feelings of increased calm.
- Patient and family members express an understanding of the causes of acute confusion.
- Patient and family members express an understanding of the importance of telling all health care providers about episodes of acute confusion.

Documentation

- Description of episodes of acute confusion
- Factors that precipitate and ameliorate periods of acute confusion
- Teaching sessions and referrals
- Evaluations for expected outcomes

REFERENCES

Brooks, P., Spillane, J. J., Dick, K., & Stuart-Shor, E. (2014). Developing a strategy to identify and treat older patients with postoperative delirium. *AORN Journal*, *99*(2), 256–276. doi:10.1016/j.aorn.2013.12.009

Hea-Jeong, H., & Yeonghee, S. (2014). Effects of nursing intervention program on reducing acute confusion in hospitalized older adults. *Korean Journal of Adult Nursing*, *26*(1), 89–97. doi:10.7475/kjan.2014.26.1.89

Ng, J., Pan, C. X., Geube, A., Tan, C., Kawai, F., & Chorost, M. (2015). Your postop patient is confused and agitated—Next steps? *Journal of Family Practice*, *64*(6), 361–366.

RISK FOR ACUTE CONFUSION

Definition

Vulnerable to reversible disturbances of consciousness, attention, cognition, and perception that develop over a short period of time, which may compromise health

Assessment

- Age, gender, level of education, occupation, and recent immigration status
- Health history, including use of medications, especially with known cognitive and psychotropic adverse effects; recent surgery; allergies; and history of alcoholism, drug abuse, and depression
- Neurologic status, including level of consciousness (LOC), orientation, thought and speech, mood, affect, memory, visual and spatial ability, judgment and insight, psychomotor activity, and perceptions; delusions, illusions, and hallucinations; pain level; recent behavioral changes; electrolyte imbalances; and history of transient ischemic attacks, head injury, early dementia, AIDS, or schizophrenia
- Cardiovascular status, including vital signs, skin color, auscultation of carotid artery and heart sounds, and history of coronary artery disease or hypertension
- Respiratory status, including rate, depth, and pattern of respirations; auscultation for breath sounds; smoking history; shortness of breath; and history of chronic obstructive pulmonary disease, cancer, or tuberculosis
- Sensory status, including results of vision and hearing examination, use of corrective lenses or hearing aid, and history of eye or ear disorders
- Nutritional status, including typical daily food intake and weight loss
- Sleep status, including recent change in sleep pattern or environment (recent hospitalization)
- Elimination status, including history of urinary tract infection (UTI) and patterns of elimination

Risk Factors

- Age ≥ 60 years
- Alteration in cognitive functioning
- Alteration in sleep–wake cycle
- Dehydration

- Dementia
- History of cerebral vascular accident
- Impaired metabolic functioning (e.g., azotemia, decreased hemoglobin, electrolyte imbalance, increase in blood urea nitrogen/creatinine)
- Impaired mobility
- Inappropriate use of restraints
- Infection
- Male gender
- Malnutrition
- Pain
- Pharmaceutical agent
- Sensory deprivation
- Substance abuse
- Urinary retention

Expected Outcomes

- Patient will remain free from injury.
- Patient's neurologic status will remain stable.
- Patient will obtain adequate amounts of sleep.
- Patient will maintain optimal hydration and nutrition.
- Family members will report an improved ability to cope with the patient's confused state.
- Patient will begin to participate in activities of daily living (ADLs).
- Patient will report feeling increasingly calm.
- Patient and family will state the causes of acute confusion.
- Patient and family will express an understanding of the importance of informing other health care providers about episodes of acute confusion.

Suggested NOC Outcomes

Cognitive Orientation; Distorted Thought Self-Control; Information Processing; Memory; Neurologic Status; Personal Safety Behavior; Sleep

Intervention and Rationales

- Assess patient's LOC and changes in behavior *to provide baseline for comparison with ongoing assessment findings.*
- Have a staff member stay at patient's bedside, if necessary, *to protect patient from harm.*
- Enlist the aid of family member *to help calm patient.*
- Limit noise and environmental stimulation *to prevent patient from becoming more confused.*
- Monitor neurologic status on a regular basis *to detect improvement or decline in patient's neurologic function.*
- Use appropriate safety measures *to protect patient from injury.* Avoid physical restraints to *prevent agitating patient.*
- Address patient by name, and mention your name *to foster patient's awareness of self and environment.*
- Give patient short, simple explanations each time you perform a procedure or task *to decrease confusion.*
- Establish or maintain elimination pattern *to assist in maintaining elimination, orientation, and patient safety.*
- Schedule nursing care to provide quiet times for patient *to help avoid sensory overload.*
- Mention time, place, and date frequently throughout day. Have a large clock and a calendar where patient can easily see them. Refer to those aids when orienting patient *to foster awareness of self and environment.*

- Keep patient's possessions in the same place as much as possible. *A consistent, stable environment reduces confusion and frustration and aids completion of ADLs.*
- Ask family to bring labeled family photos and other favorite articles *to create a more secure environment for patient.*
- Plan patient's routine, and be as consistent as possible in following it. *A consistent routine aids task completion and reduces confusion.*
- Speak slowly and clearly, and allow patient ample time to respond *to reduce sense of frustration and promote task completion.*
- PCC Encourage patient to perform ADLs, dividing tasks into small, critical units. Be patient and specific in providing instructions. Allow time for patient to perform each task. *These measures enhance self-esteem as well as help prevent complications related to inactivity.*
- PCC Encourage family to share stories and discuss familiar people and events with patient. *Sharing stories and familiar subjects promotes a sense of continuity, aids memory, and creates a sense of security and comfort.* Note that even if patient's short-term memory is impaired, remote memory still may be intact.
- PCC Confer with physician about diagnostic test results, patient's progress in behavior, and patient's LOC. *A collaborative approach to treatment helps ensure high-quality care and continuity of care.*
- Discuss episodes of acute confusion with patient and family members *to make sure they understand the cause of confusion.*
- Review supportive measures family can take at home if patient begins to exhibit signs of confusion. Tell them to give patient short explanations of activities; repeat time, place, and date frequently; speak slowly and clearly and allow patient ample time to respond; and provide patient with a consistent routine. *Teaching empowers patient and family to take greater responsibility for their health care needs.*
- Stress to patient and family that, in the future, they should inform health care providers about episodes of acute confusion *to help ensure continuity of care.*

Suggested NIC Interventions

Behavior Management: Overactivity/Inattention; Cognitive Stimulation; Delirium Management; Hallucination Management; Reality Orientation; Sleep Enhancement

Evaluations for Expected Outcomes

- Patient doesn't experience injury during episodes of acute confusion.
- Patient exhibits a mental status within his or her normal range.
- Family members report an increased ability to cope with patient's confused state.
- Patient performs ADLs to the extent possible.
- Patient reports feelings of increased calm.
- Patient and family members express an understanding of the causes of acute confusion.
- Patient and family members express an understanding of the importance of telling all health care providers about episodes of acute confusion.

Documentation

- Description of episodes of acute confusion
- Factors that precipitate and ameliorate periods of acute confusion
- Teaching sessions and referrals
- Evaluations for expected outcomes

REFERENCES

Brooks, P., Spillane, J. J., Dick, K., & Stuart-Shor, E. (2014). Developing a strategy to identify and treat older patients with postoperative delirium. *AORN Journal*, *99*(2), 256–276. doi:10.1016/j.aorn.2013.12.009

Hea-Jeong, H., & Yeonghee, S. (2014). Effects of nursing intervention program on reducing acute confusion in hospitalized older adults. *Korean Journal of Adult Nursing*, *26*(1), 89–97. doi:10.7475/kjan.2014.26.1.89

Ng, J., Pan, C. X., Geube, A., Tan, C., Kawai, F., & Chorost, M. (2015). Your postop patient is confused and agitated—Next steps? *Journal of Family Practice*, *64*(6), 361–366.

CHRONIC CONFUSION

Definition

Irreversible, longstanding, and/or progressive deterioration of intellect and personality characterized by decreased ability to interpret environmental stimuli and decreased capacity for intellectual thought processes, and manifested by disturbances or memory, orientation, and behavior

Assessment

- Age and gender
- Neurologic status, including level of consciousness (LOC), orientation, thought and speech, mood, affect, memory, visual and spatial ability, judgment and insight, psychomotor activity, and perceptions; recent behavior changes; lethargy, restlessness, short- or long-term memory loss, and sleep disturbance; and history of multiple infarctions, transient ischemic attacks, Parkinson's disease, cerebral infarctions, seizures, and alcohol or drug abuse
- Self-care status, including ability to perform instrumental or routine activities of daily living (ADLs)
- Family status, including marital status, economic status, living arrangements, presence of caregiver and relationship to patient, and caregiver's perception of patient's abilities

Defining Characteristics

- Alteration in interpretation
- Alteration in long-term memory
- Alteration in personality
- Alteration in response stimuli
- Alteration in short-term memory
- Chronic cognitive impairment
- Impaired social functioning
- Normal LOC
- Organic brain disorder
- Progressive alteration in cognitive functioning

Expected Outcomes

- Patient will remain free of injury caused by confusion.
- Patient will exhibit no signs of depression.
- Patient will maintain weight.
- Family members will discuss their ability to provide care for the patient.
- Patient will be provided with a structured environment to ensure maximum functioning.
- Family members or caregiver will describe strategies to help patient cope with chronic confusion.
- Patient will participate in selected activities to fullest extent possible.
- Family members will maintain safety of patient's home environment.

- Family members will receive information on the various options available for long-term care of the patient.
- If necessary, patient and family members will prepare for relocation to long-term care facility.
- Patient will receive adequate emotional support to help cope with stress of moving to a new environment.
- Staff at patient's new residence will receive clear instructions regarding measures to help patient cope with chronic confusion.

Suggested NOC Outcomes

Client Satisfaction: Safety; Cognition; Cognitive Orientation; Concentration; Decision-Making; Distorted Thought Self-Control; Identity; Information Processing; Memory

Interventions and Rationales

- Assess patient's cognitive abilities and changes in behavior *to provide baseline data for comparison with ongoing assessment findings.*
- Encourage family members to watch you perform mental status assessments *to give them a more accurate view of patient's abilities.*
- PCC Evaluate patient's ability in regard to self-care as well as to function alone and drive a car. *Safety is a primary concern.*
- Assess patient for depression *to determine need for treatment.*
- Weigh patient, document your findings, and include instructions for regular weighing as part of care plan *to monitor patient's nutritional status.*
- Ask family members about their ability to provide care for patient *to assess their need for assistance.* Project an attentive, nonjudgmental attitude when listening to them *to help ensure that you receive accurate information.*
- Take steps to provide a stable physical environment and consistent daily routine for patient. *Stability and consistency enhance functioning.*
- PCC Teach family members or caregiver strategies to help patient cope:
  - Place an identification bracelet on patient *to promote safety.*
  - Touch patient *to convey acceptance.*
  - Avoid unfamiliar situations when possible *to help ensure a consistent environment.*
  - Provide structured rest periods *to prevent fatigue and reduce stress.*
  - Avoid asking questions patient can't answer—for example, questions that test the patient's orientation to time, place, person, or situation—*to avoid causing frustration.*
  - Provide finger foods if patient won't sit and eat *to ensure adequate nutrition.*
  - Select activities based on patient's interests and abilities, and praise the patient for participating in activities *to enhance the sense of self-worth.*
  - Use television and radio carefully *to avoid sensory overload, which may exacerbate confusion.*
  - Limit choices patient has to make *to provide structure and avoid confusion.*
  - Label familiar photos with names of individuals pictured *to provide a sense of security.*
  - Use symbols, rather than written signs, to identify patient's room, bathroom, and other facilities *to help patient identify surroundings.*
  - Place patient's name in large block letters on clothing and other belongings *to help patient recognize personal belongings and prevent them from becoming lost.*

- **S** If possible, make a home visit *to assess safety of patient's living environment.*
- **PCC** Assist family members in contacting appropriate community services. If necessary, act as an advocate for patient within health care system *to help secure services needed for ongoing care.*
- **PCC** Provide family members with information concerning long-term health care facilities. If necessary, assist family members in moving patient to a nursing home or other long-term care setting. *A patient with chronic confusion may require ongoing skilled nursing care.*
- **PCC** If patient is to be moved to a long-term care facility, explain the reason for the decision in as simple and gentle terms as possible *to facilitate comprehension.* Allow patient to express feelings regarding the move *to facilitate grieving over loss of independence.* Provide psychological support to patient and family members *to alleviate stress they may experience during relocation.*
- **PCC** Communicate all aspects of the discharge plan to staff members at patient's new residence, including measures to ensure a stable environment and consistent routine; need to monitor patient's ongoing ability to perform ADLs; measures to ensure adequate nutrition; and interventions to provide emotional support to patient and family members. *Documenting a discharge plan and communicating it to caregivers helps ensure continuity of care. Interventions should ensure patient's dignity and rights.*

Suggested NIC Interventions

Anxiety Reduction; Area Restriction; Calming Technique; Cognitive Stimulation; Dementia Management; Emotional Support; Energy Management; Family Involvement Promotion; Medication Management; Reality Orientation; Sleep Enhancement

Evaluations for Expected Outcomes

- Patient experiences no injury because of chronic confusion.
- Patient exhibits no sign of depression.
- Patient eats enough to maintain weight.
- Family members discuss openly their ability to provide for the patient.
- Patient functions to maximum ability in a stable and structured environment.
- Family members describe strategies to help patient cope with chronic confusion.
- Patient participates in appropriate activities.
- Family maintains a safe environment in the home.
- Patient and family members receive adequate information regarding long-term care options to help them make informed decisions regarding patient's future.
- Patient expresses feelings and receives adequate emotional support before, during, and after relocation to long-term care facility.
- Care plan is communicated to staff at patient's new residence.

Documentation

- Assessment of patient's cognitive abilities, behavior, and self-care status
- Changes in patient's mental status as they occur
- Assistance given to family to help them cope with patient's confusion
- Any plans made to move patient to long-term care facility
- Teaching sessions and referrals
- Evaluations for expected outcomes

REFERENCES

Griffiths, A., Knight, A., Harwood, R., & Gladman, J. R. (2014). Preparation to care for confused older patients in general hospitals: A study of UK health professionals. *Age & Ageing*, *43*(4), 521–527. doi:10.1093/ageing/aft171

Kinnunen-Luovi, K., Saarnio, R., & Isola, A. (2014). Safety incidents involving confused and forgetful older patients in a specialized care setting—analysis of the safety incidents reported to the HaiPro reporting system. *Journal of Clinical Nursing*, *23*(17/18), 2442–2450. doi:10.1111/jocn.12364

Sampaio, F. C., & Sequeira, C. (2015). Nurses' knowledge and practices in cases of acute and chronic confusion: A questionnaire survey. *Perspectives in Psychiatric Care*, *51*(2), 98–105. doi:10.1111/ppc.12069

CONSTIPATION

related to insufficient fiber intake; insufficient fluid intake

Definition

Decrease in normal frequency of defecation accompanied by difficult or incomplete passage of stool and/or passage of excessively hard, dry stool

Assessment

- History of bowel disorder or surgery
- Gastrointestinal (GI) status, including nausea and vomiting, usual bowel elimination habits, change in bowel elimination habits, laxative use, stools characteristics (color, amount, size, and consistency), pain, inspection of abdomen, auscultation of bowel sounds, palpation for masses and tenderness, and percussion for tympany and dullness
- Nutritional status, including dietary intake, fiber intake, appetite, current weight, and change from normal weight
- Fluid status, including fluid intake, urine output, urine specific gravity, and skin turgor
- Knowledge, including ability and motivation to change current patterns and understanding of relationship between intake, bulk, and constipation

Defining Characteristics

- Abdominal pain
- Abdominal tenderness with palpable muscle resistance
- Abdominal tenderness without palpable muscle resistance
- Anorexia
- Atypical presentations in older adults (e.g., changes in mental status, urinary incontinence, unexplained falls, elevated body temperature)
- Borborygmi
- Bright red blood with stool
- Change in bowel pattern
- Decrease in stool frequency
- Decrease in stool volume
- Distended abdomen
- Fatigue
- Hard, formed stool
- Headache
- Hyperactive bowel sounds
- Hypoactive bowel sounds
- Inability to defecate
- Increase in intra-abdominal pressure
- Indigestion
- Liquid stool
- Pain with defecation
- Palpable abdominal mass
- Palpable rectal mass
- Percussed abdominal dullness
- Rectal fullness

- Rectal pressure
- Severe flatus
- Soft, paste-like stool in rectum
- Straining with defecation
- Vomiting

Expected Outcomes

- Patient's elimination pattern will return to normal.
- Patient will experience bowel movement every ____ day(s).
- Patient will consume high-fiber or high-bulk diet, unless contraindicated.
- Patient will maintain oral fluid intake of 2,500 mL daily, unless contraindicated.
- Patient will state understanding of relationship of dietary intake and bulk to constipation.
- Patient will list foods needed to prevent recurrence of problem, such as fruit, fruit juices, whole grain bread, and cereals.

Suggested NOC Outcomes

Bowel Elimination; Comfort Level; Hydration; Nutritional Status: Food & Fluid Intake; Symptom Control

Interventions and Rationales

- Monitor and record frequency and characteristics of stools. *Careful monitoring forms the basis of an effective treatment plan.*
- Record intake and output accurately *to ensure correct fluid replacement therapy.*
- Unless contraindicated, encourage fluid intake of 2,500 mL daily *to ensure correct fluid replacement therapy.*
- Place patient on bedpan or commode at specific times daily, as close as possible to usual evacuation time (if known), *to aid adaptation to routine physiologic function.*
- Administer laxative or enema, as ordered, *to promote elimination of solids and gases from GI tract.* Monitor effectiveness.
- PCC Teach patient to gently massage along the transverse and descending colon *to stimulate bowel's spastic reflex and aid stools passage.*
- PCC Consult with dietitian about increasing fiber and bulk in diet to maximum prescribed by physician. *This will improve intestinal muscle tone and promote comfortable elimination.*
- PCC Instruct patient and family in the relationship of diet, exercise, and fluid intake to constipation. Develop plan and provide for mild exercise periods. *These measures promote muscle tone and circulation and discourage deviation from prescribed diet.*

Suggested NIC Interventions

Bowel Management; Constipation/Impaction Management; Exercise Promotion; Fluid Management; Nutrition Management

Evaluations for Expected Outcomes

- Patient resumes regular bowel elimination schedule.
- Without using laxatives, enemas, or suppositories, patient has bowel movement every ____ day(s).
- Patient consumes fruit, bran, and other high-fiber foods, unless contraindicated.

- Patient drinks 2,500 mL of fluid daily, unless contraindicated.
- Patient expresses understanding of the effects of diet and fluid intake on constipation.
- Patient names foods that will help prevent recurrence of constipation.

Documentation

- Patient's expressions of concern about constipation, dietary changes, laxative use, and bowel pattern
- Observations of food and fluid intake and stools characteristics
- Patient's expression of understanding of relationship between constipation and dietary intake of fluid and bulk
- Patient's response to nursing interventions
- Evaluations for expected outcomes

REFERENCES

Bardsley, A. (2015). Approaches to managing chronic constipation in older people within the community setting. *British Journal of Community Nursing*, *20*(9), 444–450. doi:10.12968/bjcn.2015.20.9.444

Holroyd, S. (2015). How can community nurses manage chronic constipation? *Journal of Community Nursing*, *29*(5), 74–82.

Lee, A. (2015). Combating the causes of constipation. *Nursing & Residential Care*, *17*(6), 327–331.

CONSTIPATION

related to postsurgical bowel obstruction

Definition

Decrease in normal frequency of defecation accompanied by difficult or incomplete passage of stools and/or passage of excessively hard, dry stool

Assessment

- History of bowel disorder or surgery
- Gastrointestinal (GI) status, including nausea and vomiting, usual bowel elimination habits, change in bowel elimination habits, laxative use, stools characteristics (color, amount, size, and consistency), pain, inspection of abdomen, auscultation of bowel sounds, palpation for masses and tenderness, percussion for tympany and dullness, and results of upper GI series, barium enema, and sigmoidoscopy
- Nutritional status, including dietary intake, fiber intake, appetite, current weight, and change from normal weight
- Fluid and electrolyte status, including intake and output, skin turgor, urine specific gravity, and serum electrolyte level
- History of ingesting nonfood items (in psychiatric patients)

Defining Characteristics

- Abdominal pain
- Abdominal tenderness with palpable muscle resistance
- Abdominal tenderness without palpable muscle resistance
- Anorexia

- Atypical presentations in older adults (e.g., changes in mental status, urinary incontinence, unexplained falls, elevated body temperature)
- Borborygmi
- Bright red blood with stool
- Change in bowel pattern
- Decrease in stool frequency
- Decrease in stool volume
- Distended abdomen
- Fatigue
- Hard, formed stool
- Headache
- Hyperactive bowel sounds
- Hypoactive bowel sounds
- Inability to defecate
- Increase in intra-abdominal pressure
- Indigestion
- Liquid stool
- Pain with defecation
- Palpable abdominal mass
- Palpable rectal mass
- Percussed abdominal dullness
- Rectal fullness
- Rectal pressure
- Severe flatus
- Soft, paste-like stool in rectum
- Straining with defecation
- Vomiting

Expected Outcomes

- Patient will return to usual bowel pattern.
- Patient will maintain fluid balance; intake equals output.
- Patient will display normal bowel sounds.
- Patient will express pain relief or comfort.
- Patient will stop vomiting through use of antiemetics or GI tube.
- Patient will state understanding of surgical procedure.
- Patient or caregiver will demonstrate use of ileostomy or colostomy equipment.
- Patient will discuss fears and anxieties associated with bowel diversion.
- Patient or caregiver will discuss effect of bowel diversion on lifestyle.
- Patient or caregiver will state intention to contact support group.
- Patient will maintain weight.
- Patient will perform oral hygiene.

Suggested NOC Outcomes

Bowel Elimination; Comfort Level; Hydration; Medication Response; Symptom Control

Interventions and Rationales

- Carefully monitor and record frequency and characteristics of stools *to form basis of effective treatment plan.*
- Record intake and output accurately *to ensure correct fluid replacement therapy.* Report any imbalance.
- Auscultate bowel sounds and record every 4 hours. Report significant changes. *Absent or diminished bowel sounds may indicate peritoneal irritation or intestinal obstruction.*
- Record patient's weight daily *to detect possible fluid retention, food malabsorption, or increased adaptation requirements on body processes.*
- Administer pain medication and antiemetics as ordered. Monitor effectiveness *to determine need for alternative treatment.*
- PCC Promote patient comfort during vomiting episodes by providing oral care and removing vomitus promptly. Carefully record amount and characteristics of vomitus *to ensure accurate intake and output records.*

- Provide oral and nasal care every 4 hours while GI tube is present. Keep nostrils clean and moist *to prevent irritation.*
- Prepare patient for surgery:
  - Give preoperative instruction for abdominal surgery *to reduce patient's anxiety and increase trust.*
  - Inform patient about ileostomy, colostomy, or colectomy, as indicated, *to reduce anxiety.*
- PCC Instruct patient and caregivers in the use of ileostomy or colostomy equipment *to promote familiarity and establish therapeutic relationship.* Have patient and caregivers demonstrate use of equipment *to encourage feeling of shared responsibility.*
- PCC Encourage patient and family to express feelings and concerns about changes in body image *to help them learn to cope.*
- PCC Encourage visits to patient by persons from ileostomy or colostomy support groups *to provide patient with additional health care resources.*
- PCC Have the patient evaluated for home health care after discharge. The patient and family may need additional support and care after discharge. *Knowing that such help is available may enhance coping as the patient prepares to go home.*

Suggested NIC Interventions

Anxiety Reduction; Bowel Management; Fluid/Electrolyte Management; Nutrition Management; Ostomy Care; Skin Surveillance

Evaluations for Expected Outcomes

- Patient exhibits a normal bowel elimination pattern.
- Patient drinks adequate amount of fluids, with intake equal to output.
- Patient displays normal bowel sounds.
- Patient states that pain medication is effective.
- Patient doesn't vomit.
- Patient expresses understanding of surgical procedure, including need for ileostomy or colostomy.
- Patient or caregiver demonstrates care, changing, and irrigation of ileostomy or colostomy equipment.
- Patient states acceptance of bowel diversion.
- Patient comes to terms with effects of bowel diversion on lifestyle.
- Patient or caregiver identifies and contacts support group if needed.
- Patient doesn't exhibit weight loss or gain. Weight is consistent with body weight chart.
- Patient's mouth is clear and free from odor, and nostrils are clean and moist.

Documentation

- Patient's expressions of concern about vomiting, GI tube, or surgery
- Observation of characteristics of vomitus and stools, intake and output, weight, bowel sounds, and condition of oral cavity
- Patient's reaction and adaptation to ileostomy or colostomy
- Patient's and caregivers' participation in care and response to instruction
- Evaluations for expected outcomes

REFERENCES

Knowles, S., Lam, L. T., McInnes, E., Elliott, D., Hardy, J., & Middleton, S. (2015). Knowledge, attitudes, beliefs and behavior intentions for three bowel management practices in intensive care: Effects of a targeted protocol implementation for nursing and medical staff. *BMC Nursing*, *14*(1), 1–13. doi:10.1186/s12912-015-0056-z

Lee, A. (2015). Combating the causes of constipation. *Nursing & Residential Care*, *17*(6), 327–331.

Pittman, J., Beeson, T., Carter, B., & Terry, C. (2015). Implementation of a bowel management program in critical care. *Journal of Wound, Ostomy & Continence Nursing*, *42*(4), 389–394; quiz E1–E2. doi:10.1097/WON.0000000000000146

RISK FOR CONSTIPATION

Definition

Vulnerable to a decrease in normal frequency of defecation accompanied by difficult or incomplete passage of stool, which may compromise health

Assessment

- Age and gender
- Vital signs
- Health history, including bowel disorder or surgery, diabetic gastroparesis, immobility or inactivity, chronic debilitating disease, and episodes characterized by inability to swallow food and fluids
- Gastrointestinal (GI) status, including nausea and vomiting, usual bowel habits, change in bowel habits, laxative use, stools characteristics (color, amount, size, and consistency), pain, inspection of abdomen, auscultation of bowel sounds, palpation for masses and tenderness, and percussion for tympany and dullness
- Nutritional status, including dietary intake, appetite, current weight, and changes from normal diet
- Fluid status, including intake and output and skin turgor
- Musculoskeletal status, including functional mobility, joint mobility, paralysis, paresis, and activity and exercise status
- Psychosocial status, including understanding of risk of constipation; motivation to change health habits; and understanding of relationship between intake, bulk, activity and mobility, and constipation

Risk Factors

Functional

- Abdominal muscle weakness
- Average daily physical activity is less than recommended for gender and age
- Habitually ignores urge to defecate
- Inadequate toileting habits
- Irregular defecation habits
- Recent environmental change

Mechanical

- Electrolyte imbalance
- Hemorrhoids
- Hirschprung's disease
- Neurologic impairment (e.g., positive EEG, head trauma, seizure disorders)
- Obesity
- Pregnancy
- Prostate enlargement
- Rectal abscess
- Rectal anal fissure
- Rectal prolapse
- Rectal ulcer
- Rectocele
- Tumor

Pharmacologic

- Iron salts
- Laxative abuse
- Pharmaceutical agent

Physiologic

- Decrease in GI motility
- Dehydration
- Eating habit change (e.g., foods, eating times)
- Inadequate dentition
- Inadequate oral hygiene
- Insufficient dietary habits
- Insufficient fiber intake
- Insufficient fluid intake

Psychological

- Confusion
- Depression
- Emotional disturbance

Expected Outcomes

- Patient will experience no constipation.
- Patient will maintain bowel movement every ____ day(s).
- Patient will consume a high-fiber or high-bulk diet, unless contraindicated.
- Patient will maintain fluid intake of ____ mL daily (specify).
- Patient will express understanding of the relationship between constipation and dietary intake, bulk, and activity.
- Patient will express understanding of preventive measures, such as eating fruit and whole grain breads and cereals and engaging in mild activity, if appropriate.

Suggested NOC Outcomes

Bowel Elimination; Self-Care: Toileting

Interventions and Rationales

- Assess bowel sounds and check patient for abdominal distention. Monitor and record frequency and characteristics of stools *to develop an effective treatment plan for preventing constipation and fecal impaction.*
- Record intake and output accurately *to ensure accurate fluid replacement therapy.*
- Encourage fluid intake of 2.5 L daily, unless contraindicated, *to promote fluid replacement therapy and hydration.*
- Initiate bowel program. Place patient on a bedpan or commode at specific times daily, as close to usual evacuation time (if known) as possible, *to aid adaptation to routine physiologic function.*
- Administer a laxative, an enema, or suppositories, as prescribed, *to promote elimination of solids and gases from GI tract.* Monitor effectiveness.
- PCC Teach patient to gently massage along the transverse and descending colon *to stimulate the bowel's spastic reflex and aid in stool passage.*
- PCC Consult with a dietitian about how to increase fiber and bulk in patient's diet to the maximum amount prescribed by the physician *to improve intestinal muscle tone and promote comfortable elimination.*
- PCC Instruct patient, family member, or caregiver in the relationship between diet, activity and exercise, and fluid intake and constipation *to discourage departure from prescribed diet and assist in promoting elimination.*
- Include a program of mild exercise in your care plan *to promote muscle tone and circulation.*
- PCC Review care plan with patient, family member, or caregiver, emphasizing the relationship between the risk factors for constipation and preventive measures *to foster understanding.*

Suggested NIC Interventions

Anxiety Reduction; Bowel Management; Constipation/Impaction Management; Exercise Promotion; Fluid Management; Fluid Monitoring; Nutrition Management

Evaluations for Expected Outcomes

- Patient doesn't experience constipation.
- Patient has bowel movement every ____ day(s).
- Patient consumes a high-fiber or high-bulk diet, unless contraindicated.
- Patient maintains fluid intake of ____ mL daily (specify).
- Patient expresses understanding of the relationship between constipation and dietary intake, bulk, and activity.
- Patient expresses understanding of preventive measures, such as eating fruit and whole grain breads and cereals and engaging in mild activity, if appropriate.

Documentation

- Patient's, family members', or caregivers' statements regarding risk of constipation
- Presence of risk factors for constipation
- Observations of food and fluid intake, urine output, and stools characteristics
- Instructions regarding preventive care
- Patient's, family members', or caregivers' statements indicating understanding of instructions
- Patient's response to preventive interventions
- Implementation, alteration, or continuation of bowel program
- Patient's, family members', or caregivers' demonstrated ability to implement preventive measures
- Evaluations for expected outcomes

REFERENCES

Chapman, S., & Hungerford, C. (2015). Risk factors for and assessment of constipation. *Nursing Older People*, *27*(3), 16–24. doi:10.7748/nop.27.3.16.e673

Lee, A. (2015). Combating the causes of constipation. *Nursing & Residential Care*, *17*(6), 327–331.

Zanik, K., & Gray, L. (2015). Who hasn't had to deal with unanticipated constipation in the acute care setting? CRAT: Constipation Risk Assessment Tool—Why it works. *Journal of Stomal Therapy Australia*, *35*(3), 12–18.

PERCEIVED CONSTIPATION

Definition

Self-diagnosis of constipation combined with abuse of laxatives, enemas, and/or suppositories to ensure a daily bowel movement

Assessment

- Age and gender
- Family history of constipation
- History of psychiatric disorders

- Fluid and electrolyte status, including intake and output, skin turgor, urine specific gravity, and mucous membranes
- Gastrointestinal status, including bowel elimination habits, change in bowel elimination habits, stools characteristics (color, amount, size, and consistency), pain, auscultation of bowel sounds, laxative or enema use (time and duration), family habits concerning bowel movements, and rectal examination
- Nutritional status, including dietary intake and appetite
- Activity status
- Psychosocial status, including personality, stressors (finances, job, marital discord, and coping mechanisms), support systems (family and others), lifestyle, and knowledge level

Defining Characteristics

- Enema abuse
- Expects daily bowel movement
- Expects daily bowel movement at same time every day
- Laxative abuse
- Suppository abuse

Expected Outcomes

- Patient will decrease use of laxatives, enemas, or suppositories.
- Patient will state understanding of normal bowel function.
- Patient will discuss feelings about elimination pattern.
- Patient's elimination pattern will return to normal.
- Patient will experience bowel movement every _____ day(s) without laxatives, enemas, or suppositories.
- Patient will state understanding of factors causing constipation.
- Patient will get regular exercise.
- Patient will describe changes in personal habits to maintain normal elimination pattern.
- Patient will state intent to use appropriate resources to help resolve emotional or psychological problems.

Suggested NOC Outcomes

Adherence Behavior; Bowel Elimination; Health Beliefs; Health Beliefs: Perceived Threat; Knowledge: Health Behavior

Interventions and Rationales

- Modify patient's dietary habits to include adequate fluids, fresh fruits and vegetables, and whole grain cereals and breads, *which supply necessary bulk for normal elimination.*
- Encourage patient to engage in daily exercise, such as brisk walking, *to strengthen muscle tone and stimulate circulation.*
- Encourage patient to evacuate at regular times *to aid adaptation and routine physiologic function.*
- Urge patient to avoid taking laxatives, if possible, or to gradually decrease their use *to avoid further trauma to intestinal mucosa.*
- PCC Inform patient not to expect a bowel movement every day or even every other day *to avoid use of poor health practices to stimulate elimination.*

- If not contraindicated, increase patient's fluid intake to about 3 L daily *to increase functional capacity of bowel elimination.*
- PCC Explain normal bowel elimination habits so patient *can better understand normal and abnormal body functions.*
- Reassure patient that normal bowel function is possible without laxatives, enemas, or suppositories *to give patient the necessary confidence for compliance.*
- PCC Give information about self-help groups, as appropriate, *to provide additional resources for patient and family.*
- PCC Establish and implement an individualized bowel elimination regimen based on patient's needs. *Knowledge of normal body functions will improve patient's understanding of problem.*
- Instruct patient to avoid straining during elimination *to avoid tissue damage, bleeding, and pain.*
- PCC Instruct patient that abdominal massage may help relieve discomfort and promote defecation *because it triggers bowel's spastic reflex.*

Suggested NIC Interventions

Anxiety Reduction; Bowel Management; Counseling; Health Education; Nutrition Management; Teaching: Individual

Evaluations for Expected Outcomes

- Patient decreases use of laxatives, enemas, or suppositories.
- Patient describes normal bowel function and how fluid consumption, high-fiber diet, and exercise affect function.
- Patient expresses feelings about changes in elimination pattern.
- Patient's elimination pattern returns to normal.
- Without using laxatives, enemas, or suppositories, patient has bowel movement every ____ day(s).
- Patient lists factors that may cause constipation.
- Patient engages in regular exercise.
- Patient states plans to make changes in personal habits to prevent constipation.
- Patient makes contact with appropriate resources to help resolve psychological conflicts.

Documentation

- Patient's expressions of concern about change in diet, activity level, laxative and enema use, and bowel pattern
- Observations of diet, stools characteristics, and activity tolerance
- Patient teaching about diet, exercise, and constipation management
- Evaluations for expected outcomes

REFERENCES

Aschenbrenner, D. S. (2014). Overuse of certain OTC laxatives may be dangerous. *American Journal of Nursing, 114*(5), 25. doi:10.1097/01.NAJ.0000446776.76652.11

Mounsey, A., Raleigh, M., & Wilson, A. (2015). Management of constipation in older adults. *American Family Physician, 92*(6), 500–504.

Werth, B. L., Williams, K. A., & Pont, L. G. (2015). A longitudinal study of constipation and laxative use in a community-dwelling elderly population. *Archives of Gerontology & Geriatrics, 60*(3), 418–424. doi:10.1016/j.archger.2015.02.004

DEFENSIVE COPING

related to perceived threat to positive self-regard

Definition

Repeated projection of falsely positive self-evaluation based on a self-protective pattern that defends against underlying perceived threats to positive self-regard

Assessment

- Age and gender
- Family system, including marital status and sibling position
- Reason for hospitalization
- Past experience with illness
- Patient's perception of health problem
- Patient's perception of self, including self-worth, body image, problem-solving ability, and coping mechanisms
- Mental status, including general appearance, affect, mood, cognitive and perceptual functioning, and behavior
- Social interaction pattern
- Support systems, such as family and friends

Defining Characteristics

- Denial of obvious problems
- Difficulty establishing or maintaining relationships
- Difficulty in reality-testing perceptions
- Extreme sensitivity to criticism
- Grandiosity
- Lack of follow-through or participation in treatment or therapy
- Projection of blame or responsibility
- Rationalization of failures
- Reality distortion
- Ridicule of others
- Superior attitude toward and ridicule of others

Expected Outcomes

- Patient will verbally describe self, including concept, body image, successes, and positive aspects to live events.
- Patient will participate in self-care.
- Patient will engage in decision making about treatment.
- Patient will accept responsibility for own behavior.
- Patient will demonstrate follow-through in decisions related to health care.
- Patient will interact with others in a socially acceptable manner.

Suggested NOC Outcomes

Acceptance: Health Status; Coping; Self-Esteem; Social Interaction Skills

Interventions and Rationales

- PCC Encourage patient to evaluate self, possibly by making a written list of positive and negative traits. Encourage the patient to use "I" when referring to these traits. *This helps patient identify aspects of self and relate changes to specific variables.*
- Have patient perform self-care to the extent possible *to promote independence and provide a sense of control.*
- Provide a structured daily routine *to provide patient with alternatives to self-absorption.*
- PCC Help patient make treatment-related decisions, and encourage follow-through. *Ability to make decisions is principal component of autonomy.*
- Provide an opportunity for patient to meet with someone who's successfully coping with a similar problem. *This may encourage patient to work toward a positive outcome.*
- Arrange for interaction between patient and others, and observe interaction pattern. *Studying patient's verbal and nonverbal interactions with others gives clues to patient's ability to communicate effectively.*
- Provide positive feedback when patient assumes responsibility for own behavior *to reinforce effective coping behaviors.*
- PCC Refer the patient to a mental health specialist or social worker for follow-up treatment after hospitalization. *Continuing therapy is usually necessary to assist the patient to cope with health care status.*

Suggested NIC Interventions

Coping Enhancement; Counseling; Emotional Support; Patient Contracting; Self-Awareness Enhancement; Self-Responsibility Facilitation

Evaluations for Expected Outcomes

- Patient states reason for hospitalization.
- Patient uses at least two positive terms to describe self.
- Patient initiates and completes at least two self-care activities daily.
- Each day, patient makes at least one decision related to activities of daily living, self-care, or treatment.
- Patient expresses responsible attitude toward own behavior.
- Patient reports specific instances of following through on health care decisions.
- Each day, patient socializes with others in an acceptable manner.

Documentation

- Patient's perception of self
- Behavioral responses
- Social interaction patterns
- Patient's use of defense mechanisms
- Interventions used to facilitate effective coping
- Patient's responses to nursing interventions
- Evaluations for expected outcomes

REFERENCES

Fenech, G., & Thomson, G. (2015). Defense against trauma: Women's use of defense mechanisms following childbirth-related trauma. *Journal of Reproductive & Infant Psychology*, *33*(3), 268–281. doi:10.1080/02646838.2015.1030731

Kopytin, A., & Lebedev, A. (2015). Therapeutic functions of humor in group art therapy with war veterans. (2015). *International Journal of Art Therapy: Inscape*, *20*(2), 40–53. doi:10.1080/17454832.2014.1000348

Ortiz-Rivas, M. K., Moreno-Pérez, N. E., Vega-Macías, H. D., de Jesús Jiménez-González, M., & de Guadalupe Navarro-Elías, M. (2014). Adaptation of self-image level and defense mechanisms in elderly patients with complicated stoma. *Enfermeria Clinica*, *24*(6), 339–344. doi:10.1016/j.enfcli.2014.07.006

INEFFECTIVE COPING

related to situational crisis

Definition

Inability to form a valid appraisal of the stressors, inadequate choices of practiced responses, and/or inability to use available resources

Assessment

- Current health status
- Diversional activities
- Financial resources
- Occupation
- Patient's perception of present health problem or crisis
- Coping techniques that have worked for the patient in the past
- Family members' understanding of the client's health status
- Problem-solving techniques usually employed by the family to cope with life problems
- Support systems, including family, companion, friends, and clergy

Defining Characteristics

- Alteration in concentration
- Alteration in sleep pattern
- Change in communication pattern
- Destructive behavior toward others
- Destructive behavior toward self
- Difficulty organizing information
- Fatigue
- Frequent illness
- Inability to ask for help
- Inability to attend to information
- Inability to deal with a situation
- Inability to meet basic needs
- Inability to meet role expectation
- Ineffective coping strategies
- Insufficient access to social support
- Insufficient goal-directed behavior
- Insufficient problem resolution
- Insufficient problem-solving skills
- Risk-taking behavior
- Substance abuse

Expected Outcomes

- Patient will communicate feelings about the present situation.
- Patient will become involved in planning own care.
- Patient will express feeling of having greater control over present situation.
- Patient will use available support systems, such as family and friends, to aid in coping.
- Patient will identify and demonstrate ability to use at least two healthy coping behaviors.

Suggested NOC Outcomes

Aggression Self-Control; Acceptance of Health Status; Adaptation to Physical Disability; Coping; Decision-Making; Impulse Self-Control; Information Processing; Knowledge: Health Resources; Role Performance; Social Support

Interventions and Rationales

- If possible, assign a consistent care provider to patient *to provide continuity of care and promote development of therapeutic relationship.*
- PCC Arrange to spend uninterrupted periods of time with patient. Encourage expression of feelings, and accept what patient says. Try to identify factors that cause or exacerbate patient's inability to cope, such as fear of loss of health or job. *Devoting time to listening helps patient express emotions, grasp situation, and cope effectively.*
- Identify and reduce unnecessary stimuli in environment to *avoid subjecting patient to sensory or perceptual overload.*
- Initially, allow patient to depend partly on you for self-care. *Patient may regress to a lower developmental level during initial crisis phase.*
- PCC Explain all treatments and procedures, and answer patient's questions *to allay fear and allow patient to regain sense of control.*
- PCC Encourage patient to make decisions about care *to increase sense of self-worth and mastery over current situation.*
- Have patient increase self-care performance levels gradually *to allow self-paced progress.*
- Praise patient for making decisions and performing activities *to reinforce coping behaviors.*
- PCC Teach patient relaxation techniques of deep breathing and guided imagery. *Relaxation can assist to reduce anxiety and feelings of anger.*
- PCC Encourage patient to use support systems to assist with coping, *thereby helping restore psychological equilibrium and prevent crisis.*
- Help patient look at current situation and evaluate various coping behaviors *to encourage a realistic view of crisis.*
- Encourage patient to try coping behaviors. *A patient in crisis tends to accept interventions and develops new coping behaviors more easily than at other times.*
- Request feedback from patient about behaviors that seem to work *to encourage patient to evaluate effect of these behaviors.*
- PCC Refer patient for professional psychological counseling. *If patient's maladaptive behavior has high crisis potential, formal counseling helps ease nurse's frustration, increases objectivity, and fosters collaborative approach to patient's care.*

Suggested NIC Interventions

Anger Control Assistance; Anxiety Reduction; Coping Enhancement; Counseling; Decision-Making Support; Impulse Control Training; Learning Facilitation; Role Enhancement

Evaluations for Expected Outcomes

- Patient discusses recent stressful event and describes related emotions.
- Patient cooperates with nurse to plan care.
- Patient identifies problems, makes plans, and takes action.
- Patient requests assistance from family and friends.
- Patient identifies and uses at least two healthy coping behaviors such as relaxation techniques.

Documentation

- Patient's perception of present situation and what it means
- Patient's verbal expression of feelings indicating comfort or discomfort
- Observations of patient's behaviors
- Interventions to help patient cope
- Patient's responses to interventions
- Evaluations for expected outcomes

REFERENCES

Jacobs, N. L., Dehue, F., Völlink, T., & Lechner, L. (2014). Determinants of adolescents' ineffective and improved coping with cyberbullying: A Delphi study. *Journal of Adolescence*, *37*(4), 373–385. doi:10.1016/j.adolescence.2014.02.011

Meredith, P. J., Rappel, G., Strong, J., & Bailey, K. J. (2015). Sensory sensitivity and strategies for coping with pain. *American Journal of Occupational Therapy*, *69*(4), 1–10. doi:10.5014/ajot.2015.014621

Regier, N. G., & Parmelee, P. A. (2015). The stability of coping strategies in older adults with osteoarthritis and the ability of these strategies to predict changes in depression, disability, and pain. *Aging & Mental Health*, *19*(12), 1113–1122. doi:10.1080/13607863.2014.1003286

COMPROMISED FAMILY COPING

related to inadequate or incorrect information held by primary caregiver

Definition

Usually supportive primary person (family member or close friend) provides insufficient, ineffective, or compromised support, comfort, assistance, or encouragement that may be needed by the patient to manage or master adaptive tasks related to his health challenge

Assessment

- Family status, including normal pattern of interaction among family members, family's understanding and knowledge of patient's present condition, support systems available (financial, social, and spiritual), family's response to past crises, and communication patterns used to express anger, affection, confrontation, and conflict
- Patient's illness, including its progression and severity, patient's perception of health problem, and problem-solving techniques used by patient to cope with life problems

Defining Characteristics

- Family member's display of protective behavior that's disproportionate (too little or too much) to patient's abilities or need for autonomy
- Inadequate understanding or knowledge base of family member that interferes with effective assistive or supportive behaviors
- Preoccupation of family member with personal reaction (such as fear, anticipatory grief, guilt, or anxiety) to patient's illness, disability, or other situational or developmental crisis
- Family member's withdrawal from or limited communication with patient at time of need

Expected Outcomes

- Family will discuss patient's illness and its impact on family functioning.

- Family will designate a spokesperson to receive information regarding the patient's illness.
- Family will establish a visiting routine beneficial to patient and family.
- Family will state understanding of patient's health status.
- Family will identify and use available support systems.

Suggested NOC Outcomes

Caregiver Emotional Health; Caregiver–Patient Relationship; Caregiver Stressors; Family Coping; Family Normalization

Interventions and Rationales

- PCC Identify the spokesperson for the family *to avoid creating communication conflicts within family.*
- PCC Facilitate family conferences; help family members identify key issues and select support services, if needed. *Involving patient and family in care planning promotes open communication throughout illness.*
- PCC Help patient and family establish a visiting routine that won't tax their resources. Each family member may be responsible for a day or period of time, if desired. Use patient's daily routine to aid in planning; for example, no visiting during treatments or periods of uninterrupted sleep. *This enhances family's sense of contributing to patient's overall care.*
- PCC Encourage family to contact a community agency for continued support if necessary. *This is an effective health-related coping skill.*
- Provide family with clear, concise information about patient's condition. Be aware of what family has been told, and help them interpret information. *This ensures clear, uncluttered communication between patient, family, and caregivers.*
- Ensure privacy during patient and family visits. *This demonstrates respect and fosters open communication between family members.*
- PCC Help family support patient's independence. Encourage attendance at therapy sessions, and allow patient to demonstrate new skills and abilities *to help family members learn how they can help promote patient's independence and self-care.*
- PCC Provide emotional support to family by being available to answer questions. *This demonstrates your willingness to help family seek health-related information.*

Suggested NIC Interventions

Caregiver Support; Conflict Mediation; Decision-Making Support; Emotional Support; Family Involvement Promotion

Evaluations for Expected Outcomes

- Family members discuss feelings about patient's illness and its impact on family functioning.
- Family members designate spokesperson to receive and communicate information regarding the patient's illness.
- Family members agree to follow a consistent visiting routine.
- Family members accurately describe the patient's health status.
- Family member contacts at least one support person or group.

Documentation

- Family's response to patient's illness
- Family's current understanding of patient's illness
- Observations about family's interaction with patient and acceptance of current situation
- Evaluations for expected outcomes

REFERENCES

del-Pino-Casado, R., Pérez-Cruz, M., & Frías-Osuna, A. (2014). Coping, subjective burden and anxiety among family caregivers of older dependents. *Journal of Clinical Nursing*, *23*(23/24), 3335–3344. doi:10.1111/jocn.12561

Santos de Araújo Dantas, M., Amador Silva, D., Ataíde Melo de Pinho, T., Barros Torquato, I. M., Dantas de Assis, W., & dos Santos, S. R. (2015). Family coping strategies for leukemia diagnosis: Social and religious aspects. *Journal of Nursing UFPE/Revista De Enfermagem UFPE*, *9*(1), 137–142. doi:10.5205/reuol.6817-60679-1-ED.0901201519

Washington, K. T., & Rakes, C. R. (2015). Coping responses among hospice family caregivers: A confirmatory factor analysis. *Journal of Pain & Symptom Management*, *50*(6), 867–873. doi:10.1016/j.jpainsymman.2015.07.002

COMPROMISED FAMILY COPING

related to prolonged disease

Definition

Usually supportive primary person (family member or close friend) provides insufficient, ineffective, or compromised support, comfort, assistance, or encouragement that may be needed by the client to manage or master adaptive tasks related to his or her health challenge

Assessment

- Patient's illness, including course and severity and effect on family members
- Patient's health care resources, including hospital, community resources, health care providers such as therapists, and case manager (outpatient)
- Family process, including involvement with patient, quality of relationships, communication patterns, coping strategies, demands posed by patient's condition, family's understanding of patient's illness, family's feelings regarding patient's illness, willingness of family members to commit time to patient care, and family's ability to provide care

Defining Characteristics

- Significant person attempts assistive behaviors with unsatisfactory results
- Significant person attempts supportive behaviors with unsatisfactory results
- Significant person displays protective behavior disproportionate to client's abilities
- Significant person enters into limited personal communication with client
- Significant person withdraws from client
- Client expresses a complaint about significant person's response to health problem
- Significant person expresses inadequate knowledge base, which interferes with effective supportive behaviors

Expected Outcomes

- Family members will express their concerns about coping with patient's illness.
- Family members will identify their own needs for support.
- Family members will contact appropriate sources of support.
- Family members and patient will achieve better cooperation.

Suggested NOC Outcomes

Family Coping; Family Normalization

Interventions and Rationales

- Assess effects of patient's disease on family functioning *to plan interventions that enhance long-term well-being of family and patient.*
- PCC Encourage family members to hold conferences. Help them identify topics appropriate for discussion. Examples of such topics include developing coping strategies for dealing with patient's disease or resolving conflicts between meeting personal needs and meeting patient's health care needs. *Family members may find a group problem-solving approach helpful in correcting dysfunctional behaviors.*
- Evaluate and rectify any knowledge deficit that family members have about patient's disease and treatment. Experience doesn't guarantee correct knowledge. *Lack of knowledge can exacerbate frustration and tension within the family.*
- Provide an outlet for family members to express their frustrations about their present caregiving responsibilities. *Being able to talk about what they are presently experiencing will allow the opportunity to stand back and see what is happening in their relationship with the patient.*
- PCC Encourage family members to participate in appropriate support groups *to help them obtain social support and information and to provide an opportunity to express feelings.*
- PCC Encourage family members to contact and use appropriate community agencies *to help prevent burnout among family members after patient leaves the hospital.* Families may need encouragement to use support and respite care services if past efforts to use such services proved unsuccessful.

Suggested NIC Interventions

Family Involvement Promotion; Family Mobilization; Family Support; Normalization Promotion; Emotional Support; Learning Facilitation; Support Group

Evaluations for Expected Outcomes

- Family members discuss impact of patient's prolonged disease.
- Family members communicate their needs regarding the patient's prolonged care.
- Family members are aware of available sources of support, and use them appropriately.
- Family members and patient negotiate meeting patient's care needs to their mutual satisfaction.

Documentation

- Assessment of family functioning (including family's level of insight into their behavior)
- Content of family conferences

- Community resources used, their effectiveness, and recommendations for future use (indicate family's level of acceptance of nurse's recommendations)
- Evaluations for expected outcomes

REFERENCES

del-Pino-Casado, R., Pérez-Cruz, M., & Frías-Osuna, A. (2014). Coping, subjective burden and anxiety among family caregivers of older dependents. *Journal of Clinical Nursing*, *23*(23/24), 3335–3344. doi:10.1111/jocn.12561

Santos de Araújo Dantas, M., Amador Silva, D., Ataíde Melo de Pinho, T., Barros Torquato, I. M., Dantas de Assis, W., & dos Santos, S. R. (2015). Family coping strategies for leukemia diagnosis: Social and religious aspects. *Journal of Nursing UFPE/Revista De Enfermagem UFPE*, *9*(1), 137–142. doi:10.5205/reuol.6817-60679-1-ED.0901201519

Washington, K. T., & Rakes, C. R. (2015). Coping responses among hospice family caregivers: A confirmatory factor analysis. *Journal of Pain & Symptom Management*, *50*(6), 867–873. doi:10.1016/j.jpainsymman.2015.07.002

DISABLED FAMILY COPING

related to highly ambivalent family relationships

Definition

Behavior of significant person (family members or other primary person) that disables his/her capabilities and the patient's capabilities to effectively address tasks essential to either person's adaptation to the health challenge

Assessment

- Patient's illness, including its course, severity, and effect on family members
- Patient's health care resources, including hospital, community resources, and health care providers, such as therapists and case managers
- Demands on family imposed by patient's condition
- Family status, including involvement with patient, quality of relationships, communication patterns, coping strategies, family's understanding of patient's illness, family's feelings about patient's illness, willingness of family members to commit time to patient care, and family's ability to provide care

Defining Characteristics

- Abandonment
- Client's development of dependence
- Intolerance
- Agitation, depression, aggression, and hostility
- Taking on illness signs of patient
- Rejection
- Psychosomaticism
- Neglectful relationships with other family members
- Neglectful care of patient in regard to basic human needs
- Distortion of reality regarding patient
- Impaired restructuring of a meaningful life for self
- Decisions and actions by family members that are detrimental to economic or social well-being
- Carrying on usual routines without regard to patient's needs

Expected Outcomes

- To the extent possible, family members will participate in aspects of patient's care without evidence of increased conflict.
- Patient will express confidence in being able to make decisions, despite pressure from family members.
- Patient will contact appropriate sources of support outside the family.
- Patient will take steps to ensure that care needs are met despite family's shortcomings.
- Patient will express greater understanding of emotional limitations of family members.

Suggested NOC Outcomes

Caregiver Emotional Health; Caregiver–Patient Relationship; Caregiving Endurance Potential; Family Coping

Interventions and Rationales

- Assess effects of patient's disease on family functioning. *A thorough assessment of the family's coping behaviors is necessary to developing a therapeutic action plan.*
- PCC Encourage family members to participate in patient care as much as possible. *Family members should have an opportunity to overcome dysfunctional behavior.*
- Maintain objectivity when dealing with family conflicts. Don't become embroiled in the dynamics of a dysfunctional family in order *to maintain your ability to intervene objectively and effectively.*
- If patient and family members appear incapable of taking steps to heal their relationships, focus on being a patient advocate. Reaffirm patient's right to make own decisions without interference from family members. Provide necessary information to patient to facilitate decision making. *Dysfunctional family coping patterns evolve over many years and are unlikely to change just because patient has a serious illness. Accepting your limitations when working with family members will help you to avoid burnout and better meet patient's needs.*
- PCC Encourage patient to seek emotional support that the family can't provide by participating in a support group. Help patient select support group that best meets the patient's personal needs and outlook. Consider recommending Codependents Anonymous, a group for individuals who have difficulty maintaining healthy relationships as a result of being raised in a dysfunctional family. *Participation in a support group may improve patient's ability to cope as well as provide an opportunity to form meaningful relationships.*
- PCC Refer patient to a home health care agency, homemaker service, Meals on Wheels, or other appropriate outside agencies for assistance and follow-up. *Use of various community services may help to make up for shortcomings in family's ability to provide care.*
- PCC Listen openly to patient's expressions of pain over unresolved conflicts with family members. Patient may have to grieve over a future with no "ideal" family, capable of fully meeting the patient's emotional needs. *Therapeutic listening helps patient to understand self and family better and to understand how past conflicts affect present behavior.*

Suggested NIC Interventions

Anger Control Assistance; Caregiver Support; Family Involvement Promotion; Family Mobilization; Family Support

Evaluations for Expected Outcomes

- Family members demonstrate improved willingness to cooperate in patient's care.
- Patient expresses increased confidence in being able to make decisions.
- Patient contacts at least one support group in an effort to form meaningful relationships outside family.
- Patient takes steps to meet personal care needs.
- Patient indicates, either verbally or through behavior, a better understanding of family members and an increased ability to accept their emotional limitations.

Documentation

- Family's response to patient's illness
- Observations of patient's interactions with family members
- Referrals made to support groups and community services
- Patient's expressions of grief, anger, and disappointment over unresolved conflicts with family members
- Evaluations for expected outcomes

REFERENCES

Alpert, J. M., & Womble, F. E. (2015). Coping as a caregiver for an elderly family member. *Health Communication*, *30*(7), 714–721. doi:10.1080/10410236.2013.879560

Dardas, L. A., & Ahmad, M. M. (2015). Coping strategies as mediators and moderators between stress and quality of life among parents of children with autistic disorder. *Stress & Health: Journal of the International Society for the Investigation of Stress*, *31*(1), 5–12. doi:10.1002/smi.2513

Zaidman-Zait, A., Most, T., Tarrasch, R., Haddad-eid, E., & Brand, D. (2016). The impact of childhood hearing loss on the family: Mothers' and fathers' stress and coping resources. *Journal of Deaf Studies & Deaf Education*, *21*(1), 23–33. doi:10.1093/deafed/env038

DEATH ANXIETY

related to confronting the reality of terminal disease

Definition

Vague uneasy feeling of discomfort or dread generated by perceptions of a real or imagined threat to one's existence

Assessment

- Age
- History of present illness
- Mental status, including level of consciousness, orientation, cognition, memory, and insight
- Self-care status, including ability to carry out activities of daily living
- Sleep pattern
- Pain assessment, including location, quality, intensity on a scale of 1 to 10, temporal factors, sources of provocation, and relief
- Psychological status, including reaction to illness and dying, and expressions of fear, anger, hope, and anxiety
- Spiritual status, including that which gives purpose or meaning in life, religious affiliation, current perception of faith, religious practices, changes in religious beliefs or

practices brought on by illness, and evidence of unmet spiritual needs (meaning and purpose, love and relatedness, forgiveness)
- Cultural norms associated with illness and death
- Family status, including marital status, family roles, family communications, family's ability to meet patient's physical and emotional needs, extent to which religion defines family's value system, and changes patient's illness and impending death will make in family functioning

Defining Characteristics

- Concern about strain on the caregiver
- Deep sadness
- Fear of developing terminal illness
- Fear of loss of mental abilities when dying
- Fear of pain related to dying
- Fear of premature death
- Fear of prolonged dying process
- Fear of suffering related to dying
- Fear of the dying process
- Negative thoughts related to death and dying
- Powerlessness
- Worried about the impact of one's death on significant other

Expected Outcomes

- Patient will identify need for time with others and need for time alone.
- Patient will identify comfort measures that enhance feelings of well-being.
- Patient will communicate important thoughts and feelings to family members.
- Patient will obtain the requested level of spiritual support.
- Patient will use available support systems to cope with dying.
- Patient will express feelings of comfort and peacefulness.
- Patient will experience dying with dignity, sensitivity, and love.

Suggested NOC Outcomes

Acceptance: Health Status; Anxiety Level; Depression Level; Dignified Life Closure; Fear Self-Control; Hope; Spiritual Well-Being

Interventions and Rationales

PCC
- Assess how much help patient wants. *Patient may need a higher degree of independence than caregiver wants to allow.*
- Offer to spend time either reading to patient or just sitting there quietly. *Typically, patient approaching death desires the presence of another, but isn't interested in conversing.*
- If patient is confused, provide reassurance by telling the patient who's in the room. *This information may help to reduce anxiety.*
- Provide comfort measures—bathing, massage, regulation of environmental temperature, mouth care, administration of ice chips or wet washcloth—according to patient's preferences. *Some patients may prefer not to be bothered unless they specifically request comfort measures.*

PCC
- Help family members identify, discuss, and resolve issues related to patient's dying. *Patient needs the support of family members. Family members may need help removing emotional blocks that prevent them from providing full support to patient.*
- Demonstrate to patient your willingness to discuss spiritual aspects of death and dying *to foster open discussion.* Keep conversation focused on patient's spiritual values and the role they play in coping with dying *to ensure that your interaction with patient remains therapeutic.*
- Refer patient to a priest, minister, rabbi, or spiritual counselor, according to patient's preference, *to show respect for patient's beliefs and provide expert spiritual care.*

PCC
- Ask if there's a prayer or words of spiritual comfort that are especially meaningful to the patient, and recite this special prayer together if the patient seems comfortable with your request. *Doing so will demonstrate support for patient's spiritual needs and convey caring and acceptance.*
- Help patient cope by listening actively and communicating acceptance of the patient's thoughts and feelings. *Dying patients need the opportunity to express their feelings.*
- Provide simple physical gestures of support such as holding hands with patient. Encourage family members to do the same. Verify with patient that your actions aren't intrusive. *As patients begin to let go, they sometimes want to experience less touching.*
- Reassure patient that he won't be left alone; however, respect patient's requests to be alone. *For some patients, asking to be alone is part of the process of letting go.*

Suggested NIC Interventions

Active Listening; Anticipatory Guidance; Family Involvement Promotion; Pain Management; Spiritual Support; Touch

Evaluations for Expected Outcomes

- Patient expresses satisfaction with private time and time spent with others.
- Patient uses those comfort measures that enhance individual well-being and reduce physical symptoms associated with anxiety.
- Patient engages in conversation and activities with family, caregivers, and other support people.
- Patient expresses satisfaction with spiritual support that is offered.
- Patient makes appropriate use of available support systems to cope with the dying process.
- Patient exhibits sense of comfort and overall peace.
- Patient dies in a dignified manner in an environment of sensitivity and love.

Documentation

- Behavioral manifestations of anxiety
- Patient's expressions of feelings related to death and dying
- Patient's requests for visitors or expression of desire for solitude
- Conferences with family members
- Patient's requests for comfort measures and their effectiveness
- Referrals to clergy, spiritual advisors, or others
- Patient's response to nursing interventions
- Evaluations for expected outcomes

REFERENCES

Lodhi, M. K., Cheema, U. I., Stifter, J., Wilkie, D. J., Keenan, G. M., Yingwei, Y., ... Khokhar, A. A. (2014). Death anxiety in hospitalized end-of-life patients as captured from a structured electronic health record. *Research in Gerontological Nursing, 7*(5), 224–234. doi:10.3928/19404921-20140818-01

McClatchey, I. S., & King, S. (2015). The impact of death education on fear of death and death anxiety among human services students. *Omega: Journal of Death & Dying, 71*(4), 343–361. doi:10.1177/0030222815572606

Nursing care for patients developing marked anxiety on being diagnosed with cancer progression after surgery. (2015). *Cancer Nursing, 38*, S70.

Se-Young, K. (2015). Effects of death anxiety and meaning of life on somatization of grandparent raising grandchildren. *Journal of Korean Academy of Nursing, 45*(2), 262–270. doi:10.4040/jkan.2015.45.2.262

Strang, P. (2014). What is extreme death anxiety and what are its consequences? *Journal of Palliative Care, 30*(4), 321–326.

Sussman, J. C., & Liu, W. M. (2014). Perceptions of two therapeutic approaches for palliative care patients experiencing death anxiety. *Palliative & Supportive Care, 12*(4), 251–260. doi:10.1017/S1478951513000199

DECISIONAL CONFLICT

related to inexperience with decision making; insufficient support system

Definition

Uncertainty about course of action to be taken when choice among competing actions involves risk, loss, or challenge to values and beliefs

Assessment

- Age and gender
- Perception of health care options
- Developmental state
- Marital status
- Family system (nuclear, extended role, and sibling position)
- Sociocultural factors, including educational level, occupation, socioeconomic status, ethnic group, sexual preference, and religious beliefs
- Level of functioning (cognitive, emotional, and behavioral)
- Coping mechanisms
- Past experience with decision making
- Available support system

Defining Characteristics

- Delay in decision making
- Distress while attempting a decision
- Physical sign of distress (e.g., increase in heart rate, restlessness)
- Physical sign of tension
- Questioning of moral principle while attempting a decision
- Questioning of moral rule while attempting a decision
- Questioning of moral values while attempting a decision
- Questioning of personal beliefs while attempting a decision
- Questioning personal values while attempting a decision
- Recognizes undesired consequences of actions being considered
- Self-focused

- Uncertainty about choices
- Vacillating among choices

Expected Outcomes

- Patient will describe feelings about current situation.
- Patient will discuss benefits and drawbacks of treatment options.
- Patient will make minor decisions related to daily activities.
- Patient will accept assistance from family, friends, clergy, and other people.
- Patient will practice progressive muscle relaxation to decrease tension created by decisional conflict.
- Patient will report feeling comfortable about ability to make an appropriate, rational choice.

Suggested NOC Outcomes

Decision-Making; Information Processing; Participation in Health Care Decisions

Interventions and Rationales

- PCC Listen to patient's concerns about difficulties in making a decision. Use a nonjudgmental approach and encourage expression of feelings *to demonstrate acceptance of patient and respect for the patient's culture, beliefs, and value system.*
- PCC Assist the patient with the process of decision making in relation to daily activities. *Learning the process will provide the patient with a framework for decision making, and enhance the patient's feelings of self-confidence when making more difficult health care decisions.*
- PCC Help patient make decisions about daily activities *to enhance feelings of autonomy.*
- PCC Encourage visits with family, friends, and clergy; provide privacy during visits *to foster emotional support.*
- Teach progressive muscle-relaxation techniques *to decrease physical and psychological signs of tension.*
- PCC Help patient identify decision-making areas that require assistance from others, and provide appropriate referrals. *Providing referrals will ensure ongoing support. Putting patient in touch with appropriate community resources will help promote feeling that others are genuinely interested in patient's well-being.*

Suggested NIC Interventions

Active Listening; Assertiveness Training; Decision-Making Support; Learning Facilitation; Mutual Goal Setting

Evaluations for Expected Outcomes

- Patient expresses anxiety, tension, and other feelings related to difficult medical treatment decisions.
- Patient describes benefits and drawbacks of treatment options.
- Patient makes minor decisions related to daily activities.
- Patient accepts assistance from family, friends, clergy, and other people.

- Patient practices progressive muscle relaxation to decrease tension created by decisional conflict.
- Patient reports feeling at ease with ability to choose treatment option that's appropriate for him or her.

Documentation

- Patient's statements that provide insight into conflict regarding treatment options
- Cognitive, emotional, and behavioral functioning
- Interventions to assist patient with resolving decisional conflict
- Patient's response to nursing interventions
- Evaluations for expected outcomes

REFERENCES

Peccatori, F. A. (2015). Difficult choices for young patients with cancer: The supportive role of decisional counseling. *Supportive Care in Cancer*, *23*(12), 3555–3562. doi:10.1007/s00520-015-2726-5

Schubart, J. R., Levi, B. H., Dellasega, C., Whitehead, M., & Green, M. J. (2014). Factors that affect decisions to receive (or not receive) life-sustaining treatment in advance care planning. *Journal of Psychosocial Nursing & Mental Health Services*, *52*(2), 38–44. doi:10.3928/02793695-20131028-01

Meade, T., Dowswell, E., Manolios, N., & Sharpe, L. (2015). The motherhood choices decision aid for women with rheumatoid arthritis increases knowledge and reduces decisional conflict: A randomized controlled trial. *BMC Musculoskeletal Disorders*, *16*(1), 1–8. doi:10.1186/s12891-015-0713-0

INEFFECTIVE DENIAL

related to fear of death, ineffective coping strategies, or anxiety

Definition

Conscious or unconscious attempt to disavow the knowledge or meaning of an event to reduce anxiety and/or fear, leading to the detriment of health

Assessment

- Perception of present health state, including awareness of diagnosis, perception of personal relevance or impact on life pattern, and description of symptoms
- Mental status, including general appearance, affect, mood, memory, orientation, communication, thinking process, perception, abstract thinking, judgment, and insight
- Coping behaviors
- Problem-solving strategies
- Support systems, including family, friends, clergy, and financial resources
- Belief system, including values, norms, and religion
- Self-concept, including self-esteem and body image

Defining Characteristics

- Delay in seeking health care
- Denies fear of death
- Denies fear of invalidism
- Displaces fear of impact of the condition

- Displaces source of symptoms
- Does not admit impact of disease on life
- Does not perceive relevance of danger
- Does not perceive relevance of symptoms
- Inappropriate affect
- Minimizes symptoms
- Refusal of health care
- Use of dismissive gestures when speaking of distressing event
- Use of dismissive comments when speaking of distressing event
- Use of treatment not advised by health care professional

Expected Outcomes

- Patient will describe knowledge and perception of present health problem.
- Patient will describe life pattern and report any recent changes.
- Patient will express knowledge of stages of grieving.
- Patient will demonstrate behavior associated with grief process.
- Patient will discuss present health problem with physician, nurses, and family members.
- Patient will indicate, either verbally or through behavior, an increased awareness of reality.

Suggested NOC Outcomes

Acceptance: Health Status; Anxiety Level; Coping; Fear Self-Control; Health Beliefs; Health Beliefs: Perceived Threat; Symptom Control

Interventions and Rationales

- PCC Provide for a specific amount of uninterrupted, non-care-related time with patient each day. *This allows patient to discuss knowledge, feelings, and concerns.*
- PCC Encourage patient to express feelings related to present problem, its severity, and its potential impact on life pattern. *This helps patient express doubts and resolve concerns.*
- Maintain frequent communication with physician to assess what patient has been told about illness. *This fosters consistent, collaborative approach to patient's care.*
- PCC Listen to patient with nonjudgmental acceptance *to demonstrate positive regard for patient as person worthy of respect.*
- Help patient learn the stages of anticipatory grieving *to increase understanding and ability to cope.*
- As patient is ready and receptive, teach the patient about health problem and treatment regimen. Reinforce learning as patient becomes receptive. *While in a state of denial, patients are often either unwilling or unable to assimilate factual information about health issues.*
- PCC Encourage patient to communicate with others, asking questions and clarifying concerns based on readiness. *Patient fixated in denial may isolate and withdraw from others.*
- Visit more frequently as patient begins to accept reality; alleviate fears when necessary. *This helps reduce patient's fear of being alone and fosters accurate reality testing.*

Suggested NIC Interventions

Anxiety Reduction; Behavior Modification; Calming Technique; Coping Enhancement; Counseling; Decision-Making Support; Health Education; Mutual Goal Setting; Reality Orientation; Truth Telling

Evaluations for Expected Outcomes

- Patient describes present health problem.
- Patient describes life pattern and reports recent changes.
- Patient communicates understanding of stages of grieving.
- Patient demonstrates behavior appropriate to present phase of grieving process.
- When ready, patient discusses health problem with physician, nurses, and family members.
- Patient displays increasing awareness of reality, either verbally or through behavior.

Documentation

- Patient's perception of health problem
- Mental status (baseline and ongoing)
- Patient's knowledge of grief process
- Patient's behavioral responses
- Interventions implemented to assist patient
- Patient's response to nursing interventions
- Evaluations for expected outcomes

REFERENCES

Kaldy, J. (2014). Denial: When it helps, when it hurts. *Caring for the Ages, 15*(10), 1–7.

Paris, J. J., Cummings, B. M., & Moore, M. P. (2014). "Brain death," "dead," and parental denial. *Cambridge Quarterly of Healthcare Ethics, 23*(4), 371–382. doi:10.1017/S0963180114000048

Williams, A. R., Olfson, M., & Galanter, M. (2015). Assessing and improving clinical insight among patients "in denial". *JAMA Psychiatry, 72*(4), 303–304. doi:10.1001/jamapsychiatry.2014.2684

DIARRHEA

related to malabsorption, gastrointestinal inflammation, or gastrointestinal irritation

Definition

Passage of loose, unformed stools

Assessment

- History of bowel disorder or surgery
- Gastrointestinal (GI) status, including nausea and vomiting, usual bowel elimination habits, change in bowel elimination habits, stools characteristics (color, amount, size, and consistency), pain, inspection of abdomen, auscultation of bowel sounds, palpation for masses and tenderness, percussion for tympany and dullness, laxative and enema use, medications (especially antibiotics), and results of stool culture, upper GI series, and barium enema
- Nutritional status, including dietary intake, change from normal diet, appetite, current weight, change from normal weight, food irritants and contaminants, and serum albumin levels
- Fluid and electrolyte status, including intake and output, urine specific gravity, skin turgor, mucous membranes, serum potassium and sodium levels, and blood urea nitrogen
- Psychosocial status, including personality, stressors (such as finances, job, marital discord, and disease process), coping mechanisms, support systems, lifestyle, and recent travel

Defining Characteristics

- Abdominal pain
- Bowel urgency
- Cramping
- Hyperactive bowel sounds
- Loose or liquid stools >3 in 24 hours

Expected Outcomes

- Patient will control diarrhea with medication.
- Patient's elimination pattern will return to normal.
- Patient will regain and maintain fluid and electrolyte balance.
- Patient's skin will remain intact.
- Patient will discuss causative factors, preventive measures, and changed body image.
- Patient will practice stress-reduction techniques daily.
- Patient will demonstrate skill in using ostomy devices.
- Patient will seek out persons with similar conditions or join a support group.

Suggested NOC Outcomes

Bowel Elimination; Electrolyte & Acid–base balance; Fluid Balance; Hydration; Symptom Severity; Bowel Continence

Interventions and Rationales

- Monitor frequency and characteristics of stools, auscultate bowel sounds, and record results at least every shift *to monitor treatment effectiveness.*
- Tell patient to notify staff of each episode of diarrhea *to promote comfort and maintain communication.*
- Give antidiarrheal medications, as ordered, *to improve body function, promote comfort, and balance body fluids, salts, and acid–base levels.* Monitor and report efficacy.
- Monitor and record patient's intake and output, including number of stools. Report imbalances. *Monitoring ensures correct fluid replacement therapy.*
- Check skin daily *to detect and prevent breakdown.* Report decreased skin turgor or excoriation of perianal area.
- Weigh patient daily until diarrhea is controlled *to detect fluid loss or retention.*
- PCC Teach patient about:
  - causative and preventive factors *to promote understanding of problem.*
  - cleaning of perianal area, including use of powders and lotions, *to promote comfort and skin integrity.*
  - dietary restriction *to control diarrhea, such as a lactose-free diet, which reduces residual waste and decreases intestinal irritation and spasms.*
- PCC Teach stress-reduction techniques and help patient perform them daily by providing time, privacy, and needed equipment. *This temporarily relieves emotional distress.*
- S Prepare patient for surgery, and provide preoperative instruction for abdominal surgery *to reassure patient and maintain trust.*
- PCC Provide information about ileostomy or colostomy, if indicated, *to help patient understand procedure and avoid threat to health equilibrium.*
- Demonstrate use of ostomy equipment *to encourage understanding and compliance.*
- PCC Provide support and assistance while patient develops skill in caring for stoma *to improve understanding and reduce anxiety.*

PCC • Encourage expression of feelings and concerns about impact of changed body image *to allow patient to pinpoint specific fears and promote self-knowledge and growth.*

PCC • Encourage use of support groups, such as ileostomy clubs, *to provide patient with additional support and health care resources.*

Suggested NIC Interventions

Anxiety Reduction; Bowel Management; Diarrhea Management; Fluid/Electrolyte Management; Medication Management; Skin Care: Topical Treatments

Evaluations for Expected Outcomes

- Patient doesn't experience diarrhea.
- Patient's elimination pattern returns to normal.
- Patient maintains fluid and electrolyte balance.
- Patient's skin remains intact.
- Patient explains cause of diarrhea and steps to prevent recurrence.
- Patient demonstrates successful use of stress-reduction techniques.
- Patient demonstrates successful use of ostomy devices.
- Patient attends a support group for individuals with a similar condition.

Documentation

- Patient's expressions of concern about diarrhea, causative factors, surgery, and adaptation to changes in body image
- Observations of effects of medications, intake and output, weight, stools characteristics, skin condition, and stoma appearance
- Evaluations for expected outcomes

REFERENCES

Keefe, D. M., Elting, L. S., Nguyen, H. T., Grunberg, S. M., Aprile, G., Bonaventura, A., ... Sonis, S. T. (2014). Risk and outcomes of chemotherapy-induced diarrhea (CID) among patients with colorectal cancer receiving multi-cycle chemotherapy. *Cancer Chemotherapy & Pharmacology*, 74(4), 675–680. doi:10.1007/s00280-014-2526-5

Melton, E. C., & Kehl, K. A. (2015). Managing chronic diarrhea with colorectal cancer. *Journal of Hospice & Palliative Nursing*, *17*(5), 382–388. doi:10.1097/NJH.0000000000000130

Peart, J., & Richardson, A. (2015). Developing a critical care bowel management assessment tool to manage fecal incontinence. *Nursing in Critical Care*, *20*(1), 34–40. doi:10.1111/nicc.12101

DIARRHEA

related to increase in stress level and anxiety

Definition

Passage of loose, unformed stools

Assessment

- History of bowel disorder or surgery
- Gastrointestinal (GI) status, including nausea and vomiting, usual bowel elimination habits, change in bowel elimination habits, stools characteristics (color, amount, size, and

consistency), pain and discomfort, inspection of abdomen, auscultation of bowel sounds, palpation for masses and tenderness, and percussion for tympany and dullness
- Nutritional status, including dietary intake, change from normal diet, appetite, current weight, and change from normal weight
- Fluid and electrolyte status, including intake and output, urine specific gravity, skin turgor, mucous membranes, serum potassium and sodium levels, and blood urea nitrogen
- Psychosocial status, including personality, stressors (such as finances, job, and marital discord), coping mechanisms, support systems (family members and others), and lifestyle

Defining Characteristics

- Abdominal pain
- Bowel urgency
- Cramping
- Hyperactive bowel sounds
- Loose, liquid stools >3 in 24 hours

Expected Outcomes

- Patient's diarrheal episodes will decline or disappear.
- Patient will resume usual bowel pattern.
- Patient will maintain weight and fluid and electrolyte balance.
- Patient will keep skin clean and free from irritation or ulcerations.
- Patient will explain causative factors and preventive measures.
- Patient will discuss relationship of stress and anxiety to episodes of diarrhea.
- Patient will state plans to use stress-reduction techniques (specify).
- Patient will demonstrate ability to use at least one stress-reduction technique.

Suggested NOC Outcomes

Bowel Continence; Hydration; Symptom Control; Bowel Elimination

Interventions and Rationales

- Monitor and record frequency and characteristics of stools *to monitor treatment effectiveness.* Instruct patient to record diarrheal episodes and report them to staff *to promote comfort and maintain effective patient–staff communication.*
- Administer antidiarrheal medications, as ordered, *to improve body function, promote comfort, and balance body fluids, salts, and acid–base levels.* Monitor and report medications' effectiveness.
- Provide replacement fluids and electrolytes as prescribed. Maintain accurate records *to ensure balanced fluid intake and output.*
- Monitor perianal skin for irritation and ulceration; treat according to established protocol *to promote comfort, skin integrity, and freedom from infection.*
- Identify stressors and help patient solve problems *to provide more realistic approach to care.*
- PCC Encourage patient to ventilate stresses and anxiety; *release of pent-up emotions can temporarily relieve emotional distress.*
- PCC Teach patient to:
  - use relaxation techniques *to reduce muscle tension and nervousness.*
  - recognize and reduce intake of diarrhea-producing foods or substances (such as dairy products and fruit) *to reduce residual waste matter and decrease intestinal irritation.*
- Spend at least 10 minutes with patient twice daily to discuss stress-reducing techniques; *this can help patient pinpoint specific fears.*

- Encourage and assist patient to practice relaxation techniques *to reduce tension and promote self-knowledge and growth.*

Suggested NIC Interventions

Anxiety Reduction; Coping Enhancement; Diarrhea Management; Emotional Support; Energy Management; Nutrition Management; Skin Surveillance; Weight Management

Evaluations for Expected Outcomes

- Patient's diarrheal episodes decline by at least 50%.
- Patient resumes usual bowel elimination pattern.
- Patient maintains weight and fluid and electrolyte balance.
- Patient doesn't experience skin breakdown, irritation, or ulcerations.
- Patient identifies cause of diarrhea and discusses steps to prevent recurrence.
- Patient explains how stress may contribute to diarrhea.
- Patient explains plan to use stress-reduction techniques.
- Patient describes and demonstrates at least one stress-reduction technique.

Documentation

- Patient's expressions of concern and ability to manage diarrhea produced by stress and anxiety
- Observations of effects of relaxation and stress-reduction techniques and dietary management on diarrhea
- Patient's responses and skill level in carrying out stress-reduction techniques and dietary changes
- Evaluations for expected outcomes

REFERENCES

Best, C. (2015). Examining the extent to which stress contributes to disease in the gastrointestinal tract: A literature review. *Gastrointestinal Nursing*, *13*(2), 16–21.

Dainty, A. D., Allcock, N., & Cooper, J. (2014). Study of irritable bowel syndrome and co-existing psychological illness. *Nurse Researcher*, *21*(4), 27–31. doi:10.7748/nr2014.03.21.4.27.e1228

Hompson, J., & Read, N. (2015). Managing the symptoms of irritable bowel syndrome. *Nurse Prescribing*, *13*(5), 230–234.

Saito, Y., & Amit, S. (2014). Mind–body medicine and irritable bowel syndrome: A randomized control trial using stress reduction and resiliency training. *Journal of Alternative & Complementary Medicine*, *20*(5), A94–A94. doi:10.1089/acm.2014.5248.abstract

RISK FOR DISUSE SYNDROME

Definition

Vulnerable to deterioration of body systems as the result of prescribed or unavoidable musculoskeletal inactivity, which may compromise health

Assessment

- Condition leading to prolonged inactivity or immobility
- Age

- Neurologic status, including mental status, level of consciousness (LOC), and sensory and motor ability
- Cardiovascular status, including blood pressure, heart rate, temperature, peripheral pulses, capillary refill, clotting profile, skin temperature and color, presence of edema, and chest pain or discomfort
- Respiratory status, including rate and rhythm, depth of inspiration, chest symmetry, use of accessory muscles, cough and sputum, percussion of lung fields, auscultation of breath sounds, chest pain or discomfort, and arterial blood gas (ABG) levels
- Gastrointestinal (GI) status, including inspection of abdomen, auscultation of bowel sounds, palpation for tenderness and masses, percussion for areas of dullness, usual bowel habits, change in bowel habits, laxative use, pain or discomfort, and characteristics of stools (color, size, amount, and consistency)
- Nutritional status, including dietary intake, appetite, current weight, and change from normal weight
- Fluid status, including intake and output, urine specific gravity, mucous membranes, serum electrolyte levels, blood urea nitrogen (BUN), and creatinine level
- Genitourinary status, including voiding pattern, characteristics of urine (color, odor, sediment, and amount), history of urinary problems or infections, palpation of bladder, pain or discomfort, use of urinary assistive device, urinalysis, and urine cultures
- Musculoskeletal status, including range of motion (ROM); muscle size, strength, and tone; coordination; and functional mobility scale:
  0 = completely independent
  1 = requires use of equipment or device
  2 = requires help, supervision, or teaching from another person
  3 = requires help from another person and equipment or device
  4 = dependent; doesn't participate in activity
- Integumentary status, including skin color, texture, turgor, temperature, elasticity, sensation, moisture, hygiene, and lesions
- Psychosocial factors, including family support, coping style, current understanding of prescribed inactivity, willingness to cooperate with treatment, mood, behavior, motivation, and stressors (such as inactivity, finances, job, and marital discord)

Risk Factors

- Alteration in LOC
- Mechanical immobility
- Pain
- Paralysis
- Prescribed immobility

Expected Outcomes

- Patient won't display evidence of altered mental, sensory, or motor ability.
- Patient won't have evidence of thrombus formation, venous stasis, or altered cardiovascular function.
- Patient won't show evidence of decreased chest movement, cough stimulus, or depth of ventilation.
- Patient won't show pooling of secretions or signs of infection.
- Patient won't have evidence of constipation and will maintain normal bowel elimination patterns.
- Patient will maintain adequate dietary intake, hydration, and weight.
- Patient won't show evidence of urine retention, infection, or renal calculi.
- Patient will maintain muscle strength and tone and joint ROM.

- Patient won't show evidence of contractures or subluxations.
- Patient won't show evidence of skin breakdown.
- Patient will maintain normal neurologic, cardiovascular, respiratory, GI, nutritional, genitourinary, musculoskeletal, and integumentary functioning during period of inactivity.
- Patient will express feelings about prolonged inactivity.

Suggested NOC Outcomes

Comfort Level; Coordinated Movement; Endurance; Immobility Consequences: Physiologic; Immobility Consequences: Psycho-Cognitive; Mobility; Pain Level; Risk Control

Interventions and Rationales

- Provide frequent contact with staff, diversionary materials (magazines, radio, and television), and orienting mechanisms (clock and calendar). *Reality orientation fosters patient awareness of environment.*
- Avoid positions that put prolonged pressure on body parts and compress blood vessels. Patient should change positions at least every 2 hours within prescribed limits. *These measures enhance circulation and help prevent tissue or skin breakdown.*
- Inspect skin every shift, and protect areas subject to irritation. Follow facility policy for prevention of pressure ulcers *to prevent or mitigate skin breakdown.*
- Use pressure-reducing or pressure-equalizing equipment, as indicated or ordered (flotation pad, air pressure mattress, sheepskin pads, or special bed). *This helps prevent skin breakdown by relieving pressure.*
- S Apply antiembolism stockings; remove for 1 hour every 8 hours. *Stockings promote venous return to heart, prevent venous stasis, and decrease or prevent swelling of lower extremities.*
- S Monitor clotting profile. Administer and monitor anticoagulant therapy, if ordered, and monitor for signs and symptoms of bleeding *because anticoagulant therapy may cause hemorrhage.*
- S Monitor temperature, blood pressure, pulse, and respirations at least every 4 hours *to assess for indications of infection or other complications.*
- Teach and monitor deep breathing, coughing, and use of incentive spirometer. Maintain regimen every 2 hours. *These measures help clear airways, expand lungs, and prevent respiratory complications.*
- Encourage fluid intake of 2.5 to 3.5 L daily, unless contraindicated, *to maintain urine output and aid bowel elimination.* Weigh daily and monitor hydration status (serum electrolyte, BUN, creatinine levels, and intake and output).
- S Monitor breath sounds and respiratory rate, rhythm, and depth at least every 4 hours *to rule out respiratory complications.* Monitor ABG levels or pulse oximetry, if indicated, *to assess oxygenation, ventilation, and metabolic status.*
- Suction airway, as needed and ordered, *to clear airway and stimulate cough reflex;* note secretion characteristics.
- Establish baseline *to compare elimination patterns and habits.* Elevate head of bed and provide privacy to allow comfortable elimination.
- PCC Instruct patient to avoid straining during bowel movements; administer stool softeners, suppositories, or laxatives, as ordered, and monitor effectiveness. *Straining during bowel movements may be hazardous to patients with cardiovascular disorders and increased intracranial pressure.*
- Provide small, frequent meals of favorite foods to increase dietary intake. Increase fiber content to enhance bowel elimination. Increase protein and vitamin C *to promote wound healing. Limit calcium to reduce risk of renal and bladder calculi.*

- Monitor urine characteristics and patient's subjective complaints typical of urinary tract infection (UTI), such as burning, frequency, and urgency. Obtain urine cultures, as ordered. *These measures aid early detection of UTI.*
- Identify level of functioning to provide baseline for future assessment, and encourage appropriate participation in care *to prevent complications of immobility and increase patient's feelings of self-esteem.*
- Perform active or passive ROM exercises at least once per shift. Teach and monitor appropriate isotonic and isometric exercises. *These measures prevent joint contractures, muscle atrophy, and other complications of prolonged inactivity.*
- Provide or help with daily hygiene; keep skin dry and lubricated *to prevent cracking and possible infection.*
- PCC Encourage patient and family to ventilate frustration. Allow open expression of all feelings associated with prolonged inactivity *to help patient and family cope with treatment.*

Suggested NIC Interventions

Activity Therapy; Body Mechanics Promotion; Cognitive Stimulation; Energy Management; Exercise Promotion; Exercise Therapy: Ambulation; Fluid Management; Nutrition Management

Evaluations for Expected Outcomes

- Patient doesn't exhibit altered LOC, mental status, sensory ability, or motor ability.
- Patient doesn't exhibit evidence of thrombus formation, venous stasis, or altered cardiovascular function.
- Patient shows no evidence of decreased chest movement, cough stimulus, or depth of ventilation.
- Patient maintains clear breath sounds bilaterally and doesn't show evidence of fever, chills, cough, purulent sputum, pooled secretions, or rapid, shallow respirations.
- Patient's bowel elimination pattern remains normal.
- Patient maintains adequate dietary intake, daily fluid intake, and weight.
- Patient doesn't exhibit evidence of distended bladder, fever, chills, frequent burning or painful urination, urgency, hematuria, flank pain, or urine retention.
- Patient's muscle strength and tone and joint ROM remain stable.
- Patient doesn't exhibit evidence of joint contractures.
- Patient doesn't experience skin breakdown.
- Patient maintains neurologic, cardiovascular, respiratory, GI, nutritional, genitourinary, musculoskeletal, and integumentary functioning.
- Patient openly expresses frustration, anger, despondency, and other feelings associated with prolonged inactivity.

Documentation

- Patient's concerns or perceptions of circumstances necessitating inactivity; willingness to accept and participate in treatment
- Assessment of body systems at risk for deterioration
- Interventions to provide preventive or supportive care and prescribed treatment
- Treatment given to patient and patient's understanding and demonstrated ability to carry out instructions
- Patient's response to nursing interventions
- Evaluations for expected outcomes

REFERENCES

Fernandes, T., Mendes, E., Preto, L., & Novo, A. (2015). Experience of a mobilization and active exercise program on the range of motion of bedridden patients with disuse syndrome. *Journal of Rehabilitation Medicine*, *47*(8), 791–792.

Powers, S. (2014). Can antioxidants protect against disuse muscle atrophy? *Sports Medicine*, *44*, 155–165. doi:10.1007/s40279-014-0255-x

Shuval, K., Kohl, H. W., III, Bernstein, I., Cheng, D., Pettee Gabriel, K., Barlow, C. E., ... Dipietro, L. (2014). Sedentary behavior and physical inactivity assessment in primary care: The Rapid Assessment Disuse Index (RADI) study. *British Journal of Sports Medicine*, *48*(3), 250–255. doi:10.1136/bjsports-2013-092901

DEFICIENT DIVERSIONAL ACTIVITY

related to insufficient diversional activity

Definition

Decreased stimulation from (or interest or engagement in) recreational or leisure activities

Assessment

- Physical status, including mobility and activity tolerance
- Cardiovascular status, including heart rate and rhythm and blood pressure sitting and standing
- Respiratory status, including respiratory rate and rhythm—resting and with activity
- Neurologic status, including level of consciousness, orientation, mood, behavior, and memory
- Psychosocial status, including family and friends, hobbies, and interests; favorite music, television, and reading material; and changes or adaptations needed to carry out activities

Defining Characteristics

- Boredom
- Current setting does not allow engagement in activity

Expected Outcomes

- Patient will express interest in using leisure time meaningfully.
- Patient will express interest in activities that can be provided.
- Patient will participate in chosen activity.
- Patient will watch selected television program or listen to radio program or selected music daily.
- Patient will report satisfaction with use of leisure time.
- Patient or caregiver will modify environment to provide maximum stimulation, such as by hanging posters or cards and moving bed next to a window.

Suggested NOC Outcomes

Leisure Participation; Motivation; Social Involvement; Personal Well-Being

Interventions and Rationales

- PCC • Encourage discussion of previously enjoyed hobbies, interests, or skills *to direct planning of new activities.* Suggest performing an activity helpful to others or otherwise productive *to promote self-fulfillment.*
- Obtain radio, CD player, iPod, or television (if desired), and allow patient to select programs. Communicate patient's desires to coworkers. Turn on television set at ____ (time) to ____ (channel). *Use of selective television, radio, and so on can help pass time.*
- Ask volunteers (friends, family, or hospital volunteer) to read newspapers, books, or magazines to patient at specific times. *Personal contact helps alleviate boredom.*
- PCC • Work with patient and family to find ways to carry out desired activities. Use imagination and creativity; for example, a former carpenter may adapt to carving small objects rather than building large ones. *Adaptive equipment helps patient pursue previous activities within new limits.*
- PCC • Engage patient in conversation while carrying out routine care. Discuss patient's favorite topics as much as possible. *Conversation conveys caring and recognition of patient's worth.*
- Provide supplies and set time to carry out hobby; for example, give crochet hook and yarn to patient daily at ____ (time). *Specifying time for activity indicates its value.*
- Avoid scheduling procedures during patient's leisure time *to promote quality of life.*
- Provide talking books or CDs if available. *These provide low-effort sources of enjoyment for bedridden patient.*
- Obtain an adapter for television *to provide captions for hearing-impaired patient.*
- PCC • Encourage visitors to involve patient in favorite activities through discussion, reading, and attendance at programs, if appropriate, *to reduce boredom.*
- PCC • Encourage patient's family or caregiver to bring personal articles (posters, cards, and pictures) to help make environment more stimulating. *Patient may respond better to objects with personal meaning.*
- PCC • Make referral to recreational, occupational, or physical therapist for consultation on adaptive equipment to carry out desired activity; arrange for therapy sessions. *Adaptive equipment allows patient to continue enjoying activities or may stimulate interest in new activities.*
- Provide plants for patient to tend to. *Caring for live plants may stimulate interest.*
- Change scenery when possible; for example, take patient outside in wheelchair *to help reduce boredom.*
- Identify type of music patient prefers; seek help from family and hospital resources to provide selected music daily. *Music may relieve boredom and stimulate interest.*

Suggested NIC Interventions

Activity Therapy; Art Therapy; Energy Management; Recreation Therapy; Self-Responsibility Facilitation

Evaluations for Expected Outcomes

- Patient expresses desire to participate in activities during leisure time.
- Patient discusses recent activity with staff members, family, or others.
- Patient engages in activity.
- Patient discusses content of television or radio program.
- Patient reports reduced feelings of boredom.
- Patient (or caregiver) has modified environment, thereby increasing stimulation.

Documentation

- Patient's expression of boredom, frustration, and desire to carry out leisure activity
- Patient's interests and ability to carry out activity and necessary modifications required to accomplish activity
- Observations of patient's skill level and extent of participation in activity
- Patient's expression of satisfaction with use of unoccupied time
- Evaluations for expected outcomes

REFERENCES

Camic, P. M., Tischler, V., & Pearman, C. H. (2014). Viewing and making art together: A multi-session art gallery-based intervention for people with dementia and their carers. *Aging & Mental Health, 18*(2), 161–168. doi:10.1080/13607863.2013.818101

Hsin-Sing, W., Hung-Lan, W., & Hsien-Ju, L. (2014). Applying a creative art activity in care: Report on an experience with a newly admitted resident. *Journal of Nursing, 61*(5), 104–110. doi:10.6224/JN.61.5.104

Rosenbaum, S., Tiedemann, A., Ward, P. B., Curtis, J., & Sherrington, C. (2015). Physical activity interventions: An essential component in recovery from mental illness. *British Journal of Sports Medicine, 49*(24), 1544–1545. doi:10.1136/bjsports-2014-094314

RISK FOR DRY EYE

Definition

Vulnerable to eye discomfort or damage to the cornea and conjunctiva due to reduced quantity or quality of tears to moisten the eye, which may compromise health

Assessment

- Health history, including accidents, exposure to pollutants, falls, hyperthermia, hypothermia, poisoning, sensory or perceptual changes (auditory, gustatory, kinesthetic, olfactory, tactile, and visual), and trauma
- Cardiovascular status including heart rate and rhythm, blood pressure, and peripheral pulses
- Neurologic status including level of consciousness, orientation, motor activity, and strength of all extremities

Risk Factors

- Aging
- Autoimmune disease (rheumatoid arthritis, diabetes mellitus, thyroid disease)
- Contact lens wearer
- Environmental factors (e.g., air-conditioning, excessive wind, sunlight exposure, air pollution, low humidity)
- Female gender
- History of allergy
- Hormonal change
- Lifestyle choice (e.g., smoking, caffeine use, prolonged reading)
- Mechanical ventilation
- Neurologic lesion with sensory or motor reflex loss (e.g., lagophthalmos, lack of spontaneous blink reflex)
- Ocular surface damage
- Treatment regimen
- Vitamin A deficiency

Expected Outcomes

- Patient will state personal risk factors for dry eye.
- Patient will take steps to minimize risk factors.
- Patient will understand need for collaboration with health care team if signs/symptoms occur/persist.

Suggested NOC Outcomes

Risk Control; Risk Detection; Tissue Integrity: Skin/Mucous Membranes; Knowledge: Health Behavior

Interventions and Rationales

- Identify use of systemic medications that may decrease tear production, and lifestyle behaviors that may potentiate dry eye conditions. *Assessment data may influence interventions.*
- Assess for history of medical conditions *to determine underlying risks for dry eye syndrome.*
- Modify physical environment to increase humidity, minimize excessive air movement, and control dust, *which can decrease tear production.*
- Administer artificial tears as indicated *to relieve symptoms.*
- Perform protective measures such as preservative-free artificial tears or polyethylene eye cover for critically ill patients *to prevent eye damage due to dry eye syndrome.*
- PCC Teach about simple environmental modifications *to reduce evaporation of tears.* Encourage patient to take frequent breaks from visually demanding activities *to help minimize risk factors.* Suggest diet rich in omega-3 fatty acid or dietary supplement. *Diet low in omega-3 fatty acids can increase risk of dry eye syndrome.*
- PCC Instruct patient on the use of sunglasses *to limit exposure to light.*
- PCC Instruct patient to try over-the-counter artificial tears *for temporary relief of dry eye.*
- Encourage adherence to lifestyle modifications, *which will improve quality of life and decrease the risk of eye damage.*
- PCC Refer to eye specialist if symptoms persist *for further evaluation and continued care.*
- Collaborate with primary care provider regarding possible changes in medications *that may be contributing to dry eye condition.*
- Encourage annual eye exam *to monitor for any changes.*
- Offer written treatment guidelines as needed *to reinforce learning.*

Suggested NIC Interventions

Risk Management; Risk Identification; Behavior management

Evaluations for Expected Outcomes

- Patient states risk factors for dry eye.
- Patient recognizes possibility of adverse reaction to dry eye.
- Patient collaborates with health care team members.

Documentation

- Patient's expressions of concern about adverse reaction and symptoms of previous episodes of dry eye
- Observations of physiologic and behavioral manifestations of dry eye

- Interventions performed to allay adverse reaction
- Patient's response to interventions
- Evaluations for expected outcomes

REFERENCES

Ezuddin, N., Alawa, K., & Galor, A. (2015). Therapeutic strategies to treat dry eye in an aging population. *Drugs & Aging, 32*(7), 505–513. doi:10.1007/s40266-015-0277-6

Marshall, L. L., & Roach, J. M. (2016). Treatment of dry eye disease. *Consultant Pharmacist, 31*(2), 96–106. doi:10.4140/TCP.n.2016.96

Sun, H., & Kye Ha, K. (2014). Dry eye syndrome and ocular fatigue according to the status of contact lens wearing and management among female university students. *Journal of Korean Academy of Community Health Nursing/Jiyeog Sahoe Ganho Hakoeji, 25*(4), 259–269. doi:10.12799/jkachn.2014.25.4.259

RISK FOR PERIPHERAL NEUROVASCULAR DYSFUNCTION

Definition

Vulnerable to disruption in the circulation, sensation, and motion of an extremity, which may compromise health

Assessment

- History of trauma or vascular injuries
- Inspection of extremities, including signs of soft tissue injury, such as abrasions, lacerations, and contusions
- Pain sensation, including characteristics of pain (sharp, dull, constant, or intermittent), precipitating factors, and reaction to passive stretching of affected muscles
- Tactile sensation in areas innervated by major nerves of upper extremities, including deltoid, radial side of forearm, palmar surface of thumb, fingers, palmar surface of little finger, and webbed space between thumb and index finger
- Tactile sensation in lower extremities, including medial side of foot and leg, medial side of thigh, sole of foot, and lateral aspect of leg below the knee
- Motor nerve function of upper extremities, including arm abduction at shoulder, arm flexion at elbow, thumb and little finger opposition, abduction and adduction of fingers, and extension of wrist and fingers
- Motor nerve function of lower extremities, including knee extension, thigh adduction, plantar flexion and dorsiflexion of ankle, and flexion and extension of toes
- Pulses in upper and lower extremities, including radial, ulnar, brachial, femoral, popliteal, posterior tibial, and dorsalis pedis; perform bilateral comparison and rank quality using following scale:
  0 = absent
  1 = very weak, barely palpable
  2 = weak, reduced
  3 = slightly weak, easily located
  4 = normal, easily located
- Vascular status, including capillary refill time, blanching, skin temperature, and skin color
- Point tenderness, especially over bony prominences
- Edema
- Increased intracompartmental pressure
- Cranial nerves (if patient has halo cast)

Risk Factors

- Burns
- Fracture
- Immobilization
- Mechanical compression (e.g., tourniquet, cast, brace, dressing, restraint)
- Orthopedic surgery
- Trauma
- Vascular obstruction

Expected Outcomes

- Patient won't experience disability related to peripheral neurovascular dysfunction after injury or treatment.
- Patient will maintain circulation in extremities.
- Patient will feel and move each toe or finger after application of cast, brace, or splint.
- Patient will demonstrate correct body positioning techniques.
- Patient and family members will express understanding of risk of altered neurovascular status and need to report symptoms of impaired circulation.
- Patient will enroll in smoking-cessation program, as appropriate.
- Patient will not exhibit symptoms of neurovascular compromise.

Suggested NOC Outcomes

Circulation Status; Coordinated Movement; Neurologic Status: Spinal Sensory/Motor Function; Risk Control; Risk Detection; Tissue Perfusion: Peripheral

Interventions and Rationales

- S Note whether patient will undergo surgery or a procedure that increases risk of peripheral neurovascular dysfunction *to anticipate complications.*
- Immobilize the joints directly above and below the suspected fracture site, leaving room for pulse assessment *to facilitate monitoring of circulatory status.*
- As appropriate, assess circulation before the application of the cast, brace, or splint. After application of the cast, brace, or splint, have patient move fingers and toes every 4 hours until discharge *to detect signs of impaired circulation.*
- Remove the clothing around the suspected fracture site, clean the site, apply sterile dressings to open wounds, and carefully apply a cast, brace, or splint *to avoid further infection and trauma.*
- Follow facility guidelines for the application of such devices as tourniquets, restraints, and tape *to ensure adequate circulation in affected extremity.*
- If you suspect nerve compression, assess the position of the extremity that has a cast, brace, or splint. *Positioning of the extremity may affect circulation.*
- Elevate the limb above heart level after surgery or trauma *to reduce the risk of edema.* If increased intracompartmental pressure is evident, maintain the affected limb at heart level *to reduce pressure.*
- If edema appears in the affected extremity, split, bivalve, slit, or cut a window in the cast and padding according to facility protocol *to avoid neurovascular impairment.*
- Inject prescribed neurotoxic agents (such as penicillin G, hydrocortisone, tetanus toxoid, and diazepam) away from the affected extremity and major nerves *to avoid injury.*
- Avoid flexing the affected extremity. *Flexion may reduce venous circulation, increasing the risk of neurovascular complications.*
- If patient smokes, advise enrollment in a smoking-cessation program. *Quitting smoking may enhance oxygenation, decreasing the risk of peripheral neurovascular dysfunction.*

- Take steps to ease patient's anxiety. *Stress may lead to vasoconstriction.*
- Administer and monitor the effectiveness of vasodilators, as ordered, *to control vasospasm.*
- If patient requires a fasciotomy to restore circulation, provide educational material that explains this emergency procedure *to reduce patient anxiety.*
- PCC Instruct patient and family members in proper positioning when lying in bed and when sitting and in methods of obtaining pressure relief *to avoid pooling of blood and pressure ulcers.*
- If appropriate, discuss the cause of the injury and safety precautions *to avoid further injury.* Injuries to upper extremities usually result from industrial accidents; injuries to lower extremities, from automobile accidents.
- PCC Instruct patient and family members in recognizing the symptoms of peripheral neurovascular dysfunction, including numbness, pain, and tingling. Emphasize the need to report these symptoms to a physician *to prevent onset of neurovascular damage after discharge.*

Suggested NIC Interventions

Circulatory Precautions; Exercise Promotion: Strength Training; Exercise Therapy: Joint Mobility; Peripheral Sensation Management; Positioning: Neurologic; Pressure Ulcer Prevention; Skin Surveillance; Splinting

Evaluations for Expected Outcomes

- Patient doesn't experience disability related to peripheral neurovascular dysfunction.
- Patient maintains circulation in extremities.
- Patient demonstrates ability to move each toe or finger after application of cast, brace, or splint.
- Patient demonstrates correct body positioning techniques.
- Patient and family members express understanding of risk of altered neurovascular status.
- Patient enrolls in smoking-cessation program, as appropriate.
- Patient shows no symptoms of neurovascular compromise.

Documentation

- Results of neurovascular assessment (baseline and ongoing)
- Nature of injury or treatment
- History of illnesses and surgeries
- Symptoms of neurovascular dysfunction reported by patient and family members
- Patient's turning schedule
- Instructions provided to patient and family members at discharge
- Evaluations for expected outcomes

REFERENCES

Cam, R., & Korkmaz, F. D. (2014). The effect of long-term care and follow-up on complications in patients with external fixators. *International Journal of Nursing Practice, 20*(1), 89–96. doi:10.1111/ijn.12126

McKee, J., Wade, C., & McCarron, M. O. (2015). A quality improvement program with a specialist nurse in a neurovascular clinic. *Journal of Clinical Nursing, 24*(3/4), 386–392. doi:10.1111/jocn.12609

Schreiber, M. L. (2016). Evidence-based practice. Neurovascular assessment: An essential nursing focus. *MEDSURG Nursing, 25*(1), 55–57.

RISK FOR ELECTROLYTE IMBALANCE

Definition

Vulnerable to changes in serum electrolyte levels, which may compromise health

Assessment

- Fluid and electrolyte status, weight, intake and output, urine specific gravity, skin turgor, mucous membranes
- Results of laboratory tests including serum electrolytes, blood urea nitrogen
- Vital signs including heart rate and rhythm, blood pressure, pulse
- History of renal, cardiac, and gastrointestinal disorders

Risk Factors

- Compromised regulatory mechanism
- Diarrhea
- Endocrine regulatory dysfunction (e.g., glucose intolerance, increase in IGF-1, androgen, DHEA, and cortisol)
- Excessive fluid volume
- Insufficient fluid volume
- Renal dysfunction
- Vomiting
- Treatment regimen

Expected Outcomes

- Patient will maintain electrolyte levels within normal limits.
- Patient will maintain adequate fluid balance consistent with underlying disease restrictions.
- Patient will identify health situations that increase risk for electrolyte imbalance and verbalize interventions to promote balance.
- Patient will verbalize signs and symptoms that require immediate intervention by health care provider.
- Patient will remain safe from injury associated with electrolyte imbalance.

Suggested NOC Outcomes

Electrolyte & Acid–Base Balance; Fluid Balance

Interventions and Rationales

- Assess patient's fluid status. *Patients who demonstrate fluid volume alterations are likely to have electrolyte alterations as well.*
- S Monitor patient for physical signs of electrolyte imbalance. *Many cardiac, neurologic, and musculoskeletal symptoms are indicative of specific electrolyte abnormalities.*
- Collect and evaluate serum electrolyte results as ordered *to allow for prompt diagnosis and treatment of any abnormalities.*

- PCC Educate patient and family regarding risks for electrolyte disturbances associated with their particular medical condition and possible interventions if symptoms occur. *Early identification and intervention may prevent life-threatening complications of electrolyte imbalance.*
- PCC Provide support and encouragement to patient and family in their efforts to participate in the management of the condition. *Positive feedback will increase self-confidence and feeling of partnership in care.*
- PCC Coordinate care with other members of the health care team to provide safe environment. *Electrolyte imbalances can cause poor coordination, weakness, altered gait.*

Suggested NIC Interventions

Electrolyte Management; Electrolyte Monitoring; Fluid–Electrolyte Management; Laboratory Data Interpretation

Evaluations for Expected Outcomes

- Patient's electrolyte levels remain within normal limits.
- Patient's fluid balance is consistent with restrictions of underlying disease.
- Patient identifies health situations that increase the risk for electrolyte imbalance and interventions to promote balance.
- Patient verbalizes signs and symptoms that require immediate interventions by a health care provider.
- Patient remains safe from injury associated with electrolyte imbalance.

Documentation

- Record of patient's electrolyte results and interventions
- Record of patient's fluid status
- Patient's understanding of signs and symptoms that require intervention of a health care provider
- Evaluations for expected outcomes

REFERENCES

Crawford, A. H. (2014). Hyperkalemia: Recognition and management of a critical electrolyte disturbance. *Journal of Infusion Nursing*, *37*(3), 167–175. doi:10.1097/NAN.0000000000000036

Keane, M. (2014). Recognizing and managing acute hyponatremia. *Emergency Nurse*, *21*(9), 32–36.

Palmer, B. F., & Clegg, D. J. (2015). Electrolyte and acid–base disturbances in patients with diabetes mellitus. *New England Journal of Medicine*, *373*(6), 548–559. doi:10.1056/NEJMra1503102

INTERRUPTED FAMILY PROCESSES

related to power shift among family members

Definition

Change in family relationships and/or functioning

Assessment

- Family status, including normal patterns of interaction among family members, family members' and patient's understanding of present situation, and support systems available (financial, social, and spiritual)
- Family's past response to crises, including coping patterns and communication patterns to express anger, affection, and confrontation

Defining Characteristics

- Alteration in availability for affective responsiveness
- Alteration in family conflict resolution
- Alteration in family satisfaction
- Alteration in intimacy
- Alteration in participation for problem-solving
- Change in communication pattern
- Change in somatization
- Change in stress-reduction behavior
- Changes in expressions of conflict with community resources
- Changes in expressions of isolation from community resources
- Changes in participation for decision making
- Changes in available emotional support
- Decrease in mutual support
- Ineffective task completion
- Power alliance change
- Ritual change

Expected Outcomes

- Family members will agree on who's the primary decision maker.
- Family members will develop adaptive responses by assuming duties carried out by ill member; for example, meal preparation, transportation, shopping, laundry, cleaning, and providing emotional support to other family members.
- Family members will identify support systems to assist them and will participate in mobilizing those systems.
- Family members will contact a community agency or support group for continued assistance (depending on type, severity, and prognosis of illness); for example, American Cancer Society, American Lung Association, Arthritis Foundation, Hospice, Myasthenia Gravis Foundation, Multiple Sclerosis Society, or National Kidney Foundation.
- Family members will share feelings about illness.

Suggested NOC Outcomes

Coping; Decision-Making; Family Coping; Family Environment: Internal; Family Functioning; Family Normalization; Family Resiliency; Family Social Climate; Social Involvement

Interventions and Rationales

- Identify individual assuming role as head of family *to establish family hierarchy and functional ability.*
- PCC Provide head of family with information necessary for decision making, such as updated information on patient's condition. *This avoids potential for misinterpretation and places responsibility for communication within family unit.*
- PCC Help head of family decide which support systems need to be mobilized and used. *This allows opportunity to evaluate head of family's management ability and family's problem-solving ability.*

PCC
- Provide emotional support to head of family regarding altered role and additional responsibilities. *This encourages family member to express feelings, ask questions, seek help, and make decisions.*
- Expedite communication within family to allow members to express their feelings about present situation. *This encourages supportive behavior to meet reciprocal needs in a crisis.*
- Arrange with the family to spend as much time as possible with the patient to allow them to participate in providing care where it is appropriate. *This accommodation may fulfill both the patient's and the family's needs for participation.*
- Arrange for and participate in family conferences, if appropriate.

PCC
- Whenever possible, ensure privacy to family members for their discussions or conferences. *These measures allow you to help family identify and work toward mutual goals and facilitate effective family coping.*

PCC
- Make referrals to social services or community agencies, as appropriate, *to provide family with access to additional coping resources.*

PCC
- Include patient in family conferences and family interaction as often as possible.

Suggested NIC Interventions

Coping Enhancement; Counseling; Family Mobilization; Family Process Maintenance; Family Support; Family Therapy; Normalization Promotion; Spiritual Support; Support System Enhancement

Evaluations for Expected Outcomes

- Family members identify family member to be primary decision maker, serving as head of family.
- Family members assume responsibilities formerly carried out by ill member.
- Family members identify and contact available resources, as needed.
- Family members contact community support groups and associations and attend at least two meetings.
- Family members openly share feelings about present situation.

Documentation

- Observations of family's reactions to situation
- Interventions to assist family and family's responses to those interventions
- Referrals to outside agencies
- Evaluations for expected outcomes

REFERENCES

Chiao, C., Wu, H., & Hsiao, C. (2015). Caregiver burden for informal caregivers of patients with dementia: A systematic review. *International Nursing Review*, *62*(3), 340–350. doi:10.1111/inr.12194

Giovannetti, A. M., Černiauskait, M., Leonardi, M., Sattin, D., & Covelli, V. (2015). Informal caregivers of patients with disorders of consciousness: Experience of ambiguous loss. *Brain Injury*, *29*(4), 473–480. doi:10.3109/02699052.2014.990514

Kreyer, C. (2014). 'Struggling for normal in an instable situation'—informal caregivers' self-management in palliative home care. A meta-synthesis. *Pflege*, *27*(5), 307–324. doi:10.1024/1012-5302/a000378

FATIGUE

related to physical deconditioning

Definition

An overwhelming sustained sense of exhaustion and decreased capacity for physical and mental work at the usual level

Assessment

- History of underlying disease process
- Respiratory status, including dyspnea on exertion and respiratory rate and depth
- Cardiovascular status, including skin color, temperature, turgor, and blood pressure
- Age
- Sleep pattern, including hours slept at night and amount of time awake before becoming tired
- Nutritional status, including appetite, dietary intake, current weight, and change from normal weight
- Neurologic status, including headaches
- Activity status, including type and duration of exercise, occupation, and use of leisure time
- Psychosocial status, including personality stressors (finances, job, or marital discord), coping mechanisms, support systems (family members and others), and lifestyle
- Menstrual history, including length of menses and amount of menstrual flow

Defining Characteristics

- Alteration in concentration
- Alteration in libido
- Disinterest in surroundings
- Drowsiness
- Guilt about difficulty maintaining responsibilities
- Impaired ability to maintain usual physical activity
- Impaired ability to maintain usual routines
- Increase in physical symptoms
- Increase in rest requirement
- Ineffective role performance
- Insufficient energy
- Introspection
- Lethargy
- Listlessness
- Nonrestorative sleep pattern (i.e., due to caregiver responsibilities, parenting practices, sleep partner)
- Tiredness

Expected Outcomes

- Patient will identify measures to prevent or modify fatigue.
- Patient will incorporate as part of daily activities those measures necessary to modify fatigue.
- Patient will explain relationship of fatigue to disease process and activity level.
- Patient will verbally express increased energy.
- Patient will articulate plan to resolve fatigue problems.
- Patient will employ measures to prevent and modify fatigue.

Suggested NOC Outcomes

Activity Tolerance; Comfort Level; Endurance; Energy Conservation; Nutritional Status: Energy; Psychomotor Energy; Personal Health Status; Personal Well-Being

Interventions and Rationales

- Prevent unnecessary fatigue; for example, avoid scheduling two energy-draining procedures on same day. *Using energy-conserving techniques avoids overexertion and potential for exhaustion.*
- Conserve energy through rest, planning, and setting priorities *to prevent or alleviate fatigue.*
- Alternate activities with periods of rest. Encourage activities that can be completed in short periods or divided into several segments; for example, read one chapter of a book at a time. *Scheduling regular rest periods helps decrease fatigue and increase stamina.*
- PCC Discuss effect of fatigue on daily living and personal goals. Explore with patient relationship between fatigue and disease process *to help increase patient compliance with schedule for activity and rest.*
- Reduce demands placed on patient; for example, ask one family member to call at specified times and relay messages to friends and other family members *to reduce physical and emotional stress.*
- Structure patient's environment; for example, set up daily schedule based on patient's needs and desires. *This encourages compliance with treatment regimen.*
- Encourage patient to eat foods rich in iron and minerals, unless contraindicated. *This helps avoid anemia and demineralization.*
- Postpone eating when patient is fatigued *to avoid aggravating condition.*
- Provide small, frequent feedings *to conserve patient's energy and encourage increased dietary intake.*
- Establish a regular sleeping pattern. *Getting 8 to 10 hours of sleep nightly helps reduce fatigue.*
- Encourage avoidance of highly emotional situations *to minimize their impact on fatigue.*
- PCC Encourage patient to explore feelings and emotions with a supportive counselor, clergy member, or other professional *to help cope with illness.*

Suggested NIC Interventions

Activity Therapy; Coping Enhancement; Energy Management; Exercise Promotion; Nutrition Management; Mood Management; Mutual Goal Setting; Sleep Enhancement

Evaluations for Expected Outcomes

- Patient describes at least three measures to prevent or modify fatigue.
- Patient incorporates at least three measures to modify fatigue into daily routine.
- Patient discusses relationship of fatigue to disease process and activity level; for example, in heart disease, fatigue is a sign that the heart cannot meet increased oxygen demands.
- Patient reports reduced fatigue level.
- Patient describes plan to resolve fatigue problems, including both physiologic and emotional remedies.
- Patient follows measures to prevent and modify fatigue.

Documentation

- Patient's ability to describe fatigue and its relationship to disease process and condition
- Patient's ability to decrease fatigue by using various effective methods
- Patient's level of activity in relation to fatigue
- Patient's dietary intake
- Evaluations for expected outcomes

REFERENCES

Caruso, C. C. (2014). Negative impacts of shiftwork and long work hours. *Rehabilitation Nursing, 39*(1), 16–25. doi:10.1002/rnj.107

Kieft, L., & Woodward, S. (2014). Early recognition of fatigue in Parkinson's disease. *British Journal of Neuroscience Nursing, 10*(6), 281–286.

Zhu, L., Ranchor, A. V., van der Lee, M., Garssen, B., Sanderman, R., & Schroevers, M. J. (2015). The role of goal adjustment in symptoms of depression, anxiety, and fatigue in cancer patients receiving psychosocial care: A longitudinal study. *Psychology & Health, 30*(3), 268–283. doi:10.1080/08870446.2014.969263

FEAR

related to separation from support system

Definition

Response to perceived threat that is consciously recognized as a danger

Assessment

- History of experience with illness, hospitalization, and surgery
- Availability of support systems, including family members, friends, and clergy
- Financial resources
- History of coping with fear
- Physiologic manifestations of fear, including changes in pulse rate, respiratory rate, blood pressure, skin temperature, and quality and pitch of voice
- Psychological manifestations of fear, including changes in behavior, appetite, and sleep pattern

Defining Characteristics

- Apprehensiveness
- Decrease in self-assurance
- Excitedness
- Feeling dread
- Feeling of fear
- Feeling of panic
- Feeling of terror
- Feeling of alarm
- Increase in blood pressure
- Increase in tension
- Jitteriness
- Muscle tension
- Nausea
- Pallor
- Pupil dilation
- Vomiting

Cognitive

- Decrease in learning ability
- Decrease in problem-solving ability
- Decrease in productivity
- Identifies object of fear
- Stimulus believed to be a threat

Behaviors

- Attack behaviors
- Avoidance behaviors
- Focus narrowed to the source of fear
- Impulsiveness
- Increase in alertness

Physiologic

- Anorexia
- Change in physiologic response (e.g., blood pressure, heart rate, respiratory rate, oxygen saturation, and end-title CO_2)
- Diarrhea
- Dry mouth
- Dyspnea
- Fatigue
- Increase in perspiration
- Increase in respiratory rate

Expected Outcomes

- Patient will identify source of fear.
- Patient will communicate feelings about separation from support systems.
- Patient will communicate feelings of comfort or satisfaction.
- Patient will use situational supports to reduce fear.
- Patient will integrate into daily behavior at least one fear-reducing coping mechanism, such as asking questions about treatment progress or making decisions about care.

Suggested NOC Outcomes

Anxiety Control; Comfort Level; Coping; Fear Self-Control

Interventions and Rationales

- PCC Ask patient to identify source of fear; try to assess patient's understanding of situation. *Patient's perceptions may be erroneously based.*
- PCC Explain all treatments and procedures, answering any questions patient might have. Present information at patient's level of understanding or acceptance *to reduce patient's anxiety and enhance cooperation.*
- S Orient patient to surroundings. Make any adaptations to compensate for sensory deficits. *This enhances patient's ability to orient to time, place, person, and events.*
- Assign same nurse to care for patient whenever possible *to provide consistency of care, enhance trust, and reduce threat commonly associated with multiple caregivers.*
- Spend time with patient each shift *to allow time for expression of feelings, provide emotional outlet, and promote feeling of acceptance.*
- If patient has no visitors, spend an extra 15 minutes each shift in casual conversation; encourage other staff members to stop for brief visits *to help patient cope with separation.*
- Remain with the patient when he is experiencing a higher than usual level of fear *to provide a source of support.*
- PCC Encourage patient to identify source of fear. *Patient's perceptions may be erroneously based.*
- Help patient maintain daily contact with family:
  - Arrange for telephone calls.
  - Help write letters.
  - Promptly convey messages to patient from family and vice versa.
  - Encourage patient to have pictures of loved ones.
  - Provide privacy for visits; take patient to day room or other quiet area.
  These measures help patient reestablish and maintain social relationships.

- PCC Involve patient in planning care and setting goals *to renew confidence and give sense of control in a crisis situation.*
- PCC Instruct patient in relaxation techniques, such as imagery and progressive muscle relaxation, *to reduce symptoms of sympathetic stimulation.*
- Administer antianxiety medications, as ordered, and monitor effectiveness. *Drug therapy may be needed to manage high anxiety levels or panic disorders.*
- PCC Answer questions and help patient understand care *to reduce anxiety and correct misconceptions.*
- When feasible and where policies permit, relax visiting restrictions *to reduce patient's sense of isolation.*
- PCC Allow a close family member or friend to participate in care *to provide an additional source of support.*
- PCC Support family and friends in their efforts to understand patient's fear and to respond accordingly *to help them understand that patient's emotions are appropriate in context of situation.*

Suggested NIC Interventions

Active Listening; Anxiety Reduction; Cognitive Restructuring; Counseling; Coping Enhancement; Decision-Making Support; Security Enhancement; Presence; Support Group

Evaluations for Expected Outcomes

- Patient states causes of fear.
- Patient expresses distress caused by separation from support systems.
- Patient reports feeling less fearful.
- Patient reaches out to others for support through phone calls, letters, or other means.
- Patient demonstrates use of at least one coping mechanism daily to reduce fear.

Documentation

- Patient's expressions of concern about illness, hospitalization, and separation from support system, and overt expressions of fear
- Observations of physiologic and behavioral manifestations of patient's fear
- Interventions performed to allay patient's fears and encourage healthy coping mechanisms
- Patient's response to interventions
- Evaluations for expected outcomes

REFERENCES

Penman, J., & Ellis, B. (2015). Palliative care clients' and caregivers' notion of fear and their strategies for overcoming it. *Palliative & Supportive Care*, *13*(3), 777–785. doi:10.1017/S1478951514000571

Stenzel, N. M., Vaske, I., Kühl, K., Kenn, K., & Rief, W. (2015). Prediction of end-of-life fears in COPD—Hoping for the best but preparing for the worst. *Psychology & Health*, *30*(9), 1017–1034. doi:10.1080/08870446.2015.1014816

Trueland, J. (2015). When fear becomes the barrier to care. *Nursing Standard*, *30*(2), 18–20. doi:10.7748/ns.30.2.18.s21

DEFICIENT FLUID VOLUME

related to active fluid volume loss

Definition

Decreased intravascular, interstitial, and/or intracellular fluid. This refers to dehydration, water loss alone without change in sodium

Assessment

- History of fluid loss, including vomiting, nasogastric tube drainage, diarrhea, or hemorrhage
- Pulse, blood pressure, respirations, and temperature
- Fluid and electrolyte status, including weight, intake and output, urine specific gravity, skin turgor, and mucous membranes
- Laboratory studies, including serum electrolyte, blood urea nitrogen, hemoglobin levels, hematocrit (HCT), and stool cultures

Defining Characteristics

- Alteration in mental status
- Alteration in skin turgor
- Decrease in blood pressure
- Decrease in pulse pressure
- Decrease in pulse volume
- Decrease in tongue turgor
- Decrease in urine output
- Decrease in venous filling
- Dry mucous membranes
- Dry skin
- Increase in body temperature
- Increase in heart rate
- Increase in HCT
- Increase in urine concentration
- Sudden weight loss
- Thirst
- Weakness

Expected Outcomes

- Patient's vital signs will remain stable.
- Patient's skin color will be normal.
- Patient's electrolyte levels will stay within normal range.
- Patient's fluid volume will remain adequate.
- Patient will produce adequate urine volume.
- Patient will have normal skin turgor and moist mucous membranes.
- Patient's urine specific gravity will remain between 1.005 and 1.010.
- Patient's fluid and blood volume will return to normal.
- Patient will express understanding of factors that caused fluid volume deficit.

Suggested NOC Outcomes

Electrolyte & Acid–Base Balance; Fluid Balance; Hydration; Urinary Elimination; Kidney Function; Thermoregulation; Vital Signs

Interventions and Rationales

- S Monitor and record vital signs every 2 hours or as often as necessary until stable. Then monitor and record vital signs every 4 hours. *Tachycardia, dyspnea, or hypotension may indicate fluid volume deficit or electrolyte imbalance.*
- Cover patient lightly. Avoid overheating *to prevent vasodilation, blood pooling in extremities, and reduced circulating blood volume.*
- Measure intake and output every 1 to 4 hours. Record and report significant changes. Include urine, stools, vomitus, wound drainage, nasogastric drainage, chest tube drainage, and any other output. *Low urine output and high specific gravity indicate hypovolemia.*
- Administer fluids, blood or blood products, or plasma expanders as ordered *to replace fluids and whole blood loss and facilitate fluid movement into intravascular space.* Monitor and record effectiveness and any adverse effects.
- Weigh patient daily at same time to give more accurate and consistent data. *Weight is a good indicator of fluid status.*
- Assess skin turgor and oral mucous membranes every 8 hours *to check for dehydration.* Give meticulous mouth care every 4 hours *to avoid dehydrating mucous membranes.*
- Test urine specific gravity every 8 hours. *Elevated specific gravity may indicate dehydration.*
- S Don't allow patient to sit or stand up quickly as long as circulation is compromised *to avoid orthostatic hypotension and possible syncope.*
- Measure abdominal girth every 12 hours *to monitor for ascites and third-space shift.* Report changes.
- Administer and monitor medications *to prevent further fluid loss.*
- PCC Explain reasons for fluid loss, and teach patient how to monitor fluid volume; for example, by recording daily weight and measuring intake and output. *This encourages patient involvement in personal care.*

Suggested NIC Interventions

Acid–Base Management; Electrolyte Monitoring; Fluid Management; Hypovolemia Management; Nutrition Management; Swallowing Therapy; Vital Signs Monitoring

Evaluations for Expected Outcomes

- Patient's pulse rate, blood pressure, respirations, and body temperature remain within set limits.
- Patient's skin color remains normal.
- Patient's electrolyte values remain within normal range.
- Patient's fluid volume remains adequate.
- Patient's urine output remains at volume established for patient.
- Patient's skin turgor and mucous membranes remain normal.
- Patient's specific gravity remains between 1.005 and 1.010, unless specified otherwise.
- Patient's fluid volume returns to normal and remains normal, as evidenced by stable vital signs.
- Patient and caregiver demonstrate understanding of factors precipitating fluid volume deficit.

Documentation

- Patient's complaints of thirst, weakness, dizziness, and palpitations
- Observations of physical findings
- Intake and output (amount and type)

- Patient's weight and abdominal girth
- Interventions performed to control fluid loss
- Patient's response to interventions
- Evaluations for expected outcomes

REFERENCES

Bunn, D., Jimoh, F., Wilsher, S. H., & Hooper, L. (2015). Increasing fluid intake and reducing dehydration risk in older people living in long-term care: A systematic review. *Journal of the American Medical Directors Association*, *16*(2), 101–113. doi:10.1016/j.jamda.2014.10.016

McGloin, S. (2015). The ins and outs of fluid balance in the acutely ill patient. *British Journal of Nursing*, *24*(1), 14–18. doi:10.12968/bjon.2015.24.1.14

McLafferty, E., Johnstone, C., Hendry, C., & Farley, A. (2014). Fluid and electrolyte balance. *Nursing Standard*, *28*(29), 42–49. doi:10.7748/ns2014.03.28.29.42.e5531

RISK FOR DEFICIENT FLUID VOLUME

Definition

Vulnerable to experiencing decreased intravascular, interstitial, and/or intracellular fluid volumes, which may compromise health

Assessment

- History of problems that can cause fluid loss, such as vomiting, diarrhea, indwelling tubes, and hemorrhage
- Pulse, blood pressure, respirations, and temperature
- Fluid and electrolyte status, including weight, intake and output, urine specific gravity, skin turgor, and mucous membranes
- Laboratory studies, including serum electrolyte, blood urea nitrogen, and hemoglobin (Hb) levels and hematocrit (HCT)

Risk Factors

- Active fluid volume loss
- Barrier to accessing fluid
- Compromised regulatory mechanism
- Deviations affecting fluid absorption
- Deviations affecting fluid intake
- Excessive fluid loss through normal route
- Extremes of age
- Extremes of weight
- Factors influencing fluid needs
- Fluid loss through abnormal route
- Insufficient knowledge about fluid needs
- Pharmaceutical agent

Expected Outcomes

- Patient's vital signs will remain stable.
- Patient's skin color will remain normal.
- Patient will maintain urine output of at least ____ mL/hour.

- Patient's electrolyte values will remain within normal range.
- Patient will maintain intake at ____ mL/24 hours.
- Patient's intake will equal or exceed output.
- Patient will express understanding of need to maintain adequate fluid intake.
- Patient will demonstrate skill in weighing himself accurately and recording weight.
- Patient will measure and record own intake and output.
- Patient will return to normal, appropriate diet.

Suggested NOC Outcomes

Electrolyte & Acid–Base Balance; Fluid Balance; Hydration; Nausea & Vomiting Severity; Nutritional Status: Food & Fluid Intake; Risk Detection; Self-Care Status; Swallowing Status; Urinary Elimination

Interventions and Rationales

- Monitor and record vital signs every 4 hours. *Fever, tachycardia, dyspnea, or hypotension may indicate hypovolemia.*
- Maintain accurate record of intake and output *to aid estimation of patient's fluid balance.*
- Measure urine output every hour. Record and report an output of less than ____ mL/hour. *Decreased urine output may indicate reduced fluid volume.*
- Measure and record drainage from all tubes and catheters *to take such losses into account when replacing fluid.*
- When copious drainage appears on dressings, weigh dressings every 8 hours, and record with other output sources. *Excessive wound drainage causes significant fluid imbalances (1 kg dressing equals about 1 L of fluid).*
- Test urine specific gravity each shift. Monitor laboratory values, and report abnormal findings to physician. *Increased urine specific gravity may indicate dehydration. Elevated HCT and Hb level also indicate dehydration.*
- Monitor serum electrolyte levels and report abnormalities. *Fluid loss may cause significant electrolyte imbalance.*
- Obtain and record patient's weight at same time every day to help ensure accurate data. *Daily weighing helps estimate body fluid status.*
- Monitor skin turgor each shift to check for dehydration; report any decrease in turgor. *Poor skin turgor is a sign of dehydration.*
- Examine oral mucous membranes each shift. *Dry mucous membranes are a sign of dehydration.*
- Cover wounds *to minimize fluid loss and prevent skin excoriation.*
- Determine patient's fluid preferences *to enhance intake.*
- Keep oral fluids at bedside within patient's reach, and encourage patient to drink. *This gives patient some control over fluid intake and supplements parenteral fluid intake.*
- PCC Instruct patient in maintaining appropriate fluid intake, including recording daily weight, measuring intake and output, and recognizing signs of dehydration. *This encourages patient and caregiver participation and enhances patient's sense of control.*
- Force oral fluids when possible and indicated *to enhance replacement of lost fluids.* (Bowel sounds should be present and patient awake before giving oral fluids.)
- Administer parenteral fluids, as prescribed, *to replace fluid losses.* Maintain parenteral fluids or blood transfusions at prescribed rate *to prevent further fluid loss or overload.*
- Progress patient to appropriate diet, as prescribed, *to help achieve fluid and electrolyte balance.*

Suggested NIC Interventions

Acid–Base Management; Fluid Management; Fluid Monitoring; Hypovolemia Management; Nutrition Management; Intravenous (IV) Therapy; Hypovolemia Monitoring; Surveillance

Evaluations for Expected Outcomes

- Patient's temperature, pulse rate, blood pressure, and respirations are within set limits (specify).
- Patient's skin color remains normal.
- Patient's urine output remains at specified volume.
- Patient's electrolyte values remain normal.
- Patient's daily fluid intake remains within established limits (specify).
- Patient's cumulative intake equals or exceeds cumulative output.
- Patient demonstrates understanding of importance of maintaining fluid balance.
- Patient weighs himself with same scale at same time each day and records results.
- Patient measures fluid intake and output; records are reviewed to ensure accuracy.
- Patient returns to normal, appropriate diet.

Documentation

- Observations of physical findings
- Intake and output
- Drainage from indwelling tubes and catheters, including amount, color, and consistency
- Amount, color, and odor of drainage on dressings
- Patient teaching about fluid intake and diet
- Patient's response to interventions
- Evaluations for expected outcomes

REFERENCES

Bunn, D., Jimoh, F., Wilsher, S. H., & Hooper, L. (2015). Increasing fluid intake and reducing dehydration risk in older people living in long-term care: A systematic review. *Journal of the American Medical Directors Association*, *16*(2), 101–113. doi:10.1016/j.jamda.2014.10.016

McGloin, S. (2015). The ins and outs of fluid balance in the acutely ill patient. *British Journal of Nursing*, *24*(1), 14–18. doi:10.12968/bjon.2015.24.1.14

McLafferty, E., Johnstone, C., Hendry, C., & Farley, A. (2014). Fluid and electrolyte balance. *Nursing Standard*, *28*(29), 42–49. doi:10.7748/ns2014.03.28.29.42.e5531

EXCESS FLUID VOLUME

related to compromised regulatory mechanism; excessive fluid intake; excessive sodium intake

Definition

Increased isotonic fluid retention

Assessment

- Neurologic status, including level of consciousness, orientation, and mental status
- Cardiovascular status, including skin color, temperature, and turgor; jugular venous pressure; central venous pressure and pulmonary artery pressure (if available); heart rate and

rhythm; blood pressure; heart sounds, electrocardiogram (ECG) results; and hemoglobin (Hb) level and hematocrit (HCT)
- Respiratory status, including rate, depth, and pattern of respiration; breath sounds; chest X-ray; and arterial blood gas levels
- Renal status, including intake and output, urine specific gravity, weight, serum electrolyte and serum and urine osmolality levels, and blood urea nitrogen (BUN), urine and serum creatinine, and serum protein levels
- Endocrine status, including general appearance, size and body proportions, skin color and condition, and distribution of body hair

Defining Characteristics

- Adventitious breath sounds
- Alteration in blood pressure
- Alteration in mental status
- Alteration in pulmonary artery pressure (PAP)
- Alteration in respiratory pattern
- Alteration in urine specific gravity
- Anasarca
- Anxiety
- Azotemia
- Decrease in HCT
- Decrease in Hb dyspnea
- Edema
- Electrolyte imbalance
- Hepatomegaly
- Increase in central venous pressure (CVP)
- Intake exceeds output
- Jugular vein distention
- Oliguria
- Orthopnea
- Paroxysmal nocturnal dyspnea
- Pleural effusion
- Positive hepatojugular reflex
- Pulmonary congestion
- Restlessness
- Presence of S_3 heart sound
- Weight gain over short period of time

Expected Outcomes

- Patient's blood pressure and vital signs will be within normal limits.
- Patient will demonstrate no signs of hyperkalemia on ECG.
- Patient's urine specific gravity will remain within normal limits.
- Patient's HCT will be within normal limits.
- Patient's BUN, creatinine, sodium, and potassium levels will stay within acceptable range.
- Patient will plan 24-hour fluid intake, as prescribed.
- Patient will tolerate restricted intake with no physical or emotional discomfort.
- Patient will assist with activities of daily living without undue fatigue.
- Patient will demonstrate skill in selecting permitted foods, such as those low in sodium and potassium.

- Patient will describe signs and symptoms that require medical treatment.
- Patient will return to baseline weight.
- Patient will have unlabored respirations.
- Patient will have elastic skin turgor.

Suggested NOC Outcomes

Electrolyte & Acid–Base Balance; Fluid Balance; Fluid Overload Severity; Hydration; Kidney Function; Knowledge: Disease Process; Knowledge: Treatment Regimen; Nutritional Status: Food & Fluid Intake; Urinary Elimination; Vital Signs; Weight: Body Mass

Interventions and Rationales

- S Monitor blood pressure, pulse rate, heart rhythm, temperature, and breath sounds at least every 4 hours; record and report changes. *Changed parameters may indicate altered fluid or electrolyte status.*
- S Carefully monitor intake, output, and urine specific gravity at least every 4 hours. *Intake greater than output and change in specific gravity may indicate fluid retention or overload.*
- S Monitor BUN, creatinine, electrolyte, and Hb levels and HCT. *BUN and creatinine levels indicate renal function; electrolyte and Hb levels and HCT help indicate fluid status.*
- Administer diuretics *to promote fluid excretion.* Record effects.
- Assess patient daily for edema, including ascites and dependent or sacral edema. *Fluid overload or decreased osmotic pressure may result in edema, especially in dependent areas.*
- Weigh patient daily before breakfast, as ordered, *to provide consistent readings.* Check for signs of fluid retention, such as dependent edema, sacral edema, and ascites.
- Give fluids, as ordered. Monitor IV flow rate carefully *because excess IV fluids can worsen patient's condition.*
- If oral fluids are allowed, help patient make a schedule for fluid intake. *Patient involvement encourages compliance.*
- PCC Explain reasons for fluid and dietary restrictions *to enhance patient's understanding and compliance.*
- PCC Learn patient's food preferences, and plan accordingly within prescribed dietary restrictions *to enhance compliance.*
- Provide mouth care every 4 hours. Keep mucous membranes moist with water-soluble lubricant *to prevent them from dehydrating.*
- Provide sour hard candy *to decrease thirst and improve taste.*
- Support patient with positive feedback about adherence to restrictions *to encourage compliance.*
- Give skin care every 4 hours. Change patient's position at least every 2 hours. Elevate edematous extremities. *These measures enhance venous return, reduce edema, and prevent skin breakdown.*
- Alternate periods of rest and activity *to avoid worsening fatigue caused by electrolyte imbalance.*
- Increase patient's activity level, as tolerated; for example, ambulate and increase self-care measures performed by patient. *Gradually increasing activity helps body adjust to increased tissue oxygen demand and possible increased venous return.*
- Help patient into a position that aids breathing, such as Fowler's or semi-Fowler's, *to increase chest expansion and improve ventilation.*
- Administer oxygen, as ordered, *to enhance arterial blood oxygenation.*

- Apply antiembolism stockings or intermittent pneumatic compression stockings *to increase venous return.* Remove for 1 hour, and inspect skin every 8 hours or according to facility policy.
- Assess skin turgor *to monitor for edema.*
- Measure abdominal girth every shift, and report changes *to monitor for ascites.*
- Have dietitian see patient *to teach or reinforce dietary restrictions.*
- PCC Educate patient regarding
  - environmental safety measures
  - fluid restriction and diet
  - signs and symptoms requiring immediate medical treatment
  - medications (name, dosage, frequency, therapeutic effects, and adverse effects)
  - activity level
  - ways to prevent infection.

  These measures encourage patient and family members to participate more fully in care.

Suggested NIC Interventions

Acid–Base Management; Electrolyte Management; Fluid Management; Fluid Monitoring; Medication Management; Nutrition Management; Urinary Elimination Management; Vital Signs Monitoring; Weight Management

Evaluations for Expected Outcomes

- Patient's vital signs remain within established limits.
- Patient indicates, verbally and through behavior, ability to breathe comfortably.
- Signs of hyperkalemia (peaked or elevated T waves, prolonged PR intervals, widened QRS complexes, or depressed ST segments) don't appear on ECG.
- Patient's fluid intake and output remain within established limits.
- Patient's urine specific gravity remains within established limits.
- Patient's HCT remains above specified level.
- Patient's electrolyte levels remain within established limits.
- Patient plans 24-hour fluid intake.
- Patient doesn't indicate discomfort with restricted fluid intake, either verbally or through behavior.
- Patient plans own menu and selects foods low in sodium and potassium. Patient follows other dietary restrictions (specify).
- Patient expresses understanding of health problem.
- Patient demonstrates skill in health-related behaviors, such as maintaining weight and monitoring intake and output.
- Patient and caregiver list signs and symptoms that require medical attention.

Documentation

- Expression of patient's needs, desires, or perceptions of situation
- Specific changes in patient's physical status
- Observations about patient's response to treatment
- Observations about how patient appears to be coping with fluid and dietary restrictions
- Condition of skin and mucous membranes
- Interventions performed to alleviate or resolve diagnosis
- Interventions to correct fluid volume excess

- Patient's demonstration of skills
- Evaluations for expected outcomes

REFERENCES

Azzolin, K., Mussi, C. M., Ruschel, K. B., de Souza, E. N., de Fátima Lucena, A., & Rabelo-Silva, E. R. (2013). Effectiveness of nursing interventions in heart failure patients in home care using NANDA-I, NIC, and NOC. *Applied Nursing Research*, *26*(4), 239–244. doi:10.1016/j.apnr.2013.08.003

McGloin, S. (2015). The ins and outs of fluid balance in the acutely ill patient. *British Journal of Nursing*, *24*(1), 14–18. doi:10.12968/bjon.2015.24.1.14

Souza, V., Salloum Zeitoun, S., Takao Lopes, C., Dias de Oliveira, A. P., Lima Lopes, J., & Bottura Leite de Barros, A. L. (2015). Clinical usefulness of the definitions for defining characteristics of activity intolerance, excess fluid volume, and decreased cardiac output in decompensated heart failure: A descriptive exploratory study. *Journal of Clinical Nursing*, *24*(17/18), 2478–2487. doi:10.1111/jocn.12832

RISK FOR IMBALANCED FLUID VOLUME

Definition

Vulnerable to a decrease, increase, or rapid shift from one to the other of intravascular, interstitial, and/or intracellular fluid, which may compromise health. This refers to body fluid loss, gain, or both

Assessment

- Cardiovascular status including heart rate and rhythm, blood pressure, peripheral pulses
- Fluid and electrolyte status, weight, intake and output, urine specific gravity, skin turgor, mucous membranes, jugular vein distention
- Results of laboratory studies including serum electrolytes, blood urea nitrogen, hemoglobin, hematocrit
- History of cardiovascular, renal, gastrointestinal dysfunction

Risk Factors

- Apheresis
- Ascites
- Burns
- Intestinal obstruction
- Pancreatitis
- Sepsis
- Trauma
- Treatment regimen

Expected Outcomes

- Patient will remain hemodynamically stable.
- Patient will not experience electrolyte imbalance.
- Patient will maintain adequate urine output.
- Patient will identify risk factors contributing to possible imbalanced fluid volume.

Suggested NOC Outcomes

Client Satisfaction: Fluid Balance; Hydration; Vital Signs

Interventions and Rationales

- Assess for conditions that may contribute to imbalanced fluid volume. *Prompt treatment of underlying cause may prevent serious complications of fluid imbalance.*
- S Monitor vital signs and other assessment parameters frequently. *Changes in heart rate and rhythm, blood pressure, and breath sounds may indicate altered fluid status.*
- Collect and evaluate urine output frequently. Measure urine specific gravity as indicated. *Decreased urine volume and elevated urine specific gravity indicate hypovolemia.*
- Collect and evaluate serum electrolyte levels. *Fluid alterations may affect electrolyte levels.*
- Administer intravenous fluids as indicated. *Proactive fluid management may prevent serious imbalances.*
- PCC Educate patient and family regarding fluid restrictions or need for increased fluids, depending on the underlying condition. *Knowledge will enhance feeling of participation and sense of control.*
- PCC Provide encouragement and support for cooperation with prescribed treatment regimen. *Positive reinforcement will promote compliance.*
- PCC Coordinate care with other members of the health care team *to effectively manage underlying medical condition and prevent any alteration in fluid balance.*

Suggested NIC Interventions

Fluid Management; Fluid Monitoring; Intravenous (IV) Therapy

Evaluations for Expected Outcomes

- Patient remains hemodynamically stable.
- Electrolytes remain within acceptable limits.
- Patient has no electrolyte imbalances as a result of altered fluid status.
- Patient has adequate urine output.
- Patient states risk factors contributing to altered fluid status.

Documentation

- Patient's intake and output measurements
- Patient's vital signs and physical assessment findings
- Relevant lab results
- Patient's understanding of behaviors that promote fluid balance
- Evaluations for expected outcomes

REFERENCES

Elofson, K. A., Eiferman, D. S., Porter, K., & Murphy, C. V. (2015). Impact of late fluid balance on clinical outcomes in the critically ill surgical and trauma population. *Journal of Critical Care*, *30*(6), 1338–1343. doi:10.1016/j.jcrc.2015.07.009

McGloin, S. (2015). The ins and outs of fluid balance in the acutely ill patient. *British Journal of Nursing*, *24*(1), 14–18. doi:10.12968/bjon.2015.24.1.14

McLafferty, E., Johnstone, C., Hendry, C., & Farley, A. (2014). Fluid and electrolyte balance. *Nursing Standard*, *28*(29), 42–49. doi:10.7748/ns2014.03.28.29.42.e5531

IMPAIRED GAS EXCHANGE

related to alveolar–capillary membrane changes

Definition

Excess or deficit in oxygenation and/or carbon dioxide elimination at the alveolar–capillary membrane

Assessment

- Neurologic status, including level of consciousness, orientation, and mental status
- Respiratory status, including respiratory rate and depth, symmetry of chest expansion, use of accessory muscles, cough, sputum, palpation for fremitus, percussion of lung fields, auscultation of breath sounds, arterial blood gas (ABG) levels, and pulmonary function studies
- Cardiovascular status, including skin color and temperature, heart rate and rhythm, blood pressure, and complete blood count
- Activity status, including such functional capabilities as range of motion and muscle strength, activities of daily living (ADLs), and occupation

Defining Characteristics

- Abnormal ABGs
- Abnormal arterial pH
- Abnormal breathing pattern (e.g., rate, rhythm, depth)
- Abnormal skin color (e.g., pale, dusky, cyanosis)
- Confusion
- Cyanosis
- Decrease in carbon dioxide
- Diaphoresis
- Dyspnea
- Headache upon awakening
- Hypercapnia
- Hypoxemia
- Hypoxia
- Irritability
- Nasal flaring
- Restlessness
- Somnolence
- Tachycardia
- Vision disturbance

Expected Outcomes

- Patient will maintain respiratory rate within five breaths of predetermined baseline.
- Patient will express feelings of comfort in maintaining air exchange.
- Patient will cough effectively.
- Patient will expectorate sputum.
- Patient will sustain sufficient fluid intake to prevent dehydration: ___ mL/24 hours.
- Patient will perform ADLs to level of tolerance.
- Patient will have normal breath sounds.
- Patient's ABG levels will return to baselines: ___ pH; ____ partial pressure of arterial oxygen (Pa_{O_2}); ____ partial pressure of arterial carbon dioxide (Pa_{CO_2}).
- Patient will perform relaxation techniques every 4 hours.
- Patient will use correct bronchial hygiene.

Suggested NOC Outcomes

Cognition; Electrolyte & Acid–Base Balance; Respiratory Status: Gas Exchange; Respiratory Status: Ventilation; Tissue Perfusion: Pulmonary; Vital Signs

Interventions and Rationales

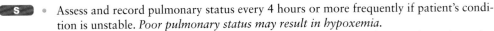

- S — Assess and record pulmonary status every 4 hours or more frequently if patient's condition is unstable. *Poor pulmonary status may result in hypoxemia.*
- S — Monitor vital signs and heart rhythm at least every 4 hours *to detect tachycardia and tachypnea, which could indicate hypoxemia.*
- Place patient in position that best facilitates chest expansion *to enhance gas exchange.*
- Change patient's position at least every 2 hours *to mobilize secretions and allow aeration of all lung fields.*
- Perform bronchial hygiene, as ordered, including coughing, percussion, postural drainage, and suctioning. *These measures promote drainage and keep airways clear.*
- Give medications, as ordered, *to improve oxygenation.* Monitor and record efficacy and adverse reactions *to guide treatment.*
- Monitor oxygen therapy, *which increases alveolar oxygen concentration and enhances arterial blood oxygenation.*
- Record intake and output *to monitor patient's fluid status.*
- S PCC — Report signs of dehydration or fluid overload immediately. *Dehydration may hinder tissue perfusion and secretion mobilization; fluid overload may cause pulmonary edema.*
- Assist patient with ADLs *to decrease tissue oxygen demand.*
- Include periods of rest in care plan *to reduce patient's tissue oxygen demand.*
- Monitor ABG levels, and notify physician immediately if Pao_2 or arterial oxygen saturation drops or $Paco_2$ rises. Administer endotracheal intubation and mechanical ventilation if needed. *This helps increase ventilation and gas exchange.*
- PCC — Teach patient relaxation techniques *to reduce tissue oxygen demand.*
- Have patient perform relaxation techniques every 4 hours *to establish routine and reduce oxygen demand.*

Suggested NIC Interventions

Airway Management; Airway Suctioning; Anxiety Reduction; Cough Enhancement; Energy Management; Mechanical Ventilation; Positioning

Evaluations for Expected Outcomes

- Patient's respiratory rate remains within established limits.
- Patient doesn't experience dyspnea.
- Patient demonstrates ability to cough and produce sputum.
- Patient expectorates sputum produced by coughing and deep breathing.
- Patient's fluid intake remains sufficient to prevent dehydration.
- Patient performs ADLs without exhibiting dyspnea or other signs of abnormal ABG levels.
- Patient has normal breath sounds.
- Patient's pH, Pao_2, and $Paco_2$ return to and remain within established limits.
- Patient performs relaxation techniques every 4 hours.
- Patient uses correct bronchial hygiene.

Documentation

- Patient's complaints of dyspnea, headache, and restlessness
- Patient's expression of well-being
- Observations of physical findings
- Effectiveness of medications
- Other treatments performed by nurse
- Evaluations for expected outcomes

REFERENCES

Casaburi, R., & Duvall, K. (2014). Improving early-stage diagnosis and management of COPD in primary care. *Postgraduate Medicine*, *126*(4), 141–154. doi:10.3810/pgm.2014.07.2792

Fratantoro, M. (2014). Reducing and preventing COPD readmissions. *RT: The Journal for Respiratory Care Practitioners*, *27*(5), 4.

Linden, A., & Butterworth, S. W. (2014). A comprehensive hospital-based intervention to reduce readmissions for chronically ill patients: A randomized controlled trial. *American Journal of Managed Care*, *20*(10), 783–792.

IMPAIRED GAS EXCHANGE

related to ventilation–perfusion imbalance

Definition

Excess or deficit in oxygenation and/or carbon dioxide elimination at the alveolar–capillary membrane

Assessment

- Neurologic status, including level of consciousness, orientation, and mental status
- Respiratory status, including respiratory rate and depth, symmetry of chest expansion, accessory muscle use, cough, sputum, palpation for fremitus, percussion of lung fields, auscultation of breath sounds, arterial blood gas (ABG) levels, and pulmonary function studies
- Cardiovascular status, including skin color and temperature, heart rate and rhythm, blood pressure, hemoglobin (Hb) level and hematocrit (HCT), red blood cell count, white blood cell count, platelet count, prothrombin time (PT), partial thromboplastin time (PTT), and serum iron level
- Activity status, including such functional capabilities as range of motion and muscle strength, activities of daily living (ADLs), and occupation

Defining Characteristics

- Abnormal ABGs
- Abnormal arterial pH
- Abnormal breathing pattern (e.g., rate, rhythm, depth)
- Abnormal skin color (e.g., pale, dusky, cyanosis)
- Confusion
- Cyanosis
- Decrease in carbon dioxide
- Diaphoresis
- Dyspnea
- Headache upon awakening
- Hypercapnia
- Hypoxemia
- Hypoxia
- Irritability

- Nasal flaring
- Restlessness
- Somnolence
- Tachycardia
- Vision disturbance

Expected Outcomes

- Patient will carry out ADLs without weakness or fatigue.
- Patient won't have signs of active bleeding.
- Patient's Hb level and HCT will return to normal (specify).
- Patient's clotting profile will remain within normal limits (specify).
- Patient will maintain adequate ventilation.
- Patient will communicate understanding of precautions needed to prevent bleeding.

Suggested NOC Outcomes

Cognition; Electrolyte & Acid–Base Balance; Respiratory Status: Gas Exchange; Respiratory Status: Ventilation; Tissue Perfusion: Pulmonary; Vital Signs

Interventions and Rationales

- Encourage patient to alternate periods of rest and activity. *Activity increases tissue oxygen demand; rest enhances tissue oxygen perfusion.*
- If patient is on bed rest, help him into a comfortable position and raise side rails *to prevent falls.*
- Have patient turn, cough, and deep breathe every 4 hours *to prevent atelectasis or fluid buildup in lungs and to enhance blood oxygen level.*
- Move patient slowly *to avoid orthostatic hypotension.*
- Assist patient when out of bed in case of dizziness. Avoid bumps and scratches *to avoid possible trauma and tissue bleeding.*
- Plan patient's activities within level of tolerance *to avoid fatigue.*
- Provide gentle oral hygiene *to avoid injuring oral mucosa.*
- Check all urine and stools for blood *to detect internal bleeding.* Check for evidence of bleeding at least once every 8 hours. *Hemorrhage or bleeding may cause anemia.*
- Administer blood or blood products, and monitor for adverse reactions *to restore fluid volume and prevent complications.*
- Consolidate laboratory work *to avoid multiple needle sticks and reduce chance of hematoma or hemorrhage in patients with altered clotting mechanisms.*
- Apply pressure for at least 1 minute after puncture *to promote clotting.*
- S Auscultate lungs every 4 hours and report abnormalities *to detect decreased or adventitious breath sounds.*
- S Monitor vital signs, heart rhythm, and ABG and Hb levels *to detect impaired gas exchange.* Report abnormalities.
- PCC Teach patient about safety at home and work, including:
  - use of soft toothbrush
  - use of an electric razor for shaving
  - careful use of sharp objects, such as knives, tweezers, and scissors
  - monitoring of urine, stools, and sputum for blood and reporting results immediately if blood is present
  - disadvantages and risks of smoking
  - using medications (name, dosage, therapeutic effect, adverse effects, and precautions).

  These measures encourage patient and caregivers to participate in care.

Suggested NIC Interventions

Acid–Base Management; Airway Management; Airway Suctioning; Anxiety Reduction; Chest Physiotherapy; Energy Management; Exercise Promotion; Fluid Management; Oxygen Therapy; Respiratory Monitoring

Evaluations for Expected Outcomes

- Patient carries out ADLs without fatigue or weakness.
- Patient doesn't exhibit signs of active bleeding, such as oozing from wounds or puncture site, bruising, petechiae, and occult blood in stools or urine.
- Patient's Hb level and HCT remain within established limits.
- Patient's clotting profile, including platelet count, PTT, PT, fibrinogen, and fibrin split products, remains within normal limits.
- Patient maintains adequate ventilation.
- Patient communicates understanding of precautions needed to prevent bleeding.

Documentation

- Patient's expression of personal feelings
- Observations about physical findings
- Results of laboratory studies that significantly affect nursing care
- Patient's response to interventions
- Evaluations for expected outcomes

REFERENCES

Ankjærgaard, K. L., Tønnesen, P., Laursen, L. C., Hansen, E. F., Andreassen, H. F., & Wilcke, J. T. (2016). Home noninvasive ventilation (NIV) treatment for COPD patients with a history of NIV-treated exacerbation; a randomized, controlled, multicenter study. *BMC Pulmonary Medicine*, 161–165. doi:10.1186/s12890-016-0184-6

Heydari, A., Farzad, M., & Ahmadi hosseini, S. (2015). Comparing inspiratory resistive muscle training with incentive spirometry on rehabilitation of COPD patients. *Rehabilitation Nursing*, *40*(4), 243–248. doi:10.1002/rnj.136

Linden, A., & Butterworth, S. W. (2014). A comprehensive hospital-based intervention to reduce readmissions for chronically ill patients: A randomized controlled trial. *American Journal of Managed Care*, *20*(10), 783–792.

DYSFUNCTIONAL GASTROINTESTINAL MOTILITY

Definition

Increased, decreased, ineffective, or lack of peristaltic activity within the gastrointestinal system

Defining Characteristics

- Abdominal cramping
- Abdominal distention
- Abdominal pain
- Absence of flatus
- Acceleration of gastric emptying
- Bile-colored gastric residual
- Change in bowel sounds
- Diarrhea
- Difficulty with defecation
- Hard, formed stool

- Increased gastric residual
- Nausea
- Regurgitation
- Vomiting

Assessment

- Health status, educational level, cultural status, requests for information; demonstrated understanding of material
- Fluid and electrolyte status, including blood urea nitrogen level, creatinine level, intake and output, mucous membranes, serum electrolyte levels, and skin turgor
- Nutritional status, including dietary patterns, laboratory tests, and serum protein level
- Neurologic status, including level of consciousness, mental status, motor function, and sensory pattern
- Gastrointestinal (GI) status, including nausea and vomiting, bowel habits, stool characteristics, history of GI problems, disease, or surgery; bowel sounds

Expected Outcomes

- Patient will verbalize strategies to promote healthy bowel function.
- Patient will acknowledge the importance of seeking medical help for persistent alteration in GI motility.
- Patient will not experience any fluid and electrolyte imbalance as a result of altered motility.
- Patient will understand the need for early ambulation following abdominal surgery.

Suggested NOC Outcomes

Bowel Elimination, Electrolyte and Acid–Base Balance, Gastrointestinal Function

Interventions and Rationales

- Assess abdomen including auscultation in all four quadrants noting character and frequency *to determine increased or decreased motility.*
- Assess current manifestations of altered GI motility *to help identify the cause of the alteration and guide development of nursing interventions.*
- Monitor intake and output *to identify need for restoration of fluid balance.*
- Collect and evaluate laboratory electrolyte specimens. *Some altered motility states may require electrolyte replacement therapy.*
- Insert nasogastric tube as prescribed for patients with absent bowel sounds *to relieve the pressures caused by accumulation of air and fluid.*
- PCC Educate patient regarding importance of maintaining diet high in natural fiber and adequate fluid intake. *Fiber increases stool bulk and softens the stool. Fluid will promote normal bowel elimination pattern.*
- Encourage activities such as walking as tolerated for patients with decreased GI motility. *Increased activity will stimulate peristalsis and facilitate elimination.*
- PCC Collaborate with dietitian and other health care professionals as needed *to meet the unique needs of each individual patient.*

Suggested NIC Interventions

Fluid/Electrolyte Management; Gastrointestinal Intubation; Tube Care: Gastrointestinal

Evaluations for Expected Outcomes

- Patient verbalizes strategies to promote healthy bowel function.
- Patient states plan to seek medical assistance for GI problems.
- Patient maintains normal electrolyte balance.
- Patient ambulates according to schedule.

Documentation

- Patient's laboratory results and bowel characteristics
- Observations of physiologic and behavioral manifestations of decreased GI motility
- Interventions performed for management of nasogastric tube
- Patient's response to interventions
- Evaluations for expected outcomes

REFERENCES

Bing, L., Sheng, T., Yan-Lan, M., Jingping, T., Bin, W., & Jian-Rong, W. (2014). Analysis of bowel sounds application status for gastrointestinal function monitoring in the intensive care unit. *Critical Care Nursing Quarterly*, *37*(2), 199–206. doi:10.1097/CNQ.0000000000000019

Neighbour, C. (2014). Improving bowel care after surgery for hip fracture. *Nursing Older People*, *26*(10), 16–22. doi:10.7748/nop.26.10.16.e649

Wallström, Å., & Frisman, G. H. (2014). Facilitating early recovery of bowel motility after colorectal surgery: A systematic review. *Journal of Clinical Nursing*, *23*(1/2), 24–44. doi:10.1111/jocn.12258

RISK FOR DYSFUNCTIONAL GASTROINTESTINAL MOTILITY

Definition

Vulnerable to a decrease in normal frequency of defecation accompanied by difficult or incomplete passage of stool, which may compromise health

Assessment

- Health status, educational level, cultural status, requests for information; demonstrated understanding of material
- Fluid and electrolyte status, including blood urea nitrogen level, creatinine level, intake and output, mucous membranes, serum electrolyte levels, and skin turgor
- Nutritional status, including dietary patterns, laboratory tests, and serum protein level
- Neurologic status, including level of consciousness, mental status, motor function, and sensory pattern
- Gastrointestinal (GI) status, including nausea and vomiting, bowel habits, stool characteristics, history of GI problems, disease, or surgery; bowel sounds

Risk Factors

- Aging
- Anxiety
- Change in water source
- Decrease in GI circulation
- Diabetes mellitus
- Eating habit change (e.g., foods, eating times)
- Food intolerance
- Gastroesophageal reflux disease (GERD)
- Immobility
- Infection
- Pharmaceutical agent
- Prematurity
- Sedentary lifestyle
- Stressors
- Unsanitary food preparation

Expected Outcomes

- Patient will maintain adequate fluid and electrolyte balance.
- Patient will identify diet selections and lifestyle changes that would promote healthy GI function.
- Patient will not experience altered GI motility related to prescribed medications.
- Patient will recognize chronic conditions that may contribute to altered GI motility, for example, diabetes, GERD.

Suggested NOC Outcomes

Electrolyte and Acid–Base Balance; Fluid Balance; Bowel Elimination

Interventions and Rationales

- Assess patient for signs of fluid or electrolyte imbalance related to increased or decreased GI motility. *Fluid and electrolyte alterations can result from either increased or decreased GI motility.*
- Assess patient for positive risk factors for altered GI motility. *This will allow for timely interventions to prevent complications associated with GI dysfunction.*
- Assist patient taking prescribed medications that affect motility with strategies to avoid GI complications. *Awareness of preventive measures will decrease GI complications.*
- Encourage early ambulation for postoperative patients receiving opioids for pain control. *Early ambulation will reduce the risk of narcotic-related constipation.*
- PCC Educate patient regarding the risk factors related to altered GI motility, including certain food choices, fluid intake, medications, and activity. *Promotion of healthy lifestyle choices will contribute to positive patient outcomes.*
- Provide encouragement and support for behaviors that enhance GI health. *Positive reinforcement results in improved confidence in self-management of health behaviors.*
- PCC Coordinate care with other disciplines as needed *to reinforce positive behaviors or to assist with complex situations.*

Suggested NIC Interventions

Diarrhea Management; Electrolyte Monitoring; Fluid Management; Nutrition Management

Evaluations for Expected Outcomes

- Patient has normal electrolyte balance.
- Patient makes dietary and fluid selections to maintain a healthy GI system.
- Patient has no adverse reaction to medications.
- Patient understands relationship of chronic conditions to GI motility.

Documentation

- Patient's expressions of concern about adverse reaction and symptoms of altered GI motility
- Observations of physiologic and behavioral manifestations of decreased GI motility
- Interventions performed to allay adverse GI reactions to medications
- Patient's response to interventions
- Evaluations for expected outcomes

REFERENCES

Bing, L., Sheng, T., Yan-Lan, M., Jingping, T., Bin, W., & Jian-Rong, W. (2014). Analysis of bowel sounds application status for gastrointestinal function monitoring in the intensive care unit. *Critical Care Nursing Quarterly*, *37*(2), 199–206. doi:10.1097/CNQ.0000000000000019

Neighbour, C. (2014). Improving bowel care after surgery for hip fracture. *Nursing Older People*, *26*(10), 16–22. doi:10.7748/nop.26.10.16.e649

Wallström, Å., & Frisman, G. H. (2014). Facilitating early recovery of bowel motility after colorectal surgery: A systematic review. *Journal of Clinical Nursing*, *23*(1/2), 24–44. doi:10.1111/jocn.12258

RISK FOR INEFFECTIVE GASTROINTESTINAL PERFUSION

Definition

Vulnerable to decrease in gastrointestinal circulation, which may compromise health

Assessment

- Health history, including history of cardiovascular disorder, gastrointestinal dysfunction, and surgical history
- Medication history
- Abdominal assessment
- Cardiovascular status, including heart rate and rhythm, blood pressure, and peripheral pulses

Risk Factors

- Abdominal aortic aneurysm
- Abdominal compartment syndrome
- Abnormal partial thromboplastin time
- Abnormal prothrombin time
- Acute gastrointestinal hemorrhage
- Age >60 years
- Anemia
- Cerebral vascular accident
- Coagulopathy (e.g., sickle cell anemia)
- Decrease in left ventricular performance
- Diabetes mellitus
- Disseminated intravascular coagulopathy
- Female gender
- Gastroesophageal varicies
- Gastrointestinal condition (e.g., ulcer, ischemic colitis, ischemic pancreatitis)
- Hemodynamic instability
- Impaired liver function (e.g., cirrhosis, hepatitis)
- Myocardial infarction
- Renal disease (e.g., polycystic kidney, renal artery stenosis, failure)
- Smoking
- Trauma
- Treatment regimen
- Vascular disease

Expected Outcomes

- Patient will acknowledge the need to report any sudden increase in abdominal pain.
- Patient will not experience any organ injury related to decrease in gastrointestinal perfusion.
- Patient will understand the rationale and need for frequent abdominal assessment.
- Patient will verbalize strategies to decrease identified individual risk factors.

Suggested NOC Outcomes

Client Satisfaction: Tissue Perfusion: Abdominal; Fluid Balance; Gastrointestinal Function

Interventions and Rationales

- Assess bowel sounds for motility. *Impaired motility can cause functional, nonmechanical obstruction, for example, ileus.*
- Assess abdomen for *distention, which can compromise blood flow and result in ischemia.*
- Monitor vital signs closely and provide early intervention for those at risk *to ensure adequate gastrointestinal perfusion.*
- PCC Educate patients at risk to promptly report any abdominal pain. *Abdominal pain is a sensitive, nonspecific indicator of gastrointestinal obstruction.*
- PCC Encourage patients at risk to ask questions and share concerns *to promote understanding and decrease anxiety.*
- PCC Coordinate care and promote early intervention for evidence of decreased gastrointestinal perfusion. *Early intervention will result in improved patient outcomes.*

Suggested NIC Interventions

Risk Identification; Circulatory Care: Arterial Insufficiency

Evaluations for Expected Outcomes

- Patient acknowledged and understood the need to report any sudden increase in abdominal pain.
- Patient did not experience any organ injury.
- Patient understood the need for frequent abdominal assessments.
- Patient verbalized strategies to decrease individual risk factors.

Documentation

- Patient's report of abdominal pain
- Vital signs and abdominal assessment findings
- Patient's verbalization of risk reduction strategies
- Evaluations for expected outcomes

REFERENCES

Chelvanayagam, S., & Newell, C. (2015). Differentiating between eating disorders and gastrointestinal problems. *Gastrointestinal Nursing, 13*(7), 56–62.

Li, G., Ren, J., Wang, G., Wu, Q., Gu, G., Ren, H., &... Li, J. (2015). Prevalence and risk factors of acute lower gastrointestinal bleeding in Crohn's disease. *Medicine, 94*(19), 1–7. doi:10.1097/MD.0000000000000804

Wani, Z. A., Bhat, R. A., Bhadoria, A. S., Maiwall, R., & Choudhury, A. (2015). Gastric varices: Classification, endoscopic and ultrasonographic management. *Journal of Research in Medical Sciences, 20*(12), 1200–1207. doi:10.4103/1735-1995.172990

GRIEVING

Definition

A normal complex process that includes emotional, physical, spiritual, social, and intellectual responses and behaviors by which individuals, families, and communities incorporate an actual, anticipated, or perceived loss into their daily lives

Assessment

- Age, gender, developmental stage
- Patient's perceived value of loss
- Emotional status including anger, denial, or hostility
- Patient's usual pattern of coping with loss
- Changes in activity level, appetite, libido, or sleep pattern
- Emotional and spiritual support systems

Defining Characteristics

- Alteration in activity level
- Alteration in dream pattern
- Alteration in immune functioning
- Alteration in neuroendocrine functioning
- Alteration in sleep pattern
- Anger
- Blaming
- Despair
- Detachment
- Disorganization
- Finding meaning in a loss
- Guilt about feeling relieved
- Maintaining a connection to the deceased
- Pain
- Panic behavior
- Personal growth
- Psychological distress
- Suffering

Expected Outcomes

- Patient will identify and acknowledge the loss.
- Patient will accept that grief is a natural response to loss and understands the grief process.
- Patient will express grief in a nondestructive manner.
- Patient will seek emotional or spiritual support.
- Patient will progress through the various stages of the grieving process.
- Patient will establish plans for the future.

Suggested NOC Outcomes

Coping; Family Coping; Grief Resolution; Life Change; Psychosocial Adjustment

Interventions and Rationales

- Assist patient to understand grieving process and accept feelings; *this enhances patient's understanding and ability to cope.*
- PCC Provide time for the patient to express feelings about death or terminal illness; *active listening helps decrease feelings of loneliness and isolation.*
- PCC Allow time for the family to express their feelings of loss or potential loss. *The family will take some consolation that they can talk to someone who has been involved in the patient's care.*
- PCC Offer the option of referral to a spiritual counselor or clergy member. *Spiritual beliefs often become stronger and occupy a more important place in the life of the patient or family during times of grieving.*
- PCC Encourage expression of grief in a support group; *comfort is received in knowing that the pain from grief is normal.*
- PCC Involve the interdisciplinary team inpatient care; *each team member offers unique training to meet patient's needs.*
- PCC Help patient make a specific plan for coping to enable patient *to integrate the loss and adjust to new lifestyle.*

Suggested NIC Interventions

Active Listening; Emotional Support; Family Support; Grief Work Facilitation; Presence; Touch; Spiritual Support

Evaluations for Expected Outcomes

- Patient identifies and acknowledges loss.
- Patient accepts that grief is a natural response to loss and understands the grief process.
- Patient is able to express grief in a nondestructive manner.
- Patient will participate in organized spiritual or emotional support systems.
- Patient progresses through the stages of grief.
- Patient describes plans for the future.

Documentation

- Patient's verbal expression of grief
- Observations of emotional responses at attempts at coping
- Interventions to assist coping with loss
- Patient's response to nursing interventions
- Evaluations for expected outcomes

REFERENCES

Miller, E. T. (2015). The grieving process: A necessary step toward healing. *Rehabilitation Nursing, 40*(4), 207–208. doi:10.1002/rnj.220

Raitio, K., Kaunonen, M., & Aho, A. L. (2015). Evaluating a bereavement follow-up intervention for grieving mothers after the death of a child. *Scandinavian Journal of Caring Sciences, 29*(3), 510–520. doi:10.1111/scs.12183

Waller, A., Turon, H., Mansfield, E., Clark, K., Hobden, B., & Sanson-Fisher, R. (2016). Assisting the bereaved: A systematic review of the evidence for grief counselling. *Palliative Medicine*, *30*(2), 132–148. doi:10.1177/0269216315588728

COMPLICATED GRIEVING

related to emotional disturbance

Definition

A disorder that occurs after the death of a significant other, in which the experience of distress accompanying bereavement fails to follow normative expectations and manifests in functional impairment

Assessment

- History of loss
- Length of grief process
- Pattern of coping (grief delayed or avoided)
- Self-destructive behaviors
- Sleep assessment
- Nutritional assessment
- Changes in presentation of self
- Social or spiritual support
- Ability to maintain roles at occupation and within family

Defining Characteristics

- Anger
- Anxiety
- Avoidance of grieving
- Decreased functioning in life roles
- Depression
- Disbelief
- Distress about the deceased person
- Excessive stress
- Experiencing symptoms the deceased experienced
- Fatigue
- Feeling dazed
- Feeling detachment from others
- Feeling shock
- Feeling stunned
- Feelings of emptiness
- Insufficient sense of well-being
- Longing for the deceased
- Low levels of intimacy
- Mistrust
- Nonacceptance of a death
- Persistent painful memories
- Preoccupation with thoughts about a deceased person
- Rumination
- Searching for a deceased person
- Self-blame
- Separation distress
- Traumatic distress
- Yearning for deceased person

Expected Outcomes

- Patient will express appropriate feelings of loss, guilt, fear, anger, or sadness.
- Patient will identify the loss and describe what it means to him.
- Patient will appropriately move through stages of grief.
- Patient will maintain healthy patterns of sleep, activity, and eating.
- Patient will verbalize understanding that grief is normal.
- Patient will use healthy coping mechanisms and social support systems.
- Patient will seek fulfillment through preferred spiritual practices.
- Patient will begin planning for future.

Suggested NOC Outcomes

Coping; Family Coping; Grief Resolution; Life Change; Psychosocial Adjustment

Interventions and Rationales

- PCC Encourage patient to express grief and feelings of anger, guilt, and sadness. *Inability to express these feelings may result in maladaptive behaviors.*
- Encourage journaling to express grief and loss. *Writing and exploring feelings is an active process, which may assist in grieving.*
- Help patient to identify an area of hope in life. *Focusing on a life purpose may decrease anger and feelings of frustration.*
- PCC Refer patient to community support systems *to help the patient deal with the bereavement and grief process.*
- Contact patient's preferred spiritual leader, if patient desires; *this may provide relief from spiritual distress.*
- Help patient to focus realistically on changes the loss has brought about. *This will assist patient in forming plans for the future and improving social relationships.*
- Encourage patient and family to engage in reminiscing; *this will give purpose and meaning to the loss and assist in maintenance of self-esteem.*
- PCC Help patient to formulate goals for the future; *this helps patient to place loss in perspective and to move on to new situations and relationships.*
- Identify previous losses and assess for depression; *in the elderly, losses frequently occur without adequate recovery time before the next loss.*

Suggested NIC Interventions

Calming Technique; Coping Enhancement; Counseling; Emotional Support; Family Therapy; Grief Facilitation Work

Evaluations for Expected Outcomes

- Patient expresses feelings, which may include grief, guilt, anger, or sadness.
- Patient verbalizes feelings and behaviors related to the grieving process and applies these behaviors and feelings to daily life.
- Patient appropriately moves through stages of grief.
- Patient maintains healthy patterns of sleep, activity, and eating.
- Patient communicates understanding that grieving is an appropriate response to loss and comes to terms with own grief response.
- Patient uses coping mechanisms and discusses loss with others, including support group and family.
- Patient experiences satisfaction and support from chosen religious practices.
- Patient begins planning for future.

Documentation

- Patient's verbal expression of grief
- Observations of emotional responses, attempts at coping, and interactions with family and staff
- Interventions to assist coping with loss

- Patient's response to nursing interventions
- Evaluations for expected outcomes

REFERENCES

Coelho, A., Delalibera, M., Barbosa, A., & Lawlor, P. (2015). Prolonged grief in palliative family caregivers. *Omega: Journal of Death & Dying*, *72*(2), 151–164. doi:10.1177/0030222815574833

Nam, I. S. (2016). Effects of psychoeducation on helpful support for complicated grief: A preliminary randomized, controlled, single-blind study. *Psychological Medicine*, *46*(1), 189–195. doi:10.1017/S0033291715001658

Supiano, K. P., & Luptak, M. (2014). Complicated grief in older adults: A randomized controlled trial of complicated grief group therapy. *Gerontologist*, *54*(5), 840–856. doi:10.1093/geront/gnt076

RISK FOR COMPLICATED GRIEVING

Definition

Vulnerable to a disorder that occurs after death of a significant other in which the experience of distress accompanying bereavement fails to follow normative expectations and manifests in functional impairment, which may compromise health.

Assessment

- History of loss
- Length of grief process
- Pattern of coping (grief delayed or avoided)
- Self-destructive behaviors
- Sleep assessment
- Nutritional assessment
- Changes in presentation of self
- Social or spiritual support
- Ability to maintain roles at occupation and within family
- Behavioral status, understanding of health problem and treatment plan, past history with health care providers, participation in health care planning and decision making; recognition and realization of potential growth, health, and autonomy

Risk Factors

- Death of a significant other
- Emotional disturbance
- Insufficient social support

Expected Outcomes

- Patient will express appropriate feelings of loss, guilt, fear, anger, or sadness.
- Patient will identify loss and describe meaning of loss.
- Patient will appropriately move through stages of grieving.
- Patient will maintain healthy patterns of sleep, activity, and eating.
- Patient will list personal strengths.
- Patient will use healthy coping mechanisms and social support systems.

- Patient will seek fulfillment through preferred spiritual practices.
- Patient will begin planning for future.

Suggested NOC Outcomes

Grief Resolution; Life Change Adjustment

Interventions and Rationales

- Identify areas of hope in patient's life *to help decrease anger and feelings of frustration.*
- Identify previous losses and assess for depression *to establish a baseline.*
- Perform interventions to promote sleep such as giving snack, pillows, backrub, or shower *to enhance rest.*
- PCC Teach patient relaxation techniques such as guided imagery, meditation, or progressive muscle relaxation *to promote feelings of comfort.*
- PCC Encourage patient to express grief and feelings of anger, guilt, and sadness. *Inability to express these feelings may result in maladaptive behaviors.*
- PCC Encourage patient to express feelings in a way the patient is most comfortable with, for example, crying, talking, writing, and/or drawing. *Dysfunctional grieving may result from an inability to express feelings freely.*
- Encourage patient to keep a journal to express feelings of grief and loss. The act of writing about feelings may aid in the grieving process. *Help patient form goals for the future to place the loss in perspective and to move on to new situations and relationships.*
- PCC Refer patient to community support systems to assist with grieving process. Contact patient's preferred spiritual leader if patient desires. *This may provide relief from spiritual distress.*

Suggested NIC Interventions

Coping Enhancement; Counseling; Emotional Support; Family Therapy; Grief Facilitation Work

Evaluations for Expected Outcomes

- Patient expresses feelings of loss and grief.
- Patient describes the impact of the loss.
- Patient articulates movement through stages of grief.
- Patient's personal strengths are sufficient for normal functioning.
- Patient uses healthy coping strategies and social support systems.
- Patient states plan for future and uses spiritual practices satisfactorily.

Documentation

- Patient's expressions of grief and loss
- Observations of physiologic and behavioral manifestations of grief
- Interventions performed to allay sleeping problems
- Patient's use of journal
- Patient's response to interventions
- Evaluations for expected outcomes

REFERENCES

Coelho, A., Delalibera, M., Barbosa, A., & Lawlor, P. (2015). Prolonged grief in palliative family caregivers. *Omega: Journal of Death & Dying*, *72*(2), 151–164. doi:10.1177/0030222815574833

Nam, I. S. (2016). Effects of psychoeducation on helpful support for complicated grief: A preliminary randomized, controlled, single-blind study. *Psychological Medicine*, *46*(1), 189–195. doi:10.1017/S0033291715001658

Supiano, K. P., & Luptak, M. (2014). Complicated grief in older adults: A randomized controlled trial of complicated grief group therapy. *Gerontologist*, *54*(5), 840–856. doi:10.1093/geront/gnt076

RISK-PRONE HEALTH BEHAVIOR

related to disability or health status change requiring change in lifestyle

Definition

Impaired ability to modify lifestyle/behaviors in a manner that improves health status

Assessment

- Nature and impact of medical diagnosis
- Behavioral responses, including verbal or nonverbal, engagement or disengagement, interest or apathy, acceptance or denial, and independence or dependence
- Knowledge of health condition
- Past experiences with family, friends, and media
- Psychosocial factors, such as age, gender, ethnic and cultural background, religious preference and beliefs, values, occupation, family support, and coping style
- Nutritional status, including modifications in diet and weight changes

Defining Characteristics

- Failure to achieve optimal sense of control
- Failure to take action that prevents health problems
- Minimizes health status change
- Nonacceptance of health status change

Expected Outcomes

- Patient will identify inability to cope and will adjust adequately.
- Patient will express understanding of the illness or disease.
- Patient will participate in health care regimen and will plan care-related activities.
- Patient will demonstrate ability to manage health problem.
- Patient will show ability to accept and adapt to a new health status and integrate learning.
- Patient will demonstrate new coping strategies.

Suggested NOC Outcomes

Acceptance: Health Status; Adaptation to Physical Disability; Coping; Health Seeking Behavior; Participation in Health Care Decisions; Psychosocial Adjustment: Life Change; Social Support; Treatment Behavior: Illness or Injury

Interventions and Rationales

- PCC Encourage patient to express feelings in a safe, private environment. *This allows patient to gain insight into and rationally define fears, goals, and potential problems.*
- Allow patient to grieve. Grieving is a normal and essential aspect with any kind of negative change in health status. *After working through denial and isolation, anger, bargaining, and depression, patient will progress toward acceptance.*
- Provide reassurance that patient's feelings, under these circumstances, are normal. *By realizing that it's acceptable to grieve, the patient will be ready to look for positive ways of coping.*
- PCC Begin teaching patient and caregivers the skills needed to adequately manage care. This will *encourage compliance and adjustment to optimum wellness.*
- PCC Spend time listening to patient's feelings. *This helps reassure patient you're interested and care.*
- PCC Help patient identify areas where it's possible to maintain control. *This prevents feelings of powerlessness and allows the patient to feel part of a team effort.*
- Encourage patient to plan for care activities, such as time of treatment, personal hygiene, and rest periods. *Doing this offers patient an opportunity to control facets of care and increases feelings of self-determination.*
- Arrange for others who have suffered similar health problems to speak with patient and family. *This exposes patient to suitable role models and may allow a trusting, supportive relationship to develop.*
- Discuss health problems and implications with family members *to enable them to participate in patient's care and to foster a trusting relationship.*
- PCC Obtain a consultation with a mental health specialist if patient develops severe depression or other psychiatric problems. *Although trauma or illness commonly causes some depression, consultation with a mental health professional may help minimize it.*

Suggested NIC Interventions

Anxiety Reduction; Behavior Modification; Coping Enhancement; Counseling; Knowledge; Decision-Making Support; Emotional Support; Mutual Goal Setting; Role Enhancement; Simple Relaxation Therapy; Support System Enhancement

Evaluations for Expected Outcomes

- Patient recognizes necessity of learning to live with impairment.
- Patient understands that grieving is a normal response to impairment.
- Patient meets learning objectives before discharge.
- Patient identifies and contacts sources of continued psychological support if needed.
- Patient identifies two areas in which he can maintain control despite altered health status.
- Patient meets with individual who has similar health problem and reports results of meeting.

Documentation

- Patient's verbalizations of specific behaviors that cause impairment of health
- Patient's nonverbal behaviors
- Patient's verbal expressions of denial, anger, or guilt because of the illness or disease process
- Patient's ability or inability to participate in care
- Evaluations for expected outcomes

REFERENCES

Leong, C. M., & Palos, G. R. (2014). Oncology nurses and indoor tanning: Stylish or risky behavior? *Clinical Journal of Oncology Nursing*, *18*(3), 363–365. doi:10.1188/14.CJON.363-365

McDonald, C. C., Sommers, M. S., & Fargo, J. D. (2014). Risky driving, mental health, and health-compromising behaviors: Risk clustering in late adolescents and adults. *Injury Prevention*, *20*(6), 365–372. doi:10.1136/injuryprev-2014-041150

Roth, A. M., Armenta, R. A., Wagner, K. D., Roesch, S. C., Bluthenthal, R. N., Cuevas-Mota, J., & Garfein, R. S. (2015). Patterns of drug use, risky behavior, and health status among persons who inject drugs living in San Diego, California: A latent class analysis. *Substance Use & Misuse*, *50*(2), 205–214. doi:10.3109/10826084.2014.962661

INEFFECTIVE HEALTH MANAGEMENT

Definition

Pattern of regulating and integrating into daily living a therapeutic regimen for the treatment of illness and its sequelae that is unsatisfactory for meeting specific health goals

Assessment

- Age
- Current health status
- History of neurologic, sensory, or psychological impairment
- Neurologic status, including level of consciousness, orientation, cognition (memory, insight, and judgment), sensory ability, and motor ability
- Knowledge of health practices, including body maintenance, preventive health care needs, health care team follow-up, and safety measures
- Personal habits, such as smoking and alcohol consumption
- Psychosocial support, including lifestyle, communication status (verbal, nonverbal, phone, and written), family members, and finances

Defining Characteristics

- Difficulty with prescribed regimen
- Failure to include treatment regimen in daily living
- Failure to take action to reduce risk factor
- Ineffective choices in daily living for meeting health goal

Expected Outcomes

- Patient will identify necessary health maintenance activities.
- Patient will make decisions about daily schedule.
- Patient will perform health maintenance activities according to level of ability (specify).
- Patient will communicate understanding of necessity for continuous self-monitoring of body functions.
- Patient will maintain muscle strength and joint mobility.
- Patient will demonstrate specific motor skills, such as brushing teeth.
- Family members will demonstrate skill in carrying out activities patient cannot perform.
- Patient will identify community and social resources available to help with health maintenance.

Suggested NOC Outcomes

Decision-Making; Health Beliefs: Perceived Resources; Health Promoting Behavior; Health Seeking Behaviors; Knowledge: Health Behavior; Knowledge: Health Promotion; Motivation; Self-Care Status; Social Support; Spiritual Health

Interventions and Rationales

- Discuss health maintenance needs with patient while carrying out routine activities *to reinforce their importance.*
- PCC Involve patient in decision making by allowing choices in determining where, when, and how activities are to be carried out. Ask, for example, "Would you like a bath or shower in the morning or evening?" *Participation in decision making increases feelings of independence.*
- Help patient perform health maintenance activities, such as daily skin inspection and weekly catheterization for residual urine. *Encouraging skill development in patient promotes continued use of those skills after discharge.*
- PCC Instruct patient in specific skills needed in monitoring health status *to prompt participation in self-care.* Allow patient to perform skills *to encourage independence.*
- Perform or help patient perform passive and active range-of-motion exercises *to help maintain joint mobility and muscle strength.*
- Identify level of mobility (independent in feeding and bathing; needs assistance to brush teeth; dependent in use of wheelchair), and communicate skill level to all personnel *to provide continuity and preserve level of independence.*
- PCC Educate family members in skills that patient cannot perform unassisted, such as bathing, maintaining hygiene, driving to appointments, transferring, or using walker. *This allows patient and family members to take active role in care.*
- PCC Consult with social services or other health care team members to identify health care resources (e.g., Meals On Wheels or homemaker services), and help patient contact and arrange for follow-up. *These resources can help patient maintain independence after discharge.*
- PCC Encourage patient and family members to verbalize feelings and concerns related to health maintenance *to help them develop greater understanding and better manage their health.*
- PCC Help family members develop coping skills necessary to deal with patient. *If patient's illness is prolonged, family members could develop maladaptive coping strategies.*
- PCC Make referrals, as appropriate, to psychiatric liaison nurse and social services *to help prevent burnout among family members.*

Suggested NIC Interventions

Anticipatory Guidance; Behavior Modification; Decision-Making Support; Health Education; Health System Guidance; Referral; Support System Enhancement; Teaching: Disease Process

Evaluations for Expected Outcomes

- Patient identifies health maintenance activities.
- Patient plans daily schedule.
- Patient's functional level is appropriate to capability level.

- Patient communicates understanding of importance of monitoring body functions, such as blood glucose levels, blood pressure, and pulse rate.
- Patient maintains muscle strength and joint mobility.
- Patient demonstrates motor skills correctly without prompting.
- Family members demonstrate skill in carrying out activities patient cannot perform.
- Patient identifies and contacts community resources to assist with health maintenance, if needed.

Documentation

- Patient's identified health needs and perceptions and limitations in achieving them
- Patient's willingness to make decisions and participate in health maintenance activities
- Observations of motor abilities, level of skill performance, and health status
- Patient's response to nursing interventions
- Evaluations for expected outcomes

REFERENCES

Risendal, B., Dwyer, A., Seidel, R., Lorig, K., Katzenmeyer, C., Coombs, L., ... Ory, M. (2014). Adaptation of the chronic disease self-management program for cancer survivors: feasibility, acceptability, and lessons for implementation. *Journal of Cancer Education*, *29*(4), 762–771. doi:10.1007/s13187-014-0652-8

Souza Carneiro, C., Dias de Oliveira, A. P., Lima Lopes, J., Bachion, M. M., Herdman, T. H., Moorhead, S. A., & Bottura Leite de Barros, A. L. (2016). Outpatient clinic for health education: Contribution to self-management and self-care for people with heart failure. *International Journal of Nursing Knowledge*, *27*(1), 49–55. doi:10.1111/2047-3095.12071

Zaldonis, J., Alrawashdeh, M., Atman, K. S., Fatigati, A., Dabbs, D., & Bermudez, C. A. (2015). Predictors and influence of goal orientation on self-management and health-related quality of life after lung transplant. *Progress in Transplantation*, *25*(3), 230–242. doi:10.7182/pit2015189

INEFFECTIVE HEALTH MANAGEMENT

related to complexity of health care system and insufficient knowledge of therapeutic regimen

Definition

Pattern of regulating and integrating into daily living a therapeutic regimen for the treatment of illness and its sequelae that is unsatisfactory for meeting specific health goals

Assessment

- Learning ability including demonstrated skills in managing health problems
- Health status including patient's understanding of health problem and treatment plan
- Past history with health care providers, participation in health care planning and decision making
- Recognition and realization of potential growth, health, and autonomy
- Support systems, relationships, and family systems
- Cultural status including affiliation with racial, ethnic, or religious groups

Defining Characteristics

- Difficulty with prescribed regimen
- Failure to include treatment regimen in daily living
- Failure to take action to reduce risk factor
- Ineffective choices in daily living for meeting health goal

Expected Outcomes

- Patient will acknowledge responsibility to manage own health condition.
- Patient will identify any barriers to optimal self-health management and determine plan to address them.
- Patient will refine problem-solving skills over time.
- Patient will increase self-efficacy, the confidence that one can carry out a behavior necessary to reach a desired goal.

Suggested NOC Outcomes

Health Status; Adherence Behavior; Compliance Behavior; Decision-Making; Health Orientation; Health-Promoting Behavior; Personal Health Status

Interventions and Rationales

- Monitor patient's self-efficacy and use of problem-solving skills as patient manages own health. *These concepts reflect a new paradigm in health management that acknowledges that patients need many skills and confidence to carry out plan of care.*
- PCC Assist patient in setting goals and making informed choices. *This patient–nurse collaborative relationship helps patient and nurse identify barriers to optimal health management and overcome them.*
- PCC Teach patient about disease states and regimens but, more importantly, teach problem-solving skills *to ensure active participation in self-health management despite any possible setbacks.*
- Provide encouragement to help motivate patient to maximize healthy behaviors. *This highlights that behavior is best changed by internal motivation rather than by external motivation.*
- PCC Coordinate care with social services and colleagues in other disciplines *to ensure that family, economic, and social barriers to optimal self-health management have been addressed.*

Suggested NIC Interventions

Behavior Modification; Complex Relationship Building; Decision-Making Support; Health Education; Learning Facilitation; Mutual Goal Setting; Self-Awareness Enhancement

Evaluations for Expected Outcomes

- Patient acknowledges responsibility for management of own health.
- Patient identifies barriers to self-health management and strategies to address them.
- Patient actively participates in problem-solving skills.
- Patient begins to develop confidence in managing own health and achieving goals.

Documentation

- Patient's statement of responsibility for self-health management
- Patient's identified barriers to self-health management and planned strategies
- Patient's use of problem-solving skills
- Evaluations for expected outcomes

REFERENCES

des Ordons, A. L. R., Sharma, N., Heyland, D. K., & You, J. J. (2015). Strategies for effective goals of care discussions and decision-making: Perspectives from a multi-centre survey of Canadian hospital-based health care providers. *BMC Palliative Care*, *14*(1), 1–10. doi:10.1186/s12904-015-0035-x

Horwood, H., Williams, M. J., & Mandic, S. (2015). Examining motivations and barriers for attending maintenance community-based cardiac rehabilitation using the health-belief model. *Heart, Lung & Circulation*, *24*(10), 980–987. doi:10.1016/j.hlc.2015.03.023

Lauritzen, C., Reedtz, C., Doesum, K., & Martinussen, M. (2015). Factors that may facilitate or hinder a family focus in the treatment of parents with a mental illness. *Journal of Child & Family Studies*, *24*(4), 864–871. doi:10.1007/s10826-013-9895-y

INEFFECTIVE FAMILY HEALTH MANAGEMENT

related to family conflict, complex treatment regimen, economically disadvantaged, or complexity of health care system

Definition

A pattern of regulating and integrating into family processes a program of treatment for illness and the sequelae that is unsatisfactory for meeting specific health goals

Assessment

- Family status, including marital status, family composition, communication patterns, coping skills, drug or alcohol abuse, psychiatric history, and beliefs and attitudes about health and illness
- Health status, including chronic or terminal illness and severely disabling physical conditions
- Socioeconomic factors, including financial status, insurance, accessibility of health care, availability of health care providers, and transportation system
- Social status, including communication skills, size of social network, degree of trust in others, self-esteem, and ability to function in social and occupational roles
- Spiritual status, including religious or church affiliation and description of faith and religious practices

Defining Characteristics

- Acceleration of illness symptoms of a family member
- Decrease in attention to illness
- Difficulty with prescribed regimen
- Failure to take action to reduce risk factor
- Inappropriate family activities for meeting health goal

Expected Outcomes

- Family members will identify behaviors that lead to conflict.
- Family members will participate in family therapy sessions and openly express feelings about illness of family member.
- Family members will express desire to have help in resolving conflicts.

- Family members will describe coping mechanisms that help reduce conflicts.
- Family members will cooperate in finding ways to incorporate therapeutic regimen into their lifestyle.
- Family members will express desire to carry out therapeutic regimen.
- Family members will plan for future course of illness.

Suggested NOC Outcomes

Compliance Behavior; Family Coping; Family Functioning; Family Normalization; Family Participation in Professional Care; Knowledge: Treatment Regimen; Risk Control; Symptom Control

Interventions and Rationales

- Spend time with family, get to know each family member individually, and establish a trusting relationship with each family member *to help identify measures that will increase family cohesiveness.*
- PCC Encourage family members to attend and participate in family therapy sessions *to strengthen family unit and promote resolution of conflict.*
- PCC Help family members describe feelings associated with the illness of their relative to bring family conflict into the open. *Unresolved family conflicts may prevent family members from fully implementing therapeutic regimen.*
- Elicit family members' personal beliefs about the illness, and review relevant information *to establish their support for improving management of therapeutic regimen.*
- PCC Educate family members about the pathophysiology of illness, and explain the relationship between the pathophysiology and the therapeutic regimen. *If family members know reasons for specific behaviors, they may be more willing to adjust their lifestyle.*
- PCC Work with family members to identify behaviors that have contributed to family conflict, and help them identify alternative behaviors *to promote resolution of the conflict.*
- Encourage family members to address individual needs assertively *to promote healthy interactions within family.*
- Help family members clarify values associated with their lifestyle *to enhance understanding of conflicts between their lifestyle and demands of therapeutic regimen.*
- PCC Work with family members to develop a daily routine for managing the therapeutic regimen that fits with their lifestyle. *Collaboration with family members makes it possible to incorporate lifestyle factors, such as culture, family dynamics, and finances, into a plan for managing the illness.*
- Assist family members in modifying factors (such as lack of supportive behaviors among family members) that interfere with treatment management *to enhance level of care.*
- PCC Work with the family in establishing goals for coping with conflicts *to focus their energy on achievable objectives and to foster hope.*
- Refer the family members to appropriate agencies, if needed. This can ensure continued family support and help reduce conflicts.
- PCC Help the family members plan for a future course of the illness. *Planning enhances family members' abilities to develop an appropriate strategy to manage the therapeutic regimen.*

Suggested NIC Interventions

Case Management; Coping Enhancement; Decision-Making Support; Family Involvement Promotion; Family Process Maintenance; Family Therapy

Evaluations for Expected Outcomes

- Family members identify unresolved conflicts.
- Family members attend and participate in family therapy sessions.
- Family members express a desire to resolve conflicts.
- Family members describe coping mechanisms that can reduce conflicts.
- Family members successfully incorporate components of therapeutic regimen into daily activities.
- Family members carry out therapeutic regimen.
- Family members establish a plan for coping with future course of illness.

Documentation

- Description of each family member's understanding of patient's illness
- Family members' expressions of feelings regarding patient's illness
- Compliance with participation in family therapy sessions
- Evaluations for expected outcomes

REFERENCES

Martinez-Marcos, M., & De la Cuesta-Benjumea, C. (2015). Women's self-management of chronic illnesses in the context of caregiving: A grounded theory study. *Journal of Clinical Nursing*, *24*(11/12), 1557–1566. doi:10.1111/jocn.12746

Saifan, A., Bashayreh, I., Batiha, A., & AbuRuz, M. (2015). Patient- and family caregiver-related barriers to effective cancer pain control. *Pain Management Nursing*, *16*(3), 400–410. doi:10.1016/j.pmn.2014.09.007

Savundranayagam, M. Y., & Orange, J. B. (2014). Matched and mismatched appraisals of the effectiveness of communication strategies by family caregivers of persons with Alzheimer's disease. *International Journal of Language & Communication Disorders*, *49*(1), 49–59. doi:10.1111/1460-6984.12043

IMPAIRED HOME MAINTENANCE

related to alteration in cognitive functioning

Definition

Inability to independently maintain a safe growth-promoting immediate environment

Assessment

- Home environment
- Financial resources
- Patient's and family's knowledge of self-care requirements
- Patient's and family's psychological status, including perception of reality, communication patterns, assignment of responsibilities, degree of awareness and concern, and history of psychiatric illness
- Drug or alcohol abuse
- Support systems, including close friends, organizations with which patient is affiliated, and community resources

Defining Characteristics

- Difficulty maintaining a comfortable environment
- Excessive family responsibilities
- Financial crisis (e.g., debt, insufficient finances)
- Insufficient clothing
- Insufficient cooking equipment
- Insufficient equipment for maintaining home
- Insufficient linen
- Pattern of disease caused by unhygienic conditions
- Pattern of infection caused by unhygienic conditions
- Request for assistance with home maintenance
- Unsanitary environment

Expected Outcomes

- Patient and family members will express concern about poor home maintenance.
- Patient and family members will verbalize plan to correct health and safety hazards in home.
- Patient and family members will identify community resources available to help maintain home.

Suggested NOC Outcomes

Family Functioning; Role Performance; Self-Care: Instrumental Activities of Daily Living (IADLs)

Interventions and Rationales

- Discuss obstacles to effective home maintenance management with patient and family *to develop understanding of potential and actual health and safety hazards.*
- Help family members assign responsibilities for household care and establish appropriate expectations *to aid communication and help set realistic goals.*
- Help family members establish daily and weekly home maintenance activities and assignments *to impose structure on family's routine and set standards for measuring progress.*
- PCC Provide family with written information on medications and various aspects of patient's treatment. *The more competent the family members feel, the greater the possibility the patient will progress without difficulty.*
- Encourage weekly discussions about progress in maintaining home maintenance *schedule to develop family unity and allow members to address problems before they become overwhelming.*
- PCC Help family members contact community resources that can assist them in their efforts to improve home maintenance management, such as self-help groups, cleaning services, and exterminators. *Community resources can lessen family's burden while members learn to function independently.*

Suggested NIC Interventions

Counseling; Emotional Support; Family Integrity Promotion; Family Support; Home Maintenance Assistance

Evaluations for Expected Outcomes

- Patient and family members establish and follow daily and weekly schedule for home maintenance.
- With the help of appropriate community resources, as needed, patient and family members clear home of clutter, debris, and waste.
- Patient and family members contact community resources.

Documentation

- Patient's and family members' expressions of difficulty in maintaining household
- Patient's and family members' mental status
- Presence of health hazards, such as filth, rodents, and waste matter
- Presence of safety hazards, such as faulty wiring
- Presence of offensive odors
- Patient's and family members' understanding of home maintenance management and resources
- Interventions to improve home maintenance skills
- Patient's and family members' responses to nursing interventions
- Evaluations for expected outcomes

REFERENCES

Jang, M., & Lee, Y. (2015). The effects of an education program on home renovation for fall prevention of Korean older people. *Educational Gerontology*, *41*(9), 653–669. doi:10.1080/03601277.2015.1033219

Kelly, A. J., Fausset, C. B., Rogers, W., & Fisk, A. D. (2014). Responding to home maintenance challenge scenarios: The role of selection, optimization, and compensation in aging-in-place. *Journal of Applied Gerontology*, *33*(8), 1018–1042. doi:10.1177/0733464812456631

Smith, L. P., Shu Wen, N., & Popkin, B. M. (2014). Resistant to the recession: Low-income adults' maintenance of cooking and away-from-home eating behaviors during times of economic turbulence. *American Journal of Public Health*, *104*(5), 840–846. doi:10.2105/AJPH.2013.301677

IMPAIRED HOME MAINTENANCE

related to insufficient support system

Definition

Inability to independently maintain a safe growth-promoting immediate environment

Assessment

- Psychosocial status
- Support systems, including family, close friends, and organizations with which patient is affiliated; if patient lives alone, access to family, friends, and pets
- Financial resources
- Home environment
- Patient's and family members' knowledge of disease and self-care requirements

Defining Characteristics

- Difficulty maintaining a comfortable environment
- Excessive family responsibilities

- Financial crisis (e.g., debt, insufficient finances)
- Insufficient clothing
- Insufficient cooking equipment
- Insufficient equipment for maintaining home
- Insufficient linen
- Pattern of disease caused by unhygienic conditions
- Pattern of infection caused by unhygienic conditions
- Request for assistance with home maintenance
- Unsanitary environment

Expected Outcomes

- Patient and family members will express need to make adjustments in home to help manage patient's condition.
- Patient and family members will identify individuals or organizations that may provide assistance.

Suggested NOC Outcomes

Family Functioning; Role Performance; Self-Care: Activities of Daily Living (ADLs)

Interventions and Rationales

- PCC Help patient and family members explore available resources *to help identify discharge problems and ease transition from hospital to home.*
- PCC Provide sufficient information to patient and family members *to ensure knowledge necessary for them to make appropriate decisions.*
- PCC Refer patient to social service department *to assist with follow-up care after discharge.*
- Suggest referral to home health agency, homemaker service, Meals On Wheels, or other appropriate outside agencies for assistance and follow-up. *Patient may need a range of community services to meet various needs.*

Suggested NIC Interventions

Caregiver Support; Family Support; Home Maintenance Assistance; Role Enhancement; Support System Enhancement

Evaluations for Expected Outcomes

- Patient and family members describe changes needed to promote maximum health and safety at home.
- Patient and family members list agencies that can assist with home care.

Documentation

- Patient's and family members' perception of problem
- Observations regarding problem's magnitude
- Interventions performed to alleviate problem
- Responses of others asked to assist with problem
- Evaluations for expected outcomes

REFERENCES

Maeder, A., Poultney, N., Morgan, G., & Lippiatt, R. (2015). Patient compliance in home-based self-care telehealth projects. *Journal of Telemedicine & Telecare, 21*(8), 439–442. doi:10.1177/1357633X15612382

Pattison, N., O'Gara, G., & Rattray, J. (2015). After critical care: Patient support after critical care. A mixed-method, longitudinal study using e-mail interviews and questionnaires. *Intensive & Critical Care Nursing, 31*(4), 213–222. doi:10.1016/j.iccn.2014.12.002

Räsänen, P. M., Kanste, O., Elo, S., & Kyngäs, H. (2014). Factors associated with the self-care of home-dwelling older people. *Journal of Nursing Education & Practice, 4*(8), 90–96. doi:10.5430/jnep.v4n8p90

HOPELESSNESS

related to lost belief in transcendent values

Definition

Subjective state in which an individual sees limited or no alternatives or personal choices available and is unable to mobilize energy on own behalf

Assessment

- Nature of chronic illness
- Patient's and family members' knowledge of illness
- Mental status, including cognitive functioning, affect, mood, and stage in grieving process
- Communication, including verbal (speech content, quality, and quantity), nonverbal (body positioning, eye contact, and facial expression), and quality of interactions with others
- Nutritional status, including alteration in appetite or body weight
- Motivation level, including personal hygiene, therapies (physical and occupational), use of diversional activities, and sense of control over current life situation
- Developmental stage, including age and role in family
- Disruption in usual roles and activities and losses (real and perceived)
- Actual or perceived self-care deficits (specify)
- Number and types of stressors
- Coping mechanisms and decision-making ability
- Support systems, including clergy, family, and friends
- Spiritual values or religious beliefs

Defining Characteristics

- Alteration in sleep pattern
- Decrease in affect
- Decrease in appetite
- Decrease in initiative
- Decrease in response to stimuli
- Decrease in verbalization
- Despondent verbal cues (e.g., "I cannot," sighing)
- Inadequate involvement in care
- Passivity

- Poor eye contact
- Shrugging in response to speaker
- Turning away from speaker

Expected Outcomes

- Patient will express feelings of hopelessness.
- Patient will recognize and accept limitations of chronic illness.
- Patient will work through stages of grieving.
- Patient will develop coping mechanisms to deal with feelings of hopelessness.
- Patient will recognize benefit of positive social interactions.
- Patient will participate in self-care activities and in decisions regarding care planning.
- Patient will resume and maintain as many former roles as possible.
- Patient will regain and maintain self-esteem.
- Patient will begin to develop feelings of hope.

Suggested NOC Outcomes

Comfort Level; Coping; Decision-Making; Depression Control; Depression Level; Hope; Mood Equilibrium; Quality of Life; Will to Live; Spiritual Health

Interventions and Rationales

- S Assess for evidence of self-destructive behavior. *Assessment for suicide potential in a depressed patient is a nursing care priority.*
- If possible, assign a primary nurse to patient to encourage establishment *of a therapeutic relationship between patient and nurse.*
- Allow for specific amount of uninterrupted, non-care-related time each shift to talk with patient. Encourage verbal response with open-ended statements and questions. If patient chooses not to talk, spend time in silence. *This establishes rapport with depressed patient even if patient talks little.*
- Provide for appropriate physical outlets for expression of feelings (punching bag, walking) *to help patient release hostilities, thereby decreasing tension and anxiety.*
- Convey belief in patient's ability to develop and use coping skills *to increase patient's self-esteem and reduce feelings of dependence.*
- Acknowledge patient's pain. Encourage patient to express feelings of depression, anger, guilt, and sadness. Convey to patient that all these feelings are appropriate. *This will help patient work through stages of coming to terms with chronic illness.*
- Identify patient's strengths, and encourage putting strengths to use *to maintain optimal functioning.*
- PCC Encourage patient's participation in self-care to fullest extent possible *to reduce feelings of helplessness.*
- Help patient to participate in usual activities as strength, energy, and time permit *to maintain a sense of being connected to others.*
- PCC Encourage patient to identify enjoyable diversions and to participate in them *to decrease negative thinking and enhance self-esteem.*
- Encourage positive thinking. Convey a sense of confidence in patient's ability to cope with illness *to promote an optimistic outlook.*
- Provide positive reinforcement for patient's efforts to participate in self-care activities *to encourage patient to participate in self-care.* Encourage patient to establish self-care schedule *to enhance feelings of usefulness and control.*

- Assist patient with hygiene and grooming needs *to help enhance patient's self-esteem.*
- Offer patient and family a realistic assessment of situation, and communicate hope for immediate future. *This facilitates acceptance, helps promote patient safety and security, and allows planning of future health care.*
- PCC Encourage patient to identify spiritual needs and facilitate fulfillment of those needs *to help patient come to terms with chronic illness and its limitations.*
- PCC Involve patient and family members in care planning, and allow patient to choose degree of self-involvement on a continuing basis. Begin by offering patient a choice between two alternatives. Increase alternatives as initiative improves. *Cognitive disturbances associated with anxiety or depression usually prevent patient from making healthy decisions.*
- PCC Teach patient and family members how to manage illness, prevent complications, and control factors in the environment that affect patient's health. *Education enables family members to become resources in patient's care.*
- PCC Refer patient and family members to other caregivers (such as dietitian, social worker, clergyman, and mental health clinical nurse specialist) or support groups, as necessary. *Referrals to outside specialists ensure continuity of care. Support groups give patient chance to discuss illness with others similarly affected.*

Suggested NIC Interventions

Coping Enhancement; Counseling; Decision-Making Support; Family Mobilization; Hope Instillation; Spiritual Growth Facilitation

Evaluations for Expected Outcomes

- Patient talks about negative feelings instead of acting on them.
- Patient expresses understanding of lifestyle changes imposed by chronic illness.
- Patient discusses impact of illness and sees future realistically.
- Patient demonstrates at least ____ (specify) coping mechanisms.
- Patient interacts with others and regains involvement in life experiences.
- Patient demonstrates understanding that involvement in self-care is necessary to maintain optimal functioning.
- Patient demonstrates involvement in as many former roles as possible.
- Patient acknowledges a belief in self and demonstrates increased energy and will to live.
- Patient states that feelings of hopelessness are less frequent and expresses feelings of hope.

Documentation

- Patient's perception of chronic illness
- Patient's responses to treatment regimen
- Patient's mental and emotional status (baseline and ongoing)
- Patient education, counseling, and precautions taken to maintain or enhance patient's level of functioning
- Interventions to help patient deal with daily stressors
- Interventions to protect patient from self-harm
- Patient's response to nursing interventions
- Evaluations for expected outcomes

REFERENCES

Gudmundsdottir, R. M., & Thome, M. (2014). Evaluation of the effects of individual and group cognitive behavioral therapy and of psychiatric rehabilitation on hopelessness of depressed adults: A comparative analysis. *Journal of Psychiatric & Mental Health Nursing*, *21*(10), 866–872. doi:10.1111/jpm.12157

Konukbay, D., & Arslan, F. (2015). The analysis of hopelessness levels and problem solving skills of parents with the disabled children. *International Journal of Caring Sciences*, *8*(2), 344–355.

Steeg, S., Haigh, M., Webb, R. T., Kapur, N., Awenat, Y., Gooding, P., … Cooper, J. (2016). The exacerbating influence of hopelessness on other known risk factors for repeat self-harm and suicide. *Journal of Affective Disorders*, *190*, 522–528. doi:10.1016/j.jad.2015.09.050

RISK FOR COMPROMISED HUMAN DIGNITY

Definition

Vulnerable for perceived loss of respect and honor, which may compromise health

Assessment

- Patient's perception of present health problem and problem-solving techniques used
- Patient health status; attitude toward and use of health care services; and beliefs, values, and attitudes about illness
- Family status, including family composition; responsibilities assumed in caring for family members (including patient); and ability of family to meet their physical, social, emotional, and economic needs
- Support systems, including family members, friends, and clergy
- Health history, including medical or mental illness, self-care abilities, and disabilities and deformities
- Legal status, including patient's authority to give consent for treatments or procedures
- Attitude of health care providers toward the patient
- Welfare and health care system and reliance on welfare for support

Risk Factors

- Cultural incongruence
- Dehumanizing treatment
- Disclosure of confidential information
- Exposure of the body
- Humiliation
- Insufficient comprehension of health information
- Invasion of privacy
- Limited decision-making experience
- Loss of control of body functions
- Stigmatization

Expected Outcomes

- Patient and family will express satisfaction with level of respect.
- Patient will identify a plan to reduce feelings of powerlessness and vulnerability and increase feelings of autonomy.
- Patient and family will develop and implement plans to protect privacy and confidentiality of patient.
- Patient and family will evaluate success of plans to protect patient privacy and confidentiality.
- Patient and family will report a reduction or elimination of compromised human dignity.

Suggested NOC Outcomes

Client Satisfaction: Protection of Rights; Coping; Personal Autonomy; Self-Esteem

Interventions and Rationales

- PCC Assess patient's satisfaction with the health care environment *to determine the extent of positive perception of the nursing staff's concern for the patient.*
- PCC Work with patient to develop a plan to increase autonomy *to promote feelings of control and independence in making life decisions.*
- PCC Include patient or patient's representative in all decision making. *This demonstrates a sense of respect for patient's right to make decisions that affect personal well-being.*
- PCC Work closely with patient and health professionals *to promote the positive perception of protection of a patient's legal and moral rights provided by nursing and other staff.*
- Implement a program to promote patient dignity that involves staff, family, and community *to assist patient in coping to manage the stressors that tax personal resources.*
- PCC Work with various health professionals, families, educators, and students *to determine the extent of the problem of protecting human dignity in the delivery of health care.*
- Encourage health professional groups and religious and social service organizations to feature guest speakers *to provide information on aspects of bioethics and human dignity in the care of patients.*
- PCC Provide education on the legal and ethical rights of patients to human dignity, and have current information available at community and senior centers. *Access to information provides patients and their families with appropriate resources to seek help.*
- PCC Encourage patient and family to participate in support networks that allow them to discuss caregiving and illness pressures and other issues related to the provision of human dignity. *This gives patient and family a chance to express their feelings openly and obtain support.*
- Develop a referral list for patient and family that includes resources that promote human dignity, including charities, clinics, support groups, and senior centers *to promote family involvement in decision making and delivery and evaluation of care.*

Suggested NIC Interventions

Body Image Enhancement; Presence; Self-Awareness Enhancement; Self-Esteem Enhancement

Evaluations for Expected Outcomes

- Patient and family express satisfaction with level of respect for the patient.
- Patient and family articulate plan to reduce feelings of powerlessness and vulnerability and increase feelings of patient autonomy.
- Patient and family develop and implement plan to protect patient privacy and confidentiality.
- Patient and family report success of plan to protect patient privacy and confidentiality.
- Patient and family report a reduction or elimination of compromised human dignity.

Documentation

- Patient and family perception of understanding of the need for human dignity
- Community resources that exist to promote human dignity

- Patient and family plans to promote human dignity
- Evaluations for expected outcomes

REFERENCES

Hurtley, R. (2015). Ensuring dignity at the end of life: a personal perspective. *Nursing & Residential Care, 17*(7), 380–384.

Råholm, M., Lillestø, B., Lohne, V., Caspari, S., Sæteren, B., Tolo Heggestad, A. K., ... Nåden, D. (2014). Perspectives of dignity of residents living in nursing homes—Experiences of family caregivers. *International Journal for Human Caring, 18*(4), 34–39.

Skorpen, F., Rehnsfeldt, A., & Thorsen, A. A. (2015). The significance of small things for dignity in psychiatric care. *Nursing Ethics, 22*(7), 754–764. doi:10.1177/0969733014551376

HYPERTHERMIA

related to increase in metabolic rate

Definition

Core body temperature above the normal diurnal range due to failure of thermoregulation

Assessment

- History of present illness
- History of exposure to communicable disease
- Health history, including chronic disease or disability, pathologic conditions known to cause dehydration, recent traumatic event, exposure to sources of infection, exposure to communicable diseases, and other related events
- Medications
- Physiologic manifestations of fever, including vital signs and skin temperature and color
- Fluid and electrolyte status, including skin turgor, intake and output, mucous membranes, serum electrolyte levels, and urine specific gravity
- Laboratory studies, including white blood cell count and culture and sensitivity findings
- Neurologic status, including level of consciousness (LOC) and orientation
- Skin integrity, including open lesions and rashes

Defining Characteristics

- Abnormal posturing
- Apnea
- Coma
- Convulsions
- Flushed skin
- Hypotension
- Infant does not maintain suck
- Irritability
- Lethargy
- Seizure
- Skin warm to touch
- Stupor
- Tachycardia
- Tachypnea
- Vasodilation

Expected Outcomes

- Patient will remain afebrile.

- Patient will maintain adequate hydration:
  - Intake and output will be balanced and within normal limits.
  - Urine specific gravity will range from 1.005 to 1.015.
- Patient will exhibit moist mucous membranes.
- Patient will exhibit good skin turgor.
- Patient will remain alert and responsive.

Suggested NOC Outcomes

Comfort Level; Hydration; Infection Severity; Thermoregulation; Vital Signs

Interventions and Rationales

- Take temperature every 1 to 4 hours *to obtain an accurate core temperature.* Identify route and record measurements. Use the same method each time temperature is taken.
- Administer antipyretics, as prescribed, and record effectiveness. *Antipyretics act on hypothalamus to regulate temperature.*
- Use nonpharmacologic measures to reduce excessive fever, such as removing sheets, blankets, and most clothing; placing ice bags on axillae and groin; and sponging with tepid water. Explain these measures to patient. *Nonpharmacologic measures lower body temperature and promote comfort. Sponging reduces body temperature by increasing evaporation from skin. Tepid water is used because cold water increases shivering, thereby increasing metabolic rate and causing temperature to rise.*
- Use a hypothermia blanket if patient's temperature rises above 103° F (39.4° C). Monitor vital signs every 15 minutes for 1 hour and then as indicated. *Temperatures that exceed 103 cannot be controlled with antipyretics alone.*
- Turn hypothermia blanket off if shivering occurs. *Shivering increases metabolic rate, increasing temperature.*
- S Monitor heart rate and rhythm, blood pressure, respiratory rate, LOC and level of responsiveness, and capillary refill time every 1 to 4 hours *to evaluate effectiveness of interventions and monitor for complications.*
- PCC Determine patient's preferences for oral fluids, and encourage patient to drink as much as possible, unless contraindicated. Monitor and record intake and output, and administer IV fluids, if indicated. *Because insensible fluid loss increases by 10% for every 1.8° F (1° C) increase in temperature, patient must increase fluid intake to prevent dehydration.*

Suggested NIC Interventions

Environmental Management; Fever Treatment; Fluid Management; Temperature Regulation

Evaluations for Expected Outcomes

- Patient remains afebrile.
- Patient maintains adequate hydration:
  - Intake and output are balanced and within normal limit for age.
  - Urine specific gravity ranges from 1.005 to 1.015.
- Patient exhibits moist mucous membranes.
- Patient exhibits good skin turgor.
- Patient remains alert and responsive.

Documentation

- Observations of physical findings
- Nursing interventions and patient's response to interventions
- Administration of medication, such as antipyretics, and patient's response
- Evaluations for expected outcomes

REFERENCES

Dam, N. M., & McCarthy, A. L. (2015). Nursing fever management in adult oncology patients: A literature review. *Australian Journal of Cancer Nursing*, *16*(2), 12–17.

Monsma, J., Richerson, J., & Sloand, E. (2015). Empowering parents for evidence-based fever management: An integrative review. *Journal of the American Association of Nurse Practitioners*, *27*(4), 222–229. doi:10.1002/2327-6924.12152

Rockett, H., Thompson, H. J., & Blissitt, P. A. (2015). Fever management practices of neuroscience nurses: What has changed? *Journal of Neuroscience Nursing*, *47*(2), 66–75. doi:10.1097/JNN.0000000000000118

HYPOTHERMIA

related to low environmental temperature

Definition

Core body temperature below the normal diurnal range due to failure of thermoregulation

Assessment

- History of present illness
- Exposure to cold
- Circumstances surrounding development of hypothermia
- Age
- Medication history
- Neurologic status, including level of consciousness, mental status, motor status, and sensory status
- Cardiovascular status, including blood pressure, capillary refill time, electrocardiogram results, heart rate and rhythm, pulses (apical, peripheral), and temperature
- Respiratory status, including arterial blood gas analysis; breath sounds; and rate, depth, and character of respirations
- Integumentary status, including color, temperature, and turgor
- Nutritional status, including current (and normal) weight and dietary pattern
- Fluid and electrolyte status, including blood urea nitrogen level, intake and output, serum electrolyte levels, and urine specific gravity
- Psychosocial status, including behavior, financial resources, mood, and occupation

Defining Characteristics

- Acrocyanosis
- Bradycardia
- Cyanotic nail beds
- Decrease in blood glucose level
- Decrease in ventilation
- Hypertension
- Hypoglycemia
- Hypoxia
- Increase in metabolic rate
- Increase in oxygen consumption
- Peripheral vasoconstriction
- Piloerection

- Shivering
- Skin cool to touch
- Slow capillary refill
- Tachycardia

Accidental Low Body Temperature in Children and Adults

- Mild hypothermia, core temperature 32° C to 35° C
- Moderate hypothermia, core temperature 30° C to 32° C
- Severe hypothermia, core temperature <30° C

Injured Adults and Children

- Hypothermia, core temperature <35° C
- Severe hypothermia, core temperature <32° C

Neonates

- Grade 1 hypothermia, core temperature 36° C to 36.5° C
- Grade 2 hypothermia, core temperature 35° C to 35.9° C
- Grade 3 hypothermia, core temperature 34° C to 34.9° C
- Grade 4 hypothermia, core temperature <34° C
- Infant with insufficient energy to maintain sucking
- Infant with insufficient weight gain (<30 g/day)
- Irritability
- Jaundice
- Metabolic acidosis
- Pallor
- Respiratory distress

Expected Outcomes

- Patient's body temperature will remain within normal range.
- Patient's skin will feel warm and dry.
- Patient's heart rate and blood pressure will remain within normal range.
- Patient won't shiver.
- Patient will express feelings of comfort.
- Patient will show no complications associated with hypothermia, such as soft tissue injury, fracture, dehydration, and hypovolemic shock, if warmed too quickly.
- Patient will understand how to prevent further episodes of hypothermia.

Suggested NOC Outcomes

Comfort Level; Neurologic Status: Autonomic; Thermoregulation; Vital Signs

Interventions and Rationales

- Monitor body temperature at least every 4 hours or more frequently, if indicated, *to evaluate effectiveness of interventions.* Record temperature and route *to allow accurate data comparison.* Baseline temperatures vary, depending on route used. If temperature drops below 95° F (35° C), use a low-reading thermometer *to obtain accurate reading.*
- Monitor and record neurologic status at least every 4 hours. *Falling body temperature and metabolic rate reduce pulse rate and blood pressure, which reduces blood perfusion to brain, resulting in disorientation, confusion, and unconsciousness.*
- Monitor and record heart rate and rhythm, blood pressure, and respiratory rate at least every 4 hours. Blood pressure and pulse decrease in hypothermia. *During rewarming, patient may develop hypovolemic shock. During warming, ventricular fibrillation and cardiac arrest may occur, possibly signaled by irregular pulse.*

- Provide supportive measures, such as placing patient in warm bed and covering with warm blankets, removing wet or constrictive clothing, and covering metal or plastic surfaces that contact patient's body. *These measures protect patient from heat loss.*
- Follow prescribed treatment regimen for hypothermia:
  - As ordered, administer medications *to prevent shivering to avoid overheating*. Monitor and record effectiveness.
  - As ordered, administer analgesic *to relieve pain associated with warming*. Monitor and record effectiveness.
  - Use hyperthermia blanket to *warm patient* if temperature drops below 95° F (35° C). Warm patient to 97° F (36.1° C).
  - As appropriate, administer fluids during rewarming *to prevent hypovolemic shock*. If administering large volumes of IV fluids, consider using a fluid warmer *to avoid heat loss.*
- Discuss precipitating factors with patient, if indicated. *Patient may require community outreach assistance with certain precipitating factors, including inadequate living conditions, insufficient finances, and abuse of medications (such as sedatives and alcohol).*
- PCC Instruct patient in precautionary measures to avoid hypothermia, such as dressing warmly even when indoors, eating proper diet, and remaining as active as possible. *Precautions help to prevent accidental hypothermia.*

Suggested NIC Interventions

Comfort Level; Fluid Management; Hypothermia Treatment; Temperature Regulation; Vital Signs Monitoring

Evaluations for Expected Outcomes

- Patient's temperature remains within normal range.
- Patient's skin is warm and dry.
- Patient's heart rate and blood pressure remain within normal range.
- Patient doesn't shiver.
- Patient voices feelings of comfort.
- Patient doesn't develop complications associated with hypothermia.
- Patient describes measures to prevent further episodes of hypothermia.

Documentation

- Patient's shivering and complaints of coldness
- Observations of physical findings
- Nursing interventions and patient's response to interventions, including physiologic, behavioral, and cognitive
- Evaluations for expected outcomes

REFERENCES

Singh, T., & Hallows, K. R. (2014). Hemodialysis for the treatment of severe accidental hypothermia. *Seminars in Dialysis*, *27*(3), 295–297. doi:10.1111/sdi.12156

Wood, T., & Thoresen, M. (2015). Physiological responses to hypothermia. *Seminars in Fetal & Neonatal Medicine*, *20*(2), 87–96. doi:10.1016/j.siny.2014.10.005

Zafren, K., Giesbrecht, G. G., Danzl, D. F., Brugger, H., Sagalyn, E. B., Walpoth, B., … Grissom, C. K. (2014). Wilderness Medical Society practice guidelines for the out-of-hospital evaluation and treatment of accidental hypothermia: 2014 Update. *Wilderness & Environmental Medicine*, *25*(4), S66–S85. doi:10.1016/j.wem.2014.10.010

BOWEL INCONTINENCE

related to impaired cognition

Definition

Change in normal bowel habits characterized by involuntary passage of stool

Assessment

- History of neurologic or psychiatric disorder
- Fluid and electrolyte status, including intake and output, skin turgor, urine specific gravity, and mucous membranes
- Gastrointestinal status, including usual bowel elimination habits, change in bowel habits, stool characteristics (color, amount, size, and consistency), pain or discomfort, inspection of abdomen, auscultation of bowel sounds, palpation for masses and tenderness, percussion for tympany and dullness, and laxative and enema use
- Characteristics of incontinence, including frequency, time of day, before or after meals, relationship to activity, and behavior pattern (restlessness)
- Neurologic status, including orientation, level of consciousness, memory, and cognitive ability

Defining Characteristics

- Bowel urgency
- Constant passage of soft stool
- Does not recognize urge to defecate
- Fecal odor
- Fecal staining of bedding
- Fecal staining of clothing
- Inability to delay defecation
- Inability to expel formed stool despite recognition of rectal fullness
- Inability to recognize rectal fullness
- Inattentive to urge to defecate
- Reddened perianal skin

Expected Outcomes

- Patient will experience bowel movement every _____ day(s) when placed on commode or toilet at _____ a.m./p.m.
- Patient's skin will remain clean and intact.
- Patient will improve control of incontinent episodes.
- Caregiver will state understanding of bowel routine.
- Caregiver will demonstrate skill in placing patient on commode.
- Caregiver will demonstrate skill in use of suppository if indicated.
- Caregiver will understand and explain relationship of food and fluid regulation to promotion of continence.
- Patient will maintain self-respect and dignity through participation and acceptance within group.

Suggested NOC Outcomes

Bowel Continence; Bowel Elimination; Cognition; Self-Care: Toileting; Tissue Integrity: Skin & Mucous Membranes

Interventions and Rationales

- Establish a regular pattern for bowel care; for example, after breakfast every other day, place patient on commode chair, and allow patient to remain upright for 30 minutes for maximum response; then clean anal area. *Following a routine encourages regular physiologic function.*
- Monitor and record incontinent episodes; keep baseline record for 3 to 7 days *to track effectiveness of toileting routine.*
- PCC Discuss bowel care routine with family or caregiver *to foster compliance.*
- Demonstrate bowel care routine to family or caregiver *to reduce anxiety from lack of knowledge or involvement in care.*
- Arrange for return demonstration of bowel care routine *to help establish therapeutic relationship with patient and family or caregiver.*
- Establish a date when family or caregiver will carry out bowel care routine with supportive assistance; *this will ensure that patient receives dependable care.*
- PCC Instruct family or caregiver on need to regulate foods and fluids that cause diarrhea or constipation *to encourage helpful nutritional habits.*
- Maintain diet log *to identify irritating foods,* and then eliminate them from patient's diet.
- Clean and dry perianal area after each incontinent episode *to prevent infection and promote comfort.*
- PCC Maintain patient's dignity by using protective padding under clothing, by removing patient from group activity after incontinent episode, and by cleaning and returning patient to group without undue attention. *These measures prevent odor, skin breakdown, and embarrassment, and promote patient's positive self-image.*

Suggested NIC Interventions

Bowel Incontinence Care; Bowel Management; Perineal Care; Skin Surveillance

Evaluations for Expected Outcomes

- Patient has one soft bowel movement every ____ day(s).
- Patient's skin remains clean, dry, and intact.
- Patient's episodes of incontinence decrease by 50%.
- Caregiver can explain bowel routine.
- Caregiver successfully demonstrates placing patient on commode.
- Caregiver successfully demonstrates insertion of suppositories.
- Caregiver explains relationship between food and fluid intake and regulation of continence, and plans appropriate diet for patient.
- Patient expresses positive self-image.

Documentation

- Patient's level of awareness, response to incontinent episodes, and acceptance of bowel care routine

- Family's or caregiver's response to incontinence and to establishment and implementation of a bowel care routine
- Observation of effects of bowel care routine, episodes of incontinence, stool characteristics, and condition of skin
- Family's or caregiver's skill in carrying out bowel care routine and modifying diet
- Evaluations for expected outcomes

REFERENCES

Collins, E., Hibberts, F., Lyons, M., Williams, A. B., & Schizas, A. P. (2014). Outcomes in nonsurgical management for bowel dysfunction. *British Journal of Nursing*, *23*(14), 776–780. doi:10.12968/bjon.2014.23.14.776

Flanagan, L., Roe, B., Jack, B., Shaw, C., Williams, K. S., Chung, A., & Barrett, J. (2014). Factors with the management of incontinence and promotion of continence in older people in care homes. *Journal of Advanced Nursing*, *70*(3), 476–496. doi:10.1111/jan.12220

Peart, J., & Richardson, A. (2015). Developing a critical care bowel management assessment tool to manage fecal incontinence. *Nursing in Critical Care*, *20*(1), 34–40. doi:10.1111/nicc.12101

BOWEL INCONTINENCE

related to lower motor nerve damage

Definition

Change in normal bowel habits characterized by involuntary passage of stool

Assessment

- History of neuromuscular disorder
- Gastrointestinal status, including usual bowel elimination pattern, history of bowel disorder, laxative or enema use, incontinence characteristics (frequency, awareness of need to defecate, and precipitating factors), presence or absence of anal sphincter reflex, and bowel sounds
- Fluid and electrolyte status, including intake and output, urine specific gravity, skin turgor, and mucous membranes
- Nutritional status, including usual dietary pattern, appetite, tolerance or intolerance for foods, current (and normal) weight
- Activity status, including type of exercise, frequency, and duration

Defining Characteristics

- Bowel urgency
- Constant passage of soft stool
- Does not recognize urge to defecate
- Fecal odor
- Fecal staining of bedding
- Fecal staining of clothing
- Inability to delay defecation
- Inability to expel formed stool despite recognition of rectal fullness
- Inability to recognize rectal fullness
- Inattentive to urge to defecate
- Reddened perianal skin

Expected Outcomes

- Patient will establish and maintain a regular pattern of bowel care.
- Patient will state understanding of bowel care routine.
- Patient or caregiver will demonstrate skill in carrying out bowel care routine with help from nurse.
- Patient or caregiver will demonstrate increasing skill in performing bowel care routine independently.
- Patient will participate in social activities.

Suggested NOC Outcomes

Bowel Continence; Bowel Elimination; Self-Care: Hygiene; Self-Care: Toileting; Tissue Integrity: Skin & Mucous Membranes

Interventions and Rationales

- For upper motor neuron lesion (anal reflex intact):
  - Establish regular pattern for bowel care; for example, after breakfast every other day, maintain patient in upright position after inserting suppository, and allow a half-hour for suppository to melt and maximum reflex response to occur. *Regular pattern encourages adaptation and routine physiologic function.*
  - PCC Discuss bowel care routine with patient and family *to promote feelings of safety, adequacy, and comfort.*
  - Demonstrate bowel care to patient and caregivers *to reduce anxiety from lack of knowledge or involvement in care.*
  - Observe return demonstration of bowel care routine by patient and caregivers *to check skills and establish a therapeutic relationship.*
  - Establish a date when patient or caregivers will carry out bowel routine independently, with supportive assistance, *to reassure patient of dependable care.*
  - PCC Instruct patient and family on need to regulate foods and fluids that cause diarrhea or constipation *to encourage good nutritional habits.*
  - Maintain dietary intake diary *to identify irritating foods;* instruct patient to avoid foods that are spicy, rich, or that produce gas *to prevent painful flatulence.*
  - Obtain order allowing modified bowel preparations for tests and procedures *to avoid interrupting routine and to encourage regular bowel function.*
  - Encourage patient to use protective padding under clothing, changing it as necessary *to prevent odor, skin breakdown, or embarrassment and to promote positive self-image.*
- For lower motor neuron lesion (flaccid sphincter):
  - Establish regular pattern for bowel care; for example, after breakfast every other day, turn patient on left side, put waterproof pads under buttocks, administer prescribed enema, and allow patient to remain in place for 2 to 5 minutes. Then perform digital removal of stool, clean perianal area, and remove soiled pads. *These procedures encourage regular physiologic function, stimulate peristalsis, minimize infection, and promote comfort and elimination.*
  - Follow interventions for upper motor neuron lesion.

Suggested NIC Interventions

Bowel Incontinence Care; Bowel Training; Emotional Support; Fluid Management; Self-Care Assistance: Toileting; Skin Surveillance; Teaching: Toilet Training

Evaluations for Expected Outcomes

- Patient establishes and maintains regular pattern of bowel care.
- Patient states understanding of bowel care routine.
- Patient or caregiver demonstrates competence in performing bowel care routine with assistance from nurse.
- Patient or caregiver carries out bowel routine independently.
- Patient attends social events without experiencing bowel incontinence.

Documentation

- Patient's feelings about problem and bowel routine
- Bowel care routine and administration of suppositories and enemas
- Description of incontinent episodes, including known precipitating factors, time of day, and other relevant details
- Patient's and caregivers' skills in bowel care
- Evaluations for expected outcomes

REFERENCES

Collins, E., Hibberts, F., Lyons, M., Williams, A. B., & Schizas, A. P. (2014). Outcomes in non-surgical management for bowel dysfunction. *British Journal of Nursing*, *23*(14), 776–780. doi:10.12968/bjon.2014.23.14.776

Flanagan, L., Roe, B., Jack, B., Shaw, C., Williams, K. S., Chung, A., & Barrett, J. (2014). Factors with the management of incontinence and promotion of continence in older people in care homes. *Journal of Advanced Nursing*, *70*(3), 476–496. doi:10.1111/jan.12220

Peart, J., & Richardson, A. (2015). Developing a critical care bowel management assessment tool to manage fecal incontinence. *Nursing in Critical Care*, *20*(1), 34–40. doi:10.1111/nicc.12101

FUNCTIONAL URINARY INCONTINENCE

related to alteration in cognitive functioning

Definition

Inability of a usually continent person to reach the toilet in time to avoid unintentional loss of urine

Assessment

- History of mental illness
- Age
- Gender
- Vital signs
- Genitourinary status, including frequency and voiding pattern

- Fluid and electrolyte status, including blood urea nitrogen level, creatinine level, intake and output, mucous membranes, serum electrolyte levels, and skin turgor
- Neuromuscular status, including activities of daily living, mental status, mobility, and sensory ability to perceive bladder fullness
- Psychosocial status, including behavior before and after voiding, support from family members, impact of incontinence on self and others, and stressors (family, job, and change in environment)

Defining Characteristics

- Completely empties bladder
- Early morning urinary incontinence
- Sensation of need to void
- Time between sensation of urge and ability to reach toilet is too short
- Voiding prior to reaching toilet

Expected Outcomes

- Patient will void at appropriate intervals.
- Patient won't void in unacceptable situations.
- Patient will have minimal, if any, complications.
- Patient and family members will demonstrate skill in managing incontinence.
- Patient will discuss impact of incontinence on self and family members.
- Patient and family members will identify resources to assist with care following discharge.

Suggested NOC Outcomes

Coordinated Movement; Self-Care: Toileting; Symptom Control; Urinary Continence; Urinary Elimination

Interventions and Rationales

- Monitor and record patient's voiding patterns *to ensure correct fluid replacement therapy.*
- Assist with specific bladder elimination procedures, such as the following:
  - Bladder training. Place patient on commode or toilet every 2 hours while awake and once during night. *Successful bladder training revolves around adequate fluid intake, muscle-strengthening exercises, and carefully scheduled voiding times.*
  - Rigid toilet regimen. Place patient on toilet at specific intervals (every 2 hours or after meals). Note whether patient was wet or dry and whether voiding occurred at each interval. *This helps patient adapt to routine physiologic function.*
  - Behavior modification. Reward continence or voiding in lavatory. Don't punish unwanted behavior such as voiding in wrong place. Reinforce behavior consistently, using social or material rewards. *This helps patient learn alternatives to maladaptive behaviors.*
  - Use of external catheter. Apply according to established procedure and maintain patency. Observe condition of perineal skin, and clean with soap and water at least twice daily. *This ensures effective therapy and prevents infection and skin breakdown.*
  - Application of protective pads and garments. Use only when interventions have failed to prevent infection and skin breakdown and promote social acceptance. Allow at least 4 to 6 weeks for trial period. *Establishing continence requires prolonged effort.*

- Maintain continence based on patient's voiding patterns and limitations.
  - Use reminders. *Reminders help limit amount of information patient must retain in memory.*
  - Orient patient to toileting environment: time, place, and activity. *A structured environment offers security and helps patient with elimination problems.*
  - Stimulate patient's voiding reflexes (give patient water to drink while on toilet, stroke area over bladder, or pour water over perineum). *External stimulation triggers bladder's spastic reflex.*
  - Provide hyperactive patient with distraction, such as a magazine, to occupy attention while on toilet. *This reduces anxiety and eases voiding.*
  - Provide privacy and adequate time *to void to allow patient to void easily without anxiety.*
  - Praise successful performance *to give patient a sense of control and to encourage compliance.*
  - Change wet clothes to accustom patient *to dry clothes.*
  - PCC Teach family members and support personnel to assist, *thus reducing anxiety that results from noninvolvement and increasing chances for successful treatment.*
  - Respond to patient's call light promptly *to avoid delays in voiding routine.*
  - Choose patient's clothing to promote easy dressing and undressing (e.g., use Velcro fasteners and gowns instead of pajamas.) *This reduces patient's frustration with voiding routine.*
- Schedule patient's fluid intake to encourage voiding at convenient times. Maintain adequate hydration up to 3,000 mL daily, unless contraindicated. *Scheduling fluid intake promotes regular bladder distention and optimal time intervals between voidings.* Limit fluid intake to 150 mL after dinner *to reduce need to void at night.*
- PCC Instruct patient and family members in continence techniques to use at home *to increase chances of successful bladder retraining.*
- Encourage patient and family members to share feelings related to incontinence. *This allows specific problems to be identified and resolved. Attentive listening conveys recognition and respect.*
- PCC Refer patient and family members to psychiatric liaison nurse, home health care agency, or support group *to provide access to additional community resources.*

Suggested NIC Interventions

Environmental Management; Pelvic Muscle Exercise; Prompted Voiding; Self-Care Assistance; Urinary Elimination Management; Urinary Habit Training

Evaluations for Expected Outcomes

- Patient voids at appropriate intervals, with minimal episodes of incontinence.
- Patient recognizes urge to void, undresses without assistance, and uses toilet.
- Patient doesn't experience urinary tract infection, skin breakdown, or other complications related to incontinence.
- Patient and family members demonstrate proper procedures for managing incontinence.
- Patient expresses feelings about condition and its effect on family. Patient and family members are neither overwhelmed nor excessively optimistic about patient's condition.
- Patient and family members contact support group or home health care agency, if needed.

Documentation

- Observations of incontinence and response to treatment regimen
- Interventions to provide supportive care and patient's response to supportive care
- Instructions given to patient and family members; return demonstration of knowledge and skills needed to carry out continence management techniques
- Patient's expression of concern about incontinence and motivation to participate in self-care
- Evaluations for expected outcomes

REFERENCES

Block, V., Rivera, M., Melnick, M., & Allen, D. D. (2015). Do physical therapy interventions affect urinary incontinence and quality of life in people with multiple sclerosis? *International Journal of MS Care*, *17*(4), 172–180. doi:10.7224/1537-2073.2014-031

Chiu, A., Huang, M., Hsu, M., Liu, J., & Chiu, J. (2015). Association of urinary incontinence with impaired functional status among older people living in a long-term care setting. *Geriatrics & Gerontology International*, *15*(3), 296–301. doi:10.1111/ggi.12272

Gosch, M., Talasz, H., Nicholas, J. A., Kammerlander, C., & Lechleitner, M. (2015). Urinary incontinence and poor functional status in fragility fracture patients: An under recognized and underappreciated association. *Archives of Orthopedic & Trauma Surgery*, *135*(1), 59–67. doi:10.1007/s00402-014-2113-6

OVERFLOW URINARY INCONTINENCE

Definition

Involuntary loss of urine associated with overdistention of the bladder

Assessment

- History of mental illness
- Age
- Gender
- Vital signs
- Genitourinary status, including frequency and voiding pattern
- Fluid and electrolyte status, including blood urea nitrogen level, creatinine level, intake and output, mucous membranes, serum electrolyte levels, and skin turgor
- Neuromuscular status, including activities of daily living, mental status, mobility, and sensory ability to perceive bladder fullness
- Psychosocial status, including behavior before and after voiding, support from family members, impact of incontinence on self and others, and stressors (family, job, and change in environment)

Defining Characteristics

- Bladder distention
- High postvoid residual volume
- Involuntary leakage of small volume of urine
- Nocturia

Expected Outcomes

- Patient will void 200 to 300 mL of clear, yellow urine every 3 to 4 hours while awake.
- Patient will have postvoid residual of less than 50 mL.
- Patient will have reduction in urinary incontinence episodes or complete absence of urinary incontinence.

- Patient will experience relief from most bothersome aspect of urinary incontinence.
- Patient will remain clean and dry without urine odor.
- Patient will express understanding of condition and activities to prevent/reduce overflow incontinence.
- Patient will express improvement in quality of life.

Suggested NOC Outcomes

Knowledge: Treatment Regimen; Urinary Continence

Interventions and Rationales

- Monitor and record patient's voiding patterns *to determine existence and extent of overflow incontinence.*
- Monitor and record patient's intake and output *to determine fluid balance.*
- Ask patient to keep a bladder diary of continent and incontinent voids to promote understanding of the extent of the problem of overflow incontinence. Discuss voiding and fluid intake patterns. *Accurate understanding of patient's pattern provides a baseline for introducing new activities.*
- Provide privacy and adequate time to void *to decrease anxiety and promote relaxation of sphincter.*
- Assist patient to assume usual position for voiding. *Some patients are unable to void while lying in bed and may develop urinary retention and overflow incontinence.*
- Massage (credé) the bladder area during urination to increase pressure in the pelvic area *to encourage drainage of urine from the bladder.*
- Institute indwelling or intermittent catheterization, as ordered. Catheterization is used as a last resort *to empty the bladder preventing overflow incontinence.*
- Assist with application of pads and protective garments (used only as a last resort) *to prevent skin breakdown and odor and to promote social acceptance.*
- PCC Teach patient and/or family to catheterize patient with chronic overflow incontinence related to urinary retention using clean technique *to manage long-term overflow incontinence.*
- PCC Teach stress management and relaxation techniques. *Stress and anxiety interfere with sphincter relaxation, causing urinary retention and overflow incontinence.*
- PCC Encourage patient to share feelings related to incontinence *to reduce anxiety.*
- Encourage patient to drink six to eight glasses of noncaffeinated, nonalcoholic, and noncarbonated liquid, preferably water, per day (unless contraindicated). *1,500 to 2,000 mL/day promotes optimal renal function and flushes bacteria and solutes from the urinary tract. Caffeine and alcohol promote diuresis and may contribute to excess fluid loss and irritation of the bladder wall.*
- Encourage patient to respond to the urge to void in a timely manner. *Ignoring the urge to urinate may cause incontinence.*
- Encourage patient to participate in regular exercise, including walking and modified sit-ups (unless contraindicated). *Weak abdominal and perineal muscles weaken bladder and sphincter control.*
- Encourage patient to avoid anticholinergics, opioids, psychotropics, α-adrenergic agonists, β-adrenergic agonists, and calcium-channel blockers (unless contraindicated), *which inhibit relaxation of the urinary sphincter and cause urinary retention.*
- PCC Provide referrals for physical therapy or psychological counseling as necessary *to enhance success.*

Suggested NIC Interventions

Urinary Incontinence Care; Urinary Retention Care

Evaluations for Expected Outcomes

- Patient voids at appropriate intervals, with minimal episodes of incontinence.
- Patient recognizes urge to void, undresses without assistance, and uses toilet.
- Patient expresses feelings about condition and its effect on family. Patient and family members are neither overwhelmed nor excessively optimistic about patient's condition.
- Patient experiences no unpleasant urine odor.

Documentation

- Observations of incontinence and response to treatment regimen
- Interventions to provide supportive care and patient's response to supportive care
- Instructions given to patient and family members; return demonstration of knowledge and skills needed to carry out continence management techniques
- Patient's expression of concern about incontinence and motivation to participate in self-care
- Evaluations for expected outcomes

REFERENCES

Fawcett, J. (2014). Effective management in male urinary incontinence. *British Journal of Community Nursing*, *19*(7), 318–321. doi:10.12968/bjcn.2014.19.7.318

Parker, W. P., & Griebling, T. L. (2015). Nonsurgical treatment of urinary incontinence in elderly women. *Clinics in Geriatric Medicine*, *31*(4), 471–485. doi:10.1016/j.cger.2015.07.003

Stanley, A. Y., & Conner, B. T. (2015). Implementing a clinical practice guideline to manage postpartum urinary retention. *Journal of Nursing Care Quality*, *30*(2), 175–180. doi:10.1097/NCQ.0000000000000087

REFLEX URINARY INCONTINENCE

related to neuromuscular impairment above level of pontine micturition center

Definition

Involuntary loss of urine at somewhat predictable intervals when a specific bladder volume is reached

Assessment

- History of sensory or neuromuscular impairment
- History of urinary tract disease, trauma, surgery, or infection
- Genitourinary status, including bladder palpation, residual urine volume after voiding, urinalysis, urine characteristics, urine culture and sensitivity, and voiding patterns
- Neuromuscular status, including anal sphincter tone, motor ability to start and stop urine stream, neuromuscular function, sensory ability to perceive bladder fullness and voiding, and involuntary voiding after stimulation of skin on abdomen, thighs, or genitals
- Fluid and electrolyte status, including blood urea nitrogen level, creatinine level, intake and output, medication history, mucous membranes, serum electrolyte levels, skin turgor, and urine specific gravity

- Sexuality status, including capability, concerns, and habits
- Psychosocial status, including coping skills, self-concept, and perception of problem by patient and family members

Defining Characteristics

- Absence of sensation of bladder fullness
- Absence of urge to void
- Absence of voiding sensation
- Inability to voluntarily inhibit voiding
- Inability to voluntarily initiate voiding
- Incomplete emptying of bladder with lesion above pontine micturition center
- Predictable pattern of voiding
- Sensation of bladder fullness
- Sensations of urgency to void without voluntary inhibition of bladder contraction

Expected Outcomes

- Patient will maintain fluid balance, with intake approximately equaling output.
- Patient will have minimal, if any, complications.
- Patient will achieve urinary continence.
- Patient and family members will demonstrate skill in managing urinary incontinence.
- Patient will discuss impact of incontinence on self and family.
- Patient and family members will identify resources to assist with care following discharge.

Suggested NOC Outcomes

Knowledge: Treatment Regimen; Nutritional Status: Food & Fluid Intake; Tissue Integrity: Skin & Mucous Membranes; Urinary Continence; Urinary Elimination

Interventions and Rationales

- Monitor intake and output *to ensure correct fluid replacement therapy.* Report output greater than intake.
- Implement and monitor effectiveness of specific bladder elimination procedure, such as the following:
  - Stimulating reflex arc. Patient who voids at somewhat predictable intervals may be able to regulate voiding by reflex arc stimulation. Trigger voiding at regular intervals (e.g., every 2 hours) by stimulating skin of abdomen, thighs, or genitals to initiate bladder contractions. Avoid stimulation at nonvoiding times. Stimulate primitive voiding reflexes by giving patient water to drink while the patient sits on toilet or by pouring water over perineum. *External stimulation triggers bladder's spastic reflex.*
  - Applying external catheter according to established procedure and maintaining patency. Observe condition of perineal skin, and clean with soap and water at least twice daily. *Cleanliness prevents skin breakdown and infection. External catheter protects surrounding skin, promotes accurate output measurement, and keeps patient dry. Applying foam strip in spiral fashion increases adhesive surface and cuts risk of impaired circulation.*
  - Inserting indwelling catheter. Monitor patency, and keep tubing free from kinks *to avoid drainage pooling and ensure accurate therapy.* Keep drainage bag below level of

bladder *to avoid urine reflux into bladder.* Perform catheter care according to established procedure. Maintain closed drainage system *to prevent bacteriuria.* Secure catheter to leg (female) or abdomen (male) *to avoid tension on bladder and sphincter.*
   - Applying suprapubic catheter. Change dressing according to established procedure *to avoid skin breakdown.* Monitor patency, and keep tubing free from kinks *to avoid drainage pooling in loops of catheter.* Keep drainage bag below bladder level *to avoid urine reflux into bladder.* Maintain closed drainage system *to prevent bacteriuria.*
   - Changing wet clothes *to prevent patient from becoming accustomed to wet clothes.*
- Encourage high fluid intake (3,000 mL daily, unless contraindicated) *to stimulate micturition reflex.* Limit fluid intake after 7 p.m. *to prevent nocturia.*
- PCC Instruct patient and family members in continence techniques to use at home. Have patient and family members return demonstrations until they can perform procedure well. *Patient education begins with assessment and depends on nurse's therapeutic relationship with patient and family.*
- PCC Encourage patient and family members to share feelings and concerns about incontinence. *A trusting environment allows nurse to make specific recommendations to resolve patient's problems.*
- PCC Refer patient and family members to psychiatric liaison nurse, home health care agency, support group, or other resources, as appropriate. *Community resources typically provide health care not available from other health agencies.*

Suggested NIC Interventions

Pelvic Muscle Exercise; Urinary Bladder Training; Urinary Elimination Management; Urinary Incontinence Care

Evaluations for Expected Outcomes

- Patient maintains fluid balance, with intake approximately equaling output.
- Patient avoids complications associated with incontinence, such as infections, swelling of penis (because of external catheter), skin breakdown, catheter obstruction, and urine odor.
- Patient achieves urinary continence.
- Patient and family members successfully demonstrate chosen technique for bladder control.
- Patient expresses both positive and negative feelings about condition. Patient can cope with dependence brought on by condition.
- Patient and family members initiate contact with support group or visiting nurse.

Documentation

- Observations of urologic condition and response to treatment regimen
- Interventions to provide supportive care and patient's response
- Instructions given to patient and family members; return demonstration of knowledge and skills needed to carry out continence management techniques
- Patient's expression of concern about incontinence and its impact on body image and lifestyle; patient's motivation to participate in self-care
- Evaluations for expected outcomes

REFERENCES

Rasmussen, M. M., Krogh, K., Clemmensen, D., Tankisi, H., Fuglsang-Frederiksen, A., Rawashdeh, Y., … Christensen, P. (2015). The artificial somato-autonomic reflex arch does not improve bowel function in subjects with spinal cord injury. *Spinal Cord, 53*(9), 705–710. doi:10.1038/sc.2015.75

Testa, A. (2015). Understanding urinary incontinence in adults. *Urologic Nursing, 35*(2), 82–86. doi:10.7257/1053-816X.2015.35.2.82
Woodward, S. (2014). Managing urinary incontinence after stroke. *British Journal of Neuroscience Nursing, 10*(Suppl 2), 25–31.

STRESS URINARY INCONTINENCE

related to weak pelvic muscles

Definition

Sudden leakage of urine with activities that increase intra-abdominal pressure

Assessment

- History of long-term use of tranquilizers, multiple pregnancies, prolonged or difficult labor, surgery, trauma, and vaginal infections
- Age
- Gender
- Vital signs
- Genitourinary status, including inspection of abdomen for scars from previous surgeries, rectal examination, vaginal examination, voiding pattern, and leakage of urine during sneezing, laughing, vomiting, coughing, defecating, physical exertion, or change from prone to upright position
- Fluid and electrolyte status, including creatinine level, blood urea nitrogen level, estrogen levels, intake and output, mucous membranes, serum electrolyte levels, and skin turgor
- Nutritional status, including appetite, dietary habits, and present weight
- Neuromuscular status, including degree of neuromuscular function, motor ability to start or stop urine stream, and sensory ability to perceive fullness
- Sexuality status, including capability, concerns, habits, and patterns
- Psychosocial status, including coping skills, self-concept, stressors (such as finances, family, and job), and perception of problem by family members

Defining Characteristics

- Involuntary leakage of small volume of urine (e.g., with coughing, laughing, sneezing, on exertion)
- Involuntary leakage of small volume of urine in the absence of detrusor contraction
- Involuntary leakage of small volume of urine in the absence of overdistended bladder

Expected Outcomes

- Patient will maintain continence.
- Patient will state increased comfort.
- Patient will state understanding of treatment.
- Patient will state understanding of surgical procedure.
- Patient and family members will demonstrate skill in managing urinary elimination problems.
- Patient and family members will identify resources to assist with care following discharge.

Suggested NOC Outcomes

Comfort Level; Referral; Tissue Integrity: Skin & Mucous Membranes; Urinary Continence; Urinary Elimination

Interventions and Rationales

- Observe patient's voiding patterns, time of voiding, amount voided, and whether voiding is provoked by stimuli. *Accurate, thorough assessment forms the basis of an effective treatment plan.*
- Provide appropriate care for patient's urologic condition, monitor progress, and report patient's responses to treatment. *Patient expects to receive adequate care and to participate in decisions regarding care.*
- Help patient to strengthen pelvic floor muscles by Kegel exercises for sphincter control. *Exercises increase muscle tone and restore cortical control.*
- PCC Promote patient's awareness of condition through education *to help patient understand illness as well as treatment.*
- Help patient reduce intra-abdominal pressure by
  - losing weight
  - avoiding heavy lifting
  - avoiding chairs or beds that are too high or too low.

  These measures reduce intra-abdominal pressure and bladder pressure.
- Provide supportive measures:
  - S PCC Respond to call bell quickly, assign patient to bed next to bathroom, put night-light in bathroom, and have patient wear easily removable clothing (gown rather than pajamas, and Velcro fasteners rather than buttons or zippers). *Early recognition of problems promotes continence; easily removed clothing reduces patient frustration and helps achieve continence.*
  - Provide privacy during toileting *to reduce anxiety and promote elimination.*
  - Have patient empty bladder before meals, at bedtime, and before leaving accessible bathroom area *to promote elimination, avoid accidents, and help relieve intra-abdominal pressure.*
  - Limit fluids to 150 mL after dinner *to reduce need to void at night.*
  - Encourage high fluid intake, unless contraindicated, *to moisten mucous membranes and maintain hydration.*
  - Suggest patient eat increased amount of salty food before going on a long trip (unless contraindicated). *Increased sodium decreases urine production.*
  - Make protective pads available for patient's undergarments, if needed, *to absorb urine, protect skin, and control odors.*
- PCC If surgery is scheduled, give attentive, appropriate preoperative and postoperative instructions and care *to reduce patient's anxiety and build trust in caregivers.*
- PCC Encourage patient to express feelings and concerns about urologic problems. *This helps patient focus on specific problem.*
- PCC Refer patient and family members to psychiatric liaison nurse, support group, or other resources, as appropriate. *Community resources typically provide health care not available from other health agencies.*
- Alert patient and family members about need for toilet schedule. Prepare for discharge according to individual needs *to ensure that patient will receive proper care.*

Suggested NIC Interventions

Pelvic Muscle Exercise; Teaching: Individual; Urinary Elimination Management; Urinary Habit Training; Urinary Incontinence Care

Evaluations for Expected Outcomes

- Patient maintains continence.
- Patient expresses satisfaction with progress in overcoming stress incontinence.
- Patient expresses understanding of techniques to reduce intra-abdominal pressure and other supportive measures.
- Patient explains surgical procedure, including risks and expected outcome.
- Patient and family members demonstrate all procedures and supportive measures to enable patient to remain continent. They also make arrangements for home care, such as providing bedroom near bathroom and purchasing easily removable clothing.
- Patient and family members contact appropriate community resources.

Documentation

- Observations of urologic condition and patient's response to treatment regimen
- Interventions to provide supportive care and patient's response to interventions
- Instructions given to patient and family members on patient's urologic problem, their response to instructions, and demonstrated ability to carry out self-care management
- Patient's expression of concern about urologic problem and its impact on body image and lifestyle
- Patient's motivation to participate in self-care
- Evaluations for expected outcomes

REFERENCES

Knarr, J., Musil, C., Warner, C., Kless, J. R., & Long, J. (2014). Female stress urinary incontinence: An evidence-based, case study approach. *Urologic Nursing*, *34*(3), 143–151. doi:10.7257/1053-816X.2014.34.3.143

Ng, S. F., Lok, M. K., Pang, S. M., & Wun, Y. T. (2014). Stress urinary incontinence in younger women in primary care: Prevalence and opportunistic intervention. *Journal of Women's Health*, *23*(1), 65–68. doi:10.1089/jwh.2013.4382

Shin, D. C., Shin, S. H., Lee, M. M., Lee, K. J., & Song, C. H. (2016). Pelvic floor muscle training for urinary incontinence in female stroke patients: A randomized, controlled, and blinded trial. *Clinical Rehabilitation*, *30*(3), 259–267. doi:10.1177/0269215515578695

URGE URINARY INCONTINENCE

related to decrease in bladder capacity

Definition

Involuntary passage of urine occurring soon after a strong sense of urgency to void

Assessment

- History of stroke, urinary tract disease, spinal cord injury, surgery, or infection
- Medication history
- Vital signs
- Genitourinary status, including cystometrogram, pain or discomfort, urinalysis, urine specific gravity, use of urinary assistive devices, and voiding pattern
- Fluid and electrolyte status, including blood urea nitrogen level, creatinine level, intake and output, mucous membranes, postvoiding residual volume, skin turgor, and serum electrolyte levels
- Neuromuscular status, including ambulation ability, degree of neuromuscular function, dexterity, and sensory ability to perceive fullness
- Sexuality status, including capability, concerns, habits, and sexual partner
- Psychosocial status, including coping skills, self-concept, stressors (such as finances, family, and job), and perception of health problem by patient and family members

Defining Characteristics

- Inability to reach toilet in time to avoid urine loss
- Involuntary loss of urine with bladder contractions
- Involuntary loss of urine with bladder spasms
- Urinary urgency

Expected Outcomes

- Patient will have fewer episodes of incontinence.
- Patient will state increased comfort.
- Patient will state understanding of treatment.
- Patient will have minimal, if any, complications.
- Patient will discuss impact of disorder on self and family members.
- Patient and family members will demonstrate skill in managing incontinence.

Suggested NOC Outcomes

Knowledge: Treatment Regimen; Self-Esteem; Tissue Integrity: Skin & Mucous Membranes; Treatment Behavior: Illness or Injury; Urinary Continence; Urinary Elimination

Interventions and Rationales

- Observe voiding pattern; document intake and output. *This ensures correct fluid replacement therapy and provides information about patient's ability to void adequately.*
- Provide appropriate care for patient's urologic condition, monitor progress, and report patient's responses to treatment. *Patient should receive adequate care and take part in decisions about care as much as possible.*
- Provide supportive measures:
  - Administer pain medication and monitor effectiveness. *Patient's knowledge that pain can be alleviated reduces tension and anxiety.*
  - Prepare pleasant toilet environment that's warm, clean, and free from odors *to promote continence.*
  - S Place commode next to bed, or assign patient bed next to bathroom. *A bedside commode or convenient bathroom requires less energy expenditure than bedpan.*
  - S Keep bed and commode at same level *to facilitate patient's movements.*

S
S

- Provide good lighting from bed to bathroom *to reduce sensory misinterpretation.*
- Remove all obstacles between bed and bathroom *to reduce chance of falling.*
- Provide clock *to help patient maintain voiding schedule through self-monitoring.*
- Unless contraindicated, maintain fluids to 3,000 mL daily *to moisten mucous membranes and ensure hydration*; limit patient to 150 mL after dinner *to reduce need to void at night.*
- Have patient wear easily removable clothes (gown instead of pajamas, and Velcro fasteners instead of buttons or zippers) *to reduce frustration and delay in voiding routine.*
- If patient loses control on way to bathroom, instruct patient to stop and take a deep breath. *Anxiety and rushing may strengthen bladder contractions.*

- Assist with specific bladder elimination procedures, such as the following:
  - Bladder training. Place patient on commode every 2 hours while awake and once during night. Provide privacy. Gradually increase intervals between toileting. *These measures aim to restore a regular voiding pattern.*
  - Rigid toilet regimen. Place patient on toilet at specific times. *This aids adaptation to routine physiologic function.* Keep baseline micturition record for 3 to 7 days *to monitor toileting effectiveness.*
- PCC Encourage patient to express feelings and concerns about the urologic problem *to identify patient's fears.*
- PCC Explain urologic condition to patient and family members; include instructions on preventive measures and established bladder schedule. *Patient education begins with educational assessment and depends on establishing a therapeutic relationship with patient and family.* Prepare patient for discharge according to individual needs *to allow patient to practice under supervision.*
- PCC Instruct patient and family members in continence techniques for home use. *This reduces fear and anxiety resulting from lack of knowledge of patient's condition, and reassures patient of continuing care.*
- PCC Refer patient and family members to psychiatric liaison nurse, support group, or other resources, as appropriate. *Community resources typically provide health care not available from other health agencies.*

Suggested NIC Interventions

Bathing; Environmental Management; Fluid Monitoring; Perineal Care; Self-Care Assistance: Toileting; Urinary Elimination Management; Urinary Habit Training; Urinary Incontinence Care

Evaluations for Expected Outcomes

- Patient maintains continence.
- Patient expresses increased comfort.
- Patient expresses understanding of treatment.
- Patient doesn't experience nighttime incontinence or other complications.
- Patient expresses feelings about condition.
- Patient and family members discuss treatment of urologic condition and home bladder schedule; they also demonstrate necessary skills.

Documentation

- Observations of urologic condition and patient's response to treatment regimen
- Interventions to provide supportive care

- Patient's response to nursing interventions
- Instructions given to patient and family members on urologic problem, their response to instructions, and their demonstrated ability to carry out self-care management
- Patient's expression of concern about urologic problem and its impact on body image and lifestyle; patient's motivation to participate in self-care
- Evaluations for expected outcomes

REFERENCES

O'Connell, K. A., Torstrick, A., & Victor, E. (2014). Cues to urinary urgency and urge incontinence. *Journal of Wound, Ostomy & Continence Nursing*, *41*(3), 259–267. doi:10.1097/WON.0000000000000023

Reid, J. (2014). Managing urinary incontinence: Guidelines for community nurses. *Journal of Community Nursing*, *28*(6), 20–26.

Weatherall, M. (2014). Current thinking about overactive bladder symptoms and urge urinary incontinence. *Australian & New Zealand Continence Journal*, *20*(2), 32–33.

RISK FOR INFECTION

related to external factors

Definition

Vulnerable to invasion and multiplication of pathogenic organisms, which may compromise health.

Assessment

- Health history, including accidents, allergies, falls, hyperthermia, hypothermia, poisoning, seizures, trauma, and exposure to pollutants
- Sensory or perceptual changes (auditory, gustatory, kinesthetic, olfactory, tactile, and visual)
- Circumstances of present situation that could lead to infection
- Neurologic status, including level of consciousness, mental status, and orientation
- Laboratory studies, including clotting factors, hemoglobin (Hb) level, hematocrit, platelet count, serum albumin level, white blood cell (WBC) count, and cultures of blood, body fluid, sputum, urine, and wound drainage

Risk Factors

- Chronic illness (e.g., diabetes mellitus)
- Inadequate vaccination
- Insufficient knowledge to avoid exposure to pathogens
- Invasive procedure
- Malnutrition
- Obesity

Inadequate Primary Defenses

- Alteration in peristalsis
- Alteration in pH of secretions
- Alteration in skin integrity
- Decrease in ciliary action
- Premature rupture of amniotic membrane
- Prolonged rupture of amniotic membrane
- Smoking
- Stasis of body fluids

Inadequate Secondary Defenses

- Decrease in Hb
- Immunosuppression
- Leukopenia

- Suppressed inflammatory response (e.g., IL-6, CRP)
- Inadequate vaccination

Increased Environmental Exposure to Pathogens

- Exposure to disease outbreak

Expected Outcomes

- Patient's temperature will stay within normal range.
- Patient's WBC count and differential will stay within normal range.
- Patient's cultures won't show evidence of pathogens.
- Patient will maintain good personal and oral hygiene.
- Patient's respiratory secretions will be clear and odorless.
- Patient's urine will remain clear, yellow, odorless, and free from sediment.
- Patient won't show evidence of diarrhea.
- Patient's wounds and incisions will appear clean, pink, and free from purulent drainage.
- Patient's IV sites won't show signs of inflammation.
- Patient won't show evidence of skin breakdown.
- Patient will take ___ mL of fluid and ___ g of protein daily.
- Patient will state infection risk factors.
- Patient will identify signs and symptoms of infection.
- Patient will remain free from signs and symptoms of infection.

Suggested NOC Outcomes

Immune Status; Infection Status; Knowledge: Treatment Procedure(s); Nutritional Status; Risk Control; Risk Detection; Wound Healing: Primary Intention

Interventions and Rationales

S

- Minimize patient's risk of infection by:
  - washing hands before and after providing care. *Hand washing is the single best way to avoid spreading pathogens.*
  - wearing gloves to maintain asepsis when providing direct care. *Gloves offer protection when handling wound dressings or carrying out various treatments.*
- Monitor temperature at least every 4 hours, and record on graph paper. Report elevations immediately. *Sustained temperature elevation after surgery may signal onset of pulmonary complications, wound infection or dehiscence, urinary tract infection, or thrombophlebitis.*
- Monitor WBC count, as ordered. Report elevations or depressions. Elevated total WBC count indicates infection. *Markedly decreased WBC count may indicate decreased production resulting from extreme debilitation or severe lack of vitamins and amino acids. Any damage to bone marrow may suppress WBC formation.*
- Culture urine, respiratory secretions, wound drainage, or blood according to facility policy and physician's order. *This identifies pathogens and guides antibiotic therapy.*
- Help patient wash hands before and after meals and after using bathroom, bedpan, or urinal. *Hand washing prevents spread of pathogens to other objects and food.*
- Assist patient when necessary to ensure that perianal area is clean after elimination. *Cleaning perineal area by wiping from area of least contamination (urinary meatus) to area of most contamination (anus) helps prevent genitourinary infections.*
- Instruct patient to report incidents of loose stools or diarrhea. Inform physician immediately. *Diarrhea or loose stools may indicate need to discontinue or change antibiotic therapy. It may also indicate need to test for Clostridium difficile.*

- Offer oral hygiene to patient every 4 hours to prevent colonization of bacteria and reduce risk of descending infection. *Disease and malnutrition may reduce moisture in mucous membranes of mouth and lips.*
- Use strict sterile technique when suctioning lower airway, inserting indwelling urinary catheters, inserting IV catheters, and providing wound care *to avoid spreading pathogens.*
- Change IV tubing, and give site care every 24 to 48 hours or as facility policy dictates *to help keep pathogens from entering body.*
- Rotate IV sites every 48 to 72 hours or as facility policy dictates *to reduce chances of infection at individual sites.*
- Have patient cough and deep-breathe every 4 hours after surgery *to help remove secretions and prevent pulmonary complications.*
- Provide tissues and disposal bags for expectorated sputum. *Convenient disposal encourages expectoration; sanitary disposal reduces spread of infection.*
- Help patient turn every 2 hours. Provide skin care, particularly over bony prominences, *to help prevent venous stasis and skin breakdown.*
- Use sterile water for humidification or nebulization of oxygen. *This prevents drying and irritation of respiratory mucosa, impaired ciliary action, and thickening of secretions within respiratory tract.*
- Encourage fluid intake of 3,000 to 4,000 mL daily, unless contraindicated, *to help thin mucus secretions.*
- Ensure adequate nutritional intake. Offer high-protein supplements, unless contraindicated. *This helps stabilize weight, improves muscle tone and mass, and aids wound healing.*
- Arrange for protective isolation if patient has compromised immune system. Monitor flow and number of visitors. *These measures protect patient from pathogens in environment.*
- PCC Teach patient about:
  - Good handwashing technique
  - Factors that increase infection risk
  - Signs and symptoms of infection.

These measures allow patient to participate in care and help patient modify lifestyle to maintain optimum health.

Suggested NIC Interventions

Incision Site Care; Infection Protection; Teaching: Procedure/Treatment; Wound Care

Evaluations for Expected Outcomes

- Patient's temperature remains within normal range.
- Patient's WBC count and differential remain within normal range.
- Patient's cultures don't exhibit pathogen growth.
- Patient demonstrates appropriate personal and oral hygiene.
- Patient's respiratory secretions remain clear and odorless.
- Patient's urine remains clear, yellow, odorless, and free from sediment.
- Patient's bowel patterns remain normal.
- Patient's incisions or wounds remain clear, pink, and free from purulent drainage.
- Patient's IV sites don't show signs of inflammation.
- Patient's skin doesn't exhibit signs of breakdown.

- Patient's fluid and protein intake remains at specified levels.
- Patient remains free from signs and symptoms of infection.

Documentation

- Temperature
- Dates, times, and sites of all cultures
- Dates, times, and sites of all catheter insertions
- Appearance of all invasive catheter sites, tube sites, and wounds
- Interventions performed to reduce infection risk
- Patient's response to nursing interventions
- Evaluations for expected outcomes

REFERENCES

Albert, N. M., Slifcak, E., Roach, J. D., Bena, J. F., Horvath, G., Wilson, S., ... Murray, T. (2014). Infection rates in intensive care units by electrocadiographic lead wire type: disposable vs. reusable. *American Journal of Critical Care*, *23*(6), 460–468. doi:10.4037/ajcc2014362

Principles of transmission-based precautions. (2015). *Nursing Times*, *111*(5), 18–19.

Spruce, L., & Wood, A. (2014). Back to basics: Environmental cleaning. *AORN Journal*, *100*(1), 54–64. doi:10.1016/j.aorn.2014.02.018

RISK FOR INFECTION

related to surgical incision

Definition

Vulnerable to invasion and multiplication of pathogenic organisms, which may compromise health

Assessment

- Age, gender, weight
- Type of surgery, reason for surgery
- Anticipated length of surgery
- Mobility status
- Current health status, including vital signs, nutritional status, and integumentary status
- Laboratory studies, including hematocrit and hemoglobin (Hb) level, complete blood count, electrolyte studies, urinalysis, blood cultures, blood coagulation studies, immunologic and serologic tests, and liver function tests
- Presence of infection (urinary, respiratory, or oral)
- Health history, including drug allergies, recent infection, substance abuse, and chronic metabolic or systemic disease (diabetes mellitus; cardiovascular, hepatic, or renal disease; coagulation disorders; and splenic or bone marrow disorders)
- Current medical treatments, including radiation therapy, chemotherapy, antibiotic or antifungal therapy, steroid treatment, anticoagulant or thrombolytic therapy, and immunosuppressive therapy
- Presence of invasive devices, including indwelling urinary catheter, endotracheal tube, tracheostomy tube, IV lines, central venous and arterial lines, drains, and gastric feeding tubes
- Wound classification (clean, clean-contaminated, contaminated, or dirty)

Risk Factors

- Chronic illness (e.g., diabetes mellitus)
- Inadequate vaccination
- Insufficient knowledge to avoid exposure to pathogens
- Invasive procedure
- Malnutrition
- Obesity

Inadequate Primary Defenses

- Alteration in peristalsis
- Alteration in pH of secretions
- Alteration in skin integrity
- Decrease in ciliary action
- Premature rupture of amniotic membrane
- Prolonged rupture of amniotic membrane
- Smoking
- Stasis of body fluids

Inadequate Secondary Defenses

- Decrease in Hb
- Immunosuppression
- Leukopenia
- Suppressed inflammatory response (e.g., IL-6, CRP)
- Inadequate vaccination

Increased Environmental Exposure to Pathogens

- Exposure to disease outbreak

Expected Outcomes

- Patient's vital signs and laboratory values will remain within normal limits.
- Patient's incision site will remain free from signs and symptoms of infection.
- Patient will not experience dehiscence.

Suggested NOC Outcomes

Immune Status; Infection Severity; Wound Healing: Secondary Intention

Interventions and Rationales

- Document and report results of preoperative nursing assessment. Identify risk factors predisposing patient to infection. *A complete nursing assessment allows development of an individualized care plan.*
- **S** Make sure all surgical team members wear appropriate operating room attire. *The human body is a major source of microbial contamination.*
- Inspect operating room for cleanliness before opening supplies and instruments *to provide a safe environment.*
- **S** Perform a surgical hand scrub. Put on sterile gown and gloves. Place sterile drapes on patient, furniture, and equipment. *Surgical hand scrub minimizes number of microorganisms on skin. Sterile gown and gloves protect against contamination. Sterile drapes create sterile field.*
- Check package integrity, chemical indicator, and, if appropriate, expiration date on all sterile items before dispensing them onto sterile field. *All items used within field must be sterile or field will become contaminated.*
- **S** Closely monitor sterile field and initiate corrective measures when a break in technique occurs. *Contamination of sterile field may lead to wound contamination and subsequent infection.*
- Use proper technique when opening items onto sterile field *to avoid contamination.*
- Perform preoperative skin preparation of surgical site. *Skin preparation reduces resident microbial count to subpathogenic amounts and inhibits rapid rebound growth of microbes.*
- Keep operating room doors closed at all times, and minimize traffic in and out. *Air turbulence caused by movement and mixing of corridor air with room air can sharply increase bacterial counts in operating room.*
- Maintain room temperature of 68° F to 75° F (20° C to 23.9° C) and relative humidity at 50% ± 10%, unless contraindicated. *Cooler air temperature and lower humidity inhibit microbial growth.*

- Classify surgical wound according to degree of contamination of wound and surrounding tissue. *Classification helps to assess risk of wound infection from an endogenous source and determine need for antibiotic therapy.*
- Wash hands following contact with patient or any object contaminated with blood or body fluids. *Handwashing is the most effective means of preventing microbial transmission.*
- Administer antibiotics, as ordered. *Intraoperative administration of antibiotics can decrease incidence of wound infection and lessen its severity.*
- Disinfect and sterilize all instruments and equipment before and immediately after surgical procedure. All instruments and equipment used during surgery must be free from microorganisms. *Sterilizing instruments and equipment after use prevents growth and spread of microorganisms during storage.*
- Promptly clean areas outside sterile field that become contaminated by blood, tissue, or body fluids with an approved disinfectant *to prevent distribution of microbes into environment.*
- Apply sterile dressing to surgical wound before removing surgical drapes *to avoid wound contamination and subsequent infection.*

Suggested NIC Interventions

Infection Control; Infection Protection; Nutrition Therapy; Wound Care

Evaluations for Expected Outcomes

- Patient's oral temperature remains below 100° F (37.8° C). Postoperative vital signs and laboratory values (especially white blood cell count) are consistent with preoperative values.
- Patient's incision site remains free from erythema, edema, undue tenderness, warmth, induration, foul odor, purulent drainage, and other signs and symptoms of infection.
- Patient's wound edges are approximated, and evidence of dehiscence is absent.

Documentation

- Results of preoperative nursing assessment
- Operative procedure
- Type of anesthesia
- Surgical times (time patient entered operating room, time incision was made, time incision was closed, and time patient left operating room)
- Wound classification
- Intraoperative administration of antibiotics
- Presence of packing, drains, indwelling urinary catheter, or other invasive devices
- Intraoperative insertion of permanent or temporary implants
- Type of wound closure method
- Type of dressing applied
- Estimated intraoperative blood loss
- Evaluations for expected outcomes

REFERENCES

Diaz, V., & Newman, J. (2015). Surgical site infection and prevention guidelines: A primer for certified registered nurse anesthetists. *AANA Journal*, *83*(1), 63–68.

Fend, J. L., Wood, F. G., Swofford, V., & Morgan, M. (2015). Avoiding surgical site infections in neurosurgical procedures. *OR Nurse*, *9*(3), 28–38. doi:10.1097/01.ORN.0000464750.00568.bb

Spruce, L. (2014). Back to basics: Surgical attire and cleanliness. *AORN Journal*, *99*(1), 138–146. doi:10.1016/j.aorn.2013.10.013

RISK FOR INJURY

Definition

Vulnerable to physical damage due to environmental conditions interacting with the individual's adaptive and defense resources, which may compromise health

Assessment

- Age
- Health history, including accidents, falls, and exposure to environmental hazards
- Environmental factors, including household layout, electrical wiring, lighting, utilities, fire precautions, presence of toxic or noxious substances, medications, special safety needs, and childproofing
- Mental status, including mood, affect, thought processes, thought content, orientation, judgment, and ability to perform activities of daily living
- Knowledge level, including understanding of household safety precautions and automobile safety
- Participation in recreational activities, such as swimming, diving, motorcycling, bicycling, and contact sports

Risk Factors

External

- Alteration in cognitive functioning
- Alteration in psychomotor functioning
- Compromised nutritional source (e.g., vitamins, food types)
- Exposure to pathogen
- Exposure to toxic chemical
- Immunization level within community
- Nosocomial agent
- Physical barrier (e.g., design, structure, arrangement of community, building, equipment)
- Unsafe mode of transport

Internal

- Abnormal blood profile
- Alteration in affective orientation
- Alteration in sensation (resulting from spinal cord injury, diabetes mellitus, etc.)
- Autoimmune dysfunction
- Effector dysfunction
- Extremes of age
- Immune dysfunction

- Impaired primary defense mechanisms (e.g., broken skin)
- Malnutrition
- Sensory integration dysfunction
- Tissue hypoxia

Expected Outcomes

- Patient and family will acknowledge presence of environmental hazards in their everyday surroundings.
- Patient and family will take safety precautions in and out of home.
- Patient and family members will develop strategy to maintain safety.
- Adults in household will childproof house to ensure safety of young children and cognitively impaired adults.
- Patient and family will optimize activities of daily living within sensorimotor limitations.

Suggested NOC Outcomes

Immune Status; Risk Control; Safety Behavior: Home Physical Environment; Safety Behavior: Personal; Safety Status: Physical Injury

Interventions and Rationales

- Help patient and family identify situations and hazards that can cause accidents *to increase patient's awareness of potential dangers.*
- S — Encourage patient to make repairs and remove potential safety hazards from environment *to decrease possibility of injury.*
- S PCC — Encourage adults to discuss safety rules with children. For example:
  - Don't play with matches.
  - Use electrical equipment carefully.
  - Know location of fire escape route.
  - Don't speak to strangers.
  - Dial 911 in an emergency.

  Teaching by parents fosters household safety.
- Improve environmental safety, as needed:
  - Orient patient to environment. Assess patient's ability to use call bell, side rails, and bed positioning controls. Keep bed at lowest level, and conduct close night watch. *These measures will help patient cope with unfamiliar surroundings.*
  - PCC — Teach patient and family about need for safe illumination. Advise patient to wear sunglasses to reduce glare. Advise using contrasting colors in household furnishings. *These measures will enhance visual discrimination.*
  - Test heating pads and bath water before using; assess extremities daily for injury *to assist patient with decreased tactile sensitivity.*
  - For patient with hearing loss, encourage use of hearing aid *to minimize deficit.*
  - S PCC — Teach patient with unstable gait correct use of adaptive devices *to decrease potential for injury.*
- PCC — Provide additional patient teaching, as needed. Possible topics may include household, automobile, and pedestrian safety. Refer patient to appropriate resources (police, fire, and home health care agency) for more information. *Health education can help patient take steps to prevent injury.*

PCC • Refer patient to appropriate community resources for more information about identifying and removing safety hazards. *This enables patient and family to alter environment to achieve optimal safety level.*

Suggested NIC Interventions

Environmental Management; Fall Prevention; Health Education; Surveillance: Safety, Home Maintenance Assistance

Evaluations for Expected Outcomes

- Patient and family identify and eliminate safety hazards in their surroundings.
- Patient and family members demonstrate prevention and safety precautions.
- Children describe safety measures they have learned.
- Patient and family point out evidence of childproofing measures in home.
- Patient increases self-care activities within limits posed by sensorimotor limitations.

Documentation

- Patient's statements about situations that cause accidents and injuries
- Patient's lack of awareness of, or disregard for, safety hazards
- Patient's cognitive deficits that inhibit learning or attention to safety hazards
- Interventions to help patient recognize and eliminate safety hazards
- Patient's or family's response to nursing interventions
- Evaluations for expected outcomes

REFERENCES

Murphy, M. P., Carmine, H., & Kolakowsky-Hayner, S. (2014). Modifiable and nonmodifiable risk factors for falls after traumatic brain injury: An exploratory investigation with implications for medication use. *Rehabilitation Nursing*, *39*(3), 113–122. doi:10.1002/rnj.89

Sherwood, G., & Zomorodi, M. (2014). A new mindset for quality and safety: The QSEN competencies redefine nurses' roles in practice. *Nephrology Nursing Journal*, *41*(1), 15–72.

Ulrich, B., & Kear, T. (2014). Patient safety and patient safety culture: Foundations of excellent health care delivery. *Nephrology Nursing Journal*, *41*(5), 447–457.

RISK FOR URINARY TRACT INJURY

Definition

Vulnerable to damage of the urinary tract structures from use of catheters, which may compromise health

Assessment

- History of urinary tract disease, trauma, surgery, or previous urethral infection
- Age
- Gender
- Vital signs
- Genitourinary status, including characteristics of urine, excretory urography, pain or discomfort, palpation of bladder, urinalysis, and voiding patterns

- Catheter placement, including securing devices
- Psychosocial status, including coping skills, patient's perception of health problem, self-concept (body image), family members, and stressors

Risk Factors

- Condition preventing ability to secure catheter (e.g., burn, trauma, amputation)
- Long-term use of urinary catheter
- Multiple catheterizations
- Retention balloon inflated to ≥30 mL
- Use of large caliber urinary catheter

Expected Outcomes

- Patient will not experience injury from urinary catheter.
- Patient will voice no discomfort with catheter placement.
- Patient will voice understanding of treatment.
- Patient will have few, if any, complications.
- Patient will discuss impact of urologic disorder on self and family members.
- Patient will demonstrate skill in managing urinary elimination problem.

Suggested NOC Outcomes

Hydration; Mobility; Physical Aging; Self-Care Toileting; Urinary Elimination

Interventions and Rationales

- Administer appropriate catheter care and monitoring of secure device. *Appropriate care prevents complications and alerts health care team to developing problems.*
- Monitor patency of indwelling urinary catheter. Keep tubing free from kinks and keep the drainage bag below the level of the bladder *to avoid urine reflux.*
- Clean the urinary meatus according to the established policy, and maintain a closed drainage system *to prevent skin irritation and bacteriuria.*
- Secure the catheter to patient's leg (female) or abdomen (male); avoid tension on the sphincter. *Anchoring the catheter avoids straining the trigone muscle of the bladder and prevents friction leading to inflammation.*
- Only use urinary catheters as necessary. Discontinue catheter if patient is able to void spontaneously. *Decreased time of use prevents injury and infection.*
- Do not overfill retention balloon of indwelling catheters. *Overfilling can lead to pressure on the bladder floor.*
- For intermittent catheterization, catheterize patient using clean or sterile technique. *These measures prevent infection, and help maintain integrity of ureterovesical function.*
- For intermittent catheterization, consider using bladder scan. *Determines if catheterization is necessary.*

Suggested NIC Interventions

Fluid Management; Perineal Care; Self-Care Assistance: Toileting; Urinary Elimination Management

Evaluations for Expected Outcomes

- Patient does not experience injury from urinary catheter.
- Patient reports no discomfort with catheter placement.
- Patient reports understanding of treatment and self-catheterization.
- Patient has no complications.
- Patient is able to discuss impact of urologic disorder on self and family members.
- Patient demonstrates skill in managing urinary elimination problem.

Documentation

- Observations of urologic condition and response to treatment regimen
- Catheter placement and patency of securing devices
- Need for continued use of catheter
- Interventions to provide supportive care and patient's response
- Instructions given to patient and family members on urologic problem, response to instructions, and demonstrated ability to manage patient's urinary elimination needs
- Patient's expression of concern about urologic problem and its impact on body image and lifestyle; patient's motivation to participate in self-care
- Evaluations for expected outcomes

REFERENCES

Esparaz, A. M., Pearl, J. A., Herts, B. R., LeBlanc, J., & Kapoor, B. (2015). Iatrogenic urinary tract injuries: Etiology, diagnosis, and management. *Seminars in Interventional Radiology*, *36*(2), 195–208. doi:10.1055/s-0035-1549378

Magers, T. L. (2013). Using evidence-based practice to reduce catheter-associated urinary tract infections. *American Journal of Nursing*, *113*(6), 34–44. doi:10.1097/01.NAJ.0000431270.01203.4b

INSOMNIA

related to anxiety

Definition

A disruption in amount and quality of sleep that impairs functioning

Assessment

- Age
- Daytime activity and work patterns
- Normal bedtime
- Number of hours of sleep patient usually needs to feel rested
- Problems associated with sleep, including early morning awakening, difficulty falling and staying asleep, nightmares, and sleepwalking
- Quality of sleep
- Sleeping environment
- Activities associated with sleep, including bath, drink, food, and medication
- Personal beliefs about sleep

Defining Characteristics

- Alteration in affect
- Alteration in concentration
- Alteration in mood
- Alteration in sleep pattern
- Compromised health status
- Decrease in quality of life
- Difficulty initiating sleep
- Difficulty maintaining sleep
- Early awakening
- Increase in absenteeism
- Increase in accidents
- Insufficient energy
- Nonrestorative sleep pattern (i.e., due to caregiver responsibilities, parenting practices, sleep partner)
- Sleep disturbance producing next-day consequences

Expected Outcomes

- Patient will identify factors that prevent or disrupt sleep.
- Patient will sleep ___ hours a night.
- Patient will express feeling of being well rested.
- Patient won't show physical signs of sleep deprivation.
- Patient won't exhibit sleep-related behavioral symptoms, such as restlessness, irritability, lethargy, and disorientation.
- Patient will perform relaxation exercises at bedtime.

Suggested NOC Outcomes

Anxiety Level; Anxiety Self-Control; Medication Response; Personal Well-Being; Rest; Sleep; Stress Level

Interventions and Rationales

- PCC Allow patient to discuss any concerns that may be preventing sleep. *Active listening helps you determine causes of difficulty with sleep.*
- Plan nursing care routines to allow ___ hours of uninterrupted sleep. *This allows consistent nursing care and gives patient uninterrupted sleep time.*
- Provide patient with usual sleep aids, such as pillows, bath before sleep, food or drink, and reading materials. Milk and some high-protein snacks, such as cheese and nuts, contain L-tryptophan, a sleep promoter. *Personal hygiene and pre-bedtime rituals precede and promote sleep in many patients.*
- Create quiet environment conducive to sleep; for example, close curtains, adjust lighting, and close door. *These measures promote rest and sleep.*
- Administer medications that promote normal sleep patterns, as ordered. Monitor and record adverse effects and effectiveness. *Hypnotic agents induce sleep; tranquilizers reduce anxiety.*
- Promote involvement in diversional activities or exercise program during day. Discuss and relate exercise and activity to improved sleep. Discourage excessive napping. *Activity and exercise promote sleep by increasing fatigue and relaxation.*
- Ask patient to describe in specific terms each morning the quality of sleep during the previous night. *This helps detect sleep-related behavioral symptoms.*
- PCC Educate patient about such relaxation and stress-reducing techniques as guided imagery, progressive muscle relaxation, aromatherapy, relaxation music, and meditation. *Purposeful relaxation efforts usually help promote sleep.*

Suggested NIC Interventions

Calming Technique; Coping Enhancement; Energy Management; Medication Management; Positioning; Simple Relaxation Therapy; Sleep Enhancement

Evaluations for Expected Outcomes

- Patient identifies factors that prevent or disrupt sleep.
- Patient sleeps specified number of hours nightly.
- Patient expresses feeling well rested.
- Patient doesn't exhibit signs of sleep deprivation.
- Patient doesn't exhibit sleep-related behavioral symptoms.
- Patient performs relaxation exercises at bedtime.

Documentation

- Patient's complaints about sleep disturbances
- Patient's report of improvement in sleep patterns
- Observations of physical and behavioral sleep-related disturbances
- Interventions to alleviate sleep disturbances
- Patient's response to nursing interventions
- Evaluations for expected outcomes

REFERENCES

Ashworth, D. K., Sletten, T. L., Junge, M., Simpson, K., Clarke, D., Cunnington, D., & Rajaratnam, S. M. (2015). A randomized controlled trial of cognitive behavioral therapy for insomnia: An effective treatment for comorbid insomnia and depression. *Journal of Counseling Psychology*, 62(2), 115–123. doi:10.1037/cou0000059

Miller, C. B., Espie, C. A., Epstein, D. R., Friedman, L., Morin, C. M., Pigeon, W. R., ... Kyle, S. D. (2014). The evidence base of sleep restriction therapy for treating insomnia disorder. *Sleep Medicine Reviews*, *18*(5), 415–424. doi:10.1016/j.smrv.2014.01.006

Richter, K., Myllymaeki, J., Scharold-Schaefer, S., Tomova, I., Mayrer, R., & Niklewski, G. (2014). Treating comorbid insomnia in older adults via cognitive–behavioral treatment, bright light, and exercise. *Health*, 6(10), 960–968. doi:10.4236/health.2014.610121

INSOMNIA

related to environmental barrier (e.g., ambient noise, daylight/darkness exposure, ambient temperature/humidity, unfamiliar setting

Definition

A disruption in amount and quality of sleep that impairs functioning

Assessment

- Daytime activity and work patterns
- Travel history
- Normal bedtime
- Detailed sleep history, including number of hours of sleep required

- Problems associated with sleep, including early morning awakening, difficulty falling and staying asleep, nightmares, and sleepwalking
- Quality of sleep
- Sleeping environment
- Activities associated with sleep
- Personal beliefs about sleep
- Chemical ingestion, including alcohol, caffeine, hypnotics, and nicotine
- Use of herbal or dietary products used to facilitate sleep
- Any illness or injury related to lack of sleep

Defining Characteristics

- Alteration in affect
- Alteration in concentration
- Alteration in mood
- Alteration in sleep pattern
- Compromised health status
- Decrease in quality of life
- Difficulty initiating sleep
- Difficulty maintaining sleep
- Early awakening
- Increase in absenteeism
- Increase in accidents
- Insufficient energy
- Nonrestorative sleep pattern (i.e., due to caregiver responsibilities, parenting practices, sleep partner)
- Sleep disturbance producing next-day consequences

Expected Outcomes

- Patient will identify factors that prevent or promote sleep.
- Patient will sleep ___ hours without interruption.
- Patient will express feeling well rested.
- Patient won't show physical signs of sleep deprivation.
- Patient will alter diet and habits to promote sleep, such as reducing caffeine and alcohol intake before bedtime.
- Patient won't exhibit sleep-related behavioral symptoms, such as restlessness, irritability, lethargy, and disorientation.
- Patient will perform relaxation exercises at bedtime.

Suggested NOC Outcomes

Anxiety Level; Fear Level; Mood Equilibrium; Personal Well-Being; Rest; Sleep

Interventions and Rationales

- Ask patient what environmental factors make sleep difficult. *Sleeping in strange or new environment tends to influence both rapid eye movement (REM) and non-REM sleep.*
- PCC Ask patient what changes would promote sleep *to allow patient to take an active role in treatment.*
- PCC Make whatever immediate changes are possible to accommodate patient; for example, reduce noise pollution, change lighting, and close door. *These measures promote rest and sleep.*
- Plan medication administration schedules to allow for maximum rest. If patient requires diuretics in the evening, give far enough in advance *to allow peak effect before bedtime. Other medications that may interfere with sleep include ß-adrenergic blockers, MAO inhibitors, and phenytoin.*

- Make a detailed plan to provide patient with a set number of hours of uninterrupted sleep, if possible. *This allows consistent nursing care and gives patient uninterrupted sleep time.*
- Provide patient with usual sleep aids, such as pillows, bath before sleep, food or drink, and reading materials. *Milk and some high-protein snacks, such as cheese and nuts, contain L-tryptophan, a sleep promoter. Personal hygiene and pre-bedtime rituals precede and promote sleep in many patients.*
- Ask patient to keep a sleep log describing sleep disturbances and the impact on daytime functioning, such as with cognition, mood, coping skills, and physical complaints. *This allows increased awareness of potential sleep disturbances.*
- Ask patient to describe in specific terms each morning the quality of sleep during the previous night. *This helps detect the presence of sleep-related behavioral symptoms.*
- PCC Teach patient such relaxation techniques as guided imagery, meditation, aromatherapy, and progressive muscle relaxation. Practice them with patient at bedtime. *Purposeful relaxation efforts usually help promote sleep.*
- Instruct patient to eliminate or reduce caffeine and alcohol intake and avoid foods that interfere with sleep (e.g., spicy foods). *Foods and beverages containing caffeine consumed fewer than 4 hours before bedtime may interfere with sleep. Alcohol disrupts normal sleep, especially when ingested immediately before retiring.*

Suggested NIC Interventions

Biofeedback; Calming Technique; Coping Enhancement; Energy Management; Security Enhancement; Simple Relaxation Therapy; Sleep Enhancement

Evaluations for Expected Outcomes

- Patient describes factors that prevent or promote sleep.
- Patient sleeps specified number of hours without interruption.
- Patient expresses feeling well rested.
- Patient shows no physical signs of sleep deprivation.
- Patient reports changing diet habits and making lifestyle changes to promote sleep.
- Patient doesn't exhibit sleep-related behavioral symptoms.
- Patient performs relaxation exercises at bedtime.

Documentation

- Patient's complaints about sleep disturbances
- Patient's verbalization of feelings about sleep
- Observations of behavior that indicate sleep deprivation
- Interventions to alleviate sleep disturbance
- Patient's response to nursing interventions
- Evaluations for expected outcomes

REFERENCES

Falbe, J., Davison, K. K., Franckle, R. L., Ganter, C., Gortmaker, S. L., Smith, L., ... Taveras, E. M. (2015). Sleep duration, restfulness, and screens in the sleep environment. *Pediatrics, 135*(2), e368–375. doi:10.1542/peds.2014-2306

Melatonin improves sleep in noisy environments. (2015). *British Journal of Hospital Medicine, 76*(4), 190–190.

Walter, E. (2015). See no lights, hear no alarms: How to sleep in the ICU environment. *Critical Care Alert, 23*(4), 25–27.

DEFICIENT KNOWLEDGE

related to alteration in cognitive functioning

Definition

Absence or deficiency of cognitive information related to a specific topic

Assessment

- Psychosocial status, including age; learning ability (affective, cognitive, and psychomotor domains); decision-making ability; developmental stage; financial resources; interest in learning, knowledge and skills related to current health problem; obstacles to learning, support systems (willingness and ability of others to help patient), and usual coping pattern
- Neurologic status, including level of consciousness, memory, mental status, and orientation

Defining Characteristics

- Inaccurate follow-through of instruction
- Inaccurate performance on a test
- Inappropriate behavior (e.g., hysterical, hostile, agitated, apathetic)
- Insufficient knowledge

Expected Outcomes

- Patient will demonstrate ability to perform simple self-care measures, such as feeding, maintaining hygiene, dressing, and toileting.
- Family members will communicate understanding of patient's cognitive impairment.
- Family members will express willingness to help patient maintain maximum independence.
- Family members will demonstrate method being used to teach patient.

Suggested NOC Outcomes

Cognition; Concentration; Information Processing; Knowledge: Disease Process; Knowledge: Health Behaviors; Knowledge: Health Resources; Knowledge: Illness Care; Stress Level

Interventions and Rationales

- Provide all equipment needed for each self-care measure patient must learn. *This reduces frustration, aids learning, and minimizes dependence by promoting self-care.*
- PCC When teaching self-care measures, go slowly and repeat frequently. Offer small amounts of information, and present it in various ways. *By building cognition, patient will be better able to complete self-care measures.*
- Have patient practice each task. Provide positive reinforcement each time patient performs task correctly. *This encourages desired behavior.*
- PCC Discuss patient's limitations with family members. *Communication promotes working relationship and reduces fear and anxiety.*
- PCC Demonstrate to family members how each self-care measure is broken down into simple tasks *to enhance patient's success and foster sense of control.*

PCC • Encourage family members to participate in patient's learning process *to help create an encouraging, therapeutic climate after discharge.*

PCC • Have family members give return demonstration of patient's methods of performing self-care measures. *This provides hands-on experience with equipment, builds confidence, and encourages compliance.*

PCC • Refer family members to outside agencies, such as a home health care organization, for assistance after patient's discharge. *This ensures continuity of care and assistance with follow-up after discharge.*

Suggested NIC Interventions

Behavior Management; Behavior Modification; Decision-Making Support; Energy Management; Family Support; Health Education; Learning Facilitation; Support System Enhancement

Evaluations for Expected Outcomes

- Patient practices simple self-care measures and demonstrates ability to perform activities of daily living.
- Family members describe cause of patient's cognitive impairment.
- Family members demonstrate willingness to help patient learn to perform self-care measures.
- Family members provide return demonstration of patient's methods of performing self-care measures.

Documentation

- Patient's abilities and limitations in performing self-care measures
- Progress made by patient in learning each specific task
- Information given to family members concerning patient's limitations and progress in learning tasks
- Family members' participation in learning process
- Referrals to outside agencies
- Evaluations for expected outcomes

REFERENCES

Fujii, M., Ishizuka, S., & Sasaki, H. (2015). Small group teaching in a psychiatric hospital for dementia patients. *Geriatrics & Gerontology International, 15*(2), 239–240. doi:10.1111/ggi.12370

Goldschmidt, J., & Song, H. (2015). Active engagement: Teaching cooking skills to young adults with autism. *Journal of Nutrition Education & Behavior*, 47(4), S29. doi:10.1016/j.jneb.2015.04.078

Meuris, K., Maes, B., & Zink, I. (2015). Teaching adults with intellectual disability manual signs through their support staff: A key word signing program. *American Journal of Speech-Language Pathology*, *24*(3), 545–560. doi:10.1044/2015_AJSLP-14-0062

DEFICIENT KNOWLEDGE

related to insufficient information

Definition

Absence or deficiency of cognitive information related to a specific topic

Assessment

- Psychosocial status, including age, learning ability (affective, cognitive, and psychomotor domains), decision-making ability, developmental stage, financial resources, health beliefs and attitudes, interest in learning, knowledge and skill regarding current health problem, obstacles to learning, support systems (willingness and ability of others to help patient), and usual coping pattern
- Neurologic status, including level of consciousness, memory, mental status, and orientation

Defining Characteristics

- Inaccurate follow-through of instruction
- Inaccurate performance on a test
- Inappropriate behavior (e.g., hysterical, hostile, agitated, apathetic)
- Insufficient knowledge

Expected Outcomes

- Patient will communicate need to know.
- Patient will state or demonstrate understanding of what has been taught.
- Patient will demonstrate ability to perform new health-related behaviors as they're taught and will list specific skills and realistic target dates for each.
- Patient will set realistic learning goals.
- Patient will state intention to make needed changes in lifestyle, including seeking help from health professional, when needed.

Suggested NOC Outcomes

Client Satisfaction: Teaching; Concentration; Knowledge: Diet; Knowledge: Disease Process; Knowledge: Energy Conservation; Knowledge: Health Behaviors; Motivation

Interventions and Rationales

- PCC Establish environment of mutual trust and respect to enhance learning. *Comfort with growing self-awareness, ability to share this awareness with others, receptiveness to new experiences, and consistency between actions and words form basis of trusting relationship.*
- PCC Negotiate with patient to develop goals for learning. *Involving patient in planning meaningful goals encourages follow-through.*
- PCC Select teaching strategies (such as discussion, demonstration, role-playing, and visual materials) appropriate for patient's individual learning style (specify) *to enhance teaching effectiveness.*
- PCC Teach skills that patient must incorporate into daily lifestyle. Have patient give return demonstration of each new skill *to help gain confidence.*
- PCC Provide written materials explaining skills patient is trying to develop and facts patient must remember. *Words and pictures will reinforce things the patient must learn to care for self.*
- Have patient incorporate learned skills into daily routine during hospitalization (specify skills). *This allows patient to practice new skills and receive feedback.*
- Provide patient with names and telephone numbers of resource people or organizations *to provide continuity of care and follow-up after discharge.*

- As needed, arrange for interpreter. *Patient who doesn't speak English may understand health-related behaviors, but may need interpreter to express them.*

Suggested NIC Interventions

Behavior Modification; Discharge Planning; Health Education; Learning Readiness Enhancement; Teaching: Prescribed Diet

Evaluations for Expected Outcomes

- Patient expresses desire to overcome lack of knowledge.
- Patient states understanding of all that has been learned.
- Patient demonstrates newly learned health-related behaviors.
- Patient develops realistic learning goals and performs new skills by target date.
- Patient identifies specific changes in lifestyle needed to promote optimal health.

Documentation

- Patient's statements of information and skills that patient knows and doesn't know
- Expressions of need to know and motivation to learn
- Learning objectives
- Methods used to teach patient
- Information imparted
- Skills demonstrated
- Patient's responses to teaching
- Evaluations for expected outcomes

REFERENCES

Kluge, A., & Frank, B. (2014). Counteracting skill decay: Four refresher interventions and their effect on skill and knowledge retention in a simulated process control task. *Ergonomics*, *57*(2), 175–190. doi:10.1080/00140139.2013.869357

Knier, S., Stichler, J. F., Ferber, L., & Catterall, K. (2015). Patients' perceptions of the quality of discharge teaching and readiness for discharge. *Rehabilitation Nursing*, *40*(1), 30–39. doi:10.1002/rnj.164

Patel, H., & Ravindra, H. N. (2016). Effectiveness of structured teaching program on knowledge regarding cardiac rehabilitation among patients undergone coronary artery bypass grafting surgery in Dhiraj General Hospital, Piparia, Vadodara. *International Journal of Nursing Education*, *8*(1), 128–134. doi:10.5958/0974-9357.2016.00023.4

LATEX ALLERGY RESPONSE

related to absent immune system response

Definition

A hypersensitive reaction to natural latex rubber products

Assessment

- Age and gender
- Weight

- Occupation
- Health history, including past episodes of latex allergy; food, pollen, or drug allergy; multiple surgical history; spina bifida; and asthma
- Current health status, including temperature, blood pressure, respiratory status, and other vital signs
- Integumentary status, including color, elasticity, hygiene, lesions, moisture, sensation, texture, and turgor
- Reports of contact with latex products, including when, where, and what
- Laboratory studies, including arterial blood gas levels, complete blood count, immunoglobulin E level, radioallergosorbent test, and scratch test

Defining Characteristics

Life-Threatening Reactions within 1 Hour of Exposure

- Bronchospasm
- Chest tightness
- Contact urticarial progressing to generalized symptoms
- Dyspnea
- Edema (i.e., lips, throat, tongue, uvula)
- Hypotension
- Myocardial infarction
- Respiratory arrest
- Syncope
- Wheezing

Type IV Reactions Occurring ≥1 Hour after Exposure

- Discomfort reaction to additives (e.g., thiurams and carbamates)
- Eczema
- Skin irritation
- Skin redness

Generalized Characteristics

- Generalized discomfort
- Generalized edema
- Reports total body warmth
- Restlessness
- Skin flushing

Gastrointestinal Characteristics

- Abdominal pain
- Nausea

Orofacial Characteristics

- Erythema (e.g., eyes, facial, nasal)
- Itching (e.g., eyes, facial, nasal, oral)
- Nasal congestion
- Periorbital edema
- Rhinorrhea
- Tearing of the eyes

Expected Outcomes

- Patient's vital signs, respiratory status, and laboratory values will return to normal.
- Patient's skin will be clear, moist, and free from erythema, edema, itching, urticaria, and breakdown.
- Patient will express awareness of allergic response to products containing latex.
- Patient will state intention to avoid contact with products containing latex.

Suggested NOC Outcomes

Comfort Level; Immune Hypersensitivity Response; Knowledge: Infection Control; Tissue Integrity: Skin & Mucous Membranes

Interventions and Rationales

- If patient exhibits compromised respiratory status, implement treatment immediately and document the findings. *Airway maintenance is a primary health consideration and must be attended to immediately.*
- Conduct a nursing assessment and document the results *to allow for development of an individualized care plan.*
- S Monitor respiratory status and document the findings *to detect changes in status and respond appropriately.* Accurate documentation is necessary to maintain continuity of care among staff.
- Administer prescribed drugs and treatments in a timely fashion. *Wheezing and shortness of breath can quickly deteriorate to respiratory distress and failure. Skin with urticaria and itching is uncomfortable and unsightly, so patients appreciate timely treatment.*
- S Become familiar with the potential adverse effects of administered drugs. Bronchodilators, antihistamines, and corticosteroids may cause systemic adverse effects; *becoming familiar with these effects and ways to respond to them may help prevent serious reactions.*
- When latex allergy is confirmed, document on the patient record, and label the record clearly *to prevent future contact with the allergen.*
- Remove all latex products from the immediate proximity of patient and the staff treating patient. *If latex products are nearby, they may be inadvertently used by the staff or patient, increasing risk for contact and allergic reaction.*
- PCC Educate patient and family about allergic reaction to latex products *to prevent future contact and allergic reactions.*
- Give patient and family a list of household items containing latex, and emphasize the importance of avoiding these. Tell them about nonlatex product substitutes. *Prevention is the foundation of treatment of latex allergy.*
- PCC Educate patient and family members about the importance of quickly seeking medical treatment for allergic reaction *to foster timely intervention.*
- Emphasize the need to inform all health care providers—including emergency medical service—about patient's latex sensitivity. Stress the importance of wearing a medical identification bracelet that specifies latex sensitivity *to prevent future contact and allergic reactions.*
- S Provide documentation of latex allergy for patient's employer. With patient's permission, communicate with the employee health department, and discuss patient's need to avoid contact with latex products *to help prevent patient's further contact with latex products and avoid latex allergy reaction.*

Suggested NIC Interventions

Allergy Management; Anaphylaxis Management; Emergency Care; Environmental Risk Protection; Latex Precautions; Skin Surveillance; Risk Identification; Teaching: Individual

Evaluations for Expected Outcomes

- Patient's vital signs, respiratory status, and laboratory values return to normal levels.
- Patient's skin is clear, moist, and free from erythema, edema, itching, urticaria, and breakdown.
- Patient expresses awareness of allergic response to products containing latex.
- Patient expresses intention to avoid contact with products containing latex.

Documentation

- Results of nursing assessment
- Diagnosis of latex allergy
- Treatment of allergic reaction, including drugs administered
- Respiratory status throughout the episode of allergic reaction
- Integumentary status throughout the episode of allergic reaction
- Evidence of refraining from latex product use during patient's care and of removal of latex products from immediate patient area; explanation of latex product substitutes
- Evidence of patient and family education regarding latex allergy and avoidance of latex products
- Evaluations for expected outcomes

REFERENCES

Hohler, S. E. (2015). Latex allergies. *OR Nurse*, *9*(1), 12–19. doi:10.1097/01.ORN.0000457107.47873.aa

Latex allergy. (2015). *Nursing*, *45*(9), 46. doi:10.1097/01.IMURSE.0000470414.79191.e8

Lowth, M. (2014). Issues in personal safety. *Practice Nurse*, *44*(4), 34–39.

Moscato, G., Pala, G., Crivellaro, M., & Siracusa, A. (2014). Anaphylaxis as occupational risk. *Current Opinion in Allergy & Clinical Immunology*, *14*(4), 328–333. doi:10.1097/ACI.0000000000000066

Packham, C. (2014). How to find the cause of skin problems at work. *Occupational Health*, *66*(12), 27–30.

Péer, L., Brezis, M. L., Shalit, M., Carvalho, B., Levin, P. D., Seri, O., & Weiniger, C. F. (2014). Evaluation of a prospectively administered written questionnaire to reduce the incidence of suspected latex anaphylaxis during elective cesarean delivery. *International Journal of Obstetric Anesthesia*, *23*(4), 335–340. doi:10.1016/j.ijoa.2014.05.009

RISK FOR LATEX ALLERGY RESPONSE

Definition

Vulnerable to a hypersensitive reaction to natural latex rubber products, which may compromise health

Assessment

- Age, gender, and weight
- Occupation
- Current health status, including vital signs, respiratory status, and integumentary status
- Health history, including drug, food, or pollen allergies; surgical history; chronic disease such as spina bifida; and previous local or systemic allergic reactions
- Laboratory studies, such as immunoglobulin E level, complete blood count, radioallergosorbent test, and scratch tests

Risk Factors

- Allergy to poinsettia plant
- Food allergy (e.g., avocado, banana, chestnut, kiwi, peanut, shellfish, mushroom, tropical fruit)
- Frequent exposure to latex product
- History of allergy
- History of asthma

- History of latex reaction
- History of surgery during infancy
- Multiple surgical procedures

Expected Outcomes

- Patient's vital signs, especially respirations, will remain within normal limits.
- Patient's skin will remain free from erythema, edema, urticaria, and breakdown.
- Patient's nasal passages and laryngeal area will remain clear and free from edema and secretions.
- Patient and family members will express understanding of risk of latex allergy.
- Patient and family members will state intention to take precautions to avoid contact with latex products.

Suggested NOC Outcomes

Allergy Response: Localized; Immune Hypersensitivity Response; Knowledge: Health Behavior; Risk Control; Risk Detection

Interventions and Rationales

- Conduct a nursing assessment to identify factors in the patient's life that set up a risk for allergy to latex products. *There may be occupational exposure or consumption of certain foods that the patient has not thought to attribute to the symptoms he is experiencing.*
- Remove all products containing latex from patient's room *to reduce risk of allergic reaction.*
- Use only nonlatex products when caring for patient *to reduce risk of latex allergy reaction in patient.*
- S Make sure all personnel are aware of the risk of latex allergy and refrain from using latex products during diagnostic procedures. *Communication with other health care personnel allows for continuity of care and reduces the risk of latex allergy reaction.*
- PCC Educate patient and family about the risk of latex allergy *to prevent allergic reaction due to contact with latex products.*
- Explain that although some reactions to latex are relatively minor (such as sneezing and runny nose), others are life-threatening. *This will foster awareness of serious nature of risk.*
- PCC Educate patient and family about the symptoms of allergic reaction and the need for quick treatment if symptoms appear. *Rapid response to allergic reaction may help prevent complications, such as skin infection (with local reaction) and respiratory failure (with systemic reaction).*
- Give patient and family a list of household items containing latex, and emphasize the importance of avoiding these. Tell them about nonlatex product substitutes. *Prevention is the foundation of treatment of latex allergy.*
- Emphasize the need to inform all health care providers—including emergency medical service—about patient's latex sensitivity. Stress the importance of wearing a medical identification bracelet that specifies latex sensitivity *to prevent future contact and allergic reactions.*
- PCC Provide emotional support to help patient cope with stress. *Fear of latex exposure can cause a high level of stress in a latex-sensitive patient. Some patients are afraid to seek medical help for fear of latex exposure.*

Suggested NIC Interventions

Allergy Management; Environmental Management; Health System Guidance; Latex Precautions; Risk Identification; Teaching: Individual

Evaluations for Expected Outcomes

- Patient's vital signs, especially respirations, remain within patient's normal limits.
- Patient's skin remains free from erythema, edema, urticaria, and breakdown.
- Patient's nasal passages and laryngeal area remain clear and free from edema and secretions.
- Patient and family members express understanding of risk of latex allergy.
- Patient and family members state intention to take precautions to avoid contact with latex products.

Documentation

- Results of nursing assessment
- Presence of risk factors
- Communication of risk factors to health care personnel involved in care or diagnostic studies of patient
- Teaching provided to patient and family members about risk factors and symptoms of allergic reactions
- Patient's and family members' statements indicating understanding of risk factors and symptoms of allergic reactions
- Evaluations for expected outcomes

REFERENCES

Hohler, S. E. (2015). Latex allergies. *OR Nurse, 9*(1), 12–19. doi:10.1097/01.ORN.0000457107.47873.aa

Latex allergy. (2015). *Nursing, 45*(9), 46. doi:10.1097/01.IMURSE.0000470414.79191.e8

Lowth, M. (2014). Issues in personal safety. *Practice Nurse, 44*(4), 34–39.

Moscato, G., Pala, G., Crivellaro, M., & Siracusa, A. (2014). Anaphylaxis as occupational risk. *Current Opinion in Allergy & Clinical Immunology, 14*(4), 328–333. doi:10.1097/ACI.0000000000000066

Packham, C. (2014). How to find the cause of skin problems at work. *Occupational Health, 66*(12), 27–30.

Péer, L., Brezis, M. L., Shalit, M., Carvalho, B., Levin, P. D., Seri, O., & Weiniger, C. F. (2014). Evaluation of a prospectively administered written questionnaire to reduce the incidence of suspected latex anaphylaxis during elective cesarean delivery. *International Journal of Obstetric Anesthesia, 23*(4), 335–340. doi:10.1016/j.ijoa.2014.05.009

SEDENTARY LIFESTYLE

related to insufficient interest in physical activity

Definition

Reports a habit of life that is characterized by a low physical activity level

Assessment

- Age, gender, and cognitive status
- Daytime activity and work patterns
- Possible precipitating factors
- Height, weight, body mass index (BMI), and muscle and weight-bearing
- Underlying conditions or medications
- Overall quality and duration of sleep
- Situational daily stressors
- Nutritional status and opportunity for exercise and social interaction
- Convenience of exercise facilities and safety of environment
- Recent changes in health status or lifestyle
- Dietary and medication history
- Culturally determined expectations of body image or dietary intake
- Risk assessment for substance abuse, smoking, and high-risk behaviors
- Disabilities

Defining Characteristics

- Average daily physical activity is less than recommended for gender and age
- Physical deconditioning
- Preference for activity low in physical activity

Expected Outcomes

- Older adult will maintain independent living status with reduced risk for falling.
- Patient will identify barriers to increasing physical activity level.
- Patient will identify health benefits to increasing physical activity level.
- Patient will increase physical activity and limit inactive forms of diversion, such as television and computer games.
- Patient will seek professional consultation to develop an appropriate plan to increase physical activity.
- Patient will identify factors that enhance readiness for sleep.
- Patient will demonstrate readiness for enhanced sleep through the use of appropriate sleep hygiene measures.
- Patient's amount of sleep and rapid eye movement (REM) sleep will be congruent with developmental needs.
- Patient will express a feeling of being rested after sleep.
- Patient will increase lean muscle and bone strength and decrease body fat.
- Patient will demonstrate weight control and, if appropriate, weight loss.
- Patient will demonstrate enhanced psychological well-being and reduced risk of depression.
- Patient will have reduced depression and anxiety and an improved mood.
- Patient with certain chronic, disabling conditions will have increased ability to perform activities of daily living (ADLs).

Suggested NOC Outcomes

Activity Intolerance; Adherent Behavior; Client Satisfaction: Teaching; Endurance; Energy Conservation; Health-promoting Behavior; Immobility Consequences: Physiologic and Psycho-cognitive; Knowledge: Diet; Knowledge: Rest; Knowledge: Risk Control; Knowledge: Sleep

Interventions and Rationales

- PCC Provide counseling tailored to patient's risk factors, needs, preferences, and abilities *to enhance emotional well-being and motivation for physical activity.*
- Discuss behavioral risk factors in lack of motivation to increase physical activity, such as ingestion of carbohydrates, caffeine, nicotine, alcohol, sedatives, and hypnotics, and fluid intake, *to focus behavior on positive outcomes of increased physical activity.*
- Instruct patient to keep a daily activity and dietary log *to help obtain a more objective view of patient's behavior.*
- Identify barriers and enhancers to increasing physical activity, including time management, access to facilities, and safe environments in which to be active. *Breaking down barriers and building opportunities for activity increase the probability of consistent physical activity.*
- PCC Educate patient about how sedentary lifestyle affects cardiovascular risk factors (such as hypertension, dyslipidemia, hyperinsulinemia, insulin resistance) *to motivate patient to be more active.*
- Discuss the need for activity that will improve psychosocial well-being.
- PCC Develop a behavior modification plan based on patient's condition, history, and precipitating factors *to maximize physical activity and compliance.*
- PCC Provide education about community resources available to increase physical activity *to decrease barriers to activity.*
- PCC Teach exercises for increasing strength and endurance *to maintain mobility and prevent musculoskeletal degeneration.*
- PCC Educate patient about using the bedroom only for sleep or sexual activity and avoiding other activities such as watching television, reading, and eating *to increase sleep efficiency.*

Suggested NIC Interventions

Activity Therapy; Body Mechanics Promotion; Energy Management; Risk Identification; Sleep Enhancement; Teaching: Prescribed Activity/Exercise

Evaluations for Expected Outcomes

- Patient seeks professional consultation to develop a plan to increase physical activity and limit inactive forms of diversion, such as watching television.
- Patient's BMI is appropriate for patient's height and weight.
- Patient verbalizes how sedentary lifestyle impacts morbidity and mortality.
- Patient reduces high-risk behaviors.
- Patient demonstrates increased ability to perform ADLs and, if appropriate, to maintain independent living status.
- Patient demonstrates motivation to increase physical activity.
- Patient demonstrates readiness for enhanced sleep through the use of appropriate sleep hygiene measures.
- Patient's amount of sleep and REM sleep matches developmental needs.
- Patient demonstrates behaviors of psychological well-being and reduced risk for developing depression.
- Patient experiences reduced depression and anxiety and improved mood.
- Change in sedentary lifestyle is congruent with cultural expectations.
- Facility policies and staff behaviors reflect opportunities to provide physical activity for patients and limit inactive forms of diversion, such as television watching and computer games.

Documentation

- Daytime activity and work patterns
- Behavioral modification plan
- Dietary and drug history
- Height, weight, and BMI
- High-risk behavior assessment
- Sleep hygiene behaviors
- Culturally determined expectations
- Nursing interventions to increase patient's physical activity
- Response to nursing interventions
- Evaluations for expected outcomes

REFERENCES

Alspach, J. G. (2015). Revisiting a familiar but lethal cardiovascular risk factor: Sedentary lifestyle. *Critical Care Nurse*, *35*(2), 14–17. doi:10.4037/ccn2015797

Saleh, Z. T., Lennie, T. A., Mudd-Martin, G., Bailey, A. L., Novak, M. J., Biddle, M., … Moser, D. K. (2015). Decreasing sedentary behavior by 30 minutes per day reduces cardiovascular disease risk factors in rural Americans. *Heart & Lung*, *44*(5), 382–386. doi:10.1016/j.hrtlng.2015.06.008

Stevens, A. B., Thiel, S., Thorud, J. L., Smith, M. L., Howell, D., Cargill, J., … Ory, M. G. (2016). Increasing the availability of physical activity programs for older adults: Lessons learned from texercise stakeholders. *Journal of Aging & Physical Activity*, *24*(1), 39–44. doi:10.1123/japa.2014-0016

RISK FOR IMPAIRED LIVER FUNCTION

Definition

Vulnerable to a decrease in liver function, which may compromise health

Assessment

- Risk management
- Pharmacologic function
- Fluid and electrolyte status, including blood urea nitrogen level, creatinine level, intake and output, mucous membranes, serum electrolyte levels, and skin turgor

Risk Factors

- HIV coinfection
- Pharmaceutical agent
- Substance abuse
- Viral infection

Expected Outcomes

- Patient will state effects of environmental and ingested chemicals and substances on health and liver function.
- Patient will work with industry managers and with public health officials to lower or eliminate the presence of environmental chemicals and substances in work or living environment.
- Patient will have liver function indicators within normal limits.

- Patient will modify lifestyle and risk behaviors to avoid behaviors leading to hepatic dysfunction and inflammation.
- Patient will manage concurrent disease processes that impact hepatic function.
- Patient will acknowledge the impact of medications on hepatic function.
- Patient will observe measures to avoid the spread of infection to self and to others.
- Patient will maintain long-term follow-up for chronic illness with health care provider.
- Patient will optimize nutritional intake for needs.

Suggested NOC Outcomes

Health-Promoting Behavior; Risk Control—Alcohol; Risk Control—Drug Use; Safe Home Environment; Substance Addiction Consequences

Interventions and Rationales

- Assist patient and family to assess workplace and home environments for potential hepatotoxic substances *to increase patient's awareness of hazards in the environment and to lower potential for hepatic injury.*
- Monitor for clinical manifestations of hepatic inflammation and dysfunction *to notify physician in order to initiate treatment if liver function is compromised.* Clinical manifestations may include fatigue, depression or mood changes, anorexia, right upper quadrant tenderness, pruritis, jaundice, bruising, or nontraumatic bleeding.
- Monitor customary clinical laboratory tests *to alert the health care provider of the status of the immune/inflammatory response, the degree of hepatic metabolic dysfunction, and the impact of concurrent disorders on liver function.* Clinical laboratory tests include complete blood cell count: lower red blood cell count, elevated WBC (increased immunocyte and inflammatory responses); basic metabolic panel—altered electrolyte balance, elevated glucose, elevated blood urea nitrogen and creatinine level, elevated HbA_{1c}; hepatic plasma markers: elevated liver enzymes (alanine aminotransferase, aspartate aminotransferase, and γ-glutamyltranspeptidase); positive immunoassays *for pathogen and viral antigens*; elevated ammonia; elevated bilirubin; low coagulation factors; low total protein/albumin; elevated lipid panel.
- Carry out postprocedure measures, as ordered, *to identify and/or minimize complications.*
- PCC Teach patient about the following: perform hand hygiene before and after personal hygiene and care; cover draining and nonhealing wounds; report to care provider; inform others of infectious condition *so that each observes barrier precautions*; adhere to prescribed plan of care and treatment with immune system modifiers (antibiotics, antivirals, interferon, others); maintain a balanced nutritional diet intake. *These measures minimize patient's risk for self-infection and spread of infection and allow the patient to help modify lifestyle to maintain optimum health level for self and for others.*
- PCC Along with health care team, prepare the patient for and later evaluate the results of liver biopsy, and provide explanation to patient and family. *The patient and family need understanding of purpose for and implications of results obtained from a liver biopsy. This support and education helps the patient understand rationale for plan of treatment and genetic counseling for genetically linked hepatic disorders.*
- Provide a nonjudgmental attitude toward patient's lifestyle choices *to promote feelings of self-worth.*
- PCC Refer patient to counseling and therapy to address lifestyle choices and risk behaviors. *Modification of behaviors will provide risk avoidance for drug and alcohol abuse and exposure to body–substance pathogen infection.*

Suggested NIC Interventions

Behavioral Modification; Environment Risk Protection; Infection Protection; Risk Identification; Risk Identification—Genetic; Self-Modification Assistance; Sports Injury Prevention; Surveillance

Evaluations for Expected Outcomes

- Patient verbalizes impact of contaminants and exposure to chemicals on health.
- Patient follows prescribed treatment plan.
- Patient expresses feelings about condition and its effect on family.
- Patient describes response to procedures.

Documentation

- Liver function tests
- Interventions to provide supportive care and patient's response to supportive care
- Instructions given to patient and family members; return demonstration of knowledge and skills needed to carry out postprocedure regimen
- Patient's expression of concern about hepatic function and motivation to participate in self-care
- Evaluations for expected outcomes

REFERENCES

McPhail, M. W., & Christopher, K. B. (2016). LiFe: A liver injury score to predict outcome in critically ill patients. *Intensive Care Medicine*, *42*(3), 361–369. doi:10.1007/s00134-015-4203–4205

Morrison, D., Sgrillo, J., & Daniels, L. H. (2014). Managing alcoholic liver disease. *Nursing*, *44*(11), 30–41. doi:10.1097/01.NURSE.0000454950.13699.e0

Soller, R. W., Ho, T., & Lightwood, J. M. (2015). Improved label and liver warning for nonprescription acetaminophen products. *Therapeutic Innovation & Regulatory Science*, *49*(6), 890–897. doi:10.1177/2168479015586002

RISK FOR LONELINESS

Definition

Vulnerable to experiencing discomfort associated with a desire or need for more contact with others, which may compromise health

Assessment

- Family status, including family composition, presence of a spouse, ability of family to meet patient's physical and emotional needs, conflicts between patient's needs and family's ability to meet them, and family members' feelings of self-worth
- Psychological status, including changes in appetite, behavior, energy level, mood, motivation, self-image, self-esteem, or sleep patterns; alcohol and drug consumption; recent death, job loss, loss of loved one, or relocation; and psychiatric history
- Social status, including interpersonal skills, size of social network, quality of relationships, degree of trust in others, level of self-esteem, and ability to function in social and occupational roles

- Health history, including medical illness, disabilities, and deformities
- Spiritual status, including religious or church affiliation, description of faith and religious practices, and support network (family, clergy, and friends)

Risk Factors

- Affectional deprivation
- Emotional deprivation
- Physical isolation
- Social isolation

Expected Outcomes

- Patient will identify feelings of loneliness and will express desire to socialize more.
- Patient will identify behaviors that lead to loneliness.
- Patient will identify people whose support and acceptance are most likely.
- Patient will spend time with others.
- Patient will be comfortable in social settings, will interact with peers, and will receive support from others.
- Patient will make specific plans to continue involvement with others, such as through recreational activities or social interaction groups.

Suggested NOC Outcomes

Grief Resolution; Loneliness Severity; Risk Control; Social Involvement; Social Support

Interventions and Rationales

- Spend sufficient time with patient to allow self-expression of feelings of loneliness *to establish trusting relationship.*
- Inform patient that you'll help with expression of feelings of loneliness and identify ways to increase social activity *to bring issue into open and help patient understand that you want to be of help.*
- PCC Work with patient to identify factors and behaviors that have contributed to loneliness *to begin changing behaviors that may have alienated others.*
- PCC Help patient identify feelings associated with loneliness *to lessen their impact and mobilize energy to counteract them.*
- Help patient curb feelings of loneliness by encouraging one-on-one interaction with others whose acceptance is likely—for example, church members or patients with similar health problems—*to promote feelings of acceptance and support.*
- PCC Encourage patient to address personal needs assertively. *By being assertive, patient assumes responsibility for meeting personal needs, without anger or guilt.*
- As patient's comfort level improves, encourage patient to attend group activities and social functions *to promote use of social skills.*
- PCC Help patient identify social activities that patient can initiate, such as becoming active in a support group or volunteer organization, *to foster feelings of control and increase social contacts.*
- PCC Help patient come to terms with being viewed differently by others because of patient's illness, and explore ways of coping with their reactions *to help patient learn to cope with stigma associated with illness.*

- PCC Work with patient to establish goals for reducing feelings of loneliness after patient leaves health care setting *to focus energy on specific objectives.*
- PCC Refer patient and family to social service agencies, mental health center, and appropriate support groups *to ensure continued care and maintain social involvement.*

Suggested NIC Interventions

Activity Therapy; Anxiety Reduction; Counseling; Emotional Support; Energy Management; Socialization Enhancement; Spiritual Support; Visitation Facilitation

Evaluations for Expected Outcomes

- Patient expresses feelings of loneliness.
- Patient describes behaviors that lead to loneliness.
- Patient lists at least _____ (specify) people whose support and acceptance are most likely.
- Patient initiates conversations with peers.
- Patient participates in group activities.
- Patient describes plans to continue involvement with others.

Documentation

- Patient's statements of loneliness
- Observations of patient's behaviors and problems associated with loneliness
- Patient's choice of activities to end isolation
- Teaching of new coping methods
- Goals established by patient
- Evidence of efforts to use new coping mechanisms
- Referral
- Evaluations for expected outcomes

REFERENCES

Dury, R. (2014). Social isolation and loneliness in the elderly: an exploration of some of the issues. *British Journal of Community Nursing, 19*(3), 125–128.

Price, B. (2015). Approaches to counter loneliness and social isolation. *Nursing Older People, 27*(7), 31–39.

Zebhauser, A., Baumert, J., Emeny, R., Ronel, J., Peters, A., & Ladwig, K. (2015). What prevents old people living alone from feeling lonely? Findings from the KORA-Age-study. *Aging & Mental Health, 19*(9), 773–780. doi:10.1080/13607863.2014.977769

IMPAIRED MEMORY

related to neurologic impairment (e.g., positive EEG, head trauma, seizure disorders)

Definition

Inability to remember or recall bits of information or behavioral skills

Assessment

- Age, gender, level of education, occupation, and living arrangements
- Cardiovascular status, including vital signs, apical pulse, pulse rate and rhythm, and heart sounds; color of skin, lips, and nails; fatigue on exertion, dyspnea, and dizziness; history

of hypertension, chest pain, or anoxia; and complete blood count and differential, thyroid studies, electrocardiography, and echocardiography
- Family status, including household composition and marital status (presence of a spouse, length of marriage, divorce, or death of spouse)
- Neurologic status, including mental status (abstract thinking, insight about present situation, judgment, long- and short-term memory, cognition, and orientation to time, place, and person); level of consciousness; sensory ability; fine and gross motor functioning; history of neurologic disorder, head injury, or psychiatric illness; medication use; and computed tomography scan, magnetic resonance imaging, cerebral angiography, electroencephalography, toxicology studies, thyroid function, and serotonin levels
- Psychological status, including changes in appetite, behavior, energy level, mood, motivation, self-image, self-esteem, and sleep patterns; alcohol and drug consumption; recent divorce, separation, death, job loss, loss of loved one, relocation, or physical or emotional trauma; and psychiatric history
- Self-care status, including ability to carry out voluntary activities and use of adaptive equipment

Defining Characteristics

- Forgetfulness
- Forgets to perform a behavior at scheduled time
- Inability to learn new information
- Inability to learn new skill
- Inability to perform a previously learned skill
- Inability to recall events
- Inability to recall factual information
- Inability to recall if a behavior was performed
- Inability to retain new information

Expected Outcomes

- Patient will express feelings about memory impairment.
- Patient will acknowledge need to take measures to cope with memory impairment.
- Patient will identify coping skills to deal with memory impairment.
- Patient and family members will state specific plans to modify lifestyle.
- Patient and family members will establish realistic goals to deal with further memory loss.

Suggested NOC Outcomes

Cognition; Cognitive Orientation; Concentration; Depression Level; Memory; Neurologic Status

Interventions and Rationales

- Observe patient's thought processes during every shift. Document and report any changes. *Changes may indicate progressive improvement or a decline in patient's underlying condition.*
- S Implement appropriate safety measures to protect patient from injury. *Patient may be unable to provide for own safety needs.*
- Call patient by name and mention your name. Provide background information (place, time, and date) frequently throughout the day *to provide reality orientation.* Use a reality orientation board *to visually reinforce reality orientation.*

- Spend sufficient time with patient to allow him or her to become comfortable discussing memory loss *to establish a trusting relationship.*
- Inform patient that you're aware of patient's memory loss and that you'll provide help in coping with the condition *to bring the issue into the open and help patient understand that your goal is to be supportive.*
- Be clear, concise, and direct in establishing goals *so that patient can maximize the use of remaining cognitive skills.*
- Offer short, simple explanations to patient each time you carry out any medical or nursing procedure *to avoid confusion.*
- Label patient's personal possessions and photos, keeping them in the same place as much as possible, *to reduce confusion and create a secure environment.*
- PCC Encourage patient to develop a consistent routine for performing activities of daily living *to enhance patient's self-esteem and increase self-awareness and awareness of patient's environment.*
- PCC Teach patient ways to cope with memory loss—for example, using an alarm to remind patient when to eat or take medications, using a pillbox organized by days of the week, keeping lists in notebooks or a pocket calendar, and having family members or friends provide reminders of important tasks. *Reminders help limit the amount of information patient must maintain in memory.*
- Encourage patient to interact with others *to increase social involvement, which may decline with memory loss.*
- PCC Encourage patient to express the feelings associated with impaired memory *to reduce the impact of memory impairment on patient's self-image and lessen anxiety.*
- PCC Help patient and family members establish goals for coping with memory loss. Discuss with family members the need to maintain the least restrictive environment possible. Instruct them on how to maintain a safe home environment for patient. *This helps ensure that patient's needs are met and promotes independence.*
- Demonstrate reorientation techniques to family members and provide time for supervised return demonstrations *to prepare them to cope with patient with memory impairment.*
- PCC Help family members identify appropriate community support groups, mental health services, and social service agencies *to assist in coping with the effects of patient's illness or injury.*

Suggested NIC Interventions

Anxiety Reduction; Calming Technique; Cerebral Perfusion Promotion; Dementia Management; Fluid/Electrolyte Management; Memory Training; Neurologic Monitoring; Reality Orientation

Evaluations for Expected Outcomes

- Patient expresses feelings about memory impairment.
- Patient acknowledges need to take measures to cope with memory impairment.
- Patient describes mechanisms for coping with memory loss.
- Patient and family members describe plans to modify lifestyle.
- Patient and family members set realistic goals to cope with further memory loss.

Documentation

- Description of patient's mental status, including documentation of changes from shift to shift
- Outline of goals for helping patient cope with memory loss

- Response of family members to techniques for keeping patient functioning at maximal level
- Referrals to community support groups
- Evaluations for expected outcomes

REFERENCES

Calev, H., Spampinato, L. M., Press, V. G., Meltzer, D. O., & Arora, V. M. (2015). Prevalence of impaired memory in hospitalized adults and associations with in-hospital sleep loss. *Journal of Hospital Medicine*, *10*(7), 439–445. doi:10.1002/jhm.2364

Merilampi, S., Sirkka, A., Leino, M., Koivisto, A., & Finn, E. (2014). Cognitive mobile games for memory-impaired older adults. *Journal of Assistive Technologies*, *8*(4), 207–223. doi:10.1108/JAT-12-2013-0033

Stout, D. M., Shackman, A. J., Johnson, J. S., & Larson, C. L. (2015). Worry is associated with impaired gating of threat from working memory. *Emotion (15283542)*, *15*(1), 6–11. doi:10.1037/emo0000015

IMPAIRED PHYSICAL MOBILITY

related to musculoskeletal impairment; neuromuscular impairment

Definition

Limitation in independent, purposeful physical movement of the body or of one or more extremities

Assessment

- History of neuromuscular disorder or dysfunction
- Musculoskeletal status, including coordination, gait, muscle size and strength, muscle tone, range of motion (ROM), and functional mobility scale:
  0 = completely independent
  1 = requires use of equipment or device
  2 = requires help, supervision, or teaching from another person
  3 = requires help from another person and equipment or device
  4 = dependent; doesn't participate in activity
- Neurologic status, including level of consciousness, motor ability, and sensory ability

Defining Characteristics

- Alteration in gait
- Decrease in fine motor skills
- Decrease in gross motor skills
- Decrease in ROM
- Decrease in reaction time
- Difficulty turning
- Discomfort
- Engages in substitutions for movement (e.g., attention to other's activity, controlling behavior, focus on preillness activity)
- Movement-induced tremor
- Postural instability
- Slowed movement
- Spastic movement
- Uncoordinated movements

Expected Outcomes

- Patient will maintain muscle strength and joint ROM.
- Patient will show no evidence of complications, such as contractures, venous stasis, thrombus formation, skin breakdown, and hypostatic pneumonia.
- Patient will achieve highest level of mobility (will transfer independently, will be wheelchair-independent, or will ambulate with such assistive devices as walker, cane, and braces).
- Patient or family member will carry out mobility regimen.
- Patient or family member will make plans to use resources to help maintain level of functioning.

Suggested NOC Outcomes

Ambulation; Ambulation: Wheelchair; Discharge Readiness: Independent Living; Discharge Readiness: Supported Living; Mobility; Transfer Performance; Activities of Daily Living

Interventions and Rationales

- Perform ROM exercises to joints, unless contraindicated, at least once every shift. Progress from passive to active, as tolerated. *This prevents joint contractures and muscular atrophy.*
- Turn and position patient every 2 hours. Establish a turning schedule for dependent patients; post at the bedside and monitor frequency of turning. *This prevents skin breakdown by relieving pressure.*
- Place joints in functional position, use trochanter roll along the thigh, abduct the thighs, use high-top sneakers, and put a small pillow under patient's head. *These measures maintain joints in a functional position and prevent musculoskeletal deformities.*
- PCC Identify the level of functioning using a functional mobility scale (see Assessment). Communicate patient's skill level to all staff members *to provide continuity and preserve identified level of independence.*
- Encourage independence in mobility by helping patient to use a trapeze and side rails, to use the unaffected leg to move the affected leg, and to perform such self-care activities as combing hair, feeding, and dressing. *This increases muscle tone and patient's self-esteem.*
- S Place items within reach of the unaffected arm if patient has one-sided weakness or paralysis *to promote patient's independence.*
- Monitor and record daily any evidence of immobility complications (such as contractures, venous stasis, thrombus, pneumonia, and urinary tract infection). *Patients with a history of neuromuscular disorders or dysfunction may be more prone to developing complications.*
- Carry out a medical regimen to manage or prevent complications; for example, administer prophylactic heparin as ordered for venous thrombosis. *This promotes patient's health and well-being.*
- Provide progressive mobilization to the limits of patient's condition (bed mobility to chair mobility to ambulation) *to maintain muscle tone and prevent complications of immobility.* Use a transfer belt, if necessary, *to support patient and prevent staff injury.*
- PCC Refer patient to a physical therapist for development of mobility regimen *to help rehabilitate musculoskeletal deficits.*
- Encourage attendance at physical therapy sessions, and support activities on the unit by using the same equipment and technique. Request written mobility plans and use as reference. *All members of the health care team should reinforce learned skills in the same manner.*
- PCC Instruct patient and family members in ROM exercises, transfers, skin inspection, and mobility regimen *to help prepare patient for discharge.*

- Demonstrate the mobility regimen and note date. Have patient and family members return mobility regimen demonstration and note date. *This ensures continuity of care and use of proper technique.*
- PCC • Assist in identifying resources to carry out the mobility regimen, such as American Heart Association and National Multiple Sclerosis Society. *These resources help provide a comprehensive approach to rehabilitation.*

Suggested NIC Interventions

Activity Therapy; Energy Management; Exercise Promotion: Strength Training; Exercise Therapy: Joint Mobility; Exercise Therapy: Muscle Control; Positioning: Wheelchair; Surveillance: Safety

Evaluations for Expected Outcomes

- Patient maintains muscle strength and joint ROM.
- Patient shows no evidence of contractures, venous stasis, thrombus formation, skin breakdown, hypostatic pneumonia, or other complications.
- Patient achieves highest mobility level possible identified by health care team (specify).
- Patient or family member carries out mobility regimen.
- Patient or family member identifies and contacts at least one resource person or group to help maintain level of functioning.

Documentation

- Patient's expression of concern about loss of mobility, current status of functional abilities, and goals set for self
- Observations of patient's mobility status, presence of complications, and response to mobility regimen
- Instruction and demonstration of skills in carrying out mobility regimen
- Patient's response to nursing interventions
- Evaluations for expected outcomes

REFERENCES

Collins, B., & O'Mahony, P. (2015). Physically disabled adults' perceptions of personal autonomy. *Occupation, Participation & Health*, *35*(3), 160–168. doi:10.1177/1539449215575264

Di Marco, F., Terraneo, S., Roggi, M. A., Repossi, A. C., Pellegrino, G. M., Veronelli, A., ... Centanni, S. (2014). Physical activity impairment in depressed COPD subjects. *Respiratory Care*, *59*(5), 726–734. doi:10.4187/respcare.02848

Donoghue, O. A., Jansen, S., Dooley, C., De Rooij, S., Van Der Velde, N., & Kenny, R. A. (2014). Atrial fibrillation is associated with impaired mobility in community-dwelling older adults. *Journal of the American Medical Directors Association*, *15*(12), 929–933. doi:10.1016/j.jamda.2014.08.005

MORAL DISTRESS

related to end-of-life decisions

Definition

Response to the inability to carry out one's chosen ethical/moral decision/action

Defining Characteristics

- Anguish about acting on one's moral choice (e.g., powerlessness, anxiety, fear)

Assessment

- Age
- Medical diagnosis
- Mental status
- Treatment options
- Cultural beliefs about illness and death
- Roles/relationship within the family
- Communication patterns
- Coping skills
- Values/beliefs
- Place of religion in patient's life

Expected Outcomes

- The patient and family will understand medical diagnosis, treatment regimen, and limitations related to extent of illness;
- The patient and family will identify ethical/moral dilemma;
- The patient and family will describe personal and family values and conflict with current situation;
- The patient and family will identify health care ethics resources to assist in resolution of conflict;
- The patient and family will verbalize relief from anguish, uneasiness, or distress.

Suggested NOC Outcomes

Acceptance: Health Status; Client Satisfaction; Communication; Decision Making; Family Integrity; Family Functioning; Family Health Status; Family Integrity; Knowledge; Spiritual Health Interventions and Rationales

Interventions and Rationales

- PCC Assess patient's and family's understanding of the diagnosis and prognosis, limitations, treatment options; description of their personal values; and their physical expressions of suffering. *Assessment factors assist in identifying appropriate interventions.*
- PCC Establish an environment in which family members can share comfortably and openly their issues and concerns.
- PCC Enlist assistance of health care ethics resources such as ethics committee or consultants. *Including experts in health care ethics will assist in identifying the patient/family values and reason for the dilemma. By identifying the source of the conflict, the process of resolution may begin, thus leading to better understanding by all parties and partial or full relief from moral suffering.*
- PCC Enlist assistance of chaplain or personal clergy *to assist in the process of resolution through clarification of values related to religious views. Chaplains and personal clergy may provide a more neutral "third party" that can help defuse the situation. Personal trusted clergy might recognize or facilitate patient/family verbal and physical expressions of suffering or relief.*
- PCC Educate patient and family about medical diagnosis, treatment regimen, and limitations *to help both patient and family understand the limits of and read about medical treatment related to medical diagnosis.*
- Provide or set aside ample time for patient and family to express their feelings about the current situation. *Open, honest communication may clear misconceptions on both sides and facilitate relief from suffering in the midst of dilemma.*

- Acknowledge ethical/moral position of the patient/family who may feel that their positions or views will go unrecognized in the midst of serious illness and high-tech treatments; they may not want to "bother" nurses and physicians with these concerns. *Acknowledging their concerns, values, and moral position allows for holistic care.*
- PCC Refer, where requested, for follow-up for a family member who needs exercise, weight management, diet assistance, health screenings, and so forth. *Assisting patient to make referrals will help ensure continued efforts on the part of the patient to live a healthier lifestyle.*

Suggested NIC Interventions

Active Listening: Anger Control Assistance; Anxiety Reduction; Conflict Mediation; Consultation; Counseling; Documentation; Family Integrity Promotion; Family support; Multidisciplinary Care Conference; Spiritual Support Family Support; Family Integrity Promotion; Family Maintenance; Truth Telling

Evaluation of Expected Outcomes

- Family members express an understanding of the patient's diagnosis, treatment options, and prognosis.
- Patient and/or family describe the ethical dilemma in a way that will allow them to arrive at practical decisions about the situation.
- Patient and/or family can articulate how options for possible resolutions are consistent with religious beliefs and personal values.
- Patient and/or family consults with clergy or other trusted advisor.

Documentation

- Current medical condition
- Changes in condition
- Patient's expressed wishes
- Discussions between nursing staff and family about the patient's condition
- Consultation with other professionals involved in the case

REFERENCES

Cavinder, C. (2014). The relationship between providing neonatal palliative care and nurses' moral distress: an integrative review. *Advances in Neonatal Care, 14*(5), 322–328. doi:10.1097/ANC.0000000000000100

Mendel, T. R. (2014). The use of neonatal palliative care: Reducing moral distress in NICU nurses. *Journal of Neonatal Nursing, 20*(6), 290–293. doi:10.1016/j.jnn.2014.03.004

Weinzimmer, S., Miller, S. M., Zimmerman, J. L., Hooker, J., Isidro, S., & Bruce, C. R. (2014). Critical care nurses' moral distress in end-of-life decision making. *Journal of Nursing Education & Practice, 4*(6), 6–12. doi:10.5430/jnep.v4n6p6

IMPAIRED ORAL MUCOUS MEMBRANE

related to dehydration

Definition

Injury to the lips, soft tissue, buccal cavity, and/or oropharynx

Assessment

- History of pathologic conditions known to cause dehydration such as diabetes mellitus
- Medications, such as diuretics and antihistamines
- Vital signs
- Fluid and electrolyte status, including blood urea nitrogen level, creatinine level, intake and output, mucous membranes, serum electrolyte levels, skin turgor, and urine specific gravity
- Oral status, including inspection of oral cavity (gums and tongue), pain or discomfort, and salivation
- Nutritional status, including current weight, change from normal weight, and dietary pattern
- Psychosocial status, including change in financial status, coping skills, habits (smoking and alcohol intake), patient's perception of health problem, and recent traumatic event

Defining Characteristics

- Bad taste in mouth
- Bleeding
- Cheilitis
- Coated tongue
- Decrease in taste sensation
- Desquamation
- Difficulty eating
- Difficulty speaking
- Enlarged tonsils
- Exposure to pathogen
- Geographic tongue
- Gingival hyperplasia
- Gingival pallor
- Gingival pocketing deeper than 4 mm
- Gingival recession
- Halitosis
- Hyperemia
- Impaired ability to swallow
- Macroplasia
- Mucosal denudation
- Oral discomfort
- Oral edema
- Oral fissure
- Oral lesion
- Oral mucosal pallor
- Oral nodule
- Oral pain
- Oral papule
- Oral ulcer
- Oral vesicles
- Presence of mass (e.g., hemangioma)
- Purulent oral–nasal drainage
- Purulent oral–nasal exudates
- Smooth atrophic tongue
- Spongy patches in mouth
- Stomatitis
- White patches in mouth
- White plaque in mouth
- White, curd-like oral exudate
- Xerostomia

Expected Outcomes

- Patient will maintain fluid balance (intake equals output).
- Patient will state increased comfort.
- Patient will have pink, moist oral mucous membranes.
- Patient will have minimal, if any, complications.
- Patient will correlate precipitating factors with appropriate oral care.
- Patient will demonstrate oral hygiene practices.

Suggested NOC Outcomes

Oral Hygiene; Tissue Integrity: Skin & Mucous Membranes

Interventions and Rationales

- Inspect patient's oral cavity every shift. Describe and document condition; report any change in status. *Regular assessments can anticipate or alleviate problems.*
- Perform the prescribed treatment regimen, including administering IV or oral fluids, *to improve the condition of patient's mucous membranes.* Monitor progress, reporting favorable and adverse responses to the treatment regimen.
- Provide supportive measures, as indicated:
  - Assist with oral hygiene before and after meals *to promote a feeling of comfort and well-being.*
  - Use a toothbrush with suction if patient can't spit out water *to minimize risk of aspiration.*
  - Provide mouthwash or gargles, as ordered, *to increase patient comfort and maintain moisture in the mouth.*
  - Lubricate patient's lips frequently with water-based lubricant *to prevent cracked, irritated skin.*
- PCC Instruct patient in oral hygiene practices, if necessary. Have patient return a demonstration of the oral care routine.
  - Use a soft-bristled toothbrush.
  - Brush with a circular motion away from the gums.
  - Include the tongue when brushing.
  - Review the need for routine visits to a dentist (annually for adults).*These measures increase patient's awareness of oral hygiene practices and reduce discomfort, resulting in increased nutrition and hydration.*
- Tell patient to chew gum or suck on sugarless hard candy *to stimulate salivation.*
- Discuss precipitating factors, if known, and work to prevent future episodes. For example, encourage patient to avoid exercising in heat and to report effects of medication. *Patient's increased awareness of causative factors will help prevent recurrence.*
- Encourage adherence to other aspects of health care management (controlling diabetes, changing dietary habits, and avoiding alcoholic beverages) *to control or minimize effects on mucous membranes.*

Suggested NIC Interventions

Fluid/Electrolyte Management; Oral Health Maintenance; Oral Health Restoration

Evaluations for Expected Outcomes

- Patient's total daily fluid intake equals total output.
- Patient chews and swallows without discomfort.
- Patient's mucous membranes remain moist, pink, and free from cuts and abrasions.
- Patient doesn't develop complications related to extended dehydration of mucous membranes.
- Patient discusses possible causes of alteration in oral mucous membranes, such as heat exhaustion and reactions to medication.
- Patient discusses and demonstrates preventive measures such as regular oral hygiene.

Documentation

- Observations of condition, healing, and response to treatment
- Interventions to provide supportive care and patient's response to supportive care

- Instructions given, patient's understanding of instructions, and patient's demonstrated skill in carrying out prescribed oral care measures
- Evaluations for expected outcomes

REFERENCES

Chipps, E., Gatens, C., Genter, L., Musto, M., Dubis-Bohn, A., Gliemmo, M., … Landers, T. (2014). Pilot study of an oral care protocol on post-stroke survivors. *Rehabilitation Nursing*, *39*(6), 294–304. doi:10.1002/rnj.154

Pai, R. R., & Ongole, R. (2015). Nurses' knowledge and education about oral care of cancer patients undergoing chemotherapy and radiation therapy. *Indian Journal of Palliative Care*, *21*(2), 225–230. doi:10.4103/0973-1075.156507

Quinn, B., & Baker, D. L. (2015). Comprehensive oral care helps prevent hospital-acquired nonventilator pneumonia. *American Nurse Today*, *10*(3), 18–23.

IMPAIRED ORAL MUCOUS MEMBRANE

related to mechanical factor (e.g., ill-fitting dentures, braces, endotracheal/nasogastric tube, oral surgery); oral trauma

Definition

Injury to the lips, soft tissue, buccal cavity, and/or oropharynx

Assessment

- History of oral surgery, dentures, braces, or dental problems
- Medications, such as diuretics and antihistamines
- Vital signs
- Fluid and electrolyte status, including blood urea nitrogen level, creatinine level, intake and output, mucous membranes, serum electrolyte levels, skin turgor, and urine specific gravity
- Oral status, including inspection of oral cavity (with gums and tongue), pain or discomfort, and salivation
- Nutritional status, including current weight, change from normal weight, and dietary pattern
- Psychosocial status, including coping skills, patient's perception of health problem, and recent traumatic event

Defining Characteristics

- Bad taste in mouth
- Bleeding
- Cheilitis
- Coated tongue
- Decrease in taste sensation
- Desquamation
- Difficulty eating
- Difficulty speaking
- Enlarged tonsils
- Exposure to pathogen
- Geographic tongue
- Gingival hyperplasia
- Gingival pallor
- Gingival pocketing deeper than 4 mm
- Gingival recession
- Halitosis
- Hyperemia
- Impaired ability to swallow
- Macroplasia
- Mucosal denudation
- Oral discomfort
- Oral edema

- Oral fissure
- Oral lesion
- Oral mucosal pallor
- Oral nodule
- Oral pain
- Oral papule
- Oral ulcer
- Oral vesicles
- Presence of mass (e.g., hemangioma)
- Purulent oral–nasal drainage
- Purulent oral–nasal exudates
- Smooth atrophic tongue
- Spongy patches in mouth
- Stomatitis
- White patches in mouth
- White plaque in mouth
- White, curd-like oral exudate
- Xerostomia

Expected Outcomes

- Patient will maintain fluid balance (intake equals output).
- Patient will have pink, moist oral mucous membranes.
- Patient will state increased comfort.
- Patient will have minimal, if any, complications.
- Patient will correlate precipitating factors with appropriate oral care.
- Patient will demonstrate correct oral hygiene practices.

Suggested NOC Outcomes

Oral Hygiene; Pain Level; Tissue Integrity: Skin & Mucous Membranes

Interventions and Rationales

- Inspect patient's oral cavity every shift. Describe and document the condition, and report any status change. *Ill-fitting dentures, jagged teeth, braces, oral surgery, and insertion of an endotracheal tube may cause mechanical trauma. Regular assessments can anticipate or alleviate problems.*
- Establish and follow a routine oral hygiene schedule. For example, soak dentures every evening, clean with denture cream, rinse, and keep them in a properly labeled container at patient's bedside. *Routine oral hygiene can improve the condition of mucous membranes.*
- Provide supportive measures, as indicated:
  - Assist with oral hygiene before and after meals *to promote a feeling of comfort and well-being.*
  - Use a toothbrush with suction if patient can't spit out water *to minimize the risk of aspiration.*
  - Provide mouthwash or gargles, as ordered, *to increase patient comfort.*
  - Lubricate patient's lips frequently with water-based lubricant. *Fluid and food intake increases when patient is more comfortable.*
- PCC Instruct patient in oral hygiene practices, if necessary. Have patient return a demonstration of the oral care routine. Tell patient to stimulate saliva by chewing gum or sucking on sugarless hard candy. *These measures increase patient's awareness of oral hygiene practices and reduce discomfort, resulting in increased nutrition and hydration.*
- Discuss precipitating factors, if known, and work to prevent future episodes (e.g., weight loss may change the contours of the oral cavity). *Patient's increased awareness of causative factors will help prevent recurrence.*
- Encourage adherence to other aspects of health care management *to control or minimize the effects on mucous membranes.* For example, encourage patients with braces to avoid popcorn, chewing gum, and caramels. *These measures reduce the risk of trauma to oral mucous membrane.*

PCC • Refer patient to a dentist, dental hygienist, or other appropriate resource to correct ill-fitting dentures, modify braces, and adjust jaw wires as needed. *Regularly scheduled dental follow-up reduces the risk of trauma to oral mucous membranes.*

Suggested NIC Interventions

Fluid/Electrolyte Management; Oral Health Maintenance; Oral Health Restoration; Nutrition Management; Pain Management

Evaluations for Expected Outcomes

- Patient's total daily fluid intake equals output.
- Patient's mucous membranes remain moist, pink, and free from cuts and abrasions.
- Patient chews and drinks without discomfort.
- Patient doesn't exhibit complications related to trauma to oral mucous membranes.
- Patient discusses possible causes of alteration in oral mucous membranes, such as ill-fitting dentures or braces.
- Patient discusses preventive measures such as regular oral hygiene, which includes cleaning of dentures.

Documentation

- Observations of condition, healing, and response to treatment
- Interventions to provide supportive care and patient's response to supportive care
- Instructions given, patient's understanding of instructions, and demonstrated skill in carrying out prescribed oral care measures
- Evaluations for expected outcomes

REFERENCES

Chipps, E., Gatens, C., Genter, L., Musto, M., Dubis-Bohn, A., Gliemmo, M., … Landers, T. (2014). Pilot study of an oral care protocol on post-stroke survivors. *Rehabilitation Nursing*, *39*(6), 294–304. doi:10.1002/rnj.154

Laverty, D., Rajaram, K., & Clark, S. (2014). Management of trauma to the palate in toddlers. *Emergency Nurse*, *22*(8), 34–38. doi:10.7748/en.22.8.34.e1382

Quinn, B., & Baker, D. L. (2015). Comprehensive oral care helps prevent hospital-acquired nonventilator pneumonia. *American Nurse Today*, *10*(3), 18–23.

IMPAIRED ORAL MUCOUS MEMBRANE

related to decrease in platelets; immunodeficiency; infection; syndrome (e.g., Sjögren's)

Definition

Injury of the lips, soft tissue, buccal cavity, and/or oropharynx

Assessment

- History of oral cavity disorder or surgery
- Medication history
- Oral status, including condition of teeth, inspection of oral cavity (including gums and tongue), oral hygiene routine, pain or discomfort, palpation of buccal mucosa, and salivation

- Nutritional status, including current weight, change from normal weight, dietary pattern, and vitamin intake
- Psychosocial status, including coping skills, family members' habits (smoking and alcohol intake), patient's perception of health problem, self-concept, and stressors (finances, family, and job)

Defining Characteristics

- Bad taste in mouth
- Bleeding
- Cheilitis
- Coated tongue
- Decrease in taste sensation
- Desquamation
- Difficulty eating
- Difficulty speaking
- Enlarged tonsils
- Exposure to pathogen
- Geographic tongue
- Gingival hyperplasia
- Gingival pallor
- Gingival pocketing deeper than 4 mm
- Gingival recession
- Halitosis
- Hyperemia
- Impaired ability to swallow
- Macroplasia
- Mucosal denudation
- Oral discomfort
- Oral edema
- Oral fissure
- Oral lesion
- Oral mucosal pallor
- Oral nodule
- Oral pain
- Oral papule
- Oral ulcer
- Oral vesicles
- Presence of mass (e.g., hemangioma)
- Purulent oral–nasal drainage
- Purulent oral–nasal exudates
- Smooth atrophic tongue
- Spongy patches in mouth
- Stomatitis
- White patches in mouth
- White plaque in mouth
- White, curd-like oral exudate
- Xerostomia

Expected Outcomes

- Patient's lesions or wounds will show improvement or heal.
- Patient will have minimal, if any, complications.
- Patient will voice increased comfort.
- Patient will demonstrate understanding of surgical measures.
- Patient will voice feelings about condition.
- Patient will explain oral care routine.
- Patient will demonstrate oral hygiene practices.

Suggested NOC Outcomes

Hydration; Oral Hygiene; Self-Care: Oral Hygiene; Tissue Integrity: Skin & Mucous Membranes

Interventions and Rationales

- Inspect patient's oral cavity every shift. Describe and document its condition, reporting any status change. *Regular assessment prevents recurrence or exacerbation of problems.*
- Perform the prescribed treatment regimen for the underlying pathologic condition. Report favorable and adverse responses to the treatment regimen. *Treating the underlying condition improves the condition of the oral mucous membranes.*

PCC
- Encourage patient to state feelings and concerns about oral condition and its impact on body image *to help accept changes in body image.*
- Provide supportive measures, as indicated:
  - Assist with oral hygiene before and after meals. Use a soft-bristled toothbrush or cotton applicator and nonalcoholic mouthwash *to minimize trauma to damaged tissues.*
  - Lubricate patient's lips frequently *to prevent cracking and irritation.*
  - Use artificial saliva solution if the mouth remains dry *to restore normal moisture.*
  - Avoid serving hot, cold, spicy, fried, or citrus foods *to avoid irritating damaged tissue.*
  - Suction the oral cavity to prevent drooling and aspiration of accumulated secretions. *Aspiration may lead to pneumonia or coughing and further trauma.*
  - Give soft or pureed foods, which don't irritate tissues, *to reduce pain.*
- If oral surgery is scheduled, give the appropriate preoperative and postoperative instruction and care. Document the response. *Instruction enhances compliance with therapy.*

PCC
- Instruct patient in oral hygiene practices, and have patient give a return demonstration. Suggest a referral to a dentist or dental hygienist. *This increases patient's awareness of oral hygiene and reduces discomfort, resulting in increased nutrition and hydration.*
- Encourage patient to stop smoking. *Smoking has been linked to mucous membrane breakdown and cancer.*

PCC
- Refer patient to a psychiatric liaison nurse or support group *to help patient cope with altered body image.*

Suggested NIC Interventions

Fluid/Electrolyte Management; Infection Protection; Nutrition Management; Oral Health Restoration; Pain Management

Evaluations for Expected Outcomes

- Patient has no lesions or wounds, or they cause patient less discomfort.
- Patient doesn't exhibit complications related to trauma to oral mucous membranes.
- Patient chews and swallows without discomfort.
- Patient discusses impending surgical procedures.
- Patient discusses fear of oral surgery and outcome.
- Patient discusses postoperative oral care routine.
- Patient demonstrates oral hygiene practices, including treatments and medications.

Documentation

- Patient's expression of concern about oral condition and its impact on body image
- Patient's willingness to join in own care
- Observations of condition, healing, and response to treatment
- Interventions to provide supportive care and patient's response to supportive care
- Instructions given, patient's understanding of instructions, and demonstrated skill in carrying out prescribed oral care measures
- Evaluations for expected outcomes

REFERENCES

Chipps, E., Gatens, C., Genter, L., Musto, M., Dubis-Bohn, A., Gliemmo, M., ... Landers, T. (2014). Pilot study of an oral care protocol on post-stroke survivors. *Rehabilitation Nursing*, 39(6), 294–304. doi:10.1002/rnj.154

Pai, R. R., & Ongole, R. (2015). Nurses' knowledge and education about oral care of cancer patients undergoing chemotherapy and radiation therapy. *Indian Journal of Palliative Care, 21*(2), 225–230. doi:10.4103/0973-1075.156507

Quinn, B., & Baker, D. L. (2015). Comprehensive oral care helps prevent hospital-acquired nonventilator pneumonia. *American Nurse Today, 10*(3), 18–23.

NAUSEA

related to gastrointestinal irritation

Definition

A subjective phenomenon of an unpleasant feeling in the back of the throat and stomach, which may or may not result in vomiting

Assessment

- Health history, including illnesses, pregnancy, and medication use
- Nutritional status, including height, weight, fluctuations in weight, food preferences, and usual dietary patterns
- Psychosocial status, including ethnic background, family dynamics, lifestyle, perception of self, recent stressful events, and coping skills

Defining Characteristics

- Aversion toward food
- Gagging sensation
- Increase in salivation
- Increase in swallowing
- Nausea
- Sour taste

Expected Outcomes

- Patient will state reasons for nausea and vomiting.
- Patient will take steps to manage episodes of nausea and vomiting.
- Patient will ingest sufficient nutrients to maintain health.
- Patient will take steps to ensure adequate nutrition when nausea abates.
- Patient will maintain weight within specified range.

Suggested NOC Outcomes

Appetite; Comfort Level; Fluid Balance; Hydration; Nausea & Vomiting Control; Nutritional Status: Food & Fluid Intake; Suffering Severity; Symptom Control

Interventions and Rationales

- Ask patient reasons for nausea or inability to eat, and document explanation in patient's own words *to plan interventions.*

- Observe patient's fluid and food intake, and document the findings *to assess nutrient consumption and the need for supplements.*
- Encourage patient to eat dry, bland foods (such as dry toast or crackers) during periods of nausea *to make it possible for patient to eat.*
- Suggest that patient avoid offensive foods and food odors, shorten food preparation time, and eat and drink slowly. *These measures may help to prevent nausea from getting worse.*
- Administer antinausea medications, as prescribed, *to provide relief from nausea and allow patient to eat.*
- PCC Teach relaxation techniques, and help patient use such techniques during mealtime *to reduce stress and divert attention from nausea, thereby helping patient eat and drink.*
- Provide distractions when patient is feeling nauseated; for example, play favorite CDs, television program, taped books, and so on. *Distraction helps to divert the patient's attention from the unpleasant feeling of nausea.*
- PCC Encourage patient to make a list of best-tolerated and least-tolerated foods *to help patient choose foods wisely when nausea abates.*
- When nausea abates, encourage patient to eat larger amounts of food *to help patient consume adequate nutrients over time.*

Suggested NIC Interventions

Diet Staging; Fluid/Electrolyte Management; Fluid Monitoring; Medication Management; Nausea Management

Evaluations for Expected Outcomes

- Patient states reasons for nausea and vomiting.
- Patient takes steps to manage episodes of nausea and vomiting.
- Patient ingests sufficient nutrients to maintain health.
- Patient takes steps to ensure adequate nutrition when nausea abates.
- Patient maintains weight within specified range.

Documentation

- Patient's statements regarding nausea and its causes
- Episodes of nausea or vomiting
- Intake and output measurements
- Types of food and fluids ingested and patient's tolerance
- Nursing interventions, including teaching provided to patient
- Patient's response to nursing interventions
- Evaluations for expected outcomes

REFERENCES

Gonella, S., Berchialla, P., Bruno, B., & Di Giulio, P. (2014). Are orange lollies effective in preventing nausea and vomiting related to dimethyl sulfoxide? A multicenter randomized trial. *Supportive Care in Cancer*, *22*(9), 2417–2424. doi:10.1007/s00520-014-2227-y

Mamaril, M. E., Windle, P. E., & Burkard, J. F. (2006). Prevention and management of postoperative nausea and vomiting: A look at complementary techniques. *Journal of PeriAnesthesia Nursing*, *21*(6), 404–410.

Moradian, S., & Howell, D. (2015). Prevention and management of chemotherapy-induced nausea and vomiting. *International Journal of Palliative Nursing*, *21*(5), 216–224.

Ng, T. L., Hutton, B., & Clemons, M. (2015). Chemotherapy-induced nausea and vomiting: Time for more emphasis on nausea? *Oncologist*, *20*(6), 576–583. doi:10.1634/theoncologist.2014-0438

NONCOMPLIANCE

related to values incongruent with plan

Definition

Behavior of person and/or caregiver that fails to coincide with a health-promoting or therapeutic plan agreed on by the person (and/or family and/or community) and health care professional. In the presence of an agreed-upon, health-promoting, or therapeutic plan, the person's or caregiver's behavior is fully or partly nonadherent and may lead to clinically ineffective or partially ineffective outcomes

Assessment

- Age
- Health beliefs
- Patient's perceptions of health problem, treatment regimen, and importance of complying with treatment regimen
- Patient's ability to learn and perform prescribed treatment (activity, diet, and medications)
- Financial resources
- Cultural and ethnic influences
- Religious influences
- Educational and language background

Defining Characteristics

- Development-related complication
- Exacerbation of symptoms
- Failure to meet outcomes
- Missing of appointments
- Nonadherence behavior

Expected Outcomes

- Patient will identify factors that influence noncompliance.
- Patient will demonstrate level of compliance that doesn't interfere with physiologic safety.
- Patient will contract with nurse to perform ____ (specify behavior and frequency).
- Patient will use support systems to modify noncompliant behavior.

Suggested NOC Outcomes

Acceptance: Health Status; Adherence Behavior; Compliance Behavior; Health Beliefs: Perceived Resources; Health Orientation; Symptom Control; Treatment Behavior: Illness or Injury

Interventions and Rationales

- Listen to patient's reasons for noncompliance. *Active listening may reveal concerns not clearly stated in words and helps individualize the teaching process.*
- Approach patient in nonjudgmental manner. *This demonstrates unconditional positive regard for patient.*

- Identify specific areas of patient's noncompliant behavior *to help develop appropriate interventions.*
- Attempt to identify influencing factors associated with noncompliant behaviors, such as lack of understanding, unrealistic expectations, and cultural differences. *Reasons for noncompliance may range widely and include lack of knowledge, forgetting, feeling better or worse, and getting contradictory advice from family, friends, and health care providers.*
- Emphasize the positive aspects of compliance. *Understanding that compliance can reduce risk factors, prevent complications, and help manage certain chronic diseases may encourage patient to comply.*
- PCC Help patient clarify personal values *to allow patient to explore the intellectual and emotional components of the values that form the basis for the behavior in question.*
- PCC Acknowledge patient's right to choose not to carry out prescribed regimen. *Patient's autonomy must be respected; control over patient's action is legitimate only if needed to prevent harm to patient, to others, or to yourself.*
- PCC Contract with patient to practice only nonthreatening behaviors. *This involves both patient and caregiver in a formal commitment and gives patient a sense of personal control.*
- Use support systems to enforce or reinforce negotiated behaviors. *Support from patient's family helps foster compliance.*
- Give positive reinforcement for compliant behavior *to encourage patient to continue such behavior.*
- As medically appropriate, support patient who chooses to follow Eastern therapies instead of traditional Western medical practices. *Such support demonstrates your respect for patient's beliefs.*
- Determine whether patient's perceived noncompliance actually stems from a lack of financial resources. Contact appropriate agencies to help patient meet the costs of medical treatment and supplies and other financial needs. *Helping patient meet the financial requirements of treatment improves compliance.*

Suggested NIC Interventions

Coping Enhancement; Counseling; Decision-Making Support; Health Education; Patient Contracting; Self-Modification Assistance; Self-Responsibility Facilitation

Evaluations for Expected Outcomes

- Patient describes factors that influence noncompliance with health care regimen.
- Patient performs daily self-care in compliance with health care regimen.
- Patient performs behaviors agreed upon in contract with nurse.
- Patient uses available support resources, as needed.

Documentation

- Patient's statements that indicate noncompliant behavior
- Direct observation of noncompliant behavior
- Statements by patient that provide insight into causes of noncompliant behavior
- Terms agreed on by patient in performing negotiated behaviors
- Patient's daily progress in complying with treatment regimen
- Evaluations for expected outcomes

REFERENCES

JaHyun, K., Engberg, S. J., & Muto, C. A. (2014). Survey on influenza vaccination noncompliance among nursing students. *Infection Control & Hospital Epidemiology*, *35*(10), 1316–1317. doi:10.1086/678076

Jancey, J., Bowser, N., Burns, S., Crawford, G., Portsmouth, L., & Smith, J. (2014). No smoking here: Examining reasons for noncompliance with a smoke-free policy in a large university. *Nicotine & Tobacco Research*, *16*(7), 976–983. doi:10.1093/ntr/ntu012
Ohri, N., Rapkin, B. D., Guha, D., Haynes-Lewis, H., Guha, C., Kalnicki, S., & Garg, M. (2015). Predictors of radiation therapy noncompliance in an urban academic cancer center. *International Journal of Radiation Oncology, Biology, Physics*, *91*(1), 232–238. doi:10.1016/j.ijrobp.2014.09.030

IMBALANCED NUTRITION: LESS THAN BODY REQUIREMENTS

related to inability to digest food; inability to absorb nutrients

Definition

Intake of nutrients insufficient to meet metabolic needs

Assessment

- Gastrointestinal (GI) assessment, including antibiotic therapy, auscultation of bowel sounds, change in bowel habits, stool characteristics (color, amount, size, and consistency), history of GI disorder or surgery, inspection of abdomen, pain or discomfort, usual bowel elimination pattern, palpation for masses and tenderness, percussion for tympany and dullness, and nausea and vomiting
- Nutritional status, including change in type of food tolerated, financial resources, height and weight, meal preparation, serum albumin level, sociocultural influences, usual dietary pattern, and weight fluctuations over past 10 years
- Change in intrapersonal or interpersonal factors, including internal or external cues that trigger desire to eat, rate of food consumption, and stated food preference
- Psychosocial status
- Activity level
- Coping behaviors
- Body image, including perception of observer and self-perception

Defining Characteristics

- Abdominal cramping
- Abdominal pain
- Alteration in taste sensation
- Body weight 20% or more below ideal weight range
- Capillary fragility
- Diarrhea
- Excessive hair loss
- Food aversion
- Food intake less than recommended daily allowance
- Hyperactive bowel sounds
- Insufficient information
- Insufficient interest in food
- Insufficient muscle tone
- Misinformation
- Misperception
- Pale mucous membranes
- Perceived inability to ingest food
- Satiety immediately upon ingesting food
- Sore buccal cavity
- Weakness of muscles required for mastication
- Weakness of muscles required for swallowing
- Weight loss with adequate food intake

Expected Outcomes

- Patient will show no further evidence of weight loss.

- Patient will tolerate oral, tube, or IV feedings without adverse effects.
- Patient will take in ___ calories daily.
- Patient will gain ___ lb weekly.
- Patient and family members will communicate understanding of preoperative instructions.
- Patient and family members will communicate understanding of special dietary needs.
- Patient and family members will demonstrate ability to plan diet after discharge.

Suggested NOC Outcomes

Nutritional Status; Nutritional Status: Nutrient Intake; Symptom Severity; Weight Control

Interventions and Rationales

- Obtain and record patient's weight at the same time every day *to obtain accurate readings.*
- Monitor fluid intake and output *because body weight may decrease as a result of fluid loss.*
- Maintain parenteral fluids, as ordered, *to provide patient with needed fluids and electrolytes.*
- Provide a diet prescribed for patient's specific condition *to improve patient's nutritional status and increase weight.*
- Determine food preferences, and provide them within the limitations of patient's prescribed diet. *This enhances compliance with diet regimen.*
- Monitor electrolyte levels and report abnormal values. *Poor nutritional status may cause electrolyte imbalances.*
- If patient vomits, record amount, color, and consistency. Keep a record of all stools. *Vomitus and stool characteristics indicate status of nutrient absorption.*
- PCC Refer patient to a dietitian or nutritional support team for dietary management (possible regimens include yogurt feedings and low-bulk diet). *Dietitian or nutritional support team can help patient and health care team individualize patient's diet within prescribed restrictions.*
- If patient is receiving tube feeding:
  - Add food coloring if patient has an altered state of consciousness or diminished gag reflex *to help detect aspiration.*
  - If possible, use a continuous infusion pump for tube feeding *to avoid diarrhea.*
  - Begin the tube feeding regimen with a small amount and diluted concentration *to decrease diarrhea and improve absorption.* Increase the volume and concentration, as tolerated.
  - Keep the head of the bed elevated during tube feeding *to reduce the risk of aspiration.*
  - Check the feeding tube placement each shift *to verify placement in the GI tract rather than in the lungs.*
- If patient is receiving total parenteral nutrition:
  - Ensure delivery, as prescribed. *Electrolytes, amino acids, and other nutrients must be tailored to patient's needs.*
  - Monitor blood glucose levels and urine specific gravity at least once each shift. *Because glucose is the main component of total parenteral nutrition, patient may become hyperglycemic if not carefully monitored.*
- Monitor bowel sounds once per shift. *Normal active bowel sounds may indicate readiness for enteral feedings; hyperactive sounds may indicate poor absorption and may be accompanied by diarrhea.*

- Reinforce the medical regimen by explaining to patient and family members the reasons for the present regimen. *Collaborative practice enhances patient's overall care.*
- PCC Teach the principles of good nutrition for patient's specific condition. *This encourages patient and family members to participate in patient's care.*
- Provide or assist with oral hygiene *to help keep patient comfortable.*
- PCC Provide preoperative teaching, if needed, *to reduce patient's fear and anxiety and promote understanding.*
- PCC Involve family members in meal planning *to encourage them to help patient comply with the diet regimen after discharge.*

Suggested NIC Interventions

Energy Management; Nutritional Counseling; Nutrition Management; Nutrition Therapy; Weight Gain Assistance

Evaluations for Expected Outcomes

- Patient remains at or above specified weight.
- Patient doesn't develop adverse reactions from feedings, such as aspiration of food particles into lungs, diarrhea, and hyperglycemia.
- Patient consumes specified number of calories daily.
- Patient's weight increases by specified amount weekly.
- Patient and family communicate understanding of preoperative instructions, either verbally or through behavior.
- Patient and family communicate understanding of special dietary needs, either verbally or through behavior.
- Patient and family plan appropriate diet for patient to follow after discharge.

Documentation

- Daily weight
- Mouth care
- Maintenance of nasogastric tube
- Intake and output
- Bowel sounds
- Blood glucose levels
- Urine specific gravity
- Patient's ability to eat
- Incidence of vomiting or diarrhea
- Presence of other complications
- Patient's statements of understanding of dietary education
- Evaluations for expected outcomes

REFERENCES

Marik, P. E. (2014). Enteral nutrition in the critically ill: Myths and misconceptions. *Critical Care Medicine*, *42*(4), 962–969. doi:10.1097/CCM.0000000000000051

Roberts, S., Desbrow, B., & Chaboyer, W. (2014). Patient perceptions of the role of nutrition for pressure ulcer prevention in hospital. *Journal of Wound, Ostomy & Continence Nursing*, *41*(6), 528–534. doi:10.1097/WON.0000000000000072

Stewart, M. L. (2014). Interruptions in enteral nutrition delivery in critically ill patients and recommendations for clinical practice. *Critical Care Nurse*, *34*(4), 14–22. doi:10.4037/ccn2014243

IMBALANCED NUTRITION: LESS THAN BODY REQUIREMENTS

related to inability to ingest food

Definition

Intake of nutrients insufficient to meet metabolic needs

Assessment

- Gastrointestinal (GI) assessment, including auscultation of bowel sounds, change in bowel habits, characteristics of stools (color, amount, size, and consistency), history of GI disorder or surgery, inspection of abdomen, pain or discomfort, palpation for masses and tenderness, percussion for tympany and dullness, nausea and vomiting, and usual bowel pattern
- Nutritional status, including financial resources, height, meal preparation, serum albumin level, sociocultural influences, usual dietary pattern, weight, and weight fluctuations over past 10 years
- Intrapersonal and interpersonal factors, including internal and external cues that trigger desire to eat, rate of food consumption, and stated food preference
- Psychosocial status
- Activity level
- Coping behaviors
- Body image, including self-perception and perception of observer

Defining Characteristics

- Abdominal cramping
- Abdominal pain
- Alteration in taste sensation
- Body weight 20% or more below ideal weight range
- Capillary fragility
- Diarrhea
- Excessive hair loss
- Food aversion
- Food intake less than recommended daily allowance
- Hyperactive bowel sounds
- Insufficient information
- Insufficient interest in food
- Insufficient muscle tone
- Misinformation
- Misperception
- Pale mucous membranes
- Perceived inability to ingest food
- Satiety immediately upon ingesting food
- Sore buccal cavity
- Weakness of muscles required for mastication
- Weakness of muscles required for swallowing
- Weight loss with adequate food intake

Expected Outcomes

- Patient will show no further evidence of weight loss.
- Patient will tolerate ___ mL of nasogastric (NG) or gastrostomy tube feedings.
- Patient will avoid aspiration, diarrhea, and hyperglycemia.
- Patient will gain ___ lb weekly.
- Patient will consume ___ calories daily.
- Patient will avoid skin breakdown and infection around tube site.
- Patient and family members will communicate understanding of special dietary needs.
- Patient and family members will demonstrate correct tube feeding procedures.

Suggested NOC Outcomes

Nutritional Status; Nutritional Status: Food & Fluid Intake; Nutritional Status: Nutrient Intake; Weight Control

Interventions and Rationales

- Obtain and record patient's weight at the same time every day *to obtain accurate readings.*
- Monitor fluid intake and output because *body weight may increase as result of fluid retention.*
- Administer the prescribed amount of food *to provide patient with needed nutrition.*
  - Begin the regimen with a small amount and diluted concentration *to decrease diarrhea and improve absorption.* Increase the volume and concentration, as tolerated.
  - Elevate the head of the bed during tube feeding *to reduce the risk of aspiration.*
  - Check the feeding tube placement at least once every shift *to verify placement in the GI tract rather than in the lungs.*
  - Give water and juices, as needed, *to maintain adequate hydration.*
  - If possible, use a continuous infusion pump *to prevent diarrhea.*
  - Put food coloring in the food *to monitor for aspiration.*
- Provide nares care every 4 hours to prevent ulceration and skin breakdown. Tape the NG tube *to prevent visual obstruction.* Use hypoallergenic tape *to minimize skin reactions.*
- Change a gastrostomy dressing daily or according to facility protocol *to prevent infection.*
- Ensure the proper temperature of each feeding (room temperature); change the feeding tube bags and tubing according to facility protocol *to maximize tolerance and minimize infection.*
- Assess and record bowel sounds once per shift *to monitor for increase or decrease.*
- S Auscultate and record breath sounds every 4 hours *to monitor for aspiration.* Report wheezes, rhonchi, crackles, or decreased breath sounds. If aspiration is suspected, stop tube feeding. Keep suction apparatus at the bedside and suction as needed. Turn patient on the side *to avoid further aspiration.*
- PCC Instruct patient and family members in tube feeding procedures. Supervise return demonstrations until competency is achieved. *This encourages patient and family members to participate in patient's care.*

Suggested NIC Interventions

Bowel Management; Enteral Tube Feeding; Fluid/Electrolyte Management; Fluid Monitoring; Nutrition Management; Positioning

Evaluations for Expected Outcomes

- Patient shows no further evidence of weight loss.
- Patient tolerates NG or gastrostomy tube feedings without adverse effects.
- Patient doesn't exhibit signs of aspiration, diarrhea, or hyperglycemia.
- Patient gains specified amount of weight weekly.
- Patient consumes specified amount of calories daily.
- Patient avoids skin breakdown and infection around tube site.
- Patient and family members communicate understanding of special dietary needs and plan appropriate diet.
- Patient and family members demonstrate correct tube feeding procedures.

Documentation

- Daily weight
- Intake and output
- Tolerance of tube feeding
- Incidents of vomiting, aspiration, and diarrhea
- Bowel sounds
- Breath sounds
- Response to instructions
- Demonstration of feeding procedures
- Evaluations for expected outcomes

REFERENCES

Bagheri, S. C., & Meyer, R. A. (2014). When to refer a patient with a nerve injury to a specialist. *Journal of the American Dental Association (JADA)*, *145*(8), 859–861. doi:10.14219/jada.2014.45

Dasgupta, M., & Brymer, C. (2015). Poor functional recovery after delirium is associated with other geriatric syndromes and additional illnesses. *International Psychogeriatrics*, *27*(5), 793–802. doi:10.1017/S1041610214002658

Jefferies, D., Johnson, M., & Langdon, R. (2015). Rekindling the role of nurses in patients' oral nutrition. *International Journal of Nursing Practice*, *21*(3), 286–296. doi:10.1111/ijn.12269

IMBALANCED NUTRITION: LESS THAN BODY REQUIREMENTS

related to psychological disorder

Definition

Intake of nutrients insufficient to meet metabolic needs

Assessment

- History of eating disorders
- Nutritional history, including financial resources, height and weight, hereditary influences, meal preparation, sociocultural influences, usual dietary pattern, and weight fluctuations over past 10 years
- Change in intrapersonal or interpersonal factors, including internal and external cues that trigger desire to eat, rate of food consumption, and stated food preference
- Activity level
- Coping behaviors
- Body image, including self-perception and perception of observer

Defining Characteristics

- Abdominal cramping
- Abdominal pain
- Alteration in taste sensation
- Body weight 20% or more below ideal weight range
- Capillary fragility
- Diarrhea
- Excessive hair loss
- Food aversion
- Food intake less than recommended daily allowance
- Hyperactive bowel sounds
- Insufficient information
- Insufficient interest in food

- Insufficient muscle tone
- Misinformation
- Misperception
- Pale mucous membranes
- Perceived inability to ingest food
- Satiety immediately upon ingesting food
- Sore buccal cavity
- Weakness of muscles required for mastication
- Weakness of muscles required for swallowing
- Weight loss with adequate food intake

Expected Outcomes

- Patient will consume at least ___ calories daily.
- Patient will gain ___ lb weekly.
- Patient will eat independently, without being prodded.
- Patient will identify emotional and psychological factors that interfere with eating.
- Patient will develop plan to monitor and maintain target weight at discharge.
- Patient will plan to use mental health resources to help resolve psychological problems.

Suggested NOC Outcomes

Adherence Behavior; Body Image; Depression Level; Nutritional Status; Nutritional Status: Food & Fluid Intake; Nutritional Status: Nutrient Intake; Weight Control

Interventions and Rationales

- Provide opportunities for patient to discuss reasons for not eating *to help assess causes of eating disorder.*
- Observe and record patient's intake (both liquid and solid) *to assess what nutrients patient consumes and what supplements patient needs.*
- PCC Determine patient's food preferences, and attempt to obtain these foods. Offer foods that appeal to olfactory, visual, and tactile senses *to enhance patient's appetite.*
- Offer high-protein, high-calorie supplements, such as milk shakes, custard, and ice cream. *Such foods prevent body protein breakdown and provide caloric energy.*
- Serve foods that require little cutting or chewing *to help prevent malingering at meals.*
- Provide a pleasant environment at mealtime *to enhance patient's appetite.*
- Keep snacks at the bedside *to give patient some control over eating time.*
- With some patients, begin with nutritious liquids, and gradually introduce solid food. *Severely malnourished patient may not be able to chew solid foods immediately.*
- Avoid asking whether patient is hungry or wants to eat. Be positive in offering food. *A positive, undemanding attitude avoids confrontation with patient.*
- Whenever possible, sit with patient for a predetermined length of time during each meal. *This inhibits patient from dawdling during the meal and from hiding or hoarding food.*
- Monitor and record elimination patterns. *Patient may be taking laxatives or diuretics to keep weight low in spite of eating.*
- Weigh patient at the same time every day. *This yields accurate data and gives patient some control over foods eaten and privileges or rewards gained.*
- Set a target weight, and have patient record daily weight *to involve patient in treatment.*
- PCC Refer patient and family members to appropriate mental health professional as most eating disorders are psychological. *Patient and family members require treatment and follow-up to prevent recurrence.*

Suggested NIC Interventions

Diet Staging; Eating Disorders Management; Fluid Monitoring; Mutual Goal Setting; Referral; Weight Gain Assistance

Evaluations for Expected Outcomes

- Patient consumes specified number of calories daily.
- Patient gains specified amount of weight weekly.
- Patient eats independently without constant encouragement.
- Patient lists emotional and psychological factors that interfere with eating.
- Patient states plan to monitor and maintain specific target weight after discharge.
- Patient contacts support groups and mental health resources, as needed.

Documentation

- Patient's expressed attitudes toward food and eating at present time
- Patient's expressed feelings about weight, body image, and emotional status
- Patient's daily intake (liquid and solid) and output (urine, stools, and vomitus)
- Daily weight and progression of weight gain
- Interventions to feed patient adequately
- Emotional support provided
- Patient's response to nursing interventions
- Evaluations for expected outcomes

REFERENCES

Brooke, J., & Ojo, O. (2015). Oral and enteral nutrition in dementia: an overview. *British Journal of Nursing*, *24*(12), 624–628.

Pilgrim, A. L., Robinson, S. M., Sayer, A. A., & Roberts, H. C. (2015). An overview of appetite decline in older people. *Nursing Older People*, *27*(5), 29–35. doi:10.7748/nop.27.5.29.e697

Zhang, F., & Meng, Z. (2014). Clinical observation of early enteral nutrition therapy for patients with severe traumatic brain injury. *Chinese Journal of Contemporary Neurology & Neurosurgery*, *14*(4), 350–352. doi:10.3969/j.issn.1672-6731.2014.04.016

OBESITY

related to average daily physical activity is less than recommended for gender and age; heritability of interrelated factors (e.g., adipose tissue distribution, energy expenditure, lipoprotein lipase activity, lipid synthesis, lipolysis); high disinhibition and restraint eating behavior score

Definition

A condition in which an individual accumulates abnormal or excessive fat for age and gender that exceeds overweight

Assessment

- Health history including smoking, medications, change-of-life events, and illnesses
- Height and weight measurements
- Waist circumference measurement

- Calculate body mass index (BMI)
- Determine whether patient was overweight as a child
- Record monthly dietary history
- Record sleep schedule and habits
- Change in intrapersonal or interpersonal factors, including internal and external cues that trigger desire to eat
- Motivation to lose weight
- Rate of food consumption and stated food preference
- Psychosocial status
- Activity level
- Coping patterns
- Body image, including self-perception and perception of observer

Defining Characteristics

- *Adult*: BMI > 30 kg/m^2
- *Child* <2 years: Term not used with children at this age
- *Child* 2 to 18 years: BMI >30 kg/m^2 or >95th percentile for age and gender

Expected Outcomes

- Patient will identify internal and external cues that increase food consumption.
- Patient will plan menus appropriate to prescribed diet.
- Patient will adhere to prescribed diet.
- Patient will state plan to monitor and maintain target weight.
- Patient will identify consequences of overeating and weight gain.
- Patient will identify controllable factors that cause overeating.
- Patient will pursue weight loss that is optimal for maintenance of health.
- Patient will lose weight reasonably: 1 to 2 lbs/week.
- Patient will state understanding of the need to increase activity level gradually.
- Patient will state sense of satisfaction with each new level of activity attained.

Suggested NOC Outcomes

Anxiety Level; Eating Disorder Self-Control; Exercise Participation; Nutritional Status; Weight: Body Mass

Interventions and Rationales

- Discuss with patient the need to lose weight. *Even a 10% decrease in body weight yields health benefits.*
- PCC Help patient set realistic goals for losing weight. *This aids positive reinforcement and reduces frustration.*
- Support and encourage healthy patient behavior. *Creates positive relationship and reinforces healthy behaviors.*
- PCC Weigh patient in a private, nonthreatening setting. *Builds trust with care team and prevents embarrassment.*
- Use medical devices and equipment specifically for obese patients. *Using equipment that is too small yields inaccurate assessment results.*
- Assess for health comorbidities, such as diabetes, skin breakdown, and hypertension. *Obesity is linked to other health concerns, which can be exacerbated by weight fluctuations.*

- PCC Encourage attendance in support groups. *Support groups offer a place to share ideas and offer emotional support.*
- Evaluate for depression and anxiety. *Eating disorders can be linked to emotion.*
- Help patient identify the problem, feelings associated with eating, and circumstances in which patient turns to food. *Permanent weight loss starts with examination of factors contributing to weight gain.*
- Discuss patient's normal food preferences *to evaluate eating habits, and include preferred foods (if nutritious) in patient's diet.*
- Evaluate nutritional status and refer to registered dietitian as needed. *Obese patients may be malnourished because of improper diet habits.*
- Discuss with patient the need for activity. *Lack of activity causes physical deconditioning and may also have a negative impact on psychological well-being.*
- Help patient select an exercise program (such as walking, jogging, aerobics, or swimming) appropriate to patient's age and physical condition. *Besides aiding weight loss, such activities offer an alternative to eating to alleviate stress.*
- PCC Teach patient exercises for increasing strength and endurance *to improve breathing and promote general physical reconditioning.*
- Support and encourage activity to patient's level of tolerance *to help foster patient's independence.*

Suggested NIC Interventions

Anxiety Reduction; Behavior Modification; Exercise Promotion; Nutrition Management; Nutritional Therapy; Risk Identification; Teaching: Prescribed Diet; Weight Reduction Assistance

Evaluations for Expected Outcomes

- Patient states a desire to lose weight.
- Patient expresses feelings about present weight.
- Patient identifies cues that increase food consumption.
- Patient and health care professional establish weekly weight-loss goal.
- Patient identifies a plan to increase activity level.
- Patient describes healthy eating pattern.
- Patient's blood pressure and pulse and respiratory rates remain within normal parameters.
- Patient expresses satisfaction with diet.
- Patient adheres to prescribed diet.
- Patient loses specified amount of weight weekly.
- Patient increases physical activity.

Documentation

- Patient's perception of weight and body image
- Patient's weekly weight
- Patient's physical measurements, especially waist circumference
- Behaviors that promote or impede weight reduction
- Observations made while patient performs physical activities
- New activities patient is able to perform
- Evaluations for expected outcomes

REFERENCES

Bray, G., Look, M., & Ryan, D. (2013). Treatment of the obese patient in primary care: Targeting and meeting goals and expectations. *Postgraduate Medicine, 125*(5), 67–77. doi:10.3810/pgm.2013.09.2692

Chacko, S. A., Chiodi, S. N., & Wee, C. C. (2015). Recognizing disordered eating in primary care patients with obesity. *Preventive Medicine*, *72*, 89–94. doi:10.1016/j.ypmed.2014.12.024

Kushner, R. F. (2012). Clinical assessment and management of adult obesity. *Circulation, 126*, 2870–2877. doi:10.1161/CIRCULATIONAHA.111.075424

Mauldin, K., & O'Leary-Kelley, C. (2015). New guidelines for assessment of malnutrition in adults: Obese critically ill patients. *Critical Care Nurse, 35*(4), 24–31. doi:10.4037/ccn2015886

National Institute of Diabetes and Digestive and Kidney Diseases. (n.d.). *Medical care for patients with obesity.* Retrieved from http://www.niddk.nih.gov/health-information/health-topics/weight-control/medical/Pages/medical-care-for-patients-with-obesity.aspx

ACUTE PAIN

related to biologic injury agent (e.g., infection, ischemia, neoplasm); chemical injury agent (e.g., burn, capsaicin, methylene chloride, mustard agent); physical injury agent (e.g., abscess, amputation, burn, cut, heavy lifting, operative procedure, trauma, overtraining)

Definition

An unpleasant sensory and emotional experience associated with actual or potential tissue damage, or described in terms of such damage (International Association for the Study of Pain); sudden or slow onset of any intensity from mild to severe with an anticipated or predictable end

Assessment

- Descriptive characteristics of pain, including location, quality, intensity on a scale of 1 to 10, temporal factors, and sources of relief
- History of exposure to physical, biologic, or chemical agents as a cause of pain
- Physiologic variables, such as age and pain tolerance
- Psychological variables, such as body image, personality, previous experience with pain, anxiety, and secondary gain
- Sociocultural variables, including cognitive style, culture or ethnicity, attitude and values, sex, and birth order
- Environmental variables, such as setting and time

Defining Characteristics

- Appetite change
- Change in physiologic parameter (e.g., blood pressure, heart rate, respiratory rate, oxygen saturation, and end-tidal CO_2)
- Diaphoresis
- Distraction behavior
- Evidence of pain using standardized pain behavior checklist for those unable to communicate verbally (e.g., Neonatal Infant Pain Scale, Pain Assessment Checklist for Seniors with Limited Ability to Communicate)
- Expressive behavior (e.g., restlessness, crying, vigilance)
- Facial expression of pain (e.g., eyes lack luster, beaten look, fixed or scattered movement, grimace)

- Guarding behavior
- Hopelessness
- Narrowed focus (e.g., time perception, thought processes, interaction with people and environment)
- Positioning to ease pain
- Protective behavior
- Proxy report of pain behavior/activity changes (e.g., family member, caregiver)
- Pupil dilation
- Self-focused
- Self-report of intensity using standardized pain scale (e.g., Wong-Baker FACES scale, visual analog scale, numeric rating scale)
- Self-report of pain characteristics using standardized pain instrument (e.g., McGill Pain Questionnaire, Brief Pain Inventory)

Expected Outcomes

- Patient will rate pain on a scale of 1 to 10.
- Patient will express relief from pain within a reasonable time after intervention.
- Patient will identify specific characteristics of pain.
- Patient will help develop a plan for pain control.
- Patient will articulate factors that intensify pain and will modify behavior accordingly.
- Patient will state and carry out appropriate interventions for pain relief.
- Patient will report more than 4 hours of sleep nightly.
- Patient will decrease amount and frequency of pain medication needed.
- Patient will state satisfaction with pain management regimen.
- Patient will use available resources to understand pain phenomenon and will cooperate with treatment plan.

Suggested NOC Outcomes

Comfort Level; Pain Control; Pain: Disruptive Effects; Pain Level; Sleep

Interventions and Rationales

- Assess patient's signs and symptoms of pain, and administer pain medication, as prescribed. Monitor and record the medication's effectiveness and adverse effects. *Assessment allows for care plan modification, as needed.*
- Use a pain scale when assessing pain. *Although pain is subjective, when using the scale you can compare the patient's perception of pain from one assessment to another.*
- Return to patient in 30 minutes to check intervention effectiveness. *This establishes trusting–caring relationship that encourages accurate communication.*
- Perform comfort measures to promote relaxation, such as massage, bathing, repositioning, and relaxation techniques. *These measures reduce muscle tension or spasm, redistribute pressure on body parts, and help patient focus on non-pain-related subjects.*
- Plan activities with patient to provide distraction, such as reading, crafts, television, and visits, *to help patient focus on non-pain-related matters.*
- PCC Provide patient with information to help increase pain tolerance; for example, reasons for pain and length of time it will last. *This educates patient and encourages compliance in trying alternative pain-relief measures.*
- Manipulate the environment to promote periods of uninterrupted rest. This promotes health, well-being, and increased energy level important to pain relief.

- Apply heat or cold, as ordered (specify), *to minimize or relieve pain.*
- Help patient into a comfortable position, and use pillows to splint or support painful areas, as appropriate, *to reduce muscle tension or spasm and to redistribute pressure on body parts.*
- PCC Collaborate with patient in administering prescribed analgesics when alternative methods of pain control are inadequate. *Gaining patient's trust and involvement helps ensure compliance and may reduce medication intake.*
- PCC Consider the services of a psychiatric mental health professional to help patient and staff members establish a realistic plan to resolve the problem. *Patients who remain helpless, unmotivated, uncooperative, and manipulative are self-destructive. Underlying causes should be explored.*
- Discuss with patient possible association between exacerbation of pain and patient's identified stressors. *This helps patient explore exacerbating emotional or environmental factors that may affect pain.*
- PCC Ask patient to help establish goals, and develop plan for pain control. *This gives patient a sense of control.*
- Provide patient with positive feedback about progress toward reaching goals *to improve motivation and encourage compliance.*
- Spend at least 15 minutes/shift allowing patient to express feelings, *which will help give patient a sense of control.*
- When possible, allow patient to use alternative pain treatments from patient's culture (such as acupuncture) as a substitute for or complement to Western treatments *to promote nonpharmacologic pain management.*

Suggested NIC Interventions

Anxiety Reduction; Coping Enhancement; Emotional Support; Hope Instillation; Medication Management; Pain Management; Positioning; Sleep Enhancement

Evaluations for Expected Outcomes

- Patient's pain rating is documented (using a scale of 1 to 10) before administering medication and 30 to 45 minutes afterward.
- Patient articulates factors that intensify pain and modifies behavior accordingly.
- Patient carries out alternative pain control measures such as heat or cold applications.
- Patient reports more than 4 hours' sleep nightly (reports of less than 4 hours require further assessment).
- Patient decreases amount and frequency of pain medication within 72 hours.
- Patient discusses characteristics of pain, including location, duration, and frequency.
- Patient reports achieving pain relief with analgesia or other measures.
- Patient participates in development of health care plan and discusses modifications.
- Patient acknowledges that pain may be related to emotional factors, and lists stressors that may exacerbate pain. Patient states satisfaction with pain management regimen.

Documentation

- Patient's description of physical pain, pain relief, and feelings about pain
- Observations of patient's physical, psychological, and sociocultural responses to pain
- Comfort measures and medications provided to reduce pain and effectiveness of interventions
- Information provided to patient about pain and pain relief

- Other interventions performed to assist patient with pain control
- Evaluations for expected outcomes

REFERENCE

Gregory, J. (2014). Dealing with acute and chronic pain: part one—assessment. *Journal of Community Nursing*, *28*(4), 83–86.
Kizza, I. B., & Muliira, J. K. (2015). Nurses' pain assessment practices with critically ill adult patients. *International Nursing Review*, *62*(4), 573–582. doi:10.1111/inr.12218
Siedlecki, S. L., Modic, M. B., Bernhofer, E., Sorrell, J., Strumble, P., & Kato, I. (2014). Exploring how bedside nurses care for patients with chronic pain: A grounded theory study. *Pain Management Nursing*, *15*(3), 565–573. doi:10.1016/j.pmn.2012.12.007
Whitaker, M. H. (2012). Sounds soothing: Music therapy for postoperative pain. *Nursing*, *146*(4), 678–679.

CHRONIC PAIN

related to muscle injury; nerve compression

Definition

Unpleasant sensory and emotional experience associated with actual or potential tissue damage, or described in terms of such damage (International Association for the Study of Pain); sudden or slow onset of any intensity from mild to severe, constant, or recurring without an anticipated or predictable end and a duration of greater than three (>3) months

Assessment

- Descriptive characteristics of pain, including location, quality, intensity on a scale of 1 to 10, temporal factors, duration, precipitating factors (food, alcohol, activity, and stress), and comfort factors
- Physiologic variables, such as general health state, length of pain, organ system involvement, pain tolerance, disability (work, family, or social), and pain interventions (such as injection, traction, ice, physical therapy, and transcutaneous electrical nerve stimulation)
- Psychological variables, such as age, self-esteem, self-worth, role (worker, husband, breadwinner), coping behavior (appropriate or inappropriate), secondary gains (disability insurance, workmen's compensation, litigation), suffering (emotional component), manipulative behavior, dependence on others or on system, and previous hospital experience
- Sociocultural variables, including educational level, motivation, culture or ethnicity, sex, values and beliefs, pain behaviors, financial distress, and religion
- Environmental variables, such as setting and time
- Pharmacologic variables, including type of drugs, amount used in 1 day, use of illicit drugs, and use of alcohol

Defining Characteristics

- Alteration in ability to continue previous activities
- Alteration in sleep pattern
- Anorexia
- Evidence of pain using standardized pain behavior checklist for those unable to communicate verbally (e.g., Neonatal Infant Pain Scale, Pain Assessment Checklist for Seniors with Limited Ability to Communicate)

- Facial expression of pain (e.g., eyes lack luster, beaten look, fixed or scattered movement, grimace)
- Proxy report of pain behavior/activity changes (e.g., family member, caregiver)
- Self-focused
- Self-report of intensity using standardized pain scale (e.g., Wong-Baker FACES scale, visual analog scale, numeric rating scale)
- Self-report of pain characteristics using standardized pain instrument (e.g., McGill Pain Questionnaire, Brief Pain Inventory)

Expected Outcomes

- Patient will identify characteristics of pain and pain behaviors.
- Patient will develop pain management program that includes activity and rest schedule, exercise program, and medication regimen that isn't pain contingent.
- Patient will carry out resocialization behavior and activities.
- Patient will state relationship of increasing pain to stress, activity, and fatigue.
- Patient will state importance of self-care behavior or activities.

Suggested NOC Outcomes

Comfort Level; Depression Level; Depression Self-Control; Pain Control; Pain Level; Quality of Life; Sleep; Symptom Control

Interventions and Rationales

- Assess patient's physical symptoms of pain, physical complaints, and daily activities. Administer pain medication, as prescribed. Monitor and record the effectiveness and adverse effects of medication. (Keep in mind that pain behavior and pain talk may be inconsistent.) *Correlating patient's pain behavior with activities, time of day, and visits may be useful in modifying tasks.*
- PCC Provide instruction about amount of pain medication needed to control symptoms, and allow the patient to remain active. *Teaching patient about medications may help to increase the accuracy of dosage necessary to provide pain relief.*
- Develop a behavior-oriented care plan; for instance, set up a plan to follow the activity schedule. *Behavioral–cognitive measures can help patient modify learned pain behaviors.*
- PCC Teach patient how to use relaxation techniques, guided imagery, massage, or music therapy to relieve pain. *These methods work as an adjunct to medications, increase self-help, and foster independence.*
- PCC Teach patient and family members such techniques as massage, application of ice, and exercise *to relieve pain and foster independence.*
- PCC Work closely with staff and patient's family *to achieve pain management goals and maximize patient's cooperation.*
- Use behavior modification; for example, spend time with patient only if the discussion includes no pain talk. Use contingency rewards for decreasing pain talk and pain behavior. *Reducing pain talk helps patient refocus on other, more important matters.*
- Encourage self-care activities. Develop a schedule. *This helps patient gain a sense of control and reduces dependence on caregivers and society.*
- Establish a specific time to talk with patient about pain and its psychological and emotional effects *to establish a trusting, supportive relationship that encompasses patient's physiologic, emotional, social, sexual, and financial concerns.*

Suggested NIC Interventions

Analgesic Administration; Behavior Modification; Biofeedback; Emotional Support; Mood Management; Pain Management; Patient Contracting; Simple Massage

Evaluations for Expected Outcomes

- Patient maintains activity diary and pain-level chart that rates severity of pain on a scale of 1 to 10.
- Patient maintains pain management program that includes activity and rest schedule, exercise program, and medication regimen.
- Patient demonstrates resocialization behavior and activities.
- Patient states that stress, activity, and fatigue may increase pain.
- Patient states that self-care activities are important.

Documentation

- Patient's description of physical pain, pain relief, and feelings about pain
- Pain talk and pain behavior and affect
- Relationship of reports of pain to activities
- Treatments and pain talk
- Time out of bed
- Comfort measures initiated by nurse, patient, or family members
- Response to interventions
- Response to pharmacologic agents
- Interaction with staff
- Evaluations for expected outcomes

REFERENCES

Barrie, J., & Loughlin, D. (2014). Managing chronic pain in adults. *Nursing Standard*, *29*(7), 50–58. doi:10.7748/ns.29.7.50.e9099

Bloot, L., Heins, M. J., Donders, R., Bleijenberg, G., & Knoop, H. (2015). The process of change in pain during cognitive-behavior therapy for chronic fatigue syndrome. *Clinical Journal of Pain*, *31*(10), 914–921. doi:10.1097/AJP.0000000000000191

Gilron, I., & Kehlet, H. (2014). Prevention of chronic pain after surgery: New insights for future research and patient care. *Canadian Journal of Anesthesia*, *61*(2), 101–111. doi:10.1007/s12630-013-0067-8

Siedlecki, S. L., Modic, M. B., Bernhofer, E., Sorrell, J., Strumble, P., & Kato, I. (2014). Exploring how bedside nurses care for patients with chronic pain: A grounded theory study. *Pain Management Nursing*, *15*(3), 565–573. doi:10.1016/j.pmn.2012.12.007

CHRONIC PAIN SYNDROME

Definition

Recurrent or persistent pain that has lasted at least three months, and that significantly affects daily functioning or well-being

Assessment

- Characteristics of pain: location, quality, intensity on a scale of 1 to 10, duration, precipitating factors (food, alcohol, activity, and stress), and comfort factors

- Physiologic variables: general health state, length of pain, organ system involvement, pain tolerance, disability (work, family, or social), and pain interventions (such as injection, traction, ice, physical therapy, and transcutaneous electrical nerve stimulation)
- Psychological variables: age, self-esteem, self-worth, depression, poor sleep quality, fatigue, decreased libido, role (worker, husband, breadwinner), coping behavior (appropriate or inappropriate), suffering (emotional component), manipulative behavior, dependence on others or on system, and previous hospital experience
- Sociocultural variables: educational level, motivation, culture or ethnicity, sex, values and beliefs, pain behaviors, financial distress, and religion
- Use of medications including type of drug, amount used in 1 day, and/or use of illicit drugs
- Use of alcohol
- Environment

Defining Characteristics

- Anxiety
- Constipation
- Deficient knowledge
- Disturbed sleep pattern
- Fatigue
- Fear
- Impaired mood regulation
- Impaired physical mobility
- Insomnia
- Obesity
- Social isolation
- Stress overload

Expected Outcomes

- Patient will develop pain management program that includes activity and rest schedule, exercise program, and medication regimen that isn't pain contingent.
- Patient will state relationship of increasing pain to stress, activity, and fatigue.
- Patient will state importance of self-care behavior or activities.

Suggested NOC Outcomes

Agitation Level; Anxiety Level; Appetite; Client Satisfaction: Pain Control; Comfort Status; Depression Level; Fatigue Level; Personal Well-Being; Quality of Life

Interventions and Rationales

- Assess patient's physical symptoms of pain, physical complaints, and daily activities. *Knowing patterns is essential in developing a pain management plan.*
- Administer pain medication, as prescribed. Monitor and record the effectiveness and adverse effects of medication. (Keep in mind that pain behavior and pain talk may be inconsistent.) *Medicating pain before it is out of control fosters better pain management.*
- PCC Provide instruction about amount of pain medication needed to control symptoms, and allow the patient to remain active. *Teaching patient about medications may help to increase the accuracy of dosage necessary to provide pain relief.*
- Develop a behavior-oriented care plan; for instance, set up a plan to follow the activity schedule. *Behavioral–cognitive measures can help patient modify learned pain behaviors.*
- PCC Teach patient how to use relaxation techniques, guided imagery, massage, or music therapy to relieve pain. *These methods work as an adjunct to medications, increase self-help, and foster independence.*
- PCC Teach patient and family members techniques such as massage, application of ice, and exercise *to relieve pain and foster independence.*

PCC
- Work closely with patient, patient's family, and staff *to achieve pain management goals and maximize patient's cooperation.*
- Encourage self-care activities. Develop a schedule. *This helps patient gain a sense of control and reduces dependence on caregivers and society.*

Suggested NIC Interventions

Analgesic Administration; Coping Enhancement; Guided Imagery; Mood management; Positioning; Relaxation Therapy

Evaluations for Expected Outcomes

- Patient maintains activity diary and pain-level chart that rates severity of pain on a scale of 1 to 10.
- Patient maintains pain management program that includes activity and rest schedule, exercise program, and medication regimen.
- Patient states that stress, activity, and fatigue may increase pain.
- Patient states that self-care activities are important.

Documentation

- Patient's description of physical pain, pain rating, pain relief, and feelings about pain
- Comfort measures initiated by nurse, patient, or family members
- Response to interventions
- Response to pharmacologic agents
- Interaction with others
- Evaluations for expected outcomes

REFERENCES

Barrie, J., & Loughlin, D. (2014). Managing chronic pain in adults. *Nursing Standard*, *29*(7), 50–58. doi:10.7748/ns.29.7.50.e9099

Bloot, L., Heins, M. J., Donders, R., Bleijenberg, G., & Knoop, H. (2015). The process of change in pain during cognitive-behavior therapy for chronic fatigue syndrome. *Clinical Journal of Pain*, *31*(10), 914–921. doi:10.1097/AJP.0000000000000191

Gilron, I., & Kehlet, H. (2014). Prevention of chronic pain after surgery: New insights for future research and patient care. *Canadian Journal of Anesthesia*, *61*(2), 101–111. doi:10.1007/s12630-013-0067-8

Siedlecki, S. L., Modic, M. B., Bernhofer, E., Sorrell, J., Strumble, P., & Kato, I. (2014). Exploring how bedside nurses care for patients with chronic pain: A grounded theory study. *Pain Management Nursing*, *15*(3), 565–573. doi:10.1016/j.pmn.2012.12.007

RISK FOR POISONING

Definition

Vulnerable to accidental exposure to, or ingestion of, drugs or dangerous products in sufficient doses, which may compromise health

Assessment

- Health history, including accidents, allergies, exposure to pollutants, falls, hyperthermia, hypothermia, poisoning, sensory or perceptual changes (auditory, gustatory, kinesthetic, olfactory, tactile, and visual), and trauma

- Circumstances surrounding present situation that might lead to injury
- Neurologic status, including level of consciousness (LOC), mental status, and orientation
- Psychosocial history, including age, habits (drug or alcohol use), occupation, and personality
- Laboratory studies, including clotting factors, hemoglobin levels and hematocrit, platelet count, white blood cell count, and toxicology screening

Risk Factors

External

- Access to dangerous product
- Access to illicit drugs potentially contaminated by poisonous additives
- Access to large supply of pharmaceutical agents in house
- Access to pharmaceutical agent

Internal

- Alteration in cognitive function
- Emotional disturbance
- Inadequate precautions against poisoning
- Insufficient knowledge of pharmacological agents
- Insufficient knowledge of poisoning prevention
- Occupational setting without adequate safeguards
- Reduced vision

Expected Outcomes

- Patient won't ingest or be exposed to dangerous substances.
- Patient will communicate an understanding of need for self-protection.
- Patient and family members will state method for safekeeping of potentially dangerous products.

Suggested NOC Outcomes

Safe Home Environment, Risk Control: Drug Use; Risk Detection

Interventions and Rationales

- Observe, record, and report falls, seizures, and unsafe practices to ensure implementation of appropriate interventions. *Overdose of certain medications (such as phenothiazines) can cause such neurologic problems as seizures.*
- S Monitor and record patient's respiratory status *because certain poisons can cause respiratory depression.*
- S Monitor and record neurologic status *because excessive toxic exposure can cause coma.* Patient may have pinpoint or dilated pupils, depending on the type of drug ingested and the length of time patient has been hypoxic.
- Monitor vital signs, intake and output, and LOC. Record and report any changes. Severe hypotension may develop following overdose. *It may be related to central nervous system defect, direct myocardial depression, or vasodilation. Marked hyperthermia can occur with salicylate overdose, which affects the metabolic rate. Dehydration may develop in some patients from an increased respiratory rate, sweating, vomiting, and urine losses.*
- S Remove dangerous or potentially dangerous products from the environment *to avoid injury.*
- Observe, record, and report falls, seizures, and unsafe practices to ensure implementation of appropriate interventions. *Overdose of certain medications can cause such neurologic problems as seizures.*

- Check the settings on oxygen flow meters every hour on patients known to retain carbon dioxide (e.g., some patients with chronic obstructive pulmonary disease). *This avoids carbon dioxide narcosis from excessive oxygen therapy in poorly ventilated patients; if unchecked, patient may stop breathing.*
- PCC Provide patient and family members with information about such specific products as medications, oxygen, and total parenteral nutrition. Tailor instructions to a specific product and patient's ability to learn self-care. *This enables patient and family members to identify and alter environmental or lifestyle factors to achieve optimum health level.*

Suggested NIC Interventions

Environmental Management: Safety; Environmental Risk Protection; Health Education; Home Maintenance Assistance; Surveillance: Safety; Vital Signs Monitoring; Medication Management; Risk Identification

Evaluations for Expected Outcomes

- Patient doesn't report or exhibit signs or symptoms resulting from exposure to or ingestion of dangerous substances.
- Patient requests information on protection from dangerous products.
- Patient and family members describe method for safekeeping of potentially dangerous products.

Documentation

- Patient's statements that indicate potential for injury
- Physical findings
- Record of falls, seizures, and unsafe practices
- Observations or knowledge of unsafe practices
- Interventions performed to prevent injury
- Patient's response to nursing interventions
- Evaluations for expected outcomes

REFERENCES

Morris, D. S., & Fiala, S. C. (2015). Online electronic cigarette retailers can do more to prevent accidental poisonings. *Tobacco Control*, *24*(4), 415–416. doi:10.1136/tobaccocontrol-2014-051779

Marcus, D. M., & Grollman, A. P. (2016). Toxicity of botanical medicines: An overlooked global health problem. *American Journal of Public Health*, *106*(1), 16–17.

Wong, C., Lin, Y., Hong, L., Chen, T., Ma, H., Hsu, Y., … Wu, M. (2016). Increased long-term risk of dementia in patients with carbon monoxide poisoning: A population-based study. *Medicine*, *95*(3), 1–5. doi:10.1097/MD.0000000000002549

RISK FOR PERIOPERATIVE-POSITIONING INJURY

Definition

Vulnerable to inadvertent anatomical and physical changes as a result of posture or equipment used during an invasive/surgical procedure, which may compromise health

Assessment

- Reason for surgery
- Type of surgery and its expected length
- Health status, including age, weight, vital signs, nutritional status, integumentary status, musculoskeletal status, hydration status, temperature, peripheral vascular status, neurologic status, and smoking history
- Laboratory studies, including hematocrit and hemoglobin levels, complete blood count, electrolyte levels, urinalysis, blood coagulation studies, and liver function tests
- Mobility status, including range of motion (ROM), presence of prosthesis, and limb abnormality, impairment, or injury
- Current medical treatments, including radiation therapy, chemotherapy, and steroid therapy

Risk Factors

- Disorientation
- Edema
- Emaciation
- Immobilization
- Muscle weakness
- Obesity
- Sensoriperceptual disturbance from anesthesia

Expected Outcomes

- Patient will maintain effective breathing patterns.
- Patient will maintain adequate cardiac output.
- Patient's surgical positioning will facilitate gas exchange.
- Patient won't show evidence of neurologic, musculoskeletal, or vascular compromise.
- Patient will maintain tissue integrity.

Suggested NOC Outcomes

Blood Coagulation; Circulation Status; Cognitive Orientation; Neurologic Status; Respiratory Status: Ventilation; Thermoregulation; Tissue Integrity: Skin & Mucous Membranes; Tissue Perfusion: Peripheral

Interventions and Rationales

- Document and report the results of the preoperative nursing assessment. Identify factors predisposing patient to tissue injury. *This information guides interventions.*
- Use the appropriate mode of patient transportation (stretcher, patient bed, wheelchair, or crib) *to ensure patient safety.*
- Make sure an adequate number of staff members assist with transferring patient—at least two for moving patient onto an operating room bed, and at least four for moving anesthetized patient off operating room bed. *Adequate staffing enhances safety.*
- Check the operating room bed before surgery for proper functioning. *Intraoperative bed malfunction can result in increased anesthesia time and a more difficult surgical approach.*
- Ensure proper positioning.

Supine Position

- Check patient's neck and spine for proper alignment *to avoid trauma.*
- Check that patient's legs are straight and ankles uncrossed. *Crossed ankles cause pressure on tissue, vessels, and nerves.*
- Place a safety strap 29 (5 cm) above patient's knees, tight enough to restrain without compromising superficial venous return. *Applied too tightly, the safety strap may cause venous thrombosis or compression of tibial, peroneal, or sciatic nerves.*
- Secure patient's arms at sides with a drawsheet, with palms down, making sure no part of the arm or hand extends over the mattress. Alternatively, secure the patient's arms on padded arm boards at less than a 90° angle from the body, with palms supinated. *Hyperextension can cause injury to the brachial plexus. Supination of palms minimizes pressure.*
- Apply eye pads if patient's eyelids won't remain closed or if surgery is being performed on the head, neck, or chest. If allowed to remain open, the eye may dry out and become infected. *Corneal abrasions may result from drapes and other foreign material rubbing against the eye.*
- If surgery is expected to last more than 2 hours or if patient is predisposed to a pressure injury, place padding under patient's occiput, scapulae, olecranon, sacrum, coccyx, and calcaneus *to protect potential pressure points.* Apply a padded footboard *to support patient's feet, avoid plantar flexion, and prevent stretching of the tibial nerve and subsequent foot drop.*
- Unless contraindicated, place a foam doughnut or small pillow under patient's head *to prevent stretching of the neck muscles.*

Prone Position

- Make sure at least four staff members assist when turning patient *to ensure safety.*
- Check the lower eye and ear for excessive pressure. Apply eye pads. *Head support helps maintain cervical and thoracic spine alignment. Checking the dependent ear and eye lowers the risk of pressure injury. Pads protect the eyes.*
- Place patient's arms on arm boards extended in front beside patient's head with the elbows slightly flexed and palms pronated *to prevent strain on the shoulder, elbows, and wrist joints.*
- Check for proper alignment of the neck and spine *to avoid trauma.*
- Check a female patient's breasts and male patient's genitalia for excessive pressure from chest rolls or a laminectomy brace *to avoid soft tissue and nerve injury.*
- Check the bilateral pulses of upper and lower extremities. *The top and bottom edges of chest rolls or a laminectomy brace may compress radial and femoral arteries.*
- Place padding under patient's knees *to avoid injury to soft tissue and knee joint.*
- Place a pillow under patient's ankles *to avoid putting pressure on toes and feet, stretching the tibial nerve, or causing plantar flexion.*

Lateral Position

- Make sure at least four staff members assist when turning patient *to ensure safety.*
- Check patient's neck and spine for proper alignment *to avoid trauma.*
- Check patient's dependent eye and ear for excessive pressure. Apply eye pads. *Head supports help maintain cervical and thoracic spine alignment. Checking the dependent ear and eye lowers the risk of pressure injury. Pads protect patient's eyes.*
- Place a small roll under patient's dependent lower axilla *to relieve pressure on chest and axilla, allow for adequate chest expansion, and prevent compression of the brachial plexus by the humeral head.*

- Place patient's lower arm on arm board at less than 90° angle from the body, with palm supinated. Place patient's upper arm on an elevated padded support at less than a 90° angle from the body, with palm pronated, and apply restraints *to avoid injury to brachial plexus.*
- Place the bottom leg flexed at the hip and knee and the top leg straight. *Flexing the bottom leg provides greater stability for the torso, decreases pressure on the lateral aspect of the lower leg, and prevents the bony areas of the knees and ankles from pressing against each other.*
- Place pillows between patient's knees and ankles *to support the top leg, prevent strain on the top hip, and pad pressure points on the medial aspects of both legs.*
- Place padding under the lateral aspects of patient's bottom knee and ankle *to reduce the risk of tissue injury to the area over the lateral malleolus of the ankle and peroneal nerve damage (foot drop).*
- Place a safety strap across patient's upper thighs or wide tape over the hips. Attach a strap or tape to the bed *to ensure safety.*

Lithotomy Position

- Secure patient's arms on arm boards or at the sides. If the arms are placed at patient's sides, position the fingers away from the break in the table *to prevent the fingers from becoming compressed in the bed mechanism.*
- Check patient's neck and spine for proper alignment *to avoid trauma.*
- Position the stirrups at equal height, and attach them to the bed securely to prevent accidental movement. *Uneven leg flexion and hip abduction can cause strain on the lumbar and sacral areas.*
- Place the loop straps of the post stirrup behind patient's ankle and under the foot. Pad the post portion of the stirrup if it could come in contact with the leg. *Loop straps support and secure the legs.*
- Pad popliteal knee support stirrups *to prevent possible thrombosis of superficial vessels and pressure injury to femoral and obturator nerves.*
- With the help of a coworker, raise and lower patient's legs simultaneously and slowly to prevent ankle and knee injury and hip dislocation. *Lowering legs too quickly may cause sudden hypotension.*
- Assess patient position following each positional change *to ensure proper body alignment and adequate padding and support.*
- Apply restraints after positioning patient *to prevent falls and injury.*

Suggested NIC Interventions

Aspiration Precautions; Bleeding Reduction: Wound; Circulatory Care: Arterial Insufficiency; Circulatory Care: Venous Insufficiency; Embolus Care: Pulmonary; Fluid Management; Hemodynamic Regulation; Infection Control: Intraoperative; Positioning: Intraoperative; Skin Surveillance; Surgical Precautions; Temperature Regulation: Intraoperative

Evaluations for Expected Outcomes

- Patient maintains effective breathing patterns. Patient's position doesn't restrict ventilation. Patient has adequate chest expansion.
- Patient maintains adequate cardiac output. Patient doesn't experience any significant episodes of hypertension or hypotension.

- Patient's positioning allows for adequate gas exchange, as evidenced by patient's ventilation–perfusion ratio and oxygen saturation.
- Patient shows no evidence of neurologic, musculoskeletal, or vascular compromise. Patient's mobility status and ROM remain at preoperative levels. Patient doesn't experience pain, numbness, tingling, or weakness in positioned body parts.
- Patient's tissue integrity remains intact; skin doesn't become reddened, discolored, ulcerated, edematous, or excoriated.

Documentation

- Results of preoperative nursing assessment
- Operative procedure, type of anesthesia, and surgical positioning
- Surgical times, including time patient entered operating room, time incision was made, time incision was closed, and time patient left operating room
- Method of patient transport and transfer
- Estimated intraoperative blood loss
- Types and placement of padding, restraints, and positional devices
- Intraoperative repositioning of patient
- Intraoperative insertion of permanent or temporary implants
- Peripheral pulses
- Evaluations for expected outcomes

REFERENCES

Innmann, M. M., Streit, M. R., Kolb, J., Heiland, J., Parsch, D., Aldinger, P. R., … Merle, C. (2015). Influence of surgical approach on component positioning in primary total hip arthroplasty. *BMC Musculoskeletal Disorders*, *16*(1), 1–7. doi:10.1186/s12891-015-0623-1

Sørensen, E. E., Kusk, K. H., & Grønkjær, M. (2015). Operating room nurses' positioning of anesthetized surgical patients. (2016). *Journal of Clinical Nursing*, *25*(5/6), 690–698. doi:10.1111/jocn.13000

Spruce, L., & Van Wicklin, S. A. (2014). Back to basics: Positioning the patient. *AORN Journal*, *100*(3), 298–305. doi:10.1016/j.aorn.2014.06.004

POSTTRAUMA SYNDROME

related to serious accident (e.g., industrial, motor vehicle)

Definition

Sustained maladaptive response to a traumatic, overwhelming event

Assessment

- History and circumstances of accident or trauma
- Physical injuries sustained, including cardiopulmonary, musculoskeletal, genitourinary, and integumentary
- Neurologic status
- Emotional reactions, including grief reaction, self-concept, and sleep pattern
- Cognitive reactions, including concentration, memory, and orientation
- Behavioral reactions, including available support systems, clergy, coping patterns, family members, problem-solving ability, and social interactions

Defining Characteristics

- Aggression
- Alienation
- Alteration in concentration
- Alteration in mood
- Anger
- Anxiety
- Avoidance behavior
- Denial
- Depression
- Dissociative amnesia
- Enuresis
- Exaggerated startle response
- Fear
- Flashbacks
- Gastrointestinal irritation
- Grieving
- Guilt
- Headache
- Heart palpitations
- History of detachment
- Hopelessness
- Horror
- Hypervigilance
- Intrusive dreams
- Intrusive thoughts
- Irritability
- Neurosensory irritability
- Nightmares
- Panic attacks
- Rage
- Reports of feeling numb
- Repression
- Shame
- Substance abuse

Expected Outcomes

- Patient will recover or be rehabilitated from physical injuries to the extent possible.
- Patient will state feelings and fears related to traumatic accident or event.
- Patient will express feelings of safety.
- Patient will use available support systems.
- Patient will use effective coping mechanisms to reduce fear.
- Patient will maintain or reestablish adaptive social interactions with family members.

Suggested NOC Outcomes

Anxiety Self-Control; Body Image; Coping; Depression Level; Fear Self-Control; Hope; Impulse Self-Control; Quality of Life; Self-Esteem; Stress Level

Interventions and Rationales

- Follow the medical regimen to manage physical injuries. *Attention to physical needs supports healing of the body.*
- Provide emotional support:
  - Visit patient frequently *to reduce patient's fear of being alone.*
  - Be available to listen *to respond empathetically to patient's feelings.*
  - Accept and encourage the statement of patient's feelings *to reassure patient that feelings are appropriate and valid.*
  - Assure patient of personal safety, and take the measures needed to ensure it. *Frequent nightmares or flashbacks may cause patient to question the safety of his or her environment.*
  - Avoid care-related activities or environmental stimuli that may intensify symptoms associated with trauma (loud noises, bright lights, abrupt entrances into patient's room, or painful procedures or treatment). *Environmental stimuli can easily intensify flashbacks to a traumatic event.*

- Reorient patient to surroundings and reality as frequently as necessary. *Posttrauma psychic numbing impairs orientation, memory, and reality perception.*
- PCC – Instruct patient in at least one fear-reducing behavior such as seeking support from others when frightened. *As patient learns to reduce fears, coping skills will increase.*

- Support patient's family members:
  - Provide time for them to express feelings.
  - Help them understand patient's reactions. *This reduces their anxiety and gives them a chance to help patient.*
- PCC Offer referrals to other support persons or groups, including clergy, mental health professionals, and trauma support groups. *Referrals help patient to regain a sense of universality, reduce isolation, share fears, and deal constructively with feelings.*
- PCC Recognize that patient's culture may affect patient's response to trauma; remain supportive and nonjudgmental *to show your support for and acceptance of patient's response to trauma.*

Suggested NIC Interventions

Active Listening; Anxiety Reduction; Coping Enhancement; Counseling; Forgiveness Facilitation; Mood Management; Security Enhancement; Socialization Enhancement; Support Group

Evaluations for Expected Outcomes

- Patient resumes usual activities of daily living to extent possible.
- Patient expresses feelings associated with traumatic event.
- Patient expresses feeling of safety.
- Patient interacts with supportive people to alleviate distress.
- Patient demonstrates use of at least one fear-reducing behavior (specify).
- Patient interacts with family members in beneficial manner.

Documentation

- Patient's perception of traumatic event
- Observations of patient's behavior
- Observations of patient's social interaction with others
- Interventions
- Patient's responses to nursing interventions
- Referrals to other support persons or groups
- Evaluations for expected outcomes

REFERENCES

Bloch, F., Blandin, M., Ranerison, R., Claessens, Y., Rigaud, A., & Kemoun, G. (2014). Anxiety after a fall in elderly subjects and subsequent risk of developing posttraumatic stress disorder at two months. A pilot study. *Journal of Nutrition, Health & Aging*, *18*(3), 303–306. doi:10.1007/s12603-013-0415-y

Rock, L. F. (2014). Sedation and its association with posttraumatic stress disorder after intensive care. *Critical Care Nurse*, *34*(1), 30–39. doi:10.4037/ccn2014209

Warlan, H., & Howland, L. (2015). Posttraumatic stress syndrome associated with stays in the intensive care unit: Importance of nurses' involvement. *Critical Care Nurse*, *35*(3), 44–54. doi:10.4037/ccn2015758

RISK FOR POSTTRAUMA SYNDROME

Definition

Vulnerable to sustained maladaptive response to a traumatic, overwhelming event, which may compromise health

Assessment

- Age and gender
- History of traumatic event, including circumstances, losses incurred (financial, property, physical integrity, close relationships), effect of trauma on social interactions, and grief reaction
- Health history, including previous traumatic events, patient's characteristic perception of such events and coping responses, and alcohol or substance abuse
- Mental status, including cognitive and emotional function, problems with concentration, memory, orientation, mood, and behavior
- Changes in appetite, self-image, sleep pattern, or sexual drive
- Available sources of support, including friends, family, caregivers, and community resources

Risk Factors

- Diminished ego strength
- Displacement for home
- Duration of traumatic event
- Environment not conducive to needs
- Exaggerated sense of responsibility
- Human service occupations (e.g., police, fire, rescue, corrections, emergency room, mental health)
- Insufficient social support
- Perceives event as traumatic
- Survivor role

Expected Outcomes

- Patient won't develop chronic posttrauma response, substance abuse, or other mental health disorders.
- Patient will express understanding of posttrauma response.
- Patient's response to trauma won't be characterized by avoidance, numbness, or intrusiveness.
- Patient will express feelings of safety.
- Patient will employ effective coping skills.
- Patient will reach out to appropriate sources of support to reduce fear.

Suggested NOC Outcomes

Coping; Depression Level; Depression Self-Control; Risk Detection; Social Support; Spiritual Health; Stress Level

Interventions and Rationales

- Follow the medical regimen *to treat medical problems associated with the traumatic event.*
- Assess patient's baseline mental status, and monitor changes in cognitive and psychosocial function *to detect the need for intervention as soon as possible.*
- Listen actively to patient's statements about the traumatic event *to encourage a trusting relationship and open discussion.*
- PCC Communicate your acceptance of patient's fears and feelings related to the traumatic event *so patient is reassured that feelings are appropriate and valid.*
- Reassure patient of safety of the environment. *Patient may be reluctant to express lingering fears and require reassurance.*
- Avoid nursing care or environmental stimuli that may worsen or initiate symptoms (such as loud noises, bright lights, and painful procedures) *to avoid triggering flashbacks to the traumatic event.* Also, warn patient to avoid disruptive stimuli.
- Caution patient before you make physical contact, and avoid approaching patient from behind *to avoid actions that may be misinterpreted and that may trigger reexperience of the traumatic event.*
- PCC Explore with patient strategies to reduce the traumatic response, such as having a support person call patient on a regular basis and using stress-reducing techniques when experiencing increased fear and anxiety, *to strengthen coping skills and foster a sense of control.*
- PCC Teach patient that a posttrauma response may occur immediately or days, weeks, or years after a trauma *to alert patient to the risk of posttrauma response.*
- PCC Help patient to increase awareness of people, places, and events that trigger or reduce a posttrauma response *to encourage patient to take an active role in treatment.*
- Provide opportunities for patient to discuss the trauma periodically, based on patient's needs and willingness to talk *to prevent the development of posttrauma response.*
- PCC Encourage family members and friends to express their perceptions and feelings about the traumatic event and reactions they see in patient *to aid assessment.*
- PCC Provide teaching to family members, friends, and caregivers about the signs and symptoms of posttrauma response and interventions they can use *to promote involvement with rather than withdrawal from patient.*
- Explore uses of appropriate community resources, and make referrals according to patient's and family members' needs *to ensure continuity of care and decrease patient's isolation.*

Suggested NIC Interventions

Coping Enhancement; Hope Instillation; Mood Management; Self-Awareness Enhancement

Evaluations for Expected Outcomes

- Patient doesn't develop chronic posttrauma response, substance abuse, or other mental health disorders.
- Patient expresses understanding of posttrauma response.
- Patient's response to trauma isn't characterized by avoidance, numbness, or intrusiveness.
- Patient expresses feelings of safety.
- Patient employs effective coping skills and reaches out to appropriate sources of support to reduce fear.

Documentation

- Patient's perception of the traumatic event
- Observation of patient's behavior, coping skills, and use of support systems
- Patient's response to nursing care activities
- Patient's communication patterns with friends, family, and others and their responses
- Teaching provided to patient and family
- Referrals for ongoing support
- Evaluations for expected outcomes

REFERENCES

Bloch, F., Blandin, M., Ranerison, R., Claessens, Y., Rigaud, A., & Kemoun, G. (2014). Anxiety after a fall in elderly subjects and subsequent risk of developing posttraumatic stress disorder at two months. A pilot study. *Journal of Nutrition, Health & Aging*, *18*(3), 303–306. doi:10.1007/s12603-013-0415-y

Rock, L. F. (2014). Sedation and its association with posttraumatic stress disorder after intensive care. *Critical Care Nurse*, *34*(1), 30–39. doi:10.4037/ccn2014209

Warlan, H., & Howland, L. (2015). Posttraumatic stress syndrome associated with stays in the intensive care unit: Importance of nurses' involvement. *Critical Care Nurse*, *35*(3), 44–54. doi:10.4037/ccn2015758

POWERLESSNESS

related to dysfunctional institutional environment

Definition

The lived experience of lack of control over a situation, including a perception that one's actions do not significantly affect an outcome

Assessment

- Nature of the medical diagnosis
- Mobility
- Behavioral responses (verbal and nonverbal), including calmness or agitation, anger, independence or dependence, interest or apathy, and satisfaction or dissatisfaction
- Usual coping strategies
- Past experiences with hospitalization
- Knowledge, including current understanding of physical condition and physical, mental, and emotional readiness to learn
- Environment, including equipment and supplies, health care professionals and personnel, lighting, location of patient's personal belongings, noise, privacy, and space

Defining Characteristics

- Alienation
- Dependency
- Depression
- Doubt about role performance
- Frustration about inability to perform previous activities
- Inadequate participation in care
- Insufficient sense of control
- Shame

Expected Outcomes

- Patient will identify feelings of powerlessness associated with the present situation.
- Patient will describe modifications or adjustments to the environment that allow feelings of control.
- Patient will participate in self-care activities (specify).
- Patient will state feelings of regained control.

Suggested NOC Outcomes

Anxiety Level; Decision-Making; Depression Self-Control; Family Participation in Professional Care; Fear Level; Health Beliefs; Self-Esteem; Social Involvement; Social Support

Interventions and Rationales

- Visit with patient 15 minutes each shift *to allow patient to express concerns and feelings.*
- Acknowledge the importance of patient's space:
  - Verbally delineate patient's space.
  - Orient patient to personal space.
  - If patient is immobilized, ask for instructions regarding placement of personal belongings.
  - If possible, allow patient to walk around the space and arrange personal belongings.*These measures enhance patient's potential for regaining sense of power.*
- S Place the call bell, television controls, bedside table, telephone, urinal, and other items within easy reach. Improvise wherever possible to give patient control over the use of these objects. Attend to patient's ability or inability to use hands and arms. *These measures help reduce patient's frustration over inability to reach items at hand.*
- Reduce irritating noises, if possible, and explain the reasons for alarms and other disturbances. *Excessive sensory stimuli can cause disorientation, hallucinations, and delusional thinking.*
- PCC Explain treatments and procedures, and encourage patient to participate in planning personal care. Provide choices for when and how activities will occur (such as bathing, eating, and getting out of bed). *This increases patient's feeling of powerfulness and reduces passivity and dependence on caregiver.*
- Provide as many situations as possible where patient can take control (such as positioning, choosing an injection site, and visiting) *to help reduce potential for maladaptive coping behaviors.*
- Encourage participation in self-care. Provide positive reinforcement for patient's activities *to encourage increasing participation in self-care in the future.*
- PCC Help patient learn as much about current health problem as possible. *The greater the patient's understanding, the more patient will feel in control.*

Suggested NIC Interventions

Anxiety Reduction; Cognitive Restructuring; Decision-Making Support; Family Presence Facilitation; Mutual Goal Setting; Presence; Self-Esteem Enhancement; Values Clarification

Evaluations for Expected Outcomes

- Patient expresses feelings of lack of control.
- Patient's environment is adjusted to enhance feelings of control.

- Patient performs self-care measures to the extent possible.
- Patient expresses feelings of regained control.

Documentation

- Patient's expressions of anger, frustration, and sense of lack of control over environment
- Patient's interest in surroundings, participation in self-care, verbalization of understanding, and demonstration of skill in relation to medical diagnosis
- Interventions to promote patient's control over environment
- Patient's response to nursing interventions
- Evaluations for expected outcomes

REFERENCES

Sheridan, N. F., Kenealy, T. W., Kidd, J. D., Schmidt-Busby, J. G., Hand, J. E., Raphael, D. L., ... Rea, H. H. (2015). Patients' engagement in primary care: Powerlessness and compounding jeopardy. A qualitative study. *Health Expectations*, *18*(1), 32–43. doi:10.1111/hex.12006

Taylor, H. (2014). Promoting a patient's right to autonomy: Implications for primary health care practitioners. Part 1. *Primary Health Care*, *24*(2), 36–41.

Uy, V., May, S. G., Tietbohl, C., & Frosch, D. L. (2014). Barriers and facilitators to routine distribution of patient decision support interventions: A preliminary study in community-based primary care settings. *Health Expectations*, *17*(3), 353–364. doi:10.1111/j.1369-7625.2011.00760.x

POWERLESSNESS

related to complex treatment regimen

Definition

Perception that one's own action won't significantly affect an outcome; a perceived lack of control over a current situation or immediate happening

Assessment

- Nature of medical diagnosis
- Mobility
- Behavioral responses (verbal and nonverbal), including calmness or agitation, anger, anxiety, depression, independence or dependence, interest or apathy, and satisfaction or dissatisfaction
- Coping strategies, including passage through grieving process
- Past experiences with illness
- Knowledge, including current understanding of physical condition and physical, mental, and emotional readiness to learn
- Environment, including equipment and supplies, health care professionals and personnel, lighting, location of patient's personal belongings, noise, privacy, and space
- Number and types of stressors
- Social factors
- Spiritual beliefs and value system

Defining Characteristics

- Alienation
- Dependency
- Depression
- Doubt about role performance

- Frustration about inability to perform previous activities
- Inadequate participation in care
- Insufficient sense of control
- Shame

Expected Outcomes

- Patient will acknowledge fears, feelings, and concerns about current situation.
- Patient will make decisions regarding course of treatment.
- Patient will decrease level of anxiety by changing response to stressors.
- Patient will participate in self-care activities (specify).
- Patient will express feelings of regained control.
- Patient will accept and adapt to lifestyle changes.

Suggested NOC Outcomes

Depression Self-Control; Family Participation in Professional Care; Health Beliefs; Health Beliefs: Perceived Ability to Perform; Participation in Health Care Decisions

Interventions and Rationales

- PCC Encourage patient to express feelings and concerns. Set aside time for discussions with patient about daily events. *This helps patient bring vaguely understood emotions into focus.*
- Accept patient's feelings of powerlessness as normal. *This indicates respect for patient and enhances feelings of self-worth.*
- Try to be present during situations where feelings of powerlessness are likely to be greatest *to help patient cope.*
- Identify and develop patient's coping mechanisms, strengths, and resources for support. *By making use of coping skills, patient can reduce anxiety and fears and successfully undergo grieving necessary to come to terms with chronic illness.*
- Discuss situations that provoke feelings of anger, anxiety, and powerlessness *to identify areas patient can control and to prevent anger from being inappropriately directed at self or others.*
- PCC Encourage participation in self-care. Provide positive reinforcement for patient's activities. Encourage patient to take an active role as a member of the health care team. *This enhances patient's sense of control and reduces passive and dependent behavior.*
- PCC Provide as many opportunities as possible for patient to make decisions about self-care (for instance, positioning, choosing an injection site, and visiting) *to communicate respect for patient and enhance feelings of independence.*
- PCC Help patient learn about the health condition, treatment, and prognosis *to help patient feel in control.*
- Modify the environment when possible to meet patient's self-care needs *to promote patient's sense of control over environment.*
- Decrease unpredictable events by discussing rules, policies, procedures, and schedules with patient. *Fear of the unknown interferes with patient's ability to cope.*
- PCC Encourage family members to support patient without taking control *to increase patient's feelings of self-worth.*
- PCC Reinforce patient's rights as stated in Patient's Bill of Rights *to protect patient's right to make decisions about health care treatment.*
- Identify and arrange to accommodate patient's spiritual needs. *Spirituality enables patient to gain courage and resist despair.*

PCC • Respect and show your acceptance of patient's cultural beliefs about health. *The belief that each patient has the personal authority and responsibility to try to reach optimal well-being is a Western value not shared by all cultures.*

Suggested NIC Interventions

Cognitive Restructuring; Decision-Making Support; Emotional Support; Health Education; Mood Management; Presence; Self-Care Assistance; Self-Responsibility Facilitation; Values Clarification

Evaluations for Expected Outcomes

- Patient verbalizes positive and negative feelings about current situation.
- Patient demonstrates increased control by participating in decisions related to health care.
- Patient describes strategies for decreasing anxiety.
- Patient actively participates in planning and executing aspects of care.
- Patient communicates renewed sense of power and control of current situation.
- Patient demonstrates ability to adapt to and accept lifestyle changes.

Documentation

- Observations and interactions related to disease process and health care environment
- Patient's responses to opportunities to participate in own care
- Patient's feelings about chronic illness and situations that can't be changed
- Teaching and counseling to enhance patient's decision-making ability
- Interventions to help patient gain sense of control
- Patient's response to nursing interventions
- Evaluations for expected outcomes

REFERENCES

de Almeida, S., Salomé, G. M., Dutra, R., & Ferreira, L. M. (2014). Feelings of powerlessness in individuals with either venous or diabetic foot ulcers. *Journal of Tissue Viability*, *23*(3), 109–114. doi:10.1016/j.jtv.2014.04.005

Taylor, H. (2014). Promoting a patient's right to autonomy: Implications for primary health care practitioners. Part 1. *Primary Health Care*, *24*(2), 36–41.

Zalonis, R., & Slota, M. (2014). The use of palliative care to promote autonomy in decision-making. *Clinical Journal of Oncology Nursing*, *18*(6), 707–711. doi:10.1188/14.CJON.707-711

RISK FOR POWERLESSNESS

Definition

Vulnerable to the lived experience of lack of control over a situation, including apperception that one's actions do not significantly affect the outcome, which may compromise health

Assessment

- Age, gender
- Nature of the medical diagnosis
- Mobility
- Behavioral responses
- Past experiences and hospitalization
- Knowledge, including understanding of present situation
- Coping skill
- Support system

Risk Factors

- Anxiety
- Caregiver role
- Economically disadvantaged
- Illness
- Ineffective coping strategies
- Insufficient knowledge to manage a situation
- Insufficient social support
- Low self-esteem
- Pain
- Progressive illness
- Social marginalization
- Stigmatization
- Unpredictability of illness trajectory

Expected Outcomes

- The patient will make decisions regarding course of action.
- The patient will decrease level of anxiety by changing response to stressors.
- The patient will participate in self-care activities.
- The patient will describe modifications or adjustments to the environment that allow feelings of control.
- The patient will discuss factors in the illness-related regimen over which control can be maintained.
- The patient will demonstrate ability to plan for controllable factors.
- The patient will express feeling of maintaining control.
- The patient will accept and adapt to lifestyle.

Suggested NOC Outcomes

Anxiety Level; Body Image; Coping; Endurance; Information Processing; Personal Autonomy; Risk Control; Social Support

Interventions and Rationales

- S Assess for high-risk behaviors; health-promoting activities; coping skills; activities of daily living, including rest and sleep; sensory perception; decision-making skills; sexuality patterns. *Assessment information helps identify appropriate interventions.*
- Modify environment when possible *to meet patient's self-care needs to promote sense of control over the environment.*
- Orient patient to space by walking with patient around space and assisting with placement of personal belongings.
- PCC Teach patient about risk factors and other aspects of the patient's medical condition *to help patient feel in control of personal care.*
- Be present when patient is facing situations in which the patient feels powerlessness *to help patient cope.*
- PCC Encourage patient to express concerns. Set aside time for discussions with the patient about daily events. *This helps the patient feel vaguely understood emotions into focus.* Discuss situations that provoke feelings of anxiety, anger, and powerlessness *to identify areas of patient concern and to prevent anger from being inappropriately directed at self.*
- Encourage participation in self-care. Provide patient with as many decisions as possible with regard to self-care (such as positioning, choosing an injection site, and receiving visitors) *to communicate respect for patient and enhance feelings of independence.*
- Provide positive environment for patient's activities. Encourage patient to take an active role as a member of patient's health care team. *This enhances patient's sense of control and reduces passive and dependent behavior.*
- PCC Encourage family members to support patient without taking control *to increase patient's feelings of self-worth.*

- Arrange to accommodate patient's spiritual needs. *Spiritual assistance may help patient gain courage and resist despair.*
- PCC Refer to mental health professional *for additional assistance with coping.* Refer patient to community resources *that may offer assistance to the patient when needed.*
- Offer written information that can be referred to when needed.

Suggested NIC Interventions

Decision-Making Support; Risk Control; Presence; Self-Assistance

Evaluation of Expected Outcomes

- Patient will be able to express feelings that may lead to powerlessness.
- Patient will identify changes in the environment that allow feelings of control.
- Patient participates regularly in self-care activities.

Documentation

- Patient's behavioral responses to current situation (e.g., anger, frustration, crying, etc.)
- Degree of independence with which patient attends to self-care activities
- Interventions to provide patient with control over the environment
- Patient's response to nursing intervention

REFERENCES

Sheridan, N. F., Kenealy, T. W., Kidd, J. D., Schmidt-Busby, J. G., Hand, J. E., Raphael, D. L., ... Rea, H. H. (2015). Patients' engagement in primary care: Powerlessness and compounding jeopardy. A qualitative study. *Health Expectations*, *18*(1), 32–43. doi:10.1111/hex.12006

Taylor, H. (2014). Promoting a patient's right to autonomy: Implications for primary health care practitioners. Part 1. *Primary Health Care*, *24*(2), 36–41.

Uy, V., May, S. G., Tietbohl, C., & Frosch, D. L. (2014). Barriers and facilitators to routine distribution of patient decision support interventions: A preliminary study in community-based primary care settings. *Health Expectations*, *17*(3), 353–364. doi:10.1111/j.1369-7625.2011.00760.x

RISK FOR PRESSURE ULCER

Definition

Vulnerable to localized injury to the skin and/or underlying tissue usually over a bony prominence as a result of pressure, or pressure in combination with shear (NPUAP, 2007)

Assessment

- Age
- Integumentary status, including color, elasticity, hygiene, lesions, moisture, sensation, temperature, texture, turgor, and quantity and distribution of hair
- Musculoskeletal status, including muscle strength and mass, joint mobility, paralysis, and range of motion
- Bowel and bladder continence
- Nutritional status, including appetite, dietary intake, hydration, current weight, and change from normal weight
- Hemoglobin and serum albumin levels and hematocrit

- Injuries
- Chronic diseases
- Circulation, especially to bony areas
- Medications
- Body type and weight
- Use of medical devices (e.g., leg braces, oxygen tubing, cervical collar)
- History of previous skin breakdown
- Risk assessment tool (Braden)

Risk Factors

- *Adult*: Braden Scale score of <18
- Alteration in cognitive functioning
- Alteration in sensation
- American Society of Anesthesiologists (ASA) Physical Status classification score ≥2
- Anemia
- Cardiovascular disease
- *Child*: Braden Q Scale of ≤16
- Decrease in mobility
- Decrease in serum albumin level
- Decrease in tissue oxygenation
- Decrease in tissue perfusion
- Dehydration
- Dry skin
- Edema
- Elevated skin temperature by 1° C to 2° C
- Extended period of immobility on hard surface (e.g., surgical procedure ≥2 hours)
- Extremes of age
- Extremes of weight
- Female gender
- Hip fracture
- History of cerebral vascular accident
- History of pressure ulcer
- History of trauma
- Hyperthermia
- Impaired circulation
- Inadequate nutrition
- Incontinence
- Insufficient caregiver knowledge of pressure ulcer prevention
- Low score on Risk Assessment Pressure Sore (RAPS) scale
- Lymphopenia
- New York Heart Association (NYHA) Functional Classification ≥ 2
- Nonblanchable erythema
- Pharmaceutical agents (e.g., general anesthesia, vasopressors, antidepressant, norepinephrine)
- Physical immobilization
- Pressure over bony prominence
- Reduced triceps skin fold thickness
- Scaly skin
- Self-care deficit
- Shearing forces
- Skin moisture
- Smoking
- Surface friction
- Use of linen with insufficient moisture wicking property

Expected Outcomes

- Patient will not experience a pressure ulcer.
- Patient's bony prominences will have limited contact with bedding and mattress.
- Patient will have adequate nutrition.
- Patient will maintain adequate circulation to skin.
- Patient will explain skin care regimen.
- Patient and family members will demonstrate skin care regimen.

Suggested NOC Outcomes

Circulation Status; Fluid Balance; Neurologic Status: Peripheral; Nutritional Status; Physical Aging; Tissue Perfusion: Peripheral

Interventions and Rationales

- Inspect patient's skin every shift; document skin condition and report status changes. *Early detection of changes prevents or minimizes skin breakdown.*
- At regular intervals, monitor skin over bony prominences for redness and blanching. *Regular monitoring of the patient's skin helps to identify problems early.*
- Use pressure redirecting devices, as needed, such as a foam mattress, alternating pressure mattress, gel headrests, sheepskin, pillows, and padding. *Devices redirect pressure and assist in avoiding discomfort and skin breakdown.*
- Keep patient's skin clean and dry; lubricate, as needed. Don't use irritating soap, and rinse skin well. *These measures alleviate skin dryness, promote comfort, and reduce the risk of irritation and skin breakdown.*
- Protect bony prominences with foam padding. *Prominences have little subcutaneous fat and are prone to breakdown; using foam padding may help promote skin integrity.*
- Lift patient's body, whenever required, using a lifting sheet, if needed. Avoid shearing force. *Shearing force results when tissues slide against each other; a lifting sheet reduces sliding.*
- Keep linen dry, clean, and free from wrinkles or crumbs. Change wet bed linens and incontinence pads immediately. *Dry, smooth linens help prevent excoriation and skin breakdown.*
- Monitor nutritional intake; maintain adequate hydration. *Anemia (less than 10 mg hemoglobin) and low serum albumin concentrations (less than 2 mg) are associated with the development of pressure ulcers. Hydration helps maintain skin integrity.*
- Use a risk assessment tool such as the Braden scale to continually assess risk as patient's condition changes. *Systematic monitoring helps to identify problems early.*
- Change patient's position at least every 2 hours; follow turning schedule posted at bedside. Monitor frequency of turning. *These measures reduce pressure on tissues, promote circulation, and help prevent skin breakdown.*
- Indicate the risk factor potential on patient's chart and care plan, and reevaluate weekly, using an accepted form such as the Braden Scale. *The risk factor score helps evaluate treatment progress.*
- PCC Explain the importance of practicing preventive skin care measures *to encourage compliance with skin care regimen.*
- PCC Supervise patient and patient's family in preventive skin care measures. Give constructive feedback. *Practice helps improve skill in managing the skin care regimen.*

Suggested NIC Interventions

Bathing; Circulatory Precautions; Electrolyte Monitoring; Positioning; Pressure Management; Skin Care: Topical Treatments

Evaluations for Expected Outcomes

- Patient's skin remains intact.
- Patient's weight remains within established limits.
- Patient maintains adequate hydration.
- Patient maintains adequate circulation to skin.
- Patient lists preventive skin care measures.
- Patient and family members demonstrate skin care measures.
- Patient and family members understand need to avoid prolonged pressure, obtain adequate nutrition, prevent incontinence, and consistently perform skin care measures.

Documentation

- Nutritional screening
- Pressure ulcer prevention plan
- Braden or other skin assessment index
- Application of barrier creams and peri care
- Use of pressure redistribution devices
- Repositioning and frequency
- Education for the patient and family regarding pressure ulcer prevention and treatment

REFERENCES

Cooper, K. L. (2013). Evidence-based prevention of pressure ulcers in the intensive care unit. *Critical Care Nurse, 33*(6), 57–67. doi:10.4037/ccn2013985

Giachetta-Ryan, D. (2015). Perioperative pressure ulcers: How can they be prevented? *OR Nurse, 9*(4), 22–28. doi:10.1097/01.ORN.0000466721.18152.14

Mallah, Z., Nassar, N., & Badr, L. K. (2015). The effectiveness of a pressure ulcer intervention program on the prevalence of hospital-acquired pressure ulcers: Controlled before and after study. *Applied Nursing Research, 28*(2), 106–113. doi:10.1016/j.apnr.2014.07.001

Moore, Z., Johansen, E., van Etten, M., Strapp, H., Solbakken, T., Smith, B. E., & Faulstich, J. (2015). Pressure ulcer prevalence and prevention practices: A cross-sectional comparative survey in Norway and Ireland. *Journal of Wound Care, 24*(8), 333–339.

Sookyung, H., Xiaobai, L., Vermillion, B., Newton, C., Fall, M., Pacharmon, K., ... Lenz, E. R. (2014). Body mass index and pressure ulcers: Improved predictability of pressure ulcers in intensive care patients. *American Journal of Critical Care, 23*(6), 494–501. doi:10.4037/ajcc2014535

INEFFECTIVE PROTECTION

related to immune disorder (e.g., HIV-associated neuropathy, varicella-zoster virus)

Definition

Decrease in the ability to guard self from internal or external threats such as illness or injury

Assessment

- Vital signs
- Health maintenance, including high-risk behaviors and health-promoting activities
- Patient's knowledge of present condition, including diagnosis, treatment, prevention of complications, and management of adverse effects
- Coping skills, including physical, psychosocial, and spiritual strengths
- Mobility status
- Comfort level, including symptom management
- Activities of daily living, including rest, sleep, and exercise
- Cardiovascular status, including heart rate, rhythm, heart sounds, blood pressure, peripheral pulses, and electrocardiogram results
- Neurologic status, including sensory perception, decision-making abilities, and thought processes
- Respiratory status, including gas exchange and breathing patterns
- Nutritional status, including food preferences, modifications in diet, and weight changes
- Bowel and bladder elimination patterns

- Protective mechanisms, including immune, hematopoietic, integumentary, and sensorimotor systems
- Laboratory studies, including white blood cell count and differential, erythrocyte sedimentation rate, immunoelectrophoresis, enzyme-linked immunosorbent assay, and cultures of blood, body fluid, sputum, urine, and wound exudate
- Sexuality patterns

Defining Characteristics

- Alteration in clotting
- Alteration in perspiration
- Anorexia
- Chilling
- Coughing
- Deficient immunity
- Disorientation
- Dyspnea
- Fatigue
- Immobility
- Insomnia
- Itching
- Maladaptive stress response
- Neurosensory impairment
- Pressure ulcers
- Restlessness
- Weakness

Expected Outcomes

- Patient won't experience chills, fever, or other signs and symptoms of illness.
- Patient will demonstrate use of protective measures, including conservation of energy, maintenance of balanced diet, and attainment of adequate rest.
- Patient will demonstrate effective coping skills.
- Patient will demonstrate personal cleanliness and will maintain clean environment.
- Patient will maintain safe environment.
- Patient will demonstrate increased strength and resistance.
- Patient's immune system response will improve.

Suggested NOC Outcomes

Abuse Protection; Immune Status; Immunization Behavior; Knowledge: Infection Control; Knowledge: Personal Safety

Interventions and Rationales

- Spend as much time as possible with patient *to provide comfort and support.*
- Promote personal and environmental cleanliness *to decrease threat from microorganisms.*
- Monitor vital signs. *This allows for early detection of complications.*
- S — Institute safety precautions *to reduce risk of falls, cuts, or other injuries and subsequent infection, bleeding, and impaired healing.*
- PCC — Teach protective measures, including the need to conserve energy, obtain adequate rest, and eat a balanced diet. Adequate sleep and nutrition enhance immune function. *Energy conservation can help decrease the weakness caused by anemia.*
- Provide relief for symptoms (fever, chills, myalgia, weakness). *Discomfort interferes with rest, disturbs nutritional intake, and places added stress on patient.*
- PCC — Teach patient coping strategies, including stress management and relaxation techniques. *Relaxation and decreased stress can increase immune function, thereby improving strength and resistance.*

Suggested NIC Interventions

Coping Enhancement; Environmental Management: Safety; Infection Control; Infection Protection; Nutritional Counseling; Positioning; Risk Identification

Evaluations for Expected Outcomes

- Patient doesn't develop petechiae, epistaxis, melena, hematuria, fever, cough, redness, drainage, pallor, headache, weakness, or dizziness. Vital signs remain within normal limits.
- Patient demonstrates a normal pattern of rest, activity, and sleep. He consumes an adequate diet.
- Patient reports being able to cope effectively.
- Patient demonstrates personal cleanliness and maintains clean environment.
- Patient uses safety precautions to avoid falls and other injuries.
- Patient demonstrates increased strength and resistance.
- Patient's immune system response improves.

Documentation

- Patient's understanding of abnormal blood profiles
- Patient's description of measures to prevent or manage complications
- Observations of patient's behavior, including health-promoting and high-risk activities
- Signs and symptoms of decreased immune resistance in body systems assessed (cardiopulmonary, neurologic, gastrointestinal, genitourinary, and integumentary)
- Observations of infection or bleeding
- Interventions to assist with coping strategies and health maintenance and promotion
- Patient's response to interventions
- Evaluations for expected outcomes

REFERENCES

Al-Jabri, A., Youssef, R., Hasson, S., Balkhair, A., Al-Belushi, M., Al-Saadoon, M., ... Idris, M. (2014). Knowledge, attitudes, and intended behaviors toward HIV testing and self-protection: A survey of Omani pregnant women. *Eastern Mediterranean Health Journal*, *20*(10), 614–622.

Belding, J. N., Naufel, K. Z., & Fujita, K. (2015). Using high-level construal and perceptions of changeability to promote self-change over self-protection motives in response to negative feedback. *Personality & Social Psychology Bulletin*, *41*(6), 822–838. doi:10.1177/0146167215580776

Barlow, M. A., Liu, S. Y., & Wrosch, C. (2015). Chronic illness and loneliness in older adulthood: The role of self-protective control strategies. *Health Psychology*, *34*(8), 870–879. doi:10.1037/hea0000182

RISK FOR ADVERSE REACTION TO IODINATED CONTRAST MEDIA

Definition

Vulnerable to noxious or unintended reaction associated with the use of iodated contrast media that can occur within seven days after contrast agent injection, which may compromise health

Assessment

- History of experience with illness, hospitalization, and surgery
- Health history, including accidents, exposure to pollutants, falls, hyperthermia, hypothermia, poisoning, sensory or perceptual changes (auditory, gustatory, kinesthetic, olfactory, tactile, and visual), and trauma

- Allergies
- Mental status, including cognitive and emotional function, problems with concentration, memory, orientation, mood, and behavior
- Risk factors
- History of previous adverse effect from iodinated contrast media
- History of allergies
- Extremes of age
- Dehydration
- Concurrent use of medications (e.g., β-blockers, interleukin-2, metformin, nephrotoxic medications)
- Fragile veins
- Underlying disease (e.g., heart disease, pulmonary disease, blood dyscrasias, endocrine disease, renal disease, pheochromocytoma, autoimmune disease)
- General debilitation

Risk Factors

- Anxiety
- Chronic illness
- Concurrent use of pharmaceutical agents (e.g., β-blockers, interleukin-2, metformin, nephrotoxins)
- Contrast media precipitates adverse event (e.g., iodine concentration, viscosity, high osmolality, ion toxicity)
- Dehydration
- Extremes of age
- Fragile vein (e.g., chemotherapy/radiation in limb to be injected, indwelling line for >24 hours, axillary lymph node dissection in limb to be injected, distal intravenous access site)
- Generalized debilitation
- History of allergy
- History of previous adverse effect from iodinated contrast media
- Unconsciousness

Expected Outcomes

- Patient will not experience an adverse reaction to iodinated contrast media.
- Patient will recognize personal risk factors for adverse reaction.
- Patient will ask questions if new information requires clarification.

Suggested NOC Outcomes

Risk Control; Risk Detection; Knowledge: Treatment procedure; Immune Hypersensitivity Response; Allergy Response

Interventions and Rationales

- Assess for any previous adverse reaction to contrast media.
- Identify preexisting disease states and current medications history that may trigger reaction to iodinated contrast media. *This is essential for the safe administration of contrast media and prevention of adverse effects.*
- Assess for history of asthma food allergies, or other allergies, *which may increase likelihood of an adverse reaction.* Assess for presence of other medical conditions including heart failure and renal insufficiency, *which may increase risk of adverse reaction.*

- Consider prehydration with normal saline solution *to decrease risk of renal damage.*
- Withhold metformin before any administration of contrast media, and resume after 48 hours once renal function has been evaluated. *This will reduce any medication-associated renal tissue damage due to contrast media.*
- Premedication with corticosteroids or antihistamines may be indicated *to reduce incidence of reaction in patients with known risk factors.*
- PCC Educate patient regarding risk factors associated with adverse reaction to iodinated contrast media. *Knowledge of risk factors is essential in preventing adverse reaction and possible organ damage.*
- Ensure patient is aware of personal risk factors to share with future providers. *This will promote continued safe administration of iodinated contrast media.*
- Encourage patient to share concerns about procedures requiring use of iodinated contrast media *to reduce anxiety.*
- PCC Collaborate with other members of the health care team regarding presence of risk factors associated with adverse reaction to iodinated contrast media. *This will allow for modifications in the preparation for the procedure and prevent complications.*

Suggested NIC Interventions

Risk Identification; Teaching: Individual

Evaluations for Expected Outcomes

- Patient has no reaction to iodinated contrast media.
- Patient recognizes possibility of adverse reaction to iodinated contrast media.
- Patient asks questions regarding the preparation for the procedure.

Documentation

- Patient's expressions of concern about adverse reaction and symptoms of previous episodes
- Observations of physiologic and behavioral manifestations of adverse reaction
- Interventions performed to allay adverse reaction
- Patient's response to interventions
- Evaluations for expected outcomes

REFERENCES

Burchardt, P., Synowiec, T., Jerzykowska, S., Angerer, D., & Zurawski, J. (2015). Early renal dysfunction after iodine contrast administration: New insight into the actual problem. *Polish Heart Journal/ Kardiologia Polska*, *73*(3), 233–234. doi:10.5603/KP.2015.0050

Egbert, R. E., De Cecco, C. N., Schoepf, U. J., McQuiston, A. D., Meinel, F. G., & Katzberg, R. W. (2014). Delayed adverse reactions to the parenteral administration of iodinated contrast media. *American Journal of Roentgenology*, *203*(6), 1163–1170. doi:10.2214/AJR.13.12310

Matthews, E. P. (2015). Adverse effects of iodine-derived intravenous radiopaque contrast media. *Radiologic Technology*, *86*(6), 623–642.

IMPAIRED RELIGIOSITY

Definition

Impaired ability to exercise reliance on beliefs and/or participate in rituals of a particular faith tradition

Assessment

- Age, gender, sex
- Religious affiliation, beliefs/values
- Usual religious practices, support system

Defining Characteristics

- Desire to reconnect with previous belief pattern
- Desire to reconnect with previous customs
- Difficulty adhering to prescribed religious beliefs
- Difficulty adhering to prescribed religious rituals (e.g., ceremonies, regulations, clothing, prayer, services, holiday observances)
- Distress about separation from faith community
- Questioning of religious belief patterns
- Questioning of religious customs

Expected Outcomes

- Patient will describe conflicts with his or her religious beliefs and the effects of his or her illness on these beliefs.
- Patient will accept counsel of a person trained in spirituality.
- Patient will engage in religious practices to the extent that it is therapeutic.
- Patient will express satisfaction with ability to practice patient's religion.

Suggested NOC Outcomes

Hope; Motivation; Quality of Life; Spiritual Health

Interventions and Rationales

- Assess spiritual or religious beliefs; religious affiliation; importance of religion in daily life; religious involvement of family; religious dietary restrictions; importance of religion in helping with usual coping. *Assessment information helps identify appropriate interventions.*
- Approach patient in a nonjudgmental way when he or she is discussing religious beliefs or spiritual needs. *The nurse's beliefs may differ radically, but it is a professional responsibility to assist the patient in an ethically sensitive way.*
- PCC Help patient list the religious practices most important to him or her *to determine what is possible to provide in the hospital.*
- Acquire simple-to-obtain items, such as books, pictures, CD, cross, *to provide comfort to the patient.*
- PCC Confirm that patient's spiritual needs are being satisfied *so that modifications can be made in the plan.*
- PCC Involve family members in helping meet patient's spiritual needs if the patient agrees. *If family members have strong spiritual beliefs, they can be a help to one another in times of pain and difficulty.*
- PCC Encourage patient and family to express feelings associated with diagnosis, treatment, and recovery. *Expression of feelings helps patient and family cope with treatment.*
- Schedule time to spend with the family. *They need time with health care providers to ask questions.*
- PCC Suggest a referral to a clergy person or faith community nurse *so that the person can discuss deeper spiritual issues.*

Suggested NIC Interventions

Religious Ritual Enhancement; Coping Enhancement; Hope Instillation Active Listening; Spiritual Growth; Spiritual Support

Evaluations for Expected Outcomes

- Patient expresses understanding about how illness impacts patient's religious beliefs.
- Patient works with staff to modify plan as needed.
- Patient requests whatever resources patient thinks will help meet present needs.
- Family and clergy visit to provide support.

Documentation

- Assessment of patient's perspectives on religiosity
- Practices that are meaningful to the patient
- Visits from clergy
- Modifications to the plan

REFERENCES

Ellington, L., Reblin, M., Ferrell, B., Puchalski, C., Otis-Green, S., Handzo, G., … Clayton, M. F. (2015). The religion of "I don't know". *Omega: Journal of Death & Dying*, *72*(1), 3–19. doi:10.1177/0030222815574689

Kuile, H. T., & Ehring, T. (2014). Predictors of changes in religiosity after trauma: Trauma, religiosity, and posttraumatic stress disorder. *Psychological Trauma: Theory, Research, Practice & Policy*, *6*(4), 353–360. doi:10.1037/a0034880

Quinlivan, M. (2014). Supporting the delivery of effective pastoral care. *British Journal of School Nursing*, *9*(8), 405–406.

READINESS FOR ENHANCED RELIGIOSITY

Definition

A pattern of reliance on religious beliefs and/or participation in rituals of a particular faith tradition, which can be strengthened

Assessment

- Age, gender, marital status
- Health history
- Support systems (family, clergy)
- Communication skills
- Cultural factors
- Religious affiliation
- Spiritual beliefs and practices that are important to patient
- Perceptions of faith, life, death, and suffering

Defining Characteristics

- Expresses desire to enhance belief patterns used in the past
- Expresses desire to enhance connection with a religious leader
- Expresses desire to enhance forgiveness
- Expresses desire to enhance participation in religious experiences
- Expresses desire to enhance participation in religious practices (e.g., ceremonies, regulations, clothing, prayer, services, holiday observances)

- Expresses desire to enhance religious customs used in the past
- Expresses desire to enhance religious options
- Expresses desire to enhance use of religious material

Expected Outcomes

- Patient will articulate all that infuses strength and hope.
- Patient will discuss aspects of religion that are important to the patient.
- Patient will list how staff can facilitate patient's participation in religious practices.
- Patient will request or agree to talk to a spiritual professional.
- Patient will express a feeling of peace with provided religious opportunities.

Suggested NOC Outcomes

Health Beliefs; Health-Promoting Behavior; Hope; Motivation; Quality of Life; Spiritual Health

Interventions and Rationales

- Perform a thorough spiritual assessment *to develop a holistic home care plan.*
- PCC Help patient list the religious practices most important to the patient *to determine what's possible to provide in the home.*
- Acquire simple-to-obtain items, such as a Bible, *to comfort patient while planning more complex support.*
- Encourage guided imagery, prayer, and meditations *as methods of enhancing spiritual experiences.*
- PCC Suggest a referral *to clergy so patient may discuss deeper spiritual issues.*
- Consider having a congregational nurse or faith community nurse visit weekly *to provide ongoing spiritual care.*
- PCC Confirm that patient's spiritual needs are being satisfied *if modifications are made to the plan.*

Suggested NIC Interventions

Presence; Religious Ritual Enhancement; Spiritual Growth Facilitation; Spiritual Support; Values Clarification

Evaluations for Expected Outcomes

- Patient describes sources of strength and hope.
- Patient discusses aspects of religion that are of deep personal importance.
- Patient receives the assistance needed to participate in religious practices.
- Patient talks to a spiritual professional.
- Patient expresses peace with the ongoing attention to personal spiritual needs.

Documentation

- Assessment of spiritual needs
- Religious practices to enjoy at home
- Efforts to obtain resources to satisfy patient's needs
- Visits by spiritual professional
- Patient's responses to interventions
- Evaluations for expected outcomes

REFERENCES

Cervelin, A. F., & Luce Kruse, M. H. (2015). Spirituality and religiosity in palliative care: Proposing a good death. *Journal of Nursing UFPE/Revista De Enfermagem UFPE*, *9*, 7615–7624. doi:10.5205/reuol.7049-61452-1-ED.0903supl201515

Kim, N. Y., Huh, H. J., & Chae, J. H. (2015). Effects of religiosity and spirituality on the treatment response in patients with depressive disorders. *Comprehensive Psychiatry*, *60*, 26–34. doi:10.1016/j.comppsych.2015.04.009

Snider, A., & McPhedran, S. (2014). Religiosity, spirituality, mental health, and mental health treatment outcomes in Australia: A systematic literature review. *Mental Health, Religion & Culture*, *17*(6), 568–581. doi:10.1080/13674676.2013.871240

RISK FOR IMPAIRED RELIGIOSITY

Definition

Vulnerable to an impaired ability to exercise reliance on religious beliefs and/or participate in rituals of a particular faith tradition, which may compromise health

Assessment

- Age, gender
- Religious affiliation, beliefs, practices; importance of religion in daily life
- Environmental assessment of present living circumstances
- Support systems (family, clergy)

Risk Factors

Developmental

- Life transition

Environmental

- Barrier to practicing religion
- Insufficient transportation

Physical

- Hospitalization
- Illness
- Pain

Psychological

- Depression
- Ineffective caregiving
- Ineffective coping strategies
- Insecurity
- Insufficient social support

Sociocultural

- Cultural barrier to practicing religion
- Insufficient social interaction

Spiritual

- Suffering

Expected Outcomes

- Patient will articulate those religious practices that are of deep personal importance.
- Patient will decide what changes to patient's practices are realistic and acceptable.
- Patient will cope with the limitations imposed by current circumstances.
- Patient will make use of the available spiritual resources.
- Patient will express satisfaction with ability to practice patient's religion.

Suggested NOC Outcomes

Health Beliefs; Health-Promoting Behavior; Hope; Motivation; Quality of Life; Spiritual Health

Interventions and Rationales

- Perform a thorough spiritual assessment *to develop a holistic care plan.*
- PCC Help patient list the religious practices that carry the most personal meaning and importance *to determine what's possible to provide for the patient.*
- If patient desires, acquire simple-to-obtain items, such as a Bible, *to comfort patient while planning more complex support.*
- Help patient explore modifications to patient's activities without compromising spiritual comfort. *Decision making promotes feelings of independence, control.*
- Explain available resources *to prepare for developing a realistic plan.*
- PCC Have patient list options for participation in religious activities *to promote optimism or acceptance in present situation.*
- Check daily, then weekly, *to assess patient's level of satisfaction with the plan.*
- PCC Work with family, friends, or clergy *to provide appropriate spiritual support.*

Suggested NIC Interventions

Active Listening; Emotional Support; Hope Instillation; Presence; Religious Addiction Prevention; Religious Ritual Enhancement; Spiritual Growth Facilitation; Spiritual Support; Values Clarification

Evaluations for Expected Outcomes

- Patient expresses satisfaction with the religious activities that are provided.
- Patient participates in practicing those religious activities that are available.
- Patient asks to modify plan as needed.
- Family and clergy visit and support.
- Patient expresses feelings of health and wholeness.

Documentation

- Thorough spiritual assessment
- Religious practices that are meaningful to patient
- Religious practices that can be provided in the present situation
- Patient's satisfaction with options
- Patient's participation in religious and other kinds of activities
- Evaluations for expected outcomes

REFERENCES

Kleebauer, A. (2014). Nurses agree religion has a place in care. *Nursing Standard*, *29*(14), 13. doi:10.7748/ns.29.14.13.s15

Mendes, A. (2015). Culture and religion in nursing: Providing culturally sensitive care. *British Journal of Nursing*, *24*(8), 459–459. doi:10.12968/bjon.2015.24.8.459

Quinlivan, M. (2014). Supporting the delivery of effective pastoral care. *British Journal of School Nursing*, *9*(8), 405–406.

RELOCATION STRESS SYNDROME

related to unpredictability of experience

Definition

Physiologic and/or psychosocial disturbance following transfer from one environment to another

Assessment

- Reason for transfer or relocation
- Nature of relocation
- Physical and mental status of patient, including health condition, cognitive functioning, and functional abilities
- Financial resources
- Support systems, including family, friends, and health care workers
- Resources available to help prepare for relocation
- Conditions in original environment versus conditions in new environment
- Coping and problem-solving abilities, including educational level, past experiences with relocation, and participation in recreational activities or hobbies

Defining Characteristics

- Alienation
- Aloneness
- Alteration in sleep pattern
- Anger
- Anxiety
- Concern over relocation
- Dependency
- Depression
- Fear
- Frustration
- Increase in illness
- Increase in physical symptoms
- Increase in verbalization of needs
- Insecurity
- Loneliness
- Loss of identity
- Loss of self-worth
- Low self-esteem
- Pessimism
- Unwillingness to move
- Withdrawal
- Worried

Expected Outcomes

- Patient will request information about new environment.
- Patient will communicate understanding of relocation.
- Patient and family members will take steps to prepare for relocation.
- Patient will use available resources.
- Patient will express satisfaction with adjustment to new environment.

Suggested NOC Outcomes

Anxiety Self-Control; Coping; Depression Level; Depression Self-Control; Loneliness Severity; Psychosocial Adjustment: Life Change; Quality of Life; Stress Level

Interventions and Rationales

- Assign a primary nurse to patient *to provide a consistent, caring, and accepting environment that enhances patient's adjustment and well-being.*
- PCC Help patient and family members prepare for relocation. Conduct group discussions, provide pictures of the new setting, and communicate any additional information that will ease transition *to help patient cope with a new environment.*
- If possible, allow patient and family members to visit the new location, and provide introductions to the new staff. *The more familiar the environment, the less stress patient will experience during relocation.*
- PCC Assess patient's needs for additional health care services before relocation *to ensure that patient receives appropriate care in the new environment.*
- PCC Communicate all aspects of patient's discharge plan to appropriate staff members at the new location *to ensure continuity of care.*
- PCC Educate family members about relocation stress syndrome and its potential effects *to encourage family members to provide needed emotional support throughout the transition period.*
- PCC Encourage patient to express emotions associated with relocation *to provide opportunity to correct misconceptions, answer questions, and reduce anxiety.*
- Reassure patient that family members and friends know the patient's new location and will continue to visit *to reduce feelings of abandonment and anxiety.*

Suggested NIC Interventions

Active Listening; Coping Enhancement; Counseling; Hope Instillation; Mood Management; Presence; Sleep Enhancement; Self-Responsibility Facilitation; Spiritual Support

Evaluations for Expected Outcomes

- Patient requests information about new environment.
- Patient expresses understanding of relocation process.
- Patient and family members complete preparations for relocation.
- Patient makes use of available resources to smooth transition to new environment.
- Patient expresses feelings associated with adjustment to new environment.

Documentation

- Evidence of patient's emotional distress over relocation
- Patient's needs in preparing for relocation
- Available resources and support systems
- Intervention to prepare patient and family members for relocation and patient's and family members' responses
- Discharge plan instructions communicated to new staff
- Evaluations for expected outcomes

REFERENCES

McGrath, P. (2015). Findings on family issues during relocation for hematology care. *Oncology Nursing Forum*, 42, E250–E256. doi:10.1188/15.ONF.E250-E256

Oh, H., Lee, S., Kim, J., Lee, E., Min, H., Cho, O., & Seo, W. (2015). Clinical validity of a relocation stress scale for the families of patients transferred from intensive care units. *Journal of Clinical Nursing, 24*(13/14), 1805–1814. doi:10.1111/jocn.12778

Yueh-Ying, Y., Shu-Ming, C., Chien-Lin, K., & Hsin-Ju, L. (2014). Exploring relocation stress and diabetes control in the elderly residents of long-term care facilities. *Journal of Nursing, 61*(6), 57–65. doi:10.6224/JN.61.6.57

RISK FOR INEFFECTIVE RENAL PERFUSION

Definition

Vulnerable to a decrease in blood circulation to the kidney, which may compromise health

Assessment

- Cardiovascular status, including heart rate and rhythm, blood pressure, and peripheral pulses
- Fluid and electrolyte status, weight, intake and output, urine specific gravity, skin turgor
- Genitourinary status, including characteristics of urine, excretory urography, pain or discomfort, palpation of bladder, urinalysis, and voiding patterns
- Results of laboratory studies, including blood urea nitrogen, creatinine, urine protein, and serum electrolytes
- History of cardiovascular or renal disorders and chronic health conditions

Risk Factors

- Abdominal compartment syndrome
- Alteration in metabolism
- Bilateral cortical necrosis
- Burns
- Cardiac surgery
- Cardiopulmonary bypass
- Diabetes mellitus
- Exposure to nephrotoxin
- Extremes of age
- Female gender
- Glomerulonephritis
- Hypertension
- Hypovolemia
- Hypoxemia
- Hypoxia
- Infection
- Interstitial nephritis
- Malignancy
- Malignant hypertension
- Polynephritis
- Renal disease (e.g., polycystic kidney, renal artery stenosis, failure)
- Smoking
- Substance abuse
- Systemic inflammatory response syndrome
- Trauma
- Treatment regimen
- Vascular embolism
- Vasculitis

Expected Outcomes

- Patient will identify risk factors that contribute to risk for decreased renal perfusion.
- Patient will make appropriate lifestyle changes to minimize risks, including careful management of chronic health conditions.
- Patient will verbalize signs and symptoms of possible renal dysfunction related to impaired perfusion.
- Patient will maintain fluid balance.

Suggested NOC Outcomes

Client Satisfaction: Cardiac Pump Effectiveness; Electrolyte & Acid–Base Balance; Kidney Function; Knowledge: Health Promotion

Interventions and Rationales

- Support patient's optimal management of preexisting health conditions that minimize the risk of decreased renal perfusion. *Effective management of chronic health conditions will help preserve kidney function.*
- Collect and evaluate lab and urine data that may indicate renal damage. *Serum creatinine levels and urine protein and creatinine are sensitive indicators of renal function.*
- Maintain mean arterial pressure of at least 60 to 70 *to provide continuous perfusion needed for renal function.*
- Observe patient's voiding pattern. Document urine color and characteristics, intake and output, and patient's daily weight. Report any changes. *Accurate intake and output measurements are essential for correct fluid replacement therapy. Urine characteristics help verify diagnosis.*
- PCC Provide patient teaching regarding the need to control modifiable risk factors and the signs and symptoms that indicate renal dysfunction. *Prevention and early intervention is essential in maintaining renal function.*
- PCC Provide patient and family with encouragement and psychological support *to reinforce positive health behaviors.*
- PCC Collaborate with other members of the health care team to develop an individualized plan of care to reduce risk factors. *A multidisciplinary approach results in positive patient outcomes.*

Suggested NIC Interventions

Electrolyte Monitoring; Hemodynamic Monitoring; Fluid Management; Urinary Elimination Management

Evaluations for Expected Outcomes

- Patient identifies risk factors that contribute to decreased renal perfusion.
- Patient identifies lifestyle changes that would minimize risks.
- Patient and family understand the need to carefully manage chronic health conditions to promote renal perfusion.
- Patient verbalizes signs and symptoms of possible renal dysfunction related to impaired perfusion.
- Patient maintains fluid balance.

Documentation

- Patient's intake and output measurements and lab values
- Patient's vital signs, including mean arterial pressure measurement
- Patient's response to teaching interventions
- Behaviors that promote renal perfusion
- Evaluations for expected outcomes

REFERENCES

Sarnak, M. J. (2014). A patient with heart failure and worsening kidney function. *Clinical Journal of the American Society of Nephrology*, *9*(10), 1790–1798. doi:10.2215/CJN.11601113

Textor, S. C., & McKusick, M. M. (2016). Renal artery stenosis: If and when to intervene. *Current Opinion in Nephrology & Hypertension*, *25*(2), 144–151. doi:10.1097/MNH.0000000000000202

Wong, B. T., Chan, M. J., Glassford, N. J., Mårtensson, J., Bion, V., Chai, S. Y., ... Bellomo, R. (2015). Mean arterial pressure and mean perfusion pressure deficit in septic acute kidney injury. *Journal of Critical Care*, *30*(5), 975–981. doi:10.1016/jjcrc.2015.05.003

INEFFECTIVE ROLE PERFORMANCE

related to physical illness

Definition

A pattern of behavior and self-expression that does not match the environmental context, norms, and expectations

Assessment

- Health history, including medical diagnosis, course and severity of illness, and reason for hospitalization
- Patient's perception of illness and its effect on social, cultural, and vocational roles
- Psychosocial status, including current stressors, support systems, hobbies, interests, work history, educational background, and changes in role function
- Family status, including roles of family members, effect of illness on patient's family, and family's understanding of patient's illness

Defining Characteristics

- Alteration in role perception
- Anxiety
- Change in capacity to resume role
- Change in others' perception of role
- Change in self-perception of role
- Change in usual pattern of responsibility
- Depression
- Discrimination
- Domestic violence
- Harassment
- Inappropriate development expectations
- Ineffective adaptation to change
- Ineffective coping strategies
- Ineffective role performance
- Insufficient confidence
- Insufficient external support for role enactment
- Insufficient knowledge of role requirements
- Insufficient motivation
- Insufficient opportunity for role enactment
- Insufficient self-management
- Insufficient skills
- Pessimism
- Powerlessness
- Role ambivalence
- Role conflict
- Role confusion
- Role denial
- Role dissatisfaction
- Role strain
- System conflict
- Uncertainty

Expected Outcomes

- Patient will express feelings about diminished ability to perform usual roles.
- Patient and family members will recognize and state feelings about limitations imposed by illness.
- Patient will make decisions about course of treatment and management of illness.
- Patient will continue to function in usual roles as much as possible.
- Patient will express feelings of making productive contribution to self-care, to others, or to environment.

Suggested NOC Outcomes

Caregiver Lifestyle Disruption; Coping; Depression Level; Psychomotor Energy; Psychosocial Adjustment: Life Change; Role Performance

Interventions and Rationales

- If possible, assign the same nurse to patient each shift *to establish rapport and foster development of a therapeutic relationship.*
- Spend ample time with patient each shift *to foster a sense of safety and decrease loneliness.*
- PCC Provide opportunities for patient to express thoughts and feelings *to help patient identify how altered role performance has affected patient's life.*
- PCC Encourage patient to explore strengths. *Having the patient talk about existing strengths will help in identifying new strengths patient needs to develop to succeed in a new role.*
- Convey a belief in patient's ability to develop the necessary coping skills. *By projecting a positive attitude, you can help patient gain confidence.*
- Be aware of patient's emotional vulnerability, and allow open expression of all emotions. *An accepting attitude will help patient deal with the effects of chronic illness and loss of functioning.*
- PCC Provide opportunities for patient to make decisions, and encourage patient to maintain personal responsibilities. *Showing respect for patient's decision-making ability enhances feelings of independence.*
- Encourage patient to participate in self-care activities, keeping in mind patient's physical and emotional limitations. *Involvement in self-care promotes optimal functioning.*
- PCC Assess patient's knowledge of illness, and educate patient about condition, treatment, and prognosis. *Education helps patient cope with effects of illness more effectively.*
- Encourage patient to recognize personal strengths and to use them. *This will help maintain optimal functioning and foster a healthier self-image.*
- PCC Encourage patient to continue to fulfill life roles within the constraints posed by illness. *This will help patient maintain a sense of purpose and preserve connections with other people.*
- PCC Encourage patient to participate in his or her care as an active member of the health care team. *This will help establish mutually accepted goals between patient and caregivers. Patient who participates in care is more likely to take an active role in other aspects of life.*
- PCC Help family members identify their feelings about patient's decreased role functioning. Encourage participation in a support group. *Relatives of patient may need social support, information, and an outlet for ventilating feelings.*
- Offer patient and family members a realistic assessment of patient's illness, and communicate hope for the immediate future. *Education helps promote patient safety and security and helps family members plan for future health care requirements.*

PCC • Educate patient and family members about managing illness, controlling environmental factors that affect patient's health, and redefining roles *to promote optimal functioning. Through education, family members may become resources in patient's care.*

Suggested NIC Interventions

Anticipatory Guidance; Caregiver Support; Coping Enhancement; Family Process Maintenance; Role Enhancement; Hope Instillation

Evaluations for Expected Outcomes

- Patient shares feelings about illness and altered role performance in constructive manner.
- Patient and family members understand role changes that are occurring because of chronic illness and express their feelings about these limitations.
- Patient demonstrates increased functioning by making decisions about health care and participating in planning and implementing aspects of personal care.
- Patient demonstrates ability to perceive options and uses options to function in usual roles as much as possible.
- Patient expresses feelings of having made productive contribution to self-care, to others, or to the environment.

Documentation

- Observations of patient's physical, emotional, and mental status
- Patient's thoughts and feelings about illness and diminished role capacity
- Nursing interventions performed to help patient understand change in role functioning
- Patient's response to nursing interventions
- Health teaching, counseling, and precautions taken to maintain or enhance patient's level of functioning
- Referrals to sources of support for patient and family members
- Evaluations for expected outcomes

REFERENCES

Cavalcanti, B. C., Marques, D. R., Guimarães, F. J., de Oliveira Mangueira, S., da Silva Frazão, I., & Perrelli, J. A. (2014). "Ineffective role performance" nursing diagnosis in postpartum women: A descriptive study. *Online Brazilian Journal of Nursing*, *13*(2), 246–254.

Chen, Y., Shaffer, M., Westman, M., Chen, S., Lazarova, M., & Reiche, S. (2014). Family role performance: Scale development and validation. *Applied Psychology: An International Review*, *63*(1), 190–218. doi:10.1111/apps.12005

Watkins, S. L., Lounsbury, P. A., & Fleming-Castaldy, R. P. (2016). The self-assessment of role performance and activities of daily living abilities (SARA™): Development and clinical utility of a client-centered screening tool and outcome measure. *Occupational Therapy in Health Care*, *30*(1), 42–57. doi:10.3109/07380577.2015.1050621

CAREGIVER ROLE STRAIN

related to increasing care needs/dependency

Definition

Difficulty in performing family/significant other caregiver role

Assessment

- Caregiver's physical and mental status, including chronic health problems, self-care abilities, mobility limitations, and level of cognitive function
- Care recipient's physical and mental status, including illness, self-care limitations, mobility limitations, and level of cognitive function
- Support systems, including financial resources, family members and friends, community services, health-related services such as geriatric day care, and home health aides
- Home environment, including layout, structural barriers, need for equipment or assistive devices, and availability of transportation
- Cultural, ethnic, and religious background
- Perceived and actual obligations of caregiver
- Caregiver's personal strengths, including coping and problem-solving abilities and participation in diversional activities or hobbies

Defining Characteristics

Caregiving Activities

- Apprehensiveness about future ability to provide care
- Apprehensiveness about future health of care receiver
- Apprehensiveness about potential institutionalization of care receiver
- Apprehensiveness about well-being of care receiver if unable to provide care
- Difficulty completing required tasks
- Difficulty performing required tasks
- Dysfunctional change to caregiving activities
- Preoccupation with care routine

Caregiver Health Status: Physiologic

- Cardiovascular disease
- Diabetes mellitus
- Fatigue
- Gastrointestinal distress
- Headache
- Hypertension
- Rash
- Weight change

Caregiver Health Status: Emotional

- Alteration in sleep pattern
- Anger
- Depression
- Emotional vacillation
- Frustration
- Impatience
- Ineffective coping strategies
- Insufficient time to meet personal needs
- Nervousness
- Somatization
- Stressors

Caregiver Health Status: Socioeconomic

- Change in leisure activities
- Low work productivity
- Refusal of career advancement
- Social isolation

Caregiver–Care Receiver Relationship

- Difficulty watching care receiver with illness
- Grieving changes in relationship with care receiver
- Uncertainty about changes in relationship with care receiver

Family Processes

- Concern about family member(s)
- Family conflict

Expected Outcomes

- Caregiver will describe current stressors.
- Caregiver will identify which stressors can and can't be controlled.
- Caregiver will identify formal and informal sources of support.

- Caregiver will show evidence of using support systems.
- Caregiver will report increased ability to cope with stress.

Suggested NOC Outcomes

Caregiver Emotional Health; Caregiver Lifestyle Disruption; Caregiver Physical Health; Caregiver Stressors; Caregiver Well-Being; Caregiving Endurance Potential; Family Support During Treatment; Role Performance

Interventions and Rationales

- PCC Help caregiver to identify current stressors in order *to evaluate the causes of role strain.*
- Using a nonjudgmental approach, help caregiver evaluate which stressors are controllable and which aren't *to begin to develop strategies to reduce stress.*
- PCC Encourage caregiver to discuss coping skills used to overcome similar stressful situations in the past *to build confidence for managing the current situation.*
- PCC Encourage caregiver to participate in a support group. Provide information on organizations such as Alzheimer's Association, Children of Aging Parents, or the referral service of the community AIDS task force *to foster mutual support and provide an opportunity for caregiver to discuss personal feelings with empathetic listeners.*
- PCC Help caregiver identify informal sources of support, such as family members, friends, church groups, and community volunteers, *to provide resources for obtaining an occasional or regularly scheduled respite.*
- PCC Help caregiver identify available formal support services, such as home health agencies, municipal or county social services, hospital social workers, physicians, clinics, and day care centers, *to enhance coping by providing a reliable structure for support.*
- If caregiver seems overly anxious or distraught, gently point out facts about care recipient's mental and physical condition. *Many times, especially when care recipient is a family member, caregiver's perspective is clouded by a long history of emotional involvement. Your input may help caregiver view the situation more objectively.* If you believe that excessive emotional involvement is hindering caregiver's ability to function, consider recommending Codependents Anonymous, a support group for people whose preoccupation with a relationship leads to chronic suffering and diminished effectiveness, *to provide support.*
- Suggest ways for caregiver to use time more efficiently. For example, caregiver may save time by filling out insurance forms while visiting and chatting with care recipient. *Better time management may help caregiver reduce stress.*

Suggested NIC Interventions

Active Listening; Caregiver Support; Coping Enhancement; Counseling; Normalization Promotion; Role Enhancement; Support Group; Home Maintenance Assistance

Evaluations for Expected Outcomes

- Caregiver identifies and develops a realistic appraisal of each stressful situation.
- Caregiver describes emotional response to each stressful situation.
- Caregiver identifies sources of support.
- Caregiver uses available support systems.
- Caregiver uses appropriate coping skills for each stressful situation.

Documentation

- Stressors (perceived and actual) identified by caregiver
- Observations of caregiver's response to stressful situations
- Referrals provided
- Caregiver's use of informal and formal support systems
- Coping strategies identified by caregiver and nurse
- Evidence of improvement in caregiver's ability to cope
- Evaluations for expected outcomes

REFERENCES

Campbell, C. L., McCoy, S., Hoffman, N., & O'Neil, P. (2014). Decreasing role strain for caregivers of veterans with dependence in performing activities of daily living. *Health & Social Work*, *39*(1), 55–62.

Ching-Tzu, Y., Hsin-Yun, L., & Yea-Ing Lotus, S. (2014). Dyadic relational resources and role strain in family caregivers of persons living with dementia at home: A cross-sectional survey. *International Journal of Nursing Studies*, *51*(4), 593–602. doi:10.1016/j.ijnurstu.2013.09.001

Li, A., Shaffer, J., & Bagger, J. (2015). The psychological well-being of disability caregivers: examining the roles of family strain, family-to-work conflict, and perceived supervisor support. *Journal of Occupational Health Psychology*, *20*(1), 40–49. doi:10.1037/a0037878

Mei Hae, O., & Kyung Min, P. (2014). The effect of a social support program on family caregivers' role strain in elderly long-term home care. *Journal of Korean Academy of Community Health Nursing/ Jiyeog Sahoe Ganho Hakoeji*, *25*(2), 137–145. doi:10.12799/jkachn.2014.25.2.137

RISK FOR CAREGIVER ROLE STRAIN

Definition

Vulnerable to difficulty in performing the family/significant other caregiver role, which may compromise health

Assessment

- Caregiver's physical and mental status, including chronic health problems, self-care abilities, mobility limitations, and level of cognitive function
- Care recipient's physical and mental status, including illness, self-care limitations, mobility limitations, and level of cognitive function
- Support systems, including financial resources, family members and friends, community services, and health-related services, such as geriatric day care and home health aides
- Home environment, including layout, structural barriers, need for equipment or assistive devices, and availability of transportation
- Cultural, ethnic, and religious background
- Perceived and actual obligations of caregiver
- Caregiver's personal strengths, including usual coping and problem-solving abilities and participation in diversional activities or hobbies

Risk Factors

- Alteration in cognitive functioning in care receiver
- Care receiver discharged home with significant needs
- Care receiver exhibits bizarre behavior
- Care receiver exhibits deviant behavior
- Caregiver health impairment
- Caregiver isolation
- Caregiver not developmentally ready for caregiver role

- Caregiver's competing role commitments
- Caregiving task complexity
- Codependency
- Congenital disorder
- Developmental delay
- Developmental delay of caregiver
- Excessive caregiving activities
- Exposure to violence
- Extended duration of caregiving required
- Family isolation
- Female caregiver
- Illness severity of care receiver
- Inadequate physical environment for providing care
- Ineffective caregiver coping pattern
- Ineffective family adaptation
- Inexperience with caregiving
- Instability in care receiver's health
- Insufficient caregiver recreation
- Insufficient respite for caregiver
- Partner as caregiver
- Pattern of family dysfunction before the caregiving situation
- Pattern of ineffective relationship between caregiver and care receiver
- Prematurity
- Presence of abuse (e.g., physical, psychological, sexual)
- Psychological disorder in caregiver
- Psychological disorder in care receiver
- Stressors
- Substance abuse
- Unpredictability of illness trajectory

Expected Outcomes

- Caregiver will identify current stressors.
- Caregiver will identify appropriate coping strategies and will state plans to incorporate strategies into daily routine.
- Caregiver will state intention to contact formal and informal sources of support.
- Caregiver will state intention to incorporate recreational activities into daily routine.
- Caregiver will report satisfaction with ability to cope with stress caused by caregiving responsibilities.

Suggested NOC Outcomes

Caregiver Emotional Health; Caregiver Home Care Readiness; Caregiver Lifestyle Disruption; Caregiver–Patient Relationship; Caregiver Physical Health; Caregiver Stressors; Caregiving Endurance Potential; Rest

Interventions and Rationales

- PCC Help caregiver identify current stressors. Ask whether stress is likely to increase or decrease in the future *to evaluate the risk of caregiver role strain.*
- PCC Encourage caregiver to discuss coping skills used to overcome similar stressful situations in the past *to bolster caregiver's confidence in ability to manage current situation and explore ways to apply coping strategies before caregiver becomes overwhelmed.*
- PCC Help caregiver identify informal sources of support, such as family members, friends, church groups, and community volunteers, *to plan for an occasional or regularly scheduled respite.*
- PCC Help caregiver identify available formal support services, such as home health agencies, municipal or county social services, hospital social workers, physicians, clinics, and day care centers, *to help lessen risk of strain on caregiver.*
- Encourage caregiver to discuss hobbies or diversional activities. *Incorporating enjoyable activities into the daily or weekly schedule will discipline caregiver to take needed breaks from caregiving responsibilities and thereby diminish stress.*

PCC
- Encourage caregiver to participate in a support group. Provide information on organizations such as Alzheimer's Association, Children of Aging Parents, or the referral service of the community task force for AIDS *to foster mutual support and provide an outlet for expressing feelings before frustration becomes overwhelming.*
- If caregiver seems overly anxious or distraught, gently point out facts about care recipient's mental and physical condition. *Many times, especially when care recipient is a family member, caregiver's perspective is clouded by a long history of emotional involvement. Your input may help caregiver view the situation more objectively.* If you believe that excessive emotional involvement is hindering caregiver's ability to function, consider recommending Codependents Anonymous, a support group for people whose preoccupation with a relationship leads to chronic suffering and diminished effectiveness, *to provide support.*
- Suggest ways for caregiver to use time efficiently; for example, caregiver may save time by filling out insurance forms while visiting and chatting with care recipient. *Better time management may help caregiver reduce stress.*

Suggested NIC Interventions

Caregiver Support; Coping Enhancement; Exercise Promotion; Home Maintenance Assistance; Referral; Respite Care; Role Enhancement; Support Group

Evaluations for Expected Outcomes

- Caregiver identifies and develops a realistic appraisal of each stressful situation.
- Caregiver describes coping strategies used in stressful situations.
- Caregiver uses available support systems.
- Caregiver incorporates recreational activities into daily routine.
- Caregiver reports satisfaction in coping with stress.

Documentation

- Current stressors identified by caregiver
- Risk factors (developmental, physiologic, psychological, and situational) for caregiver role strain identified by nurse
- Caregiver's statements indicating intention to take action to minimize stress, such as seeking help from support services, participating in a caregiver support group, and scheduling time for recreational activities
- Coping strategies identified by caregiver and nurse
- Observations of caregiver's response to stressful situations
- Referrals provided
- Evaluations for expected outcomes

REFERENCES

Campbell, C. L., McCoy, S., Hoffman, N., & O'Neil, P. (2014). Decreasing role strain for caregivers of veterans with dependence in performing activities of daily living. *Health & Social Work*, *39*(1), 55–62.

Ching-Tzu, Y., Hsin-Yun, L., & Yea-Ing Lotus, S. (2014). Dyadic relational resources and role strain in family caregivers of persons living with dementia at home: A cross-sectional survey. *International Journal of Nursing Studies*, *51*(4), 593–602. doi:10.1016/j.ijnurstu.2013.09.001

Li, A., Shaffer, J., & Bagger, J. (2015). The psychological well-being of disability caregivers: examining the roles of family strain, family-to-work conflict, and perceived supervisor support. *Journal of Occupational Health Psychology*, *20*(1), 40–49. doi:10.1037/a0037878

Mei Hae, O., & Kyung Min, P. (2014). The effect of a social support program on family caregivers' role strain in elderly long-term home care. *Journal of Korean Academy of Community Health Nursing/Jiyeog Sahoe Ganho Hakoeji*, *25*(2), 137–145. doi:10.12799/jkachn.2014.25.2.137

BATHING SELF-CARE DEFICIT

related to alteration in cognitive functioning or musculoskeletal impairment

Definition

Impaired ability to perform or complete bathing activities for self

Assessment

- History of injury or disease associated with musculoskeletal impairment, neurologic, sensory, or psychological impairment
- Self-care abilities, including knowledge and use of adaptive equipment, preparation of equipment and supplies, and technical or mechanical skills
- Musculoskeletal status, including coordination; functional ability; gait; mechanical restriction (such as cast, splint, and traction); muscle tone, size, and strength; range of motion; and tremors
- Neurologic status, including cognition, communication ability, insight or judgment, level of consciousness, memory, sensory and motor ability, and orientation
- Psychosocial status, including coping mechanisms, family members, lifestyle, patient's perceptions of health problem and self, and personality

Defining Characteristics

- Impaired ability to dry body
- Impaired ability to access bathroom
- Impaired ability to access water
- Impaired ability to gather bathing supplies
- Impaired ability to regulate bath water
- Impaired ability to wash body

Expected Outcomes

- Patient will have self-care needs met.
- Patient will have few, if any, complications.
- Patient and family members will carry out self-care program daily.
- Patient will communicate feelings about limitations.
- Patient and family members will demonstrate correct use of assistive devices.
- Patient and family members will carry out bathing and hygiene program daily.

Suggested NOC Outcomes

Adaptation to Physical Disability; Energy Conservation; Pain Level; Self-Care: Activities of Daily Living (ADLs); Self-Care: Bathing; Self-Care: Hygiene; Self-Care: Oral Hygiene

Interventions and Rationales

- Observe patient's functional, perceptual, and cognitive level every shift; document and report any changes. *Careful observation helps you adjust nursing actions to meet patient's needs.*

- Perform the prescribed treatment for underlying condition. Monitor patient's progress, reporting favorable and adverse responses to treatment. *Applying therapy consistently aids patient's independence.*
- PCC • Encourage patient to voice feelings and concerns about self-care deficits *to help patient achieve the highest functional level possible.*
- Monitor the completion of bathing and hygiene daily, offering direction and instruction as needed. Praise patient's accomplishments. *Reinforcement and rewards may encourage renewed effort.*
- Provide assistive devices, such as a long-handled toothbrush, for bathing and hygiene; instruct patient on use. *Appropriate assistive devices encourage independence.*
- Assist with or perform bathing and hygiene daily. Assist only when patient has difficulty *to promote feeling of independence.*
- PCC • Instruct patient and family members in bathing and hygiene techniques (you can give family members written instructions). Have patient and family members demonstrate bathing and hygiene under supervision. *Return demonstration identifies problem areas and increases patient's and family members' self-confidence.*
- PCC • As needed, refer patient to a psychiatric liaison nurse, support group, or home health care agency. *These extra resources will reinforce activities planned to meet patient's needs.*

Suggested NIC Interventions

Bathing; Behavior Modification; Discharge Planning; Ear Care; Foot Care; Hair Care; Nail Care; Self-Care Assistance; Teaching: Individual

Evaluations for Expected Outcomes

- Patient meets self-care needs with help of staff.
- Patient participates in activities that minimize risk of such complications as infection and skin integrity alteration.
- Patient expresses feelings about self-care deficit. If unable to meet own needs, patient seeks assistance from a family member or the staff within 24 hours.
- Patient or family members demonstrate appropriate use of assistive devices.
- Patient follows daily bathing and hygiene program. Family members assist, as needed.

Documentation

- Patient's expression of feelings and concerns about self-care limitations and their impact on body image and lifestyle
- Patient's willingness to participate in bathing and hygiene routine
- Observations of patient's impaired ability to perform self-care
- Patient's response to treatment of underlying condition
- Interventions to provide supportive care
- Patient's response to nursing interventions
- Instructions to patient and family members and their understanding of instructions and demonstrated skill in carrying out self-care functions
- Evaluations for expected outcomes

REFERENCES

Akin, S., Mendi, B., Ozturk, B., Cinper, C., & Durna, Z. (2014). Assessment of relationship between self-care and fatigue and loneliness in hemodialysis patients. *Journal of Clinical Nursing*, *23*(5/6), 856–864. doi:10.1111/jocn.12248

Cramm, J. M., & Nieboer, A. P. (2015). Disease management: The need for a focus on broader self-management abilities and quality of life. *Population Health Management*, *18*(4), 246–255. doi:10.1089/pop.2014.0120

Frost, Y., Weingarden, H., Zeilig, G., Nota, A., & Rand, D. (2015). Self-care self-efficacy correlates with independence in basic activities of daily living in individuals with chronic stroke. *Journal of Stroke & Cerebrovascular Diseases*, *24*(7), 1649–1655. doi:10.1016/j.jstrokecerebrovasdis.2015.03.054

DRESSING SELF-CARE DEFICIT

related to alteration in cognitive functioning or weakness

Definition

Impaired ability to perform or complete dressing activities for self

Assessment

- History of neurologic, sensory, psychological, or musculoskeletal impairment
- Age
- Self-care abilities, including knowledge and use of adaptive equipment, preparation of equipment and supplies, and technical or mechanical skills
- Musculoskeletal status, including coordination; functional ability; gait; mechanical restriction (such as cast, splint, and traction); muscle tone, size, and strength; range of motion; and tremors
- Neurologic status, including cognition, communication ability, insight or judgment, level of consciousness, memory, motor and sensory ability, and orientation
- Psychosocial status, including coping mechanisms, family members, lifestyle, patient's perceptions of health problem and self, and personality

Defining Characteristics

- Decrease in motivation
- Discomfort
- Environmental barrier
- Fatigue
- Impaired ability to fasten clothing
- Impaired ability to gather clothing
- Impaired ability to maintain appearance
- Impaired ability to pick up clothing
- Impaired ability to put clothing on lower body
- Impaired ability to put clothing on upper body
- Impaired ability to put on various items of clothing (e.g., shirt, socks, shoes)
- Impaired ability to remove clothing item (e.g., shirt, socks, shoes)
- Impaired ability to use assistive device
- Impaired ability to use zipper
- Musculoskeletal impairment
- Neuromuscular impairment
- Pain

Expected Outcomes

- Patient will have self-care needs met.
- Patient will have few, if any, complications.
- Patient will communicate feelings about limitations.
- Patient and family members will demonstrate correct use of assistive devices.
- Patient and family members will carry out dressing program daily.
- Patient and family members will identify resources to help cope with problems and discharge.

Suggested NOC Outcomes

Self-Care: Dressing; Self-Care: Grooming; Self-Care: Activities of Daily Living (ADLs)

Interventions and Rationales

- Observe patient's functional, perceptual, and cognitive level every shift; document and report any changes. *Careful observation helps you adjust nursing actions to meet patient's needs.*
- Perform the prescribed treatment for the underlying musculoskeletal condition. Monitor patient's progress, reporting favorable and adverse responses to treatment. *Applying therapy consistently aids patient's independence.*
- PCC Encourage patient to voice feelings and concerns about self-care deficits *to help patient achieve the highest functional level.*
- Provide privacy *to enhance patient's self-esteem.*
- Provide enough time for patient to perform dressing and grooming. *Rushing creates unnecessary stress and promotes failure.*
- Monitor patient's abilities to dress and groom daily. *This identifies problem areas before they become sources of frustration.*
- Encourage family members to provide clothing patient can easily manage. Patient may benefit from clothing slightly larger than regular size and Velcro straps. *Such clothing makes independent dressing easier.*
- Provide necessary assistive devices, such as a long-handled shoehorn and zipper pull, as needed. Instruct patient on use. *Appropriate assistive devices encourage independence.*
- Assist with or perform dressing and grooming: fasten clothes, comb hair, and clean nails. Provide help only when patient has difficulty *to promote feeling of independence.*
- PCC Instruct patient and family members in dressing and grooming techniques (you can give family members written instructions). Have patient and family members demonstrate dressing and grooming techniques under supervision. *Return demonstration reveals problem areas and increases self-confidence.*
- PCC As needed, refer patient to a psychiatric liaison nurse, support group, or home health care agency. *Extra resources reinforce activities planned to meet patient's needs.*

Suggested NIC Interventions

Body Image Enhancement; Energy Management; Self-Care Teaching: Individual; Hair Care; Self-Care Assistance: Dressing/Grooming; Skin Surveillance

Evaluations for Expected Outcomes

- Patient meets self-care needs with help of staff.
- Patient participates in activities designed to minimize risk of complications, such as complying with treatment.
- Patient expresses feelings about self-care limitations.
- Patient and family members demonstrate appropriate use of assistive devices.
- Patient follows daily dressing and grooming program. Family members assist, as needed.

Documentation

- Patient's expression of feelings and concerns about self-care limitations and their impact on body image and lifestyle

- Patient's willingness to participate in dressing and grooming
- Observations of patient's impaired ability to perform dressing and grooming
- Interventions to provide supportive care
- Patient's response to nursing interventions
- Instructions given to patient and family members, their understanding of instructions, and their demonstrated skill in carrying out self-care functions
- Evaluations for expected outcomes

REFERENCES

Akin, S., Mendi, B., Ozturk, B., Cinper, C., & Durna, Z. (2014). Assessment of relationship between self-care and fatigue and loneliness in hemodialysis patients. *Journal of Clinical Nursing*, *23*(5/6), 856–864. doi:10.1111/jocn.12248

Cramm, J. M., & Nieboer, A. P. (2015). Disease management: The need for a focus on broader self-management abilities and quality of life. *Population Health Management*, *18*(4), 246–255. doi:10.1089/pop.2014.0120

Frost, Y., Weingarden, H., Zeilig, G., Nota, A., & Rand, D. (2015). Self-care self-efficacy correlates with independence in basic activities of daily living in individuals with chronic stroke. *Journal of Stroke & Cerebrovascular Diseases*, *24*(7), 1649–1655. doi:10.1016/j.jstrokecerebrovasdis.2015.03.054

FEEDING SELF-CARE DEFICIT

related to alteration in cognitive functioning or musculoskeletal impairment

Definition

Impaired ability to perform or complete self-feeding activities

Assessment

- History of neurologic, sensory, psychological or musculoskeletal impairment
- Self-care abilities, including knowledge and use of adaptive equipment, preparation of equipment and supplies, and technical and mechanical skills
- Musculoskeletal status, including coordination; functional ability; gait; mechanical restriction (such as cast, splint, and traction); muscle tone, size, and strength; range of motion; and tremors
- Psychosocial status, including coping mechanisms, family members, lifestyle, motivation, patient's perception of health problem and self, and personality

Defining Characteristics

- Impaired ability to bring food to the mouth
- Impaired ability to chew food
- Impaired ability to get food onto utensil
- Impaired ability to handle utensils
- Impaired ability to manipulate food in mouth
- Impaired ability to open containers
- Impaired ability to pick up cup
- Impaired ability to prepare food
- Impaired ability to self-feed a complete meal
- Impaired ability to self-feed in an acceptable manner
- Impaired ability to swallow food

- Impaired ability to swallow sufficient amount of food
- Impaired ability to use assistive device

Expected Outcomes

- Patient will express feelings about feeding limitations.
- Patient will maintain weight at ___ lb.
- Patient won't have evidence of aspiration.
- Patient will consume ___ % of diet.
- Patient and family members will demonstrate correct use of assistive devices.
- Patient and family members will carry out feeding program daily.
- Patient and family members will identify resources to help cope with problems and discharge.

Suggested NOC Outcomes

Nutritional Status; Self-Care: Activities of Daily Living (ADLs); Self-Care: Eating; Swallowing Status

Interventions and Rationales

- Observe patient's functional, perceptual, or cognitive level every shift; document and report changes. *Careful observation helps you adjust nursing actions to meet patient's needs.*
- Perform the prescribed treatment for the underlying condition. Monitor patient's progress and report responses. *Applying therapy consistently aids patient's independence.*
- Weigh patient weekly and record weight. Report a change of more than 1 lb/week *to ensure adequate nutrition and fluid balance.*
- Monitor and record breath sounds every 4 hours *to check for aspiration of food.* Report crackles, wheezes, or rhonchi.
- PCC Encourage patient to express feelings and concerns about feeding deficits *to help patient achieve the highest functional level.* Provide emotional support to help patient come to terms with self-care deficit and achieve the highest functional level.
- Initiate an ordered feeding program:
  - Determine the types of food best handled by patient *to encourage patient's feelings of independence.*
  - Place patient in high Fowler's position to feed *to aid swallowing and digestion.* Support weakened extremities, and wash patient's face and hands before meals.
  - Provide assistive devices; instruct patient on their use *to allow more independence.*
  - Supervise or assist at each meal—for example, cut food into small pieces. *This aids chewing, swallowing, and digestion and reduces the risk of choking or aspiration.*
  - Feed patient slowly. *Rushing causes stress, reducing digestive activity, and causing intestinal spasms.*
  - S Keep suction equipment at the bedside *to remove aspirated foods, if necessary.*
  - PCC Instruct patient and family members in feeding techniques and equipment. *This aids understanding and encourages compliance.*
  - Record the percentage of food consumed *to ensure adequate nutrition.*
- Encourage patient to carry out the aspects of feeding according to patient's abilities. *This gives patient a sense of achievement and control.*
- PCC Refer patient to a psychiatric liaison nurse, support group, or such community agencies as Visiting Nurse Association and Meals on Wheels. *Additional resources reinforce activities planned to meet patient's needs.*

Suggested NIC Interventions

Fluid Management; Nutrition Management; Nutritional Monitoring; Self-Care Assistance: Feeding; Swallowing Therapy; Aspiration Precautions; Family Involvement Promotion

Evaluations for Expected Outcomes

- Patient expresses frustration with feeding limitations.
- Patient obtains adequate fluid and nutritional intake and maintains weight at or above established limit.
- Patient doesn't experience aspiration.
- Patient consumes established percentage of diet.
- Patient maintains weight at designated level.
- Patient and family members demonstrate proper use of assistive devices.
- Patient follows daily self-care feeding program. Family members provide assistance, as needed.
- Patient and family members identify and contact available support resources, as needed.

Documentation

- Patient's expression of feelings and concerns about inability to feed self
- Observations of patient's impaired ability to perform self-care
- Patient's response to treatment
- Patient's weight
- Patient's intake
- Interventions to provide supportive care
- Instructions given to patient and family members, their understanding of instructions, and their demonstrated skill in carrying out self-care functions
- Patient's response to interventions
- Evaluations for expected outcomes

REFERENCES

Akin, S., Mendi, B., Ozturk, B., Cinper, C., & Durna, Z. (2014). Assessment of relationship between self-care and fatigue and loneliness in hemodialysis patients. *Journal of Clinical Nursing*, *23*(5/6), 856–864. doi:10.1111/jocn.12248

Cramm, J. M., & Nieboer, A. P. (2015). Disease management: The need for a focus on broader self-management abilities and quality of life. *Population Health Management*, *18*(4), 246–255. doi:10.1089/pop.2014.0120

Frost, Y., Weingarden, H., Zeilig, G., Nota, A., & Rand, D. (2015). Self-care self-efficacy correlates with independence in basic activities of daily living in individuals with chronic stroke. *Journal of Stroke & Cerebrovascular Diseases*, *24*(7), 1649–1655. doi:10.1016/j.jstrokecerebrovasdis.2015.03.054

TOILETING SELF-CARE DEFICIT

related to alteration in cognitive functioning or musculoskeletal impairment

Definition

Impaired ability to perform or complete self-toileting activities

Assessment

- History of neurologic, sensory, psychological, or musculoskeletal impairment
- Self-care abilities, including knowledge and use of adaptive equipment, preparation of equipment and supplies, and technical or mechanical skills
- Musculoskeletal status, including coordination; functional ability; gait; mechanical restriction (such as cast, splint, and traction); muscle tone, size, and strength; range of motion; and tremors
- Neurologic status, including cognition, communication ability, insight or judgment, level of consciousness, memory, motor and sensory ability, and orientation
- Psychosocial status, including coping mechanisms, family members, lifestyle, patient's perceptions of health problem and self, and personality

Defining Characteristics

- Impaired ability to complete toilet hygiene
- Impaired ability to flush toilet
- Impaired ability to manipulate clothing for toileting
- Impaired ability to reach toilet
- Impaired ability to rise from toilet
- Impaired ability to sit on toilet

Expected Outcomes

- Patient will have self-care needs met.
- Patient will have few, if any, complications.
- Patient will communicate feelings about limitations.
- Patient will maintain continence.
- Patient and family members will demonstrate correct use of assistive devices.
- Patient and family members will carry out toileting program daily.
- Patient and family members will identify resources to help cope with problems and discharge from facility.

Suggested NOC Outcomes

Self-Care: Activities of Daily Living (ADLs); Self-Care: Hygiene; Self-Care: Toileting

Interventions and Rationales

- Observe patient's functional, perceptual, and cognitive level every shift; document and report any changes. *Careful observation helps you adjust nursing actions to meet patient's needs.*
- Perform the prescribed treatment for the underlying condition. Monitor patient's progress, reporting favorable and adverse responses to treatment. *Applying therapy consistently aids patient's independence.*
- PCC Encourage patient to voice feelings and concerns about self-care deficits *to help patient achieve the highest functional level possible.*
- Monitor intake and output and skin condition; record episodes of incontinence. *Accurate intake and output records can identify potential imbalances.*
- Use assistive devices, as needed, such as an external catheter at night, a bedpan or urinal every 2 hours during the day, and adaptive equipment for bowel care. Instruct on use.

As control improves, reduce the use of assistive devices. *Assisting at an appropriate level helps maintain patient's self-esteem.*

- Assist with toileting, only if needed. Allow patient to perform independently as much as possible *to promote independence.*
- Perform urinary and bowel care, if needed. Follow urinary or bowel elimination plans. *Monitoring success or failure of toileting plans helps identify and resolve problem areas.*
- Instruct patient and family members in toileting routine (you can give family members written instructions). Have patient and family members demonstrate toileting routine under supervision. *Return demonstration identifies problem areas and increases patient's self-confidence.*
- Provide positive, constructive feedback when assisting with toileting. *Reinforcement and rewards may enhance self-esteem.*
- Assist with toileting, giving simple instructions one at a time, *to aid comprehension.*
- Complete urinary and bowel care if patient can't do so. Follow urinary and bowel elimination plans. *Monitoring success or failure of toileting plans helps identify and resolve problem areas.*
- PCC As needed, refer patient to a psychiatric liaison nurse, support group, or home health care agency. *Extra resources reinforce activities planned to meet patient's needs.*

Suggested NIC Interventions

Bowel Training; Self-Care Assistance: Toileting; Urinary Elimination Management; Bowel Incontinence Care

Evaluations for Expected Outcomes

- Patient meets self-care needs with help of staff.
- Patient doesn't experience constipation, infection, skin integrity alteration, weight loss, or other complications of altered self-care.
- Patient and family members express feelings about self-care deficit. If unable to meet own needs, patient seeks assistance from family member or staff within 24 hours.
- Patient maintains continence.
- Patient and family members demonstrate appropriate use of assistive devices.
- Patient follows toileting program daily. Family members assist, as needed.
- Patient and family members identify and contact available support resources, as needed.

Documentation

- Patient's expression of feelings and concerns about self-care limitations and their impact on body image and lifestyle
- Patient's willingness to participate in self-care
- Observations of patient's ability to perform toileting routine and patient's response to treatment
- Patient's intake and output
- Interventions to provide supportive care
- Instructions given to patient and family members, their understanding of instructions, and their demonstrated skill in carrying out self-care functions
- Patient's response to nursing interventions
- Evaluations for expected outcomes

REFERENCES

Basak, T., Unver, V., & Demirkaya, S. (2015). Activities of daily living and self-care agency in patients with multiple sclerosis for the first 10 years. *Rehabilitation Nursing*, *40*(1), 60–65. doi:10.1002/rnj.153

Frost, Y., Weingarden, H., Zeilig, G., Nota, A., & Rand, D. (2015). Self-care self-efficacy correlates with independence in basic activities of daily living in individuals with chronic stroke. *Journal of Stroke & Cerebrovascular Diseases*, *24*(7), 1649–1655. doi:10.1016/j.jstrokecerebrovasdis.2015.03.054

Talley, K. C., Wyman, J. F., Bronas, U. G., Olson-Kellogg, B. J., McCarthy, T. C., & Hong, Z. (2014). Factors associated with toileting disability in older adults without dementia living in residential care facilities. *Nursing Research*, *63*(2), 94–104. doi:10.1097/NNR.0000000000000017

READINESS FOR ENHANCED SELF-CARE

Definition

A pattern of performing activities for oneself that helps to meet health-related goals, which can be strengthened

Assessment

- Self-care abilities, including knowledge and use of adaptive equipment, preparation of equipment and supplies, and technical and mechanical skills
- Neurologic status, including cognition, communication ability, insight or judgment, level of consciousness, memory, sensory and motor ability, and orientation
- Psychosocial status, including coping mechanisms, family members, lifestyle, patient's perceptions of self, and personality

Defining Characteristics

- Expresses desire to enhance independence with health
- Expresses desire to enhance independence with life
- Expresses desire to enhance independence with personal development
- Expresses desire to enhance independence with well-being
- Expresses desire to enhance knowledge of self-care strategies
- Expresses desire to enhance self-care

Expected Outcomes

- Patient will demonstrate positive decision making toward maximizing potential for self-care.
- Patient will express satisfaction with independence in assuming responsibility for planning self-care.
- Patient and family members will involve staff, family, and community in developing strategies for self-care.
- Patient will monitor self-care measures taken for effectiveness and make alterations as needed.

Suggested NOC Outcomes

Self-Care: Activities of Daily Living (ADLs); Adherence Behavior; Client Satisfaction: Functional Assistance; Health Beliefs: Perceived Ability to Perform

Interventions and Rationales

- PCC Assess patient's satisfaction with level of self-care *to support general well-being.*
- Assess current ability to provide self-care *to establish a baseline.*
- Assess effectiveness of self-care measures *to identify the need for adjustments.*
- PCC Assist patient to develop plan *to promote autonomous decision making to increase patient's responsibility for facilitating care.*
- PCC Provide information that supports implementation of a program to sustain health-seeking behavior *to promote patient autonomy in self-care.*
- PCC Encourage health team, family, and community efforts to participate in patient's self-care initiatives *to promote satisfactory mutual goal setting and group efforts.*
- Encourage patient and his or her family to participate in support networks that promote patient independence, where possible, *to promote patient and family resilience.*
- Develop a referral list for community resources to promote patient's enhanced self-care.

Suggested NIC Interventions

Mutual Goal Setting; Resiliency Promotion; Self-Responsibility Facilitation

Evaluations for Expected Outcomes

- Patient meets self-care needs.
- Patient makes positive decisions to maximize self-care abilities.
- Patient expresses satisfaction with independence in self-care.
- Patient monitors self-care and changes needed.

Documentation

- Patient's expression of self-care needs
- Observations of patient's impaired ability to perform self-care activities
- Interventions to provide supportive care
- Patient's response to nursing interventions
- Evaluations for expected outcomes

REFERENCES

Basak, T., Unver, V., & Demirkaya, S. (2015). Activities of daily living and self-care agency in patients with multiple sclerosis for the first 10 years. *Rehabilitation Nursing*, *40*(1), 60–65. doi:10.1002/rnj.153

Frost, Y., Weingarden, H., Zeilig, G., Nota, A., & Rand, D. (2015). Self-care self-efficacy correlates with independence in basic activities of daily living in individuals with chronic stroke. *Journal of Stroke & Cerebrovascular Diseases*, *24*(7), 1649–1655. doi:10.1016/j.jstrokecerebrovasdis.2015.03.054

Sechoaro, E. J., Scrooby, B., & Koen, D. P. (2014). The effects of rehabilitation on intellectually-disabled people—a systematic review. *Health SA Gesondheid*, *19*(1), 1–9. doi:10.4102/hsag.v19i1.693

CHRONIC LOW SELF-ESTEEM

Definition

Longstanding negative self-evaluating/feelings about self or self-capabilities

Assessment

- Reason for hospitalization or outpatient treatment

- Age
- Gender
- Developmental stage
- Family system, including marital status, role in family, and sibling position
- Perception of health problem
- Past experience with health care system
- Mental status, including abstract thinking, affect, communication, general appearance, judgment or insight, memory, mood, orientation, perception, and thinking process
- Belief system, including norms, religion, and values
- Social interaction pattern
- Social and occupational history
- Perception of self (past and present), including body image, coping mechanisms, problem-solving ability, and self-worth
- Past experience with crisis
- Past history of treatment for psychosocial disturbance, including hospitalization, medication, psychotherapy, and suicidal ideation, plans, and attempts
- Neurovegetative signs, including ability to experience pleasure, appetite, energy level, and sleep

Defining Characteristics

- Dependent on other's opinions
- Exaggerates negative feedback about self
- Excessive seeking of reassurance
- Guilt
- Hesitant to try new experiences
- Expressions of shame
- Indecisive behavior
- Nonassertive behavior
- Overly conforming
- Passivity
- Poor eye contact
- Rejection of positive feedback
- Repeatedly unsuccessful in life events
- Shame
- Underestimates ability to deal with situation

Expected Outcomes

- Patient will voice positive feelings about self.
- Patient will report feeling safe in facility environment.
- Patient will make verbal contract not to harm self while in facility.
- Patient will gradually join in self-care and decision-making process.
- Patient will engage in social interaction with others.
- Patient will demonstrate verbal and behavioral decrease in negative self-evaluation.
- Patient will voice acceptance of positive and negative feedback without exaggeration.

Suggested NOC Outcomes

Body Image; Depression Level; Mood Equilibrium; Motivation; Personal Autonomy; Quality of Life; Self-Esteem

Interventions and Rationales

- Provide for a specific amount of uninterrupted time each day to engage patient in conversation. *This time will allow the patient time for self-exploration.*
- S When appropriate, institute suicide precaution according to protocol. *Patient needs supervision until patient demonstrates adequate self-control to ensure own safety.*

- Provide patient with a simple structured daily routine. *Structured activity limits the patient's anxious behavior.*
- Spend time alone with patient listening to patient's problems that are important to him or her at this time. Have patient make a list of the three most critical issues currently in focus. *Spending this time can allow the opportunity to help patient identify strengths and begin setting some realistic goals to build self-confidence.*
- Encourage bathing, grooming, and other hygiene functions for patient every day, as needed. Encourage patient to do as much as possible independently. *Greater independence will help strengthen self-esteem.*
- PCC Teach self-healing techniques to both patient and family, such as meditation, guided imagery, yoga, and prayer, *to prevent anxiety and aid in keeping patient in a frame of mind to make positive decisions.*
- PCC Teach patient how to incorporate the use of self-healing techniques in carrying out usual daily activities.
- PCC Provide patient with concise information about decision-making skills. *This will produce benefits that can reinforce health-seeking behaviors.*
- PCC Encourage patient to express feelings about self (past and present). *Self-exploration encourages patient to consider future change.*
- Provide patient with positive feedback for verbal reports or behaviors that indicate a return to positive self-appraisal. *This gives patient feelings of significance, approval and competence, which can help cope effectively with stressful situations.*
- Encourage social interaction between patient and others. Disturbed interpersonal relationships are a direct expression of self-hate.
- Facilitate opportunities for spiritual nourishment and growth *to address patient's holistic needs for maximal therapeutic environment.*
- Encourage patient's cooperation as you continue with healing techniques, such as therapeutic touch.
- PCC Provide emotional support to family by being available to answer questions. *Accurate information will help family to cope with current situation.*
- Assist the patient to mobilize resources for assistance when discharged in order *to help the patient replace maladaptive coping behaviors with more adaptive ones.*
- Schedule time to meet with family and patient to listen to ways in which they plan to enhance their coping skills in the present situation. *Helping patient and/or family develop a realistic plan will better ensure success in meeting established goals.*
- PCC Refer family to community resources and support groups available *to assist in managing patient's illness and providing emotional and financial assistance to caregivers.*

Suggested NIC Interventions

Active Listening; Body Image Enhancement; Coping Enhancement; Decision-Making Support; Hope Instillation; Self-Esteem Enhancement; Spiritual Support; Support Group

Evaluations for Expected Outcomes

- Patient expresses feelings about self-esteem.
- Patient doesn't feel threatened by facility environment.
- At least once daily, patient reiterates commitment not to harm self.
- Patient participates in at least one aspect of self-care daily.
- Patient converses with others on daily basis.
- Patient states at least two positive aspects about self.
- Patient accepts positive feedback and constructive criticism.

Documentation

- Patient's verbal expressions and behaviors that indicate low self-esteem
- Mental status examination (baseline and ongoing)
- Suicide assessment, interventions, and patient's response
- Nursing interventions implemented to promote self-esteem
- Patient's response to interventions
- Evaluations for expected outcomes

REFERENCES

Guerrero-Escobedo, P., Tamez-Rivera, O., Amieva, H., & Avila-Funes, J. A. (2014). Frailty is associated with low self-esteem in elderly adults. *Journal of the American Geriatrics Society*, *62*(2), 396–398. doi:10.1111/jgs.12679

Noordenbos, G., Aliakbari, N., & Campbell, R. (2014). The relationship among critical inner voices, low self-esteem, and self-criticism in eating disorders. *Eating Disorders*, *22*(4), 337–351. doi:10.1080/10640266.2014.898983

Sowislo, J. F., Orth, U., & Meier, L. L. (2014). What constitutes vulnerable self-esteem? Comparing the prospective effects of low, unstable, and contingent self-esteem on depressive symptoms. *Journal of Abnormal Psychology*, *123*(4), 737–753. doi:10.1037/a0037770

SITUATIONAL LOW SELF-ESTEEM

Definition

Development of a negative perception of self-worth in response to a current situation

Assessment

- Age
- Gender
- Developmental stage
- Family system, including marital status, role in family, and sibling position
- Reason for health care visit
- Mental status, including affect, general appearance, and mood
- Cognitive ability
- Behavior
- Perception of self (past and present), including body image, coping mechanisms, and self-worth

Defining Characteristics

- Helplessness
- Indecisive behavior
- Nonassertive behavior
- Purposelessness
- Self-negating verbalizations
- Situation challenge to self-worth
- Underestimates ability to deal with situation

Expected Outcomes

- Patient will voice feelings related to current situation and its effect on self-esteem.
- Patient will verbally appraise self before and during current health problem.

- Patient will participate in decisions related to care and therapies.
- Patient will report sense of control over life events.
- Patient will articulate return to previous positive feelings about self.

Suggested NOC Outcomes

Decision-Making; Grief Resolution; Psychosocial Adjustment: Life Change; Self-Esteem

Interventions and Rationales

S
- Assess patient for suicidal ideations or thoughts of violence to self or others. *It is necessary to determine this so early intervention can be taken to prevent injury to the patient and those around.*

PCC
- Encourage patient to express feelings about self (past and present). *Self-exploration encourages patient to consider future change.*
- Provide a specific amount of uninterrupted non-care-related time to engage patient in conversation. *Such discussions help patient assume ultimate responsibility for coping responses.*
- Explore patient's usual coping mechanisms in times of stress. Suggest additional positive methods of coping. Role play with the patient in *order to help patient see what healthy coping mechanisms look like.*
- Assess patient's mental status through interview and observation at least once per day. *If anxiety resulting from self-rejection becomes severe, patient may experience disorientation and psychotic symptoms.*

PCC
- Involve patient in the decision-making process. *Making such decisions can help combat ambivalence and procrastination associated with low self-esteem.*
- Provide patient with positive feedback for verbal reports or behaviors that indicate a return to positive self-appraisal. *This gives patient feelings of significance, approval, and competence, which can help in coping effectively with stressful situations.*

Suggested NIC Interventions

Anticipatory Guidance; Decision-Making Support; Grief Work Facilitation; Self-Esteem Enhancement

Evaluations for Expected Outcomes

- Patient expresses feelings about self in relation to recent stressful events.
- Patient describes how feelings about self have changed since current health problem began.
- Patient makes decisions related to care daily.
- Patient reports feeling more self-confident and in control of current situation.
- Patient states at least two positive feelings about self.

Documentation

- Patient's expressions of lowered self-esteem
- Mental status assessment (baseline and ongoing)
- Nursing interventions directed toward return to previous positive self-esteem
- Patient's response to interventions
- Evaluations for expected outcomes

REFERENCES

Garofalo, C., Holden, C. J., Zeigler-Hill, V., & Velotti, P. (2016). Understanding the connection between self-esteem and aggression: The mediating role of emotion dysregulation. *Aggressive Behavior*, *42*(1), 3–15. doi:10.1002/ab.21601

La Mela, C., Maglietta, M., Caini, S., Casu, G. P., Lucarelli, S., Mori, S., & Ruggiero, G. M. (2015). Perfectionism, weight and shape concerns, and low self-esteem: Testing a model to predict bulimic symptoms. *Eating Behaviors*, *19*, 155–158. doi:10.1016/j.eatbeh.2015.09.002

Noser, A., & Zeigler-Hill, V. (2014). Investing in the ideal: Does objectified body consciousness mediate the association between appearance contingent self-worth and appearance self-esteem in women? *Body Image*, *11*(2), 119–125. doi:10.1016/j.bodyim.2013.11.006

RISK FOR SITUATIONAL LOW SELF-ESTEEM

Definition

Vulnerable to developing a negative perception of self-worth in response to a current situation, which may compromise health

Assessment

- Age
- Gender
- Developmental stage
- Family system, including marital status, role in family, and sibling position
- Reason for health care visit
- Mental status, including affect, general appearance, and mood
- Cognitive ability
- Behavior
- Perception of self (past and present), including body image, coping mechanisms, and self-worth

Risk Factors

- Alteration in body image
- Alteration in social role
- Behavior inconsistent with values
- Decrease in control over environment
- Developmental transition
- Functional impairment
- History of abandonment
- History of abuse (e.g., physical, psychological, sexual)
- History of loss
- History of neglect
- Inadequate recognition
- Pattern of failure
- Pattern of helplessness
- Physical illness
- Unrealistic self-expectations

Expected Outcomes

- Patient will participate in decisions related to care and therapy.
- Patient will maintain eye contact and initiate conversation.
- Patient will maintain an open and upright posture.
- Patient will verbally assess feelings about current situation and health problems and impact on lifestyle.

- Patient will express positive feelings about self (verbally or through behaviors), indicating acceptance of changes caused by health problems or situation.
- Patient will perform hygiene and self-care activities indicating attention to appearance.
- Patient will express interest in talking to others who have successfully overcome the problem of low self-esteem.

Suggested NOC Outcomes

Self-Esteem; Life Changes; Decision Making; Perceived Control; Psychosocial Adjustment

Interventions and Rationales

- Assess developmental stage; family system; role in family; sibling position; health history; mental status, including affect, general appearance, mood; cognitive ability; support systems; patient's ability to identify choices; readiness for change to occur; level of knowledge for positive decision making, coping mechanisms, environmental factors. *Information from assessment will assist the nurse to identify appropriate interventions.*
- Encourage bathing, grooming, and other hygiene functions for the patient every day, as needed. Encourage patient to do as much as possible for self. *Greater independence will help strengthen self-esteem.*
- PCC Keep patient informed about what to expect and when to expect it. *Accurate information reduces anxiety.*
- PCC Teach self-healing techniques to both the patient and family such as meditation, guided imagery, yoga, and prayer. Teach patient how to incorporate the use of self-healing techniques in carrying out usual daily activities. *These techniques help calm the mind and promote ability to cooperate with the difficulties associated with low self-esteem.*
- Encourage patient to talk about personal assets and accomplishments and about improvements in condition no matter how small these may seem. Give positive feedback. *Conversation assists you to evaluate the patient's self-concept and adaptive abilities.*
- Direct the patient's focus beyond the present state. *Focusing on the present state alone will make it difficult for the patient to plan activities that will move patient forward.*
- PCC Help patient involve the family, community, clergy, and friends with changes to the care plan *to increase the potential of the patient's control over self-care outcomes.*
- PCC Refer patient and family to other professional caregivers, for example, dietitian, social worker, clergy, and mental health professional. *Support groups such as Ostomy clubs, I Can Cope, and Reach for Recovery can provide physical, material, financial, and emotional resources to patient and the family during the recovery period.*
- PCC Assist patient to utilize appropriate resources by contacting family and scheduling follow-up appointments. *This helps give the patient a sense of direction and control over future care.*

Suggested NIC Interventions

Assertiveness Training; Coping Enhancement; Self-Modification Assistance; Self-Responsibility Facilitation

Evaluations for Expected Outcomes

- Patient expresses feelings about self in relation to recent stressful events.
- Patient describes how feelings about self have changed since current health problem began.

- Patient makes decisions related to care daily.
- Patient reports feeling more self-confident and in control of current situation.
- Patient states at least two positive feelings about self.

Documentation

- Patient's expressions of lowered self-esteem
- Mental status assessment (baseline and ongoing)
- Nursing interventions directed toward return to previous positive self-esteem
- Patient's response to interventions
- Evaluations for expected outcomes

REFERENCES

Garofalo, C., Holden, C. J., Zeigler-Hill, V., & Velotti, P. (2016). Understanding the connection between self-esteem and aggression: The mediating role of emotion dysregulation. *Aggressive Behavior*, *42*(1), 3–15. doi:10.1002/ab.21601

La Mela, C., Maglietta, M., Caini, S., Casu, G. P., Lucarelli, S., Mori, S., & Ruggiero, G. M. (2015). Perfectionism, weight and shape concerns, and low self-esteem: Testing a model to predict bulimic symptoms. *Eating Behaviors*, *19*, 155–158. doi:10.1016/j.eatbeh.2015.09.002

Noser, A., & Zeigler-Hill, V. (2014). Investing in the ideal: Does objectified body consciousness mediate the association between appearance contingent self-worth and appearance self-esteem in women? *Body Image*, *11*(2), 119–125. doi:10.1016/j.bodyim.2013.11.006

SELF-NEGLECT

related to alteration in cognitive functioning

Definition

A constellation of culturally framed behaviors involving one or more self-care activities in which there is a failure to maintain a socially accepted standard of health and well-being (Gibbons, Lauder, & Ludwick, 2006)

Assessment

- Self-care status including bathing, hygiene, grooming, feeding, and toileting
- Cultural status including cultural norms
- Patient's understanding of problem, coping mechanisms, problem-solving ability, and family system

Defining Characteristics

- Insufficient environmental hygiene
- Insufficient personal hygiene
- Nonadherence to health activity

Expected Outcomes

- Patient will demonstrate improved cognitive, functional, and mental health.
- Patient will adhere to prescribed health activities.
- Patient will experience increased safety.

- Patient will demonstrate improved coping with complex health circumstances, including personal and environmental hygiene, nutrition, and fitness.
- Patient will have fewer acute hospitalizations and emergency room visits.

Suggested NOC Outcomes

Adherence Behavior; Compliance Behavior; Decision-Making; Health Orientation; Motivation; Personal Well-Being; Risk Control; Self-Care Status

Interventions and Rationales

- Assess patient with complex health issues for adequate coping abilities. *Poor coping skills may lead to unintentional self-neglect.*
- Assess patient with failing self-care for changes in cognitive function. *Neglected self-care may be the first noticeable sign of diminishing cognitive function.*
- PCC Involve patient's family in care activities as appropriate *to improve the chance that the patient will incorporate recommended regimens into lifestyle as long-term choice.*
- PCC Teach strategies to enhance adherence to medication and other health regimens. *Some instances of self-neglect occur because the patient has not been able to incorporate recommended regimens into lifestyle.*
- PCC Encourage patient to identify internally motivating factors for adhering to health regimens. *Persons who intentionally neglect self-care as a lifestyle choice (i.e., fail to comply with medication and treatment regimens) will fare better if the decision to improve self-care is their decision.*
- PCC Refer patient demonstrating a significant decline in self-care abilities (i.e., posing a threat to self and/or community) for competency evaluation. *Unintentional self-neglect may indicate diminished competency.*

Suggested NIC Interventions

Behavior Management; Counseling; Exercise Promotion; Limit Setting; Mutual Goal Setting; Self-Care Assistance; Self-Responsibility Facilitation; Weight Management

Evaluations for Expected Outcomes

- Patient's cognitive, functional, and mental health status has improved.
- Patient adhered to prescribed regimen.
- Patient remained safe.
- Patient was able to cope with complex health situation in a positive way.

Documentation

- Patient's cognitive, functional, and mental health status
- Patient's method of coping with circumstances
- Evaluations for expected outcomes

REFERENCES

Braye, S., Orr, D., & Preston-Shoot, M. (2015). Serious case review findings on the challenges of self-neglect: Indicators for good practice. *Journal of Adult Protection*, *17*(2), 75–87. doi:10.1108/JAP-05-2014-0015

Rathbone-McCuan, E. (2014). An improved approach to treating elder self-neglect: The self-care framework. *Generations, 38*(3), 80–85.
Wilkins, S. S., Horning, S., Castle, S., Leff, A., Hahn, T. J., & Chodosh, J. (2014). Challenges and management of self-neglect in older adults with cognitive impairment. *Annals of Long-term Care, 22*(12), 30–34.

SEXUAL DYSFUNCTION

related to alteration in body function (due to anomaly, disease, medication, pregnancy, radiation, surgery, trauma, etc.)

Definition

A state in which an individual experiences a change in sexual function during the sexual response phases of desire, excitation, and/or orgasm, which is viewed as unsatisfying, unrewarding, or inadequate

Assessment

- History of problem that caused change in structure or function
- Patient's perception of change's effect
- Marital status and attitude of spouse or significant other
- Living arrangement
- Usual sexual patterns
- Sexual problems before current health problem
- Patient's attitude toward modifying sexual patterns
- Patient's present knowledge about appropriate options available

Defining Characteristics

- Alteration in sexual activity
- Alteration in sexual excitation
- Alteration in sexual satisfaction
- Change in interest toward others
- Change in self-interest
- Change in sexual role
- Decrease in sexual desire
- Perceived sexual limitation
- Seeks confirmation of desirability
- Undesired change in sexual function

Expected Outcomes

- Patient will acknowledge problem or potential problem in sexual function.
- Patient will voice feelings about changes in sexual identity.
- Patient will explain reason for sexual dysfunction.
- Patient will express willingness to obtain counseling.
- Patient will reestablish sexual activity at preillness level.

Suggested NOC Outcomes

Adaptation to Physical Disability; Body Image; Fear Level; Physical Aging; Role Performance; Sexual Functioning; Sexual Identity; Stress Level

Interventions and Rationales

- Provide a nonthreatening atmosphere and encourage patient to ask questions about personal sexuality. *A nonthreatening atmosphere encourages patient to ask questions specifically related to the current situation.*
- Allow patient to express feelings openly in a nonjudgmental atmosphere *to enhance communication and understanding between patient and caregiver.*
- PCC Provide answers to specific questions *to help patient focus on specific issues, clarify misconceptions, and build trust in the caregiver.*
- Provide time for privacy *to demonstrate respect for patient, allow time for introspection, and give patient control over time spent interacting with others.*
- Suggest that patient discuss concerns with partner. *Open discussion fosters sharing of concerns and strengthens relationships.*
- Provide support for the partner. *Supportive interventions such as active listening communicate concern, interest, and acceptance.*
- PCC Educate patient and partner about limitations imposed by patient's current physical condition. *Education about limitations imposed on sexual activity by illness helps patient avoid complications or injury.*
- PCC Suggest referral to a sex counselor or other appropriate professional for future guidance *to provide patient with a resource for postdischarge support.*

Suggested NIC Interventions

Anxiety Reduction; Emotional Support; Mutual Goal Setting; Role Enhancement; Self-Awareness Enhancement; Self-Esteem Enhancement; Sexual Counseling; Teaching: Individual; Values Clarification

Evaluations for Expected Outcomes

- Patient acknowledges existence of problem or potential problem in sexual function.
- Patient expresses anxiety, anger, depression, or frustration over changes in sexual function.
- Patient explains relationship between illness or treatment and sexual dysfunction.
- Patient expresses willingness to obtain counseling.
- Patient resumes usual level of sexual activity.

Documentation

- Patient's perception of problem
- Subtle comments made by patient about inability to cope with change in structure or function
- Observations of patient's behavior
- Interventions performed to assist patient and spouse or significant other; response to interventions
- Evaluations for expected outcomes

REFERENCES

Celik, S., Golbası, Z., Kelleci, M., & Satman, I. (2015). Sexual dysfunction and sexual quality of life in women with diabetes: The study based on a diabetic center. *Sexuality & Disability*, *33*(2), 233–241. doi:10.1007/s11195-014-9383-3

Mills, L. (2015). Sexual dysfunction in men with diabetes. *Journal of Diabetes Nursing*, *19*(9), 332–338.

Steinke, E. E., Mosack, V., & Hill, T. J. (2015). Change in sexual activity after a cardiac event: The role of medications, comorbidity, and psychosocial factors. *Applied Nursing Research*, *28*(3), 244–250. doi:10.1016/j.apnr.2015.04.011

SEXUAL DYSFUNCTION

related to misinformation about sexual function

Definition

A state in which the individual experiences a change in sexual function during the sexual response phases of desire, excitation, and/or orgasm, which is viewed as unsatisfying, unrewarding, or inadequate

Assessment

- Age
- History of impotence
  - Organic (anatomic or central nervous system defect)
  - Functional (physiologic alterations in nervous and cardiovascular systems)
  - Psychogenic (inhibition by emotions of neural transmission from brain to sexual organs)
  - Primary (failure to ever achieve satisfactory erection for coitus)
  - Secondary (at least one successful coitus)
- History of organic impotence or physiologic disorders that interfere with erection
- Anatomic anomalies of penis
- Psychological variables, including patient's perception of sexual performance, relationships, desire for erection, guilt, shame, relationship with parents (presence of overbearing mother), and family or social pressures
- Physiologic status, including medication history (response, effectiveness, and adverse reactions) and history of substance abuse (type and effect on mental status)
- Sociocultural factors, including educational level, socioeconomic status, ethnic group, and religious beliefs and practices
- Sexual history, including sexual drive, sexual preference, frequency of impotence, premature ejaculation, spontaneous morning erections, positive coital experiences, types of erotic stimulation used, past professional counseling or sex therapy, homosexual experiences, affairs (other partners or prostitutes), and feelings of anger, hostility, or disgust toward partner

Defining Characteristics

- Alteration in sexual activity
- Alteration in sexual excitation
- Alteration in sexual satisfaction
- Change in interest toward others
- Change in self-interest
- Change in sexual role
- Decrease in sexual desire
- Perceived sexual limitation
- Seeks confirmation of desirability
- Undesired change in sexual function

Expected Outcomes

- Patient will acknowledge problem in sexual function.
- Patient will voluntarily discuss the problem.
- Patient and partner will discuss their feelings and perceptions about changes in sexual performance.

- Patient will learn methods to enhance sexual pleasure for self and partner and incorporate them into sexual activities.
- Patient will continue to communicate with partner about sexual issues and needs.
- Patient will agree to obtain sexual evaluation and therapy, if needed.
- Patient will develop and maintain positive attitude toward own sexuality and sexual performance.

Suggested NOC Outcomes

Body Image; Fear Level; Physical Aging; Role Performance; Sexual Functioning; Sexual Identity; Social Interaction Skills; Stress Level

Interventions and Rationales

- Establish a therapeutic relationship with patient *to provide a safe, comfortable atmosphere for discussing sexual concerns.*
- PCC Encourage patient to discuss feelings and perceptions about sexual dysfunction *to help the patient validate perceptions and reduce emotional distress through catharsis.*
- Encourage patient and partner to discuss feelings and perceptions *to help the couple clarify issues about their relationship and improve communication.*
- PCC Educate patient and partner about alternative methods of lovemaking and expressing affection. *Alternative expressions of love and intimacy can raise patient's self-esteem until impotence is evaluated and treated.*
- Encourage use of sexual fantasies and erotica to promote sexual stimulation and erection. *This helps patient and partner achieve sexual satisfaction and decreases "spectatoring" (watching oneself during sexual activity with partner), which can inhibit performance.*
- PCC Encourage patient to seek professional evaluation and therapy *to obtain proper diagnosis and treatment.*

Suggested NIC Interventions

Active Listening; Anxiety Reduction; Behavior Management: Sexual; Counseling; Role Enhancement; Self-Awareness Enhancement; Self-Esteem Enhancement; Sexual Counseling; Teaching: Sexuality

Evaluations for Expected Outcomes

- Patient problem in sexual function.
- Patient reports feeling comfortable discussing sexual concerns.
- Patient and partner communicate with each other about their sexual relationship.
- Patient states specific ways of enhancing sexual pleasure with partner.
- Patient continues to communicate with partner about sexual issues and needs.
- Patient participates in sexual evaluation and sex therapy, if needed.
- Patient makes positive comments about self, sexuality, and sexual performance.

Documentation

- Patient's perception of sexual problem
- Overt and covert remarks made by patient that indicate personal difficulty dealing with impotence

- Observations of patient's behavior in response to patient's inability to perform
- Interventions performed to assist patient and partner
- Response to nursing interventions
- Evaluations for expected outcomes

REFERENCES

Giebink, C. B., & Alexander, I. M. (2015). Managing female sexual dysfunction. *Women's Healthcare: A Clinical Journal for NPS*, *3*(1), 41–48.

Kingsberg, S. A. (2014). Attitudinal survey of women living with low sexual desire. *Journal of Women's Health (15409996)*, *23*(10), 817–823. doi:10.1089/jwh.2014.4743

Kolzet, J., Quinn, H., Zemon, V., Tyry, T., Marrie, R., Foley, F., & Flood, S. (2015). Predictors of body image-related sexual dysfunction in men and women with multiple sclerosis. *Sexuality & Disability*, *33*(1), 63–73. doi:10.1007/s11195-014-9357-5

INEFFECTIVE SEXUALITY PATTERN

related to impaired relationship with a significant other

Definition

Expressions of concern regarding own sexuality

Assessment

- Reason for hospitalization
- Current and anticipated length of stay
- Marital status and family members
- Living arrangement
- Patient's perception of sexual identity and role
- Usual sexual activity pattern
- Patient's perception of limitation on sexual activity resulting from hospitalization
- Significance of sexual relationship to patient and partner
- Emotional reactions (affect and mood)
- Behavioral reactions (specify)

Defining Characteristics

- Alteration in relationship with significant other
- Alteration in sexual activity
- Alteration in sexual behavior
- Change in sexual role
- Difficulty with sexual activity
- Difficulty with sexual behavior
- Value conflict

Expected Outcomes

- Patient will voice feelings about changes in usual sexual activity and/or behavior.
- Patient and partner will discuss possible realistic alternatives for intimacy.
- Patient and partner will use available counseling referrals.

Suggested NOC Outcomes

Anxiety Level; Body Image; Role Performance; Self-Esteem; Sexual Identity; Stress Level

Interventions and Rationales

- Allow a specific amount of uninterrupted, non-care-related time *to talk with patient to demonstrate your comfort with sexuality issues and reassure patient that personal concerns are acceptable for discussion.*
- Display an accepting, nonjudgmental manner *to encourage patient to discuss concerns about sexuality.* Approach the partner in the same manner and include the partner in discussions with patient, if agreeable to both. *A nonjudgmental approach demonstrates unconditional positive regard for both patient and partner.*
- PCC Include patient in a plan for setting limits on inappropriate behavior, if indicated by behavioral assessment.
  - Explain aspects of patient's behavior that are inappropriate.
  - Share the proposed care plan with patient, including expectations, goals, and approaches for reducing bothersome behavior.
  - Request patient's cooperation, but be willing to compromise if the patient offers acceptable alternatives.
  - Working together to set limits allows patient to take part in planning to reduce undesirable behaviors.
- Discuss with patient and partner realistic, acceptable alternatives for intimacy needs. *Discussion encourages open communication between them as sexual partners.*
- Explain to patient and partner the limitations related to illness and facility environment *to establish a standard for realistic and acceptable behavior.*
- Provide time for privacy to allow patient and partner *to discuss feelings about sexuality and to engage in alternatives for intimacy while patient is hospitalized.*
- PCC Offer referral for counseling, such as a mental health professional and sex counselor, if indicated. *Referrals provide opportunities for additional ongoing therapy during hospitalization and after discharge.*

Suggested NIC Interventions

Anticipatory Guidance; Anxiety Reduction; Coping Enhancement; Role Enhancement; Self-Esteem Enhancement; Sexual Counseling; Teaching: Sexuality

Evaluations for Expected Outcomes

- Patient describes usual sexual activity pattern and expresses feelings resulting from changes in pattern.
- Patient and partner request privacy and seek permission to use acceptable alternatives for intimacy, such as holding and kissing.
- Patient and partner seek counseling.

Documentation

- Patient's verbal and nonverbal behaviors
- Patient's and partner's perception of current situation

- Specific nursing interventions to reduce emotional and behavioral reactions, such as active listening, limit setting, and counseling referrals
- Patient's and partner's response to nursing interventions
- Evaluations for expected outcomes

REFERENCES

Erden, S., & Kaya, H. (2015). Sexual dysfunction and anxiety levels of type 2 male diabetics. *Applied Nursing Research*, *28*(3), 239–243. doi:10.1016/j.apnr.2015.04.014

Perz, J., Ussher, J. M., & Gilbert, E. (2014). Feeling well and talking about sex: Psycho-social predictors of sexual functioning after cancer. *BMC Cancer*, *14*(1), 228–228. doi:10.1186/1471-2407-14-228

Villaamil, F. (2014). Shared embarrassment: (Not) Talking about sex in HIV-related doctor–patient encounters. *Medical Anthropology*, *33*(4), 335–350. doi:10.1080/01459740.2013.826215

INEFFECTIVE SEXUALITY PATTERN

related to skill deficit about alternatives related to sexuality

Definition

Expressions of concern regarding own sexuality

Assessment

- History of current illness
- Current treatment regimen (medications and therapies)
- Marital status and family members
- Patient's perception of sexual identity and role
- Usual sexual activity pattern
- Patient's perception of changes in sexual activity resulting from illness or treatment
- Significance of sexual relationship to patient and partner
- Emotional reactions (affect and mood)
- Behavioral reactions (specify)

Defining Characteristics

- Alteration in relationship with significant other
- Alteration in sexual activity
- Alteration in sexual behavior
- Change in sexual role
- Difficulty with sexual activity
- Difficulty with sexual behavior
- Value conflict

Expected Outcomes

- Patient will voice feelings about potential or actual changes in sexual activity.
- Patient will express concern about self-concept, self-esteem, and body image.
- Patient will state at least one effect of illness or treatment on sexual behavior.
- Patient and partner will resume effective communication patterns.
- Patient and partner will use available counseling referrals or support groups.

Suggested NOC Outcomes

Anxiety Level; Body Image; Role Performance; Self-Esteem; Sexual Identity; Stress Level

Interventions and Rationales

- Allow for a specific amount of uninterrupted time to talk with patient *to demonstrate your comfort with sexuality issues and convey reassurance that patient's concerns are acceptable for discussion.*
- Provide a nonthreatening, nonjudgmental atmosphere for patient to verbalize feelings about perceived changes in sexual identity and behaviors *to demonstrate unconditional positive regard for patient and patient's concerns about sexuality patterns.*
- PCC Provide patient and partner with information about the illness and treatment. Answer any questions and clarify any misconceptions they may have *to help them focus on specific concerns, encourage questions, and avoid misunderstandings.*
- Provide time for privacy *to demonstrate respect for patient, allow time for introspection, and give patient control over time spent interacting with others.*
- Encourage social interaction and communication between patient and partner *to foster sharing of concerns and strengthen relationship.*
- PCC Offer referral to counselors or support persons, such as a mental health professional, sex counselor, and illness-related support groups, such as "I Can Cope," Reach for Recovery, and the Ostomy Association, *to provide patient with resources for postdischarge support.*

Suggested NIC Interventions

Anticipatory Guidance; Body Image Enhancement; Coping Enhancement; Counseling; Emotional Support; Self-Awareness Enhancement; Support Group; Support System Enhancement

Evaluations for Expected Outcomes

- Patient expresses concerns and fears related to potential or actual changes in sexual activity.
- Patient expresses feelings about change in self-image resulting from illness or medical treatment.
- Patient identifies specific physical symptom that has negative effect on sexual behavior.
- Patient and partner communicate effectively.
- Patient and partner participate in therapy with appropriate counselor.

Documentation

- Patient's perception of changes in sexual patterns
- Patient's ability to interact with other people
- Interventions to support and educate patient and partner
- Response to nursing interventions
- Evaluations for expected outcomes

REFERENCES

Liu, G., Hariri, S., Bradley, H., Gottlieb, S. L., Leichliter, J. S., & Markowitz, L. E. (2015). Trends and patterns of sexual behaviors among adolescents and adults aged 14 to 59 years, United States. *Sexually Transmitted Diseases*, 42(1), 20–26. doi:10.1097/OLQ.0000000000000231

Prah, P., Copas, A. J., Mercer, C. H., Nardone, A., & Johnson, A. M. (2015). Patterns of sexual mixing with respect to social, health, and sexual characteristics among heterosexual couples in England: analyses of probability sample survey data. *Epidemiology & Infection, 143*(7), 1500–1510. doi:10.1017/S0950268814002155
Rothenbacher, D., Dallmeier, D., Mons, U., Rosamond, W., Koenig, W., & Brenner, H. (2015). Sexual activity patterns before myocardial infarction and risk of subsequent cardiovascular adverse events. *Journal of the American College of Cardiology (JACC), 66*(13), 1516–1517. doi:10.1016/j.jacc.2015.07.053

RISK FOR SHOCK

Definition

Vulnerable to an inadequate blood flow to the body's tissues that may lead to life-threatening cellular dysfunction, which may compromise health

Assessment

- Cardiovascular status including heart rate and rhythm, blood pressure, peripheral pulses
- Signs of dehydration, inflammation, or allergic responses
- Respiratory status including respiratory rate and depth, pulse oximetry
- Renal status, intake and output, urine specific gravity
- Mental status including orientation, level of consciousness

Risk Factors

- Hypotension
- Hypovolemia
- Hypoxemia
- Hypoxia
- Infection
- Sepsis
- Systemic inflammatory response syndrome

Expected Outcomes

- Patient will maintain adequate blood pressure to maintain tissue perfusion.
- Patient will not experience hemodynamic complications from underlying medical condition.
- Patient will understand the need for aggressive management of underlying medical condition in an effort to prevent shock.
- Patient will verbalize signs and symptoms of possible hypotension and hypoperfusion.

Suggested NOC Outcomes

Tissue Perfusion: Cerebral; Hydration; Fluid Balance; Vital Signs

Interventions and Rationales

- Monitor hemodynamic status frequently, including blood pressure, heart rate, oxygen saturation. *Trending of vital signs will provide database for early intervention and treatment.*
- Assess level of consciousness with each vital sign check. *Change in level of consciousness is an early indicator of cerebral hypoperfusion.*

- Administer intravenous fluids, oxygen, and medications as prescribed *to maintain fluid volume and organ perfusion.*
- Collect and evaluate serum laboratory specimens *to provide data to effectively treat underlying medical condition and avoid complication of shock.*

PCC
- Educate patient and family of reportable signs and symptoms of inadequate tissue perfusion, for example, dizziness, confusion, restlessness, and dyspnea. *Early intervention and treatment is essential in preventing permanent organ damage.*

PCC
- Encourage patient and family to express concerns and *fears to reduce anxiety.*

PCC
- Collaborate with other members of the health care team *to effectively manage underlying medical condition and prevent complications.*

Suggested NIC Interventions

Acid–Base Monitoring; Fluid/Electrolyte Management; Hypovolemia Management; Shock Management

Evaluations for Expected Outcomes

- Patient's blood pressure was adequate to maintain tissue perfusion.
- Patient did not experience any complications related to hypoperfusion.
- Patient understood the need for aggressive management of underlying medical condition to prevent hypoperfusion.
- Patient was able to verbalize reportable signs and symptoms of possible hypoperfusion and shock.

Documentation

- Patient's vital signs, intake and output, and laboratory results
- Patient's response to medical interventions to treat underlying condition
- Ability of patient to identify reportable signs and symptoms of hypoperfusion
- Evaluations for expected outcomes

REFERENCES

Gallimore, E. (2015). Clinical features and management of hemorrhagic shock. *Nursing Standard*, *30*(1), 51–58. doi:10.7748/ns.30.1.51.e9955

Hsiao, C. Y., Yang, H. Y., Chang, C. H., Lin, H. L., Wu, C. Y., Hsiao, M. C., … Yen, T. H. (2015). Risk factors for development of septic shock in patients with urinary tract infection. *BioMed Research International*, *2015*, 1–7. doi:10.1155/2015/717094

Soleimanpour, H., Safari, S., Rahmani, F., Nejabatian, A., & Alavian, S. M. (2015). Hepatic shock differential diagnosis and risk factors: A review article. *Hepatitis Monthly*, *15*(10), 9–14. doi:10.5812/hepatmon.27063

IMPAIRED SITTING

related to alteration in cognitive functioning; neurologic disorder

Definition

Limitation of ability to independently and purposefully attain and/or maintain a rest position that is supported by the buttocks and thighs, in which the torso is upright.

Assessment

- History of neuromuscular disorder or dysfunction
- Neurologic status, including level of consciousness, motor ability and sensory ability
- Musculoskeletal status, including coordination, balance, muscle size and strength, muscle tone, range of motion (ROM), and functional mobility scale:
  0 = completely independent
  1 = requires use of equipment or device
  2 = requires help, supervision, or teaching from another person
  3 = requires help from another person and equipment or device
  4 = dependent; doesn't participate in activity

Defining Characteristics

- Impaired ability to adjust position of one or both lower limbs on uneven surface
- Impaired ability to attain a balanced position of the torso
- Impaired ability to flex or move both hips
- Impaired ability to flex or move both knees
- Impaired ability to maintain the torso in balanced position
- Impaired ability to stress torso with body weight
- Insufficient muscle strength

Expected Outcomes

- Patient will achieve highest level of independence possible when sitting.
- Patient will achieve highest level of joint ROM when sitting.
- Patient will show no evidence of complications.
- Patient will achieve balance while sitting.
- Patient will maintain muscle strength.

Suggested NOC Outcomes

Activity Tolerance; Endurance; Joint Movement: Hip; Joint Movement: Spine; Neurological Status: Central Motor Control; Neurological Status: Spinal Sensory/Motor Function; Physical Fitness; Skeletal Function

Interventions and Rationales

- Perform ROM exercises to joints, unless contraindicated, at least once every shift. Progress from passive to active, as tolerated. *This prevents joint contractures and muscular atrophy.*
- Place joints in functional position. *Maintain joints in a functional position and prevent musculoskeletal deformities.*
- Identify the level of functioning using a functional mobility scale (see Assessment). Communicate patient's skill level to all staff members *to provide continuity and preserve identified level of independence.*
- Encourage independence by helping patient to use assistive devices. *This increases muscle tone and patient's self-esteem.*
- Monitor and record daily any evidence of immobility complications (such as contractures, venous stasis, thrombus, pneumonia, and urinary tract infection). *Patients with a history of neuromuscular disorders or dysfunction may be more prone to developing complications.*
- S PCC Instruct patient to call before attempting to stand without assistance. *Ensure patient safety from falls.*

- Carry out a medical regimen to manage or prevent complications; for example, administer prophylactic heparin as ordered for venous thrombosis. *This promotes patient's health and well-being.*
- S Use a transfer belt, if necessary, *to support patient and prevent staff injury.*
- S Use assistive devices as necessary, *to support patient and prevent staff injury.*
- PCC Refer patient to a physical therapist for development of sitting regimen *to help rehabilitate musculoskeletal deficits.*
- Demonstrate the sitting regimen and note date. Have patient and family members return sitting regimen demonstration and note date. *This ensures continuity of care and use of proper technique.*

Suggested NIC Interventions

Body Mechanics Promotion; Exercise Therapy: Balance; Exercise Therapy: Muscle Control; Positioning; Self-Care Assistance

Evaluations for Expected Outcomes

- Patient achievement of highest level of independence possible when sitting.
- Patient achievement of highest level of joint ROM when sitting.
- Patient has no evidence of complications.
- Patient achievement of balance while sitting.
- Patient maintains muscle strength.

Documentation

- Patient's current status of functional abilities and goals set for self
- Observations of patient's mobility status, presence of complications, and response to sitting regimen
- Instruction and demonstration of skills in carrying out sitting regimen
- Patient's response to nursing interventions
- Evaluations for expected outcomes

REFERENCES

Cabanas-Valdés, R., Cuchi, G. U., & Bagur-Calafat, C. (2013). Trunk training exercises approaches for improving trunk performance and functional sitting balance in patients with stroke: A systematic review. *Neurorehabilitation*, *33*(4), 575–592. doi:10.3233/NRE-130996

Iyengar, Y., Vijayakumar, K., Abraham, J., Misri, Z., Suresh, B., & Unnikrishnan, B. (2014). Relationship between postural alignment in sitting by photogrammetry and seated postural control in post-stroke subjects. *Neurorehabilitation*, *35*(2), 181–190. doi:10.3233/NRE-141118

Tsang, W. W., Gao, K. L., Chan, K. M., Purves, S., Macfarlane, D. J., & Fong, S. S. (2015). Sitting Tai Chi Improves the Balance Control and Muscle Strength of Community-Dwelling Persons with Spinal Cord Injuries: A Pilot Study. *Evidence-based Complementary & Alternative Medicine (eCAM)*, 1–9. doi:10.1155/2015/523852

IMPAIRED SKIN INTEGRITY

related to external or internal factors

Definition

Altered epidermis and/or dermis

Assessment

- History of skin problems, trauma, chronic debilitating disease, or immobility
- Age
- Integumentary status, including color, elasticity, hygiene, lesions, moisture, texture, turgor, sensation, temperature, and quantity and distribution of hair
- Musculoskeletal status, including joint mobility, muscle strength and mass, paralysis, and range of motion
- Nutritional status, including appetite, dietary intake, hydration, current weight, and change from normal weight
- Hemoglobin and serum albumin levels and hematocrit
- Psychosocial status, including coping patterns, family members, mental status, occupation, self-concept, and body image
- Knowledge level, including patient's current understanding of physical condition and physical, mental, and emotional readiness to learn

Defining Characteristics

- Alteration in skin integrity
- Foreign matter piercing skin

Expected Outcomes

- Patient won't show evidence of skin breakdown.
- Patient will exhibit improved or healed lesions or wounds.
- Patient will report increased comfort.
- Patient will have few, if any, complications.
- Patient will correlate precipitating factors with appropriate skin care regimen.
- Patient will explain skin care regimen.
- Patient and family members will demonstrate skin care regimen.
- Patient will voice feelings about changed body image.

Suggested NOC Outcomes

Immobility Consequences: Physiologic; Tissue Integrity: Skin & Mucous Membranes; Wound Healing: Secondary Intention

Interventions and Rationales

- Inspect patient's skin every 8 hours, describe and document skin condition, and report changes *to provide evidence of the effectiveness of skin care regimen.*
- Perform prescribed treatment regimen for the skin condition involved; monitor progress. Report favorable and adverse responses to treatment regimen *to maintain or modify current therapies, as needed.*
- Provide supportive measures, as indicated:
  - Assist with general hygiene and comfort measures *to promote comfort and general sense of well-being.*
  - Administer pain medications and monitor effectiveness. *Patient needs pain relief to maintain health.*
  - Maintain proper environmental conditions, including room temperature and ventilation. *Providing a comfortable environment promotes sense of well-being.*

- Apply a bed cradle *to protect lesions from bed covers.*
- Remind patient not to scratch *to avoid skin injury.*
- Administer and monitor effectiveness of antipruritic medications. *Antipruritics reduce the itching sensation.*
- PCC Explain dietary restrictions; for example, explain that certain foods may cause a skin allergy. *Avoiding foods that cause skin allergy helps prevent skin breakdown.*

- PCC Encourage patient to express feelings about skin condition *to enhance coping.*
- Position patient for comfort and minimal pressure on bony prominences. Change the patient's position at least every 2 hours. Monitor frequency of turning and skin condition. *These measures reduce pressure, promote circulation, and minimize skin breakdown.*
- Discuss precipitating factors, if known, and long-term effects of skin integrity interruption. *Knowledge of precipitating factors helps patient reduce their occurrence and severity.*
- Follow facility protocol for treatment of pressure ulcer or surgical wound care *to ensure provision of appropriate care.*
- PCC Instruct patient and family in the skin care regimen *to ensure compliance.*
- Supervise patient and family in the skin care regimen. Provide feedback. *Practice helps improve skill in managing patient's skin care regimen.*
- Encourage adherence to other aspects of health care management *to control or minimize effects on skin.*
- PCC Refer patient to a psychiatric liaison nurse, social service, or support group, as appropriate. *These resources provide additional support for patient and family.*

Suggested NIC Interventions

Infection Control; Nutrition Therapy; Positioning; Pressure Ulcer Prevention; Skin Surveillance

Evaluations for Expected Outcomes

- Patient's skin remains intact.
- Patient's wounds or lesions heal.
- Patient reports feeling of comfort.
- Patient doesn't experience further skin breakdown or other complications.
- Patient lists factors precipitating skin breakdown.
- Patient explains skin care regimen.
- Patient and family members demonstrate skin care regimen.
- Patient expresses feelings about changed body image.

Documentation

- Patient's concerns about skin disorder and its impact on body image and lifestyle
- Patient's willingness to participate in care
- Observations of skin condition, healing, and response to treatment regimen
- Interventions to provide supportive care
- Instructions about treatment regimen
- Patient's or family members' understanding of and skill in carrying out instructions
- Patient's response to nursing interventions
- Evaluations for expected outcomes

REFERENCES

Coyer, F., Gardner, A., Doubrovsky, A., Cole, R., Ryan, F. M., Allen, C., & McNamara, G. (2015). Reducing pressure injuries in critically ill patients by using a patient skin integrity care bundle (INSPIRE). *American Journal of Critical Care*, 24(3), 199–210. doi:10.4037/ajcc2015930

Moncrieff, G., Van Onselen, J., & Young, T. (2015). The role of emollients in maintaining skin integrity. *Wounds UK*, *11*(1), 68–74.

Weller, C. D. (2015). Wound healing and skin integrity: Principles and practice. *Wound Practice & Research*, *23*(1), 46–47.

RISK FOR IMPAIRED SKIN INTEGRITY

Definition

Vulnerable to alteration in epidermis and/or dermis, which may compromise health

Assessment

- History of skin problems, trauma, chronic debilitating disease, or immobility
- Age
- Integumentary status, including color, elasticity, hygiene, lesions, moisture, sensation, temperature, texture, turgor, and quantity and distribution of hair
- Musculoskeletal status, including muscle strength and mass, joint mobility, paralysis, and range of motion (ROM)
- Nutritional status, including appetite, dietary intake, hydration, current weight, and change from normal weight
- Hemoglobin and serum albumin levels and hematocrit
- Psychosocial status, including activities of daily living, mental status, occupation (sun exposure), and recreational activities

Risk Factors

External

- Chemical injury agent (e.g., burn, capsaicin, methylene chloride, mustard agent)
- Excretions
- Extremes of age
- Humidity
- Hyperthermia
- Hypothermia
- Mechanical factor (e.g., shearing forces, pressure, physical immobility)
- Moisture
- Radiation therapy
- Secretions

Internal

- Alteration in metabolism
- Alteration in pigmentation
- Alteration in sensation (resulting from spinal cord injury, diabetes mellitus, etc.)
- Alteration in skin turgor
- Hormonal change
- Immunodeficiency
- Impaired circulation
- Inadequate nutrition
- Pharmaceutical agent
- Pressure over bony prominence
- Psychogenetic factor

Expected Outcomes

- Patient won't experience skin breakdown.
- Patient will maintain muscle strength and joint ROM.

- Patient will sustain adequate food and fluid intake.
- Patient's mucous membranes will remain intact.
- Patient will maintain adequate skin circulation.
- Patient will communicate understanding of preventive skin care measures.
- Patient and family members will demonstrate preventive skin care measures.
- Patient and family members will correlate risk factors and preventive measures.

Suggested NOC Outcomes

Immobility Consequences: Physiologic; Nutritional Status; Physical Aging; Risk Control; Risk Detection; Tissue Integrity: Skin & Mucous Membranes

Interventions and Rationales

- Inspect patient's skin every shift; document skin condition and report status changes. *Early detection of changes prevents or minimizes skin breakdown.*
- Change patient's position at least every 2 hours; follow turning schedule posted at bedside. Monitor frequency of turning. *These measures reduce pressure on tissues, promote circulation, and help prevent skin breakdown.*
- Encourage ambulation or perform or assist with active ROM exercises at least every 4 hours while patient is awake. *Exercises prevent muscle atrophy and contracture; ambulation promotes circulation and relieves pressure.*
- Use preventive skin care devices, as needed, such as a foam mattress, alternating pressure mattress, sheepskin, pillows, and padding, *to avoid discomfort and skin breakdown.*
- Keep patient's skin clean and dry; lubricate, as needed. Don't use irritating soap, and rinse skin well. *These measures alleviate skin dryness, promote comfort, and reduce the risk of irritation and skin breakdown.*
- Protect bony prominences with foam padding. *Prominences have little subcutaneous fat and are prone to breakdown; using foam padding may help promote skin integrity.*
- Lift patient's body when moving the patient, using a lifting sheet, if needed. Avoid shearing force. *Shearing force results when tissues slide against each other; a lifting sheet reduces sliding.*
- Keep linen dry, clean, and free from wrinkles or crumbs. Change wet bed linens and incontinence pads immediately. *Dry, smooth linens help prevent excoriation and skin breakdown.*
- Monitor nutritional intake; maintain adequate hydration. *Anemia (less than 10 mg hemoglobin) and low serum albumin concentrations (less than 2 mg) are associated with the development of pressure ulcers. Hydration helps maintain skin integrity.*
- PCC Educate patient and family in preventive skin care. Teach them how to maintain good personal hygiene; use nonirritating (nonalkaline) soap; pat rather than rub skin dry; inspect skin regularly; avoid prolonged exposure to water, sun, cold, and wind; avoid rubber rings; recognize the beginning of skin breakdown (redness, blisters, and discoloration); and report signs and symptoms. *These measures encourage compliance with patient's skin care regimen.*
- Indicate the risk factor potential on patient's chart and care plan, and reevaluate weekly, using an accepted form such as the Braden Scale. *The risk factor score helps evaluate treatment progress.*
- Explain the importance of practicing preventive skin care measures *to encourage compliance with skin care regimen.*
- Supervise patient and family in preventive skin care measures. Give constructive feedback. *Practice helps improve skill in managing the skin care regimen.*

Suggested NIC Interventions

Circulatory Precautions; Infection Prevention; Positioning; Pressure Management; Pressure Ulcer Prevention; Skin Surveillance; Splinting

Evaluations for Expected Outcomes

- Patient's skin remains intact.
- Patient maintains muscle strength and joint ROM.
- Patient's weight remains within established limits.
- Patient's mucous membranes remain intact.
- Patient maintains adequate skin circulation.
- Patient lists preventive skin care measures.
- Patient and family members demonstrate skin care measures.
- Patient and family members understand need to avoid prolonged pressure, obtain adequate nutrition, prevent incontinence, and consistently perform skin care measures.

Documentation

- Patient's and family members' expressions of concern about potential skin breakdown
- Observations of risk factors and skin condition
- Use of preventive skin care devices and their effectiveness
- Instructions about preventive skin care; patient's and family members' understanding of instructions
- Patient's and family members' demonstrated skill in carrying out preventive skin care measures
- Results of Braden Scale
- Patient's response to nursing interventions
- Evaluations for expected outcomes

REFERENCES

Cowdell, F., & Garrett, D. (2014). Older people and skin: Challenging perceptions. *British Journal of Nursing*, *23*, S4–S8.

Cowdell, F., & Radley, K. (2014). What do we know about skin hygiene care for patients with bariatric needs? Implications for nursing practice. *Journal of Advanced Nursing*, *70*(3), 543–552. doi:10.1111/jan.12208

Yamaguti, W. P., Moderno, E. V., Yamashita, S. Y., Gomes, T. C., Maida, A. V., Kondo, C. S., … de Brito, C. M. (2014). Treatment-related risk factors for development of skin breakdown in subjects with acute respiratory failure undergoing noninvasive ventilation or CPAP. *Respiratory Care*, *59*(10), 1530–1536. doi:10.4187/respcare.02942

SLEEP DEPRIVATION

Definition

Prolonged periods of time without sleep (sustained natural, periodic suspension of relative consciousness)

Assessment

- Number of hours of sleep patient usually needs to feel rested
- Premorbid sleep patterns and current sleep patterns
- Daytime activity and work patterns

- Recent changes in health status or lifestyle
- Sleep environment, including recent changes to environment
- Activities that promote sleep
- Quality of sleep, as described by patient
- Dietary and drug history, including ingestion of caffeine or other stimulants, nicotine, alcohol, and sedative-hypnotics

Defining Characteristics

- Agitation
- Alteration in concentration
- Anxiety
- Apathy
- Combativeness
- Confusion
- Decrease in functional ability
- Decrease in reaction time
- Drowsiness
- Fatigue
- Fleeting nystagmus
- Hallucinations
- Hand tremors
- Heightened sensitivity to pain
- Irritability
- Lethargy
- Listlessness
- Malaise
- Perceptual disorders
- Restlessness
- Transient paranoia

Expected Outcomes

- Patient will identify factors that prevent or disrupt sleep.
- Patient will sleep ____ (specify) hours without interruption.
- Patient will express feeling well rested.
- Patient will show no physical signs of sleep deprivation.
- Patient will not exhibit complications associated with sleep deprivation, such as sleep apnea and nocturnal hypoxic episodes.
- Patient will alter diet and habits to promote sleep—for example, by reducing caffeine intake and limiting alcohol intake.
- Patient will not exhibit such sleep-related behavioral symptoms as irritability, lethargy, listlessness, restlessness, anxiety, worry, or depression.
- Patient will perform relaxation exercises at bedtime.
- Health care providers will schedule nighttime treatments to allow for maximum restful sleep.

Suggested NOC Outcomes

Concentration; Endurance; Energy Conservation; Mood Equilibrium; Rest; Sleep; Stress Level; Symptom Severity

Interventions and Rationales

- Encourage patient to identify factors in the environment that make sleeping difficult. *A strange or new environment may affect rapid eye movement and non-rapid eye movement sleep.*
- PCC Ask patient what changes would help promote sleep *to encourage patient to play an active role in care.*
- Advise patient to avoid daytime naps *to promote restful nocturnal sleep.*
- Tell patient to avoid spending long periods in bed without sleep. *Activity produces healthy fatigue, which promotes restful sleep.*

- Make immediate changes to accommodate patient—for example, reduce noise; change catheterization, medication, or treatment schedule; change lighting; and close door. *These measures promote rest and sleep.*
- Develop a plan to allow patient to have ____ hours of uninterrupted sleep, if possible. *This provides consistent nursing care and provides patient with maximum hours of uninterrupted sleep.*
- Perform interventions to promote sleep, such as giving patient a bath or back rub, ensuring that patient is positioned properly, or providing pillows, food, or drink. *Personal hygiene routine precedes sleep for many individuals. Milk and some high-protein snacks, such as cheese or nuts, contain L-tryptophan, a sleep promoter.*
- Assess patient each morning to determine quality of sleep the night before *to help detect sleep-related behavioral symptoms.*
- PCC Teach patient relaxation techniques, such as guided imagery, meditation, and progressive muscle relaxation. Practice them with patient at bedtime. *Purposeful relaxation efforts commonly promote sleep.*
- Instruct patient to limit alcohol and caffeine intake and avoid foods that interfere with sleep (such as spicy foods). Foods and beverages with caffeine should be avoided for 4 to 5 hours before bedtime. *Dietary changes may help to promote restful sleep.*
- Avoid quick, unanticipated movements when turning and positioning patients with neuromuscular dysfunction *to prevent spasticity, which may interrupt sleep.*
- In stroke patients with muscle tone problems, plan to position patient on the affected side during the last turn of the night *to promote restful sleep and help normalize patient's muscle tone for morning activities.*
- PCC Refer patient experiencing sleep deprivation to a sleep disorder center, especially if activities of daily living are affected or sleep apnea occurs. *A specialist may be required to assist in treatment.*
- Assess the daytime schedule to ensure adequate time for rest. *Excessive fatigue can result in insomnia.*
- PCC Help patient with chronic illness or disability find resources for addressing psychosocial issues. *Fears and concerns about future prevent restful sleep.*

Suggested NIC Interventions

Anxiety Reduction; Coping Enhancement; Energy Management; Environmental Management: Comfort; Progressive Muscle Relaxation; Sleep Enhancement

Evaluations for Expected Outcomes

- Patient identifies factors that prevent or disrupt sleep.
- Patient sleeps ____ (specify) hours without interruption.
- Patient expresses feeling of being well rested.
- Patient shows no physical signs of sleep deprivation.
- Patient doesn't exhibit complications associated with sleep deprivation, such as sleep apnea and nocturnal hypoxic episodes.
- Patient alters diet and habits to promote sleep—for example, by reducing caffeine intake and limiting alcohol intake.
- Patient doesn't exhibit such sleep-related behavioral symptoms, such as irritability, lethargy, listlessness, restlessness, anxiety, worry, or depression.
- Patient performs relaxation exercises at bedtime.
- Health care providers schedule nighttime treatments to allow for maximum restful sleep.

Documentation

- Patient's reports of sleep disturbances
- Patient's expressions of feelings related to sleep deprivation
- Observations of behaviors that indicate sleep deprivation
- Nursing interventions to alleviate sleep deprivation
- Patient's response to nursing interventions
- Evaluations for expected outcomes

REFERENCES

Das, S., Deepa, O. V., Pradhan, J., & Kumari, S. (2015). Factors of sleep disturbances among hospitalized patients, jeopardizing the prognosis. *Asian Journal of Nursing Education & Research, 5*(2), 302–304.

Kohansieh, M., & Makaryus, A. N. (2015). Sleep deficiency and deprivation leading to cardiovascular disease. *International Journal of Hypertension, 2015*, 1–5. doi:10.1155/2015/615681

Podgorski, T., & Wise, C. (2015). EB146 Sleep deprivation in the intensive care unit: Promoting sleep in the patients who need it most. *Critical Care Nurse, 35*(2), e73–e74.

DISTURBED SLEEP PATTERN

Definition

Time-limited interruptions of sleep amount and quality due to external factors

Assessment

- Number of hours of sleep patient usually needs to feel rested
- Premorbid sleep patterns and current sleep patterns
- Daytime activity and work patterns
- Recent changes in health status or lifestyle
- Sleep environment, including recent changes to environment
- Activities that promote sleep
- Quality of sleep, as described by patient
- Dietary and drug history, including ingestion of caffeine or other stimulants, nicotine, alcohol, and sedative-hypnotics

Defining Characteristics

- Alteration in sleep pattern
- Difficulty in daily functioning
- Difficulty initiating sleep
- Dissatisfaction with sleep
- Feeling unrested
- Unintentional awakening

Expected Outcomes

- Patient will identify factors that changed usual sleep pattern.
- Patient will sleep ____ (specify) hours without interruption.
- Patient will express feeling well rested.
- Patient will alter diet and habits to promote sleep—for example, by reducing caffeine intake and limiting alcohol intake.

- Patient will incorporate sleep preparation measures into evening routine.
- Patient will carry out relaxation exercises that promote sleep.
- Patient will express satisfaction with sleep.

Suggested NOC Outcomes

Rest; Sleep; Symptom Control; Well-Being

Interventions and Rationales

- Complete a sleep history and help the patient identify factors that may impair sleep. *Review of patterns may elicit insights that can be used to correct the problem.*
- PCC Assist the patient to identify environmental factors that make sleeping difficult. Suggest the use of "white noise" machines to mask unwanted noise. *A strange or new environment may affect rapid eye movement and non-rapid eye movement sleep.*
- PCC Ask the patient what changes would help promote sleep *to encourage the patient to play an active role in care.*
- Encourage regular evening routines that promote sleep, such as taking a warm bath or eating a small snack. *Personal hygiene routine precedes sleep for many individuals. Milk and some high-protein snacks, such as cheese or nuts, contain L-tryptophan, a sleep promoter.*
- Ask the patient to evaluate the quality of sleep the night before *to help detect sleep-related behavioral symptoms.*
- PCC Teach the patient relaxation techniques, such as guided imagery, meditation, and progressive muscle relaxation. *Purposeful relaxation efforts commonly promote sleep.*
- Instruct the patient to limit alcohol and caffeine intake and avoid foods that interfere with sleep (such as spicy foods). Foods and beverages with caffeine should be avoided for 4 to 5 hours before bedtime. *Dietary changes may help to promote restful sleep.*
- PCC Refer the patient experiencing extended sleep changes to a sleep disorder center, especially if activities of daily living are affected or sleep apnea occurs. *A specialist may be required to assist in treatment.*
- Assess the daytime schedule to ensure adequate time for rest. *Excessive fatigue can result in insomnia.*
- PCC Help the patient with chronic illness or disability find resources for addressing psychosocial issues. *Fears and concerns about future prevent restful sleep.*

Suggested NIC Interventions

Anxiety Reduction; Simple Guided Imagery; Energy Management; Environmental Management: Comfort; Progressive Muscle Relaxation; Sleep Enhancement; Anticipatory Guidance; Calming Technique; Simple Relaxation Therapy

Evaluations for Expected Outcomes

- Patient identifies factors that prevent or disrupt sleep.
- Patient sleeps ____ (specify) hours without interruption.
- Patient expresses feeling of being well rested.
- Patient alters diet and habits to promote sleep—for example, by reducing caffeine intake and limiting alcohol intake.
- Patient performs relaxation exercises at bedtime.
- Patient incorporates sleep techniques into bedtime regimen.

Documentation

- Patient's reports of sleep disturbances
- Patient's responses to sleep routine changes
- Observations of behaviors that indicate sleep deprivation
- Patient's response to guided imagery or relaxation techniques
- Patient's response to nursing interventions
- Evaluations for expected outcomes

REFERENCES

Bakken, L. N., Kim, H. S., Finset, A., & Lerdal, A. (2014). Subjective sleep quality in relation to objective sleep estimates: Comparison, gender differences, and changes between the acute phase and the six-month follow-up after stroke. *Journal of Advanced Nursing*, *70*(3), 639–650. doi:10.1111/jan.12228

Hsiao-Yean, C., Wen-Cheng, L., Yung-Hsiao, C., & Pei-Shan, T. (2014). The effects of sleep on the relationship between brain injury severity and recovery of cognitive function: A prospective study. *International Journal of Nursing Studies*, *51*(6), 892–899. doi:10.1016/j.ijnurstu.2013.10.020

Miller, N. (2015). Sleep deprivation and delirium risk in hospitalized patients. *Nursing Made Incredibly Easy*, *13*(1), 22–28. doi:10.1097/01.NME.0000457284.31841.36

IMPAIRED SOCIAL INTERACTION

related to disturbance in thought processes

Definition

Insufficient or excessive quantity or ineffective quality of social exchange

Assessment

- Reason for hospitalization (physiologic or psychiatric)
- Usual pattern of social interaction (nonverbal behaviors and verbal communication)
- Neurologic functioning, including level of consciousness, orientation, and sensory and motor ability
- Mental status, including abstract ability, affect, concentration ability, insight and judgment, memory, mood, and thought content
- History of substance abuse
- Education and intelligence level
- Sociocultural background, including beliefs, norms, religion, and values
- Support systems, including clergy, family members, and friends

Defining Characteristics

- Discomfort in social situations
- Dissatisfaction with social engagement (e.g., belonging, caring, interest, shared history)
- Dysfunctional interaction with others
- Family reports change in interaction (e.g., style, pattern,)
- Impaired social functioning

Expected Outcomes

- Patient and family members will report concern about difficulties in social interaction.
- Patient will maintain orientation to time, place, and person.
- Patient's perceptions will be reality based.

- Patient and family members will participate in care and prescribed therapies.
- Patient will verbalize perceptions of difficulty in interaction with others.
- Patient will express needs and will communicate whether needs are met.
- Patient will regain appropriate neurologic function to extent possible.
- Patient will demonstrate effective social interaction skills in one-on-one and group settings.
- Patient and family members will identify and mobilize resources for rehabilitation and discharge planning, as necessary.

Suggested NOC Outcomes

Family Social Climate; Immobility Consequences: Psycho-Cognitive; Self-Esteem; Social Interaction Skills; Social Involvement

Interventions and Rationales

- Follow the medical regimen to treat the underlying condition. *The nurse is responsible for following the medical regimen and working with the physician to plan appropriate care.*
- S Take precautions to ensure a safe and protected environment (provide side rails, help with out-of-bed activities, keep the room free from clutter, and use physical restraints, as necessary) *to reduce the potential for patient injury.*
- Assess neurologic function and mental status every shift *to monitor changes in patient's status;* reorient patient as often as necessary:
  Reorienting patient and involving family members enhances patient's reality-testing ability and overall mental status. Scheduling a daily routine narrows patient's frame of reference, thereby decreasing the potential for increased confusion.
  - Call patient by name and say your name during each interaction.
  - Tell patient the correct day, date, time, and place at least once per shift.
  - PCC Teach family members how to reorient patient, and help them do so.
  - Ask family members to bring patient familiar objects from home, such as clock, radio, and photographs.
  - Post a structured schedule of daily activities in patient's room within visual range.
  - Explain the schedule to family members and other caregivers to provide consistency and continuity.
- If delusions and hallucinations occur, don't focus on them; provide patient with reality-based information and reassure patient of safety *to increase patient's ability to grasp reality and reduce fears associated with these disturbances.*
- Provide specific, non-care-related time with patient each shift *to encourage social interaction.* Begin with one-on-one interaction and increase to group interaction as patient's skills indicate. *Gradually increasing social interaction reduces patient's feeling of being overwhelmed and eliminates sensory input that may renew a cognitive or perceptual disturbance.*
- Give positive reinforcement for appropriate and effective interaction behaviors (verbal and nonverbal) *to help patient recognize progress and enhance feelings of self-worth.*
- Assist patient and family members in progressive participation in care and therapies *to reduce feelings of helplessness and enhance patient's feeling of control and independence.*
- Initiate or participate in multidisciplinary patient-centered conferences to evaluate progress and plan discharge. In addition to patient and family members, conferences may include physical, occupational, and speech therapists; a social worker; the attending physician; and other consultants, as necessary. *These conferences involve patient and family members in a cooperative effort to develop strategies for altering the care plan, as necessary.*

Suggested NIC Interventions

Behavior Modification: Social Skills; Complex Relationship Building; Family Integrity Promotion; Family Therapy; Normalization Promotion; Support System Enhancement

Evaluations for Expected Outcomes

- Patient doesn't exhibit physical evidence of injury.
- Patient and family members express concern about patient's inability to interact normally.
- Patient remains oriented to time, place, and person.
- Patient's verbal responses and behavior don't indicate delusions or hallucinations.
- Patient and family members perform care-related procedures to extent possible.
- Patient uses words, gestures, or writing to communicate needs and whether needs are met.
- Patient maintains appropriate cognitive and perceptual functioning to extent possible.
- Patient communicates effectively in one-on-one and group settings.
- Patient and family members identify and contact available support resources, as needed.

Documentation

- Patient's verbal and nonverbal behaviors
- Neurologic and mental status assessment
- Observations of patient's social interaction skills
- Interventions to facilitate appropriate and effective social interaction
- Patient's responses to nursing interventions
- Evaluations for expected outcomes

REFERENCES

Beattie, L., Kyle, S. D., Espie, C. A., & Biello, S. M. (2015). Social interactions, emotion, and sleep: A systematic review and research agenda. *Sleep Medicine Reviews*, *24*, 83–100. doi:10.1016/j.smrv.2014.12.005

Pelzer, B., Schaffrath, S., & Vernaleken, I. (2014). Coping with unemployment: The impact of unemployment on mental health, personality, and social interaction skills. *Work*, *48*(2), 289–295. doi:10.3233/WOR-131626

Yoon, J. A., Park, S. G., & Roh, H. L. (2015). Comparisons of social interaction and activities of daily living between long-term care facility and community-dwelling stroke patients. *Journal of Physical Therapy Science*, *27*(10), 3127–3131.

IMPAIRED SOCIAL INTERACTION

related to sociocultural dissonance

Definition

Insufficient or excessive quantity or ineffective quality of social exchange

Assessment

- Reason for hospitalization (physiologic or psychiatric)
- Sociocultural background (beliefs, norms, rituals, and values)

- Usual pattern of social interaction, including dominant language, group participation, level of comprehension, nonverbal communication skills (such as drawing and gestures), and speech pattern
- Patient's position in family
- Support systems, including clergy, family members, and friends
- Education and intelligence level

Defining Characteristics

- Discomfort in social situations
- Dissatisfaction with social engagement (e.g., belonging, caring, interest, shared history)
- Dysfunctional interaction with others
- Family reports change in interaction (e.g., style, pattern,)
- Impaired social functioning

Expected Outcomes

- Patient will provide information concerning cultural background.
- Patient will identify needs and will communicate (verbally or through behavior) whether needs are met.
- Patient will express understanding of care-related instruction.
- Patient and family members will participate in planning care.
- Patient will identify effective coping techniques to deal with sociocultural differences.
- Patient will express feelings of comfort and trust in interaction with caregivers.
- Patient will use resources outside normal sociocultural group, as necessary.

Suggested NOC Outcomes

Communication; Social Interaction Skills; Social Involvement; Stress Level

Interventions and Rationales

- Assign a primary nurse to patient if possible. *Primary nursing provides consistency, enhances trust, and decreases the potential for fragmented care.*
- Provide a specific time (e.g., 10 minutes each shift) to talk with patient and family members about sociocultural background. *In many cultural groups, trust develops slowly and may be hampered by lengthy interviews.*
- Take care not to stereotype the patient into what the nurse knows about the patient's cultural background. *Stereotyping is destructive when providing individualized care to a patient. Keep in mind that not all persons in a particular culture fit a pattern.*
- PCC Explain care-related activities clearly and answer questions as accurately as possible *to enhance patient's understanding of care-related procedures and facility routine.*
- Use an interpreter when necessary *to ensure effective communication for non-English-speaking patients. The primary reasons for using an interpreter to communicate with a patient are legal, financial, and to provide quality care.*
- PCC Involve patient and family members in planning care, and continually encourage patient's participation in self-care *to increase sense of control and reduce feelings of helplessness and isolation.*
- Help patient identify and use effective social interaction behaviors, such as increased eye contact, calling people by name, and asking questions. *Teaching patient effective interpersonal communication helps in functioning more effectively in a social environment.*

- Demonstrate respect for patient's privacy, personal belongings, cultural norms, and religious beliefs and practices *to provide sensitive care to patients from varied cultural backgrounds.*
- PCC Offer a referral to other support systems (such as social services, financial counseling, home health care, mental health care, and professional care), if indicated. *This ensures comprehensive approach to patient's care.*

Suggested NIC Interventions

Active Listening; Anxiety Reduction; Coping Enhancement; Family Process Maintenance; Family Support; Mutual Goal Setting; Normalization Promotion

Evaluations for Expected Outcomes

- Patient provides information about his or her culture, including values, attitudes, roles, and beliefs.
- Patient reports needs and gratification of these needs, either verbally or through behavior.
- Patient demonstrates care-related procedures.
- Patient and family members help develop care plan.
- Patient specifies positive ways to cope with cultural differences.
- Patient communicates sense of security and demonstrates decrease in anxiety-related behaviors.
- Patient uses appropriate resources outside patient's normal sociocultural group, as needed.

Documentation

- Patient's and family members' perceptions of current situation
- Interventions to promote effective social interaction
- Patient's verbal and nonverbal responses to nursing interventions
- Evaluations for expected outcomes

REFERENCES

Beattie, L., Kyle, S. D., Espie, C. A., & Biello, S. M. (2015). Social interactions, emotion, and sleep: A systematic review and research agenda. *Sleep Medicine Reviews*, *24*, 83–100. doi:10.1016/j.smrv.2014.12.005

Pelzer, B., Schaffrath, S., & Vernaleken, I. (2014). Coping with unemployment: The impact of unemployment on mental health, personality, and social interaction skills. *Work*, *48*(2), 289–295. doi:10.3233/WOR-131626

Yoon, J. A., Park, S. G., & Roh, H. L. (2015). Comparisons of social interaction and activities of daily living between long-term care facility and community-dwelling stroke patients. *Journal of Physical Therapy Science*, *27*(10), 3127–3131.

SPIRITUAL DISTRESS

related to receiving bad news; unexpected life event

Definition

A state of suffering related to the impaired ability to experience meaning in life through connections with self, others, the world, or a superior being

Assessment

- General spiritual beliefs
- Personal spiritual beliefs
- Spiritual support systems
- Religious affiliation
- Impact of illness on spiritual beliefs

Defining Characteristics

- Anxiety
- Crying
- Fatigue
- Fear
- Insomnia
- Questioning identity
- Questioning meaning of life
- Questioning meaning of suffering

Connections to Self

- Anger
- Decrease in serenity
- Feeling of being unloved
- Guilt
- Inadequate acceptance
- Ineffective coping strategies
- Insufficient courage
- Perceived insufficient meaning in life

Connections with Others

- Alienation
- Refuses to interact with spiritual leader
- Refuses to interact with significant other
- Separation from support system

Connections with Art, Music, Literature, and Nature

- Decrease in expression of previous pattern of creativity
- Disinterest in nature
- Disinterest in reading spiritual literature

Connections with Power Greater than Self

- Anger toward power greater than self
- Feeling abandoned
- Hopelessness
- Inability for introspection
- Inability to experience the transcendent
- Inability to participate in religious activities
- Inability to pray
- Perceived suffering
- Request for a spiritual leader
- Sudden change in spiritual practice

Expected Outcomes

- Patient will express feelings and beliefs about patient's usual and current spiritual beliefs.
- Patient will identify areas of ambivalence and conflict about beliefs.
- Patient will state an understanding of grief process and its stages.
- Patient will use effective coping strategies to ease spiritual discomfort.
- Patient will seek appropriate support persons (family members, priest, minister, imam, or rabbi) for assistance.

Suggested NOC Outcomes

Hope; Personal Autonomy; Quality of Life; Spiritual Health; Suffering Severity; Will to Live

Interventions and Rationales

- Approach patient in an accepting, nonjudgmental manner *to demonstrate unconditional positive regard for patient.*

- Acknowledge patient's spiritual concerns and encourage expression of feelings *to help build a therapeutic relationship.*
- PCC Encourage patient to provide information about personal spiritual or religious beliefs and practices. *Acquiring this initial database is the first step in the nursing process.*
- PCC Instruct patient on stages of grieving and on emotions and behaviors common to each stage *to promote understanding and encourage feelings of normalcy.*
- PCC Encourage interests in art, music, nature, and so on or wherever the patient finds spiritual peace. Offer to help find books, CDs, art supplies, and so on. *Patients differ markedly in what gives them peace and promotes spiritual well-being. For many it is not religion.*
- Provide for the continuation of patient's spiritual or religious practices (allow for specific religious materials or clothing; respect dietary restrictions, if possible). *These measures demonstrate support and convey caring and acceptance to patient.*
- PCC Facilitate visits from clergy and provide privacy during visits *to demonstrate respect for patient's relationship with clergy.*
- Encourage patient to discuss concerns with clergy, *thereby using expert spiritual care resources to help patient.*

Suggested NIC Interventions

Active Listening; Anxiety Reduction; Coping Enhancement; Hope Instillation; Referral; Spiritual Growth Facilitation; Spiritual Support

Evaluations for Expected Outcomes

- Patient discusses feelings about personal spiritual or religious beliefs.
- Patient specifies areas of spiritual conflict, such as anger toward God, questioning of own usual beliefs about an afterlife, and guilt related to loss of faith.
- Patient communicates understanding of grief process and its stages.
- Patient continues religious practices that ease spiritual distress.
- Patient makes use of available resources for spiritual assistance.

Documentation

- Patient's verbal and nonverbal communication of spiritual discomfort
- Stage of anticipatory grief, as indicated by behavior
- Interventions to promote spiritual comfort
- Patient's response to interventions
- Evaluations for expected outcomes
- Observations about patient's spiritual distress or well-being

REFERENCES

Bornet, M. A., Rochat, E., Dürst, A. V., Fustinoni, S., Büla, C., von Gunten, A., & Monod, S. (2016). Instruments to assess depressive symptoms and spiritual distress investigate different dimensions. *Clinical Gerontologist*, *39*(2), 104–116. doi:10.1080/07317115.2015.1120255

Skalla, K. A., & Ferrell, B. (2015). Challenges in assessing spiritual distress in survivors of cancer. *Clinical Journal of Oncology Nursing*, *19*(1), 99–104. doi:10.1188/15.CJON.99-104

Wen-Pei, W., & Hsin-Tien, H. (2014). Applying Swanson's caring theory to manage spiritual distress in a patient with terminal lung cancer. *Journal of Nursing*, *61*(4), 97–102. doi:10.6224/JN.61.4.97

SPIRITUAL DISTRESS

related to sociocultural deprivation

Definition

A state of suffering related to the impaired ability to experience meaning in life through connections with self, others, the world, or a superior being

Assessment

- General spiritual beliefs
- Personal spiritual beliefs
- Spiritual support systems
- Religious affiliation
- Impact of illness on spiritual beliefs

Defining Characteristics

- Anxiety
- Crying
- Fatigue
- Fear
- Insomnia
- Questioning identity
- Questioning meaning of life
- Questioning meaning of suffering

Connections to Self

- Anger
- Decrease in serenity
- Feeling of being unloved
- Guilt
- Inadequate acceptance
- Ineffective coping strategies
- Insufficient courage
- Perceived insufficient meaning in life

Connections with Others

- Alienation
- Refuses to interact with spiritual leader
- Refuses to interact with significant other
- Separation from support system

Connections with Art, Music, Literature, and Nature

- Decrease in expression of previous pattern of creativity
- Disinterest in nature
- Disinterest in reading spiritual literature

Connections with Power Greater than Self

- Anger toward power greater than self
- Feeling abandoned
- Hopelessness
- Inability for introspection
- Inability to experience the transcendent
- Inability to participate in religious activities
- Inability to pray
- Perceived suffering
- Request for a spiritual leader
- Sudden change in spiritual practice

Expected Outcomes

- Patient will communicate conflict about beliefs.
- Patient will identify source of spiritual conflict.
- Patient will specify whatever spiritual assistance patient needs.
- Patient will discuss beliefs about religious practices.
- Patient will identify coping techniques to deal with spiritual discomfort.
- Patient will express feelings of spiritual comfort.

Suggested NOC Outcomes

Hope; Personal Autonomy; Quality of Life; Spiritual Health; Will to Live

Interventions and Rationales

- Listen for cues about patient's feelings. ("Why did God do this to me?" or "God is punishing me.") *Active listening demonstrates involvement with patient and allows you to hear important messages indicating spiritual distress.*
- Approach patient in a nonjudgmental way *to focus on patient's feelings without evaluating them as right or wrong, good or bad.*
- Acknowledge patient's spiritual concerns, and encourage expression of thoughts and feelings *to help build therapeutic relationship.*
- Help patient concretely define the problem causing inner conflict. *This is the first step in developing strategies for resolving conflicts.*
- For the patient whose spiritual comfort is derived from music, art, or nature, attempt to find such items (e.g., CDs, posters, or picture books) that will provide spiritual nourishment. *Not everyone finds spiritual comfort in organized religion. Indeed, each person is entitled to find spiritual hope and consolation in whatever way meets their needs.*
- Arrange for visits by clergy, as appropriate, *thereby using spiritual care resources to help patient.*
- Encourage patient to continue religious practices during hospitalization; do whatever you must to facilitate this. For example:
  These measures demonstrate support and convey caring and acceptance to patient.
  - If patient is accustomed to reading Scripture and doesn't have a Bible, try to obtain one.
  - If a Jewish male wears a yarmulke, allow him to continue wearing it, if possible.
  - In cases in which patient's religious traditions prohibit or require certain foods, make every effort to communicate these needs to the dietary department and see that they're honored.
- Communicate and collaborate with patient's clergy person or with the hospital chaplain, as appropriate. *This ensures consistent care and provides a more complete database.*
- Arrange for patient to have bedside objects that provide spiritual comfort (such as a Bible, prayer shawl, pictures, statues, and rosary beads). *Items of spiritual significance may influence patient's ability to reduce conflict.*
- Provide privacy during patient's visits with a clergy person or chaplain *to demonstrate respect for patient's relationship with clergy.*

Suggested NIC Interventions

Active Listening; Hope Instillation; Referral; Spiritual Growth Facilitation; Spiritual Support

Evaluations for Expected Outcomes

- Patient expresses feelings of uncertainty or ambivalence related to spiritual beliefs.
- Patient states specific causes of spiritual distress.
- Patient requests spiritual assistance, if needed.
- Patient discusses usual religious practices, including rituals, prayers, values, and beliefs.
- Patient reports decreased spiritual discomfort.
- Patient expresses desire to resume usual religious practices.

Documentation

- Patient's expressions of concern about spiritual matters, whether direct or indirect
- Observations about patient's spiritual distress or well-being
- Interventions carried out to promote spiritual comfort
- Observations about patient's responses to interventions
- Evaluations for expected outcomes

REFERENCES

Bornet, M. A., Rochat, E., Dürst, A. V., Fustinoni, S., Büla, C., von Gunten, A., & Monod, S. (2016). Instruments to assess depressive symptoms and spiritual distress investigate different dimensions. *Clinical Gerontologist, 39*(2), 104–116. doi:10.1080/07317115.2015.1120255

Skalla, K. A., & Ferrell, B. (2015). Challenges in assessing spiritual distress in survivors of cancer. *Clinical Journal of Oncology Nursing, 19*(1), 99–104. doi:10.1188/15.CJON.99-104

Wen-Pei, W., & Hsin-Tien, H. (2014). Applying Swanson's caring theory to manage spiritual distress in a patient with terminal lung cancer. *Journal of Nursing, 61*(4), 97–102. doi:10.6224/JN.61.4.97

RISK FOR SPIRITUAL DISTRESS

Definition

Vulnerable to an impaired ability to experience and integrate meaning and purpose in life through connectedness within self, literature, nature, and/or a power greater than oneself, which may compromise health

Assessment

- Health history, including debilitating disease (e.g., rheumatoid arthritis); terminal illness; recurrent cancer; conditions that alter body image (e.g., burns and scars); relapse or exacerbation of neurologic disease (e.g., multiple sclerosis); alcoholism, depression, and drug abuse; and major traumatic injury
- Impact of current illness, injury, or disability on lifestyle
- Spiritual status, religious affiliation, beliefs, and practices; relationship with spiritual authority (e.g., priest, rabbi); beliefs about life, death, and suffering
- Psychological status, including perception of self, body image, problem-solving ability, and coping mechanisms; sources of support (family, partner, friends, caregivers); perception of medical diagnosis or health problem (progression, severity, prognosis, treatment options); reaction to illness, injury, or disability; self-image, mood, behavior, motivation, and energy level; stressors (finances, job, marital or partner discord, losses through death or separation); expressions of grief; and changes in sleep pattern
- Family status, including socioeconomic status; quality of relationships; communication patterns; methods of conflict resolution; ability of family members to meet patient's physical, emotional, and social needs; and family goals

Risk Factors

Developmental

- Life change

Environmental

- Environmental change
- Natural disaster

Physical

- Chronic illness
- Physical illness
- Substance abuse

Psychosocial

- Anxiety
- Barrier to experiencing love
- Change in religious ritual
- Change in spiritual practice
- Cultural conflict
- Depression
- Inability to forgive
- Ineffective relationships
- Loss
- Low self-esteem
- Racial conflict
- Separation from support system
- Stressors

Expected Outcomes

- Patient will discuss current spiritual beliefs and concerns.
- Patient will discuss effects of illness, injury, or disability on personal beliefs and spiritual practices.
- Patient will use healthy coping techniques to maintain spiritual well-being.
- Patient will express feelings of spiritual well-being.
- Patient will be supported in efforts to pursue spirituality in coping with illness, injury, or disability.
- Patient will reach out to family members, partner, priest, minister, imam, rabbi, or others for assistance.

Suggested NOC Outcomes

Coping; Grief Resolution; Hope; Spiritual Health

Interventions and Rationales

- Assess the importance of spirituality in patient's life and in coping with illness. Note patient's participation in religious rituals and practices and personal desire to discuss spiritual beliefs. Assess the impact of the illness, injury, or disability on patient's spiritual outlook. *Accurate assessment of the meaning of spirituality for patient is necessary before intervening.*
- Assess patient's desire for help in coping with spiritual concerns *to determine the extent to which patient is motivated to address spiritual concerns and open to help from others.*
- Express your willingness to discuss spirituality if patient desires *to reduce isolation and to bring spiritual issues into the open.*
- PCC Encourage patient to talk about spiritual or religious beliefs and practices. Listen actively to patient's discussion of spiritual concerns *to foster open discussion.*
- PCC Encourage patient to express feelings related to recent life-threatening experience *to help patient clarify and cope with personal feelings.*
- PCC Communicate acceptance of patient's expression of spiritual concerns, even if patient's feelings are angry and negative *to reassure patient that feelings are valid.*
- Show willingness to pray with patient, if the patient wishes, *to provide spiritual support.*
- Maintain a nonjudgmental manner. Keep conversation focused on patient's spiritual values *to maintain the therapeutic value of your interaction with patient.*
- PCC Provide for continuation of patient's religious practices (e.g., help to obtain ritual items and respect dietary restrictions, if possible) *to demonstrate support and convey caring and acceptance to patient.*

PCC • Arrange for visits by clergy, as appropriate, *to provide patient with expert spiritual support.* Provide privacy during visits.

PCC • Collaborate with patient's clergyman or hospital chaplain to develop a plan to integrate spiritual interventions into patient's care *to ensure continuity of care.*

Suggested NIC Interventions

Active Listening; Anticipatory Guidance; Anxiety Reduction; Caregiver Support; Emotional Support; Hope Instillation; Spiritual Growth Facilitation; Spiritual Support

Evaluations for Expected Outcomes

- Patient discusses current spiritual or religious beliefs.
- Patient discusses effects of illness, injury, or disability on beliefs and spiritual practices.
- Patient uses healthy coping techniques to maintain spiritual well-being.
- Patient expresses feelings of spiritual well-being.
- Patient is supported in efforts to pursue spirituality in coping with illness, injury, or disability.
- Patient reaches out to family members, partner, priest, minister, rabbi, imam, or others for assistance.

Documentation

- Patient's statements regarding religious beliefs and practices
- Patient's statements indicating effect of current crisis on spiritual outlook
- Patient's statements indicating which rituals and practices help maintain spiritual well-being
- Patient's statements indicating effectiveness of interventions to promote spiritual well-being
- Visits with selected spiritual authority
- Additional referrals to clergy or chaplain
- Evaluations for expected outcomes

REFERENCES

Caldeira, S., de Carvalho, E. C., & Vieira, M. (2014). Between spiritual well-being and spiritual distress: possible related factors in elderly patients with cancer. *Revista Latino-Americana De Enfermagem (RLAE)*, *22*(1), 28–34. doi:10.1590/0104-1169.3073.2382

Daly, L., & Fahey-McCarthy, E. (2014). Attending to the spiritual in dementia care nursing. *British Journal of Nursing*, *23*(14), 787–791. doi:10.12968/bjon.2014.23.14.787

Elham, H., Hazrati, M., Momennasab, M., & Sareh, K. (2015). The effect of need-based spiritual/religious intervention on spiritual well-being and anxiety of elderly people. *Holistic Nursing Practice*, *29*(3), 136–143. doi:10.1097/HNP.0000000000000083

IMPAIRED SPONTANEOUS VENTILATION

related to respiratory muscle fatigue

Definition

Decreased energy reserves resulting in an inability to maintain independent breathing that is adequate to support life

Assessment

- Health history, including previous respiratory problems
- Respiratory status, including rate, rhythm, and depth of respirations; chest excursion and symmetry; presence of cyanosis; and use of accessory muscles
- Effectiveness of cough in clearing secretions
- Suctioning demands, including frequency and tolerance
- Sputum characteristics, including appearance, consistency, color, and odor
- Neuromuscular strength and endurance
- Mental and emotional status, including cognitive state and ability to follow directions
- Laboratory values, including arterial blood gas (ABG) levels (baseline and ongoing), complete blood count, serum electrolyte levels, coagulation studies, serum and sputum cultures, and sensitivity tests
- Vital signs
- Functional status, including ability to perform activities of daily living (ADLs)
- Related or concurrent events that may contribute to respiratory distress, such as bleeding, hypervolemia, hypovolemia, and sepsis

Defining Characteristics

- Alteration in metabolism
- Apprehensiveness
- Decrease in arterial oxygen saturation ($Sa{O_2}$)
- Decrease in cooperation
- Decrease in partial pressure of oxygen ($P{O_2}$)
- Decrease in tidal volume
- Dyspnea
- Increase in accessory muscle use
- Increase in heart rate
- Increase in partial pressure of carbon dioxide ($PC{O_2}$)
- Restlessness

Expected Outcomes

- Patient's respiratory rate will remain within 5 breaths/minute of baseline.
- Patient's ABG levels will be normal.
- Patient will indicate feeling comfortable and won't report pain, dyspnea, or fatigue.
- Patient will carry out ADLs with minimal supplemental oxygen.
- Patient's breathing pattern will return to baseline.
- Patient's $Pa{O_2}$ will remain within normal limits as activity level increases.
- Patient will breathe spontaneously after ventilator support is withdrawn.

Suggested NOC Outcomes

Anxiety Level; Endurance; Energy Conservation; Respiratory Status: Gas Exchange; Respiratory Status: Ventilation; Vital Signs

Interventions and Rationales

- S Monitor patient's vital signs every 15 minutes to 1 hour *to detect tachypnea and tachycardia, early indicators of respiratory distress.*
- S Monitor patient for nasal flaring, change in depth and pattern of breathing, use of accessory muscles, and cyanosis *to detect signs of severe respiratory distress.*
- Monitor ABG levels and report deviations promptly *to determine the need for changes to the therapeutic regimen.*

- Monitor hemoglobin (Hb) level and hematocrit (HCT). *Low Hb level and HCT indicate decreased oxygen-carrying capacity of the blood.*
- Begin oxygen support using the smallest concentration needed to make patient comfortable. Monitor closely *to avoid oxygen toxicity.*
- Elevate the head of the bed *to increase comfort and to promote adequate chest expansion and diaphragmatic excursion, thereby decreasing work of breathing.*
- Help patient progress gradually from bed rest to increased activity *to improve patient's sense of well-being.* Monitor vital signs and ABG levels closely. If respiratory status is compromised, return patient to bed rest *to decrease basal metabolic rate and lower oxygen demands.*
- PCC Explain procedures to patient. Describe specific sensations patient may experience during each procedure *to decrease anxiety.*
- S Anticipate possible complications. Keep in mind that if patient decompensates while on 100% fraction of inspired oxygen non-rebreather mask, endotracheal intubation may be required. *Anticipating complications facilitates prompt intervention.*
- If patient requires intubation, monitor for spontaneous breathing, and gradually wean the patient from the ventilator. *Progressive weaning helps patient to adjust physiologically and emotionally to increased work of breathing.*
- Avoid respiratory depressants, such as opioids, sedatives, and paralytics, *to facilitate patient's recovery.*
- PCC Provide explanations to the family. Spend time with them at the bedside, demonstrating ways in which to approach and support the patient without causing undue anxiety. *Watching someone who is having difficulty breathing makes others anxious, compounding the reaction of the patient to shortness of breath.*

Suggested NIC Interventions

Acid–Base Management; Airway Suctioning; Artificial Airway Management; Aspiration Precautions; Coping Enhancement; Mechanical Ventilation; Oxygen Therapy; Positioning; Respiratory Monitoring; Self-Care Assistance

Evaluations for Expected Outcomes

- Patient's respiratory rate is within 5 breaths/minute of baseline.
- Patient's ABG levels are normal.
- Patient indicates feeling comfortable and doesn't report pain, dyspnea, or fatigue.
- Patient carries out ADLs with minimal supplemental oxygen.
- Patient's breathing pattern returns to baseline.
- Patient's Pao_2 remains within normal limits when activity level increases.
- Patient breathes spontaneously after ventilator support is withdrawn.

Documentation

- Patient's reports of malaise, dyspnea, restlessness, chest pain, dizziness, or light-headedness
- Patient's response to nursing interventions
- Patient's response to initiation of oxygen therapy and progressive changes in therapy
- Laboratory data, including ABG levels
- Respiratory status (baseline and ongoing)
- Subtle personality changes
- Changes in breath sounds revealed by auscultation
- Evaluations for expected outcomes

REFERENCES

Buonocore, D., Wiegand, D. L., & Campbell, M. L. (2015). Caring for dying patients in the intensive care unit. *AACN Advanced Critical Care*, *26*(2), 110–122. doi:10.1097/NCI.0000000000000077

Fournier, M. (2014). Caring for patients in respiratory failure. *American Nurse Today*, *9*(11), 18–23.

Tanios, M., Epstein, S., Grzeskowiak, M., Nguyen, H. M., Hyunsoon, P., & Leo, J. (2014). Influence of sedation strategies on unplanned extubation in a mixed intensive care unit. *American Journal of Critical Care*, *23*(4), 306–315. doi:10.4037/ajcc20144446

IMPAIRED STANDING

related to injury to lower extremity; neurologic disorder

Definition

Limitation of ability to independently and purposefully attain and/or maintain the body in an upright position from feet to head

Assessment

- History of neuromuscular disorder or dysfunction
- Neurologic status, including level of consciousness, motor ability, and sensory ability
- Musculoskeletal status, including coordination, balance, muscle size and strength, muscle tone, range of motion, and functional mobility scale:
  0 = completely independent
  1 = requires use of equipment or device
  2 = requires help, supervision, or teaching from another person
  3 = requires help from another person and equipment or device
  4 = dependent; doesn't participate in activity

Defining Characteristics

- Impaired ability to adjust position of one or both lower limbs on uneven surface
- Impaired ability to attain a balanced position of the torso
- Impaired ability to extend one or both hips
- Impaired ability to extend one or both knees
- Impaired ability to flex one or both hips
- Impaired ability to flex one or both knees
- Impaired ability to maintain the torso in balanced position
- Impaired ability to stress torso with body weight
- Insufficient muscle strength

Expected Outcomes

- Patient will achieve highest level of independence possible when standing.
- Patient will show no evidence of complications.
- Patient will achieve balance while standing.
- Patient will maintain muscle strength.

Suggested NOC Outcomes

Activity Tolerance; Endurance; Joint Movement: Hip; Joint Movement: Spine; Neurological Status: Central Motor Control; Neurological Status: Spinal Sensory/Motor Function; Physical Fitness; Skeletal Function

Interventions and Rationales

- S Use a transfer belt, if necessary, *to support patient and prevent staff injury.*
- S Use assistive devices as necessary, *to support patient and prevent staff injury.*
- Identify the level of functioning using a functional mobility scale (see Assessment). Communicate patient's skill level to all staff members *to provide continuity and preserve identified level of independence.*
- Encourage independence by helping patient to use assistive devices. *This increases muscle tone and patient's self-esteem.*
- Monitor and record daily any evidence of immobility complications (such as contractures, venous stasis, thrombus, pneumonia, and urinary tract infection). *Patients with a history of neuromuscular disorders or dysfunction may be more prone to developing complications.*
- S Instruct patient to call before attempting to stand without assistance. *Ensure patient safety from falls.*
- Carry out a medical regimen to manage or prevent complications; for example, administer prophylactic heparin as ordered for venous thrombosis. *This promotes patient's health and well-being.*
- PCC Refer patient to a physical therapist *to help rehabilitate musculoskeletal deficits.*
- Demonstrate the standing procedure and note date. Have patient and family members return standing procedure demonstration and note date. *This ensures continuity of care and use of proper technique.*

Suggested NIC Interventions

Body Mechanics Promotion; Exercise Therapy: Balance; Exercise Therapy: Muscle Control; Positioning; Self-Care Assistance

Evaluations for Expected Outcomes

- Patient achievement of highest level of independence possible when standing.
- Patient has no evidence of complications.
- Patient achievement of balance while standing.
- Patient maintains muscle strength.

Documentation

- Patient's current status of functional abilities and goals set for self
- Observations of patient's mobility status, presence of complications, and response to standing
- Instruction and demonstration of skills in standing
- Patient's response to nursing interventions
- Evaluations for expected outcomes

REFERENCES

Engelhart, D., Pasma, J. H., Schouten, A. C., Meskers, C. G., Maier, A. B., Mergner, T., & van der Kooij, H. (2014). Impaired standing balance in elderly: A new engineering method helps to unravel causes and effects. *Journal of the American Medical Directors Association*, *15*(3), 227. doi:10.1016/j.jamda.2013.09.009

Pan, T., Liao, K., Roenigk, K., Daly, J. J., & Walker, M. F. (2015). Static and dynamic postural stability in veterans with combat-related mild traumatic brain injury. *Gait & Posture*, *42*(4), 550–557. doi:10.1016/j.gaitpost.2015.08.012

Travers, B., Powell, P., Klinger, L., & Klinger, M. (2013). Motor difficulties in autism spectrum disorder: Linking symptom severity and postural stability. *Journal of Autism & Developmental Disorders*, *43*(7), 1568–1583. doi:10.1007/s10803-012-1702-x

STRESS OVERLOAD

Definition

Excessive amounts and types of demands that require action

Assessment

- History or current presence of stress reactions in response to internal or external forces expressed by such physical findings as choking sensation, hyperventilation, dizziness, increased heart rate and/or blood pressure, perspiration, pupillary dilation, polyuria, and elevated blood glucose, cholesterol, and free fatty acid levels
- History or current presence of stress reactions expressed by such behavioral cues as insomnia, restlessness, "scattered" thoughts, disorganized speech, restlessness, irritability, and altered concentration
- Physical stressors, including extreme heat or cold, malnutrition, disease, infection, and pain
- Psychological stressors, including fear, sense of failure, change in company or home location, success, holiday, vacation, or promotion
- Level of stress, positive coping mechanisms, realistic thought patterns, behaviors, or energy level
- Medication history, including use of drugs, caffeine, tobacco, or alcohol that stimulates the sympathetic nervous system
- Sleep patterns or changes in daily activities that could be perceived as stressful, including too many or too few activities
- Sociologic factors, including job satisfaction, presence of support systems, family coping mechanisms, or hobbies

Defining Characteristics

- Excessive stress
- Feeling of pressure
- Impaired decision making
- Impaired functioning
- Increase in anger
- Increase in anger behavior
- Increase in impatience
- Negative impact from stress (e.g., physical symptoms, psychological distress, feeling sick)
- Tension

Expected Outcomes

- Patient will experience reduced signs of stress overload as evidenced by subjective report and observations of reduced stress, such as less facial tension and less restlessness.
- Patient will connect environmental stressors with manifestations of stress such as insomnia, tearful outbursts, irritability, or headache.
- Patients will set limits on activities assumed by saying "No" without expressions of guilt.
- Patient will develop more effective coping strategies to manage stress, such as guided imagery, exercise, healthy diet, and recreation and leisure activities.
- Patient will develop strategies to reframe distorted thinking patterns relating to internal and environmental demands, such as talking about feelings and asking for help.

Suggested NOC Outcomes

Abusive Behavior; Aggression Self-Control; Anxiety Self-Control; Coping; Self-Restraint; Stress Level

Interventions and Rationales

- Establish and promote a trusting relationship before asking patient to make any changes. *A trusting relationship can facilitate patient's attempts to make changes, whereas too many demands early in relationship can foster resistance.*
- PCC Teach prioritization of responsibilities and deadlines to facilitate patient's sense of control over stressors. *Stressors may seem overwhelming, and nurse can promote increased self-esteem when a plan is made cooperatively with nurse and patient as partners.*
- PCC Teach patient about positive self-talk. *Positive self-talk helps change and, ultimately, reverse negative emotions of guilt, fear, and worry.*
- PCC Teach coping strategies, such as reframing thoughts or using music, guided imagery, yoga, deep breathing exercises, progressive neuromuscular relaxation, or pet therapy. *Strategies that reduce tense muscles and feelings can promote deeper relaxation and reduce heart rate, respirations, and blood pressure by promoting the parasympathetic response.*
- PCC Teach assertiveness training techniques with role-play exercises. *Assertiveness training can provide a concrete way to manage stressors and enhance feeling of being empowered, such as in communicating with demanding individuals.*
- PCC Explore support systems with patient, support groups, or hobbies and outings with partner or family and friends. *Often patient is a caretaker who perceives there is little time for self and is at risk for caregiver burden. Promoting verbalization of feelings with support persons can reduce feeling of stress overload.*
- Explore role of lack of exercise and excessive intake of caffeine, alcohol, nicotine, and carbohydrates during periods of stress overload and adoption of healthier alternatives. *Inappropriate food choices, inactivity, and substance abuse can occur when patient feels stress overload.*
- Provide opportunities for patient to ventilate feelings about stressors. *Promoting a time to talk can help the patient share feelings of mounting stress before irritability and tension worsen.*

Suggested NIC Interventions

Anger Control Assistance; Assertiveness Training; Behavior Management; Behavior Modification; Calming Techniques; Cognitive Restructuring; Coping Enhancement; Impulse Control Training; Stress Management Assistance

Evaluations for Expected Outcomes

- Patient experiences reduced signs of stress overload as evidenced by subjective report and observations of reduced stress, such as less facial tension and less restlessness.
- Patient connects environmental stressors with manifestations of stress, such as insomnia, tearful outbursts, irritability, or headache.
- Patient sets limits on activities assumed by saying "No" without expressions of guilt.
- Patient addresses usual coping mechanisms for dealing with stress overload, such as increased use of alcohol, caffeine, tobacco, or carbohydrates, and adopts more effective coping strategies, such as guided imagery, exercise, healthy diet, and recreation and leisure activities.
- Patient develops strategies to reframe distorted thinking patterns relating to internal and environmental demands, such as talking about feelings and asking for help.

Documentation

- Observations of subjective and objective data
- Documentation of interventions such as yoga, guided imagery, deep breathing exercises, talking about feelings
- Patient's response to interventions
- Evaluations for expected outcomes

REFERENCES

Amirkhan, J. H., Urizar, G. G., & Clark, S. (2015). Criterion validation of a stress measure: The stress overload scale. *Psychological Assessment*, *27*(3), 985–996. doi:10.1037/pas0000081

Beattie, L., & Griffin, B. (2014). Day-level fluctuations in stress and engagement in response to workplace incivility: A diary study. *Work & Stress*, *28*(2), 124–142. doi:10.1080/02678373.2014.898712

Jess, A. (2015). Stress, coping strategies, and depression—Uninsured primary care patients. *American Journal of Health Behavior*, *39*(6), 742–750. doi:10.5993/AJHB.39.6.1

RISK FOR SUFFOCATION

related to external factors

Definition

Vulnerable to inadequate air availability for inhalation, which may compromise health

Assessment

- Health history, including accidents, allergies, exposure to pollutants, falls, hyperthermia, hypothermia, poisoning, seizures, sensory or perceptual changes (auditory, gustatory, kinesthetic, olfactory, tactile, or visual), and trauma
- Circumstances of current situation that might lead to injury
- Neurologic status, including level of consciousness, mental status, and orientation
- Laboratory studies, including clotting factors, hemoglobin level, hematocrit, platelet count, and white blood cell count

Risk Factors

- Access to empty refrigerator/freezer
- Eating large mouthfuls of food
- Gas leak
- Low-strung clothesline

- Pacifier around infant's neck
- Playing with plastic bag
- Propped bottle in infant's crib
- Small object in airway
- Smoking in bed
- Soft underlayment (e.g., loose items placed near infant)
- Unattended in water

Expected Outcomes

- Patient's airway will remain patent at all times.
- Patient's vital signs will remain within normal parameters.
- Patient and family members will demonstrate knowledge of safety measures to prevent suffocation.

Suggested NOC Outcomes

Aspiration Prevention; Personal Safety Behavior; Respiratory Status: Ventilation; Risk Control; Risk Detection

Interventions and Rationales

- S — Monitor and record patient's respiratory status. *Changes in parameters (such as respiratory rate, cough, sputum production, and skin color) may indicate airway obstruction.*
- S — Monitor and record patient's neurologic status. *Headache, depression, apathy, memory loss, poor muscle coordination, fatigue, stupor, and loss of consciousness may indicate hypoxia.*
- S — Monitor patient's vital signs and report changes. *Tachycardia and a slight rise in blood pressure may indicate hypoxia. Reduced heart rate and loss of consciousness indicate advanced hypoxia.*
- Position patient on the side, or adjust position of head and neck to prevent relaxed neck muscles from obstructing airway *to allow maximal chest expansion and prevent aspiration and airway obstruction.*
- Check all ventilator connections every 30 minutes if patient is on mechanical ventilation *to ensure patient receives proper amount of oxygen at appropriate volume and rate.*
- Check ventilator alarms every 30 minutes and after suctioning *to ensure proper alarm function.*
- Suction airway, as needed, *to prevent secretion accumulation. Do this only as needed to prevent tracheal irritation.*
- PCC — Provide patient and family members with information about safety practices *to enable them to take an active role in patient's care and ensure performance of safety measures.*

Suggested NIC Interventions

Airway Management; Aspiration Precautions; Energy Management; Respiratory Monitoring; Security Enhancement; Surveillance; Vital Signs Monitoring

Evaluations for Expected Outcomes

- Patient's airway remains free from obstruction.
- Patient's vital signs remain within normal parameters.
- Patient and family members demonstrate safety measures to prevent suffocation.

Documentation

- Patient's statements that indicate potential for injury
- Physical findings
- Observations or knowledge of unsafe practices
- Interventions performed to prevent injury
- Patient's response to nursing interventions
- Evaluations for expected outcomes

REFERENCES

Furuya, J., Hara, A., Nomura, T., & Kondo, H. (2014). Volitional chewing with a conscious effort alters and facilitates swallowing during feeding sequence. *Journal of Oral Rehabilitation*, *41*(3), 191–198. doi:10.1111/joor.12140

Lindroos, E., Saarela, R., Soini, H., Muurinen, S., Suominen, M., & Pitkala, K. (2014). Caregiver-reported swallowing difficulties, malnutrition, and mortality among older people in assisted living facilities. *Journal of Nutrition, Health & Aging*, *18*(7), 718–722. doi:10.1007/s12603-014-0506-4

RISK FOR SUFFOCATION

related to internal factors

Definition

Vulnerable to inadequate air availability for inhalation, which may compromise health

Assessment

- Health history, including accidents, allergies, exposure to pollutants, falls, hyperthermia, hypothermia, poisoning, seizures, sensory or perceptual changes (auditory, gustatory, kinesthetic, olfactory, tactile, or visual), and trauma
- Circumstances of current situation that might lead to injury
- Neurologic status, including level of consciousness, mental status, and orientation
- Laboratory studies, including clotting factors, hemoglobin level, hematocrit, platelet count, and white blood cell count

Risk Factors

- Alteration in cognitive functioning
- Alteration in olfactory function
- Emotional disturbance
- Face/neck disease
- Face/neck injury
- Impaired motor functioning
- Insufficient knowledge of safety precautions

Expected Outcomes

- Patient will avoid accidental suffocation.
- Patient's vital signs will remain within normal parameters.
- Patient and family members will demonstrate knowledge of safety measures to prevent suffocation.

Suggested NOC Outcomes

Aspiration Prevention; Neurologic Status: Consciousness; Personal Safety Behavior; Respiratory Status: Ventilation; Risk Control; Risk Detection

Interventions and Rationales

S
- Observe, record, and report falls, seizures, and unsafe practices *to ensure implementation of appropriate interventions.*

S
- Monitor and record patient's respiratory status. *Changes in parameters (such as respiratory rate, cough, sputum production, and skin color) may indicate airway obstruction.*

S
- Monitor and record patient's neurologic status. *Headache, depression, apathy, memory loss, poor muscle coordination, fatigue, stupor, and loss of consciousness may indicate hypoxia.*

S
- Monitor patient's vital signs and report changes. *Tachycardia and a slight rise in blood pressure may indicate hypoxia. Reduced heart rate and loss of consciousness indicate advanced hypoxia.*
- Position patient on the side, or adjust position of head and neck to prevent relaxed neck muscles from obstructing airway *to allow maximal chest expansion and prevent aspiration and airway obstruction.*
- Obtain suction equipment, assemble, and keep at bedside *to assure equipment readiness in case of need.*
- Suction, as needed, *to keep upper and lower airways clear and to stimulate cough reflex to enhance sputum removal.* Do this only as needed *to prevent tracheal irritation.*

PCC
- Provide patient and family members with information about safety practices *to enable patient and family members to take an active role in patient's care and ensure performance of safety measures.*

Suggested NIC Interventions

Airway Management; Aspiration Precautions; Surveillance: Safety; Vital Signs Monitoring

Evaluations for Expected Outcomes

- Patient doesn't experience accidental suffocation.
- Patient's vital signs remain within normal parameters.
- Patient or caregiver demonstrates safety measures that prevent suffocation.

Documentation

- Patient's statements about situation that indicate potential for injury
- Physical findings
- Record of falls, seizures, and unsafe practices
- Interventions that reduce risk of injury
- Patient's response to nursing interventions
- Evaluations for expected outcomes

REFERENCES

Chen, P. C., & Chuang, C. H. (2015). Accuracy of the water swallow test for dysphagia with stroke: A meta-analysis. *Journal of Nursing & Healthcare Research, 11*(2), 161–169. doi:10.6225/JNHR.11.2.161

Furuya, J., Hara, A., Nomura, T., & Kondo, H. (2014). Volitional chewing with a conscious effort alters and facilitates swallowing during feeding sequence. *Journal of Oral Rehabilitation, 41*(3), 191–198. doi:10.1111/joor.12140

Lindroos, E., Saarela, R., Soini, H., Muurinen, S., Suominen, M., & Pitkala, K. (2014). Caregiver-reported swallowing difficulties, malnutrition, and mortality among older people in assisted living facilities. *Journal of Nutrition, Health & Aging, 18*(7), 718–722. doi:10.1007/s12603-014-0506-4

DELAYED SURGICAL RECOVERY

Definition

Extension of the number of postoperative days required to initiate and perform activities that maintain life, health, and well-being

Assessment

- Age
- Gender
- Reason for surgery
- Type and length of surgical procedure
- Current health status, including weight, vital signs, temperature, nutritional status, integumentary status, neurologic status, cardiovascular status, musculoskeletal status, and pain status
- Laboratory studies, including complete blood count, electrolyte studies, urinalysis, blood cultures, blood coagulation studies, immunologic and serologic tests, liver function tests, cardiac enzyme studies, and arterial blood gas levels
- Health history, including past surgical procedures, food or drug allergies, substance abuse, mental illness, and chronic metabolic or systemic disease (diabetes mellitus; cardiovascular, hepatic, renal, or immunologic disease; coagulation disorders; and splenic or bone marrow disorders)
- Mobility status
- Complications during surgical procedure, such as hemorrhage, drop in blood pressure, and cardiac arrhythmias
- Current medical treatments, including radiation therapy, chemotherapy, antibiotic or antifungal therapy, steroid treatment, anticoagulant or thrombolytic therapy, and immunosuppressive therapy
- Social support, including family status and presence of caregiver and health care provider

Defining Characteristics

- Discomfort
- Evidence of interrupted healing of surgical area
- Excessive time required for recuperation
- Impaired mobility
- Inability to resume employment
- Loss of appetite
- Postpones resumption of work
- Requires assistance for self-care

Expected Outcomes

- Patient's vital signs and laboratory values will return to normal limits.
- Patient's wound will begin to heal; incision site will appear free from signs and symptoms of infection.
- Patient will exhibit improved nutritional status.
- Patient's postoperative complications will be resolved.
- Patient will resume normal mobility status.
- Patient will seek and obtain emotional support from family and friends.
- Patient will resume normal eating, bowel, and bladder habits.

- Patient and family members will use community resources that are available to assist after discharge.

Suggested NOC Outcomes

Ambulation; Endurance; Health Beliefs; Immobility Consequences: Physiologic; Nutritional Status; Pain Level; Wound Healing: Primary Intention

Interventions and Rationales

- Assess for factors that may be related to a delay in recovery, such as respiratory complications and infection. Document and report assessment findings *to facilitate the development of an individualized care plan.*
- Monitor wound healing. Assess the surgical site for signs of infection, such as erythema, edema, pain, drainage, odor, incision approximation, and intact sutures. *Infection may delay surgical recovery.*
- Monitor nutritional status by evaluating intake, output, and integumentary status. Consult a dietitian regarding changes to diet *to promote optimal nutritional status. Optimal nutritional status promotes wound healing and provides energy for recovery.*
- Assess all body systems *to detect signs and symptoms of postoperative complications that can delay surgical recovery.*
- Follow the prescribed pulmonary regimen *to facilitate resolution of respiratory complications, if present. Respiratory complications can lead to decreased oxygen levels, which can slow wound healing and delay mobility.*
- Following postoperative bleeding, monitor hemoglobin level and hematocrit. *Bleeding can lead to a low hemoglobin level and hematocrit, reducing the ability of red blood cells to carry oxygen, which can hinder wound healing and diminish patient's energy level.*
- If patient is suffering from psychosis, continue to reorient him during the postoperative recovery period. Report any psychological reaction, such as development of depression-like symptoms. *Psychosis or depression may delay recovery.*
- Administer pain medication, as prescribed. *A patient in pain may not move, cough, and deep-breathe as needed for timely recovery from surgery.*
- S As appropriate, make sure someone is available to walk with patient or that such devices as walkers or canes are available. Don't allow patient to ambulate alone until steady. *Assistance (from staff or with devices) enhances safety and encourages patient to improve mobility without fear of falling. Mobility will facilitate improved strength, help prevent such complications as deep vein thrombosis and, ultimately, enhance recovery.*
- Make sure patient wears support stockings or a sequential compression device as prescribed *to facilitate venous return and prevent deep vein thrombosis.*
- Monitor bowel and bladder activity. Report urine retention and absent or decreased bowel sounds. *Abnormal bowel and bladder patterns slow surgical recovery. Continual assessment ensures prompt treatment and enhances recovery.*
- Initiate a multidisciplinary care conference for patient with care providers from all disciplines as well as the patient and family. Facilitating this type of communication will help *to develop a plan that will put the patient on a faster track to recovery.*
- Make sure patient and family members have access to community resources to assist with recovery when patient returns home *to ensure ongoing recovery.*
- PCC Educate patient and family members regarding appropriate care after discharge *to help them carry out medication and treatment regimens.*

Suggested NIC Interventions

Bed Rest Care; Case Management; Discharge Planning; Energy Management; Exercise Therapy: Ambulation; Incision Site Care; Multidisciplinary Care Conference; Nutrition Management; Pain Management; Sleep Enhancement

Evaluations for Expected Outcomes

- Patient's vital signs and laboratory values return to normal limits.
- Patient's wound begins to heal; incision site appears free from signs and symptoms of infection.
- Patient exhibits improved nutritional status.
- Patient's postoperative complications are resolved.
- Patient resumes normal mobility status.
- Patient seeks and obtains emotional support from family and friends.
- Patient resumes normal eating, bowel, and bladder habits.
- Patient and family members use community resources that are available to assist after discharge.

Documentation

- Assessment findings
- Type and length of operation
- Type of anesthesia
- Intraoperative complications
- Postoperative complications (as they occur)
- Results of ongoing multisystem assessment
- Treatment regimen (for normal recovery and complications)
- Patient's and family members' progress in following treatment regimen
- Teaching provided to patient and family members
- Discharge plans
- Evaluations for expected outcomes

REFERENCE

Appoloni, A. H., Herdman, T. H., Napoleão, A. A., Campos de Carvalho, E., & Hortense, P. (2013). Concept analysis and validation of the nursing diagnosis, delayed surgical recovery. *International Journal of Nursing Knowledge*, *24*(3), 115–121. doi:10.1111/j.2047-3095.2013.01241.x

de Luis, D. A., Culebras, J. M., Aller, R., & Eiros-Bouza, J. M. (2014). Surgical infection and malnutrition. *Nutricion Hospitalaria*, *30*(3), 509–513. doi:10.3305/nh.2014.30.3.7702

Romanzini, A. E., Carvalho, E. C. D., & Galvão, C. M. (2015). Delayed surgical recovery: A concept analysis. *Revista Brasileira de Enfermagem*, *68*(5), 668–675. doi:10.1590/0034-7167.2015680526i

Santana, R. F., do Amaral, D. M., Pereira, S. K., Delphino, T. M., & Cassiano, K. M. (2014). The occurrence of the delayed surgical recovery nursing diagnosis among adults and the elderly. *Acta Paulista De Enfermagem*, *27*(1), 35–39. doi:10.1590/1982-0194201400008

RISK FOR DELAYED SURGICAL RECOVERY

Definition

Vulnerable to an extension of the number of postoperative days required to initiate and perform activities that maintain life, health, and well-being, which may compromise health

Assessment

- Age
- Gender
- Reason for surgery
- Type and length of surgical procedure
- Current health status, including weight, vital signs, temperature, nutritional status, integumentary status, neurologic status, cardiovascular status, musculoskeletal status, and pain status
- Laboratory studies, including complete blood count, electrolyte studies, urinalysis, blood cultures, blood coagulation studies, immunologic and serologic tests, liver function tests, cardiac enzyme studies, and arterial blood gas levels
- Health history, including past surgical procedures, food or drug allergies, substance abuse, mental illness, and chronic metabolic or systemic disease (diabetes mellitus; cardiovascular, hepatic, renal, or immunologic disease; coagulation disorders; and splenic or bone marrow disorders)
- Mobility status
- Complications during surgical procedure, such as hemorrhage, drop in blood pressure, and cardiac arrhythmias
- Current medical treatments, including radiation therapy, chemotherapy, antibiotic or antifungal therapy, steroid treatment, anticoagulant or thrombolytic therapy, and immunosuppressive therapy
- Social support, including family status and presence of caregiver and health care provider

Risk Factors

- American Society of Anesthesiologists Physical Status classification score ≥3
- Diabetes mellitus
- Edema at surgical site
- Extensive surgical procedure
- Extremes of age
- History of delayed wound healing
- Impaired mobility
- Malnutrition
- Obesity
- Pain
- Perioperative surgical site infection
- Persistent nausea
- Persistent vomiting
- Pharmaceutical agent
- Postoperative emotional response
- Prolonged surgical procedure
- Psychological disorder in postoperative period
- Surgical site contamination
- Trauma at surgical site

Expected Outcomes

- Patient's vital signs and laboratory values will be within normal limits.
- Patient's incision site will be free from signs and symptoms of infection.
- Patient will exhibit optimal nutritional status.
- Patient will not experience postoperative complications.
- Patient will resume normal mobility status.
- Patient will seek and obtain emotional support from family and friends.
- Patient will resume normal eating, bowel, and bladder habits.
- Patient and family members will use community resources that are available to assist after discharge.

Suggested NOC Outcomes

Ambulation; Mobility; Self-Care: Activities of Daily Living (ADLs); Knowledge: Treatment Regimen

Interventions and Rationales

- Assess for factors that may be related to a delay in recovery, such as respiratory complications and infection. Document and report assessment findings *to facilitate the development of an individualized care plan.*
- Assess preoperative nutritional status by evaluating intake, output, and integumentary status. *Optimal nutritional status promotes wound healing and provides energy for recovery.*
- Assess all body systems *to detect signs and symptoms of postoperative complications that can delay surgical recovery.*
- PCC Preprocedure, teach patient use of incentive spirometer and encourage use. *Respiratory complications can lead to decreased oxygen levels, which can slow wound healing and delay mobility.*
- Monitor hemoglobin level and hematocrit. *Bleeding can lead to a low hemoglobin level and hematocrit, reducing the ability of red blood cells to carry oxygen, which can hinder wound healing and diminish patient's energy level.*
- PCC Assess pain level. Administer as prescribed. *A patient in pain may not move, cough, and deep-breathe as needed for timely recovery from surgery.*
- Make sure patient wears support stockings or a sequential compression device as prescribed *to facilitate venous return and prevent deep vein thrombosis.*
- PCC Initiate a multidisciplinary care conference for patient with care providers from all disciplines as well as the patient and family. Facilitating this type of communication will help *to develop a plan that will put the patient on a faster track to recovery.*
- PCC Make sure patient and family members have access to community resources to assist with recovery when patient returns home *to ensure ongoing recovery.*
- PCC Educate patient and family members regarding appropriate care after discharge *to help them carry out medication and treatment regimens.*

Suggested NIC Interventions

Embolus Precautions; Exercise Therapy: Ambulation; Medication Management; Pain Management; Self-Care Assistance; vital Signs Monitoring

Evaluations for Expected Outcomes

- Patient's vital signs and laboratory values return to normal limits.
- Patient's wound begins to heal; incision site appears free from signs and symptoms of infection.
- Patient exhibits improved nutritional status.
- Patient resumes normal mobility status.
- Patient seeks and obtains emotional support from family and friends.
- Patient resumes normal eating, bowel, and bladder habits.
- Patient and family members use community resources that are available to assist after discharge.

Documentation

- Assessment findings
- Type and length of operation
- Type of anesthesia
- Intraoperative complications
- Postoperative complications (as they occur)
- Results of ongoing multisystem assessment
- Treatment regimen (for normal recovery and complications)
- Teaching provided to patient and family members
- Evaluations for expected outcomes

REFERENCES

de Luis, D. A., Culebras, J. M., Aller, R., & Eiros-Bouza, J. M. (2014). Surgical infection and malnutrition. *Nutricion Hospitalaria*, *30*(3), 509–513. doi:10.3305/nh.2014.30.3.7702

Romanzini, A. E., Carvalho, E. C. D., & Galvão, C. M. (2015). Delayed surgical recovery: A concept analysis. *Revista Brasileira de Enfermagem*, *68*(5), 668–675. doi:10.1590/0034-7167.2015680526i

Santana, R. F., do Amaral, D. M., Pereira, S. K., Delphino, T. M., & Cassiano, K. M. (2014). The occurrence of the delayed surgical recovery nursing diagnosis among adults and the elderly. *Acta Paulista de Enfermagem*, *27*(1), 35–39. doi:10.1590/1982-0194201400008

Spruce, L. (2014). Back to basics: Implementing the surgical checklist. *AORN Journal*, *100*(5), 466–476. doi:10.1016/j.aorn.2014.06.020

IMPAIRED SWALLOWING

related to neuromuscular impairment

Definition

Abnormal functioning of the swallowing mechanism associated with deficits in oral, pharyngeal, or esophageal structure or function

Assessment

- History of neuromuscular, cerebral, or respiratory disease
- Age
- Gender
- Nutritional status, including appetite, dietary intake, hydration, current weight, and change from normal weight
- Neurologic status, including barium swallow; chest X-ray; cognition; esophageal video fluoroscopy; gag reflex; level of consciousness; memory; motor ability; orientation; symmetry of face, mouth, and neck; sensory function; and tongue movement

Defining Characteristics

First Stage: Oral

- Abnormal oral phase of swallow study
- Chocking prior to swallowing
- Coughing prior to swallowing
- Drooling
- Food falls from mouth
- Food pushed out of mouth
- Gagging prior to swallowing
- Inability to clear oral cavity
- Incomplete lip closure
- Inefficient nippling
- Inefficient suck
- Insufficient chewing
- Nasal reflux
- Piecemeal deglutition
- Pooling of bolus in lateral sulci
- Premature entry of bolus

- Prolonged bolus formation
- Prolonged meal time with insufficient consumption
- Tongue action ineffective in forming bolus

Second Stage: Pharyngeal

- Abnormal pharyngeal phase of swallow study
- Alteration in head position
- Chocking
- Coughing
- Delayed swallowing
- Fevers of unknown etiology
- Food refusal
- Gagging sensation
- Gurgly voice quality
- Inadequate laryngeal elevation
- Nasal reflux
- Recurrent pulmonary infection
- Repetitive swallowing

Third Stage: Esophageal

- Abnormal esophageal phase of swallow study
- Acidic-smelling breath
- Bruxism
- Difficulty swallowing
- Epigastric pain
- Food refusal
- Heartburn
- Hematemesis
- Hyperextension of head
- Nighttime awakening
- Nighttime coughing
- Odynophagia
- Regurgitation
- Repetitive swallowing
- Reports "something stuck"
- Unexplained irritability surrounding mealtimes
- Volume limiting
- Vomiting
- Vomitus on pillow

Expected Outcomes

- Patient won't show evidence of aspiration pneumonia.
- Patient will achieve adequate nutritional intake.
- Patient will maintain weight.
- Patient will maintain oral hygiene.
- Patient and caregiver will demonstrate correct feeding techniques to maximize swallowing.
- Patient and caregiver will list strategies to prevent aspiration.

Suggested NOC Outcomes

Appetite; Aspiration Prevention; Cognition; Nutritional Status: Food & Fluid Intake; Swallowing Status; Swallowing Status: Esophageal Phase; Swallowing Status: Oral Phase; Swallowing Status: Pharyngeal Phase

Interventions and Rationales

- Elevate the head of the bed 90° during mealtimes and for 30 minutes after the completion of a meal *to decrease the risk of aspiration.*
- Position patient on the side when recumbent *to decrease the risk of aspiration.*
- S Keep suction apparatus at the bedside; observe and report instances of cyanosis, dyspnea, or choking. *Symptoms indicate the presence of material in the lungs.*
- Monitor intake and output and weight daily until stabilized. Establish an intake goal—for example, "Patient consumes ____mL of fluid and ____ % of solid food." Record and report any deviation from this. *Evaluating calorie and protein intake daily allows any necessary modifications to begin quickly.*
- PCC Consult with a dietitian to modify patient's diet, and conduct a calorie count, as needed, *to establish nutritional requirements.*

- PCC Consult with a dysphagia rehabilitation team, if available, *to obtain expert advice.*
- Provide mouth care three times daily *to promote comfort and enhance appetite.*
- Keep the oral mucous membrane moist by frequent rinses; use a bulb syringe or suction, if necessary, *to promote comfort.*
- Lubricate patient's lips *to prevent cracking and blisters.*
- Encourage patient to wear properly fitted dentures *to enhance chewing ability.*
- Serve food in attractive surroundings; encourage patient to smell and look at food. Remove soiled equipment, control smells, and provide a quiet atmosphere for eating. *A pleasant atmosphere stimulates appetite; food aroma stimulates salivation.*
- PCC Teach patient and family members about positioning, dietary requirements, and specific feeding techniques, including facial exercises (such as whistling), using a short straw to provide sensory stimulation to patient's lips, tipping the head forward to decrease aspiration, applying pressure above the lip to stimulate mouth closure and the swallowing reflex, and checking the oral cavity frequently for food particles (remove if present). *These measures allow patient to take an active role in maintaining health.*

Suggested NIC Interventions

Airway Suctioning; Aspiration Precautions; Feeding; Positioning; Referral; Risk Identification; Swallowing Therapy

Evaluations for Expected Outcomes

- Patient shows no evidence of aspiration pneumonia. Breath sounds remain bilaterally clear; fever, chills, purulent sputum, and rapid shallow respirations are absent.
- Patient's fluid and dietary intake remains within established daily limits.
- Patient's weight remains stable.
- Patient demonstrates appropriate oral hygiene practices.
- Patient and caregiver demonstrate feeding techniques to maximize swallowing and minimize risk of complications.
- Patient and caregiver list strategies to prevent aspiration.

Documentation

- Patient's expressions of feelings about current situation
- Observations of weight, swallowing ability, intake and output, and oral hygiene
- Patient's response to nursing interventions
- Instructions about diet monitoring and feeding techniques
- Evaluations for expected outcomes

REFERENCES

Clayton, N. A., Carnaby, G. D., Peters, M. J., & Ing, A. J. (2014). Impaired laryngopharyngeal sensitivity in patients with COPD: The association with swallow function. *International Journal of Speech-Language Pathology*, *16*(6), 615–623. doi:10.3109/17549507.2014.882987

Crary, M. A., & Carnaby, G. D. (2014). Adoption into clinical practice of two therapies to manage swallowing disorders: Exercise-based swallowing rehabilitation and electrical stimulation. *Current Opinion in Otolaryngology & Head & Neck Surgery*, 22(3), 172–180. doi:10.1097/MOO.0000000000000055

Szczesniak, M., Maclean, J., Zhang, T., Graham, P., & Cook, I. (2014). Persistent dysphagia after head and neck radiotherapy: A common and under-reported complication with significant effect on non-cancer-related mortality. *Clinical Oncology*, 26(11), 697–703. doi:10.1016/j.clon.2014.08.009

RISK FOR THERMAL INJURY

Definition

Vulnerable to extreme temperature damage to skin and mucous membranes, which may compromise health.

Assessment

- Cardiovascular status, including blood pressure, capillary refill time, electrocardiogram results, heart rate and rhythm, pulses (apical, peripheral), and temperature
- Health history, including past episodes of allergy; food, pollen, or drug allergy; multiple surgical history; spina bifida; and asthma
- Current health status, including temperature, blood pressure, respiratory status, and other vital signs
- Knowledge level, including patient's current understanding of physical condition and physical, mental, and emotional readiness to learn
- Self-care abilities, including knowledge and use of adaptive equipment, preparation of equipment and supplies, and technical or mechanical skills

Risk Factors

- Alteration in cognitive functioning
- Extremes of age
- Extremes of environmental temperature
- Fatigue
- Inadequate protective clothing (e.g., flame-retardant sleepwear, gloves, ear covering)
- Inadequate supervision
- Inattentiveness
- Insufficient knowledge of safety precautions (patient, caregiver)
- Intoxication (alcohol, drugs)
- Neuromuscular impairment
- Neuropathy
- Smoking
- Treatment regimen
- Unsafe environment

Expected Outcomes

- Patient will not experience thermal injury.
- Patient will acknowledge presence of environmental hazards in home.
- Patient will take safety precautions to prevent injury.

Suggested NOC Outcomes

Risk Control; Risk Detection; Safe Home Environment; Knowledge: Personal Safety

Interventions and Rationales

- S Assess environment for potential risks for thermal injury *to prevent accidents.*
- Assess patient for any cognitive impairment *that would increase risk for thermal injury.*
- PCC Assess knowledge of fire safety and emergency response *to ensure rapid notification of emergency personnel.*
- S Remove dangerous or potentially dangerous items from the environment *to avoid injury.*
- Suggest a decrease in the maximum water temperature *to decrease potential scalding.*
- S Ensure proper functioning of all fire/smoke alarms *to provide quick intervention in case of fire.*

- PCC Encourage adults/family member to discuss fire safety measures with children and elderly family members *to promote household safety.*
- Encourage use of flame-retardant sleepwear *to minimize injury in the event of a fire.*
- Encourage patient/family to report any potential safety hazards *to decrease chance of thermal accident.*
- PCC Refer patient/family to community resources for fire safety to ensure all possible precautions have been identified and implemented.
- PCC Refer at-risk patients who are living alone to home health services *for follow-up home safety evaluation.*

Suggested NIC Interventions

Environmental Management: Safety; Fire Setting Precautions; Risk Identification; Surveillance: Safety

Evaluations for Expected Outcomes

- Patient has no incidents of thermal injury.
- Patient removes environmental hazards from home.
- Patient uses appropriate safety measures.

Documentation

- Patient's expressions of concern about risk for thermal injury
- Observations of measures taken to minimize environmental hazards
- Interventions performed to allay thermal injury risk
- Patient's response to interventions
- Evaluations for expected outcomes

REFERENCES

McWilliams, T., Hendricks, J., Twigg, D., & Wood, F. (2015). Burns education for non-burn specialist clinicians in Western Australia. *Burns*, *41*(2), 301–307. doi:10.1016/j.burns.2014.06.015

Olszewski, A., Yanes, A., Stafford, J., Greenhalgh, D. G., Palmieri, T. L., Sen, S., & Tran, N. (2016). Development and implementation of an innovative burn nursing handbook for quality improvement. *Journal of Burn Care & Research*, *37*(1), 20–24. doi:10.1097/BCR.0000000000000299

Scanavacca, M., & Pisani, C. F. (2015). Monitoring risk for oesophageal thermal injury during radiofrequency catheter ablation for atrial fibrillation: does the characteristic of the temperature probe matter? *EP: Europace*, *17*(6), 835–837. doi:10.1093/europace/euv101

INEFFECTIVE THERMOREGULATION

related to trauma or illness

Definition

Temperature fluctuation between hypothermia and hyperthermia

Assessment

- History of current illness
- Medication history

- Neurologic status, including level of consciousness (LOC), mental status, motor status, and sensory status
- Cardiovascular status, including blood pressure, capillary refill time, electrocardiogram, heart rate and rhythm, pulses (apical and peripheral), and temperature
- Respiratory status, including arterial blood gas measurements, breath sounds, and rate, depth, and character of respirations
- Integumentary status, including color, temperature, and turgor
- Fluid and electrolyte status, including blood urea nitrogen level, intake and output, serum electrolyte levels, and urine specific gravity
- Laboratory studies, including clotting factors, hemoglobin level, hematocrit, platelet count, and white blood cell count

Defining Characteristics

- Cyanotic nail beds
- Fluctuations in body temperature above or below normal range
- Flushed skin
- Hypertension
- Increase in body temperature above normal range
- Increase in respiratory rate
- Mild shivering
- Moderate pallor
- Piloerection
- Reduction in body temperature below normal range
- Seizures
- Skin cool to touch
- Skin warm to touch
- Slow capillary refill
- Tachycardia

Expected Outcomes

- Patient will maintain body temperature at normothermic levels.
- Patient won't shiver.
- Patient will express feelings of comfort.
- Patient will have warm, dry skin.
- Patient will maintain heart rate, respiratory rate, and blood pressure within normal range.
- Patient won't exhibit signs of compromised neurologic status.
- Patient and family members will voice an understanding of health problem.

Suggested NOC Outcomes

Hydration; Thermoregulation; Vital Signs

Interventions and Rationales

- Monitor patient's body temperature every 4 hours, or more often if indicated. Record the temperature and route (keep in mind that the baseline depends on the route). *Monitoring determines the effectiveness of therapy or whether intervention is required and allows accurate comparison of data.*
- Monitor and record patient's neurologic status every 8 hours. Report any changes to the physician. *Changes in LOC can result from tissue hypoxia related to altered tissue perfusion. Hyperthermia increases cerebral edema and thus intracranial pressure (ICP); hypothermia depresses metabolic rate.*
- Monitor and record patient's heart rate and rhythm, blood pressure, and respiratory rate every 4 hours. *Hyperthermia may create hypoxia by increasing oxygen demand, which results from increased tissue metabolism (metabolism increases 7% with each increase of 1° F [0.6° C]). This, in turn, results in faster breathing and a rising pulse rate.*

- Administer analgesics, antipyretics, and medications that prevent shivering, as prescribed. Monitor and record their effectiveness. *Antipyretics help reduce fever. Shivering tends to retard the lowering of body temperature.*
- If patient develops excessive fever, take the following steps following institutional protocol:
  - Remove blankets; place a loincloth over patient.
  - Apply ice bags to the axilla and groin.
  - Initiate a tepid water sponge bath.
  - Use a hypothermia blanket if temperature rises above ____. Cool patient to ____.

  These measures help reduce excessive fever.
- Maintain hydration.
  - Monitor intake and output.
  - Administer parenteral fluids, as ordered.
  - Determine patient's fluid preference. Keep oral fluids at the bedside and encourage patient to drink.

  These measures help maintain fluid balance. Keeping preferred fluids at the bedside allows patient to actively participate in the prescribed treatment.
- Maintain the environmental temperature at a comfortable setting.
  - Ensure that all metal and plastic surfaces that come into contact with patient's body are covered.
  - Use or remove blankets as necessary for comfort.
  - Make sure that linens and clothing are clean and dry.

  The temperature of the external environment affects ease of body temperature regulation.
- PCC Instruct patient and family members about:
  - signs and symptoms of altered body temperature
  - precautionary measures to avoid hypothermia or hyperthermia
  - adherence to other aspects of health care management to help normalize patient's temperature (such as dietary habits and measures to prevent increased ICP)
  - rationale for treatment.

  These measures allow patient to take an active role in health maintenance.

Suggested NIC Interventions

Bathing; Environmental Management; Fever Treatment; Fluid Management; Fluid Monitoring; Temperature Regulation; Vital Signs Monitoring

Evaluations for Expected Outcomes

- Patient's temperature remains within normal parameters.
- Patient doesn't shiver.
- Patient indicates feelings of comfort, either verbally or through behavior.
- Patient's skin remains warm and dry.
- Patient's heart rate and blood pressure remain within normal range.
- Patient and family state understanding of health problem.

Documentation

- Patient's needs and perceptions of current problem
- Physical findings
- Intake and output
- Patient's response to nursing interventions
- Evaluations for expected outcomes

REFERENCES

Gaither, J. B., Galson, S., Curry, M., Mhayamaguru, M., Williams, C., Keim, S. M., … Spaite, D. W. (2015). Environmental hyperthermia in prehospital patients with major traumatic brain injury. *Journal of Emergency Medicine (0736-4679)*, *49*(3), 375–381. doi:10.1016/j.jemermed.2015.01.038

Griggs, K. E., Leicht, C. A., Price, M. J., & Goosey-Tolfrey, V. L. (2015). Thermoregulation during intermittent exercise in athletes with a spinal cord injury. *International Journal of Sports Physiology & Performance*, *10*(4), 469–475. doi:10.1123/ijspp.2014-0361

Lee, S. J., Jeung, K. W., Lee, B. K., Min, Y. I., Park, K. N., Suh, G. J., … Kang, G. H. (2015). Impact of case volume on outcome and performance of targeted temperature management in out-of-hospital cardiac arrest survivors. *American Journal of Emergency Medicine*, *33*(1), 31–36. doi:10.1016/j.ajem.2014.10.003

IMPAIRED TISSUE INTEGRITY

related to impaired circulation

Definition

Damage to the mucous membranes, cornea, integumentary system, muscular fascia, muscle, tendon, bone, cartilage, joint capsule, and/or ligament

Assessment

- History of peripheral vascular disease or surgery
- Age
- Gender
- Integumentary status, including color, skin care practices, temperature, tenderness, texture, turgor, and edema
- Cardiovascular status, including blood pressure, cardiac output, patient and family history of cardiovascular disease, peripheral pulses, and smoking history
- Nutritional status, including dietary patterns, laboratory tests, serum lipid level, serum protein level, and change from normal weight
- Neurologic status, including motor function and sensory pattern

Defining Characteristics

- Damaged tissue
- Destroyed tissue

Expected Outcomes

- Patient will attain relief from immediate signs and symptoms (pain, ulcers, color changes, and edema).
- Patient will maintain collateral circulation.
- Patient will voice intent to stop smoking.
- Patient will voice intent to follow specific management routines after discharge.

Suggested NOC Outcomes

Knowledge: Treatment Regimen; Self-Care Hygiene; Tissue Integrity: Skin & Mucous Membranes; Tissue Perfusion: Peripheral; Wound Healing: Secondary Intention

Interventions and Rationales

- Provide scrupulous foot care. Administer and monitor treatments according to institutional protocols. *Foot care prevents fungal infections and ingrown toenails, stimulates circulation, and allows detection of signs and symptoms you should immediately report to the physician.*
- PCC Instruct patient to avoid pressure on popliteal space. For example, say "Don't cross your legs or wear constrictive clothing," *to avoid reducing arterial blood supply and increasing venous congestion.*
- Encourage adherence to an exercise regimen, as tolerated. *Exercise improves arterial circulation and venous return by promoting muscle contraction and relaxation.*
- PCC Educate patient about risk factors and prevention of injury. Refer patient to a smoking cessation program. *Teaching about factors influencing peripheral vascular disease and prevention of tissue damage helps prevent complications.*
- Maintain adequate hydration. Monitor intake and output and record daily weight. *Adequate hydration reduces blood viscosity and decreases the risk of clot formation.*
- If patient has venous insufficiency, apply antiembolism stockings or intermittent pneumatic compression stockings as prescribed, removing them for 1 hour every 8 hours or according to institutional protocol. Elevate patient's feet when he's sitting and elevate foot of bed 69 to 89 (15 to 20.5 cm) when he's lying down. *These measures promote venous return and decrease venous congestion in lower extremities.*

If patient has arterial insufficiency, elevate the head of the bed 6 to 9 in (15 to 20.5 cm) when he's lying down *to increase arterial blood supply to extremities.*

Suggested NIC Interventions

Circulatory Care: Arterial Insufficiency; Circulatory Precautions; Nutrition Management; Oral Health Maintenance; Positioning; Pressure Management; Pressure Ulcer Prevention; Skin Surveillance; Teaching: Foot Care

Evaluations for Expected Outcomes

- Patient attains relief from immediate symptoms.
  - Patient's feet show no signs of infection, ingrown toenails, or impaired circulation.
  - Patient maintains normal skin turgor.
  - Patient's mucous membranes remain moist.
  - Patient maintains balanced intake and output.
  - Patient's weight remains stable.
- Patient's vital signs remain within normal parameters.
- Patient uses interventions (antiembolism stockings or intermittent pneumatic compression stockings, elevation of feet, and elevation of head of bed) to promote arterial and venous circulation.
- Patient states rationale for quitting smoking and begins smoking cessation program.
- Patient describes plan to incorporate prescribed treatment program into postdischarge routine, including avoiding risk factors and activities that contribute to vascular compression (such as popliteal compression, leg crossing, and wearing constrictive clothing), following exercise program, and practicing foot care.

Documentation

- Patient's expressions of feelings about current situation
- Observations of skin color, turgor, temperature, and ulcer size

- Patient's response to nursing interventions
- Evaluations for expected outcomes

REFERENCES

da Silva, N. M., de Cássia Lopes Chaves, É., de Carvalho, E. C., & Iunes, D. H. (2013). Instrument for assessing tissue integrity of the feet of patients with diabetes mellitus. *Acta Paulista de Enfermagem*, *26*(6), 535–541.

Lundgren, J. (2015). Evolution of a deep tissue injury or a declining pressure ulcer? *Wound Care Advisor*, *4*(5), 18–19.

Malaquias, S. G., Bachion, M. M., Martins, M. A., de Barros Nunes, C. A., de Vasconcelos Torres, G., & Pereira, L. V. (2014). Impaired tissue integrity-related factors and defining characteristics in persons with vascular ulcers. *Texto & Contexto Enfermagem*, *23*(2), 434–442. doi:10.1590/0104-07072014001090013

IMPAIRED TISSUE INTEGRITY

related to surgical procedure

Definition

Damage to the mucous membranes, cornea, integumentary system, muscular fascia, muscle, tendon, bone, cartilage, joint capsule, and/or ligament

Assessment

- Reason for, type of, and anticipated length of surgery
- Health status, including age, sex, weight, vital signs, and nutritional, integumentary, cardiovascular, neurologic, respiratory, and psychosocial status
- Mobility status, including range of motion
- Patient's description of pain, numbness, and tingling
- Laboratory studies, including hematocrit, hemoglobin level, complete blood count, blood coagulation studies, immunologic and serologic tests, electrolyte levels, urinalysis, liver function tests, and serum protein levels
- Wound classification (clean, clean-contaminated, contaminated, or dirty)
- Allergies to medications, irrigation solutions, or cleaning solutions
- Health history, including altered immunologic status, malnutrition, and chronic metabolic or systemic disease (diabetes mellitus; cancer; cardiovascular, renal, or hepatic diseases; coagulation disorders; blood dyscrasias; or hematopoietic diseases)
- Current medical treatments, including chemotherapy and radiation, steroid, immunosuppressive, anticoagulant, thrombolytic, and antibiotic therapy
- Presence of infection, draining wounds, bruises, shear ulcers, or pressure ulcers

Defining Characteristics

- Damaged tissue
- Destroyed tissue

Expected Outcomes

- Patient will express feelings of comfort.
- Patient will remain free from alteration in tissue integrity related to physical hazards.

- Patient will remain free from alteration in tissue integrity related to chemical hazards.
- Patient will remain free from alteration in tissue integrity related to electrical hazards.

Suggested NOC Outcomes

Hydration; Infection Severity; Sensory Function: Cutaneous; Thermoregulation; Tissue Integrity: Skin & Mucous Membranes; Wound Healing: Secondary Intention

Interventions and Rationales

- Document and report the results of the preoperative nursing assessment. Identify factors that predispose patient to impaired tissue integrity. *A complete nursing assessment allows the development of an individualized care plan.*
- Classify the surgical wound according to the degree of contamination of the wound and surrounding tissue. *Classifying the surgical wound facilitates the assessment of the risk of wound infection and subsequent tissue injury.*
- Use padding, special mattresses, and support devices during surgery. *These measures reduce undue pressure and decrease the risk of impaired tissue integrity.*
- Maintain the environmental temperature at a comfortable setting. Offer blankets, if needed. *A comfortable environment reduces shivering, muscle tension, and reactive pain. These metabolic stressors can affect the rate of cellular repair.*
- Monitor patient for signs of hypothermia (shivering, cool skin, pallor, piloerection, and increased heart rate) *to determine the need to implement warming measures.*
- Warm prepping and irrigation solutions *to prevent a reduction in patient's temperature.*
- For infants (aged 1 year or younger), use a warming unit and head covering. *Infants have immature thermoregulatory mechanisms and don't retain adequate body heat.*
- When using pneumatic tourniquets, pad the skin, place the cuff so the skin is free from wrinkles, set to proper pressure, and monitor inflation time. *Improper tourniquet use can impair the circulatory status of the affected limb.*
- Check patient history for a sensitivity or allergy to prepping solution. Clean and prepare the skin incision site with nonirritating solutions. *Hypoallergenic, physiologic prepping and cleaning solutions reduce the risk of tissue reaction and injury.*
- To avoid the pooling of solutions, use towels or pads during prep. When using sprays, shield patient's face and eyes. *Pooled solutions can produce skin maceration. Sprays can damage the cornea and mucous membranes.*
- Ensure adequate aeration of items sterilized by ethylene oxide gas. *Residual gas is toxic to tissue.*
- Rinse chemosterilized items adequately. *Residual chemosterilization solutions are toxic to tissue.*
- Remove powder from gloves. *Glove powder can cause granulomas and other reactions.*
- Perform sponge, sharp, and instrument counts according to protocol, account for other items (such as bulldogs, umbilical tapes, and vessel loops), and document results. *Retained objects can produce a foreign body reaction or injury to tissue.*
- Follow the manufacturer's instructions for applying medications and chemical agents, such as glutaraldehyde and methylmethacrylate. *Agents can be toxic when applied directly to tissue.*
- Use physiologic solutions or prescribed medications for irrigation or topical application. *Nonphysiologic solutions can cause interstitial edema and cellular injury or death.*
- Check the label, route, dose, and expiration date of each medication with the scrub nurse *to reduce the risk of error.*
- When administering medications, record the drug, dosage, and route. Document verbal orders and have the physician cosign. *Documentation helps reduce medication errors.*

- Inspect all electrical, mechanical, and air-powered equipment before use. Operate equipment according to manufacturers' instruction *to reduce the chances of patient injury.*
- Apply an electrosurgical dispersive pad to clean, dry skin near the operative site. Avoid bony prominences, hairy surfaces, scar tissue, and areas of poor circulation. *Proper placement reduces the risk of burn injury.*
- When using a hypothermia or hyperthermia blanket, avoid creases, place a sheet between the skin and the blanket, and set and maintain the correct temperature. Pad the extremities during hypothermia therapy. *Proper use protects against tissue injury.*

Suggested NIC Interventions

Hemorrhage Control; Incision Site Care; Infection Control: Intraoperative; Infection Protection; Medication Management; Positioning; Pressure Ulcer Prevention

Evaluations for Expected Outcomes

- Patient has minimal or no shivering, muscle tension, or reactive pain.
- Patient doesn't develop rash, edema, bruises, discoloration, redness, skin breakdown, or other signs of altered tissue integrity related to physical hazards.
- Patient doesn't develop allergic or toxic reaction to sterilizing agents, glove powder, irrigating solutions, medications, or chemical agents and has little or no reaction to cleaning procedure.
- Patient doesn't develop reddened or discolored areas at site of electrosurgical grounding pad or adjacent tissue or any other signs of postoperative alteration in tissue integrity related to electrical hazards.

Documentation

- Results of preoperative nursing assessment
- Surgical procedure
- Type of anesthesia
- Preoperative and postoperative diagnosis
- Wound classification
- Preexisting conditions that increase risk of tissue injury
- Nursing interventions performed to protect tissue integrity
- Medications administered
- Patient's status on discharge to postanesthesia care unit (PACU)
- Skin condition on discharge to PACU
- Presence of lines, tubes, catheters, and drains
- Type of wound closure and dressing
- Evaluations for expected outcomes

REFERENCES

da Silva, N. M., de Cássia Lopes Chaves, É., de Carvalho, E. C., & Iunes, D. H. (2013). Instrument for assessing tissue integrity of the feet of patients with diabetes mellitus. *Acta Paulista de Enfermagem*, *26*(6), 535–541.

Lundgren, J. (2015). Evolution of a deep tissue injury or a declining pressure ulcer? *Wound Care Advisor*, *4*(5), 18–19.

Malaquias, S. G., Bachion, M. M., Martins, M. A., de Barros Nunes, C. A., de Vasconcelos Torres, G., & Pereira, L. V. (2014). Impaired tissue integrity-related factors and defining characteristics in persons with vascular ulcers. *Texto & Contexto Enfermagem*, *23*(2), 434–442. doi:10.1590/0104-07072014001090013

RISK FOR IMPAIRED TISSUE INTEGRITY

Definition

Vulnerable to damage to the mucous membrane, cornea, integumentary system, muscular fascia, muscle, tendon, bone, cartilage, joint capsule, and/or ligament, which may compromise health

Assessment

- History of peripheral vascular disease or surgery
- Age
- Gender
- Integumentary status, including color, skin care practices, temperature, tenderness, texture, turgor, and edema
- Cardiovascular status, including blood pressure, cardiac output, patient and family history of cardiovascular disease, peripheral pulses, and smoking history
- Mobility status, including range of motion
- Nutritional status, including dietary patterns, laboratory tests, serum lipid level, serum protein level, and change from normal weight
- Neurologic status, including motor function and sensory pattern
- Current medical treatments, including surgery, chemotherapy and radiation, steroid, immunosuppressive, anticoagulant, thrombolytic, and antibiotic therapy

Risk Factors

- Alteration in metabolism
- Alteration in sensation
- Chemical injury agent (e.g., burn, capsaicin, methylene chloride, mustard agent)
- Excessive fluid volume
- Extremes of age
- Extremes of environmental temperature
- High voltage power supply
- Humidity
- Imbalanced nutritional state (e.g., obesity, malnutrition)
- Impaired circulation
- Impaired mobility
- Insufficient fluid volume
- Insufficient knowledge about maintaining tissue integrity
- Insufficient knowledge about protecting tissue integrity
- Mechanical factor
- Peripheral neuropathy
- Pharmaceutical agent
- Radiation therapy
- Surgical procedure

Expected Outcomes

- Patient will not experience tissue impairment.
- Patient will maintain collateral circulation.
- Patient will describe measures to protect tissue.
- Patient will have adequate hydration.

Suggested NOC Outcomes

Body Positioning: Self-Initiated; Circulation Status; Hydration; Mobility; Nutritional Status; Tissue Perfusion: Peripheral

Interventions and Rationales

- Inspect patient's skin every shift; document skin condition and report status changes. *Early detection of changes prevents or minimizes skin breakdown.*
- Monitor any wounds and surrounding tissue. *Allows for individualized care.*
- Monitor placement of tubing and devices. *Correct placement and frequent inspection of devices prevents skin breakdown.*
- Evaluate need to specialty pressure redirecting devices. *Pressure redirecting devices help to eliminate pressure points on skin and tissue.*
- Provide scrupulous foot care. Administer and monitor treatments according to institutional protocols. *Foot care prevents fungal infections and ingrown toenails, stimulates circulation, and allows detection of signs and symptoms you should immediately report to the physician.*
- PCC Instruct patient to avoid pressure on popliteal space. For example, say "Don't cross your legs or wear constrictive clothing," *to avoid reducing arterial blood supply and increasing venous congestion.*
- Encourage exercise, as tolerated. *Exercise improves arterial circulation and venous return by promoting muscle contraction and relaxation.*
- PCC Educate patient about risk factors and prevention of injury. Refer patient to a smoking cessation program. *Teaching about factors influencing peripheral vascular disease and prevention of tissue damage helps prevent complications.*
- Maintain adequate hydration. Monitor intake and output and record daily weight. *Adequate hydration reduces blood viscosity and decreases the risk of clot formation.*
- Identify and document factors that predispose patient to impaired tissue integrity. *A complete nursing assessment allows the development of an individualized care plan.*

Suggested NIC Interventions

Electrolyte Monitoring; Fluid Monitoring; Nutrition Management; Positioning; Pressure Ulcer Prevention; Skin Surveillance

Evaluations for Expected Outcomes

- Patient's tissue remains intact.
- Patient's mucous membranes remain moist.
- Patient's weight remains stable.
- Patient's vital signs remain within normal parameters.
- Patient uses interventions (antiembolism stockings or intermittent pneumatic compression stockings, elevation of feet, and elevation of head of bed) to promote arterial and venous circulation.
- Patient states rationale for quitting smoking and begins smoking cessation program.
- Patient doesn't develop rash, edema, bruises, discoloration, redness, skin breakdown, or other signs of altered tissue integrity related to physical hazards.
- Patient maintains adequate circulation to tissue.

Documentation

- Observations of skin color, turgor, and temperature
- Preexisting conditions that increase risk of tissue injury
- Nursing interventions performed to protect tissue integrity
- Medications administered

- Presence of lines, tubes, catheters, and drains
- Evaluations for expected outcomes

REFERENCES

da Silva, N. M., de Cássia Lopes Chaves, É., de Carvalho, E. C., & Iunes, D. H. (2013). Instrument for assessing tissue integrity of the feet of patients with diabetes mellitus. *Acta Paulista de Enfermagem*, *26*(6), 535–541.

Lundgren, J. (2015). Evolution of a deep tissue injury or a declining pressure ulcer? *Wound Care Advisor*, *4*(5), 18–19.

Malaquias, S. G., Bachion, M. M., Martins, M. A., de Barros Nunes, C. A., de Vasconcelos Torres, G., & Pereira, L. V. (2014). Impaired tissue integrity-related factors and defining characteristics in persons with vascular ulcers. *Texto & Contexto Enfermagem*, *23*(2), 434–442. doi:10.1590/0104-07072014001090013

RISK FOR DECREASED CARDIAC TISSUE PERFUSION

Definition

Vulnerable to a decrease in cardiac (coronary) circulation, which may compromise health

Assessment

- Cardiovascular status including blood pressure, heart rate and rhythm, skin color, temperature, and peripheral pulses
- Results of echocardiogram and other diagnostic tests
- Medical history including family history, history of cardiovascular disease, and medication history

Risk Factors

- Cardiac tamponade
- Cardiovascular surgery
- Coronary artery spasm
- Diabetes mellitus
- Family history of cardiovascular disease
- Hyperlipidemia
- Hypertension
- Hypovolemia
- Hypoxemia
- Hypoxia
- Increase in C-reactive protein
- Insufficient knowledge about modifiable risk factors (e.g., smoking, sedentary lifestyle, obesity)
- Pharmaceutical agent
- Substance abuse

Expected Outcomes

- Patient will remain hemodynamically stable.
- Patient will not experience any signs or symptoms of decreased cardiac tissue perfusion.
- Patient will verbalize modifiable risk factors for decreased cardiac perfusion.
- Patient will identify reportable symptoms of possible decreased cardiac perfusion.

Suggested NOC Outcomes

Knowledge: Cardiac Disease Management; Cardiac Pump Effectiveness; Circulation Status; Tissue Perfusion: Cardiac

Interventions and Rationales

- S • Assess hemodynamic status, including blood pressure, heart rate, oxygen saturation, and respiratory rate for any abnormalities *that may be early indicators of altered perfusion.*
- S • Monitor cardiac rhythm for any irregularities *that may indicate cardiac irritability.*
- Assist with preparation and completion of diagnostic tests and the postprocedural care. *Safe completion of diagnostic tests will result in improved patient outcomes.*
- Treat episodes of tachycardia promptly. *Cardiac tissue is perfused during diastole and perfusion is decreased if tachycardia is not treated.*
- PCC • Provide patient with information regarding modifiable risk factors. *Knowledge of risk factors will contribute to informed decisions about lifestyle changes.*
- PCC • Encourage patient and family to share concerns regarding outcomes of tests *to reduce anxiety.*
- PCC • Collaborate with other members of the health care team to ensure that all underlying medical conditions are being managed effectively. *This will minimize the possibility of cardiac perfusion complications.*

Suggested NIC Interventions

Risk Identification; Teaching: Disease Process; Cardiac Care; Hemodynamic Regulation

Evaluations for Expected Outcomes

- Patient remained hemodynamically stable.
- Patient did not experience any signs or symptoms of decreased cardiac tissue perfusion.
- Patient verbalized modifiable risk factors for decreased cardiac perfusion.
- Patient identified reportable symptoms of possible decreased cardiac perfusion.

Documentation

- Hemodynamic status including vital signs and physical assessment findings
- Patient's report of any symptoms related to decreased cardiac tissue perfusion
- Patient's understanding of risk reduction interventions
- Evaluation of expected outcomes

REFERENCES

Duruturk, N., Tonga, E., Karatas, M., & Doganozu, E. (2015). Activity performance problems of patients with cardiac diseases and their impact on quality of life. *Journal of Physical Therapy Science, 27*(7), 2023–2028.

Ramos, L. M. (2014). Cardiac diagnostic testing: what bedside nurses need to know. *Critical Care Nurse, 34*(3), 16–28. doi:10.4037/ccn2014361

ter Hoeve, N., Huisstede, B., Stan, H. J., van Domburg, R. T., Sunamura, M., & van den Berg-Emons, R. G. (2015). Does cardiac rehabilitation after an acute cardiac syndrome lead to changes in physical activity habits? Systematic review. *Physical Therapy, 95*(2), 167–179. doi:10.2522/ptj.20130509

RISK FOR INEFFECTIVE CEREBRAL TISSUE PERFUSION

Definition

Vulnerable to a decrease in cerebral tissue circulation, which may compromise health

Assessment

- Cardiovascular status including heart rate and rhythm, blood pressure, and peripheral pulses
- Neurologic status including level of consciousness, orientation, motor activity, and strength of all extremities
- History of recent trauma, injury
- Results of diagnostic and laboratory tests

Risk Factors

- Abnormal partial thromboplastin time
- Abnormal prothrombin time
- Akinetic left ventricular wall segment
- Aortic atherosclerosis
- Arterial dissection
- Atrial fibrillation
- Atrial myxoma
- Brain injury (e.g., cerebrovascular impairment, neurologic illness, trauma, tumor)
- Brain neoplasm
- Carotid stenosis
- Cerebral aneurysm
- Coagulopathy (e.g., sickle cell anemia)
- Dilated cardiomyopathy
- Disseminated intravascular coagulopathy
- Embolism
- Hypercholesterolemia
- Hypertension
- Infective endocarditis
- Mechanical prosthetic valve
- Mitral stenosis
- Pharmaceutical agent
- Recent myocardial infarction
- Sick sinus syndrome
- Substance abuse
- Treatment regimen

Expected Outcomes

- Patient will understand the need for frequent neurologic assessments to assess for any changes.
- Patient will experience adequate cerebral perfusion evidenced by normal neurologic checks.
- Patient will remain hemodynamically stable.
- Patient will participate in diagnostic testing when necessary.
- Patient will verbalize strategies to minimize or decrease modifiable risk factors.

Suggested NOC Outcomes

Tissue Perfusion: Cerebral; Neurologic Status; Circulation Status

Interventions and Rationales

- Assess patient for positive risk factors for decrease in cerebral perfusion, including carotid stenosis, hypertension, coagulopathies, atrial fibrillation, and smoking. *Risk factor reduction will result in positive patient outcomes.*
- Facilitate completion of diagnostic tests and provide postprocedural care to prevent complications *to ensure accurate, safe, and timely diagnosis and treatment.*
- Maintain adequate oxygenation *to ensure cerebral perfusion.*
- PCC Educate at-risk patients of the signs of decreased cerebral perfusion about the importance of timely medical intervention for positive symptoms. *Change in mental status is a sensitive indicator for decreased cerebral perfusion.*

- PCC • Encourage at-risk patient and family to ask questions and share concerns *to increase their confidence and ability to recognize and respond to warning signs of decreased cerebral perfusion.*
- PCC • Collaborate with community organizations to educate public on risk factors for and symptoms of decreased cerebral perfusion and the appropriate response. *Increased community awareness may result in a more timely intervention for decreased cerebral perfusion conditions.*

Suggested NIC Interventions

Cerebral Perfusion Promotion; Neurologic Monitoring

Evaluations for Expected Outcomes

- Patient accepts the need for frequent neurologic assessments to evaluate changes in condition.
- Patient condition reflects normal cerebral perfusion.
- Patient's hemodynamic status supports adequate cerebral perfusion.
- Patient participates in diagnostic testing.
- Patient identifies modifiable risk factors for decreased cerebral perfusion.

Documentation

- Trending of neurologic assessments
- Vital sign results, including blood pressure, heart rate, and oxygenation status
- Patient tolerance and results of diagnostic tests
- Evaluations for expected outcomes

REFERENCES

de Abreu Almeida, M., Barragan da Silva, M., Paulsen Panato, B., de Oliveira Siqueira, A. P., Palma da Silva, M., Engelman, B., ... Gaedke Nomura, A. T. (2015). Clinical indicators to monitor patients with risk for ineffective cerebral tissue perfusion. *Investigacion & Educacion En Enfermeria, 33*(1), 155–163. doi:10.1590/S0120-53072015000100018

Høiseth, L. Ø., Hisdal, J., Hoff, I. E., Hagen, O. A., Landsverk, S. A., & Kirkebøen, K. A. (2015). Tissue oxygen saturation and finger perfusion index in central hypovolemia: Influence of pain. *Critical Care Medicine, 43*(4), 747–756. doi:10.1097/CCM.0000000000000766

Lipp, L. L. (2014). Brain perfusion and oxygenation. *Critical Care Nursing Clinics of North America, 26*(3), 389–398. doi:10.1016/j.ccell1.2014.04.008

RISK FOR INEFFECTIVE PERIPHERAL TISSUE PERFUSION

Definition

Vulnerable to a decrease in blood circulation to the periphery, which may compromise health

Assessment

- Pain sensation, including characteristics (sharp, dull, constant, or intermittent); precipitating factors
- Psychosocial status, including age, learning ability, decision-making ability, developmental stage, financial resources, health beliefs, knowledge and skill regarding current health problem, usual coping patterns

- Cardiovascular status including heart rate and rhythm, blood pressure, and peripheral pulses
- Neurologic status including level of consciousness, orientation, motor activity, and strength of all extremities
- Behavioral status, understanding of health problem and treatment plan, past history with health care providers, participation in health care planning and decision making; recognition and realization of potential growth, health, autonomy

Risk Factors

- Diabetes mellitus
- Endovascular procedure
- Excessive sodium intake
- Hypertension
- Insufficient knowledge of aggravating factors (e.g., smoking, sedentary lifestyle, trauma, obesity, salt intake, immobility)
- Insufficient knowledge of disease process
- Insufficient knowledge of risk factors
- Sedentary lifestyle
- Smoking
- Trauma

Expected Outcomes

- Patient will be free from tissue injury due to decreased peripheral perfusion.
- Patient will understand the need for smoking cessation
- Patient will understand the need for moderate activity to promote circulation.
- Patient will state reportable changes that indicate decreased peripheral perfusion.

Suggested NOC Outcomes

Activity Tolerance; Tissue Integrity: Skin and Mucous Membranes; Tissue Perfusion: Peripheral

Interventions and Rationales

- Assess lower extremities for early signs of ineffective peripheral perfusion. *Early identification and intervention will improve patient outcomes.*
- Assess patient's history for presence of heart disease, hyperlipidemia, diabetes, and smoking, *which are significant risk factors for impaired peripheral tissue perfusion.*
- PCC Evaluate patient's understanding of lifestyle modifications *to enable patient participation in risk factor reduction.*
- Administer and evaluate effectiveness of medications to treat underlying medical conditions that place patient at risk for decreased peripheral perfusion. C*ontrol of risk factors will prevent or delay onset of tissue hypoperfusion.*
- Position extremity at or lower than level of the heart *to promote peripheral perfusion.*
- PCC Instruct patient to initiate a regular walking program *to promote collateral circulation* and improve perfusion.
- PCC Teach patient to avoid crossing of the legs *to avoid constriction.*
- Encourage patient to carefully follow treatment regimens for existing medical conditions *that are risk factors for decreased peripheral tissue perfusion.*
- PCC Refer patients who smoke to smoking cessation program *because continued smoking will significantly increase risks for development of peripheral tissue damage.*

Suggested NIC Interventions

Circulatory Care: Arterial Insufficiency, Exercise Promotion, Positioning, Skin Surveillance

Evaluations for Expected Outcomes

- Patient has no tissue injury due to decreased peripheral perfusion.
- Patient understands need for smoking cessation.
- Patient understands need for moderate activity.
- Patient states changes that may indicate poor peripheral perfusion.

Documentation

- Observations of lower extremity status
- Interventions performed to manage decreased peripheral perfusion
- Interventions performed to manage decreased peripheral perfusion
- Patient's response to interventions
- Evaluations for expected outcomes

REFERENCES

Ait-Oufella, H., Bige, N., Boelle, P. Y., Pichereau, C., Alves, M., Bertinchamp, R., … Guidet, B. (2014). Capillary refill time exploration during septic shock. *Intensive Care Medicine*, *40*(7), 958–964. doi:10.1007/s00134-014-3326-4

Garg, P. K., Biggs, M. L., Carnethon, M., Ix, J. H., Criqui, M. H., Britton, K. A., … Mukamal, K. J. (2014). Metabolic syndrome and risk of incident peripheral artery disease: The cardiovascular health study. *Hypertension (0194911X)*, *63*(2), 413–419. doi:10.1161/HYPERTENSIONAHA.113.01925

Piller, L. B., Simpson, L. M., Baraniuk, S., Habib, G. B., Rahman, M., Basile, J. N., … Davis, B. R. (2014). Characteristics and long-term follow-up of participants with peripheral arterial disease during ALLHAT. *JGIM: Journal of General Internal Medicine*, *29*(11), 1475–1483. doi:10.1007/s11606-014-2947-1

INEFFECTIVE PERIPHERAL TISSUE PERFUSION

related to insufficient knowledge of disease process

Definition

Decrease in blood circulation to the periphery, which may compromise health

Assessment

- Cardiovascular status including blood pressure, heart rate, and rhythm
- Peripheral vascular assessment, peripheral pulses, temperature and color of extremities, skin integrity
- Activity status
- Pain assessment

Defining Characteristics

- Absence of peripheral pulses

- Alteration in motor functioning
- Alteration in skin characteristic (e.g., color, elasticity, hair, moisture, nails, sensation, temperature)
- Ankle-brachial index <0.90
- Capillary refill time >3 seconds
- Color does not return to lowered limb after 1 minute leg elevation
- Decrease in blood pressure in extremities
- Decrease in pain-free distances achieved in the 6-minute walk test
- Decrease in peripheral pulses
- Delay in peripheral wound healing
- Distance in the 6-minut walk test below normal range (400 to 700 m in adults)
- Edema
- Extremity pain
- Femoral bruit
- Intermittent claudication
- Paresthesia
- Skin color pales with limb elevation

Expected Outcomes

- Patient will understand the need to maintain moderate activity level to promote circulation.
- Patient will articulate the need and rationale for smoking cessation.
- Patient will not experience ischemic damage to involved extremity.
- Patient will experience adequate perfusion to promote wound healing.
- Patient will acknowledge the importance of protecting involved extremity from injury.
- Patient will recognize reportable changes in skin characteristics to the involved extremity that indicate decreased perfusion.

Suggested NOC Outcomes

Activity Tolerance; Tissue Integrity: Skin and Mucous Membranes; Tissue Perfusion: Peripheral

Interventions and Rationales

- Evaluate involved extremity for clinical signs (pain, decreased temperature, pallor, delayed capillary refill, weak or absent pulse, decreased sensation, and decreased pulse oximetry), *which are indicators of ineffective peripheral perfusion.*
- Protect the extremity from injury using sheepskin or bed cradle and position extremity at or lower than level of heart *to promote collateral blood flow.*
- PCC Instruct patient to increase walking activity *to promote collateral circulation and improve blood supply to the extremity.*
- Encourage patient to protect extremity from injury or extreme hot or cold temperatures. *Infection or ulcer formation may develop more easily due to decreased blood supply.*
- PCC Refer patients who smoke to smoking cessation program *since continued smoking will significantly increase risks for further damage.*

Suggested NIC Interventions

Circulatory Care: Arterial Insufficiency; Exercise Promotion; Positioning; Skin Surveillance

Evaluations for Expected Outcomes

- Patient understands the need to maintain moderate activity to promote blood flow to extremity.
- Patient states the need for smoking cessation.
- Patient's involved extremity is free of injury or ischemic damage.
- Patient recognizes reportable changes to involved extremity that indicate decreased perfusion.

Documentation

- Patient's understanding of need for moderate activity and implementation plan
- Patient's plan for smoking cessation
- Assessment of involved extremity
- Assessment of peripheral pain
- Evaluations for expected outcomes

REFERENCES

Ait-Oufella, H., Bige, N., Boelle, P. Y., Pichereau, C., Alves, M., Bertinchamp, R., ... Guidet, B. (2014). Capillary refill time exploration during septic shock. *Intensive Care Medicine*, *40*(7), 958–964. doi:10.1007/s00134-014-3326-4

Forsythe, R. O., & Hinchliffe, R. J. (2016). Assessment of foot perfusion in patients with a diabetic foot ulcer. *Diabetes/Metabolism Research & Reviews*, *32*, 232–238. doi:10.1002/dmrr.2756

Høiseth, L. Ø., Hisdal, J., Hoff, I. E., Hagen, O. A., Landsverk, S. A., & Kirkebøen, K. A. (2015). Tissue oxygen saturation and finger perfusion index in central hypovolemia: Influence of pain. *Critical Care Medicine*, *43*(4), 747–756. doi:10.1097/CCM.0000000000000766

IMPAIRED TRANSFER ABILITY

related to neuromuscular impairment

Definition

Limitation of independent movement between two nearby surfaces

Assessment

- Age
- Gender
- Vital signs
- Drug history
- History of neuromuscular disorder or dysfunction
- Musculoskeletal status, including coordination, muscle size and strength, muscle tone, range of motion (ROM), functional mobility as follows:
  0 = completely independent
  1 = requires use of equipment or device
  2 = requires help, supervision, or teaching from another person
  3 = requires help from another person and equipment or device
  4 = dependent; doesn't participate in activity
- Neurologic status, including level of consciousness, motor ability, and sensory ability
- Endurance, for example, how long patient can remain sitting in wheelchair before becoming fatigued
- Knowledge of wheelchair transfer techniques

Defining Characteristics

- Impaired ability to transfer between bed and chair
- Impaired ability to transfer between bed and standing position
- Impaired ability to transfer between car and chair
- Impaired ability to transfer between chair and floor
- Impaired ability to transfer between chair and standing position
- Impaired ability to transfer between floor and standing position
- Impaired ability to transfer between uneven levels
- Impaired ability to transfer in or out of bath tub
- Impaired ability to transfer in or out of shower
- Impaired ability to transfer on or off a commode
- Impaired ability to transfer on or off a toilet

Expected Outcomes

- Patient won't exhibit complications associated with impaired wheelchair transfer mobility, such as depression, altered health maintenance, and falls.
- Patient will maintain or improve muscle strength and joint ROM.
- Patient will achieve highest level of mobility possible (independence with regard to wheelchair transfer, ability to transfer to wheelchair with assistance, verbalization of needs regarding wheelchair transfer).
- Patient will maintain safety during wheelchair transfer.
- Patient will adapt to alteration in ability to perform wheelchair transfer.
- Patient will demonstrate understanding of wheelchair transfer techniques.
- Patient will participate in social and occupational activities to the greatest extent possible.

Suggested NOC Outcomes

Balance; Body Positioning: Self-Initiated; Transfer Performance; Coordinated Movement; Mobility

Interventions and Rationales

- Perform ROM exercises to the joints of affected limbs, unless contraindicated, at least once every 8 hours. Progress from passive to active ROM, as tolerated, *to prevent joint contractures and muscle atrophy.*
- Identify patient's level of independence using the functional mobility scale. Report the findings to the staff *to provide continuity and preserve or improve the documented level of independence.*
- Monitor and record daily evidence of complications related to altered mobility or decreased ability to perform wheelchair transfer (contractures, venous stasis, skin breakdown, thrombus formation, depression, altered health maintenance, or self-care deficit). *Patients with neuromuscular dysfunction are at risk for complications.*
- PCC Teach patient wheelchair transfer techniques, such as performing a standing or sitting transfer, *to maintain muscle tone, prevent complications of immobility, and promote independence.* Adapt teaching to the limits imposed by the patient's condition *to prevent injury.*
- PCC Refer patient to a physical therapist for the development of a wheelchair mobility program *to assist with rehabilitation of musculoskeletal deficits.*

- Encourage patient to attend physical therapy. Request a written copy of wheelchair transfer instructions to use as a reference *to maintain continuity of care and foster safety.*
- Assess patient's skin upon return to bed and request a wheelchair cushion, if necessary, *to maintain skin integrity.*
- PCC As part of your teaching plan, demonstrate transfer techniques to family members and note the date. Have them perform a return demonstration *to ensure the use of proper technique and to promote continuity of care.*
- PCC Identify resources (stroke program, sports association for disabled, National Multiple Sclerosis Society) *to promote patient's reintegration into the community.*

Suggested NIC Interventions

Body Mechanics Promotion; Energy Management; Exercise Promotion: Strength Training; Exercise Therapy: Balance; Fall Prevention; Self-Care Assistance: Transfer

Evaluations for Expected Outcomes

- Patient doesn't exhibit complications associated with impaired wheelchair transfer mobility, such as depression, altered health maintenance, and falls.
- Patient maintains or improves muscle strength and joint ROM.
- Patient achieves highest level of mobility possible (independence with regard to wheelchair transfer, ability to transfer to wheelchair with assistance, verbalization of needs regarding wheelchair transfer).
- Patient maintains safety during wheelchair transfer.
- Patient adapts to alteration in ability to perform wheelchair transfer.
- Patient demonstrates understanding of wheelchair transfer techniques.
- Patient participates in social and occupational activities to the greatest extent possible.

Documentation

- Patient's mobility status
- Presence of complications
- Evidence of alterations in patient's ability to perform wheelchair transfer
- Patient's statements regarding difficulties in wheelchair transfer
- Instruction of transfer techniques
- Patient's and family members' return demonstration of skills
- Patient's response to nursing interventions
- Evaluations for expected outcomes

REFERENCES

Kent-Braun, J. A., Callahan, D. M., Fay, J. L., Foulis, S. A., & Buonaccorsi, J. P. (2014). Muscle weakness, fatigue, and torque variability: Effects of age and mobility status. *Muscle & Nerve*, *49*(2), 209–217. doi:10.1002/mus.23903

Peterson, M. J., Williams, N., Caves, K., & Morey, M. C. (2014). A pilot study of partial unweighted treadmill training in mobility-impaired older adults. *Biomed Research International*, *2014*, 321048. doi:10.1155/2014/321048

Ursin, M. H., Ihle-Hansen, H., Fure, B., Tveit, A., & Bergland, A. (2014). Balance and mobility in acute stroke: Association with subgroups of stroke and socio-demographic characteristics. *European Journal of Physiotherapy*, *16*(4), 230–237. doi:10.3109/21679169.2014.934280

RISK FOR TRAUMA

related to external factors (chemical, environmental, physical agents)

Definition

Vulnerable to accidental tissue injury (e.g., wound, burn, fracture), which may compromise health

Assessment

- Health history, including accidents, allergies, exposure to pollutants, falls, hyperthermia, hypothermia, poisoning, sensory or perceptual changes (auditory, gustatory, kinesthetic, olfactory, tactile, and visual), seizures, and trauma
- Circumstances of current situation that might lead to injury from surgery or from chemical, physical, or human agents
- Neurologic status, including level of consciousness, mental status, and orientation
- Laboratory studies, including clotting factors, hemoglobin level, hematocrit, and platelet and white blood cell counts

Risk Factors

External

- Absence of call-for-aid device
- Absence of stairway gate
- Absence of window guard
- Access to weapon
- Bathing in very hot water
- Bed in high position
- Children riding in front seat of car
- Defective appliance
- Delay in ignition of gas appliance
- Dysfunctional call-for-aid device
- Electrical hazard (e.g., faulty plug, frayed wire, overloaded outlet/fuse box)
- Exposure to corrosive product
- Exposure to dangerous machinery
- Exposure to radiation
- Exposure to toxic chemical
- Extremes of environmental temperature
- Flammable object (e.g., clothing, toys)
- Gas leak
- Grease on stove
- High crime neighborhood
- Icicles hanging from roof
- Inadequate stair rails
- Inadequately stored combustible (e.g., matches, oily rags)
- Inadequately stored corrosive (e.g., lye)
- Insufficient protection from heat source
- Misuse of headgear (e.g., hard hat, motorcycle helmet)
- Misuse of seat restraint
- Insufficient anti-slip material in bathroom
- Nonuse of seat restraints
- Obstructed passageway
- Playing with dangerous object
- Playing with explosive
- Pot handle facing front of stove
- Proximity to vehicle pathway (e.g., driveway, railroad track)
- Slippery floor
- Smoking in bed
- Smoking near oxygen
- Struggling with restraints
- Unanchored electric wires
- Unsafe operation of heavy equipment (e.g., excessive speed, while intoxicated, without required eyewear)
- Unsafe road
- Unsafe walkway
- Use of cracked dishware
- Use of throw rugs
- Use of unstable chair
- Use of unstable ladder
- Wearing loose clothing around open flames

Internal

- Alteration in cognitive functioning
- Alteration in sensation (resulting from spinal cord injury, diabetes mellitus, etc.)
- Decrease in eye-hand coordination

- Decrease in muscle coordination
- Economically disadvantaged
- Emotional disturbance
- History of trauma (e.g., physical, psychological, sexual)
- Impaired balance
- Insufficient knowledge of safety precautions
- Insufficient Vision
- Weakness

Expected Outcomes

- Patient will avoid injury.
- Patient will state understanding of safety precautions.
- Patient will use assistive devices correctly (e.g., walker or cane).

Suggested NOC Outcomes

Balance; Coordinated Movement; Fall Prevention Behavior; Knowledge: Fall Prevention; Risk Control; Safe Home Environment

Interventions and Rationales

- Observe, record, and report falls, seizures, and unsafe practices. *Accurate assessment promotes appropriate interventions; documentation ensures continuity of care.*
- Monitor and record patient's respiratory status. *Trauma increases respiratory rate; other respiratory effects depend on the nature of the trauma.*
- Monitor and record patient's neurologic status *to detect changes and to report deteriorated status.*
- Remain with the patient in case of a seizure; loosen restrictive clothing, and protect the patient from environmental hazards. Don't restrain the patient or pry the mouth open. Keep an oral airway at the bedside and maintain a patent airway. Turn patient to the side after the seizure stops and suction if secretions occlude the airway. Record seizure characteristics, including onset, duration, and body movements. Reorient patient to surroundings and allow a rest period. *Remaining with patient provides safety and information for accurate documentation of the event. Loosening clothing and proper positioning may prevent further harm.*
- S Keep the side rails up at all times *to protect patient and provide a sense of security.*
- S Keep the bed in a low position except when providing direct care *to minimize the effects of a possible fall.*
- PCC S Emphasize the importance of asking for help before getting up. *Illness or injury may have weakened patient.*
- Help debilitated, weak, or unsteady patient to get out of bed. Ensure that the floor is dry and that furniture and litter don't block patient's way *to help prevent falls.*
- When using soft restraints, don't secure them too tightly *to avoid skin burns.*
- Use leather restraints following facility policy; pad them well before applying. Release each extremity on a rotation basis every hour; check for skin burns. *Such restraints should be used only when other kinds are ineffective.*
- PCC S Instruct patient and family members on safety practices such as correct use of a walker, crutches, or cane. *These enable patient and family members to take an active role in health care and maintain a safe environment.*

Suggested NIC Interventions

Environmental Management: Safety; Fall Prevention; Health Education; Pressure Ulcer Prevention; Seizure Precautions; Surveillance: Safety; Teaching: Disease Process

Evaluations for Expected Outcomes

- Patient remains free from injury.
- Patient identifies specific safety precautions.
- Patient demonstrates proper use of assistive devices (specify).

Documentation

- Patient's statements that indicate potential for injury
- Physical findings
- Observations or knowledge of unsafe practices
- Interventions performed to prevent injury
- Patient's response to nursing interventions
- Evaluations for expected outcomes

REFERENCES

Cordovilla-Guardia, S., Guerrero-López, F., Maldonado, A., Vilar-López, R., Salmerón, J., Romero, I., … Fernández-Modéjar, E. (2014). Trauma risk perception related to alcohol, cannabis, and cocaine intake. *European Journal of Trauma & Emergency Surgery*, *40*(6), 693–699. doi:10.1007/s00068-014-0384-9

Newgard, C. D., Holmes, J. F., Haukoos, J. S., Bulger, E. M., Staudenmayer, K., Wittwer, L., … Western Emergency Services Translational Research Network (WESTRN) Investigators. (2016). Improving early identification of the high-risk elderly trauma patient by emergency medical services. *Injury*, *47*(1), 19–25. doi:10.1016/j.injury.2015.09.010

Silverstein, M., Kistin, C., Bair-Merritt, M., Wiltsey-Stirman, S., Feinberg, E., Diaz-Linhart, Y., … Cabral, H. (2016). Avoidance as an obstacle to preventing depression among urban women at high risk for violent trauma. *Archives of Women's Mental Health*, *19*(1), 63–70. doi:10.1007/s00737-015-0521-4

RISK FOR VASCULAR TRAUMA

Definition

Vulnerable to damage to vein and its surrounding tissues related to the presence of a catheter and/or infused solutions, which may compromise health

Assessment

- Integumentary status including color, turgor, lesions, and wounds
- Fluid and electrolyte and medication therapies
- Mobility status

Risk Factors

- Difficulty visualizing artery or vein
- Inadequate anchoring of catheter
- Inappropriate catheter type
- Inappropriate catheter width
- Insertion site
- Irritating solution (e.g., concentration, temperature, pH)
- Length of time catheter is in place
- Rapid infusion rate

Expected Outcomes

- Patient will not experience vascular trauma as a result of catheter or infused solution.
- Patient will communicate reportable signs and symptoms indicating possible catheter infusion-related problems.
- Patient will maintain recommended position of extremity during treatment.

Suggested NOC Outcomes

Tissue Integrity: Skin & Mucous Membranes; Comfort Status: Physical; Knowledge: Treatment Procedure

Interventions and Rationales

- Assess patient for pain at insertion site. *Pain is often the first symptom of vascular trauma.*
- Use transparent dressing over the insertion site. *This will secure the catheter and facilitate frequent assessment of the insertion site.*
- Perform prescribed insertion site checks and progress of the infusion *to ensure early identification of problems and timely interventions to avoid vascular trauma.*
- PCC Educate patient about the purpose of the infusion and reportable symptoms indicative of trauma, for example, burning, swelling, and warmth. *Prompt termination of the infusion and the catheter will minimize damage to the tissue.*
- Support patient throughout intravenous therapy *to decrease anxiety and promote positive patient outcomes.*
- PCC Collaborate with experienced team members in the management of complex intravenous therapy *to ensure all possible steps are taken to minimize complications.*

Suggested NIC Interventions

Intravenous Therapy; Medication Administration: Intravenous (IV); Skin Surveillance; Teaching: Procedure/Treatment

Evaluations for Expected Outcomes

- Patient did not experience vascular trauma as a result of intravenous therapy.
- Patient was able to maintain proper position of the extremity during treatment.
- Patient was able to identify reportable signs and symptoms of infusion-related problems.

Documentation

- Intravenous site checks and interventions
- Patient reports of possible complications of intravenous therapy
- Intake and output including type of intravenous fluid and rate of infusion
- Evaluations for expected outcomes

REFERENCES

Higgins, N., Keogh, S., & Rickard, C. (2015). Evaluation of a pilot educational program on safe and effective insertion and management of peripheral intravenous catheters. *Journal of the Association for Vascular Access*, *20*(1), 37–42. doi:10.1016/j.java.2014.12.001

Schreiber, M. L. (2016). Evidence-based practice. Neurovascular assessment: An essential nursing focus. *MEDSURG Nursing*, *25*(1), 55–57.

Weir, G. R., Smart, H., van Marie, J., & Cronje, F. J. (2014). Arterial disease ulcers, part 1: Clinical diagnosis and investigation. *Advances in Skin & Wound Care*, *27*(9), 422–430. doi:10.1097/01.ASW.0000453095.19109.5c

UNILATERAL NEGLECT

related to brain injury (e.g., cerebrovascular impairment, neurologic illness, trauma, tumor)

Definition

Impairment in sensory and motor response, mental representation, and spatial attention of the body, and the corresponding environment, characterized by inattention to one side and overattention to the opposite side. Left-side neglect is more severe and persistent than right-side neglect

Assessment

- History of neurologic impairment
- Age
- Neurologic status, including awareness of body parts, cognition, level of consciousness, mental status, memory, sensory function, orientation, position sense, visual acuity, visual fields, ability to communicate (verbally and nonverbally), and bowel and bladder control
- Musculoskeletal status, including coordination, muscle size and strength, muscle tone, range of motion (ROM), and functional mobility scale:
  0 = completely independent
  1 = requires use of equipment or device
  2 = requires help, supervision, or teaching from another person
  3 = requires help from another person and equipment or device
  4 = dependent; doesn't participate in activity
- Integumentary status, including color, texture, turgor, temperature, elasticity, sensation, moisture, hygiene, and lesions
- Psychosocial status, including coping mechanisms, support systems (family and others), lifestyle, and understanding of physical condition
- Self-care abilities, including preparation of equipment and supplies, technical or mechanical skills, and use of assistive devices

Defining Characteristics

- Alteration in safety behavior on neglected side
- Disturbance of sound lateralization
- Failure to dress neglected side
- Failure to eat food from portion of plate on neglected side
- Failure to groom neglected side
- Failure to move eyes in the neglected hemisphere
- Failure to move head in the neglected hemisphere
- Failure to move limbs in the neglected hemisphere
- Failure to move trunk in the neglected hemisphere
- Failure to notice people approaching from the neglected side
- Hemianopsia
- Impaired performance on line cancellation, line bisection, and target cancellation tests
- Left hemiplegia from cerebrovascular accident
- Marked deviation of the eyes to stimuli on the nonneglected side
- Marked deviation of the trunk to stimuli on the nonneglected side
- Omission of drawing on the neglected side
- Perseveration
- Representational neglect (e.g., distortion of drawing on the neglected side)
- Substitution of letters to form alternative words when reading

- Transfer of pain sensation to the nonneglected limb
- Unaware of positioning of neglected limb
- Unilateral visuospatial neglect
- Use of vertical half of page only when writing

Expected Outcomes

- Patient will avoid injury to affected body part.
- Patient will avoid skin breakdown.
- Patient will avoid contractures.
- Patient will recognize neglected body part.
- Patient and family members will demonstrate exercises for affected body part.
- Patient and family members will demonstrate measures for maximum functioning and arrange environment to protect affected body part.
- Patient and family members will express feelings about altered state of health and neurologic deficits.
- Patient and family members will identify community resources and support groups to help cope with the effects of illness.

Suggested NOC Outcomes

Adaptation to Physical Disability; Body Image; Body Mechanics Performance; Body Positioning: Self-Initiated; Self-Care: Activities of Daily Living (ADLs)

Interventions and Rationales

- Place a sling on the affected arm *to prevent dangling or injury.* Support the affected leg and foot while in bed, place a foot strap on the wheelchair, and perform other measures, as appropriate, *to keep patient's limbs in functional position and avoid contractures.* Use a drawsheet to move patient up in bed *to avoid skin abrasions.*
- Touch the affected limb. Describe it in conversation with patient *to remind patient of neglected body part.*
- Direct patient to perform activities that require the use of the affected limb. *A patient who uses a paretic or paralyzed limb will more easily integrate the affected limb into his or her body image.*
- Encourage patient to check the position of the affected body part with each repositioning or transfer *to reestablish awareness of the body part.*
- Establish and follow a regular turning schedule *to maintain skin integrity.*
- PCC Request consultations with occupational and physical therapists about adaptive equipment, exercise program, and other recommendations *to increase patient's awareness of the affected limb.*
- S Use safety belts or protective devices according to facility policy. *Safety devices remind patient of self-limitations and help prevent falls.*
- Remove splints and other devices at least every 2 hours. Inspect the skin for pressure areas. Reapply the splint. *Proper use of splints and other devices prevents deformities and maintains skin integrity.*
- Perform ROM exercises on the affected side at least once every shift, unless medically contraindicated, *to maintain joint flexibility and prevent contractures.*
- PCC Instruct family and nursing personnel to observe the position of the affected body part frequently. Remove food or drainage from the face if unnoticed by patient. Place the arm or leg in the proper position as often as necessary *to prevent injury.*

- When approaching the patient, do so from the nonneglected side in order that the patient will see you and not become startled. *The patient will not move the eyes in the neglected hemisphere and so will not see you.*
- Arrange the environment for maximum functioning; for example, place water, television controls, and the call bell within reach on the nonneglected side. *These measures enhance orientation and encourage independence.*
- Assist with ADLs or provide supervision, as appropriate, *to protect patient's affected side.* Teach the family the reasons for unilateral neglect. Help them to understand how they can work with the patient to minimize frustration. *Families not understanding can challenge the patient inappropriately by ignoring the patient's ability to use the neglected side.*
- PCC Encourage patient and family members to express their feelings regarding patient's condition and level of functioning *to release tension and enhance coping.*
- PCC Refer patient and family members to appropriate support groups and other community resources *to assist patient and family in adjusting to patient's altered state of health.*

Suggested NIC Interventions

Anticipatory Guidance; Body Image Enhancement; Coping Enhancement; Exercise Therapy: Joint Mobility; Mutual Goal Setting; Self-Care Assistance; Unilateral Neglect Management

Evaluations for Expected Outcomes

- Patient doesn't experience injury.
- Patient's skin doesn't show signs of breakdown.
- Patient doesn't show evidence of contractures.
- Patient recognizes and protects neglected body part when carrying out ADLs.
- Patient and family members demonstrate exercise routine for affected body part.
- Patient and family members demonstrate measures for maximum functioning and arrange environment to protect affected body part.
- Patient and family members openly express fear and other feelings associated with patient's neurologic deficits and altered level of functioning.
- Patient and family members identify and contact appropriate community resources and support groups.

Documentation

- Patient's expressions of feelings about neglected side of body
- Safety measures taken to prevent injury
- Patient's ability to perform ADLs and nursing measures taken to overcome deficits
- Observations of patient's and family's coping skills
- Patient's response to nursing interventions, including verbal expressions or behavior that indicates increased awareness of affected limb
- Evaluations for expected outcomes

REFERENCES

Chin-Ying, D., & Li-Chan, L. (2015). Nursing care of unilateral neglect patients. *Journal of Nursing*, 62(1), 92–97. doi:10.6224/JN.62.1.92

Park, J. H., & Lee, J. H. (2015). The effects of mental practice on unilateral neglect in patients with chronic stroke: A randomized controlled trial. *Journal of Physical Therapy Science*, 27(12), 3803–3805.

Patole, R. R., Kulkarni, V. N., Rairikar, S. A., Shyam, A. K., & Sancheti, P. K. (2015). Effect of task-specific treatment in patients with unilateral neglect. *Indian Journal of Physiotherapy & Occupational Therapy*, 9(1), 74–77. doi:10.5958/0973-5674.2015.00016.7

IMPAIRED URINARY ELIMINATION

related to anatomic obstruction or sensory motor impairment

Definition

Dysfunction in urinary elimination

Assessment

- History of urinary tract disease, trauma, surgery, or previous urethral infection
- Age
- Gender
- Vital signs
- Genitourinary status, including characteristics of urine, excretory urography, pain or discomfort, palpation of bladder, urinalysis, and voiding patterns
- Fluid and electrolyte status, including blood urea nitrogen and creatinine levels, intake and output, mucous membranes (inspection), serum electrolyte levels, skin turgor, and urine specific gravity
- Nutritional status, including appetite, constipation, dietary intake, elimination habits, current weight and change from normal, and rectal examination
- Sexuality status, including capability, concerns, habits, and sexual partners
- Psychosocial status, including coping skills, patient's perception of health problem, self-concept (body image), family members, and stressors (such as finances and job)

Defining Characteristics

- Dysuria
- Frequent voiding
- Hesitancy
- Nocturia
- Urinary incontinence
- Urinary retention
- Urinary urgency

Expected Outcomes

- Patient will maintain fluid balance; intake will equal output.
- Patient will voice increased comfort.
- Patient will voice understanding of treatment.
- Patient will have few, if any, complications.
- Patient will discuss impact of urologic disorder on self and family members.
- Patient will demonstrate skill in managing urinary elimination problem.
- Patient will maintain urinary continence.
- Patient and family members will identify resources to assist with care following discharge.

Suggested NOC Outcomes

Urinary Continence; Urinary Elimination

Interventions and Rationales

- Observe patient's voiding pattern. Document urine color and characteristics, intake and output, and patient's daily weight. Report any changes. *Accurate intake and output measurements are essential for correct fluid replacement therapy. Urine characteristics help verify diagnosis.*
- Administer appropriate care for the urologic condition and monitor progress (e.g., strain urine). Report favorable and adverse responses to the treatment regimen. *Appropriate*

care helps patient recover from the underlying disorder. Reporting responses to treatment allows modification of the treatment, as needed.

- Observe bowel habits.
  - Check for constipation.
  - Check for fecal impaction; if present, disimpact and institute a bowel regimen. These measures promote comfort and prevent loss of rectal muscle tone from prolonged distention.

PCC

- If patient requires surgery, give appropriate preoperative and postoperative instructions and care. *Accurate information allows patient to understand the procedure and builds trust in caregivers.*

PCC

- Explain reasons for therapy and intended effects to patient and family members *to increase patient's understanding and build trust in caregivers.* If patient needs urinary diversion, prepare him for a change in body appearance (instruct patient and family members how to care for the ostomy site postoperatively). *Preparation and appropriate information helps patient and family members cope with changes.*
- Assist with bladder elimination procedure, as indicated.
  - For bladder training, place patient on the commode or toilet every 2 hours while awake and once during the night. Maintain regular fluid intake while patient is awake. Provide privacy. Teach patient how to perform Kegel exercises to strengthen sphincter control. *These measures aid adaptation to routine physiologic function. Women with good muscle tone can improve levator muscle action significantly if they perform Kegel exercises regularly.*
  - For intermittent catheterization, catheterize patient using clean or sterile technique every 2 hours. Record amount voided spontaneously and amount obtained with catheterization (e.g., 7 a.m., spontaneous void of 200 mL; catheter void of 150 mL). Record bladder balance daily. *These measures promote normal voiding, prevent infection, and help maintain integrity of ureterovesical function. Catheterization schedule is based on flow sheet data and can provide a baseline chart.*
  - Bladder balance for amount of residual urine/amount of voided urine
  - For external catheterization (in a male patient), monitor patency. Apply a condom catheter according to the established policy. *Applying a foam strip in a spiral fashion increases the adhesive surface and reduces the risk of impairing circulation.* Avoid constriction. Observe the skin condition of the penis, and clean with soap and water at least twice daily. *These measures prevent infection and ensure therapeutic effectiveness.*
  - For an indwelling urinary catheter, monitor patency. Keep the tubing free from kinks, and keep the drainage bag below the level of the bladder *to avoid urine reflux.* Clean the urinary meatus according to the established policy, and maintain a closed drainage system *to prevent skin irritation and bacteriuria.* Secure the catheter to patient's leg (female) or abdomen (male); avoid tension on the sphincter. *Anchoring the catheter avoids straining the trigone muscle of the bladder and prevents friction leading to inflammation.*
  - For a suprapubic catheter, monitor patency. Change the dressing and clean the catheter site according to policy. Keep the tubing free from kinks; keep the drainage bag below bladder level. Maintain a closed drainage system. *Suprapubic drainage allows increased patient mobility and reduces the risk of bladder infection.*
- Provide supportive measures, as indicated:
  - Administer pain medication and monitor patient to reduce pain and assess the effects of medication.
  - Encourage fluids, as ordered, to moisten mucous membranes and dilute chemical materials within the body.

PCC

  - Refer patient to a dietitian for instructions on diet. Dietary changes may decrease urinary infections.

- Assist with general hygiene and comfort measures, as needed. Cleanliness prevents bacterial growth and promotes comfort.
- Maintain the patency of catheters, drainage bags, and other urinary elimination equipment to avoid reflux and risk of infection and ensure the effectiveness of therapy.
- Provide meatal care according to facility policy to promote cleanliness and comfort and reduce the risk of infection.
- Provide privacy during the toileting procedure to avoid inhibiting elimination.
- Respond to patient's call bell quickly, assign patient to the bed next to the bathroom and have patient wear easily removed clothing (such as a gown rather than pajamas). These measures reduce delay and impediments to the voiding routine.

PCC • Alert patient and family members to the signs and symptoms of a full bladder: restlessness, abdominal discomfort, sweating, and chills. *Adequate education increases patient's and family members' ability to maintain health level and to prevent patient from harming himself.*

PCC • Instruct patient and family members on catheterization techniques to be used at home; provide time for return demonstrations until they can perform the procedure well. *Knowledge of procedures and rationales reduces anxiety and promotes comfort. Demonstrations may progress through several sessions until patient can perform independently.*

PCC • Encourage patient to ventilate feelings and concerns related to his or her urologic problem. *Active listening conveys respect for patient; ventilation helps pinpoint patient's fears.*

PCC • Refer patient and family members to a psychiatric liaison nurse, sex counselor, or support group, when appropriate. *These resources help patient gain knowledge of self and the situation, reduce anxiety, and promote personal growth. Community resources usually provide support and care not available in other health agencies.*

PCC • Explain the urologic condition to patient and family members, including instructions on preventive measures, if appropriate. Prepare for discharge according to individual needs. *Accurate health knowledge increases patient's ability to maintain health. Involving family members assures patient of continued care.*

Suggested NIC Interventions

Anxiety Reduction; Fluid Management; Urinary Elimination Management; Urinary Retention Care; Weight Management; Urinary Bladder Training; Urinary Catheterization

Evaluations for Expected Outcomes

- Patient's fluid intake equals output.
- Patient expresses feelings of comfort.
- Patient voices understanding of treatment, including urinary diversion therapy, if appropriate.
- Patient doesn't show evidence of skin breakdown, infection, or other complications.
- Patient discusses disease, signs and symptoms, complications, treatments, and adjustments to lifestyle caused by altered urinary pattern.
- Patient and family members demonstrate skill in managing urinary elimination problem, including catheterization techniques to be used at home.
- Patient demonstrates proficiency in steps necessary to manage urinary elimination problems.
- Patient maintains urinary continence.
- Patient and family members identify and contact home health care agency, support group, or other resources, as needed.

Documentation

- Observations of urologic condition and response to treatment regimen
- Interventions to provide supportive care and patient's response
- Instructions given to patient and family members on urologic problem, response to instructions, and demonstrated ability to manage patient's urinary elimination needs
- Patient's expression of concern about urologic problem and its impact on body image and lifestyle; patient's motivation to participate in self-care
- Evaluations for expected outcomes

REFERENCES

Patel, J. A., Kaufman, A. S., Howard, R. S., Rodriguez, C. J., & Jessie, E. M. (2015). Risk factors for urinary retention after laparoscopic inguinal hernia repairs. *Surgical Endoscopy*, *29*(11), 3140–3145. doi:10.1007/s00464-014-4039-z

Sung, K. H., Lee, K. M., Chung, C. Y., Kwon, S. S., Lee, S. Y., Ban, Y. S., & Park, M. S. (2015). What are the risk factors associated with urinary retention after orthopedic surgery? *BioMed Research International*, *2015*, 1–5. doi:10.1155/2015/613216

Wilson, M. (2015). Assessing and treating urinary incontinence in men. *British Journal of Community Nursing*, *20*(6), 268–270. doi:10.12968/bjcn.2015.20.6.268

READINESS FOR ENHANCED URINARY ELIMINATION

Definition

A pattern of urinary functions for meeting eliminatory needs, which can be strengthened

Assessment

- Nutritional status: weight (compare to normal chart); laboratory studies: serum albumin, glucose; daily food intake, usual dietary patterns, food preferences, food allergies, changes in weight
- Patient's perception of health problem, coping mechanisms, problem-solving ability, decision-making competencies, relationships, family system, self-worth
- Reproductive status, maternal history, number of pregnancies, live births, abortions or miscarriages.
- Genitourinary status, including frequency and voiding pattern
- Fluid and electrolyte status, including blood urea nitrogen level, creatinine level, intake and output, mucous membranes, serum electrolyte levels, and skin turgor
- Neuromuscular status, including activities of daily living, mental status, mobility, and sensory ability to perceive bladder fullness
- Psychosocial status, including behavior before and after voiding, support from family members, and stressors (family, job, and change in environment)

Defining Characteristics

- Expresses desire to enhance urinary elimination

Expected Outcomes

- Patient will maintain urine output that is clear and straw colored with no odor.
- Patient will drink 64 oz of noncaffeinated, nonalcoholic beverages per day (unless contraindicated).

- Patient will maintain blood pressure in normal range.
- Patient will avoid use of nonsteroidal anti-inflammatory drugs (NSAIDs), analgesics, and anticholinergics.
- Patient will express understanding of health promotion activities to enhance urinary elimination.
- Patient will express improvement in quality of life.

Suggested NOC Outcomes

Urinary Continence; Urinary Elimination

Interventions and Rationales

- Assess that weight is within established norms *to prevent pressure on bladder, which contributes to incontinence.*
- Monitor and record patient's intake and output *to determine fluid balance.*
- Assess that blood pressure is within norms; *elevated ranges contribute to renal failure.*
- Discuss voiding and fluid intake patterns *to provide a baseline for introducing new activities.*
- Discuss foods that increase acidity in the urine (cranberries, meats, eggs, whole grains, and prunes) and foods that are low in sodium. *Increased acidity in the urine impedes bacterial growth. Foods high in sodium cause fluid retention and decreased urine output.*
- PCC Discuss hygiene practices, including hand hygiene, wiping and cleaning from front to back, and taking showers rather than baths (females). *Cleaning from front to back prevents transferring microorganisms from the bowel to the urinary meatus. Showering flushes microorganisms away from the urinary meatus, preventing UTIs.*
- PCC Teach female patient to perform Kegel exercises *to strengthen pelvic muscles and prevent development of incontinence (which occurs in 20% to 40% of elderly women). Assist with application of pads and protective garments (used only as a last resort) to prevent skin breakdown and odor and to promote social acceptance.*
- Assist with application of pads and protective garments (used only as a last resort) *to prevent skin breakdown and odor and to promote social acceptance.*
- PCC Teach stress management techniques. *Stress stimulates release of antidiuretic hormones and interferes with sphincter relaxation, which causes urine retention.*
- Explain reasons for activities that enhance urinary elimination *to patient to promote understanding and compliance.*
- Encourage patient to drink six to eight glasses of noncaffeinated, nonalcoholic, noncarbonated liquid, preferably water, per day (unless contraindicated). *1,500 to 2,000 mL/day promotes optimal renal function and flushes bacteria and solutes from the urinary tract. Caffeine and alcohol promote diuresis and may contribute to excess fluid loss. Caffeine, alcohol, and carbonation are irritating to the bladder wall.*
- Encourage patient to respond to the urge to void in a timely manner. *Ignoring the urge to urinate may cause incontinence.*
- Encourage patient to participate in regular exercise, including walking and modified situps (unless contraindicated). *Weak abdominal and perineal muscles weaken bladder and sphincter control.*
- For female patient, encourage her to void before and after intercourse *to flush microorganisms away from the urinary meatus, preventing UTI; to avoid bubble baths that may cause chemical irritation to urinary meatus, increasing the risk of UTI; and to wear cotton underpants as cotton is an absorbent fabric that prevents perineal moisture retention.*

- Encourage patient to avoid NSAIDs, analgesics, and anticholinergics. *NSAIDs and analgesics impair renal blood flow. Anticholinergic drugs inhibit relaxation of urinary sphincter and cause urine retention.*
- Encourage patient to stop smoking (if applicable) or refrain from starting. *Smoking contributes to renal and bladder cancer. Nicotine is a potent vasoconstrictor.*
- Encourage patient to avoid exposure to petroleum, heavy metals, asbestos, dyes, rubber, leather, ink, and paint. *Exposure to carcinogens increases the risk of renal and bladder cancer.*

Suggested NIC Interventions

Urinary Elimination Management

Evaluations for Expected Outcomes

- Patient maintains adequate intake.
- Patient carries out Kegel exercises.
- Patient expresses satisfaction with stress reduction techniques, avoidance of carcinogens.
- Patient experiences satisfaction with urinary elimination.

Documentation

- Observations of intake and output
- Interventions to provide supportive care and patient's response to supportive care
- Instructions given to patient; return demonstration of knowledge and skills needed to carry out exercise and stress management techniques
- Evaluations for expected outcomes

REFERENCES

Rahman, A. N., Schnelle, J. F., & Osterweil, D. (2014). Implementing toileting trials in nursing homes: Evaluation of a dissemination strategy. *Geriatric Nursing*, *35*(4), 283–289. doi:10.1016/j.gerinurse.2014.03.002

Testa, A. (2015). Understanding urinary incontinence in adults. *Urologic Nursing*, *35*(2), 82–86. doi:10.7257/1053-816X.2015.35.2.82

Vickerman, J. (2014). Practical tips for promoting continence in the care home. *Nursing & Residential Care*, *16*(5), 250–254.

URINARY RETENTION

related to blockage in urinary tract; high urethral pressure; reflex arc inhibition; strong sphincter

Definition

Incomplete emptying of the bladder

Assessment

- History of sensory or neuromuscular impairment, prostate enlargement, surgery, urethral trauma or tumor, or urinary tract disease
- Age
- Gender

- Vital signs
- Genitourinary status, including pain or discomfort, palpation of bladder, residual urine volume after voiding, urethral obstruction (prostate hyperplasia or masses, fecal impaction, masses, and swelling), urinalysis, urine characteristics, and voiding patterns
- Fluid and electrolyte status, including inspection of mucous membranes, intake and output, skin turgor, urine specific gravity, and serum electrolyte, blood urea nitrogen, and creatinine levels
- Medication history
- Neuromuscular status, including anal sphincter tone, motor ability to start and stop stream, neuromuscular function, and sensory ability to perceive bladder fullness and voiding
- Sexuality status, including capability and concerns or partner's concerns
- Psychosocial status, including coping skills, patient's or family members' perception of problem, self-concept, and stressors (such as finances and job)

Defining Characteristics

- Absent urinary output
- Bladder distention
- Dribbling of urine
- Dysuria
- Frequent voiding
- Overflow incontinence
- Residual urine
- Sensation of bladder fullness
- Small voiding

Expected Outcomes

- Patient will maintain fluid balance, with intake equal to output.
- Patient will voice increased comfort.
- Patient will voice understanding of treatment.
- Patient will have few, if any, complications.
- Patient's urinalysis will remain normal.
- Patient will avoid bladder distention.
- Patient and family members will demonstrate skill in managing urine retention.
- Patient will discuss impact of urologic disorder on self and family members.
- Patient and family members will identify resources to assist with care following discharge.

Suggested NOC Outcomes

Knowledge: Treatment Regimen; Symptom Control; Symptom Severity; Urinary Continence; Urinary Elimination

Interventions and Rationales

- Monitor intake and output. Report if intake exceeds output. *Accurate intake and output measurements are essential for correct fluid replacement therapy.*
- Monitor voiding pattern. *Data on time, place, amount, and patient's awareness of micturition are needed to establish a pattern of incontinence.*
- Assist with the ordered bladder elimination procedure as follows:
  - Voiding techniques. Perform Credé's or Valsalva's maneuver every 2 to 3 hours *to increase bladder pressure to pass urine.* Repeat until empty.

  - Intermittent catheterization. Catheterize using clean or sterile technique every 2 hours. Record amount voided spontaneously and amount obtained with catheterization. *These measures promote normal voiding, prevent infection, and help maintain the integrity of ureterovesical function.*
  - Use of an indwelling urinary catheter. Monitor patency and avoid kinks in tubing. Keep the drainage bag below bladder level *to avoid urine reflux*. Perform catheter care according to established policy and maintain a closed drainage system *to prevent skin irritation and bacteriuria*. Secure the catheter to patient's leg (female) or abdomen (male), avoiding tension on the sphincter. *Anchoring the catheter prevents straining of the bladder's trigone muscle and prevents friction leading to inflammation.*
  - Use of a suprapubic catheter. Change dressings according to facility policy. Monitor patency and avoid kinks in the tubing. Keep drainage bag below bladder level. Maintain closed drainage system. *Suprapubic drainage allows for increased mobility and reduces the risk of bladder infection.*
  - Administer pain medication, as ordered, and monitor patient *to reduce pain and assess the medication's effects.*
- For fecal impaction, disimpact and institute a bowel regimen *to promote comfort and prevent the loss of rectal muscle tone from prolonged distention.*
- Encourage a high fluid intake 2 L/day, unless contraindicated, *to moisten mucous membranes and dilute chemical materials within the body.* Limit fluid intake after 7 p.m. *to prevent nocturia.*
- Monitor therapeutic and adverse effects of prescribed medications *for early recognition and treatment of drug reactions.*
- PCC If patient requires surgery, give appropriate preoperative and postoperative instructions and care *to increase patient's understanding*. If urinary diversions are being considered, prepare the patient for a change in body image. *Preparation and appropriate information helps patient and family members cope with changes.*
- PCC Instruct patient and family members on voiding techniques to be used at home. Provide for return demonstrations until they can perform the procedure well. *Knowledge of procedures and rationales reduces anxiety and promotes comfort. Demonstrations may progress through several sessions until patient can perform independently.*
- PCC Encourage patient and family members to share feelings and concerns related to urologic problems. *Ventilation helps pinpoint patient's fears and establishes an environment of trust in which patient and family members can begin to deal with the situation.*
- PCC Refer patient and family members to a psychiatric liaison nurse, enterostomal therapist, sex counselor, support group, or home health care agency, when appropriate. *These resources help patient gain knowledge of self and situation, reduce anxiety, and help promote personal growth. Community resources usually provide services not available at other health agencies.*

Suggested NIC Interventions

Distraction; Perineal Care; Urinary Bladder Training; Urinary Catheterization: Intermittent; Urinary Elimination Management

Evaluations for Expected Outcomes

- Patient's fluid intake equals output.
- Patient expresses feelings of comfort.
- Patient expresses understanding of treatment, including ordered bladder elimination procedure and surgery, if appropriate.

- Patient doesn't experience skin breakdown or other complications.
- Patient's urinalysis remains normal.
- Patient avoids bladder distention.
- Patient and family members demonstrate skill in managing urine retention, including voiding techniques to be used at home.
- Patient expresses at least one fear, one concern, and one positive feeling about urologic problem. If appropriate, patient expresses feelings and fears about surgery.
- Patient or family contacts home health care agency, support group, or other resources, as needed.

Documentation

- Observations of urologic condition and response to treatment regimen
- Interventions to provide supportive care and patient's response
- Instructions given to patient and family members on urologic problem and their returned response and demonstrated ability to manage patient's urinary elimination
- Patient's concerns about urologic problem and its impact on body image and lifestyle; motivation to participate in self-care
- Evaluations for expected outcomes

REFERENCES

Oh, J. J., Kim, S. H., Shin, J. S., & Shin, S. J. (2016). Risk factors for acute postpartum urinary retention after vaginal delivery: Focus on episiotomy direction. *Journal of Maternal-Fetal & Neonatal Medicine*, *29*(3), 408–411. doi:10.3109/14767058.2014.1002395

Patel, J. A., Kaufman, A. S., Howard, R. S., Rodriguez, C. J., & Jessie, E. M. (2015). Risk factors for urinary retention after laparoscopic inguinal hernia repairs. *Surgical Endoscopy*, *29*(11), 3140–3145. doi:10.1007/s00464-014-4039-z

Sung, K. H., Lee, K. M., Chung, C. Y., Kwon, S. S., Lee, S. Y., Ban, Y. S., & Park, M. S. (2015). What are the risk factors associated with urinary retention after orthopedic surgery? *BioMed Research International*, *2015*, 1–5. doi:10.1155/2015/613216

DYSFUNCTIONAL VENTILATORY WEANING RESPONSE

Definition

Inability to adjust to lowered levels of mechanical ventilator support that interrupts and prolongs the weaning process

Assessment

- Health history, including previous respiratory problems
- Nutritional status, including caloric intake and type of and tolerance for feeding
- Neurologic status, including mental status and level of consciousness
- Emotional status, including signs of anxiety or stress
- Laboratory values, including arterial blood gas (ABG) levels (baseline and ongoing), serum electrolyte and blood glucose levels, complete blood count, blood and sputum culture, and sensitivity tests
- Weaning parameters and current ventilator settings
- Respiratory status, including respiratory rate, pattern, character, and depth; chest expansion and symmetry; sputum characteristics (color, amount, odor, and consistency); cough

effectiveness; presence of cyanosis in mucous membranes and nail beds; and auscultation of breath sounds
- Need for suctioning, including frequency and patient's response
- Musculoskeletal status, including muscle mass, strength, and endurance level
- Cognitive state, including patient's ability to follow directions and readiness to learn
- Recent administration of potential respiratory-depressant medications, such as opioids, sedatives, and neuromuscular blockers
- Vital signs
- Pulse oximetry readings

Defining Characteristics

Mild

- Breathing discomfort
- Fatigue
- Fear of machine malfunction
- Increase in focus on breathing
- Mild increase of respiratory rate over baseline
- Perceived need for increase in oxygen
- Restlessness
- Warmth

Moderate

- Abnormal skin color (e.g., pale, dusky, cyanosis)
- Apprehensiveness
- Decrease in air entry on auscultation
- Diaphoresis
- Facial expression of fear
- Hyperfocused on activities
- Impaired ability to cooperate
- Impaired ability to respond to coaching
- Increase in blood pressure from baseline (≤20 mm Hg)
- Increase in heart rate from baseline (≤20 beats/min)
- Minimal use of respiratory accessory muscles
- Moderate increase in respiratory rate over baseline

Severe

- Abnormal skin color (e.g., pale, dusky, cyanosis)
- Adventitious breath sounds
- Agitation
- Asynchronized breathing with the ventilator
- Decrease in level of consciousness
- Deterioration in ABGs from baseline
- Gasping breaths
- Increase in blood pressure from baseline (≥20 mm Hg)
- Increase in heart rate from baseline (≥20 beats/min)
- Paradoxical abdominal breathing
- Profuse diaphoresis
- Shallow breathing
- Significant increase in respiratory rate above baseline
- Use of significant respiratory accessory muscles

Expected Outcomes

- Patient will maintain respiratory rate within 5 breaths/minute of baseline during weaning period.
- Patient's ABG levels will remain within acceptable limits (specify).
- Patient's mental status and emotional state will remain stable during gradual withdrawal of ventilatory support.
- Patient will express comfort with progressive ventilator changes.
- Patient will experience no dyspnea, fatigue, or pain during progressive ventilator changes.
- Patient will remain within adequate weaning parameters:
  - Tidal volume: 4 to 5 cc/kg
  - Negative inspiratory force: greater than or equal to –20 cm H_2O

  - Vital capacity: 10 to 15 cc/kg
  - Minute ventilation: 6 to 10 L
- Patient's cough will effectively clear secretions.

Suggested NOC Outcomes

Anxiety Self-Control; Client Satisfaction: Technical Aspects of Care; Depression Self-Control; Respiratory Status: Gas Exchange; Respiratory Status: Ventilation; Risk Control; Vital Signs

Interventions and Rationales

S
- Monitor patient's vital signs every hour when changing ventilator settings. *Fever, tachycardia, tachypnea, and elevated blood pressure may indicate hypoxemia.*
- Auscultate for breath sounds every 2 hours and report deviations. *Adventitious sounds may precede respiratory failure.*
- Place patient in a comfortable position (preferably Fowler's) *to facilitate adequate chest expansion and drainage.*

PCC
- Describe all weaning procedures to patient. Explain that he may experience changes in breathing rate and pattern, increased difficulty breathing, and fatigue *to decrease anxiety.*
- If patient is receiving intermittent mandatory ventilation (IMV), begin to decrease IMV by increments of 2 breaths/minute. This process may take place over days or weeks. *Lowering IMV encourages patient to take own breaths, thereby exercising respiratory muscles.*
- Monitor ABG levels with every ventilator change *to assess for adequate oxygenation and acid–base balance.*
- Include periods of rest between ventilator changes, especially at night, *to reduce tissue oxygen demand.*
- If patient tolerates IMV of 2 to 4 breaths/minute, try pressure support ventilation (PSV). *PSV prolongs positive airway pressure during inspiration, allowing patient to regulate own respiratory rate and tidal volume.*
- When patient is breathing adequately without IMV, place the patient on continuous positive airway pressure (CPAP) of 5 cm H_2O *to prevent alveolar collapse.*
- When patient tolerates CPAP, place on T-piece (T-bar) of 30% to 50% fraction of inspired oxygen. *This allows patient to breathe independently, continue to receive oxygen, and remain intubated in the event of respiratory compromise.*
- When patient tolerates longer weaning periods, incorporate activities of daily living into patient's daily routine *to increase muscular strength and endurance.*
- When patient has satisfactory respiratory status, weaning parameters, and ABG levels, assist with the removal of the ventilator tubes and keep the oxygen mask on hand *to prevent respiratory compromise.*
- Assess patient for stridor, respiratory distress, and dysphonia and report these findings to the physician *to monitor the need for renewed ventilatory assistance.*
- Perform chest physiotherapy and suctioning, as needed, *to maintain a patent airway.*
- Monitor the respiratory effects of medications closely and evaluate the response to bronchodilators *to detect respiratory status compromise.* Avoid respiratory depressants.

Suggested NIC Interventions

Acid–Base Management; Airway Management; Anxiety Reduction; Aspiration Precautions; Mechanical Ventilatory Weaning; Respiratory Monitoring; Support System Enhancement; Teaching: Procedure/Treatment; Vital Signs Monitoring

Evaluations for Expected Outcomes

- Patient's respiratory rate is within 5 breaths/minute of baseline during weaning period.
- Patient's ABG levels are within specified acceptable limits.
- Patient maintains stable mental and emotional status during withdrawal of ventilatory support.
- Patient expresses comfort with progressive ventilator changes.
- Patient doesn't experience dyspnea, fatigue, or pain during progressive ventilator changes.
- Patient remains within adequate weaning parameters.
- Patient's cough effectively clears secretions.

Documentation

- Patient's reports of malaise, anxiety, restlessness, breathlessness, and unusual pain
- Patient's response to ventilator changes
- Subtle changes in patient's mental or emotional status
- Laboratory data, including ABG levels
- Patient's response to nursing interventions, including positioning, chest physiotherapy, and suctioning
- Patient's response to medications, including opioids, bronchodilators, and neuromuscular blockers
- Respiratory rate, pattern, and depth, including changes from baseline
- Evaluations for expected outcomes

REFERENCES

Hetland, B., Lindquist, R., & Chlan, L. L. (2015). The influence of music during mechanical ventilation and weaning from mechanical ventilation: A review. *Heart & Lung*, *44*(5), 416–425. doi:10.1016/j.hrtlng.2015.06.010

Peñuelas, O., Thille, A. W., & Esteban, A. (2015). Discontinuation of ventilatory support: New solutions to old dilemmas. *Current Opinion in Critical Care*, *21*(1), 74–81. doi:10.1097/MCC.0000000000000169

Rose, L., Dainty, K. N., Jordan, J., & Blackwood, B. (2014). Weaning from mechanical ventilation: A scoping review of qualitative studies. *American Journal of Critical Care*, *23*(5), e54–e71. doi:10.4037/ajcc2014539

IMPAIRED VERBAL COMMUNICATION

related to physiologic condition (e.g., brain tumor, decreased circulation to brain, weakened musculoskeletal system)

Definition

Decreased, delayed, or absent ability to receive, process, transmit, and/or use a system of symbols

Assessment

- Neurologic status, including level of consciousness, orientation, cognition, memory (recent and remote), insight, and judgment
- Speech characteristics, including pattern (garbled, incomprehensible, difficulty forming words), language and vocabulary, level of comprehension and expression, and ability to use other forms of communication (such as eye blinks, gestures, pictures, and nods)
- Motor ability

- Circulatory status, including a history of cardiac and circulatory problems, pulse, blood pressure, arteriogram, electroencephalography, and computed tomography scan
- Respiratory status, including dyspnea and use of accessory muscles

Defining Characteristics

- Absence of eye contact
- Difficulty comprehending communication
- Difficulty expressing thoughts verbally (e.g., aphasia, dysphasia, apraxia, dyslexia)
- Difficulty forming sentences
- Difficulty forming words (e.g., aphonia, dyslalia, dysarthria)
- Difficulty in selective attending
- Difficulty in use of body expressions
- Difficulty in use of facial expressions
- Difficulty maintaining communication
- Difficulty speaking
- Difficulty verbalizing
- Disoriented to person
- Disoriented to place
- Disoriented to time
- Does not speak
- Dyspnea
- Inability to speak
- Inability to speak language of caregiver
- Inability to use body expressions
- Inappropriate verbalization
- Partial visual deficit
- Refusal to speak
- Slurred speech
- Stuttering
- Total visual deficit

Expected Outcomes

- Patient's self-care needs will be met by staff members.
- Patient and family members will express satisfaction with level of communication ability.
- Patient will maintain orientation.
- Patient will maintain effective level of communication.
- Patient will answer direct questions correctly.

Suggested NOC Outcomes

Cognition; Communication; Communication: Expressive; Communication: Receptive; Information Processing; Sensory Function Status

Interventions and Rationales

PCC
- Observe patient closely for cues to personal needs and desires, such as gestures, pointing to objects, looking at items, and pantomime *to enhance understanding*. Don't continually respond to gestures if the potential exists to improve speech *to avoid discouraging improvement*.

S
- Monitor and record changes in patient's speech pattern or level of orientation. *Changes may indicate improvement or deterioration of condition.*
- Speak slowly and distinctly in a normal tone when addressing patient, and stand where patient can see and hear you. *These actions promote comprehension and active participation.*
- Reorient patient to reality:
  - Call patient by name.
  - Tell patient your name.
  - Give patient background information (place, date, and time).

  - Use television or radio to augment orientation.
  - Use large calendars and reality orientation boards.

  These measures develop orientation skills through repetition and recognition of familiar objects.
- Use short, simple phrases and yes-or-no questions when patient is very frustrated *to reduce frustration.*
- Encourage attempts at communication and provide positive reinforcement *to aid comprehension.*
- PCC Allow ample time for a response. Don't answer questions yourself if patient has the ability to respond. *This improves patient's self-concept and reduces frustration.*
- Repeat or rephrase questions, if necessary, *to improve communication.* Don't pretend to understand if you don't *to avoid misunderstanding.*
- Remove distractions from the environment during attempts at communication. *Reduced distractions improve comprehension.* Use communication boards (including alphabet and some common words and pictures), if appropriate, *to aid comprehension.*
- Review diagnostic test results *to determine improvement or deterioration of the disease process.* Adjust the care plan accordingly.

Suggested NIC Interventions

Active Listening; Anxiety Reduction; Communication Enhancement: Hearing Deficit; Communication Enhancement: Speech Deficit; Energy Management; Learning Facilitation; Touch

Evaluations for Expected Outcomes

- Patient's needs are met by staff members.
- Patient and family members communicate at satisfactory level.
- Patient demonstrates orientation by consistently communicating thoughts to family and staff.
- Patient communicates effectively ____ times every 8 hours (specify).
- Patient correctly answers ____ direct questions (specify).

Documentation

- Patient's current level of communication, orientation, and satisfaction with communication efforts
- Observations of speech deficits, expressiveness and receptiveness, and ability to communicate
- Interventions carried out to promote effective communication
- Patient's response to nursing interventions
- Evaluations for expected outcomes

REFERENCES

Cheba, M., Żuralska, R., & Skrzypek-Czerko, M. (2014). Difficulties related to the communication with the patient with aphasia according to the nursing staff. *Journal of Neurological & Neurosurgical Nursing, 3*(2), 75–80. doi:10.15225/PNN.2014.3.2.4

Dark, J., & Sander, R. (2014). An overview of communication, movement and perception difficulties after stroke. *Nursing Older People, 26*(5), 32–37. doi:10.7748/nop.26.5.32.e567

Johnson, M., & Feng, L. (2014). Communication difficulty and relevant interventions in mild cognitive impairment: Implications for neuroplasticity. *Topics in Geriatric Rehabilitation, 30*(1), 18–34. doi:10.1097/TGR.0000000000000001

IMPAIRED VERBAL COMMUNICATION

related to physical barrier (e.g., tracheostomy, intubation)

Definition

Decreased, delayed, or absent ability to receive, process, transmit, and/or use a system of symbols

Assessment

- History of respiratory, neurologic, or musculoskeletal disorder or surgery
- Respiratory status, including dyspnea, use of accessory muscles, and respiratory pattern
- Neurologic status, including mental status (level of consciousness, orientation, cognition, memory, insight, and judgment) and speech (pattern, signing, and such communication aids as artificial larynx, computer-assisted speech device, pen and pencil, slate, picture board, and alphabet board)
- Musculoskeletal status, including range of motion and manual dexterity

Defining Characteristics

- Absence of eye contact
- Difficulty comprehending communication
- Difficulty expressing thoughts verbally (e.g., aphasia, dysphasia, apraxia, dyslexia)
- Difficulty forming sentences
- Difficulty forming words (e.g., aphonia, dyslalia, dysarthria)
- Difficulty in selective attending
- Difficulty in use of body expressions
- Difficulty in use of facial expressions
- Difficulty maintaining communication
- Difficulty speaking
- Difficulty verbalizing
- Disoriented to person
- Disoriented to place
- Disoriented to time
- Does not speak
- Dyspnea
- Inability to speak
- Inability to speak language of caregiver
- Inability to use body expressions
- Inappropriate verbalization
- Partial visual deficit
- Refusal to speak
- Slurred speech
- Stuttering
- Total visual deficit

Expected Outcomes

- Patient will communicate needs and desires without undue frustration.
- Patient will use alternate means of communication.
- Patient will demonstrate correct use of adaptive equipment.
- Patient will express plans to use appropriate resources to maximize communication skills.

Suggested NOC Outcomes

Client Satisfaction: Communication; Communication; Communication: Expressive; Communication: Receptive

Interventions and Rationales

- Maintain a consistent daily schedule of activities as much as possible. Observe patient closely for cues to needs and desires, such as gestures, pointing to or looking at objects, and pantomime, *to enhance understanding.*

- PCC • Obtain communication aids for patient's use, such as an alphabet board, slate, pen, paper, and picture board, *to provide alternative communication methods.*
- Use short, simple phrases and yes-or-no questions *to reduce frustration and anxiety.*
- PCC • Encourage communication attempts; allow time to select or write words or draw pictures *to reduce pressure and improve interaction with others.*
- Allow ample time for a response; don't answer questions for patient *to reduce frustration.*
- PCC • Consult with a speech therapist to suggest such communication aids as an artificial larynx. Assist with its use. *Appropriate early referral encourages the use of communication aids.*
- Demonstrate communication techniques, such as gestures, sign language, and eye blinking, to patient and family members *to develop alternative communication skills.*
- Assist patient in energy-conserving techniques *to allow maximum breath for speech or use of communication aids.*
- Use a tracheostomy plug *to facilitate speech,* if tolerated by patient.
- S • Provide patient with emergency call system (bell or call light), and respond to all calls immediately and in person. Place a sign over the intercom to alert all staff members of the need to respond quickly. *Prompt responses reduce patient's fear and anxiety.*
- PCC • Encourage attendance at a laryngectomy club or other appropriate support groups *to provide additional support.*

Suggested NIC Interventions

Active Listening; Anxiety Reduction; Communication Enhancement: Speech Deficit; Energy Management; Environmental Management; Learning Facilitation; Referral

Evaluations for Expected Outcomes

- Patient consistently communicates needs without frustration.
- Patient successfully uses alternate means of communication (specify).
- Patient uses adaptive equipment ____ times daily to improve communication (specify).
- Patient identifies and contacts appropriate support resources, such as speech therapist and laryngectomy club.

Documentation

- Patient's feelings about inability to communicate
- Observations of patient's attempts to communicate, response to and ability to use alternate communication means, and level of frustration or fatigue
- Patient's response to nursing interventions
- Patient's preferences in daily care activities, such as when to shave or bathe and what kind of razor to use
- Evaluations for expected outcomes

REFERENCES

Bird, J., & Parente, R. (2014). Recognition of nonverbal communication of emotion after traumatic brain injury. *Neurorehabilitation, 34*(1), 39–43. doi:10.3233/NRE-131006

Dark, J., & Sander, R. (2014). An overview of communication, movement and perception difficulties after stroke. *Nursing Older People, 26*(5), 32–37. doi:10.7748/nop.26.5.32.e567

Johnson, M., & Feng, L. (2014). Communication difficulty and relevant interventions in mild cognitive impairment: Implications for neuroplasticity. *Topics in Geriatric Rehabilitation, 30*(1), 18–34. doi:10.1097/TGR.0000000000000001

IMPAIRED WALKING

related to neuromuscular impairment

Definition

Limitation of independent movement within the environment on foot

Assessment

- Age
- Gender
- Vital signs
- History of stroke, spinal cord injury, head injury, multiple sclerosis, Guillain–Barré syndrome, or Parkinson's disease
- Medication history
- Musculoskeletal status, including coordination, gait, muscle size and strength, muscle tone, range of motion (ROM), and functional mobility as follows:
  0 = completely independent
  1 = requires use of equipment or device
  2 = requires help, supervision, or teaching from another person
  3 = requires help from another person and equipment or device
  4 = dependent; doesn't participate in activity
- Neurologic status, including level of consciousness, motor ability, and sensory ability
- Endurance level—for example, how far the patient can walk before tiring

Defining Characteristics

- Impaired ability to climb stairs
- Impaired ability to navigate curbs
- Impaired ability to walk on decline
- Impaired ability to walk on incline
- Impaired ability to walk on uneven surface
- Impaired ability to walk required distance

Expected Outcomes

- Patient won't exhibit complications associated with impaired walking, such as alteration in skin integrity, contractures, venous stasis, or thrombus formation.
- Patient will maintain or improve muscle strength and joint ROM.
- Patient will achieve highest level of ambulation possible (independence using wheelchair, ambulation with device, ambulation without device).
- Patient will maintain safety during ambulation.
- Patient will demonstrate ability to use equipment or devices safely.
- Patient will adapt to alteration in walking.
- Patient will participate in social and occupational activities.
- Patient will demonstrate understanding of specific interventions related to coping with alteration in walking.
- Patient will utilize community resources to promote and maintain highest level of mobility.

Suggested NOC Outcomes

Ambulation; Balance; Coordinated Movement; Endurance; Fall Prevention Behavior; Mobility; Safe Home Environment; Self-Care: Activities of Daily Living (ADLs)

Interventions and Rationales

- Perform ROM exercises for joints of affected limbs, unless contraindicated, at least once per shift. Progress from passive to active ROM, as tolerated, *to prevent joint contractures and muscle atrophy.*
- Make sure that patient maintains anatomically correct and functional body positioning. Encourage repositioning every 2 hours when patient is in bed. Establish a turning schedule for dependent patients. *Proper positioning relieves pressure, thereby preventing skin breakdown and fluid accumulation in dependent extremities.*
- Identify and record patient's level of independence using the functional mobility scale. Communicate the findings to the staff *to provide continuity and preserve documented level of independence.*
- Implement a preambulation program (e.g., turning in bed, sitting on the side of the bed, sitting up in a chair) *to increase independence and patient's self-esteem.*
- Monitor and record daily evidence of complications related to altered walking, such as contractures, venous stasis, skin breakdown, or thrombus formation. *Patient with a history of neuromuscular dysfunction is at risk for complications.*
- Follow the prescribed medical regimen to manage or prevent complications (e.g., administration of prophylactic heparin for venous thrombosis) *to promote patient's health and well-being.*
- Provide progressive ambulation up to the limits imposed by patient's condition *to maintain muscle tone and prevent complications associated with immobility.*
- PCC Refer patient to a physical therapist for development of a program to promote walking *to assist with rehabilitation of musculoskeletal deficits.*
- PCC Encourage attendance at physical therapy sessions and reinforce prescribed activities by using the same equipment, devices, and techniques used in therapy sessions. Request a written copy of patient's ambulation program to use as a reference. *These measures maintain continuity and help ensure patient's safety.*
- PCC Instruct patient and family members in ambulation techniques and measures *to prevent complications to help prepare patient and family for discharge.*
- Demonstrate ambulation regimen and note the date. Have patient and family members perform a return demonstration *to ensure continuity of care and use of proper technique.*
- PCC Assist in identifying resources, such as a community stroke program, sports associations for the disabled, or the National Multiple Sclerosis Society, *to promote patient's reintegration into the community.*

Suggested NIC Interventions

Energy Management; Exercise Promotion: Strength Training; Exercise Therapy: Ambulation; Self-Care Assistance

Evaluations for Expected Outcomes

- Patient doesn't exhibit complications associated with impaired walking, such as alteration in skin integrity, contractures, venous stasis, or thrombus formation.
- Patient maintains or improves muscle strength and joint ROM.

- Patient achieves highest level of ambulation possible (independence using wheelchair, ambulation with device, ambulation without device).
- Patient maintains safety during ambulation.
- Patient demonstrates ability to use equipment or devices safely.
- Patient adapts to alteration in walking.
- Patient participates in social and occupational activities.
- Patient demonstrates understanding of specific interventions related to coping with alteration in walking.
- Patient utilizes community resources to promote and maintain highest level of mobility.

Documentation

- Patient's ambulation status, presence of complications, and response to ambulation program
- Patient's statements regarding loss of ambulation ability, current ambulation ability, and goals set for improved ambulation ability
- Patient teaching
- Return demonstration of skills for carrying out ambulation program
- Patient's response to nursing interventions
- Evaluations for expected outcomes

REFERENCES

Brach, J. S., Lowry, K., Perera, S., Hornyak, V., Wert, D., Studenski, S. A., & VanSwearingen, J. M. (2015). Improving motor control in walking: A randomized clinical trial in older adults with subclinical walking difficulty. *Archives of Physical Medicine & Rehabilitation*, *96*(3), 388–394. doi:10.1016/j.apmr.2014.10.018

Eronen, J., Bonsdorff, M., Rantakokko, M., & Rantanen, T. (2014). Environmental facilitators for outdoor walking and development of walking difficulty in community-dwelling older adults. *European Journal of Aging*, *11*(1), 67–75. doi:10.1007/s10433-013-0283-7

Iskander, M. (2015). A woman with difficulty walking and multiple falls. *JAAPA: Journal of the American Academy of Physician Assistants (Lippincott Williams & Wilkins)*, *28*(5), 54–56. doi:10.1097/01.JAA.0000464281.30655.93

WANDERING

Definition

Meandering, aimless, or repetitive locomotion that exposes the individual to harm; frequently incongruent with boundaries, limits, or obstacles

Defining Characteristics

- Continuous movement from place to place
- Eloping behavior
- Frequent movement from place to place
- Fretful locomotion
- Haphazard locomotion
- Hyperactivity
- Impaired ability to locate landmarks in a familiar setting
- Locomotion into unauthorized spaces
- Locomotion resulting in getting lost
- Locomotion that cannot be easily dissuaded
- Long periods of locomotion without an apparent destination

- Pacing
- Periods of locomotion interspersed with periods of nonlocomotion (e.g., sitting, standing, sleeping)
- Persistent locomotion in search of something
- Scanning behavior
- Searching behavior
- Shadowing a caregiver's locomotion
- Trespassing

Assessment

- Age and gender
- Neurologic status, including level of consciousness, orientation, thought and speech, mood, affect, memory, visual and spatial ability, judgment and insight, psychomotor activity, and perceptions; recent behavior changes; lethargy, restlessness, short- or long-term memory loss, and sleep disturbance; and history of multiple infarctions, transient ischemic attacks, Parkinson's disease, cerebral infarctions, seizures, and alcohol or drug abuse
- Self-care status, including ability to perform instrumental or routine activities of daily living (ADLs)
- Musculoskeletal status, including range of motion (ROM); muscle size, strength, and tone; coordination; and functional mobility scale:
  0 = completely independent
  1 = requires use of equipment or device
  2 = requires help, supervision, or teaching from another person
  3 = requires help from another person and equipment or device
  4 = dependent; doesn't participate in activity

Expected Outcomes

- Patient will participate in physical or other __________ (specify) activities to minimize wandering behavior.
- Patient will ambulate safely.
- Patient will not have unplanned exits or elopements.
- Patient and the family will anticipate patient's wandering behavior or ambulation patterns and provide gratification before onset of wandering behavior.
- Patient and the family will identify factors that contribute to wandering behaviors.

Suggested NOC Outcomes

Elopement Occurrence; Elopement Propensity Risk; Safe Wandering; Personal Safety Behavior; Safe Home Environment; Ambulation

Interventions and Rationales

- Assess characteristics of wandering behavior, *to determine severity of problem and plan interventions.*
- Assess reasons for specific behavior problems *to determine possible triggers for wandering behaviors.*
- Determine how family members or partner handles wandering behavior *to provide a comprehensive database for planning care.*
- Assess patient's hobbies and previous social, leisure, and exercise activities and patterns *to assist in planning interventions.*

S
- Provide safe and structured daily routine (including regular exercise, walking, and ROM exercises) and *environment to decrease wandering behavior and minimize caregiver stress.*
- Avoid using physical or chemical restraints to control patient's wandering behavior. *Restraints may increase agitation, anxiety, sensory deprivation, falls, and wandering behavior.*
- Check patient for hunger, thirst, discomfort, or need for toileting. *These needs may precipitate wandering.*

PCC
- Instruct patient and/or family about the following:
  - Use dead bolt locks on doors and keep a key accessible for quick exit *to prevent unplanned exits and facilitate entrance and exit in emergency situations.*
  - Use fences and hedges around patios or yards and lock gates *to prevent unsafe exits.*
  - Install electronic devices with buzzers or bells *to alert others when door or window is open.*
- Encourage participation in activities (e.g., dancing) and simple household chores (e.g., raking leaves, folding laundry) *to reduce anxiety and restlessness.*

PCC
- Notify neighbors, local police department, and staff in retirement communities about patient's condition. Keep a list of neighbors' names and phone numbers handy. *Awareness by others can prevent patient from becoming lost or injured.*

PCC
- Utilize community resources, such as the Alzheimer's Association's Safe Return Program, *to assist in identification, location, and return of individuals with disorders characterized by wandering behaviors.*

Suggested NIC Interventions

Activity Therapy; Surveillance: Safety; Environmental Management: Safety; Home Maintenance Management; Elopement Precautions

Evaluations for Expected Outcomes

- Patient's participation in activities.
- Patient ambulatory efforts.
- Patient has no episodes of elopement.
- Patient performs ADLs to the extent possible.
- Patient and family members express an understanding of the causes of wandering.
- Patient and family members express knowledge of factors that lead to wandering.

Documentation

- Description of episodes of wandering
- Factors that precipitate and ameliorate episodes of wandering
- Teaching sessions and referrals
- Evaluations for expected outcomes

REFERENCES

Bantry White, E., & Montgomery, P. (2015). Dementia, walking outdoors and getting lost: Incidence, risk factors and consequences from dementia-related police missing person reports. *Aging & Mental Health, 19*(3), 224–230. doi:10.1080/13607863.2014.924091

Feldkamp, J. K. (2015). Implement safety measures to avoid resident elopements. *Caring For the Ages, 16*(5), 14–14.

Futrell, M., Devereaux Melillo, K., & Remington, R. (2014). Wandering. *Journal of Gerontological Nursing, 40*(11), 16–23. doi:10.3928/00989134-20140911-01

Sheth, H. S., Krueger, D., Bourdon, S., & Palmer, R. M. (2014). A new tool to assess risk of wandering in hospitalized patients. *Journal of Gerontological Nursing, 40*(3), 28–33. doi:10.3928/00989134-20140128-06

PART II

Adolescent Health

APPLYING EVIDENCE-BASED PRACTICE

The Question

What risk factors should be targeted when developing educational programs for teen sexuality?

Evidence-Based Resources

Centers for Disease Control and Prevention. (n.d.). *Schools play a key role in HIV/STD and teen pregnancy prevention*. Retrieved March 1, 2016, from http://www.cdc.gov/features/hivstdprevention/

Centers for Disease Control and Prevention. (2013). *MMWR weekly: Youth risk behavior surveillance—United States, 2013*. Retrieved from http://www.cdc.gov/mmwr/pdf/ss/ss6304.pdf

Danawi, H., Bryant, Z., & Hasbini, T. (2016). Targeting unintended teen pregnancy in the U.S. *International Journal of Childbirth Education*, *31*(1), 28–31.

Goesling, B., Colman, S., Trenholm, C., Terzian, M., & Moore, K. (2014). Programs to reduce teen pregnancy, sexually transmitted infections, and associated sexual risk behaviors: A systematic review. *Journal of Adolescent Health*, *54*(5), 499–507. doi:10.1016/j.jadohealth.2013.12.004

Helfrich, C. M., & McWey, L. M. (2014). Substance use and delinquency: High-risk behaviors as predictors of teen pregnancy among adolescents involved with the child welfare system. *Journal of Family Issues*, *35*(10), 1322–1338. doi:10.1177/0192513X13478917

Jackson, J. M., Seth, P., DiClemente, R. J., & Lin, A. (2015). Association of depressive symptoms and substance use with risky sexual behavior and sexually transmitted infections among African American female adolescents seeking sexual health care. *American Journal of Public Health*, *105*(10), 2137–2142. doi:10.2105/AJPH.2014.302493

Lee, Y. M., Cintron, A., & Kocher, S. (2014). Factors related to risky sexual behaviors and effective STI/ HIV and pregnancy intervention programs for African American adolescents. *Public Health Nursing*, *31*(5), 414–427. doi:10.1111/phn.12128

Negriff, S., Schneiderman, J. U., & Trickett, P. K. (2015). Child maltreatment and sexual risk behavior: Maltreatment types and gender differences. *Journal of Developmental & Behavioral Pediatrics*, *36*(9), 708–716. doi:10.1097/DBP.0000000000000204

New teen data—What it means for your practice. (2015). *Contraceptive Technology Update, 36*(10), 113–115.

The National Campaign to Prevent Teen Unplanned Pregnancy. (n.d.). *National and state data*. Retrieved March 1, 2016, from http://thenationalcampaign.org/data/landing

Pazol, K., Whiteman, M. K., Folger, S. G., Kourtis, A. P., Marchbanks, P. A., & Jamieson, D. J. (2015). Sporadic contraceptive use and nonuse: Age-specific prevalence and associated factors. *American Journal of Obstetrics & Gynecology, 212*(3), 324.e1–324.e8. doi:10.1016/j.ajog.2014.10.004

Evaluating the Evidence

Teen pregnancy rates in the United States have declined over the last two decades. In 2013, 47% of high school students reported being sexually active. Of those sexually active teens, 86% reported they used a method of contraception (Centers for Disease Control and Prevention [CDC], 2013; National Campaign, n.d.). Unfortunately, despite the growing use of contraceptives among teens, the United States continues to have higher rates of teen pregnancy, abortion, and sexually transmitted disease than do comparable countries (Goesling, Colman, Trenholm, Terzian, & Moore, 2014). Around half of all reported sexually transmitted infections (STIs) in the United States are adolescents aged 15 to 24 years (Jackson, Seth, DiClemente, & Lin, 2015). Because of the high incidence of STIs, it is beneficial to identify factors associated with high-risk behaviors in the adolescent population.

Several studies (Danawi, Bryant, & Hasbini, 2016; Jackson et al., 2015; Lee, Cintron, & Kocher, 2014; Negriff, Schneiderman, & Trickett, 2015) have examined the challenges adolescents experience that increase behaviors leading to increased risks of pregnancy and STIs over other age groups. As adolescents begin to lose support systems from structured environments, the outcomes are not always positive.

Social determinants of health affecting teen sexual behavior include poverty, education, social support networks, and living environment (Danawi et al., 2016). Lee et al. (2014) explored factors related to risky sexual behaviors of African American adolescents in a south Chicago, IL, community to determine which preventive strategies for reduction of STI/HIV transmission and pregnancy would be most effective. The study identified five factors that contribute to risky sexual behavior: substance use, gender roles, peer influence, parental involvement, and knowledge about sex and STIs. Relationships between substance use and depression (Jackson et al., 2015), substance use and sexual abuse (Negriff et al., 2015), and substance use and delinquency (Helfrich & McWey, 2014) have also been identified as factors.

Teens report the highest rate of contraceptive use; however, data indicate that use is sporadic. Two out of three teens report using at least one contraceptive method during their first sexual encounter ("Teen Data", 2015). Although 79% of females aged 15 to 19 years report using contraceptives regularly, contraceptive use is often abandoned due to difficulty of use, dissatisfaction, or difficulty finding a stable method for use over time. Teens may be vulnerable to higher risk of STIs and unwanted pregnancy while they search for a contraceptive method suited to their needs (Pazol et al., 2015).

Applying the Results and Making a Decision

The frequency of adolescent pregnancy and transmission of sexually transmitted disease is alarmingly high. The statistics compel that intervention programs aimed at adolescents must stay relevant with associated risk factors. Program content should also include education about contraceptives and safe sexual practices. With teens aged 15 to 24 years comprising around half of all reported STIs in the United States, the statistical results are clear that current interventions must be updated to improve the future health of adolescents.

Reevaluating Process and Identifying Areas for Improvement

Reduction in the rate of STIs in the adolescent population will require a multifaceted approach. Education for the prevention of STI will have to be initiated in the areas of highest structured support: clinics, physician offices, and schools. According to the CDC (n.d.), "research shows that well-designed, well-implemented school-based HIV/STD prevention programs can significantly reduce sexual risk behaviors among students" (para. 5). With formally structured programs implemented by well-qualified instructors, this initiative could show significant success.

INTRODUCTION

This section focuses on providing nursing care for adolescent patients. The tremendous physiologic and cognitive changes that occur between ages 10 and 18 are commonly accompanied by overpowering emotional turmoil.

Because the adolescent patient commonly struggles with issues of independence and identity, be particularly sensitive to individual needs when taking the health history. Be alert to language; adolescents particularly resent being "talked down to." Although some adolescents prize their independence, others still need parental support during physical examination and history taking. If possible, perform at least part of the nursing assessment in private to allow for open discussion of highly personal issues such as sexuality.

Many adolescents feel invulnerable, placing them at high risk of health problems such as drug and alcohol abuse, sexually transmitted diseases, and trauma. When talking with the adolescent patient, explore feelings of personal invulnerability and discuss potential consequences.

Interventions should foster independence and promote self-esteem while helping the adolescent obtain needed support from parents and health care providers. Care plans included in the Adult Health and Child Health sections of this manual may also be useful. Use every opportunity to teach the adolescent patient about health promotion. Increased knowledge allows the adolescent to assume responsibility for self-care.

Adolescence can also be a trying time for families. In addition to asking direct questions about family relationships, be alert to nonverbal and verbal indications of conflict. Also, be aware that parents may have needs while struggling with their adolescent's newly found independence.

DISTURBED BODY IMAGE

related to an eating disorder

Definition

Confusion in mental picture of one's physical self

Assessment

- Age
- Gender
- Health history, including previous eating disorders; dieting; physical, emotional, or sexual abuse; and episodes of emesis and self-induced emesis
- History of weight loss or gain of 2 lb/week
- Exercise pattern, including type and duration
- Cardiovascular status, including skin color and temperature, heart rate and rhythm, blood pressure, and complete blood count
- Nutritional status, including daily food intake, food likes and dislikes, meal preparation, and knowledge of dietary requirements; height and weight (and weight fluctuations) over past year; serum albumin, lymphocyte, and electrolyte levels; and signs of malnutrition or dehydration
- Psychological status, including expressions of need for control or perceived loss of self-control, behavioral changes, expressions of helplessness, recent emotional crisis, stress, and body image

- Perception of ideal feminine or masculine form
- Family status, including role performance, perception of role within family, and attitudes and perceptions related to food, body image, success, and control
- Use of diuretics and laxatives
- Medication use, either prescription or over the counter

Defining Characteristics

- Absence of body part
- Alteration in body function
- Alteration in body structure
- Alteration in view of one's body (e.g., appearance, structure, function)
- Avoids looking at one's body
- Avoids touching one's body
- Behavior of acknowledging one's body
- Behavior of monitoring one's body
- Change in ability to estimate spatial relationship of body to environment
- Change in lifestyle
- Change in social involvement
- Depersonalization of body part by use of impersonal pronouns
- Emphasis on remaining strengths
- Extension of body boundary (e.g., includes external object)
- Fear of reaction by others
- Focus on past appearance
- Focus on past function
- Heightened achievement
- Hiding of body part
- Negative feeling about body
- Nonverbal response to change in body (e.g., appearance, structure, function)
- Overexposure of body part
- Perceptions that reflect an altered view of one's body appearance
- Personalization of body part by name
- Personalization of loss by name
- Preoccupation with change
- Preoccupation with loss
- Refusal to acknowledge change
- Trauma to nonfunctioning body part

Expected Outcomes

- Adolescent will
  - comply with prescribed treatment;
  - express feelings associated with food, exercise, weight loss, and medical condition;
  - describe perception of personal daily caloric needs;
  - express understanding that current eating and exercise patterns are self-destructive;
  - consume appropriate number of calories each day;
  - ask for help in controlling destructive behavior;
  - participate in decisions about care and participate in support group for people with eating disorders;
  - express insight into reasons behind current eating patterns and other self-destructive behaviors;

- learn and implement new coping behaviors;
- express positive feelings about self;
- express satisfaction with parental involvement in care.

Suggested NOC Outcomes

Body Image; Child Development: Adolescence; Nutritional Status; Psychosocial Adjustment: Life Change; Self-Esteem; Weight: Body Mass

Interventions and Rationales

- Implement the adolescent's prescribed therapy *to help restore health and body function.*
- Monitor and record the adolescent's vital signs, weight, and electrolyte levels *to detect abnormal values and prevent complications.*
- Obtain a referral for dietary consultation *to identify caloric intake, necessary diet modifications, and goals for weight gain and stabilization.*
- PCC Obtain a referral for psychiatric evaluation *to identify problems related to altered body image, poor self-esteem, and inappropriate coping.*
- Convey a positive, caring attitude to the adolescent, and take steps to ensure continuity of care throughout treatment *to ensure safety and foster a trusting therapeutic relationship.*
- PCC Encourage the adolescent to participate in self-care and, as appropriate, to make decisions about therapy *to foster a sense of control and involvement in restoring health.*
- Express acceptance of the adolescent as a person and provide reassurance of the ability to overcome problems *to validate self-perception and enhance confidence.*
- PCC Maintain communication throughout the adolescent's course of treatment *to assess coping mechanisms and level of self-esteem.*
- PCC Encourage the adolescent to express feelings about self, eating, exercise, hospitalization, and medical condition *to correct misconceptions, help the adolescent clarify thoughts, and reinforce realistic self-appraisal.*
- Reinforce appropriate behaviors *to encourage the adolescent to comply with therapy and to participate in care.*
- Use behavior modification strategies consistently *to enable the adolescent to predict consequences of behavior.*
- Avoid using coercive techniques to make the adolescent participate in care or adhere to rules. *Use of coercion may encourage the adolescent to view manipulative behavior as acceptable.*
- S Monitor food consumption and record intake *to ensure that the adolescent consumes prescribed calories.*
- Monitor the adolescent in the bathroom *to detect episodes of purging.*
- Without conveying an attitude of distrust, watch for signs of noncompliance with the medical regimen. Emphasize that prescribed caloric intake is necessary to maintain health and it won't lead to obesity. *This promotes early detection of self-destructive behavior and may improve the adolescent's sense of control.*
- Report progress to the adolescent throughout hospitalization *to increase motivation and awareness of achievements.*
- Assist in identifying positive aspects of adolescent's appearance *to improve self-esteem by correcting distorted perceptions about body image.*
- Help direct the adolescent's need for control away from body image and eating behaviors by encouraging participation in appropriate diversional activities *to channel energies into new areas in which the adolescent can take pride.*
- PCC Encourage the adolescent's participation in group discussions with peers who also have eating disorders *to foster insight and group support.*

- Help the adolescent identify appropriate coping strategies. Discuss previously effective strategies *to help the adolescent substitute them for maladaptive ones.*
- Encourage parents to demonstrate emotional support for the adolescent throughout the course of treatment *to strengthen the family support system.*
- PCC Encourage parents to participate in a support group with other parents of children with eating disorders *to provide a forum for expressing feelings and obtaining support from individuals who can understand their concerns.*
- Teach parents how to detect signs that their child may be relapsing into self-destructive behaviors *to help them identify the need for early assistance and enhance their confidence in their ability to protect their child from harm.*

Suggested NIC Interventions

Active Listening; Body Image Enhancement; Coping Enhancement; Counseling; Developmental Enhancement: Adolescent; Parent Education: Adolescent; Support Group; Therapy Group

Evaluations for Expected Outcomes

- Adolescent complies with prescribed treatment regimen.
- Adolescent expresses feelings associated with food, exercise, weight loss, and medical condition.
- Adolescent describes perception of personal daily caloric needs.
- Adolescent expresses understanding that current eating and exercise patterns are self-destructive.
- Adolescent consumes appropriate number of calories each day.
- Adolescent asks for help in controlling destructive behavior.
- Adolescent participates in decisions related to care and treatment.
- Adolescent participates in support group for people with eating disorders.
- Adolescent expresses insight into reasons behind eating patterns and other self-destructive behaviors.
- Adolescent learns and implements new coping behaviors.
- Adolescent expresses positive feelings about self.
- Adolescent expresses satisfaction with parental involvement in care.

Documentation

- Vital signs
- Weight (recorded daily or weekly according to facility's protocol)
- Amount of food consumed at each meal
- Adolescent's description of himself or herself
- Observations of rituals related to food and exercise
- Adolescent's participation in and response to support group
- Observations of self-destructive behaviors, such as forced emesis or use of laxatives or diuretics
- Observations of manipulative behaviors
- Coping mechanisms
- Exercise patterns
- Behavior modification techniques used by caregivers
- Adolescent's response to treatment protocol
- Adolescent's response to nursing interventions

- Evidence of changes in adolescent's self-perception
- Evaluations for expected outcomes

REFERENCES

Alegría, C. A., & Larsen, B. (2015). 'That's who I am: A fat person in a thin body': Weight loss, negative self-evaluation, and mitigating strategies following weight loss surgery. *Journal of the American Association of Nurse Practitioners*, *27*(3), 137–144. doi:10.1002/2327-6924.12158

Černelič-Bizjak, M., & Jenko-Pražnikar, Z. (2014). Impact of negative cognitions about body image on inflammatory status in relation to health. *Psychology & Health*, *29*(3), 264–278. doi:10.1080/08870446.2013.844807

Jones, M., Kass, A. E., Trockel, M., Glass, A. I., Wilfley, D. E., & Taylor, C. B. (2014). A population-wide screening and tailored intervention platform for eating disorders on college campuses: The healthy body image program. *Journal of American College Health*, *62*(5), 351–356. doi:10.1080/07448481.2014.901330

DECISIONAL CONFLICT

related to conflict with moral obligation; inexperience with decision making

Definition

Uncertainty about course of action to be taken when choice among competing actions involves risk, loss, or challenge to values and beliefs

Assessment

- Age
- Gender
- Developmental stage, including physical maturity, cognition, beliefs, values, and ethics
- Family system, including nuclear family, extended family, birth order, family roles, and evidence of conflict
- History of sexual experiences, including experimentation, trauma, and other experiences
- Psychological status, including level of function, coping mechanisms, support systems, self-image, self-esteem, and attitude toward physical appearance
- Sociocultural status, including level of education, ethnicity, and religious affiliation
- Sexual orientation

Defining Characteristics

- Delay in decision making
- Distress while attempting a decision
- Physical sign of distress (e.g., increase in heart rate, restlessness)
- Physical sign of tension
- Questioning of moral principle while attempting a decision
- Questioning of moral rule while attempting a decision
- Questioning of moral values while attempting a decision
- Questioning of personal beliefs while attempting a decision
- Questioning of personal values while attempting a decision
- Recognizes undesired consequences of actions being considered
- Self-focused
- Uncertainty about choices
- Vacillating among choices

Expected Outcomes

- Adolescent will express feelings about morals and decision making.
- Adolescent will discuss conflicts between personal values and social pressures.
- Adolescent will identify desirable and undesirable consequences of undesired activity.
- Adolescent will describe family conflicts and will explore their potential effect on sexual conduct.
- Adolescent will accept help from parents, other family members, friends, and health professionals.
- Adolescent will report confidence in choosing behavior consistent with personal values.

Suggested NOC Outcomes

Coping; Decision-Making; Information Processing; Participation in Health Care Decisions; Personal Autonomy

Interventions and Rationales

- Visit the adolescent frequently, and encourage frequent visits by family members *to promote a trusting therapeutic relationship and ease anxiety and fears.*
- Encourage expressions of feelings about social patterns *to improve recognition of feelings and foster open discussion.*
- Assess the adolescent's knowledge of sex and sexuality. Discuss sexual behavior and its potential consequences. Provide information about safer sex practices, birth control, and abstinence. *Correct information about sexual practices reduces the adolescent's confusion about whether to be sexually active.*
- Listen attentively and remain nonjudgmental as the adolescent describes personal fears, values, and desires. *Nonjudgmental, active listening demonstrates your unconditional positive regard for the adolescent.*
- Provide guidance as the adolescent explores options for alternate behaviors *to promote confidence in decision-making capabilities.*
- Discuss peer pressure. Ask if the adolescent feels strong social. Ask about other ways peers exert influence and explore ways of coping with peer pressure. *The adolescent must learn to deal with peer pressure.*
- Discuss family conflicts. Ask the adolescent if troubled family relationships are pushing him or her to become sexually active or participate in undesirable activity. *The adolescent may seek in sexual relationships love or attention in undesirable behavior the adolescent doesn't receive from family members.*
- PCC Respect the adolescent's right to make choices based on personal values, desires, religious beliefs, cultural norms, and sexual preference *to foster autonomy and self-confidence.*
- PCC Help the adolescent identify a support network (friends, family, community services, and church or synagogue groups), and encourage their use in decision making *to help the adolescent make decisions and resolve conflicts in an emotionally supportive environment.*

Suggested NIC Interventions

Counseling; Decision-Making Support; Mutual Goal Setting; Self-Responsibility Facilitation; Teaching: Individual

Evaluations for Expected Outcomes

- Adolescent expresses feelings related to morals and decision making.
- Adolescent describes conflicts between personal values and social pressure.
- Adolescent expresses increased understanding of options regarding undesired activity and their potential consequences.
- Adolescent discusses possible influences, including peer pressure and conflicts with family, on decision to be sexually active.
- Adolescent identifies support network and uses it to aid decision making.
- Adolescent reports feeling more comfortable with ability to make decisions regarding sexuality and sexual activity.

Documentation

- Adolescent's statements indicating conflict over decision about whether to be sexually active
- Adolescent's cognitive, emotional, and behavioral functioning
- Adolescent's knowledge of birth control and safer sex practices
- Nursing interventions to help adolescent make choices regarding sexuality and sexual conflict
- Adolescent's response to interventions
- Evaluations for expected outcomes

REFERENCES

Callister, M., Coyne, S. M., Stern, L. A., Stockdale, L., Miller, M. J., & Wells, B. M. (2012). A content analysis of the prevalence and portrayal of sexual activity in adolescent literature. *Journal of Sex Research*, *49*(5), 477–486. doi:10.1080/00224499.2011.572306

Jenkins, M. (2015). A concept analysis of self-efficacy and adolescent sexual risk-taking behavior. *Nursing Forum*, *50*(1), 31–36. doi:10.1111/nuf.12070

Ong, J., Wong, W., Lee, A., Holroyd, E., & Huang, S. Y. (2013). Sexual activity and adolescent health risk behaviours amongst high school students in three ethnic Chinese urban populations. *Journal of Clinical Nursing*, *22*(23/24), 3270–3279. doi:10.1111/jocn.12267

Whitfield, C., Jomeen, J., Hayter, M., & Gardiner, E. (2013). Sexual health information seeking: A survey of adolescent practices. *Journal of Clinical Nursing*, *22*(23/24), 3259–3269. doi:10.1111/jocn.12192

DECISIONAL CONFLICT

related to unclear personal beliefs; unclear personal values

Definition

Uncertainty about course of action to be taken when choice among competing actions involves risk, loss, or challenge to values and beliefs

Assessment

- Age
- Physical maturity
- Sociocultural factors, including level of education, financial status, and ethnic group
- Family history, including family roles, coping patterns, family's ability to meet adolescent's physical and emotional needs, and history of substance abuse in family members

- Level of functioning (cognitive, emotional, and behavioral)
- Coping mechanisms
- Available support systems
- Evidence of drug use, including drug toxicology screening, urinalysis, personality changes, and social withdrawal

Defining Characteristics

- Delay in decision making
- Distress while attempting a decision
- Physical sign of distress (e.g., increase in heart rate, restlessness)
- Physical sign of tension
- Questioning of moral principle while attempting a decision
- Questioning of moral rule while attempting a decision
- Questioning of moral values while attempting a decision
- Questioning of personal beliefs while attempting a decision
- Questioning of personal values while attempting a decision
- Recognizes undesired consequences of actions being considered
- Self-focused
- Uncertainty about choices
- Vacillating among choices

Expected Outcomes

- Adolescent will discuss conflict.
- Adolescent will describe conflict between personal values and options and external value systems (parental, societal, peer, and legal).
- Adolescent will identify perceived desirable and undesirable consequences.
- Adolescent will accept assistance from parents, other family members, friends, and health care providers.
- Adolescent will report increased comfort with making choices that are consistent with personal values.

Suggested NOC Outcomes

Decision-Making; Family Functioning; Personal Autonomy; Information Processing; Participation in Health Care Decisions

Interventions and Rationales

- Visit the adolescent frequently, scheduling a specific amount of time each day, *to promote trust and provide time when the adolescent can discuss feelings confidentially.*
- Make the adolescent aware that you're willing to discuss all topics, including substance use. Assure the adolescent that all information will be kept confidential *to encourage honest discussion of concerns.*
- Encourage the adolescent to explore feelings related to drug use, school, family, friends, and other vital topics. Remain nonjudgmental and be willing to listen to the adolescent's values, beliefs, and concerns *to demonstrate that you regard the adolescent as a worthwhile person with valid values and beliefs.*
- Ask the adolescent to describe family and home life *to assess for family conflict that may be creating emotional distress.* Provide referrals for family counseling if needed.

- Ask the adolescent about peer pressure. Explore ways of coping with peer pressure. *The adolescent must learn to deal with peer pressure.*
- Discuss the adolescent's self-esteem, and explore ways of building self-esteem *to strengthen the adolescent's ability to deal with peer pressure.*
- PCC Help the adolescent explore alternative recreational activities, such as sports, art, music, community service, or participation in church or synagogue groups, *to help develop alternatives to substance use.*
- Teach the adolescent about the health and legal consequences of substance abuse. *Accurate information will help the adolescent make informed, rational decisions.*
- PCC Encourage the adolescent to identify and use a support network (family, friends, clinics, school nurse, or other health care providers). *A support network can help the adolescent make decisions and resolve conflicts in an emotionally supportive environment.*
- PCC Refer the adolescent for long-term counseling if necessary. *Long-standing emotional conflicts may require in-depth intervention.*

Suggested NIC Interventions

Counseling; Decision-Making Support; Learning Facilitation; Patient Contracting; Support System Enhancement

Evaluations for Expected Outcomes

- Adolescent discusses conflict over decision-making process.
- Adolescent discusses peer pressure, family conflict, or other factors that may be influencing undesirable behaviors.
- Adolescent identifies health and legal consequences of drug use.
- Adolescent identifies available sources of emotional support and requests help, if needed.
- Adolescent reports increased self-esteem and ability to deal with peer pressure.

Documentation

- Evidence of drug use
- Adolescent's stated feelings about drug use
- Adolescent's level of cognitive, emotional, and behavioral functioning
- Interventions performed to help adolescent make choices about drug use
- Adolescent's response to interventions
- Evaluations for expected outcomes

REFERENCES

Atilola, O., Stevanovic, D., Balhara, Y. S., Avicenna, M., Kandemir, H., Knez, R., . . . Vostanis, P. (2014). Role of personal and family factors in alcohol and substance use among adolescents: An international study with focus on developing countries. *Journal of Psychiatric & Mental Health Nursing*, *21*(7), 609–617. doi:10.1111/jpm.12133

Lamont, A., Woodlief, D., & Malone, P. (2014). Predicting high-risk versus higher-risk substance use during late adolescence from early adolescent risk factors using latent class analysis. *Addiction Research & Theory*, *22*(1), 78–89.

Roy, É., Nolin, M., Traoré, I., Leclerc, P., & Vasiliadis, H. (2015). Nonmedical use of prescription medication among adolescents using drugs in Quebec. *Canadian Journal of Psychiatry*, *60*(12), 556–563.

INEFFECTIVE HEALTH MAINTENANCE

related to impaired decision making

Definition

Inability to identify, manage, and/or seek out help to maintain health

Assessment

- Age
- Gender
- Developmental stage, including cognitive ability and physical maturity
- Level of knowledge about type 1 diabetes mellitus, routine health practices, preventive needs and safety measures, and treatment and follow-up
- Level of motivation to perform self-care
- Current health status, including height, weight, recent illnesses, and adolescent's perception of personal health status
- Social status, including lifestyle, activity level, sports, interests, and socioeconomic status
- Family health history, including history of diabetes mellitus

Defining Characteristics

- Absence of adaptive behaviors to environmental changes
- Absence of interest in improving health behaviors
- Inability to take responsibility for meeting basic health practices
- Insufficient knowledge about basic health practices
- Insufficient social support
- Pattern of lack of health-seeking behavior

Expected Outcomes

- Adolescent will describe feelings about self-management disease.
- Adolescent will describe disease process.
- Adolescent will describe influence of peer pressure on health care practices.
- Adolescent will describe proper techniques for managing signs and symptoms of disease.
- Adolescent will demonstrate ability to perform self-care activities, such as properly administering medications and choosing appropriate foods.
- Adolescent won't exhibit signs or symptoms of complications.

Suggested NOC Outcomes

Health Beliefs: Perceived Resources; Health-Promoting Behavior; Health-Seeking Behavior; Knowledge: Health Behavior; Knowledge: Treatment Regimen; Risk Detection; Symptom Control

Interventions and Rationales

- Evaluate the adolescent's understanding of disease and attitude about the need to manage it. *This will help you determine which teaching interventions to use.*

- Correct any misconceptions about disease and the therapeutic regimen. Use teaching materials appropriate for the adolescent's age *to increase knowledge and instill confidence in management ability.*
- Discuss peer pressure. Ask the adolescent if social pressure contributes to ignoring diet or avoiding self-administering medications. Ask if the adolescent feels embarrassed about the eating disorder. Explore ways of coping with peer pressure. *The adolescent must learn to deal with peer pressure.*
- Observe as the adolescent performs self-care activities *to assess skills and overall progress.*
- Teach the adolescent how to interpret test results and correlate these values with the degree of disease control *to increase autonomy and decision-making skills.*
- Provide written materials that cover each teaching topic. *These materials help reinforce learning and can refresh the adolescent's memory later.*
- Describe resources available to help the adolescent manage the disorder. Consider arranging a visit with the other members of the health care team *to reinforce teaching.*
- PCC Work with the adolescent to develop an exercise plan *to promote health.* The plan should identify a support person capable of assisting during an emergency. *This ensures the adolescent's safety while allowing participation in activities.*
- Discuss how to manage disease during illness. Also, explain that fever, nausea, vomiting, and diarrhea require modifications in the prescribed diet, such as substituting juice for raw fruits. Teach the adolescent to check over-the-counter medications, such as cold remedies, for sugar content and to avoid products high in sugar. Explain the importance of following the prescribed regimen. *These measures help provide a sense of control, ensure safety, and prevent complications.*
- S Teach the adolescent to recognize signs and symptoms that must be reported to the health care provider *to improve management skills and ensure safety.*
- S Discuss possible complications. *Understanding possible major complications may encourage the adolescent to adhere to the prescribed regimen.*
- PCC Encourage the adolescent to contact a support group *to provide peer support.*

Suggested NIC Interventions

Health Education; Patient Contracting; Self-Modification Assistance; Self-Responsibility Facilitation; Support System Enhancement; Teaching: Disease Process

Evaluations for Expected Outcomes

- Adolescent expresses feelings about self-management of disease.
- Adolescent accurately describes disease process.
- Adolescent discusses influence of peer pressure on health care practices.
- Adolescent demonstrates techniques for managing signs and symptoms of disease.
- Adolescent demonstrates proficiency in self-care activities, including administering medications and selecting appropriate foods.
- Adolescent doesn't exhibit signs or symptoms of complications.

Documentation

- Adolescent's statements that indicate understanding of disease, health-promoting activities, management techniques during exercise and illness, and necessary self-care skills
- Adolescent's statements indicating disregard for consequences of failing to properly manage disease

- Adolescent's response to interventions and teaching
- Literature provided to adolescent about managing the disorder
- Observations of adolescent's demonstrations of self-care techniques
- Referrals to community resources or hospital services
- Evaluations for expected outcomes

REFERENCES

Larson, N., Davey, C. S., Coombes, B., Caspi, C., Kubik, M. Y., & Nanney, M. S. (2014). Food and beverage promotions in Minnesota secondary schools: Secular changes, correlates, and associations with adolescents' dietary behaviors. *Journal of School Health, 84*(12), 777–785. doi:10.1111/josh.12209

Melnyk, B., Kelly, S., Jacobson, D., Arcoleo, K., & Shaibi, G. (2014). Improving physical activity, mental health outcomes, and academic retention in college students with freshman 5 to thrive: COPE/Healthy lifestyles. *Journal of the American Association of Nurse Practitioners, 26*(6), 314–322. doi:10.1002/2327-6924.12037

Viggiano, A., Viggiano, E., Costanzo, A., Viggiano, A., Andreozzi, E., Romano, V., . . . Amaro, S. (2015). Kaledo, a board game for nutrition education of children and adolescents at school: Cluster randomized controlled trial of healthy lifestyle promotion. *European Journal of Pediatrics, 174*(2), 217–228. doi:10.1007/s00431-014-2381-8

RISK FOR POISONING

Definition

Vulnerable to accidental exposure to, or ingestion of, drugs or dangerous products in sufficient doses, which may compromise health

Assessment

- Age
- Gender
- Developmental stage, including cognitive ability and physical maturity
- Medication history (prescription and over the counter)
- Physical status, including evidence or history of renal or hepatic impairment, eating disorders, or substance abuse
- Family status, including living arrangement, family dynamics, history or current evidence of substance abuse, and financial status
- Social status, including peer group and related social pressures and level of activity
- Knowledge of risks associated with use of drugs, alcohol, or other potentially hazardous substances (such as fumes from glue, nitrous oxide propellants, or lighter fuel gases)
- Psychological status, including evidence of depression or depressive disorder, feelings of isolation, history of attempted suicide, and level of self-esteem
- Results of laboratory tests

Risk Factors

External

- Access to dangerous product
- Access to illicit drugs potentially contaminated by poisonous additives
- Access to large supply of pharmaceutical agents in house
- Access to pharmaceutical agent

Internal

- Alteration in cognitive functioning
- Emotional disturbance
- Inadequate precautions against poisoning
- Insufficient knowledge of pharmacologic agents
- Insufficient knowledge of poisoning prevention
- Occupational setting without adequate safeguards
- Reduced vision

Expected Outcomes

- Adolescent will express understanding of harmful and potentially lethal effects of substance abuse.
- Adolescent will remain free from toxicity and other injuries during hospital stay.
- Adolescent will identify stressors and feelings that precipitate episodes of substance abuse.
- Adolescent will demonstrate two or more constructive techniques for coping with stressors.
- Adolescent will describe prescribed medication regimen, including dosage and administration schedule, and will demonstrate compliance.
- Adolescent will describe available community resources and will express intention to contact them.

Suggested NOC Outcomes

Family Physical Environment; Personal Safety Behavior; Risk Control; Risk Control: Drug Use; Safe Home Environment

Interventions and Rationales

- S Follow a medical regimen to treat toxicity or other injury caused by substance abuse *to ensure the adolescent's safety and promote recovery.*
- Teach the adolescent about the harmful and potentially lethal effects of abusing drugs, alcohol, or other dangerous substances *to enhance knowledge and foster better informed decisions*. Provide appropriate written materials. *Written materials reinforce teaching and allow review after discharge.*
- PCC Help the adolescent identify stressors, such as depression, peer pressure, or family dysfunction, that may precipitate substance abuse *to provide a basis for developing strategies to prevent future episodes.*
- Describe available community resources to help prevent or treat substance abuse. *Support services and groups can provide the adolescent with safe settings in which to explore problems and feelings and develop adaptive methods of coping.*
- S If medication is prescribed for the adolescent, explain the reason for the medication. Discuss administration techniques, schedule, dosage, cautions, and possible adverse effects *to promote compliance with the medication regimen.*

Suggested NIC Interventions

Environmental Risk Protection; Health Education; Substance Use Prevention; Surveillance: Safety

Evaluations for Expected Outcomes

- Adolescent describes harmful and potentially lethal effects of substance abuse.
- Adolescent remains free from toxicity caused by use of drugs, alcohol, or other hazardous substances.
- Adolescent describes stressors and feelings that precipitate episodes of substance abuse.
- Adolescent demonstrates two or more constructive techniques for coping with such stressors as depression, peer pressure, and family dysfunction.
- Adolescent describes prescribed medication regimen and demonstrates compliance.
- Adolescent describes available community resources and expresses intention to contact appropriate support services.

Documentation

- Interventions to treat toxicity or other injury
- Factors that increase adolescent's risk of drug toxicity
- Knowledge deficits and learning objectives
- Teaching topics, materials, and methods
- Adolescent's response to nursing interventions
- Indications that adolescent is using adaptive techniques to cope with stress, anxiety, peer pressure, or dysfunctional family
- Referrals to community resources or professionals for ongoing counseling
- Evaluations for expected outcomes

REFERENCES

Coalition addresses ADHD meds misuse among college students. (2015). *Brown University Child & Adolescent Behavior Letter, 31*(9), 3.

Houle, K. M., & Simonian, S. J. (2014). Adolescent swimmers: Breathing complaints and prescription asthma medication use and misuse. *Children's Health Care, 43*(2), 96–109. doi:10.1080/02739615.2013.867787

Kaye, S., Darke, S., & Torok, M. (2014). Diversion and misuse of pharmaceutical stimulants among illicit drug users. *Addiction Research & Theory, 22*(2), 109–116. doi:10.3109/16066359.2013.779677

Knopf, A. (2015). Study: Peak age for initiating prescription stimulant abuse is 16–19. *Alcoholism & Drug Abuse Weekly, 27*(26), 6. doi:10.1002/adaw.20480

RISK FOR CAREGIVER ROLE STRAIN

Definition

Vulnerable to difficulty in performing the family/significant other caregiver role, which may compromise health

Assessment

- Adolescent caregiver's physical and mental status, including age, sex, and developmental stage; level of cognitive functioning; emotional functioning; and self-care abilities
- Care recipient's physical and mental status, including age, sex, illness, self-care limitations, mobility limitations, level of cognitive functioning, and relationship to adolescent (parent, sibling, or other)
- Family status, including role performance and perception of role within family
- Available resources, including finances, emotional support system, community services, and health-related services, such as geriatric day care and home health nursing assistants

- Home environment, including structural barriers, layout of home, need for medical equipment or devices, and availability of transportation
- Cultural, ethnic, and religious background
- Perceived and actual obligations of adolescent
- Effect of caregiver responsibilities on adolescent
- Adolescent's coping skills, problem-solving abilities, and ability to participate in hobbies and preferred activities

Risk Factors

- Alteration in cognitive functioning in care receiver
- Care receiver discharged home with significant needs
- Care receiver exhibits bizarre behavior
- Care receiver exhibits deviant behavior
- Caregiver health impairment
- Caregiver isolation
- Caregiver not developmentally ready for caregiver role
- Caregiver's competing role commitments
- Caregiving task complexity
- Codependency
- Congenital disorder
- Developmental delay
- Developmental delay of caregiver
- Excessive caregiving activities
- Exposure to violence
- Extended duration of caregiving required
- Family isolation
- Female caregiver
- Illness severity of care receiver
- Inadequate physical environment for providing care
- Ineffective caregiver coping pattern
- Ineffective family adaptation
- Inexperience with caregiving
- Instability in care receiver's health
- Insufficient caregiver recreation
- Insufficient respite for caregiver
- Partner as caregiver
- Pattern of family dysfunction prior to the caregiving situation
- Pattern of ineffective relationship between caregiver and care receiver
- Prematurity
- Presence of abuse (e.g., physical, psychological, sexual)
- Psychological disorder in caregiver
- Stressors
- Substance abuse
- Unpredictability of illness trajectory

Expected Outcomes

- Adolescent will identify current stressors.
- Adolescent will identify and implement adaptive coping strategies.
- Adolescent will identify personal developmental needs and tasks.

- Adolescent will contact sources of support to help provide care.
- Adolescent will allot time each day for respite, recreation, and personal developmental activities.
- Adolescent will report reduced stress related to caregiver duties.

Suggested NOC Outcomes

Caregiver Emotional Health; Caregiver Home Care Readiness; Caregiver Lifestyle Disruption; Caregiver–Patient Relationship; Caregiver Physical Health; Caregiver Stressors; Stress Level

Interventions and Rationales

- Assess developmental stage and needs of the adolescent caregiver *to provide a basis for developing interventions that reduce caregiver role strain. During adolescence, individuals begin establishing their identity by trying various roles without assuming complete responsibility for them. The imposed role of caregiver impedes this developmental task.*
- PCC Help the adolescent identify current stressors. Discuss how the adolescent's responsibility to act as a caregiver places limits on lifestyle *to evaluate the degree of caregiver role strain.*
- PCC Encourage the adolescent to discuss coping skills used previously *to reinforce confidence in ability to manage the current situation and explore new ways to apply coping strategies.*
- PCC Help the adolescent identify informal sources of support, such as family members, support groups, or church groups that can help with caregiver tasks, *to provide opportunities for respite from caregiver activities.*
- Teach the adolescent about formal sources of support, such as home health care agencies, social workers, physicians, clinics, and day care centers, *to allow the adolescent to fulfill other obligations such as attending school.*
- Encourage regular participation in enjoyable activities, such as sports, hobbies, reading, or social gatherings. *Incorporating enjoyable activities into the daily schedule helps discipline the adolescent to take needed breaks from caregiver responsibilities.*
- Provide the adolescent with information about available support groups and encourage participation. *Support groups provide an outlet for expressing feelings and foster a sense of support and belonging.*
- Assess the adolescent's view of actual and perceived responsibilities as a caregiver and correct any misconceptions. *Emotional ties to the care recipient, confusion about roles within the family, or codependence may cloud the adolescent caregiver's perceptions. Your input helps the adolescent develop a more objective view of the situation.*

Suggested NIC Interventions

Caregiver Support; Coping Enhancement; Decision-Making Support; Family Involvement Promotion; Family Mobilization; Referral; Spiritual Support; Support Group

Evaluations for Expected Outcomes

- Adolescent describes emotional response to life stressors.
- Adolescent identifies and uses adaptive coping strategies.
- Adolescent identifies personal developmental needs and tasks.

- Adolescent uses available support systems.
- Adolescent schedules respite periods for personal developmental needs and recreation.
- Adolescent reports reduced stress from caregiver responsibilities.

Documentation

- Care recipient's physical and mental status and adolescent caregiver's responsibility for providing care
- Current stressors identified by adolescent
- Risk factors (developmental, situational, psychological, and pathophysiologic) for caregiver role strain
- Adolescent's statements indicating intention to take actions to minimize stress, such as joining support group, seeking help from support services, and scheduling periods of respite
- Observations of adolescent's response to stress
- Coping strategies identified by adolescent and nurse
- Referrals provided
- Evaluations for expected outcomes

REFERENCES

Paidipati, C. P., & Deatrick, J. A. (2015). The role of family phenomena in children and adolescents with attention deficit hyperactivity disorder. *Journal of Child & Adolescent Psychiatric Nursing*, *28*(1), 3–13. doi:10.1111/jcap.12097

Rissanen, M., Kylmä, J., Hintikka, J., Honkalampi, K., Tolmunen, T., & Laukkanen, E. (2013). Factors helping adolescents to stop self-cutting: Descriptions of 347 adolescents aged 13–18 years. *Journal of Clinical Nursing*, 22(13/14), 2011–2019.

Woodman, A. C., & Hauser-Cram, P. (2013). The role of coping strategies in predicting change in parenting efficacy and depressive symptoms among mothers of adolescents with developmental disabilities. *Journal of Intellectual Disability Research*, *57*(6), 513–530.

RISK FOR SELF-DIRECTED VIOLENCE

Definition

Vulnerable to behaviors in which an individual demonstrates that he or she can be physically, emotionally, and/or sexually harmful to self

Assessment

- Age
- Gender
- Developmental stage
- Availability of weapons or toxic substances
- Mood and affect, including persistent depression; feelings of worthlessness, hopelessness, helplessness, isolation, inadequacy, and humiliation; deterioration in school work; and flat, distant, remote affect
- Behavioral changes, including loss of interest in personal appearance, overeating or eating too little, verbal or written cues or preoccupation with death, threats of suicide, acting out (such as sexual promiscuity, delinquency, or running away), low energy level, sleep disturbances, frequent naps, irritability, somatic and physical complaints,

antisocial or self-destructive behavior, tendency to be accident-prone, and acts of self-mutilation
- Psychological status, including loss of interest in hobbies and preferred activities, refusal to attend school (cutting class and truancy), social withdrawal and isolation, academic problems, and feelings of rejection by peers and social group

Risk Factors

- Age ≥ 45 years
- Age 15 to 19 years
- Behavioral cues (e.g., writing forlorn love notes, directing angry messages at a significant other who has rejected the person, giving away personal items, taking out a large life insurance policy)
- Conflict about sexual orientation
- Conflict in interpersonal relationship(s)
- Employment concern (e.g., unemployed, recent job loss/failure)
- Engaged in autoerotic sexual acts
- History of multiple suicide attempts
- Insufficient personal resources (e.g., achievement, insight, affect unavailable and poorly controlled)
- Marital status (e.g., single, widowed, divorced)
- Mental health issue (e.g., depression, psychosis, personality disorder, substance abuse)
- Occupation (e.g., executive, administrator/owner of business, professional, semi-skilled worker)
- Pattern of difficulties in family background (e.g., chaotic or conflictual, history of suicide)
- Physical health issue
- Psychological disorder
- Social isolation
- Suicidal ideation
- Suicidal plan
- Verbal cues (e.g., talking about death, "better off without me," asking about lethal dosage of medication)

Expected Outcomes

- Adolescent won't harm self while in hospital.
- Adolescent will recover from suicidal episode.
- Adolescent will discuss feelings that precipitated suicide attempt.
- Adolescent will attend therapy sessions with mental health professional.
- Adolescent will describe available resources for crisis prevention and management.
- Adolescent will report improved feelings of self-worth.

Suggested NOC Outcomes

Depression Self-Control; Impulse Self-Control; Mood Equilibrium; Quality of Life; Self-Mutilation Restraint; Suicide Self-Restraint; Will to Live

Interventions and Rationales

PCC
- Take all suicide threats seriously. *Early intervention reduces the likelihood of a suicide attempt.*

- PCC Ask the adolescent directly, "Have you thought about killing yourself?" If the adolescent says yes, ask, "What do you plan to do?" *Suicide risk increases if the adolescent has a definite plan.*
- S Remove any objects that the adolescent could use for self-inflicted injury, such as razors, belts, glass objects, and pills, *to ensure safety.*
- S Arrange supervision (preferably one-on-one) for the adolescent according to facility policy. This ensures compliance with legal requirements *to protect the adolescent while demonstrating staff concern.*
- PCC Make a contract with the adolescent against self-harm for a specific period. Continue negotiating until there's no evidence of suicidal ideation. *A contract puts the subject of suicide in the open, places some responsibility for safety on the adolescent, and demonstrates your regard for the adolescent as worthwhile.*
- S Supervise administration of all prescribed medications and be aware of their actions and possible adverse effects. *Medications may be a treatment alternative. By watching as they're administered, you prevent the adolescent from hoarding doses (sometimes called* "cheeking"), *thus ensuring the adolescent's safety.*
- Convey a caring, nonjudgmental attitude when talking with the adolescent. *This demonstrates your unconditional positive regard and helps establish a trusting relationship.*
- PCC Listen carefully as the adolescent talks. Don't challenge the adolescent's statements or reinforce denial of the current situation. *This communicates caring, support, and understanding without reinforcing denial, which usually masks underlying suicidal feelings.*
- PCC Encourage the adolescent to set a goal of cooperating with psychiatric intervention. *Ambivalence about psychiatric care or refusal to attend sessions indicates that the adolescent is still in denial.*
- Provide the adolescent and the adolescent's family members with telephone numbers for crisis prevention centers, suicide hotlines, counselors, and other community support services. *Having many alternatives for support helps reduce the adolescent's anxiety.*

Suggested NIC Interventions

Behavior Management: Self-Harm; Counseling; Crisis Intervention; Family Involvement Promotion; Mutual Goal Setting; Suicide Prevention; Support Group

Evaluations for Expected Outcomes

- Adolescent doesn't harm self during hospital stay.
- Adolescent recovers from suicide attempt.
- Adolescent discusses feelings and reasons for attempting suicide.
- Adolescent attends counseling sessions with mental health professional.
- Adolescent describes crisis prevention resources, such as hotline telephone number, local crisis center, or name of therapist.
- Adolescent expresses improved sense of self-worth.

Documentation

- Adolescent's description of feelings before and after suicide attempt
- Observations of adolescent's behavior, mood, and affect
- Nursing interventions to reduce or prevent self-destructive behavior
- Adolescent's response to interventions
- Evaluations for expected outcomes

REFERENCES

Kaess, M., Durkee, T., Brunner, R., Carli, V., Parzer, P., Wasserman, C., . . . Kahn, J. (2014). Pathological internet use among European adolescents: Psychopathology and self-destructive behaviours. *European Child & Adolescent Psychiatry*, *23*(11), 1093–1102.

McAndrew, S., & Warne, T. (2014). Hearing the voices of young people who self-harm: Implications for service providers. *International Journal of Mental Health Nursing*, *23*(6), 570–579. doi:10.1111/inm.12093

Zhang, W., Finy, M., Bresin, K., & Verona, E. (2015). Specific patterns of family aggression and adolescents' self- and other-directed harm: The moderating role of personality. *Journal of Family Violence*, *30*(2), 161–170. doi:10.1007/s10896-014-9662-x

SITUATIONAL LOW SELF-ESTEEM

related to alteration in social role; developmental transition

Definition

Development of a negative perception of self-worth in response to a current situation

Assessment

- Age
- Gender
- Level of education
- Family history, including marital status of parents, financial status, family rules, ability of family to modify rules, consequences when rules are broken, how family members communicate, quality of communication, methods of conflict resolution, family alliances, family stability, ability of family to meet adolescent's physical and emotional needs, and disparities between adolescent's needs and family's ability to meet them
- Goals and values, including extent to which family permits adolescent to pursue individual goals and values
- Family genogram
- Parental status, including level of education, knowledge of normal growth and development, ability to agree on appropriate discipline, stability of parental relationship, and understanding of adolescent's self-esteem disturbance
- Adolescent's psychological status, including changes in appetite, energy level, motivation, personal hygiene, self-image, self-esteem, and sleep patterns; alcohol or drug abuse; reaction to puberty; quality of relationships with authority figures; and scholastic performance

Defining Characteristics

- Helplessness
- Indecisive behavior
- Nonassertive behavior
- Purposelessness
- Self-negating verbalizations
- Situational challenge to self-worth
- Underestimates ability to deal with situation

Expected Outcomes

- Adolescent and parents will describe areas of conflict.
- Adolescent will begin to express feelings openly to family members.

- Parents will encourage and support adolescent's attempt at expression of feelings.
- Adolescent will describe positive qualities about self.
- Parents will describe positive qualities of adolescent and family unit.
- Adolescent and parents will state plans for continued outpatient family treatment.

Suggested NOC Outcomes

Body Image; Child Development: Adolescence; Depression Level; Motivation; Quality of Life; Self-Esteem

Interventions and Rationales

- Provide a secure, structured environment for the adolescent and the adolescent's parents *to foster open discussion of family conflicts.*
- PCC Educate all family members about the schedule, purpose, and goals of individual and family treatment. *Awareness of expectations and rationale for treatment will enhance cooperation.*
- PCC Encourage the adolescent to participate in group activities, group therapy, and individual counseling *to provide opportunities to develop enhanced self-esteem.*
- PCC Encourage the adolescent to express feelings directly, such as "I'm mad because of my curfew." *Such statements help the adolescent recognize and talk about feelings.*
- Tell parents that their child is learning to directly express feelings. *Because family communication patterns are deeply ingrained, parents may need time to adjust to their child's assertiveness.*
- Help parents understand the value of talking about feelings *to encourage them to express emotions appropriately and to discourage them from punishing their child for expressing feelings toward them.*
- Provide the adolescent with a small notebook in which to write positive events as they occur *to encourage focus on strengths and to enhance self-esteem.*
- Teach parents to reward and praise the adolescent for expressing feelings *to enhance self-esteem.*
- Use role-playing to teach the adolescent different ways to respond to specific family conflicts. *This will help the adolescent develop problem-solving and negotiating skills.*
- PCC Communicate with the outpatient clinician *to plan continued treatment for family.*
- Emphasize to the adolescent and parents the need for continued support and family therapy after discharge *to enhance compliance.*

Suggested NIC Interventions

Developmental Enhancement: Adolescent; Family Support; Hope Instillation; Mood Management; Self-Esteem Enhancement; Values Clarification

Evaluations for Expected Outcomes

- Adolescent and parents begin to talk about difficulties at home.
- Adolescent begins to express feelings directly to family members.
- Parents demonstrate support for adolescent's expression of feelings.
- Adolescent uses positive statements about self.
- Parents make positive statements about adolescent and family as a whole.
- Parents and adolescent agree to participate in outpatient treatment.

Documentation

- Specific family conflicts as described by adolescent and parents
- Adolescent's and parents' behavior when interacting with each other
- Nursing interventions to facilitate family communication and expression of feelings
- Frequency of family visits and therapy appointments
- Adolescent's description of own strengths
- Referrals for continued treatment after discharge
- Evaluations for expected outcomes

REFERENCES

Ahmann, E. (2014). Encouraging positive behavior in 'challenging' children: The nurtured heart approach™. *Pediatric Nursing*, *40*(1), 38–42.

Altıntaş, A., Aşçı, F. H., Kin-İşler, A., Güven-Karahan, B., Kelecek, S., Özkan, A., . . . Kara, F. M. (2014). The role of physical activity, body mass index and maturity status in body-related perceptions and self-esteem of adolescents. *Annals of Human Biology*, *41*(5), 395–402. doi:10.3109/03014460.2013.857721

Greenleaf, C., Petrie, T. A., & Martin, S. B. (2014). Relationship of weight-based teasing and adolescents' psychological well-being and physical health. *Journal of School Health*, *84*(1), 49–55. doi:10.1111/josh.12118

SOCIAL ISOLATION

related to social behavior incongruent with norms

Definition

Aloneness experienced by the individual and perceived as imposed by others and as a negative or threatening state

Assessment

- Age
- Gender
- Developmental stage
- Level of education
- Reason for hospitalization (physiologic or psychiatric)
- Attitudes of family, friends, teachers, and other important individuals toward adolescent
- Available support systems
- Factors contributing to social isolation, including delayed physical development, immaturity, altered mental status, changes in behavior or cognition, illness, and history of trauma
- Self-esteem
- Coping and problem-solving ability
- Evidence of substance abuse
- Current and past stressors
- Sociocultural factors, including ethnic and religious background

Defining Characteristics

- Absence of support system
- Aloneness imposed by others
- Cultural incongruence

- Desire to be alone
- Developmental delay
- Developmentally inappropriate interests
- Disabling condition
- Feeling different from others
- Flat affect
- History of rejection
- Hostility
- Illness
- Inability to meet expectations of others
- Insecurity in public
- Meaningless actions
- Member of a subculture
- Poor eye contact
- Preoccupation with own thoughts
- Purposelessness
- Repetitive actions
- Sad affect values incongruent with cultural norms
- Withdrawn

Expected Outcomes

- Adolescent will express feelings of social isolation.
- Adolescent will identify causes of social isolation.
- Adolescent will participate in planning social activities.
- Adolescent will identify personal behaviors that are considered socially unacceptable and will acknowledge the need for change.
- Adolescent will demonstrate more socially acceptable behaviors.
- Adolescent will exhibit effective interpersonal communication skills.
- Adolescent will report feeling less isolated as social interaction improves and will report improved sense of self-esteem.

Suggested NOC Outcomes

Family Social Climate; Personal Well-Being: Leisure Participation; Loneliness Severity; Social Interaction Skills; Social Involvement; Social Support

Interventions and Rationales

- Assign a primary nurse to the adolescent *to enhance continuity of care, establish a trusting relationship, and provide an opportunity to practice developing a one-on-one relationship.*
- PCC Arrange uninterrupted time to talk with the adolescent during each visit. Listen to the adolescent's concerns and feelings. Provide honest feedback (positive and negative) about the adolescent's behavior *to encourage appropriate behaviors and reinforce awareness of inappropriate ones. Feedback is essential to behavior modification.*
- Provide guidance as the adolescent explores possible causes for feelings of social isolation. Help the adolescent identify inappropriate behaviors, and and provide education about ways to improve communication and interpersonal skills *to foster socially acceptable behavior. The adolescent may be more willing to learn new skills and behaviors after becoming aware of the connection between unacceptable behavior patterns and feelings of isolation.*

- Make a contract with the adolescent that requires demonstration of one new behavior within a specific period. Reward successful changes in behavior. *Contracts can enhance self-esteem by giving the adolescent responsibility for making constructive changes and allowing enough time to practice new behavior and communication skills without fear of criticism. Successful completion of the contract provides positive reinforcement.*
- Demonstrate appropriate communication skills and behaviors in all interactions with the adolescent *to provide an example of appropriate behavior and reinforce teaching concepts.*
- PCC Engage the adolescent in role-playing activities that simulate social situations. Provide encouragement and positive reinforcement, and avoid criticism *to provide an opportunity to rehearse new skills in a safe environment, which reduces anxiety and boosts self-confidence.*
- PCC Encourage the adolescent to participate in group activities and one-on-one interactions with staff members. *Gradual increases in social interaction help reduce the adolescent's feelings of social isolation and instill confidence in newly developed communication and interpersonal skills.*
- Talk to the adolescent about community resources, such as social services or support groups, that can provide ongoing support. Provide names, addresses, and phone numbers whenever possible. *This provides the adolescent with ongoing opportunities for social interaction in a supportive environment.*

Suggested NIC Interventions

Behavior Modification: Social Skills; Coping Enhancement; Counseling; Emotional Support; Socialization Enhancement; Support Group; Support System Enhancement; Therapy Group

Evaluations for Expected Outcomes

- Adolescent expresses feelings of social isolation and desire for help.
- Adolescent identifies causes of social isolation.
- Adolescent takes part in planning social activities.
- Adolescent identifies socially unacceptable personal behaviors and acknowledges the need for change.
- Adolescent demonstrates more socially appropriate behaviors.
- Adolescent exhibits effective communication skills.
- Adolescent reports increased social interaction, decreased feelings of isolation, and improved self-esteem.

Documentation

- Observations of adolescent's behavior and communication skills
- Adolescent's description of causes for impaired social interaction
- Nursing interventions to promote behavior modification and improved socialization
- Adolescent's response to interventions
- Resources and referrals provided to adolescent or family members
- Evaluations for expected outcomes

REFERENCES

Cantrell, K. A., & Boles, J. (2015). The children's corner: Perspectives on supportive care. Bridging isolation for youth with chronic conditions: Are we thinking virtually? *Pediatric Nursing*, *41*(5), 254–256.

Jackson, S. L., & Cunningham, S. A. (2015). Social competence and obesity in elementary school. *American Journal of Public Health*, *105*(1), 153–158. doi:10.2105/AJPH.2014.302208
McCarthy, A. (2015). Summer camp for children and adolescents with chronic conditions. *Pediatric Nursing*, *41*(5), 245–250.

RISK FOR TRAUMA

Definition

Vulnerable to accidental tissue injury (e.g., wound, burn, fracture), which may compromise health

Assessment

- Age
- Gender
- Level of education
- Developmental factors, including tendency to test independence and take risks (especially in company of peers), feelings of indestructibility, high level of energy, need for peer approval, and access to potential safety hazards (such as complex machinery or tools, farm equipment, car, motorcycle, jet ski, or snowmobile)
- Health history, including allergies, sports accidents, auditory or visual impairments, and seizure disorders
- Social history, including academic performance, sports, hobbies, social activities, and occupation
- Neurologic status, including level of consciousness and orientation

Risk Factors

External

- Absence of call-for-aid device
- Absence of stairway gate
- Absence of window guard
- Access to weapon
- Bathing in very hot water
- Bed in high position
- Children riding in front seat of car
- Defective appliance
- Delay in ignition of gas appliance
- Dysfunctional call-for-aid device
- Electrical hazard (e.g., faulty plug, frayed wire, overloaded outlet/fuse box)
- Exposure to corrosive product
- Exposure to dangerous machinery
- Exposure to radiation
- Exposure to toxic chemical
- Extremes of environmental temperature
- Flammable object (e.g., clothing, toys)
- Gas leak
- Grease on stove
- High-crime neighborhood

PART III

Child Health

APPLYING EVIDENCE-BASED PRACTICE

The Question

Will increasing sleep duration prevent obesity in children?

Evidence-Based Resources

American Academy of Sleep Medicine. (2008). *Obstructive sleep apnea*. Retrieved from http://www.aasmnet.org/resources/factsheets/sleepapnea.pdf

Centers for Disease Control and Prevention. (2015, August 27). *Childhood obesity facts*. Retrieved from http://www.cdc.gov/healthyschools/obesity/facts.htm

Chaput, J. (2016). Is sleep deprivation a contributor to obesity in children? *Eating & Weight Disorders*, *21*(1), 5–11. doi:10.1007/s40519-015-0233-9

Jarrin, D., McGrath, J., Poirier, P., & Quality Cohort Collaborative Group. (2015). Autonomic dysfunction: A possible pathophysiological pathway underlying the association between sleep and obesity in children at risk for obesity. *Journal of Youth & Adolescence*, *44*(2), 285–297. doi:10.1007/s10964-014-0235-3

Kong, I. G., Lee, H. J., Kim, S. Y., Sim, S., & Choi, H. G. (2015). Physical activity, study sitting time, leisure sitting time, and sleep time are differently associated with obesity in Korean adolescents: A population-based study. *Medicine*, *94*(44), 1–6. doi:10.1097/MD.0000000000001965

McDonald, L., Wardle, J., Llewellyn, C. H., & Fisher, A. (2015). Nighttime sleep duration and hedonic eating in childhood. *International Journal of Obesity*, *39*(10), 1463–1466. doi:10.1038/ijo.2015.132

Morrissey, B., Malakellis, M., Whelan, J., Millar, L., Swinburn, B., Allender, S., & Strugnell, C. (2016). Sleep duration and risk of obesity among a sample of Victorian school children. *BMC Public Health*, *16*, 1–8. doi:10.1186/s12889-016-2913-4

Neal, J. E. (2015). Childhood obesity and sleep disturbances. *NASN School Nurse*, *30*(6), 322–324. doi:10.1177/1942602X15608922

Roberts, R. E., & Duong, H. T. (2015). Is there an association between adolescent sleep restriction and obesity? *Journal of Psychosomatic Research*, *79*(6), 651–656. doi:10.1016/j.jpsychores.2015.05.012

Evaluating the Evidence

Childhood obesity has steadily increased over the last 30 years. The Centers for Disease Control and Prevention (CDC) data indicates 18% of children aged 6 to 11 years are obese. Overweight and obesity in children is measured by body mass index (BMI), a calculation based on the height and weight of the child. Obesity is defined as a BMI at or above the 95th percentile for children of the same age and sex (CDC, 2015). Because obesity increases the risk for many serious health conditions, understanding factors that increase the risk for obesity is necessary to improve the future health of children.

The relationship between sleep and obesity in children was the focus of several studies (Chaput, 2016; Jarrin, McGrath, Poirier, & Quality Cohort Collaborative Group, 2015; Kong, Lee, Kim, Sim, & Choi, 2015; Morrissey et al., 2016; Roberts & Duong, 2015). Busy lifestyles can lead to earlier wake times and later bedtimes. The evidence suggests that sleep duration of less than 8 hours/night may be a contributing factor to obesity and to other health concerns.

Modernized societies increasingly use technology to save time and make tasks easier. Unfortunately, the development of these tools has decreased the need for physical activity. A study conducted by Kong et al. (2015) examined the relationships between study sitting time, leisure sitting time, and sleep time with obesity in Korean adolescents. The results indicated to maintain a healthy weight; physical activity of more than 2 days/week and sleep time greater than 8 hours/night are recommended.

Lack of sleep can lead to poor eating habits, which contribute to obesity. Shorter sleeping time, poor quality of sleep, and later bedtimes are associated with increased snacking and increased number of meals/day (Chaput, 2016). A study conducted by McDonald, Wardle, & Fisher (2015) examined the relationship between sleep and food responsiveness in children aged 5 years. Results suggested that poor sleep may increase overeating due to a response to food cues rather than a response to hunger.

Childhood obesity may affect the quality of sleep. Obstructive sleep apnea (OSA) is defined as a breathing disorder in which there is prolonged partial upper airway obstruction (American Academy of Sleep Medicine, 2008). Around 60% of overweight and obese children are affected by OSA. The resulting poor quality sleep can cause daytime hyperactivity, reduced concentration and focus, anxiety, and depression (Neal, 2015).

Applying the Results and Making a Decision

The literature provides evidence that there is a relationship between sleep and obesity. Sleep duration is a possible contributing factor for the development of obesity. Physical activity, eating habits, and nutrition are also linked with obesity. Medical intervention is necessary to screen children for factors that contribute to decreased sleep duration, such as OSA, when obesity is recognized.

Re-Evaluating Process and Identifying Areas for Improvement

Recognizing contributing factors and providing education to the community are critical in preventing childhood obesity. Although the primary causes of childhood obesity are lack of physical activity and unhealthy dietary intake, sleep habits and sleep duration may also have a significant effect. Obesity in children must be recognized early in order to avoid complications such as diabetes, hypertension, and cardiovascular disease.

INTRODUCTION

This section focuses on facilitating the achievement of full developmental potential and optimal health of children. When talking to children, show understanding by using simple language and establishing a rapport. To calm a frightened child, turn portions of your examination into a game, talk about toys, hobbies, or other subjects of interest, and be generous with compliments.

Your care plan should emphasize working with the entire family. Obtaining accurate assessment information, for example, usually requires the cooperation and trust of family members.

During each stage of growth and development, the child must master specific physical, cognitive, and developmental tasks. Assessment should include an evaluation of the child's growth and developmental level as well as an examination of body systems. Other assessment areas include family roles and relationships, parenting style, stressors, coping patterns, religion, cultural background, living conditions, and financial status. You'll also want to explore how the child and family members perceive any health problems.

After analyzing the assessment data, you'll formulate a problem statement. Use the nursing diagnoses in this section to build problem statements that include the child's actual health problems or health problems for which the child is at risk. Be sure to take into account physiologic, psychosocial, or cognitive aspects of the child's well-being.

Encourage the child and family members to participate when developing interventions. Some family members may need encouragement to ask questions about the child's status; others may want to become involved in treatment-related decisions. To foster participation, be sensitive to the family's values, ideas, and beliefs. Provide referrals to appropriate social service agencies and other community resources.

Remember to evaluate goals after the implementation of your care plan. By carefully monitoring the effectiveness of interventions, you'll readily see where revisions are needed to meet outcomes.

RISK FOR ASPIRATION

Definition

Vulnerable to entry of gastrointestinal secretions, oropharyngeal secretions, solids, or fluids to the tracheobronchial passages, which may compromise health

Assessment

- Respiratory status, including rate, depth, and pattern of respirations; auscultation of breath sounds; frequency and effectiveness of cough; ability to handle secretions; palpation for fremitus; percussion of lung fields; and sputum characteristics (color, consistency, amount, and odor)
- Neurologic status, including mental status and level of consciousness (LOC)
- Gastrointestinal status, including presence or absence of gag and swallowing reflex, gastroesophageal reflux, and continuous or intermittent tube feedings
- Diagnostic studies, including arterial blood gas levels, chest X-rays, and cardiorespiratory monitoring

Risk Factors

- Barrier to elevating upper body
- Decrease in gastrointestinal motility
- Decrease in LOC
- Delayed gastric emptying
- Depressed gag reflex
- Enteral feedings
- Facial surgery
- Facial trauma
- Impaired ability to swallow
- Incompetent lower esophageal sphincter
- Increase in gastric residual
- Increase in intragastric pressure
- Ineffective cough
- Neck surgery
- Neck trauma
- Oral surgery
- Oral trauma
- Presence of oral/nasal tube (e.g., tracheal, feeding)
- Treatment regimen
- Wired jaw

Expected Outcomes

- Auscultation will reveal clear breath sounds.
- Auscultation will reveal presence of bowel sounds.
- Child will maintain patent airway.
- Child will breathe easily, cough effectively, and show no signs of respiratory distress or infection.
- Family members will demonstrate measures to prevent aspiration.
- Child's respiratory rate will remain within normal limits for age.
- Family members will describe plan for home care (e.g., removing objects that a child could choke on).

Suggested NOC Outcomes

Aspiration Prevention; Knowledge: Treatment Procedure(s); Respiratory Status: Ventilation; Risk Control; Swallowing Status

Interventions and Rationales

- Assess the child for gag and swallowing reflexes. *Impaired reflexes may cause aspiration.*
- Assess respiratory status at least every 4 hours or according to established standards; begin cardiopulmonary monitoring *to detect signs of possible aspiration (increased respiratory rate, cough, sputum production, and diminished breath sounds).*
- Auscultate bowel sounds every 4 hours and reports changes. *Delayed gastric emptying may cause regurgitation of stomach contents.*
- Elevate the head of the bed or place the child in Fowler's position *to aid breathing.*
- Help the child turn, cough, and deep breathe every 2 to 4 hours. Perform postural drainage, percussion, and vibration every 4 hours, or as ordered. Suction, as needed, *to stimulate cough and clear upper and lower airways. These measures promote drainage of secretions and full expansion of lungs.*
- Perform chest physiotherapy before feeding the child *to decrease the risk of emesis leading to aspiration.*
- Hold an infant with head elevated during feeding, and position in an infant seat after feeding. *Such positioning uses gravity to prevent regurgitation of stomach contents and promotes lung expansion.*
- Recognize the progression of airway compromise and report your findings *to detect complications early.*

- Encourage fluids within prescribed restrictions. Provide humidification, as ordered (such as an oxygen tent or nebulizer). *Fluids and humidification liquefy secretions.*
- Place the child in the lateral position. Change the child's position at least every 2 hours *to reduce the potential for aspiration by allowing secretions and blood to drain.*

PCC
- Instruct the child and family members in the home care plan. *The child and family members must demonstrate the ability to ensure adequate home care before discharge.*

PCC
- Refer to outside agency for assistance after discharge. *Family members may need support to continue care and perceive themselves capable of acting quickly if aspiration occurs.*

Suggested NIC Interventions

Airway Management; Aspiration Precautions; Feeding; Positioning; Respiratory Monitoring; Vital Signs Monitoring; Vomiting Management

Evaluations for Expected Outcomes

- Auscultation reveals clear breath sounds.
- Auscultation reveals presence of bowel sounds.
- Child maintains airway patency.
- Child breathes easily, coughs effectively, and shows no signs of respiratory distress or infection.
- Family members demonstrate measures to prevent aspiration in child (e.g., correct positioning of infant during and after feeding).
- Child's respiratory rate remains within normal limits for age.
- Family members describe plan for home care.

Documentation

- Child's ability to handle oral secretions and feedings
- Observation of respiratory status and response to treatment regimen
- Child's and family members' abilities to carry out home care plan
- Evaluations for expected outcomes

REFERENCES

Bamber, A. R., Pryce, J., Ashworth, M., & Sebire, N. J. (2014). Fatal aspiration of foreign bodies in infants and children. *Fetal & Pediatric Pathology, 33*(1), 42–48. doi:10.3109/15513815.2013.846446

Irving, S. Y., Lyman, B., Northington, L., Bartlett, J. A., & Kemper, C. (2014). Nasogastric tube placement and verification in children: Review of the current literature. *Critical Care Nurse, 34*(3), 67–78. doi:10.4037/ccn2014606

Kelly, C. J., & Walker, R. M. (2015). Perioperative pulmonary aspiration is infrequent and low risk in pediatric anesthetic practice. *Pediatric Anesthesia, 25*(1), 36–43. doi:10.1111/pan.12549

RISK FOR IMPAIRED ATTACHMENT

Definition

Vulnerable to disruption of the interactive process between parent/significant other and child that fosters the development of a protective and nurturing reciprocal relationship

Assessment

- Family status, including marital status, composition of family, ages of family members, ability of family to meet physical and emotional needs of its members, evidence of abuse, and health history
- Parental status, including level of education, knowledge of normal growth and development, stability of relationship, and available support systems
- Parents' psychological status, including energy level, motivation, recent life changes, psychiatric history, maternal history of drug abuse, and alcohol or antidepressant use by either partner
- Child's neurologic status, including muscle tone and reflexes; infant lethargy, irritability, seizures, or tremors; and Brazelton Neonatal Behavioral Assessment, Dubowitz Gestational Age Assessment, and Bayley Scales of Infant Development
- Child's sensory status, including vision or hearing loss, visual and auditory-evoked potentials, and audiometric tests
- Sleep pattern, including infant's usual hours of sleep

Risk Factors

- Anxiety
- Child's illness prevents effective initiation of parental contact
- Disorganized infant behavior
- Inability of parent to meet personal needs
- Insufficient privacy
- Parental conflict resulting from disorganized infant behavior
- Parent–child separation
- Physical barrier (e.g., infant in isolette)
- Prematurity
- Substance abuse

Expected Outcomes

- Parents will initiate positive interaction with child.
- Parents will hold child and talk to him.
- Parents will express confidence in their ability to respond to child's needs.
- Parents will respond appropriately to child.
- Parents will express positive feelings about child.
- Parents will express confidence in their ability to care for child.
- Parents will recognize when they need assistance.
- Child will respond positively to parents, show interest in their faces, and become calm when soothed by them.

Suggested NOC Outcomes

Parenting Performance; Role Performance

Interventions and Rationales

- Perform an ongoing assessment of parent and child interaction *to evaluate whether parent–child attachment is proceeding normally.*
- Speak positively about the child in the parents' presence *to encourage the parents to develop positive view of the child.*

- Maintain eye contact with the child while providing care, talk to the child, and touch appropriately *to demonstrate healthy interactions with the child.*
- Help the parents learn to understand behavioral cues from the child. For example, the child may become fussy when ready for a nap or may pull the ear if there is an earache. *Developing better understanding of their child's behavior will decrease the parents' frustration and help them care more effectively for the child.*
- Provide the parents and the child with privacy *to promote attachment.*
- Assess the parents' knowledge of child care and development *to develop an appropriate teaching plan.*
- PCC Teach the parents to provide physical care for the child *to increase their sense of competence and self-confidence.*
- PCC Encourage the parents to make eye contact with the child, caress and talk to the child in soothing tone, call by name, and make positive remarks *to foster a healthy parent–child attachment and to help ensure the child's well-being.*
- Observe the parents; note whether their responses to the child are appropriate. Compliment them when they exhibit successful parenting skills *to increase their confidence.*
- Discuss life changes precipitated by birth *to help the parents express their frustrations and feelings about role changes.* Topics may include altered finances, changes in living space, care-taking arrangements, and new roles and responsibilities for parents and siblings.
- Provide the parents with sources of ongoing support and care *to ensure adequate follow-up.*
- S Assess the home environment. Discuss adaptations the parents need to make. *Adaptations in the home environment may be needed to help the parents properly care for their child.*

Suggested NIC Interventions

Abuse Protection Support: Child; Coping Enhancement; Developmental Enhancement: Child; Parenting Promotion

Evaluations for Expected Outcomes

- Parents initiate positive interactions with child.
- Parents make eye contact with child, caress and talk to child, and call by name.
- Parents express confidence in their ability to meet child's needs.
- Parents respond appropriately to child's behavioral cues, provide stimulation when he's alert and ready, don't overstimulate him, and recognize when he needs to nap.
- Parents express positive feelings about child.
- Parents express confidence in ability to care for child at home.
- Parents recognize when they need assistance and make plans to contact appropriate resources.
- Child responds positively to parents, shows interest in their faces, and becomes calm when soothed by them.

Documentation

- Description of parent and child interactions
- Nursing interventions to promote attachment
- Parents' response to nursing interventions
- Child's response to modifications in parents' behavior
- Evaluations for expected outcomes

REFERENCES

Falk, N., Norris, K., & Quinn, M. (2014). The factors predicting stress, anxiety, and depression in the parents of children with autism. *Journal of Autism & Developmental Disorders*, *44*(12), 3185–3203. doi:10.1007/s10803-014-2189-4

Lawless, A., Coveney, J., & MacDougall, C. (2014). Infant mental health promotion and the discourse of risk. *Sociology of Health & Illness*, *36*(3), 416–431. doi:10.1111/1467-9566.12074

Milan, S., & Acker, J. C. (2014). Early attachment quality moderates eating disorder risk among adolescent girls. *Psychology & Health*, *29*(8), 896–914. doi:10.1080/08870446.2014.896463

DISTURBED BODY IMAGE

related to surgical procedure

Definition

Confusion in mental picture of one's physical self

Assessment

- Physiologic changes
- Behavioral changes
- Child's and family members' perceptions of health problem
- Child's developmental stage
- Child's eating pattern, sleeping pattern, and usual play activities

Defining Characteristics

- Absence of body part
- Alteration in body function
- Alteration in body structure
- Alteration in view of one's body (e.g., appearance, structure, function)
- Avoids looking at one's body
- Avoids touching one's body
- Behavior of acknowledging one's body
- Behavior of monitoring one's body
- Change in ability to estimate spatial relationship of body to environment
- Change in lifestyle
- Change in social involvement
- Depersonalization of body part by use of impersonal pronouns
- Emphasis on remaining strengths
- Extension of body boundary (e.g., includes external object)
- Fear of reaction by others
- Focus on past appearance
- Focus on past function
- Heightened achievement
- Hiding or body part
- Negative feeling about body
- Nonverbal response to change in body (e.g., appearance, structure, function)
- Overexposure of body part
- Perceptions that reflect an altered view of one's body appearance
- Personalization of body part by name
- Personalization of loss by name
- Preoccupation with change
- Preoccupation with loss
- Refusal to acknowledge change
- Trauma to nonfunctioning body part

Expected Outcomes

- Child will acknowledge change in body appearance or function.
- Child will express positive feelings about self.
- Family members will acknowledge change in child's appearance or body functioning and will verbalize acceptance of child.

Suggested NOC Outcomes

Acceptance: Health Status; Body Image; Child Development: Middle Childhood; Coping; Psychosocial Adjustment: Life Change; Self-Esteem

Interventions and Rationales

- Hold, rock, or touch the child frequently *to give the child awareness of body integrity.*
- Provide an opportunity for the child to interact with peers who have experienced similar health problem *to decrease the child's feelings of isolation and sense of being different from others.*
- Give the child as much freedom as possible. If restraints are called for, use the minimum restraint necessary to prevent injury. *Providing the least restrictive environment enhances the child's control over own surroundings and provides an opportunity to release feelings through physical activity.*
- PCC Explain medical procedures in age-appropriate language. For a child younger than age 7, use dolls and actual medical equipment to describe procedures. *A child in the preoperational stage of development understands best by seeing and manipulating objects.* For an older child, use body diagrams to illustrate what changes will and won't appear in the body as a result of medical treatment or disease progression. *Illustration is one technique to reinforce learning.*
- For a young child, cover injection sites with adhesive bandages. *A child in the preoperational stage of development may hold the misconception that injections create holes that allow blood to drain out. Adhesive bandages may help reinforce the child's sense of body integrity.*
- PCC Encourage a young child to participate in play activities *to allow the child to act out feelings that may not have the verbal or cognitive skills to express.*
- Set aside time with the older school-age child to discuss feelings *to assess perceptions, clarify misconceptions, and provide an opportunity to ventilate emotions.*
- PCC Ensure privacy during procedures *to accommodate the heightened sense of modesty that children develop beginning in early school-age years.*
- PCC Encourage family members to express feelings and concerns about changes in the child's body appearance or function. Provide accurate information and answer questions thoroughly. *Encouraging open discussion enables you to provide emotional support and may help ease family members' anxiety.*

Suggested NIC Interventions

Coping Enhancement; Developmental Enhancement: Child; Parent Education: Childrearing Family; Risk Identification; Self-Esteem Enhancement

Evaluations for Expected Outcomes

- Child expresses understanding of changes in body.
- Child expresses positive feelings about self.
- Family members acknowledge change, verbalize positive feelings about child, and display warmth and affection by holding, comforting, and hugging child as appropriate for child's age.

Documentation

- Child's statements about appearance
- Family members' statements about changes in child's body structure or function

- Account of child's behavior during medical procedures and in play activities
- Observations of family members' behavior toward child and participation in care
- Evaluations for expected outcomes

REFERENCES

Kjölhede, E. A., Gustafsson, P., Gustafsson, P., & Nelson, N. (2014). Overweight and obese children have lower cortisol levels than normal weight children. *Acta Paediatrica*, *103*(3), 295–299. doi:10.1111/apa.12499

Martin, G. M. (2015). Obesity in question: Understandings of body shape, self, and normalcy among children in Malta. *Sociology of Health & Illness*, *37*(2), 212–226. doi:10.1111/1467-9566.12216

McCarthy, A. (2015). Summer camp for children and adolescents with chronic conditions. *Pediatric Nursing*, *41*(5), 245–250.

RISK FOR IMBALANCED BODY TEMPERATURE

Definition

Vulnerable to failure to maintain body temperature within normal parameters, which may compromise health

Assessment

- Age
- Vital signs, including pattern of temperature fluctuation
- Hydration status, including mucous membranes, skin turgor, and fontanels (in infants)
- Respiratory status, including respiratory rate and depth, dyspnea, and use of accessory muscles
- Neurologic status, including incidence of seizures, cerebrospinal fluid infection, abscess, hemorrhage, and history of trauma or cranial surgery
- Nutritional status, including decreased intake and vomiting
- Medication history, including effects of drugs or toxins
- Evidence of disturbance in the temperature-regulating centers of brain

Risk Factors

- Acute brain injury
- Alteration in metabolic rate
- Condition affecting temperature regulation
- Decreased sweat response
- Dehydration
- Extremes of age
- Extremes of environmental temperature
- Extremes of weight
- Inactivity
- Inappropriate clothing for environmental temperature
- Increase in oxygen demand
- Increased body surface area to weight ratio
- Inefficient nonshivering thermogenesis
- Insufficient supply of subcutaneous fat
- Pharmaceutical agent
- Sedation
- Sepsis
- Vigorous activity

Expected Outcomes

- Child will maintain body temperature of 98.6° F to 99.5° F (37° C to 37.5° C).
- Child will maintain weight within 5% of baseline.

- Child will maintain balanced intake and output within normal limits for age.
- Child's urine specific gravity will remain between 1.010 and 1.015.

Suggested NOC Outcomes

Hydration; Medication Response; Thermoregulation

Interventions and Rationales

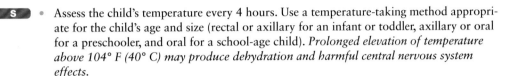

- S Assess the child's temperature every 4 hours. Use a temperature-taking method appropriate for the child's age and size (rectal or axillary for an infant or toddler, axillary or oral for a preschooler, and oral for a school-age child). *Prolonged elevation of temperature above 104° F (40° C) may produce dehydration and harmful central nervous system effects.*
- Weigh the child daily every morning and record the results. *A decrease in weight may indicate dehydration.*
- S Maintain adequate fluid intake by offering small amounts of flavored fluids at frequent intervals; record intake and output in every shift. *Fever increases the child's fluid requirements by increasing the metabolic rate. High-calorie liquids, such as colas, fruit juices, and flavored water sweetened with corn syrup, help prevent dehydration.*
- Administer antipyretics, as ordered, and monitor effectiveness. *Antipyretics act on the hypothalamus to regulate body temperature.*
- Check and record urine specific gravity with each voiding. *Urine specific gravity increases with dehydration.* Adequate urine output and urine specific gravity between 1.010 and 1.015 indicates sufficient hydration for children.
- Give a tepid sponge bath for increased temperature *to increase vaporization from skin and decrease body temperature.*
- PCC Teach parents to dress the child in lightweight clothing when the child has elevated body temperature *to allow perspiration to evaporate, thereby releasing body heat.*

Suggested NIC Interventions

Fever Treatment; Medication Management; Temperature Regulation; Vital Signs Monitoring

Evaluations for Expected Outcomes

- Child maintains body temperature of 98.6° F to 99.5° F (37° C to 37.5° C).
- Child maintains baseline weight.
- Child maintains balanced intake and output within normal limits for age.
- Child maintains urine specific gravity of 1.010 to 1.015.

Documentation

- Observation of physical findings
- Nursing interventions, including administration of medications
- Child's body temperature (recorded every 4 hours)
- Child's weight, urine output, and urine specific gravity
- Child's response (behavioral, cognitive, and physiologic) to interventions, including administration of antipyretics
- Evaluations for expected outcomes

REFERENCES

Knight, A. (2015). Clinical update. Triage nurse's assessment of a child with a fever. *Australian Nursing & Midwifery Journal*, *22*(10), 28–31.

Lowth, D. M. (2014). The child with a temperature. *Practice Nurse*, *44*(11), 26–30.

Purssell, E. (2014). Fever in children—A concept analysis. *Journal of Clinical Nursing*, *23*(23/24), 3575–3582. doi:10.1111/jocn.12347

Vermeulen, S., Barreto, M., La Penna, F., Prete, A., Martella, S., Biagiarelli, F., & Villa, M. P. (2014). Exhaled breath temperature in children: Reproducibility and influencing factors. *Journal of Asthma*, *51*(7), 743–750. doi:10.3109/02770903.2014.906606

INEFFECTIVE BREATHING PATTERN

related to fatigue

Definition

Inspiration and/or expiration that doesn't provide adequate ventilation

Assessment

- Age
- Allergies
- History of respiratory disorders
- Respiratory status, including rate and depth of respiration, symmetry of chest expansion, use of accessory muscles, nasal flaring, presence of cough, anteroposterior chest diameter, palpation for fremitus, percussion of lung fields, auscultation of breath sounds, pulmonary function studies, arterial blood gas (ABG) monitoring, and pulse oximetry readings
- Cardiovascular status, including history of congenital or acquired heart disease
- Neurologic status, including mental status and level of consciousness
- Emotional well-being
- Knowledge, including understanding of physical condition and physical, mental, and emotional readiness to learn

Defining Characteristics

- Abnormal breathing pattern (e.g., rate, rhythm depth)
- Altered chest excursion
- Bradypnea
- Decrease in expiratory pressure
- Decrease in inspiratory pressure
- Decrease in minute ventilation
- Decrease in vital capacity
- Dyspnea
- Increase in anterior–posterior chest diameter
- Nasal flaring
- Orthopnea
- Prolonged expiration phase
- Pursed-lip breathing
- Tachypnea
- Use of accessory muscles to breathe
- Use of three-point position

Expected Outcomes

- Auscultation won't reveal abnormal breath sounds.
- Child's oxygen saturation (Sa_{O_2}) level will remain above 95%.
- Child's respiratory status will remain within normal limits for age.
- Child will demonstrate adequate breathing pattern, with easy, unlabored respirations.

- Child will demonstrate correct technique in pursed-lip breathing, abdominal breathing, and relaxation techniques.
- Child or family member will demonstrate correct technique to use in medication administration, oxygen administration, and airway suctioning.
- Child will participate in age-appropriate play activities without increased respiratory difficulty.
- Family members will develop effective care plan for child's return home.

Suggested NOC Outcomes

Anxiety Level; Energy Conservation; Respiratory Status: Airway Patency; Respiratory Status: Ventilation; Vital Signs

Interventions and Rationales

- Assess respiratory rate and depth every 2 to 4 hours; monitor for nasal flaring, chest retractions, and cyanosis *to detect early signs of respiratory compromise.*
- Monitor ABG values and pulse oximetry readings *to evaluate oxygenation and respiratory status.*
- Auscultate breath sounds every 2 to 4 hours *to detect decreased or adventitious breath sounds;* report changes.
- Administer oxygen, as ordered, *to help reduce hypoxemia and relieve respiratory distress.*
- Force fluids *to liquefy secretions and prevent dehydration related to increased respiratory rate.*
- Provide nebulizer treatment, vaporizer, or mist tent therapy, as ordered, *to liquefy secretions.*
- Provide postural drainage and chest percussion every 4 hours before meals *to facilitate removal of secretions.*
- Suction airway, as needed, *to remove secretions.*
- S Place the child in Fowler's position, raising the head of the bed. Place an overbed table padded with a pillow in front of the child and have the child extend arms over the table *to promote lung expansion.*
- PCC Remain with the child and offer reassurance during periods of respiratory difficulty *to relieve anxiety.*
- Administer bronchodilators and antibiotics, as ordered. *Dilation of bronchi allows greater passageway for air. Antibiotics treat infection.* Monitor effectiveness and check for adverse reactions *to ensure the safety and efficacy of therapy.*
- S Prohibit parents and other visitors from smoking in the child's room and explain why. *Smoking depletes the room of its natural oxygen supply and poses a serious fire hazard in a room with oxygen equipment.*
- PCC Schedule necessary care activities to provide frequent rest periods *to prevent fatigue and reduce oxygen demand.* Allow adequate playtime. *All children require play for normal growth and development.*
- Assist with activities of daily living, as necessary, *to help the child conserve energy and avoid fatigue.*
- Identify the child's developmental level and select appropriate teaching methods. For a preschooler or early school-age child, use stuffed animals, puppets, and drawings. *A preschooler uses sensory experiences to understand information.* For an older school-age child, use demonstration and audiovisual materials such as body outline. *A child in this age group has the ability to think logically but not abstractly.*

- Limit the number of new skills taught each day according to the child's age and ability. Teach a preschooler 1 skill/day and a school-age child, 2 skills/day. *Limiting daily teaching avoids overloading the child with new information and enhances learning.*
- Teach the child pursed-lip breathing, abdominal breathing, and relaxation techniques. *These measures allow the child to participate in maintaining own health status and improve ventilation.*
- Discuss with the child and family members ways to conserve energy while carrying out the daily routine *to prepare the child for discharge from the hospital.*
- PCC Help the family plan for care at home. Discuss medication administration, use of assistive equipment, and available community resources. Also discuss the signs and symptoms of complications and when to report them. *Increasing the family's knowledge improves the likelihood of compliance with medical treatment, thereby decreasing the risk of recurrence of breathing problems.*

Suggested NIC Interventions

Acid–Base Management; Airway Management; Chest Physiotherapy; Energy Management; Oxygen Therapy; Positioning; Respiratory Monitoring; Smoking Cessation Assistance

Evaluations for Expected Outcomes

- Auscultation reveals normal breath sounds.
- Pulse oximetry readings reveal Sao_2 above 95%.
- Child's respiratory status remains within normal limits for age.
- Child demonstrates adequate breathing pattern and unlabored respirations.
- Child demonstrates correct technique in pursed-lip breathing, abdominal breathing, and relaxation techniques.
- Family members demonstrate correct technique in medication administration, oxygen administration, and suctioning.
- Child participates in age-appropriate play activities without increased respiratory difficulty.
- Family members describe care plan they'll implement upon child's return home.

Documentation

- Child's expressions of comfort in breathing
- Child's and family members' understanding of medical diagnosis and readiness to learn
- Child's and family members' responses to teaching
- Physical findings from pulmonary assessment
- Interventions performed
- Child's and family members' responses to nursing interventions
- Evaluations for expected outcomes

REFERENCES

Booker, R. (2014). Asthma in children: Diagnostic and management dilemmas. *Practice Nurse*, *44*(11), 13–18.

Pascoal, L. M., Lopes, M. O., da Silva, V. M., Beltrão, B. A., Chaves, D. R., de Santiago, J. V., & Herdman, T. H. (2014). Ineffective breathing pattern: Defining characteristics in children with acute respiratory infection. *International Journal of Nursing Knowledge*, *25*(1), 54–61.

Stores, R. J., & Stores, G. (2014). The significance of aspects of screening for obstructive sleep apnea in children with Down Syndrome. *Journal of Intellectual Disability Research*, *58*(4), 381–392. doi:10.1111/jir.12033

CHRONIC FUNCTIONAL CONSTIPATION

related to autonomic neuropathy; habitually ignores urge to defecate; insufficient fluid intake

Definition

Infrequent or difficult evacuation of feces, which has been present for at least three of the prior 12 months

Assessment

- Health history, including history of bowel disorder or surgery and age onset of symptoms.
- Gastrointestinal status, including nausea and vomiting, usual bowel elimination habits, changes in bowel elimination habits, laxative use, stool characteristics (color, amount, size and consistency), duration of symptoms and pain.
- Abdominal assessment, including inspection of abdomen, auscultation of bowel sounds, percussion for tympany or dullness, and palpation for tenderness or masses. Results of diagnostic test such as X-ray, anorectal manometry, colonic manometry, barium enema, and sigmoidoscopy.
- Nutritional status, including dietary intake, fiber intake, and appetite, current weight, and change from normal weight.
- Fluid and electrolyte status, including intake and output, skin turgor, urine specific gravity, and serum electrolytes.
- Detailed medication history.
- Activity status.

Defining Characteristics

- Abdominal distention
- ADULT: Presence of ≥2 of the following symptoms of Rome III classification system:
  - Lumpy or hard stools in ≥25% defecations
  - Straining during ≥25% of defecations
  - Sensation of incomplete evacuation for ≥25% of defecations
  - Sensation of anorectal obstruction/blockage for ≥25% of defecations
  - Manual maneuvers to facilitate ≥25% of defecations (digital manipulation, pelvic floor support)
  - ≤3 evacuations/week
- CHILD ≤4 years: Presence of ≥2 criteria on Roman III Pediatric classification system for ≥1 month:
  - ≤2 defecations/week
  - ≥1 episode of fecal incontinence/week
  - Stool retentive posturing
  - Painful or hard bowel movements
  - Presence of large fecal mass in the rectum
  - Large diameter stools that may obstruct the toilet
- CHILD ≥4 years: Presence of ≥2 criteria on Roman III Pediatric classification system for ≥2 months:
  - ≤2 defecations/week
  - ≥1 episode of fecal incontinence/week
  - Stool retentive posturing

  - Painful or hard bowel movements
  - Presence of large fecal mass in the rectum
  - Large diameter stools that may obstruct the toilet
- Fecal impaction
- Fecal incontinence (in children)
- Leakage of stool with digital stimulation
- Pain with defecation
- Palpable abdominal mass
- Positive fecal occult blood test
- Prolonged straining
- Type 1 or 2 on Bristol Stool Chart

Expected Outcomes

- Child will maintain a normal bowel pattern.
- Child will maintain fluid balance
- Child will display normal bowel sounds
- Child will express adequate pain relief
- Parent will identify measures to maintain normal bowel pattern in child
- Parent will demonstrate willingness to adhere to treatment measures

Suggested NOC Outcomes

Adherence Behavior; Bowel Elimination; Comfort Level; Health Beliefs; Hydration; Knowledge: Health Behavior; Nutritional Status: Food & Fluid Intake; Symptom Control

Interventions and Rationales

- Monitor and record frequency and characteristics of stool *to determine extent of the problem.*
- Instruct the child, or parents if child is too young, to keep a daily bowel diary *to gather more reliable information about the child's bowel habits since memory recall can be inaccurate.*
- Assure child is getting the recommended amounts of fiber in diet *as fiber intake below normal limits has been associated with functional constipation.*
- Keep an accurate intake and output record *to evaluate fluid intake status.*
- Assure child is receiving recommended daily fluid intake as per age and weight. *Adequate hydration aids in normal bowel elimination pattern.*
- PCC Encourage daily physical activity *to strengthen muscles and promote circulation.*
- Instruct parents to begin a toilet training system. This involves sitting on the toilet for 5 minutes after each meal to actively try to defecate. *This takes advantage of the gastrocolic reflex that increases colonic peristalsis, facilitating defecation.*
- A footstool may be necessary for children whose feet do not touch the floor to facilitate a relaxed posture during defecation. *This ensures the child has the best posture to aid in defecation.*
- PCC Educate parents and child on any prescribed pharmacologic treatments. *It is important for the parents to understand how and when to administer the prescribed medications and any side effects to watch for.*

Suggested NIC Interventions

Bowel Management; Bowel Training; Constipation/Impaction Management; Counseling; Exercise Promotion; Fluid Management; Health Education; Nutrition Management; Nutrition Management

Evaluations for Expected Outcomes

- Child exhibits a normal bowel pattern.
- Child drinks adequate amount of fluids.
- Child displays normal bowel sounds.
- Child states pain relief measures are adequate.
- Parent identifies measures to maintain normal bowel pattern in child.
- Parent states willingness to adhere to treatment measures.

Documentation

- Physical assessment findings of the abdomen, including bowel sounds and inspection, palpation and percussion findings
- Fluid balance status, including intake and output, skin turgor, specific gravity, and mucous membranes
- Frequency and characteristics of stool
- Child and parent participation in care
- Evaluation for expected outcomes

REFERENCES

Gijsbers, C., Kneepkens, C., Vergouwe, Y., & Büller, H. (2014). Occult constipation: Fecal retention as a cause of recurrent abdominal pain in children. *European Journal of Pediatrics*, *173*(6), 781–785. doi:10.1007/s00431-013-2257-3

Guidance on severe constipation in children released. (2014). *Emergency Nurse*, *22*(3), 7.

Koppen, I. J. N., Lammers, L. A., Benninga, M. A., & Tabbers, M. M. (2015). Management of functional constipation in children: Therapy in practice. *Pediatric Drugs*, *17*, 349–360.

Lowth, M. (2014). The child with abdominal pain. *Practice Nurse*, *44*(9), 10–13.

Rivi, E., Filippi, M., Fornasari, E., Mascia, M. T., Ferrari, A., & Costi, S. (2014). Effectiveness of standing frame on constipation in children with cerebral palsy: A single-subject study. *Occupational Therapy International*, *21*(3), 115–123. doi:10.1002/oti.1370

DISABLED FAMILY COPING

Definition

Behavior of primary person (family member, significant other, or close friend) that disables his or her capabilities and the client's capabilities to effectively address tasks essential to either person's adaptation to the health challenge

Assessment

- Child's illness, including severity, duration, and impact on family
- Family process, including number and ages of children, usual patterns of interaction, roles of parents and children, communication patterns, relationship changes (such as separation, divorce, or remarriage), and past response to crisis
- Family members' understanding of child's present health status

- Family resources (financial, social, and spiritual)
- Parental status, including perception of child's behavior, past responses to stress, child care provisions, history of inappropriate parenting, and history of destructive behavior or substance abuse
- Alteration in child's growth and development resulting from illness or dysfunctional parenting
- Transportation limitations, including geographic distances to health resources

Defining Characteristics

- Abandonment
- Adopts illness symptoms of client
- Aggression
- Agitation
- Client dependence
- Depression
- Desertion
- Disregard for client' needs
- Distortion of reality about client's health problem
- Family behaviors detrimental to well-being
- Hostility
- Impaired ability to structure a meaningful life
- Impaired individualism
- Intolerance
- Neglect of basic needs of client
- Neglect of relationship with family member
- Neglect of treatment regimen
- Performing routines without regard for client's needs
- Prolonged hyperfocus on client
- Psychosomatic symptoms
- Rejection

Expected Outcomes

- Family members will identify factors that trigger stress and inappropriate behavior.
- Family members will make use of appropriate sources of support.
- Family members will interact appropriately with staff members and each other.
- Parents will meet their children's developmental needs.
- Family members will express feelings and individual needs.
- All children in the family will meet developmental milestones appropriate for their ages.
- Family members will meet child's health care needs.

Suggested NOC Outcomes

Caregiver Emotional Health; Caregiver–Patient Relationship; Caregiving Endurance Potential; Family Coping; Family Health Status; Family Social Climate; Family Support During Treatment

Interventions and Rationales

- Assess the family history *to identify the family's strengths and limitations.*
- Determine if family members are prepared to accept help. *Changes in behavior won't take place until family members are ready.*
- Communicate only brief amounts of information to family members at any one time. *Family members under stress usually can't grasp large amounts of information.*
- Help the family identify which tasks to tackle now and which to put off until the stress level decreases. *Performing easy, familiar activities decreases discomfort during times of stress.*

- PCC • Encourage family members to allow open expression of feelings and to avoid passing judgment on one another. *Family members need to be able to communicate openly without putting each other on the defensive.*
- Identify instances of successful communication among family members *to single out and encourage positive behavior.*
- Use play activity to promote self-esteem in children. *Parents commonly forget the developmental needs of children during crisis. If one child is seriously ill, parents may ignore siblings.*
- Help family members identify situations that trigger inappropriate behavior. *Family members must learn to recognize their tolerance threshold to react appropriately.*
- Help family members identify coping mechanisms used successfully in the *past to enable them to develop appropriate responses without learning new behaviors.*
- PCC • Help family members identify options when confronted with difficult decisions. *Members of dysfunctional families commonly believe they lack choices.*
- PCC • Teach parents about the health care and developmental needs of their child. *Family-centered care is essential for an ill child.*
- PCC • Provide referrals to appropriate social service agencies in order *to help family members find additional resources.*

Suggested NIC Interventions

Anger Control Assistance; Caregiver Support; Family Involvement Promotion; Family Therapy; Mutual Goal Setting; Normalization Promotion; Support Group

Evaluations for Expected Outcomes

- Family members state specific factors that lead to inappropriate behavior.
- Family members state their plans for contacting sources of support.
- Family members interact (with each other and staff) with appropriate verbal and nonverbal behavior.
- Parents meet their children's developmental needs.
- Family members express feelings and try to meet each other's emotional needs.
- Children show evidence of achieving age-appropriate developmental tasks.
- Family members meet chronically ill child's health care needs.

Documentation

- Observation of family members' interactions with each other and with outsiders
- Observations of family members' reactions to stress
- Examples of communication between family members
- Parents' understanding of normal childhood growth and development
- Interventions performed to help improve family members' coping skills
- Family members' level of participation in the care of ill child
- Referrals to community resources
- Evaluations for expected outcomes

REFERENCES

Bello-Utu, C. F., & DeSocio, J. E. (2015). Military deployment and reintegration: A systematic review of child coping. *Journal of Child & Adolescent Psychiatric Nursing*, *28*(1), 23–34. doi:10.1111/jcap.

Butler, M. P., Begley, M., Parahoo, K., & Finn, S. (2014). Getting psychosocial interventions into mental health nursing practice: A survey of skill use and perceived benefits to service users. *Journal of Advanced Nursing*, *70*(4), 866–877. doi:10.1111/jan.12248

Wu, L., Chiou, S., Sheen, J., Lin, P., Liao, Y. M., Chen, H., & Hsiao, C. (2014). Evaluating the acceptability and efficacy of a psycho-educational intervention for coping and symptom management by children with cancer: A randomized controlled study. *Journal of Advanced Nursing*, *70*(7), 1653–1662. doi:10.1111/jan.12328

IMPAIRED DENTITION

related to insufficient oral hygiene

Definition

Disruption in tooth development/eruption patterns or structural integrity of individual teeth

Assessment

- Child's age (chronological and developmental) and gender
- Dental health history, including primary and secondary tooth development; frequency of visits to the dentist; frequency of brushing; condition of teeth (such as presence of caries, extractions, plaque, malocclusion, and evulsion), gums, lips, tongue, and mucous membranes; and signs of salivary dysfunction (such as fissuring at corners of mouth, sore mucous membranes, dryness and cracking of lips, crusting of tongue and palate, and paresthesia of tongue or mucous membrane)
- Health history, including medication history, X-ray treatments, infection, allergies, trauma, lead poisoning, rubella, nephrotic illness, and malnutrition
- Nutritional status, including amount of sugar in diet
- Socioeconomic conditions, including access to dental health care
- Environmental conditions, including lack of fluoride in drinking water
- Family status, including willingness and ability of child's primary caregiver to supervise or perform dental health measures and to take child to dental appointments

Defining Characteristics

- Abraded teeth
- Absence of teeth
- Dental caries
- Enamel discoloration
- Erosion of enamel
- Excessive oral calculus
- Excessive oral plaque
- Facial asymmetry
- Halitosis
- Incomplete tooth eruption for age
- Loose tooth
- Malocclusion
- Premature loss of primary teeth
- Root caries
- Tooth fracture
- Tooth misalignment
- Toothache

Expected Outcomes

- Child will brush teeth with minimal supervision.
- Child will demonstrate good brushing technique.
- Child won't show evidence of dental caries, periodontal disease, or malocclusion.
- Child will reduce quantity of cariogenic food in diet.
- Child's teeth will show evidence of good daily oral hygiene.

Suggested NOC Outcomes

Oral Hygiene; Self-Care: Oral Hygiene

Interventions and Rationales

- PCC Teach the child principles of good dental hygiene using teaching methods appropriate to age group *to foster compliance.*
- Demonstrate good brushing technique. Stress the importance of having teeth feel clean rather than the need to follow a specific procedure. Help the child establish a schedule for brushing. If necessary, provide direct assistance as well as demonstrations *to reinforce good dental hygiene habits.*
- PCC Teach the child and parents or caregiver, if necessary, about the relationship between diet and dental health. For example, show the child pictures of foods that promote good dental health (such as milk) and pictures of foods that promote tooth decay (such as those containing refined sugar, honey, or molasses). If the child can read food labels, teach the child to identify and avoid products with excessive sucrose *to increase the child's awareness of cariogenic foods and encourage better eating habits and more frequent brushing.*
- If assessment reveals evidence of dental caries, periodontal disease, malocclusion, or other conditions requiring dental care, contact the child's parents *to ensure they're aware of impaired dentition and the need for follow-up care.* Provide a referral to a dentist *to ensure professional care.*
- Assess whether the child's parents are able and willing to assist in meeting the child's needs regarding dental health. Provide referrals to community resources that may help family members obtain dental care. *The high cost of dental care may cause some families to neglect dental care needs.*
- If the child is prone to dental problems, emphasize the need for more meticulous home dental care *to avoid further deterioration of the child's teeth and gums.*
- Schedule an appointment to determine whether the child's parents or caregiver have followed up on your referral to a dentist *to ensure continuity of care.*

Suggested NIC Interventions

Oral Health Maintenance; Oral Health Promotion; Teaching: Individual

Evaluations for Expected Outcomes

- Child assumes responsibility for brushing teeth with minimal supervision.
- Child demonstrates good brushing technique.
- Child shows no evidence of dental caries, periodontal disease, or malocclusion.
- Child reduces quantity of cariogenic foods in diet.
- Child's teeth show evidence of good daily oral hygiene.

Documentation

- Dental health history
- Evidence of dental problems
- Teaching sessions with child and parents or caregiver
- Evidence of improvement in child's dental hygiene
- Child's response to nursing interventions
- Evaluations for expected outcomes

REFERENCES

Chi, D., McManus, B., & Carle, A. (2014). Caregiver burden and preventive dental care use for US children with special health care needs: A stratified analysis based on functional limitation. *Maternal & Child Health Journal*, *18*(4), 882–890

Friedman, J. W., & Mathu-Muju, K. R. (2014). Dental therapists: Improving access to oral health care for underserved children. *American Journal of Public Health*, *104*(6), 1005–1009. doi:10.2105/AJPH.2014.301895

Masterson, E. E., & Sabbah, W. (2015). Maternal allostatic load, caretaking behaviors, and child dental caries experience: A cross-sectional evaluation of linked mother–child data from the third national health and nutrition examination survey. *American Journal of Public Health*, *105*(11), 2306–2311. doi:10.2105/AJPH.2015.302729.

RISK FOR DELAYED DEVELOPMENT

Definition

Vulnerable to delay of 25% or more in one or more of the areas of social or self-regulatory behavior, or in cognitive, language, gross, or fine motor skills, which may compromise health

Assessment

- Family process, including number and ages of children, usual patterns of interaction, roles of parents and children, communication patterns, relationship changes (such as separation, divorce, or remarriage), and past response to crisis
- Parental status, including perception of child's behavior, past responses to stress, child care provisions, history of inappropriate parenting, and history of destructive behavior or substance abuse
- Alteration in child's growth and development resulting from illness or dysfunctional parenting
- Developmental level (physical, cognitive, psychosocial, and linguistic) and learning needs
- Growth history, including changes in child's size and form, current height and weight, percentile on pediatric growth grid, body proportions, bone development (determined through X-ray examination), tooth development, organ systems development, neuroendocrine function (growth hormone, thyroid hormone, and androgen levels), genetic abnormalities that may affect growth, prenatal influences (fetal exposure to alcohol or illicit drugs, maternal smoking, or malnutrition), birth trauma (possible oxygen deprivation or nerve injuries), and breast-feeding or bottle-feeding
- Cultural information, including nationality, ethnicity, religious affiliation, and beliefs and practices regarding health and child rearing
- Psychosocial status, including family's resources, health beliefs and attitudes, interest in learning, knowledge and skill regarding current health problem, obstacles to learning, support systems (willingness and ability of others to help the child), and usual coping pattern

Risk Factors

Prenatal

- Economically disadvantaged
- Endocrine disorder
- Functional illiteracy
- Genetic disorder
- Infection
- Inadequate nutrition
- Insufficient prenatal care
- Late-term prenatal care
- Maternal age ≤15 years
- Maternal age ≥35 years
- Substance abuse
- Unplanned pregnancy
- Unwanted pregnancy

Individual

- Behavior disorder (e.g., attention deficit, oppositional defiant)
- Brain injury (e.g., abuse, accident, hemorrhage, shaken baby syndrome)
- Chronic illness
- Congenital disorder
- Failure to thrive
- Genetic disorder
- Hearing impairment
- History of adoption
- Inadequate nutrition
- Involvement with the foster care system
- Lead poisoning
- Natural disaster
- Positive drug screen
- Prematurity
- Recurrent otitis media
- Seizure disorder
- Substance abuse
- Technology dependence (e.g., ventilator, augmentative communication)
- Treatment regimen
- Visual impairment

Environment

- Economically disadvantaged
- Exposure to violence
- Learning disability
- Mental health issue (e.g., depression, psychosis, personality disorder, substance abuse)
- Presence of abuse (e.g., physical, psychological, sexual)

Caregiver

- Learning disability
- Mental health issue (e.g., depression, psychosis, personality disorder, substance abuse)
- Presence of abuse (e.g., physical, psychological, sexual)

Expected Outcomes

- Child will continue to grow and gain weight in accordance with growth chart of age and sex.
- Child will consume _____ calories and ________ mL of fluids representing ________ servings (specify for each food group).
- Child will participate in activities and be provided with a supervised, unconfined environment that includes age-appropriate toys and fosters interaction with child's development.
- Parents will express understanding of measures to reduce child's risk for delayed development.
- Parents will identify risk factors that may interfere with child's development.

Suggested NOC Outcomes

Family Functioning; Growth; Parenting Performance; Personal Health Status; Risk Control

Interventions and Rationales

- Assess family's developmental stage; family roles; family rules; socioeconomic status; family health history; history of substance abuse; history of sexual abuse of spouse or children; problem-solving and decision-making skills; religious affiliation; ethnicity. *Assessment information will aid in developing a workable plan of care.*
- Weigh and measure child. Review growth chart *to establish current height and weight values.* Establish a meal program *to meet the child's nutritional needs.*
- Create an environment in which family members can express themselves openly and honestly. Establish rules for communication during meetings with the family. *Having rules allows everyone to participate and keep the discussion on the designated topic.*

PCC • Teach parents about nutritional requirements needed for child of specific weight and age. Discuss various meal choices available to the child. *Providing instruction in writing simplifies the parents' role in selecting healthy foods.*

PCC • Educate parents about child's need for quality interaction with family members and others.

- Inform parents about age-appropriate activities and toys as well as potential playmates for a child of specific age. Emphasize importance of providing an unconfined, supervised environment in which the child can *play to encourage play that encourages the child to move freely.*

PCC • Educate parents about risk factors that may lead to delayed development, such as lack of supportive interactions or age-appropriate activities. *The ability to recognize risk factors will promote getting help for the parents and child sooner.*

PCC • Teach coping skills to parents *to enable them to deal effectively with the child's needs.*

PCC • Encourage parents to listen to the child and communicate in a loving, supportive way *in order to allow the child to maintain a positive attitude.*

PCC • Encourage parents to identify preventive measures they may initiate at home to ensure continuity of care. *Consistency in providing care will help the child understand that the plan carries over to all aspects of child's life.*

- Provide parents with a copy of child's teaching plan. *This helps to reinforce what the child is learning.*

PCC • Refer to case manager/social worker *to ensure that a home assessment is done.*

PCC • Refer to nutritionist *for follow-up with food issues.*

Suggested NIC Interventions

Nutrition Management; Family Process Maintenance; Coping Enhancement; Family Integrity Promotion; Maintenance; Normalization Promotion; Substance Use Prevention; Substance Use Treatment; Risk Identification

Evaluations for Expected Outcomes

- Child meets developmental milestones.
- Child consumes adequate food and fluid to maintain normal weight.
- Child participates in activities appropriate for age and developmental stage.
- Parents' expression of normal developmental stages and measures to reduce developmental delays.

Documentation

- Observations of developmental assessments
- Interventions to provide supportive care and patient's response
- Instructions given to patient and family members on developmental stages and measures to reduce developmental delay
- Child's weight
- Evaluations for expected outcomes

REFERENCES

Attaway, J., Stone, C. L., Sendor, C., & Rosario, E. R. (2015). Effect of amplification on speech and language in children with aural atresia. *American Journal of Audiology*, 24(3), 354–359. doi:10.1044/2015_AJA-15-0021

Mulrine, C., & Kollia, B. (2015). Speech, language, hearing delays: Time for early intervention? *Journal of Family Practice*, *64*(3), E1–E9.
Tiesler, C., & Heinrich, J. (2014). Prenatal nicotine exposure and child behavioral problems. *European Child & Adolescent Psychiatry*, *23*(10), 913–929. doi:10.1007/s00787-014-0615-y
Van der Linde, B. W., van Netten, J. J., Otten, B., Postema, K., Geuze, R. H., & Schoemaker, M. M. (2015). Activities of daily living in children with developmental coordination disorder: Performance, learning, and participation. *Physical Therapy*, *95*(11), 1496–1506. doi:10.2522/ptj.20140211

DIARRHEA

related to malabsorption

Definition

Passage of loose, unformed stools

Assessment

- History of bowel disorder or surgery
- Gastrointestinal status, including nausea and vomiting, usual bowel patterns, changes in bowel patterns, stool characteristics (color, amount, consistency, and presence of blood or mucus), pain, inspection of abdomen, auscultation of bowel sounds, and palpation for masses and tenderness
- Medication history, including use of antibiotics
- Nutritional status, including dietary intake, appetite, weight, and changes to usual diet
- Fluid and electrolyte status, including intake and output, urine specific gravity, skin turgor, mucous membranes, and serum potassium and sodium levels
- Skin integrity

Defining Characteristics

- Abdominal pain bowel urgency
- Cramping
- Hyperactive bowel sounds
- Loose liquid stools >3 in 24 hours

Expected Outcomes

- Child will exhibit normal elimination pattern for age.
- Child will maintain balanced intake and output within normal limits for age.
- Auscultation will reveal normal bowel sounds.
- Child will maintain body temperature of 98.6° F to 99.5° F (37° C to 37.5° C).
- Child's urine specific gravity will be between 1.010 and 1.015.
- Child's skin will remain intact.
- Caregivers will demonstrate appropriate skin care techniques.

Suggested NOC Outcomes

Bowel Continence; Bowel Elimination; Electrolyte & Acid/base balance; Fluid Balance; Hydration; Symptom Severity

Interventions and Rationales

- Assess the frequency and characteristics of stools, and auscultate bowel sounds every 4 hours *to monitor the treatment's effectiveness.*
- Monitor and record intake and output, urine specific gravity (with each voiding), skin turgor, condition of mucous membranes, presence of tears, and condition of fontanels (in infants) *to monitor hydration status and the need for fluid replacement.*
- Record daily weight before the first feeding each morning *to determine if the child is suffering from dehydration. Weight loss of 5% or more in 1 day may indicate dehydration.*
- As ordered, offer an oral replacement solution such as dextrose and electrolytes (Pedialyte) or clear liquids in small amounts (5 to 15 mL) every 10 to 15 minutes, waiting 20 to 30 minutes after voiding of loose stools, *to decrease intestinal irritation and the likelihood of further diarrhea.*
- Don't offer fruit juices or carbonated fluids. *The high glucose content and osmolar load associated with these beverages may stimulate further episodes of diarrhea.*
- Offer the child the BRAT (banana, rice, apple, and toast) diet, as ordered, 4 hours after last loose stool *to help meet the child's nutritional needs without exacerbating diarrhea.*
- Check the skin in the perianal area after each stool. Change the diaper frequently and clean skin thoroughly *to prevent skin breakdown.*
- Apply protective ointment to the diaper area *to provide a barrier between the child's skin and stools.*
- Monitor the child's temperature every 2 to 4 hours *to detect fever, which may be associated with fluid loss and inflammation.* Measure the temperature using axillary or oral routes *because the use of a rectal thermometer may stimulate further diarrhea.*
- PCC Teach caregivers the importance of frequent diaper changes and meticulous skin care for the child. Instruct them not to use powder in the diaper area *to avoid caking and subsequent skin breakdown.*

Suggested NIC Interventions

Diarrhea Management; Electrolyte Management; Fluid Management; Nutrition Management; Skin Care: Topical Treatments; Skin Surveillance

Evaluations for Expected Outcomes

- Child regains normal elimination pattern.
- Child maintains balanced intake and output within normal limits for age.
- Auscultation reveals normal bowel sounds.
- Child remains afebrile.
- Child's urine specific gravity remains between 1.010 and 1.015.
- Child's skin remains intact, without signs of redness or irritation.
- Caregivers demonstrate appropriate skin care techniques.

Documentation

- Frequency and characteristics of stool
- Appearance of skin
- Intake and output
- Weight (recorded daily)
- Evidence of caregivers' knowledge of dietary management and skin care techniques
- Evaluations for expected outcomes

REFERENCES

Ehsanur Rahman, A., Moinuddin, M., Molla, M., Worku, A., Hurt, L., Kirkwood, B., . . . Muhe, L. (2014). Childhood diarrheal deaths in seven low- and middle-income countries. *Bulletin of the World Health Organization*, *92*(9), 664–671. doi:10.2471/BLT.13.134809

Lohner, S., Küllenberg, D., Antes, G., Decsi, T., & Meerpohl, J. J. (2014). Prebiotics in healthy infants and children for prevention of acute infectious diseases: A systematic review and meta-analysis. *Nutrition Reviews*, 72(8), 523–531. doi:10.1111/nure.12117

Sarmin, M., Ahmed, T., Bardhan, P. K., & Chisti, M. J. (2014). Specialist hospital study shows that septic shock and drowsiness predict mortality in children under five with diarrhea. *Acta Paediatrica*, *103*(7), e306-e311. doi:10.1111/apa.12640

DEFICIENT DIVERSIONAL ACTIVITY

related to prolonged hospitalization

Definition

Decreased stimulation from (or interest or engagement in) recreational or leisure activities

Assessment

- Level of comfort, including mobility and activity tolerance
- Cardiovascular status, including heart rate and rhythm, blood pressure, history of murmurs, cardiac disease
- Respiratory status, including respiratory rate at rest and during activity, shortness of breath, cyanosis, and wheezing
- Neurologic status, including level of consciousness, orientation, mood, behavior, memory, and coordination
- Psychosocial status, including presence of family members, social interaction, cultural and ethnic background, hobbies, interests, and changes or adaptations needed to carry out activities
- Environment, including isolation and availability of diversional activities
- Developmental level (physical, cognitive, psychosocial, and linguistic) and learning needs

Defining Characteristics

- Boredom
- Current setting does not allow engagement in activity

Expected Outcomes

- Child will select and participate in age-appropriate play.
- Child will express enjoyment in selected play activity.
- Child will achieve age-appropriate developmental tasks.

Suggested NOC Outcomes

Leisure Participation; Motivation; Play Participation; Social Involvement

Interventions and Rationales

- Provide various toys, supplies, and activities for the child's use. Make sure items are appropriate to the child's age, developmental level, and environment. *Ready access to diversional activities entices the child to make use of time alone. Age-appropriate items are geared to the child's cognitive, motor, and safety needs.*
- PCC Encourage family members to bring the child's favorite toys, family pictures, or other objects from home. Provide space in the child's room for cards and gifts from family and friends. Encourage the parents to tape-record stories for their child and provide a tape player so the child can listen *to maintain a sense of attachment with the family and provide a sense of security.*
- PCC Encourage the child to visit the playroom and participate in individual and group activities. *Participating in play activities helps the child meet developmental needs.*
- Discuss the child's diversional activity deficit with a play therapist *to enable the play therapist to better address the child's special needs.*
- Schedule time to personally engage the child in therapeutic or developmental play. Schedule play periods for day and evening shifts. *This ensures that the child has ample opportunity for diversional activity and prevents the child from being isolated for prolonged periods. Participation in play will also strengthen your relationship with the child.*
- PCC For a child confined to bed, provide creative, challenging games. For example, make a fishing pole with large safe hook and challenge the child to pick up items around the room; glue Velcro on soft balls and create a "dart board" on the wall; or make string-and-paper-cup "telephones" to use with other patients in the room. *Creative play encourages age-appropriate behavior, helps make the environment more enjoyable and challenging, and gives the child greater control and independence.*
- Provide opportunities for therapeutic play. For example, encourage the child to play with safe hospital equipment, play nurse or doctor, play house, pound clay, or perform "procedures" on a doll. *Therapeutic play offers the child an opportunity to express fears, fantasies, sadness, and misconceptions; to learn more about illness and its treatment; and to release pent-up feelings safely. This helps the child develop a better sense of control and enhances the child's ability to cope with hospitalization and treatment.*
- Provide art and craft supplies for the preschool or school-age child *to enhance the child's creativity, provide an emotional outlet, and encourage the development of initiative and industry.*

Suggested NIC Interventions

Energy Management; Recreation Therapy; Self-Responsibility Facilitation; Socialization Enhancement; Therapeutic Play; Visitation Facilitation

Evaluations for Expected Outcomes

- Child voluntarily participates in age-appropriate activities.
- Child expresses contentment with activities.
- Child achieves age-appropriate developmental tasks.

Documentation

- Child's expressions of boredom and desire for activity
- Assessment of child's physical, cognitive, and psychosocial developmental abilities
- Evaluation of child's physical, educational, and psychosocial need for activity
- Nursing interventions directed at providing diversional activity
- Child's response to play
- Evaluations for expected outcomes

REFERENCES

Bailey, C. G., & DiPerna, J. C. (2015). Effects of classroom-based energizers on primary grade students' physical activity levels. *Physical Educator*, 72(3), 480–495.

Behrens, T. K., Wegner, R. L., Miller, D. J., Liebert, M. L., & Smith, J. H. (2015). Parents' and children's perceptions of the keep it moving! after-school physical activity program. *Physical Educator*, 72(3), 445–459.

Jun, Z., Shoham, D. A., Tesdahl, E., & Gesell, S. B. (2015). Network interventions on physical activity in an afterschool program: An agent-based social network study. *American Journal of Public Health*, *105*(S2), S236–S243. doi:10.2105/AJPH.2014.302277

FEAR

related to separation from support system; unfamiliar setting

Definition

Response to perceived threat that is consciously recognized as a danger

Assessment

- Age
- Psychosocial factors, including child's understanding of own illness and treatment plan, verbal and nonverbal indicators of fear, and availability of family and friends
- Changes in behavior, eating, or sleeping patterns
- Physiologic manifestations of fear, including temperature, pulse rate, blood pressure, respiratory rate, and skin color and temperature

Defining Characteristics

- Apprehensiveness
- Decrease in self-assurance
- Excitedness
- Feeling dread
- Feeling of fear
- Feeling of panic
- Feeling of terror
- Feeling of alarm
- Increase in blood pressure
- Increase in tension
- Jitteriness
- Muscle tension
- Nausea
- Pallor
- Pupil dilation
- Vomiting

Cognitive

- Decrease in learning ability
- Decrease in problem-solving ability
- Decrease in productivity
- Identifies object of fear
- Stimulus believed to be a threat

Behaviors

- Attack behaviors
- Avoidance behaviors
- Focus narrowed to the source of fear
- Impulsiveness
- Increase in alertness

Physiologic

- Anorexia
- Change in physiologic response (e.g., blood pressure, heart rate, respiratory rate, oxygen saturation, and end-title CO_2)
- Diarrhea
- Dry mouth
- Dyspnea
- Fatigue
- Increase in perspiration
- Increase in respiratory rate

Expected Outcomes

- Child will identify sources of fear.
- Child will demonstrate effective use of coping mechanisms.
- Child will seek comfort from parents.
- Child will express understanding of medical procedures.
- Child's vital signs will remain within normal limits for age.
- Child will exhibit fewer physiologic or behavioral manifestations of fear.

Suggested NOC Outcomes

Anxiety Self-Control; Comfort Level; Coping; Fear Level; Fear Self-Control

Interventions and Rationales

- Acknowledge the child's fear. *Bringing feelings out allows for discussion and identification of coping strategies.*
- Don't dismiss fear or blithely reassure the child that "everything will be all right." *Refusing to acknowledge fear or giving false reassurance impairs coping.*
- PCC Spend as much time as possible talking with the child. For infants and toddlers, use nonverbal communication, such as holding and rocking. *Establishing rapport encourages the child to express own feelings and provides comfort.*
- Help the child identify sources of *fear to enable the child to put emotions into perspective.*
- Provide the child with accurate information about the child's condition and scheduled procedures and treatments. Orient the child to the facility's sights and sounds. *Accurate information dispels misconceptions that can fuel fear.*
- PCC Encourage the parents and family members to stay with the child as much as possible and participate in child's care, as appropriate, *to enhance the child's ability to cope and decrease fear caused by separation.*

Suggested NIC Interventions

Coping Enhancement; Counseling; Emotional Support; Presence; Security Enhancement

Evaluations for Expected Outcomes

- Child verbalizes known sources of fear.
- Child demonstrates effective use of coping mechanisms.
- Child expresses feelings of comfort.
- Child expresses understanding of medical procedures.
- Child's vital signs remain within normal limits for age.
- Child exhibits marked decrease in physiologic and behavioral manifestations of fear.

Documentation

- Child's verbal and behavioral expressions of fear
- Physiologic manifestations of fear
- Interventions performed to reduce fear
- Child's response to interventions
- Family's involvement in child's care

- Child's response to family involvement
- Evaluations for expected outcomes

REFERENCES

Dougherty, J. P. (2015). The experience of siblings of children with type 1 diabetes. *Pediatric Nursing, 41*(6), 279–305.

Foster, J. M., & Hagedorn, W. B. (2014). A qualitative exploration of fear and safety with child victims of sexual abuse. *Journal of Mental Health Counseling, 36*(3), 243–262.

Sparapani, V. C., Jacob, E., & Nascimento, L. C. (2015). What is it like to be a child with type 1 diabetes mellitus? *Pediatric Nursing, 41*(1), 17–22.

DEFICIENT FLUID VOLUME

related to active fluid volume loss

Definition

Decreased intravascular, interstitial, and/or intercellular fluid. This refers to dehydration, water loss alone without change in sodium

Assessment

- Age
- Height and weight
- History of diarrhea or vomiting
- Gastrointestinal (GI) status, including usual bowel patterns, changes in bowel patterns, stool characteristics (color, amount, size, consistency, and frequency), auscultation of bowel sounds, and inspection of abdomen
- Stool culture, ova, and parasites
- Nutritional status, including dietary intake, changes from usual pattern, appetite, current weight, and recent weight changes
- Fluid and electrolyte status, including intake and output, urine specific gravity, skin turgor, mucous membranes, serum sodium and potassium and blood urea nitrogen levels, and hematocrit (HCT)
- Medication history, including use of laxatives, enemas, and antibiotics
- Neurologic status, including level of consciousness
- Presence of sick children or adults at home, school, or day care
- Respiratory status, including increased respiratory rate
- Child's and family members' knowledge of factors that cause vomiting or diarrhea

Defining Characteristics

- Alteration in mental status
- Alteration in skin turgor
- Decrease in blood pressure
- Decrease in pulse pressure
- Decrease in pulse volume
- Decrease in tongue turgor
- Decrease in urine output
- Decrease in venous filling
- Dry mucous membranes
- Dry skin
- Increase in body temperature
- Increase in heart rate
- Increase in HCT
- Increase in urine concentration
- Sudden weight loss
- Thirst
- Weakness

Expected Outcomes

- Child will maintain normal weight.
- Child's intake and output will be balanced and within normal limits for age.
- Child's electrolyte values will remain within normal limits for age.
- Child will maintain urine specific gravity of 1.010 to 1.015.
- Child will exhibit moist mucous membranes, good skin turgor, and flat fontanels (in infant).
- Child will exhibit normal elimination patterns for age.
- Child will retain feedings and won't experience emesis.

Suggested NOC Outcomes

Electrolyte and Acid/Base Balance; Fluid Balance; Hydration; Nutritional Status: Food & Fluid Intake; Vital Signs

Interventions and Rationales

- Record intake and output in every shift. Include urine, stools, vomitus, nasogastric, or chest tube drainage, and any other output *to obtain fluid status. Increased output and decreased intake indicate fluid deficit.*
- Weigh the child each morning before the first feeding. *Weight loss of 5%/day indicates fluid deficit.*
- Assess skin turgor, mucous membranes, and fontanels (in infant) in every shift. *Fluid loss occurs first in extracellular spaces, resulting in poor skin turgor, dry mucous membranes, and sunken fontanels.*
- Monitor vital signs every 4 hours or more frequently, if needed. *Fever and increased respiratory rate contribute to fluid loss. A weak, thready pulse and a drop in blood pressure indicate dehydration.*
- Check urine specific gravity every voiding. *Increased specific gravity indicates lack of fluids to dilute urine.*
- Monitor laboratory study results (electrolytes, pH, and HCT). *During fluid loss, electrolytes are excreted, which may lead to electrolyte imbalance.*
- Assess the child's behavior and activity level in every shift. *A child with dehydration may develop anorexia, decreased activity level, and general malaise.*
- After diarrhea and vomiting have decreased, offer small amounts (5 to 15 mL) of clear fluids frequently *to replace fluid loss without causing further GI irritation.*
- If the child is permitted nothing by mouth, provide mouth care every 4 hours, or as needed, *to help keep mucous membranes moist. In infants, oral care and a pacifier help meet the developmental need for sucking.*
- Monitor IV fluid infusion every hour. *Because fluid balance is less stable in young children, an infusion rate that's too fast or too slow can lead to fluid imbalance more rapidly than in adults.*
- Secure the IV site by wrapping it in a soft bandage *to protect the site and allow the child free movement of the extremity.*

Suggested NIC Interventions

Fluid/Electrolyte Management; Intravenous (IV) Therapy; Urinary Elimination Management; Vital Signs Monitoring

Evaluations for Expected Outcomes

- Child maintains normal weight.
- Child exhibits balance of intake and output within normal limits for age.
- Child's electrolyte levels, pH, and HCT remain within age-appropriate ranges.
- Child's urine specific gravity remains between 1.010 and 1.015.
- Child exhibits moist mucous membranes, good skin turgor, and flat fontanels (in infant).
- Child experiences normal elimination patterns for age.
- Child retains feedings without emesis.

Documentation

- Intake and output
- Weight (recorded daily)
- Skin turgor, mucous membranes, vital signs, and other physical findings
- Urine specific gravity and other laboratory values
- Interventions and child's response
- Evaluations for expected outcomes

REFERENCES

Bontant, T., Matrot, B., Abdoul, H., Aizenfisz, S., Naudin, J., Jones, P., & Dauger, S. (2015). Assessing fluid balance in critically ill pediatric patients. *European Journal of Pediatrics*, *174*(1), 133–137. doi:10.1007/s00431-014-2372-9

Hew-Butler, T., Kenney, E. L., Long, M. W., Cradock, A. L., & Gortmaker, S. L. (2015). Inadequate hydration or normal body fluid homeostasis? *American Journal of Public Health*, *105*(10), e5–e7. doi:10.2105/AJPH.2015.302825

Kenney, E. L., Long, M. W., Cradock, A. L., & Gortmaker, S. L. (2015). Prevalence of inadequate hydration among US children and disparities by gender and race/ethnicity: National health and nutrition examination survey, 2009–2012. *American Journal of Public Health*, *105*(8), e113–e118. doi:10.2105/AJPH.2015.302572

RISK FOR DEFICIENT FLUID VOLUME

Definition

Vulnerable to experiencing decreased intravascular, interstitial, and/or intracellular fluid volumes, which may compromise health

Assessment

- Age
- History of problems that can cause excessive fluid loss, such as vomiting, diarrhea, hemorrhage, and ketoacidosis
- Vital signs
- Level of consciousness
- Fluid and electrolyte status, including intake and output, urine specific gravity, skin turgor, mucous membranes, fontanels (in infant), electrolyte levels, and blood urea nitrogen levels
- Gastrointestinal (GI) status, including usual bowel patterns, changes in bowel patterns, stool characteristics (color, amount, consistency, and frequency), auscultation of bowel sounds, and inspection of abdomen

- Nutritional status, including dietary intake, changes from usual pattern, appetite, current weight, and recent weight changes
- Psychosocial status, including developmental level, stressors (such as school, disease process, family discord, or separation from family), and coping mechanisms
- Respiratory status, including increased respiratory rate
- Child's and family members' knowledge of factors that cause vomiting or diarrhea

Risk Factors

- Active fluid volume loss
- Barrier to accessing fluid
- Compromised regulatory mechanism
- Deviations affecting fluid absorption
- Deviation affecting fluid intake
- Excessive fluid loss through normal route
- Extremes of age
- Extremes of weight
- Factors influencing fluid needs
- Fluid loss through abnormal route
- Insufficient knowledge about fluid needs
- Pharmaceutical agent

Expected Outcomes

- Child will maintain weight.
- Child's urine specific gravity will remain between 1.010 and 1.015.
- Child's intake and output will be balanced and within normal limits for age.
- Child will exhibit good skin turgor, moist mucous membranes, and flat fontanels (in infant).
- Child will exhibit appropriate elimination patterns for age.
- Child won't show signs of fluid and electrolyte imbalance.
- Child will retain feedings without experiencing emesis.

Suggested NOC Outcomes

Appetite; Electrolyte & Acid/Base Balance; Fluid Balance; Hydration; Nutritional Status: Food & Fluid Intake; Urinary Elimination

Interventions and Rationales

- Record intake and output in every shift. Include urine, stools, vomitus, nasogastric or chest tube drainage, and any other output *to obtain fluid status. Increased output and decreased intake result in fluid deficits.*
- Weigh the child each morning before the first feeding. *Weight loss of 5%/day indicates fluid deficit.*
- Assess skin turgor, mucous membranes, and fontanels (in infant) in every shift. *Fluid loss first occurs in extracellular spaces, resulting in poor skin turgor, dry mucous membranes, and sunken fontanels.*
- Monitor vital signs at least every 4 hours or more frequently, if needed. *Increased temperature and increased respiratory rate contribute to fluid loss. A weak, thready pulse and drop in blood pressure indicate dehydration.*
- Check urine specific gravity every voiding. *Increased specific gravity indicates lack of fluids to dilute urine.*
- S Monitor laboratory studies (electrolytes, pH, and hematocrit [HCT]). *During fluid loss, electrolytes are excreted, which may lead to electrolyte imbalance.*
- Assess the child's behavior and activity level in every shift. *A child with dehydration may develop anorexia, decreased activity level, and general malaise.*

- When diarrhea and vomiting have decreased, offer small amounts (5 to 15 mL) of clear fluids *to replace fluid loss without causing further GI irritation.*
- If the child is permitted nothing by mouth, provide mouth care every 4 hours, and as needed, *to help keep mucous membranes moist. In infants, oral care and pacifier help meet the developmental need for sucking.*
- S Monitor IV fluid infusion every hour. *Because fluid balance is less stable in young children, infusing too rapidly or too slowly can lead to fluid imbalance more quickly than in adults.*
- Secure the IV site by wrapping it in a soft bandage *to protect the site and allow the child to move hand or arm freely.*

Suggested NIC Interventions

Electrolyte Management; Fluid Management; Intravenous (IV) Therapy; Nutrition Management; Vital Signs Monitoring

Evaluations for Expected Outcomes

- Child maintains weight.
- Child's urine specific gravity remains between 1.010 and 1.015.
- Child exhibits balanced intake and output within normal limits for age.
- Child exhibits good skin turgor, moist mucous membranes, and flat fontanels (in infant).
- Child has appropriate elimination patterns for age.
- Child's electrolyte values, pH, and HCT remain within age-appropriate ranges.
- Child retains feedings without experiencing emesis.

Documentation

- Intake and output
- Weight (recorded daily)
- Skin turgor, mucous membranes, vital signs, and other physical findings
- Urine specific gravity and other laboratory values
- Interventions and child's response
- Evaluations for expected outcomes

REFERENCES

Bontant, T., Matrot, B., Abdoul, H., Aizenfisz, S., Naudin, J., Jones, P., & Dauger, S. (2015). Assessing fluid balance in critically ill pediatric patients. *European Journal of Pediatrics, 174*(1), 133–137. doi:10.1007/s00431-014-2372-9

Pooling resources to boost fluid intake among patients. (2014). *Nursing Management—UK, 21*(5), 7.

Smith, T. S. (2014). Decreased solid food intake in a toddler: Is that a problem? *Pediatric Nursing, 40*(4), 199–200.

GRIEVING

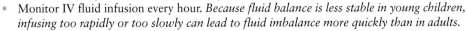

related to anticipatory loss of significant object (e.g., possession, job, status)

Definition

A normal complex process that includes emotional, physical, spiritual, social, and intellectual responses and behaviors by which individuals, families, and communities incorporate an actual, anticipated, or perceived loss into their daily lives

Assessment

- Child's state of grief and mourning
- Child's developmental level
- Perceived value of loss
- Usual patterns of coping with loss
- Behavioral manifestations of grieving
- Somatic problems associated with grieving process, including changes in appetite, sleep pattern, and activity level
- Available support systems

Defining Characteristics

- Alteration in activity level
- Alteration in dream pattern
- Alteration in immune functioning
- Alteration in neuroendocrine functioning
- Alteration in sleep pattern
- Anger
- Blaming
- Despair
- Detachment
- Disorganization
- Finding meaning in a loss
- Guilt about feeling relieved
- Maintaining a connection to the deceased
- Pain
- Panic behavior
- Personal growth
- Psychological distress
- Suffering

Expected Outcomes

- Child will express feelings in nondestructive manner.
- Child will seek emotional support from family members to help cope with loss.
- Child will take advantage of available resources, such as participation in play therapy, to help cope with loss.
- Parents will express understanding of grieving process.
- Parents will participate in care of child and interact positively with child.

Suggested NOC Outcomes

Communication; Coping; Depression Level; Family Coping; Family Integrity; Grief Resolution; Psychosocial Adjustment: Life Change

Interventions and Rationales

- PCC Encourage the child to express feelings through drawing, puppetry, or gross motor play *to provide a safe outlet for pent-up emotions. A child doesn't have the verbal and cognitive skills to express feelings and needs alternative means of expression. Allow the child to express grief in own way; intervene only to prevent physically destructive behavior.*
- PCC Plan to spend time in each shift with the child. If the child doesn't wish to talk, spend the time in silence *to convey concern, understanding, and support.*
- Reassure the child that it's all right to be angry or sad. Assess whether the child feels responsible for the loss, and clear up misconceptions *to help alleviate guilt feelings.*
- Reassure the family that grief is a normal reaction to loss; explain the stages of the grieving process and normal responses. Help parents understand that the child's feelings and behavior are normal under the present circumstances. *Understanding the grieving process will enhance the family's ability to cope.*

PCC • Encourage parents and siblings to participate in the care of the child. Remind them of child's need for emotional support at this time. *The child may fear about no longer being loved or cared for after the loss. It's crucial that the child receives emotional reassurance.*
- Offer the child simple choices related to care issues *to give the child a sense of control to meet developmental needs for initiative and industry.*

PCC • Encourage the child and family members to develop coping strategies for dealing with loss, such as participating in diversional activities, reminiscing, or seeking out support groups *to facilitate the grieving process.*
- Provide positive feedback for effective coping behavior *to help the child and family members regain self-confidence.*

Suggested NIC Interventions

Active Listening; Anticipatory Guidance; Coping Enhancement; Family Support; Family Therapy; Grief Work Facilitation; Hope Instillation; Spiritual Support

Evaluations for Expected Outcomes

- Child expresses feelings in nondestructive manner.
- Child's verbal expressions and behavior indicate knowing that the child will receive emotional support from family and won't be blamed, punished, or abandoned because of the loss.
- Child uses available resources to help cope with loss.
- Parents express understanding of grieving process.
- Parents participate in care of child and interact positively with child.

Documentation

- Child's verbal expressions and behavior
- Child's eating, sleeping, and activity patterns
- Observation of emotional responses
- Child's attempts to gain control, such as making decisions and using support systems
- Interaction between parents and child
- Nursing interventions and child's response to them
- Evaluations for expected outcomes

REFERENCES

Bugge, K. E., Darbyshire, P., Røkholt, E. G., Haugstvedt, K. S., & Helseth, S. (2014). Young children's grief: Parents' understanding and coping. *Death Studies*, *38*(1), 36–43. doi:10.1080/07481187.2012.718037

Burger, K. J., & Watson, L. (2014). A blue shell. *Critical Care Nurse*, *34*(3), 86–87. doi:10.4037/ccn2014545

Mullen, J. E., Reynolds, M. R., & Larson, J. S. (2015). Caring for pediatric patients' families at the child's end of life. *Critical Care Nurse*, *35*(6), 46–56. doi:10.4037/ccn2015614

RISK FOR DISPROPORTIONATE GROWTH

Definition

Vulnerable to growth above the 97th percentile or below the 3rd percentile for age, crossing two percentile channels, which may compromise health

Assessment

- Age
- Gender
- Physiologic status, including basal metabolic rate, temperature, motor development, sleep patterns (time and quality of sleep), activity level, and vision and hearing screening
- Growth history, including changes in child's size and form, current height and weight, percentile on pediatric growth grid, body proportions, bone development (determined through X-ray examination), tooth development, organ systems development, neuroendocrine function (growth hormone, thyroid hormone, and androgen levels), genetic abnormalities that may affect growth, prenatal influences (fetal exposure to alcohol or illicit drugs, maternal smoking, or malnutrition), birth trauma (possible oxygen deprivation or nerve injuries), and breast-feeding or bottle-feeding
- Environmental factors, including chemical or radiation exposure, lead exposure, passive inhalation of tobacco smoke, and exposure to water, air, or food contaminants
- Nutritional status, including dietary intake, appetite, ability to feed self or availability of feeding assistance, and consumption of adequate calories and appropriate number and size of servings for child's age and sex (based on the U.S. Department of Agriculture's Food Guide Pyramid)
- Social status, including family structure, type and quality of parents' or guardian's interactions with child, peer relationships (if age appropriate), and socioeconomic status
- Cultural information, including nationality, ethnicity, religious affiliation, and beliefs and practices regarding health and child rearing
- Health history, including psychiatric or medical diagnoses and use of over-the-counter or prescription medications

Risk Factors

Caregiver

- Alteration of cognitive functioning
- Learning disability
- Mental health issue (e.g., depression, psychosis, personality disorder, substance abuse)
- Presence of abuse (e.g., physical, psychological, sexual)

Environmental

- Deprivation
- Economically disadvantaged
- Exposure to teratogen
- Exposure to violence
- Lead poisoning
- Natural disaster

Individual

- Anorexia
- Chronic illness
- Infection
- Insatiable appetite
- Maladaptive feeding behavior by caregiver
- Maladaptive self-feeding behavior
- Malnutrition
- Prematurity
- Substance abuse

Prenatal

- Congenital disorder
- Exposure to teratogen
- Genetic disorder
- Inadequate maternal nutrition
- Maternal infection
- Multiple gestation
- Substance abuse

Expected Outcomes

- Child will grow and gain weight as expected based on growth chart norms for age and gender.
- Child will consume ______ calories and _____ mL of fluids representing ____ servings (specify for each food group).
- Child will sleep _____ hours daily.
- Child will maintain age-appropriate activity level.
- Child and parents or guardian will identify risk factors that may lead to disproportionate growth.
- Child and parents or guardian will state understanding of preventive measures to reduce risk of disproportionate growth.

Suggested NOC Outcomes

Appetite; Body Image; Child Development: Middle Childhood; Growth; Risk Control; Weight: Body Mass

Interventions and Rationales

- Weigh and measure the child and review the growth chart curve *to establish current height and weight values and compare the results with growth history.*
- Collaborate with the dietary department to establish a meal program that meets the child's nutritional needs. Educate the child and parents or guardian on nutritional requirements for the child's age and gender. Discuss the various meals available to the child at *home to promote growth.*
- Establish a routine sleep schedule for the child. Provide a comfortable environment that promotes rest *to ensure adequate duration and quality of sleep and to initiate a routine sleep pattern that may be continued when the child returns home.* Naps may be recommended, depending on the child's age.
- Identify age-appropriate activities and exercises for the child *to stimulate bone growth and muscle development and to promote cardiovascular health.*
- PCC Teach the child and parents or guardian about risk factors associated with disproportionate growth, such as poor nutrition, lack of regular sleep, environmental hazards, or lack of age-appropriate activities. Help them identify preventive measures to be taken at home *to promote continuity of care.*
- PCC Encourage healthy, loving interactions between the child and family. Model healthy, positive interactions with the child for parents. *Disproportionate growth may be associated with emotional deprivation.*
- If a medical or psychiatric illness places the child at risk for disproportionate growth, make sure the child gets adequate follow-up medical care *to ensure appropriate, professional care.* If the parents or guardian can't afford care, assist with obtaining access to community resources *to promote continuity of care.*
- PCC If financial hardship interferes with the family's ability to provide for the child, offer a referral to a social worker *to improve the family's access to community resources.*

Suggested NIC Interventions

Active Listening; Behavior Modification; Coping Enhancement; Counseling; Nutritional Management; Patient Contracting; Weight Management

Evaluations for Expected Outcomes

- Child continues to grow and gain weight as expected based on growth chart norms for age and gender.
- Child consumes ______ calories and _____ mL of fluids representing ____ servings (specify for each food group).
- Child sleeps _____ hours daily.
- Child maintains activity level appropriate for age.
- Child and parents or guardian identify risk factors that may lead to disproportionate growth.
- Child and parents or guardian express understanding of preventive measures to reduce risk of disproportionate growth.

Documentation

- Child's age, gender, height, and weight
- Growth history
- Presence of risk factors for disproportionate growth
- Input and output
- Daily appetite level
- Duration of sleep (including any disruptions in sleep cycle)
- Child's level of participation in activities and the type of activities
- Teaching provided to child and parents or guardian regarding disproportionate growth
- Parents' or guardian's response to teaching, including statements indicating understanding of disproportionate growth, ability to identify risk factors for disproportionate growth, and understanding of need to make alterations in child's environment and daily schedule
- Follow-up care plan and referrals
- Evaluations for expected outcomes

REFERENCES

Allvin, K., Hellström, A., Dahlgren, J., & Andersson Grönlund, M. (2014). Birth weight is the most important predictor of abnormal retinal vascularization in moderately preterm infants. *Acta Paediatrica*, *103*(6), 594–600. doi:10.1111/apa.12599

Knopf, A. (2015). Growth chart for the mind may be able to detect psychosis early. *Brown University Child & Adolescent Behavior Letter*, *31*(7), 1–2.

Michaelsen, K. F. (2014, May). Are the new Danish 2014 growth references really more appropriate than the World Health Organization standards? *Acta Paediatrica*, *103*(5), 464–465. doi:10.1111/apa.12586.

HYPERTHERMIA

related to illness

Definition

Core body temperature above the normal diurnal range due to failure of thermoregulation

Assessment

- History of present illness
- Age, gestational age at birth

- Health history, including chronic disease or disability, pathologic conditions known to cause dehydration, recent traumatic event, exposure to sources of infection (intrauterine or extrauterine), exposure to communicable diseases, and other related events
- Medication history
- Physiologic manifestations of fever, including vital signs, skin temperature, and skin color
- Fluid and electrolyte status, including skin turgor, intake and output, mucous membranes, serum electrolyte levels, and urine specific gravity
- Laboratory studies, including white blood cell count and culture and sensitivity findings
- Neurologic status, including level of consciousness (LOC) and history of seizures
- Skin integrity, including presence of open lesions and rashes

Defining Characteristics

- Abnormal posturing
- Apnea
- Coma
- Convulsions
- Flushed skin
- Hypotension
- Infant does not maintain such
- Irritability
- Lethargy
- Seizure
- Skin warm to touch
- Stupor
- Tachycardia
- Tachypnea
- Vasodilation

Expected Outcomes

- Child will remain afebrile.
- Child will maintain adequate hydration, with balanced intake and output within normal limits for age, urine specific gravity between 1.010 and 1.015, and moist mucous membranes, skin turgor within normal limits, and flat fontanels (in infant).
- Child will remain alert and responsive and won't show evidence of seizure activity or decreased LOC.
- Parents will identify risk factors for infection and state measures to prevent infection.
- Parents will demonstrate correct technique for assessing temperature.
- Parents will identify appropriate measures to reduce fever and prevent dehydration.

Suggested NOC Outcomes

Hydration; Infection Severity; Thermoregulation; Vital Signs

Interventions and Rationales

- Take an axillary or oral temperature every 1 to 4 hours and 1 hour after administration of antipyretics. Record measurements and identify the route *to obtain an accurate core temperature.* Use same site and method with each measurement *to maintain accuracy of results.*
- Administer antipyretics, as ordered, and record effectiveness. *Antipyretics act on the hypothalamus to regulate temperature.* Avoid using aspirin. *Aspirin use in children with viral symptoms, especially with flulike symptoms or varicella (chickenpox), has been linked to Reye's syndrome.*
- Use nonpharmacologic measures to reduce high fever, such as removing sheets, blankets, and most clothing (except diapers and underwear); placing cool cloths on the axillae and groin; and sponging with tepid water. Explain these measures to the child and family

members. *Nonpharmacologic measures lower body temperature and promote comfort. Sponging reduces body temperature by increasing evaporation from skin. Tepid water is used because cold water increases shivering, thereby increasing metabolic rate and causing the temperature to rise.*

- S Use a hypothermia blanket, as ordered, if the child's temperature rises above 103° F (39.4° C). Monitor vital signs every 15 minutes for 1 hour and then as indicated. *Too rapid reduction of fever can cause vascular collapse in young children.* Turn off the blanket if shivering occurs. *Because shivering increases metabolic rate, it's counterproductive to cooling therapy.*
- S Monitor heart rate and rhythm, blood pressure, respiratory rate, LOC and responsiveness, and capillary refill time every 1 to 4 hours *to evaluate the effectiveness of interventions and monitor for complications such as seizures.*
- Determine the child's preferences for oral fluids and encourage the child to drink as much as possible, unless contraindicated. Monitor and record intake and output, and administer IV fluids, if indicated. *Because insensible fluid loss increases by 10% for every 0.5° F (1° C) increase in temperature, the child must increase fluid intake to prevent dehydration.*
- Discuss precipitating factors with the parents or primary caregiver. Teach the parents
  - how to take a temperature correctly
  - ways to prevent fever, such as increased fluid intake
  - not to overdress a young child

  Effective teaching will help prevent future episodes of hyperthermia.
- Describe the complications of fever to the parents and explain which signs and symptoms they need to report to a physician. *Early recognition and treatment of fever reduces the risk of complications, such as dehydration and febrile seizures.*

Suggested NIC Interventions

Fever Treatment; Fluid Management; Infection Control; Temperature Regulation; Vital Signs Monitoring

Evaluations for Expected Outcomes

- Child remains afebrile.
- Child maintains adequate hydration.
- Child remains alert and responsive and doesn't exhibit evidence of seizure activity.
- Parents identify risk factors for infection and state measures to prevent infection.
- Parents demonstrate correct technique for assessing temperature.
- Parents identify appropriate measures to reduce fever and prevent dehydration.

Documentation

- Observations of physical assessment findings
- Nursing interventions, including administration of medications
- Child's response (behavioral, cognitive, and physiologic) to interventions, including administration of antipyretics
- Evaluations for expected outcomes

REFERENCES

Niven, D. J., Gaudet, J. E., Laupland, K. B., Mrklas, K. J., Roberts, D. J., & Stelfox, H. T. (2015). Accuracy of peripheral thermometers for estimating temperature: A systematic review and meta-analysis. *Annals of Internal Medicine*, *163*(10), 768–777.

Saliba, E. (2015). Should we extend the indications for therapeutic hypothermia? *Acta Paediatrica, 104*(2), 114–115. doi:10.1111/apa.12891
Vilinsky, A., & Sheridan, A. (2014). Hypothermia in the newborn: An exploration of its cause, effect, and prevention. *British Journal of Midwifery, 22*(8), 557–562.

RISK FOR INJURY

Definition

Vulnerable to physical damage due to environmental conditions, interacting with the individual's adaptive and defensive resources, which may compromise health

Assessment

- Age
- Environmental factors, including toxic substances within the reach of child, stairs not blocked, and unsafe play equipment
- Developmental status, including cognitive abilities (language and reasoning), sensory perception, response to stimuli (pain, touch, and warmth), level of independence, and motor skills
- Child's and family members' understanding of safety practices
- Behavior
- Laboratory studies, including toxicology screening

Risk Factors

External

- Alteration in cognitive functioning
- Alteration in psychomotor functioning
- Compromised nutritional source (e.g., vitamins, food types)
- Exposure to pathogen
- Exposure to toxic chemical
- Immunization level within community
- Nosocomial agent
- Physical barrier (e.g., design, structure, arrangement of community, building equipment)
- Unsafe mode of transport

Internal

- Abnormal blood profile
- Alteration to affective orientation
- Alteration in sensation (resulting from spinal cord injury, diabetes mellitus, etc.)
- Autoimmune dysfunction
- Biochemical dysfunction
- Extremes of age
- Immune dysfunction
- Impaired primary defense mechanisms (e.g., broken skin)
- Malnutrition
- Sensory integration dysfunction
- Tissue hypoxia

Expected Outcomes

- Child will remain free from physical injury.
- During hospitalization, staff members will keep toxic substances out of child's reach, have equipment inspected for safety, and remove unsafe equipment.
- Child and family members will express understanding of safety measures.
- Family members will take action to eliminate household safety hazards.

Suggested NOC Outcomes

Immune Status; Parenting: Psychosocial Safety; Risk Control; Risk Detection; Safe Home Environment

Interventions and Rationales

- Assess and document any motor, mental, or sensory deficits *to identify specific safety needs.*
- Keep frequently used items within the child's easy reach *to help prevent falls.*
- S Encourage the use of necessary assistive devices, such as hearing aids, glasses, and leg braces, *to enhance safety and help prevent injury.*
- S Orient the child to own immediate environment, as necessary, *to promote mobility and improve safety.*
- S Assess the amount of supervision the child needs to ensure safety. *Maintaining supervision is especially important if the child is hyperactive, disoriented, or unconscious.*
- S Keep the bed side rails up at all times *to prevent falls.*
- S Keep the bed in low position except when providing direct care *to ease getting in and out of bed and to reduce the danger of falling.*
- S Use locks on wheelchairs, stretchers, and beds, when appropriate, *to immobilize equipment and enhance safety.*
- S Ensure that all equipment, medical supplies, and toys in the child's room are appropriate for the child's developmental age. Make sure the infant's or toddler's room doesn't contain small objects, sharp instruments, or sharp furniture corners *to reduce the risk of injury.*
- S Promote electrical safety. Apply electrical outlet covers to all unused outlets. Inspect all electrical appliances brought from home and have them approved by a safety officer before use. Don't place liquids, jellies, or creams on electrical appliances. Finally, test all electrical equipment before using on a child. *Electrical appliances pose potential hazards for child and staff members.*
- PCC S Instruct the child and family members in standard safety practices, including
  - wiping up spills immediately.
  - providing nonslip surfaces in hallways, on stairs, and in bathtubs and shower stalls.
  - draining all water from bathtubs immediately after a bath.
  - placing toxic substances in locked cabinets or out of reach of the child. *Teaching promotes household safety.*

Suggested NIC Interventions

Health Education; Parent Education: Childrearing Family; Risk Identification

Evaluations for Expected Outcomes

- Child remains free from physical injury.
- During hospitalization, staff members keep toxic substances out of the child's reach, have equipment inspected for safety, and remove unsafe equipment.
- Child and family members express understanding of safety measures.
- Family members eliminate elements of safety hazards from home.

Documentation

- Statements by child or family members that indicate high risk of injury
- Assessment of home environment

- Observation of physical findings
- Child's and family members' knowledge of safety practices
- Nursing interventions to reduce the risk of injury
- Child's and family members' responses to interventions
- Evaluations for expected outcomes

REFERENCES

Dryden, E. M., Desmarais, J., & Arsenault, L. (2014). Effectiveness of the IMPACT: Ability program to improve safety and self-advocacy skills in high school students with disabilities. *Journal of School Health*, *84*(12), 793–801. doi:10.1111/josh.1221

McClure, R., Kegler, S., Davey, T., & Clay, F. (2015). Contextual determinants of childhood injury: A systematic review of studies with multilevel analytic methods. *American Journal of Public Health*, *105*(12), e37–e43. doi:10.2105/AJPH.2015.302883

Taylor, W. C., Upchurch, S. L., Brosnan, C. A., Selwyn, B. J., Nguyen, T. Q., Villagomez, E. T., & Meininger, J. C. (2014). Features of the built environment related to physical activity friendliness and children's obesity and other risk factors. *Public Health Nursing*, *31*(6), 545–555. doi:10.1111/phn.12144

RISK FOR CORNEAL INJURY

Definition

Vulnerable to infection of inflammatory lesion in the corneal tissue that can affect superficial or deep layers, which may compromise health

Assessment

- Neurologic status, including level of consciousness, orientation, motor activity, and strength in all extremities.
- Glasgow Coma Scale score.
- Detailed eye assessment, including blinking rate, amount of moisture in the eye, quality of the eye moisture, ability or inability to maintain eyelid closure.

Risk Factors

- Blinking <5 times/minute
- Exposure of the eyeball
- Glasgow Coma Scale score <7
- Intubation
- Mechanical ventilation
- Periorbital edema
- Pharmaceutical agent
- Prolonged hospitalization
- Tracheostomy
- Use of supplemental oxygen

Expected Outcomes

- Child will not develop dry eyes.
- Child's eyes will not become infected.
- Child will not develop corneal abrasion or injury.

Suggested NOC Outcomes

Risk Control; Risk Detection; Tissue Integrity: Skin/Mucous Membranes; Knowledge: Health Behavior

Interventions and Rationales

- Assess the eyes with each head-to-toe assessment *to identify any changes as soon as they occur.*
- S • Complete hand hygiene prior to performing eye care. *This reduces the potential for infection.*
- Perform eye care as indicated by hospital policy or protocol *to keep eyes clean.*
- When performing eye care, wipe eye from nasal edge and outward *to avoid whipping discharge into the lacrimal duct.*
- S • When performing eye care, use a new sterile gauze for the second eye *to reduce the risk for infection.*
- Implement prescribed treatments to protect the eyes such as prescribed eye drops or hydrogel dressings *to maintain the moisture in the eyes.*
- PCC • Educate parents on prescribed eye care regimen *to alleviate fears.*

Suggested NIC Interventions

Risk Management; Risk Identification; Behavior management

Evaluations for Expected Outcomes

- Moisture maintained in child's eyes.
- Child shows no signs of infection in eyes.
- Child's corneas are free from injury.

Documentation

- Observations of the eye, including blink rate, moisture, and ability to maintain eye lid closure.
- Interventions performed.
- Patient response to interventions.
- Evaluations for expected outcomes.

REFERENCES

Banks, K., & Bevan, A. (2014). Predictors for somatic symptoms in children. *Nursing Children & Young People, 26*(1), 16–20.

Casale, M., Wild, L., Cluver, L., & Kuo, C. (2014). The relationship between social support and anxiety among caregivers of children in HIV-endemic South Africa. *Psychology, Health & Medicine, 19*(4), 490–503. doi:10.1080/13548506.2013.832780

Douglas, L. & Berry, S. (2011). Developing clinical guidelines in eye care for intensive care units. *Nursing Children and Young People, 23*(5), 14–20.

Witham, G., Haigh, C., & Foy, S. (2014). The challenges of health professionals in meeting the needs of vulnerable patients undergoing chemotherapy: A focus group study. *Journal of Clinical Nursing, 23*(19/20), 2844–2853. doi:10.1111/jocn.12583

DEFICIENT KNOWLEDGE

related to insufficient knowledge of resources

Definition

Absence or deficiency of cognitive information related to a specific topic

Assessment

- Age
- Developmental status, including learning ability (affective, cognitive, and psychomotor domains), decision-making ability, and developmental stage
- Psychosocial status, including family's resources, health beliefs and attitudes, interest in learning, knowledge and skill regarding current health problem, obstacles to learning, support systems (willingness and ability of others to help the child), and usual coping pattern
- Neurologic status, including level of consciousness, memory, mental status, and orientation
- Parents' understanding of child's illness, including severity, prescribed treatment, and overall health needs

Defining Characteristics

- Inaccurate follow-through of instruction
- Inaccurate performance on a test
- Inappropriate behavior (e.g., hysterical, hostile, agitated, apathetic)
- Insufficient knowledge

Expected Outcomes

- Child and family members will communicate the need to gain knowledge and establish realistic learning goals.
- Child and family members will demonstrate understanding of what they have been taught.
- Child and family members will demonstrate ability to perform recently learned health-related behaviors.
- Child and family members will verbalize their intention to make needed changes in lifestyle.

Suggested NOC Outcomes

Information Processing; Knowledge: Child Physical Safety; Knowledge: Energy Conservation; Knowledge: Health Behavior; Knowledge: Health Resources

Interventions and Rationales

- Establish an environment of mutual trust and respect *to enhance learning.*
- Communicate openly and honestly with the child and encourage the parents and others to visit regularly *to enhance the child's feelings of trust in the staff and comfort within the hospital environment.*
- Identify the child's level of cognitive, physical, linguistic, and perceptual development *to establish appropriate learning goals.*
- PCC Select teaching methods appropriate to the child's developmental level:
  - For a preschooler or early school-age child, use stuffed animals or puppets. *A child in this age group uses own senses and manipulation of objects to learn.*
  - For an older school-age child, use demonstration techniques, role playing, and illustrations. Relate new terms and concepts to the child's experiences. For example, to explain ventricular septal defect, you might say "your heart is like a house with four

rooms and a door to one of the rooms isn't working right." *At this age, a child thinks concretely and best understands explanations related to past experiences.*

- Limit the number of new skills taught each day according to the child's age and ability. *Limiting daily teaching helps to avoid overloading the child with new information.* Keep in mind that a young child who successfully learns single concepts may still have difficulty determining when to apply learned rules.
- Develop a daily schedule for the hospitalized child with plans for rest, meals, play, and performing learned skills. *Establishing routines provides a more controlled, pleasant environment for the child and thereby fosters learning. Play is a valuable component of any child's life.*
- PCC Encourage family members to participate in planning the child's daily schedule, making it as similar as possible to a typical day at home. *Involving the child's family helps reinforce the skills necessary for home care after discharge.*
- Regularly discuss progress toward goal achievement with the child and family members. Make changes in the care plan as necessary. *Evaluation helps to reinforce effective learning techniques and identify ineffective techniques. It allows analysis of progress and redirection of activities as necessary.*
- Have the child and family members demonstrate learned skills. *Return demonstration allows you to evaluate learning and helps the child and family members gain confidence in new skills.*

Suggested NIC Interventions

Discharge Planning; Family Support; Health Education; Health System Guidance; Learning Facilitation; Learning Readiness Enhancement; Parent Education: Childrearing Family; Support System Enhancement

Evaluations for Expected Outcomes

- Child and family members communicate need to gain knowledge and establish realistic learning goals.
- Child and family members express understanding of material being taught.
- Child and family members demonstrate ability to perform new health-related behaviors correctly.
- Child and family members express intention to institute needed changes in child's lifestyle.

Documentation

- Child's and family members' knowledge and skills
- Child's and family members' statements that indicate knowledge deficit
- Child's and family members' expressions that indicate motivation to learn
- Learning objectives
- Teaching methods used
- Information taught
- Skills demonstrated
- Response to teaching
- Evaluations for expected outcomes

REFERENCES

Bostock-Cox, B. (2016). Choosing and using inhalers: What's the formula? *Practice Nurse*, 46(2), 22–28.

O'Neal, C. W., Lucier-Greer, M., Mancini, J. A., Ferraro, A. J., Ross, D. B., & O'Neal, C. W. (2016). Family relational health, psychological resources, and health behaviors: A dyadic study of military couples. *Military Medicine*, *181*(2), 152–160. doi:10.7205/MILMED-D-14-00740

Schlucter, J., Dokken, D., & Ahmann, E. (2015). Family matters. Transitions from pediatric to adult care: Programs and resources. *Pediatric Nursing*, *41*(2), 85–88.

IMBALANCED NUTRITION: LESS THAN BODY REQUIREMENTS

related to inability to absorb nutrients or insufficient dietary intake

Definition

Intake of nutrients insufficient to meet metabolic needs

Assessment

- Age
- Developmental level
- Gastrointestinal (GI) status, including usual bowel patterns, change in bowel habits, stool characteristics (color, amount, size, and consistency), pain or discomfort, nausea and vomiting, history of GI disorder or surgery, presence of colic, inspection of abdomen, palpation for masses and tenderness, percussion for tympany and dullness, auscultation of bowel sounds, and sucking and swallowing ability (of infants)
- Medication history, including use of antibiotics
- Nutritional status, including dietary history, change in type of food tolerated, height, weight, physical growth percentile (from pediatric growth grid), meal preparation, sociocultural influences, usual dietary pattern, weight fluctuations in past year, and weight maintenance as height increases
- Change in intrapersonal or interpersonal factors, including desire to eat and rate of food consumption
- Psychosocial status, including body image (perception of observer and self-perception), level of attachment with primary caregiver, and family's financial resources
- Laboratory studies, including hemoglobin levels and hematocrit
- Health status, including heart rate, respiratory status, integumentary status, and oral mucosa
- Presence and type of tube feedings
- Activity level and mood

Defining Characteristics

- Abdominal cramping
- Abdominal pain
- Alteration in taste sensation
- Body weight 20% or more below ideal weight range
- Capillary fragility
- Diarrhea
- Excessive hair loss
- Food aversion
- Food intake less than recommended daily allowance
- Hyperactive bowel sounds
- Insufficient information
- Insufficient interest in food
- Insufficient muscle tone
- Misinformation
- Misperception
- Pale mucous membranes

- Perceived inability to ingest food
- Satiety immediately upon ingesting food
- Sore buccal cavity
- Weakness of muscles required for mastication
- Weakness of muscles required for swallowing
- Weight loss with adequate food intake

Expected Outcomes

- Child will exhibit no further weight loss and, if malnourished, will gain 2.2 lb (1 kg)/week.
- Child will take in ____ calories/day and will retain feedings without emesis.
- Child and family members will express understanding of total parenteral nutrition (TPN), if appropriate, or demonstrate understanding of other feeding techniques essential to daily nutritional requirements.
- Family members will express willingness to continue feeding regimen at home.

Suggested NOC Outcomes

Appetite; Health Beliefs; Nutritional Status; Nutritional Status: Food & Fluid Intake; Nutritional Status: Nutrient Intake; Self-Care: Eating; Weight Control

Interventions and Rationales

- Provide a diet that meets child's daily caloric requirements. Daily caloric intake depends on age, metabolic status, and activity level. General guidelines include
  - younger than age 6 months—108 kcal/kg/day
  - ages 6 to 12 months—98 kcal/kg/day
  - ages 1 to 3—1,300 kcal/day
  - ages 4 to 6—1,800 kcal/day
  - ages 7 to 10—2,000 kcal/day
  - ages 11 to 14—2,500 kcal/day
  - ages 15 to 18—3,000 kcal/day

  A diet meeting the child's caloric requirements helps meet the child's maintenance and growth needs.
- Provide small, frequent feedings *to reduce fatigue and improve intake.*
- For infants older than age 6 months, offer solid foods before formula or breast milk. Place solid foods in the center of the tongue, using a small spoon to press downward slightly *to facilitate swallowing. Older infants and young toddlers may resist solid foods, preferring milk or formula.*
- Record and describe food intake. Refer family members to a dietitian or nutritional support team for dietary management. *A dietitian or nutritional support team can individualize the child's diet within prescribed restrictions.*
- Promote adequate rest *to reduce fatigue and improve the child's ability and desire to eat.*
- Obtain and record the child's weight each morning before the first feeding *to accurately monitor the response to therapy.*
- Provide parenteral fluids, as ordered, *to ensure adequate fluid and electrolyte levels.*
- S Monitor electrolyte values and report abnormalities. *Poor nutritional status may cause electrolyte imbalances.*
- Monitor and record the amount, color, consistency, and presence of occult blood in emesis and stools. *Characteristics of vomitus and stools provide clues to nutrient absorption.*

- If the child is receiving tube feedings:
  - Use a continuous infusion pump, if possible, *to help prevent diarrhea, fatigue, and stimulation of vagal response. A continuous infusion pump also helps prevent reduction in the cough or gag reflex and overstimulation of the stomach.*
  - Provide an infant with opportunities to suck on a pacifier *to satisfy oral needs.*
  - S Check feeding tube placement before each feeding *to verify tube placement in the GI tract rather than in the lung.*
  - Begin the regimen with small amounts and diluted concentrations *to decrease diarrhea and improve absorption.* Increase volume and concentration, as tolerated.
  - S Keep the head of the bed elevated during feedings *to reduce the risk of aspiration.*
  - PCC Teach the parents the correct technique for tube feeding *to ensure compliance with the feeding regimen at home.*
- If the child is receiving TPN:
  - S Carefully monitor delivery of TPN *to promote effective therapy and prevent circulatory overload.*
  - S Monitor blood glucose level, urine specific gravity, and urine glucose, protein, and metabolite levels at least in every shift *to detect metabolic complications, osmotic diuresis, hypoglycemia, and pulmonary edema.*
  - Provide or assist with oral hygiene *to enhance the child's comfort and improve appetite.*
  - PCC Teach the parents the correct technique for maintaining TPN infusion at home *to ensure the parents continue the feeding regimen after discharge.*

Suggested NIC Interventions

Enteral Tube Feeding; Nutrition Management; Referral; Total Parenteral Nutrition (TPN) Administration; Weight Gain Assistance; Weight Management

Evaluations for Expected Outcomes

- Child's weight stabilizes or increases.
- Child takes in enough calories and essential nutrients and retains feedings.
- Child and family members demonstrate understanding of nutritional principles and requirements, feeding techniques, and special needs.
- Family members express willingness to continue feeding regimen at home.

Documentation

- Child's weight (recorded daily)
- Child's sucking and swallowing reflexes
- Intake and output
- Incidence of emesis or diarrhea
- Characteristics of emesis or stools
- Presence of complications
- Statements by child and family members that indicate understanding of feeding protocol
- Evaluations for expected outcomes

REFERENCES

Nehring, I., Kewitz, K., von Kries, R., & Thyen, U. (2014). Long-term effects of enteral feeding on growth and mental health in adolescents with anorexia nervosa—results of a retrospective German cohort study. *European Journal of Clinical Nutrition*, *68*(2), 171–177

Rocks, T., Pelly, F., & Wilkinson, P. (2014). Nutritional management of anorexia nervosa in children and adolescent inpatients: The current practice of Australian dietitians. *Nutrition & Dietetics*, *71*(2), 100–107. doi:10.1111/1747-0080.12058

Rossler, L. (2014). Eating disorders and artificial re-feeding. *Mental Health Practice*, *17*(9), 21–26.

OVERWEIGHT

related to average daily physical activity is less than recommended for gender and age; heritability of interrelated factors (e.g., adipose tissue distribution, energy expenditure, lipoprotein lipase activity, lipid synthesis, lipolysis); high disinhibition and restraint eating behavior score

Definition

A condition in which an individual accumulates abnormal or excessive fat for age and gender

Assessment

- Health history, including family history of overweight.
- Body measurements, including height, weight, and body mass index (BMI) or percentile on growth chart.
- Dietary habits including food preferences and normal dietary intake.
- Activity level.
- Sedentary level.
- Psychosocial status, including behavior, mood, stressors, coping mechanisms, and support systems (family, friends).

Defining Characteristics

- Adult: BMI >25 kg/m^2
- Child <2 years: Weight-for-length >95th percentile
- Child 2 to 18 years: BMI >85th but <95th percentile, or 25 kg/m^2 (whichever is smaller)

Expected Outcomes

- Child will identify internal and external factors contributing to weight gain.
- Child will state need to lose weight.
- Child will lose weight.
- Child with help from parent will plan to monitor weight and sustain target weight.
- Child will express feelings regarding dietary regimen and current weight.
- Child will identify internal and external cues that lead to increased food consumption.
- Child with help from parent will plan meals appropriate for prescribed diet.
- Child will adhere to prescribed diet.
- Child will participate in regular physical activity
- Child will achieve weight goal.
- Parents will state understanding of dietary and physical activity recommendations.
- Parents participate in meal and activity planning and weight monitoring.

Suggested NOC Outcomes

Anxiety Level; Eating Disorder Self-Control; Exercise Participation; Nutritional Status; Weight: Body Mass

Interventions and Rationales

- With input from parent and child, set a realistic weight goal. *Involvement in the decision-making process improves compliance with plan of care.*
- Instruct child, with help from parent to keep a food diary, *to have an accurate record of intake.*
- Have a dietitian calculate caloric intake the child will require to reach a healthy weight *to allow planning of appropriate diet.*
- Determine child's food preferences *to evaluate eating habits and to include preferred foods, if nutritional, in child's diet.*
- Weigh child weekly or as prescribed *to monitor the effectiveness of the diet.*
- Encourage a diet of foods low in calories and fat; high in complex carbohydrates and fiber, and rich in lean proteins and fruits and vegetables. *This encourages child to eat food that provides energy without causing weight gain.*
- PCC Encourage child and parents to express feelings about dietary changes to assess their perception of the problem. Help child identify emotions associated with food and situations that trigger eating episodes. *Permanent weight maintenance requires an understanding of the risk factors that contribute to weight gain.*
- Give patient emotional support and positive feedback for adhering to the prescribed diet. *This will foster compliance and help ensure adherence to the diet.*
- Discuss the importance of incorporating physical activity into lifestyle. Help child select activities appropriate for age and physical condition. *Physical activity aids in weight loss and offers an alternative to eating to alleviate stress.*
- PCC Refer child as appropriate to resources for health coaching, behavior modification, or cognitive therapy *to prevent relapse into high-risk eating behaviors.*

Suggested NIC Interventions

Anxiety Reduction; Behavior Modification; Exercise Promotion; Nutrition Management; Nutritional Therapy; Risk Identification; Teaching: Prescribed Diet; Weight Reduction Assistance

Evaluations for Expected Outcomes

- Child identifies internal and external factors contributing to weight gain.
- Child states need to lose weight.
- Child loses weight.
- Child with help from parent monitors weight and sustains target weight.
- Child expresses feelings regarding dietary regimen and current weight.
- Child identifies internal and external cues that lead to increased food consumption.
- Child with help from parent plans meals appropriate for prescribed diet.
- Child adheres to prescribed diet.
- Child participates in regular physical activity
- Child achieves weight goal.
- Parents state understanding of dietary and physical activity recommendations.
- Parents participate in meal and activity planning and weight monitoring.

Documentation

- Child's expression of feelings about weight, eating, and dietary regimen.
- Child's weight and height.
- Child's body measurements plotted on growth chart.

- Ability of child to maintain target weight.
- Foods consumed by child.
- Physical activity performed by child.
- Behaviors that promote or impede weight maintenance.
- Parental participation in care.
- Evaluations for expected outcomes.

REFERENCES

Bleich, S. N., Jones-Smith, J., Jones, H., O'Hara, M., & Rutkow, L. (2016). The voices for healthy kids campaign and US state legislation to prevent childhood obesity. *American Journal of Public Health*, *106*(3), 436–439. doi:10.2105/AJPH.2015.303002

Gilliland, J., Clark, A. F., Kobrzynski, M., & Filler, G. (2015). Convenience sampling of children presenting to hospital-based outpatient clinics to estimate childhood obesity levels in local surroundings. *American Journal of Public Health*, *105*(7), 1332–1335. doi:10.2105/AJPH.2015.302622

Subica, A. M., Grills, C. T., Douglas, J. A., & Villanueva, S. (2016). Communities of color creating healthy environments to combat childhood obesity. *American Journal of Public Health*, *106*(1), 78–86. doi:10.2105/AJPH.2015.302887

RISK FOR OVERWEIGHT

Definition

Vulnerable to abnormal or excessive fat accumulation for age and gender, which may compromise health

Assessment

- Health history, including family history of overweight.
- Body measurements, including height, weight, and body mass index (BMI) or percentile on growth chart.
- Dietary habits, including food preferences and normal dietary intake.
- Activity level.
- Sedentary level.
- Psychosocial status, including behavior, mood, stressors, coping mechanisms, and support systems (family, friends).

Risk Factors

- Adult: BMI approaching 25 kg/m^2
- Average daily physical activity is less than recommended for gender and age
- Child <2 years: Weight-for-length approaching 95th percentile
- Child 2 to 18 years: BMI approaching 85th percentile, or 25 kg/m^2 (whichever is smaller)
- Children who are crossing BMI percentiles upward
- Children with high BMI percentiles
- Consumption of sugar-sweetened beverages
- Disordered eating behaviors (e.g., binge eating, extreme weight control)
- Disordered eating perceptions
- Eating in response to external cues (e.g., time of day, social situations)
- Eating in response to internal cues other than hunger (e.g., anxiety)
- Economically disadvantaged
- Energy expenditure below energy intake based on standard assessment (e.g., WAVE assessment*)
- Excessive alcohol consumption
- Fear regarding lack of food supply

*WAVE assessment = Weight, activity, variety in diet, excess.

- Formula- or mixed-fed infants
- Frequent snacking
- Genetic disorder
- Heritability of interrelated factors (e.g., adipose tissue distribution, energy expenditure, lipoprotein lipase activity, lipid synthesis, lipolysis)
- High disinhibition and restraint eating behavior score
- High frequency of restaurant or fried food
- Higher baseline weight at beginning of each pregnancy
- Low dietary calcium intake in children
- Maternal diabetes mellitus
- Maternal smoking
- Obesity in childhood
- Parental obesity
- Portion sizes larger than recommended
- Premature pubarche
- Rapid weight gain during childhood
- Rapid weight gain during infancy, including the first week, first 4 months, and first year
- Sedentary behavior occurring for >2 hours/day
- Shortened sleep time
- Sleep disorder
- Solid foods as major food source at <5 months of age

Expected Outcomes

- Child will identify internal and external factors contributing to potential weight gain.
- Child with help from parent will plan to monitor weight and sustain target weight.
- Child will express feelings regarding dietary regimen and current weight.
- Child will identify internal and external cues that lead to increased food consumption.
- Child with help from parent will plan meals appropriate for prescribed diet.
- Child will adhere to prescribed diet.
- Child will participate in regular physical activity
- Child will maintain weight goal.
- Parents will state understanding of dietary and physical activity recommendations.
- Parents participate in meal and activity planning and weight monitoring.

Suggested NOC Outcomes

Anxiety Level; Eating Disorder Self-Control; Exercise Participation; Nutritional Status; Weight: Body Mass

Interventions and Rationales

- With input from parent and child, set a realistic weight goal. *Involvement in the decision-making process improves compliance with plan of care.*
- Instruct child, with help from parent to keep a food diary, *to have an accurate record of intake.*
- Have a dietitian calculate caloric intake child will require to reach a healthy weight *to allow planning of appropriate diet.*
- Determine child's food preferences *to evaluate eating habits and to include preferred foods, if nutritional, in child's diet.*
- Weigh child weekly or as prescribed *to monitor the effectiveness of the diet.*
- Encourage a diet of foods low in calories and fat; high in complex carbohydrates and fiber, and rich in lean proteins and fruits and vegetables. *This encourages child to eat food that provides energy without causing weight gain.*
- PCC Encourage child and parents to express feelings about dietary changes to assess their perception of the problem. Help child identify emotions associated with food and situations

that trigger eating episodes. *Permanent weight maintenance requires an understanding of the risk factors that contribute to weight gain.*
- Give patient emotional support and positive feedback for adhering to the prescribed diet. *This will foster compliance and help ensure adherence to the diet.*
- Discuss the importance of incorporating physical activity into lifestyle. Help child select activities appropriate for age and physical condition. *Physical activity aids in weight loss and offers an alternative to eating to alleviate stress.*
- PCC Refer child as appropriate to resources for health coaching, behavior modification, or cognitive therapy *to prevent relapse into high-risk eating behaviors.*

Suggested NIC Interventions

Anxiety Reduction; Behavior Modification; Exercise Promotion; Nutrition Management; Nutritional Therapy; Risk Identification; Teaching: Prescribed Diet; Weight Reduction Assistance

Evaluations for Expected Outcomes

- Child identifies internal and external factors contributing to potential weight gain.
- Child with help from parent monitors weight and sustains target weight.
- Child expresses feelings regarding dietary regimen and current weight.
- Child identifies internal and external cues that lead to increased food consumption.
- Child with help from parent plans meals appropriate for prescribed diet.
- Child adheres to prescribed diet.
- Child participates in regular physical activity
- Child maintains weight goal.
- Parents state understanding of dietary and physical activity recommendations.
- Parents participate in meal and activity planning and weight monitoring.

Documentation

- Child's expression of feelings about weight, eating, and dietary regimen.
- Child's weight and height.
- Child's body measurements plotted on growth chart.
- Ability of child to maintain target weight.
- Foods consumed by child.
- Physical activity performed by child.
- Behaviors that promote or impede weight maintenance.
- Parental participation in care.
- Evaluations for expected outcomes.

REFERENCES

Bleich, S. N., Jones-Smith, J., Jones, H., O'Hara, M., & Rutkow, L. (2016). The voices for healthy kids campaign and US state legislation to prevent childhood obesity. *American Journal of Public Health, 106*(3), 436–439. doi:10.2105/AJPH.2015.303002

Gilliland, J., Clark, A. F., Kobrzynski, M., & Filler, G. (2015). Convenience sampling of children presenting to hospital-based outpatient clinics to estimate childhood obesity levels in local surroundings. *American Journal of Public Health, 105*(7), 1332–1335. doi:10.2105/AJPH.2015.302622

Strong, G., & Lee, S. (2014). Breast-feeding to reduce the risks of childhood obesity: Recommendations for childbirth educators. *International Journal of Childbirth Education, 29*(2), 26–30.

Subica, A. M., Grills, C. T., Douglas, J. A., & Villanueva, S. (2016). Communities of color creating healthy environments to combat childhood obesity. *American Journal of Public Health, 106*(1), 78–86. doi:10.2105/AJPH.2015.302887

ACUTE PAIN

related to biologic injury agent (e.g., infection, ischemia, neoplasm); chemical injury agent (e.g., burn, capsaicin, methylene chloride, mustard agent); physical injury agent (e.g., abscess, amputation, burn, cut, heavy lifting, operative procedure, trauma, overtraining)

Definition

An unpleasant sensory and emotional experience associated with actual or potential tissue damage, or described in terms of such damage (International Association for the Study of Pain); sudden or slow onset of any intensity from mild to severe with an anticipated or predictable end

Assessment

- Age
- Gender
- Descriptive characteristics of pain, including location, quality, intensity rated on a pictorial assessment scale, temporal factors, and sources of relief
- Physiologic variables, including pain tolerance
- Psychological variables, such as body image, personality, previous experience with pain, anxiety, and secondary gain
- Sociocultural variables, including cognitive style, culture, ethnicity, attitude, values, and birth order
- Environmental variables, such as setting and time

Defining Characteristics

- Appetite change
- Change in physiologic parameter (e.g., blood pressure, heart rate, respiratory rate, oxygen saturation, and end-tidal CO_2)
- Diaphoresis
- Distraction behavior
- Evidence of pain using standardized pain behavior checklist for those unable to communicate verbally (e.g., Neonatal Infant Pain Scale, Pain Assessment Checklist for Seniors with Limited Ability to Communicate)
- Expressive behavior (e.g., restlessness, crying, vigilance)
- Facial expression of pain (e.g., eyes lack luster, beaten look, fixed or scattered movement, grimace)
- Guarding behavior
- Hopelessness
- Narrowed focus (e.g., time perception, thought processes, interaction with people and environment)
- Positioning to ease pain
- Protective behavior
- Proxy report of pain behavior/activity changes (e.g., family member, caregiver)
- Pupil dilation
- Self-focused
- Self-report of intensity using standardized pain scale (e.g., Wong-Baker FACES scale, visual analog scale, numeric rating scale)
- Self-report of pain characteristics using standardized pain instrument (e.g., McGill Pain Questionnaire, Brief Pain Inventory)

Expected Outcomes

- Child will express feeling of improved comfort or demonstrate pain relief through playful, smiling, responsive behavior.

- Child will identify measures effective in relieving pain.
- Parents will express awareness of the child's pain and will perform measures to comfort the child.

Suggested NOC Outcomes

Anxiety Level; Comfort Level; Pain Control; Pain Level; Stress Level; Symptom Control

Interventions and Rationales

- Assess the child's physical symptoms and behavioral cues. If appropriate, encourage the child to describe pain on a pictorial scale depicting a happy face (no pain) and a series of grimacing faces gradually increasing to a sad face with tears (worst pain possible). *A young child lacks verbal skills to describe variations in pain sensation. Pain scales and observation of nonverbal behavior provide alternative means to assess pain in a young child.*
- PCC Administer analgesics, as ordered, and document the effectiveness and adverse effects. *Analgesics depress the central nervous system, thereby reducing pain.*
- Using a pain flow chart, record the time of medication administration and results of pain assessment every hour until the next dose *to monitor the therapy's effectiveness.*
- Demonstrate acceptance when the child reveals pain. *This helps establish a trusting relationship with the child and encourages open expression of feelings. A child may deny pain to appear "good."*
- PCC Provide comfort measures, such as massage, repositioning, and instruction in deep breathing and relaxation techniques. *Nonpharmacologic techniques decrease the focus on pain and may enhance the effectiveness of analgesics by reducing muscle tension.*
- Apply heat or cold, as appropriate, to the pain site. *Applying heat relaxes muscles and decreases pain. Applying cold results in vasoconstriction, decreasing the inflammatory response, and reducing pain.*
- Provide diversional activities, such as books, toys, and arts and crafts. *Because of their immature cognitive functioning and short attention span, young children may be distracted from pain by diversional activities. Older children are less easily distracted.*
- Provide honest information to the child before potentially painful procedures. Tell the child the reasons for the pain and how long it should last. *Honest information builds trust and fosters a sense of control over pain.*
- Help the child obtain uninterrupted rest periods. *Adequate rest promotes the child's well-being and enhances the effectiveness of pain medication.*
- Discuss the child's pain with parents or primary caregiver and enlist their help in pain assessment and management. Ascertain the parents' usual means of providing comfort to the child. *Because parents are most familiar with a child's usual behavior, they can offer valuable information to assist pain assessment and management.*
- Try to anticipate the onset of pain. Provide prescribed medication before painful procedures such as dressing changes or activities such as deep breathing. *Careful pain management can improve relief and may enable the child to cope better with procedures.*
- PCC Encourage the child to report which pain relief measures prove most effective *to give the child a sense of control and promote effective modification of therapy.*

Suggested NIC Interventions

Analgesic Administration; Coping Enhancement; Emotional Support; Medication Management; Mood Management; Pain Management; Sleep Enhancement

Evaluations for Expected Outcomes

- Child demonstrates reduced pain, as evidenced by verbal reports of pain relief, absence of behavioral signs of pain, and resumption of activities of daily living (age-appropriate diversional activities, social interaction, and adequate nutritional intake and rest).
- Child identifies most effective pain relief measures.
- Parents respond to child's expression of pain and provide comfort to child.

Documentation

- Child's description of pain, feelings about pain, and statements about pain relief
- Observations of child's physical and psychological responses to pain
- Comfort measures and medications provided to reduce pain
- Effectiveness of interventions
- Information taught to child and family members about pain and pain relief
- Additional interventions provided to assist child with pain control
- Evaluations for expected outcomes

REFERENCES

Hill, J. J., & Keating, J. L. (2015). Research report. Daily exercises and education for preventing low back pain in children: Cluster randomized controlled trial. *Physical Therapy*, *95*(4), 507–516. doi:10.2522/ptj.20140273

Lowth, M. (2014). The child with abdominal pain. *Practice Nurse*, *44*(9), 10–13.

Roberts-Turner, R. (2016). Quality improvement. Pain management: An evidence-based approach. *Pediatric Nursing*, *42*(1), 39–49

IMPAIRED PARENTING

related to insufficient knowledge about parenting skills

Definition

Inability of the primary caretaker to create, maintain, or regain an environment that promotes the optimum growth and development of the child

Assessment

- Parental status, including age, degree of apprehension, developmental state, family roles, and relationship with spouse or significant other
- Gender and health status of other children
- Parents' knowledge of child care and normal growth and development
- Previous bonding history
- Interaction of parent and infant or child, including care practices, eye contact, smiling, touching, verbalization, visual and voice responses, and response to appearance, disabilities, and gender of child

- Psychosocial status, including financial stressors and previous experience, work demands, and support of family, friends, and significant other

Defining Characteristics

Infant of Child

- Behavior disorder (e.g., attention deficit, oppositional defiant)
- Delay in cognitive development
- Diminished separation anxiety
- Failure to thrive
- Frequent accidents
- Frequent illness
- History of abuse (e.g., physical, psychological, sexual)
- History of trauma (e.g., physical, psychological, sexual)
- Impaired social functioning
- Insufficient attachment behavior
- Low academic performance
- Runaway

Parental

- Abandonment
- Decrease in ability to manage child
- Decrease in cuddling
- Deficient parent–child interaction
- Frustration with child
- History of childhood abuse (e.g., physical psychological, sexual)
- Hostility
- Inadequate child health maintenance
- Inappropriate care-taking skills
- Inappropriate child care arrangements
- Inappropriate stimulation (e.g., visual, tactile, auditory)
- Inconsistent behavior management
- Inconsistent care
- Inflexibility in meeting needs of child
- Neglects needs of child
- Perceived inability to meet child's needs
- Perceived role inadequacy
- Punitive
- Rejection of child
- Speaks negatively about child
- Unsafe home environment

Expected Outcomes

- Parents will establish eye, physical, and verbal contact with infant or child.
- Parents will voice satisfaction with infant or child.
- Parents will demonstrate correct feeding, bathing, and dressing techniques.
- Parents will express willingness to work to maintain relationship with each other.
- Parents will state plans for well-child care.
- Parents will express knowledge of developmental norms.
- Parents will provide play activities for child.
- Parents will identify ways to express anger and frustration that don't harm child.

Suggested NOC Outcomes

Caregiver Performance: Direct Care; Child Development: Middle Childhood; Family Coping; Family Functioning; Parenting: Early/Middle Childhood Physical Safety; Parenting Performance

Interventions and Rationales

PCC

- Involve parents in the care of the infant or child immediately *to promote attachment to the child.*
- Provide opportunities for caretaking by allowing parents to share a room with their infant or child or by extending visitation periods. *Participation in care increases a parent's feeling of self-esteem and self-worth.*

- Educate parents about
  - normal growth and development
  - breast-feeding or bottle-feeding techniques
  - infant care, such as bathing and dressing
  - routine well-child care
  - signs and symptoms of illness
  - the child's need for tactile and sensory stimulation

  Knowledge of normal growth and development may decrease unrealistic expectations and increase chances of successful parenting.
- When caring for the child in the parents' presence, act as a role model for effective parenting skills. *Lack of knowledge of routine child care practices and growth and developmental norms significantly contributes to child abuse. Demonstration is a more effective means of teaching parenting skills than lecturing.*
- PCC Encourage questions about care taking and provide appropriate information *to allay anxiety and monitor knowledge retention.*
- Praise parents when they display appropriate parenting skills *to provide positive reinforcement.*
- PCC Refer parents to a family support group and other community resources such as Parents Anonymous. *Battering parents typically lack a support system and have a sense of being alone. A support group may help ease isolation.*
- PCC Encourage verbalization of the infant's or child's impact on family life. *Ventilation of feelings helps parents deal more effectively with the stress of child care.*
- S Be alert for signs and symptoms of child abuse, including neglect, uncleanliness, and frequent accidents or withdrawn, fearful behavior on the part of the child. Report actual or suspected child abuse to appropriate authorities. *Reporting child abuse is your professional duty. The United States legally requires nurses to report abuse.*

Suggested NIC Interventions

Coping Enhancement; Family Process Maintenance; Family Support; Mutual Goal Setting; Parent Education: Childrearing Family; Role Enhancement

Evaluations for Expected Outcomes

- Parents make appropriate physical, verbal, and eye contact when interacting with infant or child.
- Parents make statements indicating satisfaction with infant or child.
- Parents demonstrate correct feeding, bathing, and dressing techniques.
- Parents express willingness to maintain their relationship with each other.
- Parents bring infant for routine well-child care.
- Parents verbalize knowledge of developmental norms.
- Parents provide play activities for child.
- Parents identify ways to express anger and frustration that don't harm child.

Documentation

- Parents' expressions of feelings about child
- Parents' expressions of concern about their performance as parents
- Observation of parental visits, bonding, care taking, and knowledge level
- Instructions given to parents and parents' understanding of their responsibilities
- Infant's weight
- Evaluations for expected outcomes

REFERENCES

Reed, L. (2015). Early socialization. *International Journal of Childbirth Education, 30*(2), 31–34.
Revell, M. A. (2015). The African American father does matter in parenting. *International Journal of Childbirth Education, 30*(1), 25–29.
Wilson, S., McKenzie, K., Quayle, E., & Murray, G. (2014). A systematic review of interventions to promote social support and parenting skills in parents with an intellectual disability. *Child: Care, Health & Development, 40*(1), 7–19. doi:10.1111/cch.12023

RISK FOR IMPAIRED PARENTING

Definition

Vulnerable to inability of the primary caretaker to create, maintain, or regain an environment that promotes the optimum growth and development of the child, which may compromise the well-being of the child

Assessment

- Ages of caregiver and child
- Caregiver's psychosocial status, including developmental state, educational level, family roles, presence or absence of spouse or significant other, financial stressors, previous parenting experience, work demands, and support of family, friends, or significant other
- Interaction between caregiver and infant or child, including care practices, eye contact, response to appearance and gender of infant, smiling, touching, verbalization, and visual and voice responses

Risk Factors

Infant or Child

- Alteration in perceptual abilities
- Behavior disorder (e.g., attention deficit, oppositional defiant)
- Developmental delay
- Difficult temperament
- Disabling condition
- Gender other than desired
- Illness
- Multiple births
- Prematurity
- Prolonged separation from parent
- Temperament conflicts with parental expectations

Knowledge

- Alteration in cognitive functioning
- Ineffective communication skills
- Insufficient cognitive readiness for parenting
- Insufficient knowledge about child development
- Insufficient knowledge about child health maintenance
- Insufficient knowledge about parenting skills
- Insufficient response to infant cues
- Low educational level
- Preference for physical punishment
- Unrealistic expectations

Physiologic

- Physical illness

Psychological

- Closely spaced pregnancies
- Depression
- Difficult birthing process
- Disabling condition
- High number of pregnancies

- History of mental illness
- History of substance abuse
- Nonrestorative sleep pattern (i.e., due to caregiver responsibilities, parenting practices, sleep partner)
- Sleep deprivation
- Young parental age

Social

- Change in family unit
- Compromised home environment
- Conflict between partners
- Economically disadvantaged
- Father of child not involved
- History of abuse (e.g., physical, psychological, sexual)
- History of being abusive
- Inadequate child care arrangements
- Ineffective coping strategies
- Insufficient access to resources
- Insufficient family cohesiveness
- Insufficient parental role model
- Insufficient problem-solving skills
- Insufficient resources (e.g., financial, social, knowledge)
- Insufficient social support
- Insufficient transportation
- Insufficient valuing of parenthood
- Late-term prenatal care
- Legal difficulty
- Low self-esteem
- Mother of child not involved
- Parent–child separation
- Relocation
- Role strain
- Single parent
- Social isolation
- Stressors
- Unemployment
- Unplanned pregnancy
- Unwanted pregnancy
- Work difficulty

Expected Outcomes

- Caregiver will establish eye, physical, and verbal contact with infant or child.
- Caregiver will demonstrate correct feeding, bathing, and dressing techniques.
- Caregiver will state plans to bring infant or child to clinic for routine physical and psychological examinations.
- Caregiver will express understanding of developmental norms.
- Caregiver will provide age-appropriate play activities.

Suggested NOC Outcomes

Caregiver Performance: Direct Care; Family Coping; Family Functioning; Parenting Performance

Interventions and Rationales

- Assess the amount of developmental stimulation provided by the caregiver. For example, use the Home Observation for Measurement of the Environment (HOME) Inventory on a home visit *to assess whether the home environment is developmentally stimulating.*
- PCC Instruct the caregiver in the basics of infant and child care. *Research shows that the primary source of information about parenting is the caregiver's own parents. If a caregiver lacks an effective role model, you may need to supply basic information about parenting.*
- When caring for the child in the caregiver's presence, act as a role model for effective parenting skills. Demonstrate comfort measures, such as rocking the infant, and show the caregiver how to hold the infant in an *en face* position *to familiarize the caregiver with routine child care practices.*
- PCC Teach the caregiver about normal growth and development, and identify ages at which the child should master developmental tasks such as rolling over, crawling, and walking.

This will help the caregiver monitor the child's growth and development and practice appropriate safety precautions, such as blocking stairways, securing crib side rails, and preventing other accidents. Also, discuss problematic behaviors associated with specific ages, such as colic, temper tantrums, and sleeping difficulties, *to further enhance the caregiver's understanding of developmental norms.*

- Discuss the child's need for tactile and sensory stimulation. Demonstrate play activities that promote developmental skills, such as shaking a rattle in front of an infant to build eye-and-hand coordination or placing a mobile above an infant to encourage visual tracking and trunk and head control. *Sensory experiences promote cognitive development.*
- Familiarize the caregiver with techniques for detecting symptoms of illness in an infant or child, including
  - taking temperatures and reading thermometers
  - assessing the child's respiratory status
  - observing for behavioral cues of illness, such as increased crying, rubbing ears, or drawing legs to abdomen.

  Knowledge of how to monitor the child's health status will assist in the diagnosis and early treatment of problems.
- PCC Encourage the caregiver to ask questions about infant and child care. Identify the questions parents commonly ask about infant care, such as cord care, feeding techniques, and bathing. Reassure the caregiver that other parents also need to ask basic questions. *A caregiver who lacks effective parenting role models may not know what questions to ask or may hesitate to ask questions because of embarrassment.*
- Praise the caregiver for display of appropriate parenting skills *to provide positive reinforcement.*
- Emphasize the importance of making regular visits to a health care professional, even when the child appears healthy. *Routine visits allow early detection of developmental delays and provision of preventive care, such as immunizations.*
- PCC As necessary, refer the caregiver and family to a physician, nurse practitioner, or social services for follow-up *to ensure continuity of care.*

Suggested NIC Interventions

Counseling; Family Integrity Promotion: Childbearing Family; Family Process Maintenance; Family Support; Parenting Promotion

Evaluations for Expected Outcomes

- Caregiver makes appropriate eye, physical, and verbal contact with infant or child.
- Caregiver demonstrates correct feeding, bathing, and dressing techniques.
- Caregiver brings infant or child to clinic for routine examinations.
- Caregiver expresses understanding of developmental norms and accurately assesses child's developmental status and needs.
- Caregiver provides age-appropriate play activities.

Documentation

- Evidence of neglect of infant or child
- Observations of caregiver's skills and knowledge level
- Presence or absence of caregiver–child bonding behaviors
- Questions asked by caregiver about care of infant or child

- Instructions given to caregiver and caregiver's response
- Evaluations for expected outcomes

REFERENCES

Bello-Utu, C. F., & DeSocio, J. E. (2015). Military deployment and reintegration: A systematic review of child coping. *Journal of Child & Adolescent Psychiatric Nursing*, *28*(1), 23–34. doi:10.1111/jcap.12099
Reed, L. (2015). Early socialization. *International Journal of Childbirth Education*, *30*(2), 31–34.
Revell, M. A. (2015). The African American father does matter in parenting. *International Journal of Childbirth Education*, *30*(1), 25–29.
Seay, A., Freysteinson, W. M., & McFarlane, J. (2014). Positive parenting. *Nursing Forum*, *49*(3), 200–208. doi:10.1111/nuf.12093

PARENTAL ROLE CONFLICT

related to parent–child separation

Definition

Parental experience of role confusion and conflict in response to crisis

Assessment

- Parental status, including age and maturity; apprehension, fear, and guilt; coping mechanisms employed; developmental state of family and other children; knowledge of normal growth and development of children; past response to crises; understanding of child's present condition; previous parent–child relationship; spiritual practices of parents and family; stability of parental relationship; and support systems available to parent
- Parent–child interaction, including eye contact, response to appearance (such as bandages, deformities, and hospital equipment), smiling, touching, and verbalization
- Child's health status, including severity of illness and health care needs
- Child's level of development

Defining Characteristics

- Anxiety
- Concern about change in parental role
- Concern about family (e.g., functioning, communication, health)
- Disruption in caregiver routine
- Fear
- Frustration
- Guilt
- Perceived inadequacy to provide for child's needs (e.g., physical, emotional)
- Perceived loss of control over decisions relating to child
- Reluctance to participate in usual caregiving activities

Expected Outcomes

- Parents will communicate feelings about present situation.
- Parents will participate in their child's daily care.

- Parents will express feelings of greater control and ability to contribute more to child's well-being.
- Parents will express knowledge of child's developmental needs.
- Parents will hold, touch, and convey warmth and affection to child.
- Parents will use available support systems or agencies to assist in coping.

Suggested NOC Outcomes

Caregiver Adaptation to Patient Institutionalization; Caregiver Home Care Readiness; Coping; Family Coping; Family Normalization

Interventions and Rationales

- S Orient the parents or primary caregivers to the hospital environment, visiting procedures, medical equipment, and staff. *Familiarity decreases anxiety.*
- PCC Provide family-centered care by obtaining the parents' input for the child's care. *Parents can meet many of the child's needs better than staff.* Involve the parents in the child's care conferences and in the physical care of the child. *Participation may decrease the parents' feelings of helplessness.*
- PCC Teach the parents normal childhood physical and psychological development *to prepare the parents to deal with changes.*
- PCC Encourage parental involvement in appropriate support groups or agencies when necessary or ordered. *Such groups can provide emotional support and help reduce feelings of being overwhelmed.*
- Ask the parents if they have questions about the child's status and provide information, as requested, *to reduce feelings of helplessness.*
- Provide for the needs of the parents, as appropriate. Offer facilities for showering, sleeping, and eating. Be available to care for the child if the parents need an opportunity to rest. *Helping the parents meet their needs will empower them to meet child care demands.*

Suggested NIC Interventions

Caregiver Support; Coping Enhancement; Family Involvement Promotion; Family Presence Facilitation; Family Process Maintenance; Role Enhancement

Evaluations for Expected Outcomes

- Parents communicate feelings about present situation.
- Parents participate in their child's daily care.
- Parents express feelings of control in present situation.
- Parents communicate knowledge of child's developmental needs.
- Parents hold, touch, and express warmth and affection to child.
- Parents contact support systems or community agencies to assist in coping.

Documentation

- Observations of parents' ability to cope and their level of involvement in child's hospital care and daily needs
- Interventions performed to help parents lower stress and cope with situation
- Referrals to outside agencies or support groups

- Child's medical and emotional state
- Evaluations for expected outcomes

REFERENCES

Macías, M. (2015). Impact of hospital admission care at a pediatric unit: A qualitative study. *Pediatric Nursing*, *41*(6), 285–294.
Noyes, J., Brenner, M., Fox, P., & Guerin, A. (2014). Reconceptualizing children's complex discharge with health systems theory: Novel integrative review with embedded expert consultation and theory development. *Journal of Advanced Nursing*, *70*(5), 975–996. doi:10.1111/jan.12278
Pieper, P., & Garvan, C. (2014). Health-related quality of life in the first year following a childhood concussion. *Brain Injury*, *28*(1), 105–113. doi:10.3109/02699052.2013.847208

PARENTAL ROLE CONFLICT

related to home care of a child with special needs

Definition

Parental experience of role confusion and conflict in response to crisis

Assessment

- Extent of child's special needs
- Parental status, including age and maturity, developmental state of family, authority within family, employment status, financial needs, marital status, stability of parental relationship, knowledge of normal growth and development, understanding of child's condition and prognosis, expectations regarding child, participation in community, past response to crises, and coping mechanisms
- Available support systems, including other family members, friends, visiting nurses, and community resources
- Parent–child interaction
- Parent–child relationship before development of special needs and any changes that have occurred
- Religious practices of parents and family
- Presence of conflict between family's lifestyle and child's needs
- Home environment

Defining Characteristics

- Anxiety
- Concern about change in parental role
- Concern about family (e.g., functioning, communication, health)
- Disruption in caregiver routine
- Fear
- Frustration
- Guilt
- Perceived inadequacy to provide for child's needs (e.g., physical, emotional)
- Perceived loss of control over decisions relating to child
- Reluctance to participate in usual caregiving activities

Expected Outcomes

- Parents will seek out and accept external support, education, and assistance in caring for child at home.
- Parents will demonstrate knowledge of child's developmental needs.
- Parents will begin to provide physical, emotional, and developmental care to child at home.
- Parents will seek assistance in meeting their own emotional and developmental needs.
- Parents will express feelings of greater control and capability in meeting their child's needs.
- Siblings will voice their emotional needs.

Suggested NOC Outcomes

Caregiver Home Care Readiness; Coping; Family Coping; Family Functioning; Family Resiliency; Parenting Performance

Interventions and Rationales

- PCC Provide family-centered care by involving parents in their child's care. Explain their rights as primary caregivers. Provide information to help them make informed decisions. Give them an opportunity to support the child during painful procedures. *Parents can meet the needs of their child better than staff members can. Parents need to receive proper information and have their own needs met before they can meet the child's needs.*
- Promote the emotional well-being of parents by providing respite care, encouraging parents to spend time away from the child to enhance their marital relationship, and providing information about additional sources of support. *Encouraging parents to pay attention to their own emotional needs will enhance their ability to care for their child.*
- Listen to the parents, child, and siblings openly and without passing judgment *to gain their trust.*
- PCC Help parents develop realistic expectations of their child and formulate achievable short-term goals based on the child's needs and abilities *to reduce frustration and feelings of helplessness.*
- Ensure attention to all of the child's normal health needs, including dental care, immunizations, safety, and educational and nutritional needs. *A chronically ill child needs total health care, not just illness-related interventions.*
- Pay attention to the needs of siblings at home. Devote time to discussing their feelings about having a brother or sister with special needs. How do their friends react? Contact their school nurse for assistance. Encourage them to help care for their brother or sister, but make sure activities are age-appropriate. *Becoming involved will help siblings achieve greater self-esteem and enhance their sense of control.*
- Advocate normal growth and development for the child with special needs. Encourage visits by friends and discourage overprotective behavior *to help the child obtain social acceptance. Increased social interaction will encourage parents, siblings, and others to view the child as a unique individual instead of a burden. This, in turn, will help promote the child's self-esteem.*
- PCC Act as a liaison between the family and the multidisciplinary health care team, equipment vendors, community agencies, and third-party payers. *An organized approach with one central coordinator decreases stress for the family and enhances continuity of care.*

Suggested NIC Interventions

Crisis Intervention; Decision-Making Support; Family Process Maintenance; Limit Setting; Mutual Goal Setting; Parenting Promotion; Role Enhancement

Evaluations for Expected Outcomes

- Parents seek out and use community resources to assist in meeting child's physical, psychological, and educational needs.
- Parents express increased knowledge of their child's needs and demonstrate comfort in caring for child at home.
- Parents provide appropriate physical, emotional, and developmental care to child at home.
- Parents seek help to meet their own emotional and developmental needs.
- Parents express feelings of greater control and capability in meeting child's needs.
- Siblings come to terms with having brother or sister with special needs.

Documentation

- Family members' expressions of feelings about their role in caring for child at home
- Observations of parent–child interaction
- Physical and psychological status of child with special needs
- Nursing interventions to resolve parental role conflict at home
- Parents,' child's, and siblings' responses to interventions
- Evaluations for expected outcomes

REFERENCES

Alsem, M. W., Siebes, R. C., Gorter, J. W., Jongmans, M. J., Nijhuis, B. J., & Ketelaar, M. (2014). Assessment of family needs in children with physical disabilities: Development of a family needs inventory. *Child: Care, Health & Development*, *40*(4), 498–506. doi:10.1111/cch.12093

Smalley, L., Kenney, M., Denboba, D., & Strickland, B. (2014). Family perceptions of shared decision making with health care providers: Results of the national survey of children with special health care needs, 2009–2010. *Maternal & Child Health Journal*, *18*(6), 1316–1327. doi:10.1007/s10995-013-1365-z

Tétreault, S., Blais-Michaud, S., Marier Deschênes, P., Beaupré, P., Gascon, H., Boucher, N., & Carrière, M. (2014). How to support families of children with disabilities? An exploratory study of social support services. *Child & Family Social Work*, *19*(3), 272–281.

BATHING SELF-CARE DEFICIT

related to alteration in cognitive functioning

Definition

Impaired ability to perform or complete bathing activities for self

Assessment

- Age
- History of neurologic, sensory, or developmental impairment
- Self-care abilities, including knowledge and use of adaptive equipment, preparation of equipment and supplies, and technical or mechanical skills

- Musculoskeletal status, including range of motion, muscle tone, gait, muscle size and strength, functional capabilities, and mechanical restrictions (such as splints, casts, or traction)
- Neurologic status, including cognition, communication ability, insight or judgment, level of consciousness, memory, motor ability, orientation, and sensory ability
- Psychosocial status, including child's affective reaction to imbalances between motor abilities and cognitive reasoning abilities, usual lifestyle, and parents' perception of developmental delay

Defining Characteristics

- Impaired ability to dry body
- Impaired ability to access bathroom
- Impaired ability to access water
- Impaired ability to gather bathing supplies
- Impaired ability to regulate bath water
- Impaired ability to wash body

Expected Outcomes

- Child's skin will remain clean, dry, and intact.
- Child and family members will voice feelings about self-care deficit.
- Child or family member will demonstrate ability to perform bathing.
- Child or family member will perform self-care program daily.

Suggested NOC Outcomes

Coordinated Movement; Psychomotor Energy; Self-Care: Bathing; Self-Care: Hygiene

Interventions and Rationales

- Assess the child's functional, cognitive, and perceptual level at established intervals. Document and report any changes. *Ongoing assessment allows you to identify changing needs and adjust interventions accordingly.*
- Provide the prescribed treatment for the child's underlying condition. Monitor and report progress *to provide a basis for the care plan.*
- Monitor completion of bathing *to evaluate self-care abilities and identify areas of need.* Provide help only when the child has difficulty.
- PCC Teach the child and family members bathing techniques. Have them perform return demonstrations *to identify problem areas and build self-confidence.*
- Allow ample time to perform self-care. Encourage the child to complete each task. Provide constructive feedback. *Rushing creates unnecessary stress and promotes failure. Completing a task without assistance promotes self-confidence. Positive feedback encourages progress.*
- Provide privacy for self-care activities. *Modesty becomes important to children around age 6.*
- S Provide safety equipment such as nonslip mats, grab bars, shower seats *to promote safety.*
- PCC Refer the child and family to support groups or community services *to provide continued assistance for efforts to promote self-care independence.*

Suggested NIC Interventions

Bathing; Decision-Making Support; Energy Management; Self-Care Assistance: Bathing; Teaching: Individual

Evaluations for Expected Outcomes

- Child's skin remains clean, dry, and intact.
- Child and family members voice feelings about self-care deficit.
- Child or family member displays competence in performing bathing through return demonstration.
- Child or family member performs self-care program daily.

Documentation

- Child's expressions of frustration or feelings of inadequacy
- Family members' expressions of concern regarding child's inability to carry out bathing
- Child's response to treatment of underlying condition
- Child's motor and sensory status
- Observations of child's impaired self-care ability
- Interventions to promote self-care skills and provide supportive care
- Instructions to child and family members, their understanding of instructions, and their demonstrated ability to carry out bathing
- Child's and family members' responses to nursing interventions
- Evaluations for expected outcomes

REFERENCES

Greener, M. (2015). Bath time: More than good clean fun. *British Journal of Midwifery*, *23*(6), 402–405.
Hugill, K. (2014). Neonatal skin cleansing revisited: Whether or not to use skin cleansing products. *British Journal of Midwifery*, *22*(10), 694–698.
Watkins, J. (2016). Common skin complaints in neonates. *British Journal of Midwifery*, *24*(1), 12–16. doi:10.12968/bjom.2016.24.1.12

DRESSING SELF-CARE DEFICIT

related to alteration in cognitive functioning

Definition

Impaired ability to perform or complete dressing activities for self

Assessment

- Age
- History of neurologic, sensory, or developmental impairment
- Self-care abilities, including knowledge and use of adaptive equipment, preparation of equipment and supplies, and technical or mechanical skills
- Musculoskeletal status, including range of motion, muscle tone, gait, muscle size and strength, functional capabilities, and mechanical restrictions (such as splints, casts, or traction)

- Neurologic status, including cognition, communication ability, insight or judgment, level of consciousness, memory, motor ability, orientation, and sensory ability
- Psychosocial status, including child's affective reaction to imbalances between motor abilities and cognitive reasoning abilities, usual lifestyle, and parents' perception of developmental delay

Defining Characteristics

- Decrease in motivation
- Discomfort
- Environmental barrier
- Fatigue
- Impaired ability to fasten clothing
- Impaired ability to gather clothing
- Impaired ability to maintain appearance
- Impaired ability to pick up clothing
- Impaired ability to put clothing on lower body
- Impaired ability to put clothing on upper body
- Impaired ability to put on various items of clothing (e.g., shirt, socks, shoes)
- Impaired ability to remove clothing item (e.g., shirt, socks, shoes)
- Impaired ability to use assistive device
- Impaired ability to use zipper
- Musculoskeletal impairment
- Neuromuscular impairment
- Pain

Expected Outcomes

- Child will be dressed each day.
- Child and family members will express feelings and concerns regarding child's self-care deficit.
- Child or family member will display competence in performing dressing skills through return demonstration.
- Child or family member will perform self-care program daily.

Suggested NOC Outcomes

Body Image; Energy Conservation; Self-Care: Dressing; Self-Care: Hygiene

Interventions and Rationales

- Assess the child's functional, cognitive, and perceptual level at periodic intervals. Document and report any changes. *Ongoing assessment allows you to identify changing needs and adjust interventions accordingly.*
- Provide the prescribed treatment for the child's underlying condition. Monitor and report progress *to provide a basis for the care plan.*
- Monitor completion of dressing *to evaluate self-care abilities and identify areas of need.* Provide help only when the child has difficulty. *Appropriate assistance provides an opportunity to teach self-care and promote good habits.*
- Suggest clothing that the child can manage easily, such as clothing slightly larger than regular size or pants and shoes with Velcro fasteners *to foster independence and improve self-esteem.*
- PCC Instruct the child and family members in dressing techniques. Have them perform return demonstrations *to identify problem areas and build self-confidence.*
- Allow ample time to perform self-care. Encourage the child to complete each task. Provide constructive feedback. *Rushing creates unnecessary stress and promotes failure.*

Completing a task without help promotes self-confidence. Positive feedback encourages progress.

- Provide privacy for dressing. *Modesty becomes important to children around age 6.*
- PCC Refer the child and family to support groups or community services *to provide ongoing assistance.*

Suggested NIC Interventions

Body Image Enhancement; Dressing; Energy Management; Self-Care Assistance: IADL

Evaluations for Expected Outcomes

- Child is dressed each day.
- Child and family members voice feelings regarding deficit in dressing skills.
- Child or family member displays competence in performing dressing skills through return demonstration.
- Child or family member performs self-care program daily.

Documentation

- Child's expressions of frustration or feelings of inadequacy
- Family members' expressions of feelings and concerns regarding child's inability to carry out dressing
- Child's response to treatment of underlying condition
- Child's motor and sensory status
- Interventions to promote self-care skills and provide supportive care
- Instructions provided to child and family members, their understanding of instructions, and their demonstrated ability to carry out dressing
- Child's and family members' responses to nursing interventions
- Evaluations for expected outcomes

REFERENCES

Harris, S. R., Mickelson, E. C., & Zwicker, J. G. (2015). Diagnosis and management of developmental coordination disorder. *Canadian Medical Association. Journal, 187*(9), 659–665.

Schreibman, L., Dawson, G., Stahmer, A. C., Landa, R., Rogers, S. J., Mcgee, G. G., . . . Halladay, A. (2015). Naturalistic developmental behavioral interventions: Empirically validated treatments for autism spectrum disorder. *Journal of Autism and Developmental Disorders, 45*(8), 2411–2428. doi:10.1007/s10803-015-2407-8

Van der Linde, B. W., van Netten, J. J., Otten, B., Postema, K., Geuze, R. H., & Schoemaker, M. M. (2015). Activities of daily living in children with developmental coordination disorder: Performance, learning, and participation. *Physical Therapy, 95*(11), 1496–1506.

FEEDING SELF-CARE DEFICIT

related to alteration in cognitive functioning

Definition

Impaired ability to perform or complete self-feeding activities

Assessment

- Age
- History of injury or disease associated with musculoskeletal impairment
- Self-care abilities, including knowledge and use of adaptive equipment, preparation of equipment and supplies, and technical and mechanical skills
- Musculoskeletal status, including coordination, functional ability, muscle tone and strength, range of motion, and mechanical restrictions (such as cast, splint, or traction)
- Neurologic status, including cognition, communication ability, level of consciousness, motor ability, and sensory status
- Nutritional status, including weight and food preferences
- Psychosocial status, including child's affective reaction to imbalances between motor abilities and cognitive reasoning abilities, usual lifestyle, and parents' perception of developmental delay

Defining Characteristics

- Impaired ability to bring food to the mouth
- Impaired ability to chew food
- Impaired ability to get food onto utensil
- Impaired ability to handle utensils
- Impaired ability to manipulate food in mouth
- Impaired ability to open containers
- Impaired ability to pick up cup
- Impaired ability to prepare food
- Impaired ability to self-feed a complete meal
- Impaired ability to self-feed in an acceptable manner
- Impaired ability to swallow food
- Impaired ability to swallow sufficient amount of food
- Impaired ability to use assistive device

Expected Outcomes

- Child will consume adequate calories and maintain desired weight.
- Auscultation will reveal clear breath sounds.
- Child and family members will express feelings and concerns.
- Child or family member will demonstrate correct feeding technique.

Suggested NOC Outcomes

Appetite; Cognition; Nutritional Status; Nutritional Status: Food & Fluid Intake; Self-Care Status; Self-Care: Eating; Swallowing Status

Interventions and Rationales

- Assess the child's functional, cognitive, and perceptual level at periodic intervals. Document and report any changes. *Ongoing assessment allows you to identify changing needs and adjust interventions accordingly.*
- Provide the prescribed treatment for the child's underlying condition. Monitor and report progress *to provide a basis for the care plan.*
- Weigh the child daily and record results *to assess nutritional status.*

- Determine the type of food the child handles most and tolerates best (finger foods, soft or liquid diet) *to enhance self-feeding ability.*
- Monitor and record breath sounds every 4 hours. Report any evidence of crackles, wheezing, or rhonchi *to detect aspiration.*
- Monitor the feeding routine *to evaluate self-care abilities and identify areas of need.* Assist only if necessary; for example, cut food into bite-size portions. *Appropriate assistance provides an opportunity to teach self-care and promote good habits.*
- Instruct the child and family members in the feeding routine. Have them perform return demonstrations *to build self-confidence.*
- Allow ample time to perform self-care activities. Encourage the child to complete each task. Provide constructive feedback. *Rushing creates unnecessary stress and promotes failure. Completing a task without assistance promotes self-confidence. Positive feedback encourages progress.*
- S Position the child in the upright sitting position. Use supportive devices, as needed, to maintain the child's posture. Sit at eye level with the child. *These measures help decrease the risk of aspiration. Sitting at eye level helps prevent the child from hyperextending the neck, which may increase the risk of aspiration.*
- PCC Teach specific tasks (such as grasping a spoon, opening the mouth, closing the lips around a utensil, or swallowing) rather than the total feeding skill. Use behavior modification techniques of praise and reward to mark accomplishments. *Children may not have cognitive or motor abilities to complete the total skill. Breaking down behavior into smaller units increases the likelihood of success.*

Suggested NIC Interventions

Energy Management; Nutrition Management; Nutritional Counseling; Self-Care Assistance: Feeding

Evaluations for Expected Outcomes

- Child maintains weight above fifth percentile on pediatric growth charts.
- Aspiration doesn't occur as evidenced by clear breath sounds heard during auscultation.
- Child and family members voice feelings regarding feeding routine.
- Child or family member demonstrates correct feeding technique.

Documentation

- Child's expressions of frustration or feelings of inadequacy
- Family members' expressions of concern
- Child's response to treatment of underlying condition
- Child's motor and sensory status
- Interventions performed to promote self-care skills and provide supportive care
- Instructions provided to child and family members, their understanding of instructions, and their demonstrated ability to carry out feeding routine
- Child's and family members' responses to nursing interventions
- Evaluations for expected outcomes

REFERENCES

Brown, L. F., Pickler, R. H., & Wetzel, P. A. (2014). Maternal attention and preterm infant feeding. *Journal for Specialists in Pediatric Nursing*, 19(3), 257–265. doi:10.1111/jspn.12077

Thoyre, S. M., Pados, B. F., Jinhee, P., Estrem, H., Hodges, E. A., McComish, C., . . . Murdoch, K. (2014). Development and content validation of the pediatric eating assessment tool (Pedi-EAT). *American Journal of Speech-Language Pathology, 23*(1), 46–59. doi:10.1044/1058-0360(2013/12-0069)

Wieringa, J., Stok, J., Rossum, A., & Filippini, L. (2014). Feeding problems in a lethargic infant (Case Presentation). *Acta Paediatrica, 103*(3), 236–237. doi:10.1111/apa.12508

TOILETING SELF-CARE DEFICIT

related to alteration in cognitive functioning

Definition

Impaired ability to perform or complete self-toileting activities

Assessment

- Developmental factors, including age, maturity, and smooth-muscle control
- History of neurologic, sensory, or developmental impairment
- Self-care abilities, including knowledge and use of adaptive equipment, preparation of equipment and supplies, and technical or mechanical skills
- Musculoskeletal status, including range of motion, muscle tone, gait, muscle size and strength, functional capabilities, and mechanical restrictions (such as splints, casts, or traction)
- Neurologic status, including cognition, communication ability, insight or judgment, level of consciousness, memory, motor ability, orientation, and sensory ability
- Psychosocial status, including child's affective reaction to imbalances between motor abilities and cognitive reasoning abilities, usual lifestyle, and parents' perception of developmental delay

Defining Characteristics

- Impaired ability to complete toilet hygiene
- Impaired ability to flush toilet
- Impaired ability to manipulate clothing for toileting
- Impaired ability to reach toilet
- Impaired ability to rise from toilet
- Impaired ability to sit on toilet

Expected Outcomes

- Child will maintain normal urine and bowel elimination patterns for age.
- Child and family members will voice feelings about impaired toileting ability.
- Child and family members will demonstrate correct toileting activities.
- Child's skin will remain clean, dry, and intact.

Suggested NOC Outcomes

Balance; Coordinated Movement; Self-Care: Hygiene; Self-Care: Toileting; Self-Direction of Care

Interventions and Rationales

- Observe the child's functional, cognitive, and perceptual level. Document and report any changes. *Ongoing assessment allows you to identify changing needs and adjust interventions accordingly.*
- Provide the prescribed treatment for the child's underlying condition. Monitor and report progress *to provide a basis for the care plan.*
- Monitor intake and output *to detect fluid and electrolyte imbalances.*
- Assess skin condition, especially in the perianal area, *to detect evidence of skin breakdown.*
- Assist with toileting when necessary. As much as possible, allow the child to perform the toilet routine independently *to enhance toileting ability and promote feelings of control.*
- PCC Teach the child and family members the toileting routine. Have the child and family members demonstrate the toileting routine under supervision. *Return demonstration allows you to evaluate learning and increases the child's and family members' confidence.*
- Provide privacy for toileting activities. *Modesty becomes important to children around age 6.*
- Assist with specific bladder elimination procedures, such as intermittent self-catheterization, as prescribed. Assess the child's readiness to learn self-catheterization. Instruct the child or family members in the technique and request a return demonstration *to evaluate understanding and ability.* Maintain sterile technique in the hospital and clean technique at home *to prevent infection.*
- Assist with the use of incontinence aids, such as diapers, pads, and pants, which may be prescribed as an alternative to indwelling devices. *Incontinence aids prevent the soiling of clothes and linen, reduce embarrassment, and draw urine away from skin.*
- Establish a regular pattern for bowel care. For example, after breakfast, place the child on the toilet or commode for 1 hour after inserting a glycerin suppository; allow the child to remain upright for 30 minutes, and then clean the anal area. *Regular bowel care encourages routine physiologic function.*
- PCC Teach the parents the bowel care routine *to foster compliance.*
- Maintain a diet log *to identify irritant foods,* and then eliminate such foods from the child's diet *to promote regular bowel function.* Teach parents the need to regulate the child's intake of foods and fluids that cause diarrhea or constipation *to encourage healthful nutritional patterns.*
- PCC Teach parents to regulate the child's fluid intake according to a specific schedule and to limit fluid intake after dinner *to encourage voiding at appropriate times.*

Suggested NIC Interventions

Bowel Training; Self-Care Assistance: Bathing/Hygiene; Urinary Elimination Management

Evaluations for Expected Outcomes

- Child maintains normal elimination patterns for age.
- Child and family members express feelings associated with child's toileting routine.
- Child and family members demonstrate correct toileting activities.
- Child's skin remains intact with no evidence of breakdown.

Documentation

- Child's expressions of feelings of inadequacy or depression
- Family members' concerns about child's inability to carry out toileting activities

- Child's response to treatment of underlying condition
- Child's motor and sensory status
- Interventions to promote self-care skills and to provide supportive care
- Child's and family members' responses to nursing interventions
- Instructions to child and family members, their understanding of instructions, and demonstrated ability to carry out toileting routine
- Evaluations for expected outcomes

REFERENCES

Ghanma, A., Puttemans, K., Deneyer, M., Benninga, M., & Vandenplas, Y. (2014). Amsterdam infant stool scale is more useful for assessing children who have not been toilet trained than Bristol stool scale. *Acta Paediatrica*, *103*(2), e91–e92. doi:10.1111/apa.12422

Ladi Seyedian, S., Sharifi-Rad, L., Ebadi, M., & Kajbafzadeh, A. (2014). Combined functional pelvic floor muscle exercises with Swiss ball and urotherapy for management of dysfunctional voiding in children: A randomized clinical trial. *European Journal of Pediatrics*, *173*(10), 1347–1353. doi:10.1007/s00431-014-2336-0

Smith, J. (2015). Oh crap! Potty training: Everything modern parents need to know to do it once and do it right. *Library Journal*, *140*(13), 74–76.

INEFFECTIVE THERMOREGULATION

related to illness; trauma

Definition

Temperature fluctuations between hypothermia and hyperthermia

Assessment

- Age
- History of illness or injury, including related events, such as exposure to infection (intrauterine or extrauterine)
- Perinatal history, including asphyxia
- Health history, including chronic disease or disability
- Medication history, including antibiotics, steroids, nonsteroidal anti-inflammatory drugs
- Vital signs, including temperature, pulse, blood pressure, and respirations
- Skin color and temperature
- Fluid and electrolyte status, including skin turgor, intake and output, mucous membranes, serum electrolyte levels, and urine specific gravity
- Neurologic status, including level of consciousness
- Nutritional status, including willingness and ability to eat, current weight, and weight gain pattern (on growth chart)

Defining Characteristics

- Cyanotic nail beds
- Fluctuations in body temperature above and below the normal range
- Flushed skin
- Hypertension
- Increase in body temperature above the normal range
- Increased respiratory rate
- Mild shivering
- Moderate pallor

- Piloerection
- Reduction in body temperature below normal range
- Seizures
- Skin cool to touch
- Skim warm to touch
- Slow capillary refill
- Tachycardia

Expected Outcomes

- Child will maintain body temperature at normal levels (96.8° F to 99° F [36° C to 37.2° C]).
- Child's fluid intake and output will remain balanced and within normal limits for age.
- Child will maintain adequate glucose intake and will consume ___ calories/day.
- Child and family members will identify risk factors and describe measures to prevent dehydration.
- Family members will demonstrate procedure for assessing axillary or oral temperature accurately.
- Family members will demonstrate measures to care for child with fever.

Suggested NOC Outcomes

Hydration; Thermoregulation; Vital Signs

Interventions and Rationales

- Take an axillary or oral temperature every 1 to 4 hours. Avoid taking rectal temperatures. Record the temperature and route. *Physically and psychologically safer than rectal thermometers, axillary and oral thermometers provide an accurate core temperature.*
- If the child has a fever, remove sheets, blankets, and most clothing (except diapers and underwear). Place cool cloths on the axilla and groin. Perform a tepid sponging procedure. Use a hypothermia blanket, as ordered, for temperature above 103° F (39.4° C). Set the blanket temperature at 41° F (5° C). Discontinue if shivering occurs *because shivering increases the metabolic rate and supports fever.* Monitor vital signs every 15 minutes for 1 hour, and as indicated, *because decreasing body temperature too rapidly can cause vascular collapse. These steps reduce excessive fever.*
- S Monitor heart rate, rhythm, and respiratory rate. *Careful monitoring determines the need for more aggressive intervention.*
- Calculate the child's fluid, glucose, and electrolyte requirements. Administer IV fluids as indicated. Monitor and record intake and output *to compensate for an increase in metabolic rate and to prevent dehydration. Insensible fluid losses increase by 10% for every 0.5° F (1° C) rise in temperature.*
- If the child's body temperature is below 96.8° F (36° C), use a warming blanket. Set the blanket temperature at 100.4° F (38° C). Keep the child wrapped in blankets and cover the child's head. *The body surface area, particularly the head, is proportionately larger in a young child; adequate covering will prevent heat loss. These steps combat hypothermia.*
- PCC Teach parents how to take an accurate temperature and have parents provide a return demonstration *to ensure accurate monitoring after discharge.*
- Determine the child's preferences for oral fluids. Push fluids in a manner appropriate to the child's age and level of development. *A well-hydrated child's temperature returns to normal range more quickly.*
- Discuss factors that precipitate neurogenic temperature drift with family members *to prevent future episodes.*

Suggested NIC Interventions

Environmental Management; Fever Treatment; Fluid Management; Temperature Regulation; Vital Signs Monitoring

Evaluations for Expected Outcomes

- Child's temperature remains within normal limits.
- Child maintains balanced fluid intake and output within normal limits for age.
- Child maintains adequate glucose and caloric intake.
- Child and family members identify risk factors and describe measures to prevent dehydration.
- Family members demonstrate ability to measure axillary or oral temperature accurately.
- Family members demonstrate measures to care for child with fever.

Documentation

- Observations of physical findings
- Nursing interventions performed
- Medications administered
- Child's response to nursing interventions
- Evaluations for expected outcomes

REFERENCES

Joseph, R. A. (2015). Neonatal care. Prolonged mechanical ventilation: Challenges to nurses and outcome in extremely preterm babies. *Critical Care Nurse*, *35*(4), 58–66. doi:10.4037/ccn2015396

Lowth, D. M. (2014). The child with a temperature. *Practice Nurse*, *44*(11), 26–30.

Vilinsky, A., & Sheridan, A. (2014). Hypothermia in the newborn: An exploration of its cause, effect, and prevention. *British Journal of Midwifery*, *22*(8), 557–562.

IMPAIRED VERBAL COMMUNICATION

related to alteration in development

Definition

Decreased, delayed, or absent ability to receive, process, transmit, and/or use a system of symbols

Assessment

- Age
- Health history, including past respiratory, neurologic, or musculoskeletal disorders or surgery
- Respiratory status, including dyspnea, use of accessory muscles, and respiratory pattern
- Neurologic status, including mental status and speech (pattern, signing, and such communication aids as artificial larynx, computer-assisted speech device, pen and pencil, picture board, and alphabet board)
- Musculoskeletal status, including range of motion and manual dexterity
- Parental status, including understanding of normal speech development, level of frustration with child's speech impairment, and coping skills

Defining Characteristics

- Absence of eye contact
- Difficulty comprehending communication
- Difficulty expressing thoughts verbally (e.g., aphasia, dysphasia, apraxia, dyslexia)
- Difficulty forming sentences
- Difficulty forming words (e.g., aphonia, dyslalia, dysarthria)
- Difficulty in selective attending
- Difficulty in use of body expressions
- Difficulty in use of facial expressions
- Difficulty maintaining communication
- Difficulty speaking
- Difficulty verbalizing
- Disoriented to person
- Disoriented to place
- Disoriented to time
- Does not speak
- Dyspnea
- Inability to speak
- Inability to speak language of caregiver
- Inability to use body expressions
- Inappropriate verbalization
- Partial visual deficit
- Refusal to speak
- Slurred speech
- Stuttering
- Total visual deficit

Expected Outcomes

- Family members will express desire to better understand child's communication impairment.
- Family members will demonstrate understanding of verbal development in children and alternative communication techniques.
- Child will communicate needs.

Suggested NOC Outcomes

Cognition; Information Processing

Interventions and Rationales

PCC
- Teach parents to:
  - talk to, read to, and play music for the child
  - repeat the sounds the child makes
  - point to objects and name them
  - use generative speech ("What would you like to wear today?") rather than directive speech ("Do you want to wear the red shirt?").

  These measures stimulate language development. Generative speech requires the child to generate words rather than simply responding with yes or no.
- Describe to family members the alternative methods of assessing the needs of a speech-delayed child. A toddler or preschooler may communicate needs through role playing with dolls and stuffed animals. A preschooler or school-age child may communicate through drawing. Parents may use pictorial (faces) pain scale to assess an ill child's level of discomfort. *These techniques will enable the family to better understand their speech-impaired child.*
- Assess the family members' level of understanding of the speech development process. Tell them that a toddler has limited receptive language skills and should be given one direction at a time. A preschooler has limited vocabulary and may communicate through gestures and symbols. Further explain that each child develops speech at a different rate. *These measures increase family members' understanding of the child's speech impairment.*

Suggested NIC Interventions

Anxiety Reduction; Communication Enhancement: Speech Deficit; Presence; Touch

Evaluations for Expected Outcomes

- Family members describe stages of speech development.
- Family members demonstrate alternative methods of assessing needs of speech-delayed child.
- Child communicates needs.

Documentation

- Family members' understanding of speech development process
- Family members' demonstration of alternative methods of assessing needs of speech-delayed child
- Family members' understanding of alternative methods of communicating with child
- Nursing interventions and family's and child's response to them
- Evaluations for expected outcomes

REFERENCES

Cascella, P. W., Bruce, S. M., & Trief, E. (2015). Sign language, speech, and communication repair abilities by children with congenital deaf-blindness. *Journal of Visual Impairment & Blindness*, *109*(2), 141–146.

Mulrine, C., & Kollia, B. (2015). Speech, language, hearing delays: Time for early intervention? *Journal of Family Practice*, *64*(3), E1–E9.

Ramkissoon, I., Estis, J. M., & Flagge, A. G. (2014). Digit speech recognition threshold (SRT) in children with normal hearing, ages 5–8 years. *American Journal of Audiology*, *23*(2), 182–189. doi:10.1044/2014_AJA-13-0039

Tong, X., Tong, X., & McBride-Chang, C. (2015). Tune in to the tone: Lexical tone identification is associated with vocabulary and word recognition abilities in young Chinese children. *Language & Speech*, *58*(4), 441–458. doi:10.1177/0023830914562988

PART IV

Maternal–Neonatal Health

APPLYING EVIDENCE-BASED PRACTICE

The Question

Does delayed clamping of the umbilical cord have a significant benefit for the term infant?

Evidence-Based Resources

Are there long-term benefits of delayed cord clamping? (2014). *Journal of Paediatrics & Child Health, 50*(12), 1027–1028. doi:10.1111/jpc.12767_3

Bechard, J. L. (2015). Delayed umbilical cord clamping: Is it necessary to wait? *International Journal of Childbirth Education, 30*(2), 14–16.

Conner, S. N., & Macones, G. A. (2014). Delayed umbilical cord clamping. *Contemporary OB/GYN, 59*(6), 46–49.

Holvey, N. (2014). The imperative of implementing delayed cord clamping to improve maternal and neonatal outcomes. *British Journal of Midwifery, 22*(9), 651–656.

Nakagawa, M., Ishida, Y., Nagaoki, Y., Ohta, H., Shimabukuro, R., Hirata, M., . . . Kusakawa, I. (2015). Correlation between umbilical cord hemoglobin and rate of jaundice requiring phototherapy in healthy newborns. *Pediatrics International, 57*(4), 626–628. doi:10.1111/ped.12583

Ranjit, T., Nesargi, S., Rao, P. N. S., Sahoo, J. P., Ashok, C., Chandrakala, B. S., & Bhat, S. (2015). Effect of early versus delayed cord clamping on hematological status of preterm infants at 6 wk of age. *Indian Journal of Pediatrics, 82*(1), 29–34. doi:10.1007/s12098-013-1329-8

Evaluating the Evidence

The debate is ongoing as to whether the timing of cord clamping is detrimental or beneficial to the infant after delivery. The standard practice in many hospital facilities is to clamp the cord immediately after delivery; then to avoid cold stress, place the infant in a warmer or skin-to-skin on the mother. Bechard (2015) describes delayed or late cord clamping as occurring 2 or 3 minutes after delivery of the infant, or at the point at which the cord is no longer pulsating. Early cord clamping occurs when the cord is clamped within the first 15 seconds after delivery of the infant.

Conner and Macones (2014) completed a systematic review to examine current practice related to delayed umbilical cord clamping. The review was divided by preterm and term deliveries. Outcomes for 738 neonates delivered either vaginally or cesarean between 24 and 36 weeks revealed fewer transfusions for anemia, less intraventricular hemorrhage, better circulatory stability, and a lower risk of necrotizing enterocolitis. Outcomes for 3,911 term neonates revealed higher neonatal hemoglobin concentration and a lower probability of iron deficiency at 3 to 6 months. Both groups associated delayed cord clamping with an increased incidence of jaundice.

Ranjit et al. (2015) completed a study with preterm infants that compared the effects of early cord clamping versus delayed cord clamping on hematocrit (HCT) and serum ferritin at 6 weeks. Results indicated that delayed cord clamping offered significant benefits of raised HCT and ferritin levels. Both groups had similar incidence of jaundice; however, the delayed cord clamp group required longer duration of phototherapy.

A study conducted by Nakagawa et al. (2015) examined the correlation between umbilical cord hemoglobin and rate of jaundice requiring phototherapy. Of the infants studied, those with high cord blood hemoglobin were more likely to develop jaundice, requiring phototherapy. The authors noted that severity of neonatal jaundice differed with race. Peak bilirubin levels of Asian-American newborns were 10 to 14 mg/dL 72 to 120 hours after birth, while white and African-American newborns were 5 to 6 mg/dL 72 to 96 hours after birth.

Applying the Results and Making a Decision

The literature supports delayed cord clamping as beneficial to the term newborn. Because of the benefits of delayed cord clamping identified in current research, the standard practice of immediate cord clamping after birth of the infant should be reevaluated globally. One concern that has caused practitioners to avoid the practice of delayed cord clamping is the possibility that the delay may contribute to neonatal jaundice. According to Bechard (2015), because the decision to delay cord clamping is currently determined by the health care provider, the provider must weigh the benefits and risks to provide optimal care.

Re-Evaluating Process and Identifying Areas for Improvement

The current standard of practice should be reevaluated globally. Parents should be given the facts about the benefits of delayed cord clamping when devising the birth plan and be allowed to make an informed choice prior to the birthing process (Holvey, 2014). Practitioners should be made aware of the benefits of increased transfusion of blood from the placenta to the newborn as well as the prolonged benefit of added iron stores ("Are there long-term benefits of delayed cord clamping?", 2014).

INTRODUCTION

This section covers maternal, fetal, and neonatal care, with an emphasis on meeting the changing needs of the mother, child, and family. Because of the dynamic nature of pregnancy and childbirth, you'll need to be flexible in planning care. Expect to revise your care plans continually during the time that you're providing care.

During pregnancy, you'll assess maternal factors, such as age, past experience with pregnancy and delivery, health history, reaction to fetal movement, and nutritional status. Keep in mind that the mother's health status directly affects the fetus' well-being.

After birth, you'll assess neonatal factors such as Apgar scores, gestational age, weight in relation to gestational age, vital signs, feeding patterns, muscle tone, condition of fontanels, and characteristics of the neonate's cry.

Throughout your assessment, maintain a family-centered, holistic approach. When assessing, be aware of how pregnancy and the neonate's arrival affects the entire family. Evaluate how the mother, father, siblings, and other family members bond with the neonate.

The nursing diagnoses included in this section relate to actual or potential health problems of the developing family and focus on the physiologic and psychosocial needs of family members. Use information gathered during assessment to develop appropriate plans of care for the prenatal period, labor and delivery, the postpartum period, and for the neonate.

When implementing your care plan, reinforce interventions through teaching. Encourage family members to become involved in the planning and implementation of care. Stay attentive to changing educational needs of the new mother and remain sensitive and supportive of her emotional concerns.

Inform other members of the health care team of your nursing goals and enlist their support as needed. Keep colleagues informed about the family's progress in attaining goals.

Evaluate goals frequently. Thoughtful evaluation will allow you to promptly determine the need for revisions, thereby ensuring that the plan of care accurately reflects the developing family's current needs.

ANXIETY

related to major change (e.g., economic status, environment, health status, role function, role status); situation crisis

Definition

Vague, uneasy feeling of discomfort or dread accompanied by an autonomic response (the source is often nonspecific or unknown to the individual); a feeling of apprehension caused by anticipation of danger. It is an alerting sign that warns of impending danger and enables the individual to take measures to deal with threat

Assessment

- History of stress-related signs or symptoms
- Cultural influences
- Current worries, fears, and concerns
- Expectations of labor experience, including knowledge and past experience
- Behavior, including reaction to fetal movement and uterine activity, motor activity, excessive or extraneous movements, and interactions with nurse and significant others
- Cognitive status, including ability to concentrate, learn, and remember

- Physiologic status
- Usual coping methods
- Mood
- Personality
- Progress of labor

Defining Characteristics

Behavioral

- Decrease in productivity
- Extraneous movement
- Fidgeting
- Glancing about
- Hypervigilance
- Insomnia
- Poor eye contact
- Restlessness
- Scanning behavior
- Worried about change in life event

Affective

- Anguish
- Apprehensiveness
- Distress
- Fear
- Feeling of inadequacy
- Helplessness
- Increase in wariness
- Irritability
- Jitteriness
- Overexcitement
- Rattled
- Regretful
- Self-focused
- Uncertainty
- Worried

Physiologic

- Facial tension
- Hand tremors
- Increase in perspiration
- Increase in tension
- Shakiness
- Trembling
- Voice quivering

Sympathetic

- Alteration in respiratory pattern
- Anorexia
- Brisk reflexes
- Cardiovascular excitation
- Diarrhea
- Dry mouth
- Facial flushing
- Heart palpitations
- Increase in blood pressure
- Increase in heart rate
- Increase in respiratory rate
- Pupil dilation
- Superficial vasoconstriction
- Twitching
- Weakness

Parasympathetic

- Abdominal pain
- Alteration in sleep pattern
- Decrease in heart rate
- Decreased blood pressure
- Diarrhea
- Faintness
- Fatigue
- Nausea
- Tingling in extremities
- Urinary frequency
- Urinary hesitancy
- Urinary urgency

Cognitive

- Alteration in attention
- Alteration in concentration
- Awareness of physiologic symptoms
- Blocking of thoughts
- Confusion
- Decrease in perceptual field
- Diminished ability to learn
- Diminished ability to problem-solve
- Fear
- Forgetfulness
- Preoccupation
- Rumination
- Tendency to blame others

Expected Outcomes

- Patient will express feelings of anxiety.
- Patient will identify causes of anxiety.
- Patient will make use of available emotional support.
- Patient will show fewer signs of anxiety.
- Patient will identify positive aspects of her efforts to cope during childbirth.
- Patient will acquire increased knowledge about childbirth and will be better prepared to cope with future births.

Suggested NOC Outcomes

Anxiety Self-Control; Concentration; Coping; Social Interaction Skills; Symptom Control

Interventions and Rationales

- Assess the patient's knowledge, experience, and expectations of labor *to learn the precise source of anxiety and increase the effectiveness of interventions.*
- Discuss normal labor progression with the patient, and explain what to expect during labor *to increase the patient's knowledge about normal progression of labor and understanding of her own experience.*
- PCC Involve the patient in making decisions about care *to reduce the sense of powerlessness that some women experience during labor.*
- Share information on labor progression, vital signs, and the neonate's condition with the patient to provide reassurance of normality and increase her sense of participation.
- Interpret environmental sights and sounds (electronic fetal monitor strip, fetal monitor sounds, and activities on unit) for the patient to make the environment seem less threatening.
- PCC Attend to the patient's comfort needs to increase trust and reduce anxiety.
- Encourage the patient to employ coping skills used successfully in the past to enhance her sense of control.
- PCC Teach new coping skills (relaxation, breathing techniques, and positioning) to diminish anxiety by increasing the patient's sense of power and control. Review these skills with the patient periodically because anxiety impairs recall.
- PCC Organize your work to spend as much time as possible with the patient to provide comfort and assistance, thereby promoting the patient's sense of security.
- PCC Allow family members to participate in care to provide comfort and help the patient cope with labor.

Suggested NIC Interventions

Anxiety Reduction; Calming Technique; Simple Relaxation Therapy; Spiritual Support

Evaluations for Expected Outcomes

- Patient expresses feelings of anxiety about pregnancy or birth.
- Patient identifies causes of anxiety.
- Patient communicates with nurse or family members to gain reassurance, information, or emotional support.
- Patient's physiologic or behavioral signs return to normal.
- Patient, verbally or nonverbally, indicates that giving birth was a positive experience and expresses satisfaction with her behavior while giving birth.

- Patient verbalizes increased knowledge about childbirth and displays confidence in her ability to cope with future births.

Documentation

- Patient's expressions of anxiety
- Patient's statements of reasons for anxiety
- Observation of physical or behavioral signs of anxiety
- Interventions to assist patient with coping
- Patient's response to interventions
- Evaluations for expected outcomes

REFERENCES

Burke, C. T., & Perndorfer, C. C. (2015). Negative emotional responses to motherhood-related support receipt during pregnancy predict postpartum depressive symptoms. *Anxiety, Stress, & Coping*, 1–9.

Caldwell, B. A., & Redeker, N. S. (2015). Maternal stress and psychological status and sleep in minority preschool children. *Public Health Nursing, 32*(2), 101–111. doi:10.1111/phn.12104

Kisvetrová, H., Klugar, M., & Kabelka, L. (2013). Spiritual support interventions in nursing care for patients suffering death anxiety in the final phase of life. *International Journal of Palliative Nursing, 19*(12), 599–605.

Rossman, B., Greene, M. M., & Meier, P. P. (2015). The role of peer support in the development of maternal identity for 'NICU moms'. *Journal of Obstetric, Gynecologic & Neonatal Nursing, 44*(1), 3–16. doi:10.1111/1552-6909.12527

RISK FOR ASPIRATION

Definition

Vulnerable to entry of gastrointestinal secretions, oropharyngeal secretions, solids, or fluids to the tracheobronchial passages, which may compromise health

Assessment

- Gestational age
- Neonate's weight in relation to gestational age
- Maternal sedation before delivery and effects of maternal sedation on labor
- Neonate's health status, including preexisting conditions, anomalies, intrauterine environment, urologic status, cardiovascular status, respiratory status, and GI status
- Laboratory studies of neonate, including fluid, electrolyte, and arterial blood gas levels
- Neonate's vital signs
- Neonate's nutritional status, including continuous or intermittent gavage feeding

Risk Factors

- Barrier to upper body
- Decrease in gastrointestinal (GI) motility
- Decrease in level of consciousness
- Delayed gastric emptying
- Decreased gag reflex
- Enteral feedings
- Facial surgery
- Facial trauma
- Impaired ability to swallow
- Incompetent lower esophageal sphincter
- Increase is gastric residual
- Increase in intragastric pressure
- Ineffective cough

- Neck surgery
- Neck trauma
- Oral surgery
- Oral trauma
- Presence of oral/nasal tube (e.g., tracheal, feeding)
- Treatment regimen
- Wired jaw

Expected Outcomes

- Neonate will receive suctioning, as needed, and will maintain clear airway.
- Neonate won't exhibit gastric distention.
- Neonate will demonstrate minimal to moderate quantity of nasopharyngeal and oropharyngeal secretions.
- Neonate will tolerate initial feeding.
- Neonate won't demonstrate any color changes during feeding.
- Neonate will demonstrate appropriate suck and swallow reflex.
- Neonate will have no adventitious breath sounds.
- Neonate won't exhibit signs and symptoms of aspiration.

Suggested NOC Outcomes

Aspiration Prevention; Respiratory Status: Airway Patency; Respiratory Status: Ventilation; Risk Detection; Swallowing Status

Interventions and Rationales

- Regularly assess the neonate's respiratory status until stable *to evaluate respiratory system transition to extrauterine life.*
- Monitor vital signs, according to facility protocol, and report changes *to determine multisystem adjustment to extrauterine existence.*
- Suction as needed *to keep the upper and lower airways clear.* If the neonate aspirates meconium, assist the physician with laryngoscopy to suction below the vocal cords. If you're in the delivery room, suction the oropharynx and nasopharynx with a bulb syringe, DeLee catheter, or suction catheter attached to wall suction. *These measures may prevent additional respiratory compromise.*
- Perform a head-to-toe physical assessment *to detect abnormalities in other body systems that may affect respiratory effort.*
- Withhold oral feedings if signs of respiratory distress occur. Provide IV fluids, as ordered. *Sucking may place additional stress on the neonate in respiratory distress and may lead to aspiration.*
- When offering the initial feeding, observe for suck and swallow reflex, gag and cough reflex, and color changes. Have suction equipment available and ready to use. *Early detection of difficulty may prevent neonatal morbidity and mortality.*
- If the neonate is receiving gavage feeding:
  - Keep the head of the bed elevated during and after feedings, unless contraindicated.
  - Ensure proper positioning of the neonate before feeding or administering medication.
  - Monitor residual gastric contents and follow parameters for withholding feedings.
  - Once per shift, measure abdominal girth to check for distention; stop gavage feeding immediately if you suspect aspiration. Keep suction apparatus at the bedside and suction, as needed. Turn the neonate on his right side.

  Preventive measures reduce the risk of aspiration.
- Review laboratory results and report abnormalities. *Early identification of abnormal laboratory values reduces the risk of aspiration.*

- PCC • Explain to the parents the reasons for these interventions *to gain parental understanding and cooperation, which contributes to a positive outcome.*
- PCC • Instruct the parents in feeding techniques that will help prevent a distended abdomen leading to aspiration. Tell them to avoid overfeeding and to burp the neonate at frequent intervals (after intake of ½ to 1 oz [14.5 to 29.5 mL]). Instruct the parents to position the neonate on his right side with the head of the bed elevated for 30 to 60 minutes after feeding. *Providing instructions encourages parental understanding and cooperation.*

Suggested NIC Interventions

Aspiration Precautions; Positioning; Respiratory Monitoring; Vital Signs Monitoring; Vomiting Management

Evaluations for Expected Outcomes

- Neonate receives suctioning as needed and maintains patent airway.
- Neonate doesn't exhibit gastric distention.
- Neonate has minimal to moderate nasopharyngeal and oropharyngeal secretions.
- Neonate tolerates initial feeding.
- Neonate doesn't demonstrate color changes during feeding.
- Neonate has appropriate suck and swallow reflex.
- Neonate has no adventitious breath sounds.
- Neonate shows no signs or symptoms of aspiration.

Documentation

- Neonate's tolerance of initial feeding and of gavage feeding
- Residual gastric contents after gavage feeding
- Incidents of vomiting, aspiration, or both
- Breath sounds
- Observations of physical findings
- Interventions performed to prevent aspiration
- Evaluations for expected outcomes

REFERENCES

Louis, D., Sundaram, V., Mukhopadhyay, K., Dutta, S., & Kumar, P. (2014). Predictors of mortality in neonates with meconium aspiration syndrome. *Indian Pediatrics, 51*(8), 637–640.

Mallick, M. S. (2014). Tracheobronchial foreign body aspiration in children: A continuing diagnostic challenge. *African Journal of Pediatric Surgery, 11*(3), 225–228. doi:10.4103/0189-6725.137330

Sharma, P., Nangia, S., Tiwari, S., Goel, A., Singla, B., & Saili, A. (2014). Gastric lavage for prevention of feeding problems in neonates with meconium-stained amniotic fluid: A randomised controlled trial. *Paediatrics and International Child Health, 34*(2), 115–119. doi:10.1179/2046905513Y.0000000103

DISORGANIZED INFANT BEHAVIOR

related to pain, prematurity, oral impairment, impaired motor functioning, feeding intolerance, environmental overstimulation, or insufficient sensory stimulation

Definition

Disintegrated physiological and neurobehavioral response of infant to the environment

Assessment

- Cardiovascular status, including pulse and respirations
- Gastrointestinal (GI) status, including feeding pattern, food tolerance, defecation pattern, ability to maintain adequate weight, and abdominal bloating and distention
- Neurologic status, including muscle tone, neonatal reflexes, excessive crying, lethargy, irritability, seizures, tremors, and assessments such as Brazelton Neonatal Behavioral Assessment and Dubowitz Gestational Age Assessment
- Sensory status, including responsiveness to visual, tactile, and auditory stimuli and experience with pain
- Parental status, including knowledge of normal growth and development
- Sleep status, including sleep patterns and usual hours of sleep
- Parents' psychological status, including energy level, motivation, self-image, competence, recent life changes, experience with children, and eye contact and interaction with infant

Defining Characteristics

Attention–Interaction System

- Impaired response to sensory stimuli (e.g., difficult to soothe, unable to sustain alertness)

Motor System

- Alteration in primitive reflexes
- Exaggerated startle response
- Finger splaying
- Fisting
- Hands to face
- Hyperextension of extremities
- Impaired motor tone
- Jitteriness
- Tremor
- Twitching
- Uncoordinated movements

Physiologic

- Abnormal skin color (e.g., pale, dusky, cyanosis)
- Arrhythmia
- Bradycardia
- Desaturation
- Feeding intolerance
- Tachycardia
- Time-out signals (e.g., gaze, hiccough, sneeze, slack jaw, open mouth, tongue thrust)

Regulatory Problems

- Inability to inhibit startle reflex
- Irritability

State-Organization System

- Active-awake (e.g., fussy, worried gaze)
- Diffuse alpha EEG activity with eyes closed
- Irritable crying
- Quiet-awake (e.g., starting, gaze aversion)
- State oscillation

Expected Outcomes

- Parents will learn to identify and understand infant's behavioral cues.
- Parents will identify their own emotional responses to infant's behavior.
- Parents will identify means to help infant overcome behavioral disturbance.
- Parents will identify ways to improve their ability to cope with infant's responses.
- Infant will begin to show appropriate signs of maturation.
- Parents will express positive feelings about their ability to care for infant.
- Parents will identify resources for help with infant.

Suggested NOC Outcomes

Knowledge: Infant Care; Neurological Status; Preterm Infant Organization; Sleep

Interventions and Rationales

- Explain to the parents that infant maturation is a developmental process and that their participation is crucial *to help them understand the importance of nurturing the infant.*
- Explain to the parents that their actions can help modify some of their infant's behavior. However, make it clear that infant maturation isn't completely within their control. *This explanation may help decrease the parents' feelings of incompetence.*
- Explain to the parents that infants give behavioral cues that indicate their needs. Discuss appropriate ways to respond to these behavioral cues—for example, providing stimulation that doesn't overwhelm the infant, stopping stimulation when the infant gives behavioral cues (such as yawning, looking away, or becoming agitated), and finding methods to calm the infant if the infant becomes agitated (such as swaddling, gentle rocking, and quiet vocalizations). Help the parents identify and cope with their responses to the infant's behavioral disturbance *to help them recognize and adjust their response patterns. When the infant doesn't respond positively to them, the parents may feel inadequate or become frustrated. They need to understand that these reactions are normal.*
- PCC Explore with the parents ways to cope with stress imposed by the infant's behavior *to help them develop better coping skills.*
- Praise the parents when they demonstrate appropriate methods of interacting with the infant *to provide positive reinforcement.*
- Provide the parents with information on sources of support and special infant services *to help them cope with their infant's long-term needs.*

Suggested NIC Interventions

Environmental Management; Neurologic Monitoring; Newborn Care; Parent Education: Infant; Positioning; Sleep Enhancement

Evaluations for Expected Outcomes

- Parents state their understanding of infant's behavioral cues.
- Parents discuss appropriate ways of responding to infant's behavior and exhibit decreased frustration with infant's behavior.
- Parents identify ways to help infant overcome behavioral disturbance by recognizing infant's needs and responding appropriately.
- Parents report improved ability to cope with stress of caring for infant.
- Infant begins to show appropriate signs of maturation, such as longer periods of sleep, shorter periods of crying, longer periods of being awake and alert, smoother transitions between behavioral states, and positive responses to parents' interventions.
- Parents express positive feelings about their ability to care for infant.
- Parents identify resources for help with infant.

Documentation

- Assessment of factors that may enhance or retard infant behavioral development
- Parents' expressed feelings about caring for infant
- Nursing interventions and infant's response to them
- Evaluations for expected outcomes

REFERENCES

Brown, L. F., Pridham, K. A., & Brown, R. (2014). Sequential observation of infant regulated and dysregulated behavior following soothing and stimulating maternal behavior during feeding. *Journal for Specialists in Pediatric Nursing, 19*(2), 139–148. doi:10.1111/jspn.12062

Heun, N. (2014). Improving newborn pain management: Systematic pain assessment and operators' compliance with potentially better practices. *Journal of Clinical Nursing, 23*(3/4), 596–599. doi:10.1111/jocn.12036
Lopez, O., Subramanian, P., Rahmat, N., Theam, L. C., Chinna, K., & Rosli, R. (2015). The effect of facilitated tucking on procedural pain control among premature babies. *Journal of Clinical Nursing, 24*(1/2), 183–191. doi:10.1111/jocn.12657

READINESS FOR ENHANCED ORGANIZED INFANT BEHAVIOR

Definition

A pattern of modulation of the physiological and behavioral systems of functioning (i.e., autonomic, motor, state-organizational, self-regulatory, and attentional–interactional systems) in an infant, which can be strengthened

Assessment

- Cardiovascular status, including pulse and respirations
- Gastrointestinal status, including feeding and defecation patterns, food tolerance, ability to maintain adequate weight, and abdominal distention and bloating
- Neurologic status, including excessive crying, poor sleep patterns, lethargy, irritability, seizures, tremors, muscle tone, neonate reflexes, and assessments such as Brazelton Neonatal Behavioral Assessment and Dubowitz Gestational Age Assessment
- Sensory status, including responsiveness to visual, tactile, and auditory stimuli and experience with pain
- Sleep status, including usual hours of sleep
- Parental status, including knowledge of normal growth and development
- Parents' psychological status, including energy level, motivation, experience with children, eye contact and interaction with infant, and Home Observation Measurement of the Environment results

Defining Characteristics

- Parent expresses desire to enhance cue recognition
- Parent expresses desire to enhance recognition of infant's self-regulatory behaviors

Expected Outcomes

- Parents will express understanding of their role in infant's behavioral development.
- Parents will express confidence in their ability to interpret infant's behavioral cues.
- Parents will identify means to promote infant's behavioral development.
- Parents will express positive feelings about their ability to care for infant.
- Parents will identify resources for help with infant.

Suggested NOC Outcomes

Child Development: 2 Months; Knowledge: Infant Care; Neurological Status; Sleep

Interventions and Rationales

- Explain to the parents that infant maturation is a developmental process. Further explain that infants exhibit three behavioral states: sleeping, crying, and being awake and alert. Also explain that infants provide behavioral cues that indicate their needs. *Education will help parents understand the importance of nurturing the infant and prepare them to respond to the infant's behavioral cues.*
- Explain to the parents that their actions can help promote infant development. Make it clear, however, that infant maturation isn't completely within their control. *This explanation may decrease feelings of anxiety and incompetence and help to prevent unrealistic expectations.*
- Demonstrate appropriate ways of interacting with the infant, such as moderate stimulation, gentle rocking, and quiet vocalizations, *to help the parents identify the most effective methods of interacting with their child.*
- Help the parents interpret behavioral cues from their infant *to foster healthy parent–child interaction.* For example, help them recognize when the infant is awake and alert, and point out to them that this is a good time to provide stimulation.
- Help the parents identify ways they can promote the infant's development, such as providing stimulation by shaking a rattle in front of the infant, talking to the infant in a gentle voice, and looking at the infant when feeding him, *to encourage practices that promote the infant's development. Sensory experiences promote cognitive development.*
- PCC Explore with the parents ways to cope with stress caused by the infant's behavior *to increase their coping skills.*
- Praise the parents for their attempts to enhance their interaction with the infant *to provide positive reinforcement.*
- PCC Provide the parents with information on sources of support and special infant services *to encourage them to continue to foster their infant's development.*

Suggested NIC Interventions

Attachment Promotion; Developmental Care; Family Integrity Promotion: Childbearing Family; Infant Care; Sleep Enhancement

Evaluations for Expected Outcomes

- Parents express understanding of their role in infant's behavioral development.
- Parents express confidence in their ability to recognize infant's behavioral cues.
- Parents identify activities that foster positive responses from infant and provide appropriate sensory and tactile stimulation.
- Parents express positive feelings about their ability to care for infant.
- Parents identify resources for help with infant.

Documentation

- Assessment of factors that may enhance infant's behavioral development
- Parents' expressed feelings about caring for their infant
- Nursing interventions and infant's response to them
- Evaluations for expected outcomes

REFERENCES

Greener, M. (2015). Bath time: More than good clean fun. *British Journal of Midwifery*, *23*(6), 402–405.

Heun, N. (2014). Improving newborn pain management: Systematic pain assessment and operators' compliance with potentially better practices. *Journal of Clinical Nursing, 23*(3/4), 596–599. doi:10.1111/jocn.12036
Ward, T. (2015). Reasons for mother–infant bed-sharing: A systematic narrative synthesis of the literature and implications for future research. *Maternal & Child Health Journal, 19*(3), 675–690. doi:10.1007/s10995-014-1557-1

RISK FOR DISORGANIZED INFANT BEHAVIOR

Definition

Vulnerable to alteration in integration and modulation of the physiological and behavioral systems of functioning (i.e., autonomic, motor, state-organization, self-regulatory, and attentional–interactional systems, which may compromise health

Assessment

- Cardiovascular status, including pulse and respirations
- Gastrointestinal status, including feeding and defecation patterns, food tolerance, ability to maintain adequate weight, and abdominal bloating and distention
- Neurologic status, including muscle tone, neonate reflexes, excessive crying, lethargy, irritability, seizures, tremors, and assessments such as Brazelton Neonatal Behavioral Assessment and Dubowitz Gestational Age Assessment
- Sensory status, including infant's responsiveness to visual, tactile, and auditory stimuli and experience with pain
- Sleep status, including sleep pattern and usual hours of sleep
- Parental status, including knowledge of normal growth and development
- Parents' psychological status, including energy level, motivation, experience with children, and eye contact and interaction with infant

Risk Factors

- Impaired motor functioning
- Insufficient containment within environment
- Invasive procedure
- Oral impairment
- Pain
- Parent expresses desire to enhance environmental conditions
- Prematurity
- Procedure

Expected Outcomes

- Parents will identify factors that place infant at risk for behavioral disturbance.
- Parents will identify potential signs of behavioral disturbance in infant.
- Parents will identify appropriate ways to interact with infant.
- Parents will identify their reactions to infant (including ways of coping with occasional frustration and anger).
- Parents will express positive feelings about their ability to care for infant.
- Parents will identify resources for help with infant.

Suggested NOC Outcomes

Child Development: 2 Months; Knowledge: Infant Care; Knowledge: Parenting; Preterm Infant Organization

Interventions and Rationales

- Explain to the parents that infant maturation is a developmental process and that their participation is crucial *to help them understand the importance of nurturing the infant.*
- Explain to the parents that their actions can help modify some of their infant's behavior. However, make it clear that infant maturation isn't completely within their control. *This explanation may decrease the parents' feelings of incompetence.*
- Explain to the parents that certain risk factors may interfere with the infant's ability to achieve optimal development. These risk factors include overstimulation, lack of stimulation, lack of physical contact, and painful medical procedures. *Educating the parents will help them understand their role in interpreting the infant's behavioral cues and providing appropriate stimulation.*
- Describe for the parents the potential signs of a behavioral disturbance in the infant: inappropriate responses to stimuli, such as the failure to respond to human contact or tendency to become agitated with human contact; physiologic regulatory problems, such as a breathing disturbance in a premature infant; and apparent inability to interact with the environment. *Education will help the parents recognize if the infant has a problem in behavioral development.*
- Demonstrate appropriate ways of interacting with the infant *to help the parents identify and interpret the infant's behavioral cues and respond appropriately.* For example, help them recognize when the infant is awake and alert, and help them understand when the infant needs more stimulation, such as being spoken to or held.
- PCC Explore with the parents ways to cope with the stress imposed by the infant's behavior *to increase their coping skills.* Help them identify their emotional responses to the infant's behavior *to help them recognize and adjust their response patterns.* Explain that it's normal for parents to experience feelings of inadequacy, frustration, or anger if the infant doesn't respond positively to them.
- Praise the parents when they demonstrate appropriate methods of interacting with the infant *to provide positive reinforcement.*
- PCC Provide the parents with information on sources of support and special infant services *to help them cope with the infant's long-term needs.*

Suggested NIC Interventions

Infant Care; Newborn Monitoring; Parent Education: Infant; Positioning; Surveillance

Evaluations for Expected Outcomes

- Parents identify risk factors for behavioral disturbance.
- Parents identify potential signs of behavioral disturbance in infant.
- Parents identify actions that promote their infant's development.
- Parents report improvement in their ability to cope with the stress of raising an infant.
- Parents express positive feelings about their ability to care for infant.
- Parents identify resources for help with infant.

Documentation

- Assessment of factors that could disturb infant's behavioral development
- Parents' expression of feelings about caring for infant
- Nursing interventions and infant's response to them
- Evaluations for expected outcomes

REFERENCES

Baylis, R., Ewald, U., Gradin, M., Hedberg Nyqvist, K., Rubertsson, C., & Thernström Blomqvist, Y. (2014). First-time events between parents and preterm infants are affected by the designs and routines of neonatal intensive care units. *Acta Paediatrica (Oslo, Norway: 1992), 103*(10), 1045–1052. doi:10.1111/apa.12719

Colditz, P., Sanders, M. R., Boyd, R., Pritchard, M., Gray, P., O'Callaghan, M. J., . . . Jardine, L. (2015). Prem baby triple P: A randomised controlled trial of enhanced parenting capacity to improve developmental outcomes in preterm infants. *BMC Pediatrics*, 1515. doi:10.1186/s12887-015-0331-x

Poehlmann, J., Burnson, C., & Weymouth, L. A. (2014). Early parenting, represented family relationships, and externalizing behavior problems in children born preterm. *Attachment & Human Development, 16*(3), 271–291. doi:10.1080/14616734.2014.884610

INSUFFICIENT BREAST MILK

Definition

Low production of maternal breast milk

Assessment

- Maternal status, including age and maturity, parity, level of prenatal breast-feeding preparation, past breast-feeding experience, previous postpartum history, physical condition (actual or perceived inadequate milk supply and comfort level), and psychosocial factors (apprehension level, body image, stress from family and career, sociocultural views of breastfeeding, and emotional support from significant others)
- Neonatal status, including satisfaction and contentment, growth rate, age–weight relationship, urine output, quantity and characteristics of stools, and ability to latch onto breasts

Defining Characteristics

Infant

- Constipation
- Frequent crying
- Frequently seeks to suckle at breast
- Prolonged breast-feeding time
- Voids small amounts of concentrated urine
- Weight gain is <500 g in a month

Mother

- Absence of milk production with nipple stimulation
- Delay in milk production
- Expresses breast milk less than prescribed volume

Expected Outcomes

- Mother will produce sufficient milk to satisfy the growth needs of the neonate.
- Mother will *perceive* that she is producing sufficient milk for her baby.
- Mother and baby will achieve successful and sustained breast-feeding sessions.
- Mother will be free of emotions related to low self-esteem, poor body image, and guilt.

Suggested NOC Outcomes

Knowledge: Infant Care; Newborn Adaptation; Breastfeeding Establishment: Infant; Breastfeeding Establishment: Maternal; Nutritional Status: Nutrition Intake; Parent-Infant Attachment; Self-Esteem

Interventions and Rationales

- Position the mother/baby properly for baby to latch to nipple and suckle. *The couplet may need direction in assuming the best position of comfort for suckling.*
- Assess to see if the neonate is able to latch properly to the nipple to suckle. *Ensuring the baby has latched to the nipple instead of the areola aids in milk expression.*
- Evaluate whether there is adequate milk removal from each breast at each session. *Milk production is stimulated and increases by suckling and milk removal.*
- Do a physical examination of the breast every shift; check nipples for inversion and for pore openings, *as anatomic conditions will limit the ability of the milk to flow to the newborn.*
- Examine the breasts for engorgement, inflammation, infection, or pain. *These conditions cause discomfort and limit the tolerance of the mother to breast-feed; the mother must remain healthy to continue breast-feeding; inflammation and infection need to be treated.*
- Assess exhaustion level and the rest and sleep patterns of mother. *Exhaustion and inability to rejuvenate depresses milk production.*
- Assess the neonate's mouth to determine normal anatomy of tongue and palate; assess the neonate's mouth for Candida infection. *Anatomic imperfections and thrush infection affect the neonate's ability to suckle.*
- Assess the neonate's nose for patency to allow for breathing during suckling. *Neonates are nose breathers and must have patent nares in order to suckle.*
- Monitor the neonate's weight gain daily. *Sufficient nutrition from breast milk will allow weight gain.* Weigh the neonate before and after breast-feeding session. *When used, this can provide an indicator that the breast milk is sufficient.*
- Monitor the neonate's diaper for urine output (number per day, concentration of urine). *Urine output amount and color are indicators of hydration.* Check fluid–electrolyte status of neonate (urine characteristics and amount; stool output). *These measures guide the health care provider in determining the hydration status of the neonate.*
- Monitor the neonate for clinical presence of jaundice. *Breastfed neonates have lower rates of jaundice; if jaundice develops, it may be an indicator of insufficient milk intake.*
- Provide adequate nourishment and fluid intake to the mother (>150 mL/kg/day). *This is the minimum amount of fluid intake to sustain the mother and provide extra fluid for milk production.*
- Provide quiet uninterrupted time for breast- feeding. *Distractions and interruptions interfere with milk production, milk ejection, and the neonate's focus on suckling.*
- PCC Encourage the mother to talk about emotions, including frustration and disappointment. *Allowing others to help the mother through emotional barriers may assist in creating*

peaceful emotions that aid in milk production and milk let down. Listen carefully to the mother's concerns for clues to emotions and coping with disappointment and guilt; early signs of depression and stress. *Early intervention allows emotional healing and allows the mother to focus on the neonate and breast- feeding.*

- Provide rest and sleep intervals for the mother. *Rest and sleep rejuvenate the mother and promote milk production*
- Reduce nipple pain; ensure proper position as the neonate latches to the nipple; check for candidal infection—apply prescribed medication and nipple ointment; air-dry nipples. *Identifying and treating common conditions in the mother who is breast-feeding are important to sustain breast-feeding.*
- PCC Instruct the mother about the following:
  - Milk production may take a week before a sufficient amount is produced. *Understanding expectations improves confidence and reduces anxiety.*
  - Suckle the neonate at least eight times a day to stimulate milk production; goal is 8 to 12 times daily. *Understanding expectations improves confidence and reduces anxiety.*
  - Express milk or pump breasts regularly if the neonate is unable to suckle. *The breasts must be stimulated frequently to stimulate milk production.*
  - Provide the mother and family unit nutritional instructions for best foods and fluids for intake to support breast milk production. *Adequate and proper nutrition will aid the mother in recovery from labor and delivery and provide important nutrients to the neonate.*
  - Teach the mother techniques to keep the neonate awake during the feeding sessions. *The neonate often needs stimulation to remain awake at the breast to suckle sufficient milk.*
- Check with health care provider about substances and medications that can suppress milk production (i.e., caffeine, tobacco, nicotine, pseudoephedrine, diuretics, contraception pills). *To improve and sustain milk production, avoidance of substances that depress or limit milk production is important.*
- PCC Use a multidisciplinary team approach to support the mother for breast milk production—registered nurse, lactation specialist, certified nurse midwife, pediatrician, registered dietitian, social worker. *A team approach brings expertise to address the needs of the mother and promotes health and well-being for the family unit.*

Suggested NIC Interventions

Breastfeeding Assistance; Active Listening; Newborn Care; Parent Education: Infant; Teaching: Infant Nutrition; Lactation Counseling; Sleep Enhancement

Evaluations for Expected Outcomes

- Mother's production of breast milk becomes sufficient.
- Neonate experiences no loss of weight, jaundice, or dehydration.
- Mother expresses satisfaction with breast-feeding.
- Parents report improved ability to cope with stress of caring for infant.
- Mother–infant experience success in breast-feeding.

Documentation

- Assessment of factors that may enhance or retard breast-feeding
- Mother's expressions of satisfaction or problems with breast-feeding
- Nursing interventions and mother–infant's response to them
- Evaluations for expected outcomes

REFERENCES

Briere, C., Lucas, R., McGrath, J. M., Lussier, M., & Brownell, E. (2015). Establishing breast-feeding with the late preterm infant in the NICU. *Journal of Obstetric, Gynecologic & Neonatal Nursing, 44*(1), 102–113. doi:10.1111/1552-6909.12536

Munblit, D., Boyle, R. J., & Warner, J. O. (2015). Factors affecting breast milk composition and potential consequences for development of the allergic phenotype. *Clinical and Experimental Allergy, 45*(3), 583–601. doi:10.1111/cea.12381

Niannì, M. L., Roggero, P., Amato, O., Orsi, A., Garbarino, F., Garavaglia, E., . . . Mosca, F. (2014). Intervention for promoting breast milk use in neonatal intensive care unit: A pilot study. *The Journal of Maternal–Fetal & Neonatal Medicine, 27*(5), 475–478. doi:10.3109/14767058.2013.818971

Walker, T. C., Keene, S. D., & Patel, R. M. (2014). Early feeding factors associated with exclusive versus partial human milk feeding in neonates receiving intensive care. *Journal of Perinatology, 34*(8), 606–610. doi:10.1038/jp.2014.63

INEFFECTIVE BREAST-FEEDING

related to insufficient parental knowledge regarding breast-feeding techniques; maternal anxiety; poor infant sucking reflex

Definition

Difficulty providing milk to an infant or young child directly from the breasts, which may compromise nutritional status of the infant/child

Assessment

- Maternal status, including age and maturity, relationships with significant others, previous bonding history, parity, level of prenatal breast-feeding preparation, knowledge or previous breast-feeding experience, physical condition (actual or perceived inadequate milk supply, nipple shape, and comfort level), and psychosocial factors (apprehension level, body image and perceptions, stress from family and career, sociocultural views of breast-feeding, and emotional support from significant others)
- Neonatal status, including satisfaction and contentment, growth rate, and age–weight relationship

Defining Characteristics

- Inadequate infant stooling
- Infant arching at breast
- Infant crying at the breast
- Infant crying within the first hour after breast-feeding
- Infant fussing within 1 hour of breast-feeding
- Infant inability to latch on to maternal breast correctly
- Infant resisting latching on to breast
- Infant unresponsive to other comfort measures
- Insufficient emptying of each breast per feeding
- Insufficient infant weight gain
- Insufficient signs of oxytocin release
- Perceived inadequate milk supply
- Sore nipples persisting beyond first week
- Sustained infant weight loss
- Unsustained suckling at the breast

Expected Outcomes

- Mother will express physical and psychological comfort with breast-feeding techniques and practice.
- Mother will show decreased anxiety and apprehension.
- Neonate will feed successfully on both breasts and appear satisfied for at least 2 hours after feeding.
- Neonate will grow and thrive.
- Mother will state at least one resource for breast-feeding support.

Suggested NOC Outcomes

Breastfeeding Establishment: Infant; Breastfeeding Establishment: Maternal; Breastfeeding Maintenance; Fluid Balance; Hydration; Knowledge: Breastfeeding

Interventions and Rationales

- PCC Educate the mother in breast care and breast-feeding techniques. *This reduces anxiety and enhances proper nutrition of the neonate.*
- Be available, yet discreet, during breast-feeding. *Assessment of the mother's technique can reveal problem areas.* Encourage the mother to ask questions *to increase understanding and reduce anxiety.*
- PCC Teach techniques for encouraging the let down reflex, including:
  - warm shower
  - breast massage
  - physically caring for the neonate
  - holding the neonate close to the breasts.

  These measures reduce anxiety and promote the let down reflex.
- Provide the mother and infant with a quiet, private, comfortable environment with decreased external stressors *to promote successful breast-feeding.*
- PCC Encourage the expression of fears and anxieties between the mother and significant other *to reduce anxiety and increase the mother's sense of control.*
- Offer information about the importance of adequate nutrition and fluid intake while breast-feeding *in order to meet the infant's demand for breast milk.*
- Offer written information, a reading list, or information about breast-feeding support groups *to help meet the mother's emotional and learning needs.*

Suggested NIC Interventions

Breastfeeding Assistance; Emotional Support; Lactation Counseling; Nutrition Management; Parent Education: Infant; Support Group

Evaluations for Expected Outcomes

- Mother expresses physical and psychological comfort with breast-feeding techniques and practice.
- Mother displays decreased anxiety and apprehension.
- Neonate feeds successfully on both breasts and appears satisfied for at least 2 hours after feeding.
- Neonate grows and thrives.
- Mother states at least one available resource for breast-feeding support.

Documentation

- Mother's expressions of comfort with breast-feeding ability
- Observations of bonding and breast-feeding process
- Teaching and instructions given
- Referrals to support groups
- Neonate growth and weight
- Evaluations for expected outcomes

REFERENCES

The Association of Women's Health, Obstetric, and Neonatal Nurses. (2015). Breast-feeding. *Journal of Obstetric, Gynecologic, & Neonatal Nursing*, 44, 145–150.

Cordero, L., Thung, S., Landon, M. B., & Nankervis, C. A. (2014). Breast-feeding initiation in women with pregestational diabetes mellitus. *Clinical Pediatrics, 53*(1), 18–25. doi:10.1177/0009922813496455

Otsuka, K., Taguri, M., Dennis, C., Wakutani, K., Awano, M., Yamaguchi, T., & Jimba, M. (2014). Effectiveness of a breast-feeding self-efficacy intervention: Do hospital practices make a difference? *Maternal and Child Health Journal, 18*(1), 296–306. doi:10.1007/s10995-013-1265-2

Ozlüses, E., & Celebioglu, A. (2014). Educating fathers to improve breast-feeding rates and paternal–infant attachment. *Indian Pediatrics, 51*(8), 654–657.

INTERRUPTED BREAST-FEEDING

related to contraindications to breast-feeding (e.g., pharmaceutical agents); maternal–infant separation

Definition

Break in the continuity of providing milk to an infant or young child directly from the breasts, which may compromise breastfeeding success and/or nutritional status of the infant/child.

Assessment

- Maternal status, including age and maturity, employment hours, relationship with significant other, parity, level of prenatal breast-feeding knowledge or experience, and physical condition (comfort level, nipple shape, presence of infection, and use of medication)
- Neonatal status, including age–weight relationship, growth rate, neurologic status, respiratory status, suck reflex, and factors that interfere with proper sucking (such as cleft lip or palate)

Defining Characteristics

- Nonexclusive breast-feeding

Expected Outcomes

- Mother will express her understanding of factors that necessitate interruption in breast-feeding.
- Mother will express comfort with her decision about whether to resume breast-feeding.
- Mother will express and store breast milk appropriately.
- Mother will resume breast-feeding when interfering factors cease.
- Mother will have adequate milk supply when breast-feeding resumes.

- Mother will obtain relief from discomfort associated with engorgement.
- Infant's nutritional needs will be met.

Suggested NOC Outcomes

Breastfeeding Maintenance; Knowledge: Breastfeeding; Motivation; Parent–Infant Attachment; Parenting Performance; Role Performance

Interventions and Rationales

- Assess the mother's understanding of reasons for interrupting breast-feeding *to evaluate the need for additional instruction.*
- Reassure the mother that the neonate's nutritional needs will be met through other methods *to allay her anxiety.*
- Assess the mother's desire to resume breast-feeding *to help plan interventions.*
- PCC Provide appropriate educational materials, including audiovisual aids and written materials. *Audiovisual aids demonstrate proper expressing and storing techniques; written material allows the mother to review information at her own pace.*
- PCC Instruct the mother in techniques for expressing and storing breast milk *to ensure adequate milk supply.*
- Recommend the use of a breast pump according to the following guidelines *to provide maximum stimulation and prolactin production*:
  - Initiate pumping 24 to 48 hours after delivery.
  - Pump a minimum of five times a day.
  - Pump a minimum of 100 minutes/day.
  - Pump long enough to soften the breasts each time, regardless of duration.
- Encourage the mother to save her breast milk in a sterile container and store it in the refrigerator or freezer for future feedings. *Preserving breast milk ensures that the neonate receives maternal antibodies and helps to encourage maternal involvement in neonatal care.*
- If the mother must pump for a prolonged period, encourage her to use a piston-style electric pump. *Using an electric pump rather than a hand pump produces milk with a higher fat content.*
- PCC If the mother intends to resume breast-feeding, instruct her in ways to relieve breast engorgement *to prevent discomfort that may keep the neonate from sucking effectively.*
- If appropriate, instruct the mother in the use of devices such as a nipple shield, *which is designed to alter flat or inverted nipples, a condition that may interfere with successful breast-feeding.*
- Review the mother's daily routine *to advise her how to incorporate breast-feeding into her schedule.*
- PCC Provide the mother with information about breast-feeding support groups. *A support group can help the mother obtain needed emotional support and continue learning.*
- If the mother doesn't intend to resume breast-feeding, advise her to wear a supportive bra, apply ice, and take a mild analgesic, such as acetaminophen, *to alleviate discomfort associated with engorgement.*

Suggested NIC Interventions

Attachment Promotion; Bottle-Feeding; Emotional Support; Lactation Counseling; Parent Education: Infant; Teaching: Individual

Evaluations for Expected Outcomes

- Mother describes factors that necessitate interruption in breast-feeding.
- Mother expresses comfort with her decision about whether to resume breast-feeding.
- Mother demonstrates proper milk expression and storage techniques.
- Mother resumes breast-feeding when interrupting factors are eliminated.
- Mother has adequate milk supply when breast-feeding resumes.
- Mother obtains relief from discomfort associated with engorgement.
- Infant's nutritional needs are met, as evidenced by appropriate weight gain (e.g., 1 oz [28.3 g]/day for first 6 months of life).

Documentation

- Factors that necessitated interruption in breast-feeding (reassessed periodically to determine status)
- Mother's expression of feelings about the need to interrupt breast-feeding
- Mother's decision whether to continue breast-feeding when possible
- Mother's efforts to ensure adequate milk supply
- Mother's responses to nursing interventions
- Neonate's growth, weight, and output
- Referrals to support groups
- Evaluations for expected outcomes

REFERENCES

The Association of Women's Health, Obstetric, and Neonatal Nurses. (2015). Breast-feeding. *Journal of Obstetric, Gynecologic, & Neonatal Nursing*, 44, 145–150.

Jenkins, J. M., & Foster, E. M. (2014). The effects of breast-feeding exclusivity on early childhood outcomes. *American Journal of Public Health, 104*(Suppl 1), S128–S135. doi:10.2105/AJPH.2013.301713

Ozlüses, E., & Celebioglu, A. (2014). Educating fathers to improve breast-feeding rates and paternal–infant attachment. *Indian Pediatrics, 51*(8), 654–657.

Tang, L., Lee, A. H., & Binns, C. W. (2015). Predictors of early introduction of complementary feeding: longitudinal study. *Pediatrics International, 57*(1), 126–130. doi:10.1111/ped.12421

READINESS FOR ENHANCED BREAST-FEEDING

Definition

A pattern of providing milk to an infant or young child directly from the breasts, which may be strengthened

Assessment

- Maternal status, including age and maturity, parity, level of prenatal breast-feeding preparation, past breast-feeding experience, previous postpartum history, physical condition (actual or perceived inadequate milk supply and comfort level), and psychosocial factors (apprehension level, body image, stress from family and career, sociocultural views of breast-feeding, and emotional support from significant others)
- Neonatal status, including satisfaction and contentment, growth rate, age–weight relationship, urine output, quantity and characteristics of stools, and ability to latch onto breasts

Defining Characteristics

- Mother expresses desire to enhance ability to provide breast milk for child's nutritional needs
- Mother expresses desire to enhance ability to exclusively breast-feed

Expected Outcomes

- Mother will breast-feed neonate successfully and will experience satisfaction with breast-feeding process.
- Neonate will feed successfully on both breasts and appear satisfied.
- Neonate will grow and develop in pace with accepted standards.
- Mother will continue breast-feeding neonate after early postpartum period.

Suggested NOC Outcomes

Breastfeeding Establishment: Infant; Breastfeeding Establishment: Maternal; Breastfeeding Maintenance; Breastfeeding Weaning; Hydration; Knowledge: Breastfeeding

Interventions and Rationales

- Assess the mother's knowledge and experience of breast-feeding *to focus teaching on specific learning needs.*
- PCC Educate the mother and selected support person about breast-feeding techniques:
  - Clean hands and breasts before nursing.
  - Position the neonate for feeding (the neonate should be able to grasp most of the areola).
  - Change positions to decrease nipple tenderness and use both breasts at each feeding.
  - Remove the neonate from the breast by breaking suction; avoiding setting time limits in the early stage.

  Greater understanding of techniques improves chances for success.
- PCC Teach the mother how to use warm showers and compresses, relaxation and guided imagery, infant suckling, holding the infant close to breasts, and listening to the infant cry *to stimulate letdown.*
- PCC Educate the mother about nutritional needs. She requires a well-balanced diet plus an additional 500 calories and two extra glasses of fluid each day *to maintain an adequate milk supply.* She should limit caffeine and avoid foods that make her uncomfortable.
- PCC Teach the mother what to expect from a breast-feeding neonate *to prepare the mother for care of the neonate at home.* The neonate should pass one to six stools and wet six to eight diapers per day. Stools should be soft to liquid and nonodorous. The neonate should feed every 2 to 3 hours, or as needed, and appear content and satisfied after feeding. Explain that the neonate also requires nonnutritive sucking.
- Assist the mother and family in planning for home care. The mother needs to rest when the neonate sleeps, practice self-care, learn techniques for expressing and storing breast milk, and recognize signs of engorgement and infection. Family members should understand the importance of helping and supporting the mother in her desire to breast-feed. *A mother who stops breast-feeding after she returns home and resumes work usually does so because of fatigue.*
- Provide quiet environment and privacy *to enhance development of breast-feeding skills.*
- PCC Encourage mother to express concerns about breast-feeding *to reduce anxiety.*
- PCC Offer mother information about breast-feeding support groups *to help meet emotional and learning needs.*

Suggested NIC Interventions

Breastfeeding Assistance; Family Support; Lactation Counseling; Nutrition Management; Parent Education: Infant

Evaluations for Expected Outcomes

- Mother breast-feeds neonate successfully and expresses satisfaction with breast-feeding.
- Neonate feeds on both breasts and appears satisfied.
- Neonate's weight and length remain consistent and within 10th and 19th percentiles on pediatric growth grid.
- Mother continues to breast-feed infant after discharge from hospital.

Documentation

- Mother's expressions about breast-feeding experience
- Observations of breast-feeding techniques and mother–infant interaction during breast-feeding
- Teaching and instructions given
- Neonate's growth and weight
- Referrals to support groups
- Mother's plans for breast-feeding after discharge
- Evaluations for expected outcomes

REFERENCES

Brown, C. L., Dodds, L., Legge, A., Bryanton, J., & Semenic, S. (2014). Factors influencing the reasons why mothers stop breastfeeding. *Canadian Journal of Public Health, 105*(3), e179–e185.

Fugate, K., Hernandez, I., Ashmeade, T., Miladinovic, B., & Spatz, D. L. (2015). Improving human milk and breastfeeding practices in the NICU. *Journal of Obstetric, Gynecologic & Neonatal Nursing, 44*(3), 426–438. doi:10.1111/1552-6909.12563

Lopes, T. P., Moura, L. D., & Lima, M. P. (2014). Breastfeeding and sucking habits in children enrolled in a mother–child health program. *BMC Research Notes, 7*, 362. doi:10.1186/1756-0500-7-362

Moss, B. G., & Yeaton, W. H. (2014). Early childhood healthy and obese weight status: Potentially protective benefits of breastfeeding and delaying solid foods. *Maternal and Child Health Journal, 18*(5), 1224–1232. doi:10.1007/s10995-013-1357-z

INEFFECTIVE BREATHING PATTERN

related to neurologic immaturity

Definition

Inspiration and/or expiration that does not provide adequate ventilation

Assessment

- Gestational age
- Weight in relation to gestational age
- Maternal sedation before delivery
- Preexisting conditions, including anomalies, adverse intrauterine environment, and prematurity

- Health assessment, including laboratory studies and neurologic, cardiovascular, respiratory, integumentary, Gastrointestinal, and fluid and electrolyte status

Defining Characteristics

- Abnormal breathing pattern (e.g., rate, rhythm, depth)
- Altered chest excursion
- Bradypnea
- Decrease in expiratory pressure
- Decrease in inspiratory pressure
- Decrease in minute ventilation
- Decrease in vital capacity
- Dyspnea
- Increase in anterior–posterior chest diameter
- Nasal flaring
- Orthopnea
- Prolonged expiration phase
- Pursed-lip breathing
- Tachypnea
- Use of accessory muscles to breathe
- Use of three- point position

Expected Outcomes

- Neonate will establish normal respiratory rate (40 to 60 breaths/minute) within 1 hour of birth.
- Neonate will have no signs of respiratory distress 1 hour after birth.
- Neonate won't require assisted ventilation or supplemental oxygen.
- Neonate will have Apgar score of 8 to 10 at 5 minutes after birth.
- Neonate will make successful transition to extrauterine life with adequate respiratory function.

Suggested NOC Outcomes

Respiratory Status: Airway Patency; Respiratory Status: Ventilation; Vital Signs

Interventions and Rationales

- Immediately after delivery:
  - Vigorously dry the neonate and place him under a radiant warmer.
  - Suction the oropharynx and nasopharynx, as needed, with a bulb syringe, DeLee catheter, or suction catheter connected to wall suction.
  - Obtain 1-minute and 5-minute Apgar scores.
  - Provide whiffs of oxygen, if indicated.
  - Remove wet blankets and replace them with dry ones.
  - Observe for signs of respiratory distress (nasal flaring, tachypnea, retractions, grunting, and use of accessory muscles for breathing).
  - S Provide or assist with resuscitative measures, as indicated, including bag and mask; naloxone (Narcan) administration, as ordered, if respiratory distress is secondary to maternal sedation; intubation; and suctioning below the vocal cords under direct visualization. *Respiratory difficulties are responsible for most morbidity and mortality during the neonatal period. Accurate assessment and prompt intervention at delivery are critical to sustaining life.*
- Transfer the neonate to the nursery when stable or if the neonate needs more extensive resuscitation measures *to help improve transition to extrauterine life.*
- On admission to the nursery:
  - Obtain the neonate's vital signs. Observe central and peripheral color. Note signs of respiratory distress.

- Perform a physical assessment, noting anomalies or other abnormal findings.
- Maintain a neutral thermal environment.
- Obtain a brief obstetric history, including the course of labor and delivery and condition of the neonate before his arrival in the nursery. Note the presence of risk factors.
- Obtain laboratory studies, as ordered.
- Provide resuscitative measures, if needed.
- Continue monitoring vital signs until stable, then routinely or as ordered.

Obtaining baseline data and identifying risk factors will help direct interventions.

- Perform chest physiotherapy, as indicated, *to clear the lungs of fluid.*
- Continually assess the need to repeat suctioning to maintain a patent airway. *Repeated pharyngeal suctioning can prevent aspiration caused by the neonate's immature glottal reflex.*

Suggested NIC Interventions

Airway Management; Aspiration Precautions; Respiratory Monitoring; Ventilation Assistance

Evaluations for Expected Outcomes

- Neonate establishes respiratory rate of 40 to 60 breaths/minute within 1 hour of birth.
- Neonate has no signs of respiratory distress 1 hour after birth.
- Neonate doesn't require assisted ventilation or supplemental oxygen.
- Neonate has Apgar score of 8 to 10 at 5 minutes after birth.
- Neonate makes successful transition to extrauterine life with adequate respiratory function.

Documentation

- Vital signs
- Physical findings
- Interventions performed to enhance neonate's ability to breathe effectively
- Neonate's responses to nursing interventions
- Evaluations for expected outcomes

REFERENCES

Branson, R. D., Gomaa, D., & Rodriquez, D., Jr. (2014). Management of the artificial airway. *Respiratory Care, 59*(6), 974–990. doi:10.4187/respcare.03246

El-Radhi, A. S. (2015). Management of common neonatal problems. *British Journal of Nursing, 24*(5), 258–265. doi:10.12968/bjon.2015.24.5.258

Ivanov, V. A. (2016). Reduction of endotracheal tube connector dead space improves ventilation: A bench test on a model lung simulating an extremely low birth weight neonate. *Respiratory Care, 61*(2), 155–161. doi:10.4187/respcare.04076

INEFFECTIVE CHILDBEARING PROCESS

Definition

Pregnancy and childbirth process and care of the newborn that does not match the environmental context, norms, and expectations

Assessment

- Age of patient and partner
- Availability of family members or friends to help
- Planned or unplanned pregnancy
- Family status, including number and ages of other children, usual patterns of interaction among family members, family members' assumed or expected roles, communication patterns, support systems, financial resources, past responses to change, spiritual resources, and living conditions
- Perceived impact of pregnancy on the family unit
- Psychosocial status, including developmental stage, previous experience with childbearing, expectations of the birth process, interest in learning, and current level of knowledge about pregnancy, birth, and recovery
- Ability to learn, including cognitive domain, intellectual and conceptual skills, and attention span
- Support systems, including presence of support person and support person's interest in helping patient and ability to participate in doing so

Defining Characteristics

During Pregnancy

- Inadequate prenatal care
- Inadequate prenatal lifestyle (e.g., elimination, exercise, nutrition, personal hygiene, sleep)
- Inadequate preparation of newborn care items
- Inadequate preparation of the home environment
- Ineffective management of unpleasant symptoms in pregnancy
- Insufficient access of support system
- Insufficient respect for unborn baby
- Unrealistic birth plan

During Labor and Delivery

- Decrease in proactivity during labor and delivery
- Inadequate lifestyle for stage of labor (e.g., elimination, exercise, nutrition, personal hygiene, sleep)
- Inappropriate response to onset of labor
- Insufficient access of support system
- Insufficient attachment behavior

After Birth

- Inadequate baby care techniques
- Inadequate postpartum lifestyle (e.g., elimination, exercise, nutrition, personal hygiene, sleep)
- Inappropriate baby feeding techniques
- Inappropriate breast care
- Insufficient access of support system
- Insufficient attachment behavior
- Unsafe environment for an infant

Expected Outcomes

- Mother will demonstrate a willingness to improve her lifestyle and adhere to medical recommendations for optimal prenatal health.
- Mother will seek and convey confidence in knowledge about pregnancy, the labor delivery process, and newborn care.
- Mother will cooperate and follow the care directives of the health care team during labor and delivery and the postpartum period.
- Mother will demonstrate coping and emotional strength to adapt to emergent situations during the prenatal, intrapartal, postpartal, and newborn care periods
- Mother will exhibit maternal interest, attachment, and bonding with the newborn
- Mother will perform skills for self-care and newborn care, including breast-feeding skills

- Mother will seek to meet positive self-care needs and to meet the newborn's physical, social, nutritional, and safety needs.

Suggested NOC Outcomes

Fetal Status: Antepartum; Fetal Status: Intrapartum; Newborn Adaptation; Breastfeeding Establishment: Infant; Breastfeeding Establishment: Maternal; Parent-Infant Attachment; Role Performance; Prenatal Health Behavior; Knowledge: Breastfeeding; Knowledge: Infant Care; Knowledge: Labor and Delivery; Maternal Status: Antepartum; Maternal Status: Intrapartum; Maternal Status: Postpartum

Interventions and Rationales

- Assess baseline knowledge of prenatal self-care, labor and delivery process, and newborn care *to identify and resolve knowledge deficits.*
- Assess physical and psychological states of the mother during pregnancy *in order to treat medical conditions and develop a patient-centered plan to address needs and deficits.*
- Monitor physiologic vital signs and parameters at each phase of childbearing, *as these aid the clinicians in determining courses of action in response to evolving pathophysiologic needs.*
- Monitor the emotional baseline of the mother/family unit *to identify strengths needed to cope with unknown, rapidly changing conditions.*
- Anticipate needs and provide for opportunities for the mother to reach out for assistance and knowledge for her self-care and expectations of labor and delivery and newborn care. *The mother's engagement in the processes demonstrates interest and initiates autonomy.*
- PCC Teach the mother self-care for common prenatal discomforts *to promote patient comfort and autonomy.*
- PCC Teach the mother about the pregnancy process and the labor and delivery. *Understanding expectations improves confidence, reduces anxiety, and aids in creating a trusting relationship.*
- Demonstrate comfort techniques that aid in labor management and delivery. *As the individual is free from discomfort, she can be more accepting of instruction and assist in the labor–delivery processes.*
- PCC Include the mother in planning for changes in the treatment plan during labor and delivery to *indicate respect, reduce anxiety and fear of the unknown.*
- Provide accurate information to the mother/family unit during crisis/emergent situations. *This aids in anxiety reduction, trust establishment, and the family unit's ability to cooperate with the treatment team for the safety of mother and fetus/newborn.*
- Demonstrate techniques that match the mother's abilities to care for the newborn while the newborn is undergoing therapeutic care. *Demonstrate respect and individualization of the plan of care for the mother to meet the physical and emotional needs of the newborn.*
- Provide supportive environment during prenatal, intrapartum, and postpartum periods; *when the mother feels comfortable and cared for, she can focus on self-care, healing, and care of newborn undergoing intensive care management.*
- Provide bonding time between the newborn and mother/family unit; skin-to-skin cuddling; and encourage breast-feeding at delivery *to enhance critical bond development between mother/family unit and newborn.*

- Support the mother/family unit in the recovery and healing process for the mother and the neonate following unplanned, emergent stressful events. *Allowing the mother/family unit to verbalize and explore feelings and emotions aids in the integration process of healing.*
- Arrange for transportation to provider for clinic visit. *Nonadherence to prenatal and postpartum visits may be related to transportation issues.*
- Provide antenatal and postnatal classes on self-care and care of the newborn by a certified childbirth educator. *Advanced knowledge of the childbearing process promotes empowerment and positive maternal outcomes.*
- PCC Coordinate multidisciplinary team—registered nurse, nurse midwife, physician, lactation consultant, registered dietitian, and social worker. *These professionals assess and uniquely meet the needs of the mother and newborn when there have been events that interfered with the childbearing process.*
- PCC Assist the family unit to develop the support system/network if management of medical and neonatal conditions warrants extended hospitalization. *Anticipatory guidance in seeking resources and assistance will aid the family to cope and provide autonomy in supporting the family as it supports its members in the hospital.*

Suggested NIC Interventions

Role Enhancement; Parent Education: Infant; Teaching: Infant Safety; Birthing; Infant Care; Family Involvement Promotion; Coping Enhancement

Evaluations for Expected Outcomes

- Mother expresses knowledge of prenatal, labor and delivery, and postnatal processes.
- Mother incorporates suggestions provided.
- Mother/infant bond is established.
- Parents express increased confidence in their ability to perform appropriate feeding techniques.
- Mother demonstrates correct breast-feeding techniques.
- Mother provides adequate care for self and newborn.
- Mother and infant's needs are met.

Documentation

- Results of assessment
- Instructions given to mother
- Neonate's daily weight
- Parents' knowledge of feeding techniques, involvement with caregiving, and bonding with neonate
- Parents' and neonate's responses to nursing interventions
- Evaluations for expected outcomes

REFERENCES

Noseff, J. (2014). Theory usage and application paper: Maternal role attainment. *International Journal of Childbirth Education, 29*(3), 58–61.

Ordway, M. R., Sadler, L. S., Dixon, J., & Slade, A. (2014). Parental reflective functioning: Analysis and promotion of the concept for paediatric nursing. *Journal of Clinical Nursing, 23*(23/24), 3490–3500. doi:10.1111/jocn.12600

Pei-Jung, L., Jen-Jiuan, L., & Chin-Mi, C. (2015). Concept analysis of postpartum depression. *Journal of Nursing, 62*(3), 66–71. doi:10.6224/JN.62.3.66

RISK FOR INEFFECTIVE CHILDBEARING PROCESS

Definition

Vulnerable to not matching environmental context, norms, and expectations of pregnancy, childbirth process, and the care of the newborn

Assessment

- Age of patient and partner
- Planned or unplanned pregnancy
- Family status, including number and ages of other children, usual patterns of interaction among family members, family members' assumed or expected roles, communication patterns, support systems, financial resources, past responses to change, spiritual resources, and living conditions
- Perceived impact of pregnancy on the family unit
- Psychosocial status, including developmental stage, previous experience with childbearing, expectations of the birth process, interest in learning, and current level of knowledge about pregnancy, birth, and recovery
- Ability to learn, including cognitive domain, intellectual and conceptual skills, and attention span
- Support systems, including presence of support person and support person's interest in helping patient and ability to participate in doing so

Risk Factors

- Domestic violence
- Inconsistent prenatal health visits
- Insufficient cognitive readiness for parenting
- Insufficient knowledge of childbearing process
- Inadequate maternal nutrition
- Insufficient parental role model
- Insufficient prenatal care
- Insufficient support system
- Low maternal confidence
- Maternal powerlessness
- Maternal psychological distress
- Substance abuse
- Unplanned pregnancy
- Unrealistic birth plan
- Unwanted pregnancy

Expected Outcomes

- Patient demonstrates a willingness to improve her lifestyle for optimal prenatal health.
- Patient seeks and conveys confidence in knowledge about pregnancy, the labor delivery process, and newborn care.
- Patient cooperates and follows the care directives of the health care team during labor and delivery and the postpartum period.
- Patient exhibits maternal interest, attachment, and bonding with the newborn
- Patient performs skills for self-care and newborn care
- Patient seeks to meet positive self-care needs and to meet the newborn's physical, social, nutritional, and safety needs.

Suggested NOC Outcomes

Fetal Status: Antepartum; Fetal Status: Intrapartum; Newborn Adaptation; Breastfeeding Establishment: Infant; Breastfeeding Establishment: Maternal; Parent-Infant Attachment; Role Performance; Prenatal Health Behavior; Knowledge: Breastfeeding; Knowledge: Infant Care; Knowledge: Labor and Delivery; Maternal Status: Antepartum; Maternal Status: Intrapartum; Maternal Status: Postpartum

Interventions and Rationales

- Assess baseline knowledge of prenatal self-care, labor and delivery process, and newborn care *to identify and resolve knowledge deficits.*
- Assess physical and psychological states of the mother during pregnancy *in order to treat medical conditions and develop plan to address deficits.*
- Analyze cultural beliefs contributing to mother's behavior *since understanding by the health care team can aid in determining a plan of approach and treatment that is patient-centered.*
- Convey a nonjudgmental attitude *to allow a trusting relationship to develop.*
- Anticipate needs and provide for opportunities for the mother to reach out for assistance and knowledge for her self-care and expectations of labor and delivery and newborn care. *Mother's engagement in the processes demonstrates interest and initiates autonomy.*
- Monitor intrapartal parameters according to accepted standard of practice *to maintain physiologic needs and respond to evolving pathophysiologic needs.*
- Implement treatment plan prenatally or intrapartum to alleviate medical conditions *to enhance the physiologic condition of the mother.*
- PCC Teach the mother self-care for common prenatal discomforts *to promote patient autonomy.*
- PCC Teach the mother about the pregnancy process and the labor and delivery. *Understanding expectations improves confidence, reduces anxiety, and aids in creating a trusting relationship.*
- Demonstrate comfort techniques that aid in labor management and delivery. *As the individual is free from discomfort, she can be more accepting of instruction and assist in the labor–delivery processes.*
- PCC Include the mother in planning for changes in treatment plan during labor and delivery *to indicate respect and reduce anxiety and fear of the unknown.*
- Demonstrate techniques that match the mother's abilities to care for the newborn. *Demonstrate respect and individualization of the plan of care for the mother.*
- Provide supportive environment during prenatal, intrapartum, and postpartum periods. *When the mother feels comfortable and cared for, she can focus on self-care and care of newborn*
- Provide bonding time between newborn and mother; skin-to-skin cuddling; and encourage breastfeeding at delivery. *These and other actions enhance critical bond development between mother and newborn.*
- PCC Provide antenatal and postnatal classes on self-care and care of the newborn by a certified childbirth educator. *Advanced knowledge of the childbearing process promotes empowerment and positive maternal outcomes.*
- PCC Coordinate multidisciplinary team—registered nurse, nurse midwife, physician, lactation consultant, registered dietitian, and social worker. *These professionals assess and uniquely meet the needs of the mother and newborn.*

Suggested NIC Interventions

Role Enhancement; Parent Education: Infant; Teaching: Infant Safety; Birthing; Infant Care; Family Involvement Promotion; Coping Enhancement

Evaluations for Expected Outcomes

- Mother expresses knowledge of prenatal, labor and delivery, and postnatal processes.
- Mother incorporates suggestions provided.
- Mother–infant bond is established.
- Parents express increased confidence in their ability to perform appropriate feeding techniques.
- Mother demonstrates correct breast-feeding techniques.
- Mother provides adequate care for self and newborn.
- Mother and infant's needs are met.

Documentation

- Results of assessment
- Instructions given to mother
- Neonate's daily weight
- Parents' knowledge of feeding techniques, involvement with caregiving, and bonding with neonate
- Parents' and neonate's responses to nursing interventions
- Evaluations for expected outcomes

REFERENCES

Biro, M. A., Yelland, J. S., & Brown, S. J. (2014). Why are young women less likely to breast-feed? Evidence from an Australian population-based survey. *Birth: Issues in Perinatal Care, 41*(3), 245–253. doi:10.1111/birt.12112

Karlsdottir, S. I., Halldorsdottir, S., & Lundgren, I. (2014). The third paradigm in labour pain preparation and management: the childbearing woman's paradigm. *Scandinavian Journal of Caring Sciences, 28*(2), 315–327. doi:10.1111/scs.12061

Metcalfe, A., Vekved, M., & Tough, S. (2014). Educational attainment, perception of workplace support and its influence on timing of childbearing for Canadian women: A cross-sectional study. *Maternal & Child Health Journal, 18*(7), 1675–1682. doi:10.1007/s10995-013-1409-4

INEFFECTIVE COPING

related to inadequate opportunity to prepare for stressor; situation crisis

Definition

Inability to form a valid appraisal of the stressors, inadequate choices of practiced responses, and/or inability to use available resources

Assessment

- Psychosocial status, including age, developmental stage, health beliefs, and attitudes, feelings about pregnancy, decision-making ability, usual coping patterns, support systems, income, ability to learn (cognitive, affective, and psychomotor domains), motivation to learn, and obstacles to learning

- Neurologic status, including level of consciousness, orientation, memory, and mental status
- Pain threshold, perception of pain, and response to analgesia or anesthesia
- Labor, including stage and length of labor, complications, patient's ability to concentrate, patient's ability to use breathing techniques, and presence and effectiveness of support person
- Circumstances surrounding delivery, including method of delivery (vaginal [complicated or uncomplicated], cesarean [elective or nonelective], or vaginal birth after previous cesarean delivery), analgesia or anesthesia, presence and effectiveness of support person, and outcome (actual and perceived)
- Previous experience with pregnancy, labor, and delivery and knowledge of birth process
- Medical history, including preexisting and pregnancy-induced conditions

Defining Characteristics

- Alteration in concentration
- Alteration in sleep pattern
- Change in communication pattern
- Destructive behavior toward others
- Destructive behavior toward self
- Difficulty organizing information
- Fatigue
- Frequent illness
- Inability to ask for help
- Inability to attend to information
- Inability to deal with a situation
- Inability to meet basic needs
- Inability to meet role expectation
- Ineffective coping strategies
- Insufficient access of social support
- Insufficient goal-directed behavior
- Insufficient problem resolution
- Insufficient problem-solving skills
- Risk-taking behavior
- Substance abuse

Expected Outcomes

- Patient will express need to develop better coping behaviors.
- Patient will set realistic learning goals.
- Patient will demonstrate ability to use newly learned coping skills.
- Patient will communicate feelings about pregnancy, labor, and delivery.
- Patient will maintain appropriate sense of control throughout course of labor and delivery.
- Patient will enlist help from support person and nurses to obtain physical and psychological comfort.
- Patient will demonstrate ability to cope with unexpected change.

Suggested NOC Outcomes

Anxiety Self-Control; Coping; Decision-Making; Information Processing; Role Performance; Social Interaction Skills; Social Support

Interventions and Rationales

- Establish an environment of mutual trust and respect *to enhance the patient's learning.*
- Negotiate with the patient to develop learning goals *to promote cooperation and foster a sense of control.*
- PCC Select teaching strategies (discussion, demonstration, role playing, and visual materials) appropriate for the patient's learning style *to encourage compliance.*

PCC
- Teach skills that the patient can use during labor and delivery. Have her give a return demonstration of each new skill. *The patient must thoroughly understand these skills before labor begins because painful contractions will reduce her attention span.*
- During the first (latent) phase of labor (dilation 1 to 4 cm), take these steps:
  - PCC Encourage the patient to ventilate her feelings and to participate in her own care. Offer diversions such as reading materials. Review breathing techniques she can use during labor. *These measures help allay the patient's fears and help her achieve a sense of control.*
  - PCC Involve the support person in care and comfort measures *to allay the patient's fears.*
  - Provide continuous monitoring *to identify deviations from normal.*
- During the active phase of labor (dilation 4 to 8 cm), take these steps:
  - Encourage the patient to assume a comfortable position *to promote relaxation between contractions.*
  - Assist the patient with breathing techniques *to reduce anxiety and prevent hyperventilation.*
  - PCC Encourage the support person to participate in patient care and comfort. Allow involvement to the extent that is comfortable to both the woman and the support person (e.g., give back rub, provide ice chips, assist with walking) *to provide continuity of care and encourage a therapeutic relationship.*
  - PCC Provide encouragement and instruction between contractions *to foster a sense of control.*
  - Administer analgesia, as ordered, *to reduce pain.*
  - Provide opportunities for rest between contractions, when appropriate. Reassure the patient about fetal status. *These measures reinforce the patient's ability to cope.*
- During the transitional phase of labor (dilation 8 to 10 cm), take these steps:
  - Assist the patient with breathing during contractions. Advise her not to push until complete dilation occurs.
  - Encourage rest between contractions.
  - Identify and reduce unnecessary stimuli in the environment.
  - Explain all treatments and procedures and answer the patient's questions.

  These measures help allay fear and reduce sensory overload.
- During delivery, provide these measures:
  - PCC Instruct the patient in effective pushing techniques *to promote the effectiveness of her bearing-down efforts.*
  - Continue to reassure the patient and provide encouragement. Explain the physiologic changes and procedures being performed *to prepare the patient psychologically for delivery.*
  - Escort the support person to the delivery room. Explain each step of the process. Instruct the support person in how to effectively coach the patient *to provide further support for the patient and strengthen her ability to cope.*
- During delivery of the placenta, take these steps:
  - Enlist the patient's cooperation in maintaining her position *to facilitate delivery of the placenta.*
  - Show the neonate to the patient and explain the care being provided. Reassure the patient about the neonate's condition *to provide emotional support.*
  - If permitted, allow the patient and support person to hold the neonate. If the patient desires, allow her to breast-feed the neonate *to promote bonding.*
- In a cesarean delivery, allow the patient to express her feelings. Explain the procedure and care being provided. Allow the support person to be present before and during delivery, if permitted. *Failure to provide the patient with a source of support and opportunity to express negative feelings may interfere with her ability to cope with the impending tasks of motherhood.*

Suggested NIC Interventions

Anticipatory Guidance; Anxiety Reduction; Calming Technique; Coping Enhancement; Decision-Making Support; Emotional Support; Patient Contracting

Evaluations for Expected Outcomes

- Patient states need for better coping behaviors.
- Patient participates in establishing learning goals.
- Patient successfully uses breathing and relaxation techniques during labor and delivery.
- Patient becomes more comfortable with expressing feelings about pregnancy, labor, and delivery.
- Patient maintains appropriate sense of control during labor and delivery.
- Support person and nurses provide effective comfort to patient during labor and delivery.
- Patient demonstrates ability to cope with unexpected change.

Documentation

- Patient's previous knowledge of labor and delivery
- Patient's expressions indicating her motivation to learn
- Patient's learning objectives
- Methods used to teach patient
- Information taught and skills demonstrated to patient
- Patient's response to nursing interventions
- Patient's and support person's level of satisfaction with delivery
- Patient's expressions of comfort, discomfort, or both
- Evaluations for expected outcomes

REFERENCES

Drayton, V., Walker, D., & Mikolowsky, K. (2015). Indicators of successful implementation of programs to promote healthy weight among women. *Maternal & Child Health Journal, 19*(3), 429–437. doi:10.1007/s10995-014-1538-4

Mood and anxiety disorders in pregnant and postpartum women. (2015). *Journal of Obstetric, Gynecologic & Neonatal Nursing, 44*(5), 687–689. doi:10.1111/1552-6909.12734

Rossman, B., Greene, M. M., & Meier, P. P. (2015). The role of peer support in the development of maternal identity for 'NICU moms'. *Journal of Obstetric, Gynecologic & Neonatal Nursing, 44*(1), 3–16. doi:10.1111/1552-6909.12527

COMPROMISED FAMILY COPING

related to exhaustion of support person's capacity; situational crisis faced by support person

Definition

A usually supportive primary person (family member, significant other, or close friend) provides insufficient, ineffective, or compromised support, comfort, assistance, or encouragement that may be needed by the client to manage or master adaptive tasks related to the his or her health challenge

Assessment

- Family process, including normal pattern of interaction among family members; family's understanding and knowledge of neonate's condition; support systems available (financial, social, and spiritual); family's response to past crises, including coping behaviors and problem-solving techniques; recreational activities; and communication patterns used to express anger, affection, and confrontation
- Neonate's health status
- Family's perception of present situation
- Degree of difficulty imposed by care of neonate
- Possible impact of neonate's health status on family's future structure and lifestyle

Defining Characteristics

- Assistive behaviors by support person produce unsatisfactory results
- Client complaint about support person's response to health problem
- Client concern about support person's response to health problem
- Limitation in communication between support person and client
- Protective behavior by support person incongruent with client's abilities
- Protective behavior by support person incongruent with client's need for autonomy
- Support person reports inadequate understanding that interferes with effective behaviors
- Support person reports insufficient knowledge that interferes with effective behaviors
- Support person reports preoccupation with own reaction to client's need
- Support person withdrawn from client

Expected Outcomes

- Family members will communicate feelings about neonate's condition.
- Family members will engage in healthy coping behaviors.
- Family members will become involved in planning for and providing neonate's care.
- Family members will identify and use available support systems.
- Family members will set realistic goals for neonate.
- Family members will express feeling of having greater control over their situation.

Suggested NOC Outcomes

Caregiver Emotional Health; Caregiver–Patient Relationship; Caregiver Stressors; Caregiving Endurance Potential; Family Coping; Parent–Infant Attachment; Parenting Performance

Interventions and Rationales

- PCC Encourage family members to voice their feelings about the neonate's condition *to decrease tension by clearing up misunderstandings and misconceptions.*
- Identify and reduce unnecessary environmental stimuli *to enhance family members' ability to focus on caring for the neonate.*
- Assess family members' understanding of the neonate's condition. Help them view the situation realistically and understand its future implications. *Setting realistic goals helps the family plan for the future and avoid unnecessary disappointment.*
- PCC Actively involve family members in learning to care for the neonate *to decrease feelings of helplessness and isolation from the neonate.*

- Explain the rationale for all treatments and procedures to family members *to help reduce anxiety and enhance cooperation.*
- Involve the family members in decision making when possible *to increase their feelings of involvement and control.*
- Provide positive feedback when family members care for the neonate *to increase self-esteem and reinforce their ability to care for the neonate successfully.*
- PCC Encourage family members to identify and contact support systems and resources, such as extended family, friends, clergy, and community groups, *to decrease the sense of being overwhelmed.*
- Help family members identify and use appropriate coping behaviors *to reduce anxiety and tension.*
- PCC Coordinate referrals to other health care professionals, such as a social worker or physical therapist, *to ensure clear communication among health care providers, which enables the neonate to receive appropriate comprehensive care.*
- Provide family members with up-to-date reports on the neonate's condition *to ease anxiety and help the family plan for future needs.*

Suggested NIC Interventions

Caregiver Support; Coping Enhancement; Emotional Support; Family Involvement Promotion; Family Mobilization; Family Support; Spiritual Support

Evaluations for Expected Outcomes

- Family members voice their feelings about neonate's condition.
- Family members identify and use at least two healthy coping behaviors.
- Family members demonstrate ability to plan for and provide neonate's care.
- Family members identify and use available support systems.
- Family members set realistic goals for neonate.
- Family members express feeling of increased control over their situation.

Documentation

- Family members' perceptions of neonate's health and long-term implications
- Observations of family members' behaviors, including interactions with neonate
- Family members' statements indicating their feelings toward neonate
- Teaching and referrals given to family members
- Family members' abilities to meet neonate's physical and emotional needs
- Consultations with other health care team members
- Interventions to help family members cope
- Family members' responses to nursing interventions
- Evaluations for expected outcomes

REFERENCES

Chrupcala, K. A., Edwards, T. M., & Spatz, D. L. (2015). A continuous quality improvement project to implement infant-driven feeding as a standard of practice in the newborn/infant intensive care unit. *Journal of Obstetric, Gynecologic & Neonatal Nursing, 44*(5), 654–664. doi:10.1111/1552-6909.12727

Rossman, B., Greene, M. M., & Meier, P. P. (2015). The role of peer support in the development of maternal identity for 'NICU moms'. *Journal of Obstetric, Gynecologic & Neonatal Nursing, 44*(1), 3–16. doi:10.1111/1552-6909.12527

Samra, H. A., McGrath, J. M., Fischer, S., Schumacher, B., Dutcher, J., & Hansen, J. (2015). The NICU parent risk evaluation and engagement model and instrument (PREEMI) for neonates in intensive care units. *Journal of Obstetric, Gynecologic & Neonatal Nursing*, *44*(1), 114–126. doi:10.1111/1552-6909.12535

INTERRUPTED FAMILY PROCESSES

related to situational transition

Definition

Change in family relationships and/or functioning

Assessment

- Age of patient and partner
- Availability of family members or friends to help
- Planned or unplanned pregnancy
- Family status, including number and ages of other children, usual patterns of interaction among family members, family members' assumed or expected roles, communication patterns, support systems, financial resources, past responses to change, spiritual resources, and living conditions
- Perceived impact of pregnancy on family unit
- Presence of obstetric or fetal complications or other medical conditions

Defining Characteristics

- Alteration in availability for affective responsiveness
- Alteration in family conflict resolution
- Alteration in family satisfaction
- Alteration in intimacy
- Alteration in participation for problem solving
- Change in communication pattern
- Change in somatization
- Change in stress-reduction behavior
- Changes in expressions of conflict with community resources
- Changes in expressions of isolation from community resources
- Changes in participation for decision making
- Changes in available emotional support
- Decrease in mutual support
- Ineffective task completion
- Power alliance change
- Ritual change

Expected Outcomes

- Family members will take on portion of duties carried out by patient, such as housecleaning, heavy lifting, and meal preparation.
- Patient and family members will voice realistic expectations about pregnancy's impact on their future.
- Patient and family members will share their feelings about pregnancy with each other.
- Family members will identify and contact appropriate support systems.
- Family will welcome new member of the family.

Suggested NOC Outcomes

Family Coping; Family Functioning; Family Normalization; Family Resiliency; Parenting Performance

Interventions and Rationales

PCC
- Encourage family members to express their feelings about the pregnancy. Tell them that a wide range of emotions, ranging from fear to excitement, may accompany a diagnosis of pregnancy. *Pent-up feelings can lead to misunderstanding and resentment.*
- Provide emotional support to the patient and family members *to help them come to terms with altered roles and responsibilities.*

PCC
- Encourage the pregnant woman to voice her concerns about the pregnancy's potential impact on family structure and finances *to identify unrealistic fears and decrease anxiety.*
- Arrange and participate in family conferences, as needed. *Some families may require help to improve interpersonal communication.*
- Refer family members to classes in prepared childbirth or parenting, psychological counseling, or social service and health care agencies, as appropriate, *to provide additional information and support.*
- Periodically assess the woman's acceptance of pregnancy *to determine the need for further interventions. The mother usually grows to accept the pregnancy as the uterus develops and she feels the fetus kick. She may also fantasize about what the neonate will look like and begin preparing for birth.*

Suggested NIC Interventions

Coping Enhancement; Family Integrity Promotion; Family Process Maintenance; Family Support; Normalization Promotion; Parent Education: Childrearing Family

Evaluations for Expected Outcomes

- Family members take on portion of patient's duties.
- Patient and family members voice realistic expectations about emotional and financial impact of pregnancy on family structure.
- Patient and family members honestly communicate feelings about pregnancy.
- Patient and family members identify and contact potential support groups or organizations.
- Neonate is successfully integrated into family.

Documentation

- Reactions of patient and partner to diagnosis of pregnancy
- Referrals to outside agencies
- Patient's adherence to prescribed medical practices
- Observations of patient's acceptance of and interest in pregnancy as it progresses
- Interventions to assist patient and family
- Patient's and family's responses to nursing interventions
- Evaluations for expected outcomes

REFERENCES

Feldman, R. (2014). When maternity doesn't matter: Dispersing pregnant women seeking asylum. *British Journal of Midwifery, 22*(1), 23–28.

Gazmararian, J., Elon, L., Yang, B., Graham, M., & Parker, R. (2014). Text4baby program: An opportunity to reach underserved pregnant and postpartum women? *Maternal & Child Health Journal, 18*(1), 223–232. doi:10.1007/s10995-013-1258-1

Webb, M. S., Passmore, D., Cline, G., & Maguire, D. (2014). Ethical issues related to caring for low birth weight infants. *Nursing Ethics, 21*(6), 731–741. doi:10.1177/0969733013513919

Zani, A. V., Pamplona Tonete, V. L., & de Lima Parada, C. G. (2014). Maternal representations about the provision of care to newborns at risk: a collective discourse. *Online Brazilian Journal of Nursing, 13*(3), 321–331.

INTERRUPTED FAMILY PROCESSES

related to shift in family roles

Definition

Change in family relationships and/or functioning

Assessment

- Family status, including assumed or expected roles, communication patterns, developmental stage of family members, number and ages of other children, financial resources, past responses to change, available support systems, significant others, and spiritual practices
- Family members' perceptions of impact of birth on their assumed roles

Defining Characteristics

- Alteration in availability for affective responsiveness
- Alteration in family conflict resolution
- Alteration in family satisfaction
- Alteration in intimacy
- Alteration in participation for problem solving
- Change in communication pattern
- Change in somatization
- Change in stress-reduction behavior
- Changes in expressions of conflict with community resources
- Changes in expressions of isolation from community resources
- Changes in participation for decision making
- Changes in available emotional support
- Decrease in mutual support
- Ineffective task completion
- Power alliance change
- Ritual change

Expected Outcomes

- Family members will voice feelings about neonate.
- Family members will express need to assume new or altered roles and adapt to changes within family structure.
- Family members will contact support groups for help, if needed.
- Neonate will be successfully welcomed into family structure.

Suggested NOC Outcomes

Family Coping; Family Functioning; Family Normalization; Parenting Performance; Social Support

Interventions and Rationales

- PCC Encourage family members to express their feelings about the arrival of the neonate and altered roles and responsibilities *to help clear up misunderstandings and misconceptions.*
- Explore with family members the ways the neonate will affect family structure and functioning. Topics may include changes in finances and living space, caretaking arrangements, and new roles or responsibilities for parents and siblings. *Discussing legitimate concerns may improve family members' attitudes toward the neonate.*

- Discuss with family members the degree of sibling preparation and the possibility of sibling rivalry. *Siblings must be reassured that they're still vital members of the family.* Encourage siblings to visit the neonate at the hospital *to decrease separation anxiety, foster a sense of family, and facilitate bonding.*
- Assess measures taken to prepare the home for the arrival of the neonate. *Lack of preparation may indicate limited financial resources or difficulty accepting the neonate.*
- Assess the need for help from social services or community agencies and coordinate referrals *to ensure ongoing comprehensive care.*

Suggested NIC Interventions

Coping Enhancement; Emotional Support; Family Integrity Promotion; Family Process Maintenance; Family Support; Normalization Promotion; Support System Enhancement

Evaluations for Expected Outcomes

- Family members share feelings about neonate with each other.
- Family members assume new or additional responsibilities, as needed, such as preparing meals, assisting with transportation, shopping, cleaning, and providing child care.
- Family members contact community agencies or support groups for assistance, if needed.
- Family members come to terms with arrival of neonate.

Documentation

- Observations of family members' reactions to neonate
- Family members' statements indicating attitudes toward neonate
- Interventions performed to help family cope with new arrival
- Family members' responses to nursing interventions
- Referrals to outside agencies
- Evaluations for expected outcomes

REFERENCES

Barkin, J. L., Bloch, J. R., Hawkins, K. C., & Thomas, T. S. (2014). Barriers to optimal social support in the postpartum period. *Journal of Obstetric, Gynecologic & Neonatal Nursing, 43*(4), 445–454. doi:10.1111/1552-6909.12463

Lindberg, L., & Kost, K. (2014). Exploring U.S. men's birth intentions. *Maternal & Child Health Journal, 18*(3), 625–633. doi:10.1007/s10995-013-1286-x

Taubman–Ben-Ari, O., & Spielman, V. (2014). Personal growth following the first child's birth: A comparison of parents of pre- and full-term babies. *Social Work Research, 38*(2), 91–106.

READINESS FOR ENHANCED FAMILY PROCESSES

Definition

A pattern of family functioning to support the well-being of family members, which can be strengthened

Assessment

- Family structure, including perception of self and family, family composition, social roles of family members, family developmental stages, socioeconomics, education, occupation, ethnicity, and cultural and religious beliefs

- Family health pattern, including perception of health, health management, family developmental tasks, coping mechanisms, health beliefs and values, health status, stressors, and safety
- Family function, including family interactions, use of resources, decision making, growth and development, responses to affection and concerns

Defining Characteristics

- Expresses desire to enhance balance between autonomy and cohesiveness
- Expresses desire to enhance communication pattern
- Expresses desire to enhance energy level of family to support activities of daily living
- Expresses desire to enhance family adaptation to change
- Expresses desire to enhance family dynamics
- Expresses desire to enhance family resilience
- Expresses desire to enhance growth of family members
- Expresses desire to enhance interdependence with community
- Expresses desire to enhance maintenance of boundaries between family members
- Expresses desire to enhance respect for family members
- Expresses desire to enhance safety of family members

Expected Outcomes

- Family members will identify family goals and structured directions.
- Family members will express enjoyment and satisfaction in their roles in the family.
- Family members will regularly participate in traditional family activities.
- Family members will maintain open and positive communications.
- Family members will maintain a safe home environment.
- Family members will contact community resources for help, if needed.
- Family members will seek regular health screenings and immunizations.
- Family members will identify and acknowledge risk factors.
- Family members will make plans for dealing with life changes and unexpected events.
- Family members will maintain healthy lifestyles by exercising regularly, eating a well-balanced diet, avoiding substance abuse, and using proven holistic health strategies.

Suggested NOC Outcomes

Community Competence; Community Health Status; Compliance Behavior; Decision-Making; Family Coping; Family Functioning; Family Health Status; Family Integrity; Family Normalization; Family Participation in Professional Care; Health Beliefs: Perceived Ability to Perform; Health Beliefs: Perceived Control; Health Orientation; Health Promoting Behavior; Hope; Identity; Risk Detection

Interventions and Rationales

- PCC Encourage family members to identify individual and family goals and structured directions. *Individual and family goals set the boundaries that are respected by the family members. Family functioning with structured direction should enhance family members' ability to meet their physical, social, and psychological needs.*
- PCC Encourage family members to express enjoyment and satisfaction in their roles in the family *to enhance family dynamics and strengthen family bonds.*

- Assist the family members in coping with changes related to growth and development. *Each transition stage of growth and development is a stressful life event.*
- Explore with the family members traditional activities that all family members will enjoy doing together. *Sharing traditional family activities increases loyalty, security, and a sense of belonging for family members.*
- Assess measures taken to maintain open and positive communications. *Healthy communications bridge the gap between members of the family.*
- Assist family to clarify family values and beliefs regarding health and health practices by helping the family identify their values, restate the values, and identify conflicts between values and action. *Values guide actions and have power to motivate behaviors. Value conflicts could lead to noncompliant health practices and interrupt the well-being of family members.*
- PCC Assess measures taken to maintain safety in the home environment. *Environments that are free from environmental hazards, both chemical and physical, assure a sense of security.*
- Assess the stress-coping ability of the family members, individually and as a whole, to determine the strength and weakness status of the individual's and family's stress-coping pattern. Help the family make realistic plans for dealing with life changes and unexpected events. *Preparation for stress enhances the use of coping mechanisms and minimizes the threat.*
- PCC Provide the family with information on social support and community resources. *Social support and community resources enhance the family process, reinforce family strength, and assist when families are experiencing stresses.*
- PCC Provide the family with information on recommended health screenings and immunizations, and encourage them to schedule regular checkups according to their growth and developmental stages. *Screening is a valuable tool to enhance preventive interventions.*
- Help the family develop a Genogram to identify genetic risk factors. *Information from a Genogram highlights a family's health patterns, provides knowledge leading to early identification of genetically related diseases, and may delay disease onset.*
- PCC Educate and encourage family members to exercise regularly, eat a well-balanced diet, avoid substance abuse, and use proven holistic health strategies. *Health-promotion behaviors could maintain optimum health.*

Suggested NIC Interventions

Active Listening; Anticipatory Guidance; Attachment Promotion; Behavior Modification: Social Skills; Coping Enhancement; Emotional Support; Environmental Management: Attachment Process; Environmental Management: Comfort; Environmental Management: Safety; Environmental Management: Violence Prevention; Exercise Promotion; Family Involvement Promotion; Family Mobilization; Family Process Maintenance; Family Support; Health Education; Health Screening; Health System Guidance; Hope Instillation; Humor; Meditation Facilitation; Risk Identification; Role Enhancement; Security Enhancement; Self-Esteem Enhancement; Self-Responsibility Facilitation; Socialization Enhancement; Spiritual Support; Support System Enhancement; Truth Telling; Values Clarification

Evaluations for Expected Outcomes

- Family functions in a structured and goal-oriented direction.
- Family members state enjoyment and satisfaction in their roles in the family.

- Family members regularly participate in traditional family activities.
- Family members maintain open and positive communications.
- Family members maintain a safe home environment.
- Family utilizes various available social support venues as well as community resources to meet the needs of the family and individual family members.
- Family members participate in regular health screenings and immunizations.
- Family members identify and acknowledge risk factors.
- Family members have plans for dealing with life changes and unexpected events.
- Family members maintain healthy lifestyle by exercising regularly, eating a well-balanced diet, avoiding substance abuse, and using proven holistic health strategies.

Documentation

- Identification of goals and activities carried out
- Satisfaction level of family members
- Use of support services
- Health visits, patterns of exercise and diet, use of other health-promoting strategies
- Evaluations for expected outcomes

REFERENCES

Alhusen, J. L., Bullock, L., Sharps, P., Schminkey, D., Comstock, E., & Campbell, J. (2014). Intimate partner violence during pregnancy and adverse neonatal outcomes in low-income women. *Journal of Women's Health, 23*(11), 920–926. doi:10.1089/jwh.2014.4862

Edéll-Gustafsson, U., Angelhoff, C., Johnsson, E., Karlsson, J., & Mörelius, E. (2015). Hindering and buffering factors for parental sleep in neonatal care. A phenomenographic study. *Journal of Clinical Nursing, 24*(5/6), 717–727. doi:10.1111/jocn.12654

Levin, A., & Chalmers, B. (2014). Family-centered neonatal intensive care. *Birth: Issues in Perinatal Care, 41*(3), 300. doi:10.1111/birt.12129

Rossman, B., Greene, M. M., & Meier, P. P. (2015). The role of peer support in the development of maternal identity for 'NICU moms'. *Journal of Obstetric, Gynecologic & Neonatal Nursing, 44*(1), 3–16. doi:10.1111/1552-6909.12527

INEFFECTIVE INFANT FEEDING PATTERN

related to neurologic impairment (e.g., positive EEG, head trauma, seizure disorders) or neurologic delay

Definition

Impaired ability of an infant to suck or coordinate the suck/swallow response resulting in inadequate oral nutrition for metabolic needs.

Assessment

- Perinatal history, including gestational age and Apgar score
- Suck and swallow reflex, including condition of lip and palate
- Nutritional status, including intake (type, amount, and frequency of feedings), output (frequency, amount, and characteristics of urine), current weight, weight change since birth, skin turgor, and signs of dehydration
- Laboratory studies, including glucose and bilirubin levels
- Parental status, including age, maturity level, and previous experience with infant feeding

Defining Characteristics

- Inability to coordinate sucking, swallowing, and breathing
- Inability to initiate an effective suck
- Inability to sustain an effective suck

Expected Outcomes

- Neonate won't lose more than 10% of birth weight within first week of life.
- Neonate will gain 4 to 7 oz (113.5 to 198.5 g)/week after first week of life.
- Parents or caregivers will identify factors that interfere with neonate establishing effective feeding pattern.
- Parents will express increased confidence in their ability to perform appropriate feeding techniques.
- Neonate won't become dehydrated.
- Neonate will receive adequate supplemental nutrition until able to suckle sufficiently.
- Neonate will establish effective suck and swallow reflexes that allow for adequate intake of nutrients.

Suggested NOC Outcomes

Breastfeeding Establishment: Infant; Breastfeeding Maintenance; Nutritional Status: Food & Fluid Intake

Interventions and Rationales

- Weigh the neonate at the same time each day on the same scale *to detect excessive weight loss early.*
- Assess the neonate's sucking pattern *to monitor for ineffective patterns.*
- Assess the parents' knowledge of feeding techniques *to help identify and clear up misconceptions.*
- Assess the parents' level of anxiety about the neonate's feeding difficulty. *Anxiety may interfere with the parents' ability to learn new techniques.*
- Remain with the parents and neonate during the feeding *to identify problem areas and direct interventions.*
- PCC Teach the parents to place the neonate in the upright position during feeding *to prevent aspiration.*
- PCC Teach the parents to unwrap and position a sleepy neonate before feeding *to ensure that the neonate is awake and alert enough to suckle sufficiently.*
- Provide positive reinforcement for the parents' efforts to improve their feeding technique *to decrease anxiety and enhance feelings of success.*
- For bottle-feeding, record the amount ingested at each feeding; for breast-feeding, record the number of minutes the neonate nurses at each breast and the amount of any supplement ingested *to monitor for inadequate caloric and fluid intake.*
- Provide an alternative nipple, such as a preemie nipple. *A preemie nipple has a larger hole and softer texture, which makes it easier for the neonate to obtain formula.*
- For breast-feeding, ensure the neonate's tongue is properly positioned under the mother's nipple *to promote adequate sucking.*
- Monitor the neonate for poor skin turgor, dry mucous membranes, decreased or concentrated urine, and sunken fontanels and eyeballs *to detect possible dehydration and allow for immediate intervention.*

- Record the number of stools and amount of urine voided each shift. *An altered bowel elimination pattern may indicate decreased food intake; decreased amounts of concentrated urine may indicate dehydration.*
- Assess the need for gavage feeding. *The neonate may temporarily require alternative means of obtaining adequate fluids and calories.*
- Alternate oral and gavage feeding *to conserve the neonate's energy.*
- S If the neonate requires IV nourishment, assess the insertion site, amount infused, and infusion rate every hour *to monitor fluid intake and identify possible complications, such as infiltration and phlebitis.*
- Assess the neonate for neurologic deficits or other pathophysiologic causes of ineffective sucking *to identify the need for more extensive evaluation.*

Suggested NIC Interventions

Attachment Promotion; Breastfeeding Assistance; Lactation Counseling; Nonnutritive Sucking

Evaluations for Expected Outcomes

- Neonate doesn't lose more than 10% of birth weight within first week of life.
- Neonate gains 4 to 7 oz/week after first week of life.
- Parents identify factors that interfere with effective feeding.
- Parents express increased confidence in their ability to perform appropriate feeding techniques.
- Neonate maintains urine output of 1 mL/kg/day, urine specific gravity of 1.003 to 1.013, good skin turgor, moist mucous membranes, and soft, flat fontanels.
- Neonate receives adequate nutrition.
- Neonate establishes effective sucking reflex and coordinated suck and swallow response.

Documentation

- Frequency, amount, and type of fluid ingested by neonate
- Effectiveness of suck reflex
- Neonate's daily weight
- Parents' knowledge of feeding techniques, involvement with caregiving, and bonding with neonate
- Frequency of neonate's bowel elimination and urination
- Signs of dehydration
- Nursing interventions
- Use of special feeding techniques and equipment
- Parents' and neonate's responses to nursing interventions
- Evidence of neurologic or other physical impairment in neonate
- Evaluations for expected outcomes

REFERENCES

Chung, J., Lee, J., Spinazzola, R., Rosen, L., & Milanaik, R. (2014). Parental perception of premature infant growth and feeding behaviors: Use of gestation-adjusted age and assessing for developmental readiness during solid food introduction. *Clinical Pediatrics, 53*(13), 1271–1277. doi:10.1177/0009922814540039

Gibertoni, D., Corvaglia, L., Vandini, S., Rucci, P., Savini, S., Alessandroni, R., . . . Faldella, G. (2015). Positive effect of human milk feeding during NICU hospitalization on 24 month neurodevelopment of very low birth weight infants: An Italian cohort study. *Plos One, 10*(1), e0116552. doi:10.1371/journal.pone.0116552

Pickler, R. H., Wetzel, P. A., Meinzen-Derr, J., Tubbs-Cooley, H. L., & Moore, M. (2015). Patterned feeding experience for preterm infants: Study protocol for a randomized controlled trial. *Trials, 16*, 255. doi:10.1186/s13063-015-0781-3

DEFICIENT FLUID VOLUME

related to compromised regulatory mechanism

Definition

Decreased intravascular, interstitial, and/or intracellular fluid. This refers to dehydration, water loss alone without change in sodium

Assessment

- Vital signs, including temperature, pulse rate, blood pressure, and respirations
- Fluid and electrolyte status, including weight, intake and output, urine specific gravity, skin turgor, mucous membranes, and electrolyte and blood urea nitrogen levels

Defining Characteristics

- Alteration in mental status
- Alteration in skin turgor
- Decrease in blood pressure
- Decrease in pulse pressure
- Decrease in pulse volume
- Decrease in tongue turgor
- Decrease in urine output
- Decrease in venous filling
- Dry mucous membranes
- Dry skin
- Increase in body temperature
- Increase in heart rate
- Increase in hematocrit
- Increase in urine concentration
- Sudden weight loss
- Thirst
- Weakness

Expected Outcomes

- Patient will maintain fluid balance.
- Patient will demonstrate optimal hydration.
- Patient will show no signs of dehydration.

Suggested NOC Outcomes

Electrolyte and Acid/Base Balance; Fluid Balance; Hydration; Nausea and Vomiting Severity; Urinary Elimination

Interventions and Rationales

- Monitor vital signs as often as policy dictates. *Decreased blood pressure and increased pulse rate may be late signs of fluid volume loss. With gestational hypertension, increased blood pressure may occur.*

- Assess skin turgor and examine oral mucous membranes for dryness. *Dehydration can cause dry mucous membranes, skin tenting, and dry, cracked lips.*
- Continuously monitor intake and output. Administer and monitor parenteral fluids. Maintain intake according to order or protocol (usually 125 to 175 mL/hour). Output should approximate intake. *These measures help ensure adequate hydration.*
- Monitor electrolyte values and report abnormalities. *Hypernatremia may indicate dehydration, requiring IV volume replacement. Hypernatremia may also be related to excessive insensible water loss.*
- Provide the patient with ice chips or a cool, damp, 4 3 4 gauze compress *to increase patient comfort and decrease mouth dryness, especially if the patient breathes through her mouth.*
- Measure the amount and character of vomitus to assess the need for an antiemetic. *When labor begins, blood is rerouted to serve the energy needs of the contracting uterus and blood flow to the gastrointestinal (GI) tract decreases. GI motility and absorption also decrease so that food may remain in the stomach for up to 12 hours. These factors predispose the patient to nausea and vomiting, especially during the transition phase of labor.*
- As ordered, administer an antiemetic, and evaluate its effectiveness *to help control emesis and prevent excessive fluid loss.*
- Keep the patient cool and comfortable. Change her gown, as indicated, and apply cool compresses to her face and body *to reduce discomfort caused by diaphoresis.*
- Position the patient on her left side *to aid kidney perfusion and increase cardiac and urine output.*
- If urine output is reduced, carefully assess the patient for peripheral edema, hyperreflexia, increased blood pressure, and presence of urine protein. *Decreased urine output, increased blood pressure, hyperreflexia, and peripheral edema may indicate intrapartal gestational hypertension. Proteinuria may result from dehydration, exhaustion, or preeclampsia.*

Suggested NIC Interventions

Electrolyte Management: Hypernatremia; Fluid/Electrolyte Management; Fluid Monitoring; Hemodynamic Regulation; Hypovolemia Management; Medication Management

Evaluations for Expected Outcomes

- Patient maintains fluid balance, with intake approximately equaling output.
- Patient maintains optimal hydration.
- Patient has no signs of dehydration; her mucous membranes remain pink and moist; skin turgor remains optimal; vital signs stay within normal limits; and urine output is at least 30 mL/hour or 100 mL in 4 hours.

Documentation

- Patient's vital signs
- Observation of patient's fluid volume status
- Intake and output
- Nursing interventions performed to maintain adequate fluid intake
- Patient's response to nursing interventions
- Evaluations for expected outcomes

REFERENCES

Czeizel, A. E., & Puhó, E. (2004). Association between severe nausea and vomiting in pregnancy and lower rate of preterm births. *Paediatric and Perinatal Epidemiology, 18*(4), 253–259.

IV fluids given to women during labour may over-hydrate baby. (2011). *Nursing Standard, 26*(3), 16.
Lothian, J. A. (2014). Healthy birth practice #4: Avoid interventions unless they are medically necessary. *Journal of Perinatal Education, 23*(4), 198–206. doi:10.1891/1058-1243.23.4.198
Shennan, A., Thallon, A., Hart, D., & O'Sullivan, G. (2005). Caesarean section and calorific intake in labour; the influence of carbohydrate solution intake during labour. *International Journal of Obstetrics and Gynaecology, 112*(10), 1454.

DEFICIENT FLUID VOLUME

related to active fluid volume loss

Definition

Decreased intravascular, interstitial, and/or intracellular fluid. This refers to dehydration, water loss alone without change in sodium

Assessment

- History of problems that can cause fluid loss, such as hemorrhage, vomiting, diarrhea, and indwelling catheters
- Vital signs
- Fluid and electrolyte status, including weight, intake and output, urine specific gravity, skin turgor, mucous membranes, and serum electrolyte and blood urea nitrogen levels
- Laboratory studies, including hemoglobin (Hb) level and hematocrit (HCT)
- Factors that place patient at high risk for postpartum hemorrhage, including grand multipara, overdistended uterus, prolonged labor, previous history of postpartum hemorrhage, traumatic delivery, uterine fibroids, overstimulation with oxytocin, and bleeding disorders

Defining Characteristics

- Alteration in mental status
- Alteration in skin turgor
- Decrease in blood pressure
- Decrease in pulse pressure
- Decrease in pulse volume
- Decrease in tongue turgor
- Decrease in urine output
- Decrease in venous filling
- Dry mucous membranes
- Dry skin
- Increase in body temperature
- Increase in heart rate
- Increase in HCT
- Increase in urine concentration
- Sudden weight loss
- Thirst
- Weakness

Expected Outcomes

- Patient's vital signs will remain stable.
- Patient's hematology studies will be within normal range.
- Patient's uterus will remain firm.
- Medical personnel will quickly identify signs of possible shock and initiate treatment.
- Patient's bladder won't become distended.
- Patient's blood volume will return to normal.

Suggested NOC Outcomes

Blood Loss Severity; Electrolyte & Acid/Base Balance; Fluid Balance; Hydration; Risk Detection; Urinary Elimination

Interventions and Rationales

- Immediately after delivery, monitor the color, amount, and consistency of the lochia every 15 minutes for 1 hour, then every 4 hours for 24 hours, then every shift until discharge. Weigh or count sanitary pads if the lochia is excessive. *Hemorrhage is the most common cause of mortality during childbirth.*
- Monitor and record vital signs every 15 minutes for 1 hour, then every 4 hours for 24 hours, then every shift until discharge *to detect signs of hemorrhage and shock, such as increased pulse and respiratory rates and decreased blood pressure.*
- Immediately after delivery, palpate the fundus every 15 minutes for 1 hour, then every 4 hours for 24 hours, then every shift until discharge. Note its location and tone. *Palpation of the fundus will enable you to detect uterine atony (lack of normal uterine muscle tone or strength), the most common cause of postpartum hemorrhage.*
- Gently massage a boggy fundus; avoid overstimulation. *Gentle stimulation can help the fundus to become firm; overstimulation can cause relaxation.*
- Explain to the patient the process of involution and the need to palpate the fundus. Teach the patient to assess and gently massage the fundus and to notify you if bogginess persists. *Explaining normal postpartum physiologic adjustments can decrease the patient's anxiety and increase cooperation.*
- Evaluate postpartum hematology studies and report abnormal results. Consider whether the patient needs typing and crossmatching for transfusion. *Comparison of postdelivery Hb and HCT with previous results provides information about the amount of blood loss and allows time to plan interventions, such as requesting blood from a blood bank.*
- Administer fluids, blood or blood products, or plasma expanders, as ordered, *to replace lost blood volume.* Monitor for adverse reactions.
- Monitor the patient's intake and output every shift. Note bladder distention and catheterize, as ordered. *A distended bladder interferes with the involution of the uterus.*
- Administer oxytocic agents, such as oxytocin (Pitocin), methylergonovine (Methergine), and ergonovine (Ergotrate), as ordered, and evaluate their effectiveness. *Oxytocic agents stimulate uterine musculature, controlling postpartum hemorrhage and atony.*
- S Regularly assess the patient for signs and symptoms of shock, including rapid thready pulse, increased respiratory rate, decreased blood pressure and urine output, and cold, clammy, pale skin. *Prompt recognition and treatment of shock limits the amount of fluid lost and the impact on other body systems.*

Suggested NIC Interventions

Acid-Base Management; Bleeding Reduction: Antepartum Uterus; Blood Products Administration; Electrolyte Management; Fluid Monitoring; Hemodynamic Regulation; Intravenous (IV) Therapy; Medication Management; Shock Management; Vital Signs Monitoring

Evaluations for Expected Outcomes

- Patient's vital signs remain stable.
- Results of patient's hematology studies are within normal range.
- Patient's uterus remains firm.

- If patient develops shock, medical personnel identify it quickly and promptly start treatment.
- Patient doesn't develop distended bladder.
- Patient's blood loss after delivery is less than 500 mL and fluid volume is replenished.

Documentation

- Estimation of blood loss
- Signs of possible shock
- Location and tone of fundus
- Laboratory results
- Replacement of lost fluid
- Nursing interventions to control active blood loss
- Patient's response to nursing interventions
- Evaluations for expected outcomes

REFERENCES

Gandhi, H. (2014). Prevention of postpartum hemorrhage: Exogenous oxytocin in the third stage of labor. *Kentucky Nurse, 62*(3), 4.

Guidelines for oxytocin administration after birth: AWHONN practice brief number 2. (2015). *Journal of Obstetric, Gynecologic & Neonatal Nursing, 44*(1), 161–163. doi:10.1111/1552-6909.12528

Williams, C. (2014). Should midwives measure blood loss in the fourth stage of labour? *British Journal of Midwifery, 22*(6), 394–398.

HYPOTHERMIA

related to ineffective vascular control; ineffective nonshivering thermogenesis

Definition

Core body temperature below the normal diurnal range due to failure of thermoregulation.

Assessment

- History of present illness
- Gestational age
- Prenatal and intrapartal history
- Presence of maternal risk factors, such as fever, diabetes mellitus, drug use, dystocia, and history of perinatal asphyxia
- Neurologic status, including level of consciousness (LOC) and sensory status
- Cardiovascular status, including core temperature, heart rate and rhythm, blood pressure, and capillary refill time
- Respiratory status, including rate, rhythm, and depth; breath sounds; and arterial blood gas values
- Integumentary status, including temperature, color (central vs. peripheral), and turgor
- Nutritional status, including dietary pattern, birth weight, current weight, and recent weight changes
- Fluid and electrolyte status, including intake and output, serum glucose and electrolyte levels, and urine specific gravity
- Psychosocial status, including behavior, parental stressors, parental coping skills, and financial resources

Defining Characteristics

- Acrocyanosis
- Bradycardia
- Cyanotic nail beds
- Decrease in blood glucose level
- Decrease in ventilation
- Hypertension
- Hypoglycemia
- Hypoxia
- Increase in metabolic rate
- Increase in oxygen consumption
- Peripheral vasoconstriction
- Piloerection
- Shivering
- Skin cool to touch
- Slow capillary refill
- Tachycardia

Accidental Low Body Temperature in Children and Adults

- Mild hypothermia, core temperature 32° C to 35° C
- Moderate hypothermia, core temperature 30° C to 32° C
- Severe hypothermia, core temperature <30° C

Injured Adults and Children

- Hypothermia, core temperature <35° C
- Severe hypothermia, core temperature <32° C

Neonates

- Grade 1 hypothermia, core temperature 36° C to 36.5° C
- Grade 2 hypothermia, core temperature 35° C to 35.9° C
- Grade 3 hypothermia, core temperature 34° C to 34.9° C
- Grade 4 hypothermia, core temperature <34° C
- Infant with insufficient energy to maintain sucking
- Infant with insufficient weight gain (<30 g/day)
- Irritability
- Jaundice
- Metabolic acidosis
- Pallor
- Respiratory distress

Expected Outcomes

- Neonate will exhibit body temperature within normal limits.
- Neonate will have warm, dry skin and capillary refill time within normal limits.
- Neonate's cardiovascular status will be within normal limits.
- Neonate won't develop complications of hypothermia.
- Neonate won't shiver.
- Neonate won't develop signs of hyperthermia related to radiant heat source.
- Neonate will be weaned from self-contained incubation unit or radiant warmer bed, as tolerated.
- Family members will verbalize knowledge of how hypothermia develops and will state measures to prevent recurrent hypothermia.
- Family members will demonstrate ability to measure neonate's temperature accurately.
- Family members will demonstrate willingness to provide adequate home care for neonate.

Suggested NOC Outcomes

Thermoregulation: Newborn; Vital Signs

Interventions and Rationales

- Monitor body temperature every 1 to 3 hours by axillary or inguinal route (avoid rectal measurement). Record temperature and route. *Monitoring body temperature helps to detect developing complications*. If using an electronic heat source, such as a radiant warmer, monitor the device's temperature reading hourly and compare it with the neonate's body temperature *to evaluate the effectiveness of interventions.*

- Monitor and record neurologic status every 1 to 4 hours. *Falling body temperature and slowed metabolic rate may cause decreased LOC.*
- Monitor and record vital signs every 1 to 4 hours. As ordered, initiate and maintain continuous electronic cardiorespiratory monitoring. *These measures help avert metabolic acidosis and respiratory arrest.*
- Provide supportive measures:
  - Maintain a neutral thermal environment—a narrow range of environmental temperatures that maintain a stable core temperature with minimal caloric and oxygen expenditure. Determination of a neutral thermal environment depends on the neonate's age and weight.
  - If indicated, place the neonate in an open crib. For mild hypothermia, dress the neonate with an undershirt, diaper, and knitted or stockinette cap and cover him with double blankets.
  - Avoid overheating the neonate.
  - Keep the diaper area dry.
  - Keep head covered.
  - Cover all metal or plastic surfaces that could come in contact with the neonate.
  - Maintain the room temperature between 75° F and 78° F (23.9° C and 25.6° C).
  - Perform all procedures under a radiant warmer, if possible. Postpone bathing the neonate.

  These measures protect the neonate from heat loss.
- For severe hypothermia, place the neonate in an isolette or overhead radiant warmer bed, providing these supportive measures:
  - Keep the neonate undressed.
  - Set the mechanism to the desired skin temperature (96.8° F to 97.8° F [36° C to 36.6° C]).
  - If the neonate is under a radiant warmer, use plastic wrap placed like a blanket to prevent heat and fluid loss. Use a sheet large enough to cover only the neonate. Border it with tape.
  - Attach a skin probe to the right upper quadrant of the neonate's abdomen. Don't place it over bone or the rib cage.
  - Use a heat shield for a very unstable neonate inside an isolette.
  - Monitor carefully for evaporative loss and insensible fluid loss. Keep in mind that radiant warmer and isolette therapy increase fluid maintenance needs.

  These measures help ensure safe use of a radiant warmer or isolette.
- Follow the prescribed treatment regimen for hypothermia, which may include administering an antibiotic in cases of sepsis, administering IV fluids, and feeding the neonate small, frequent portions, if appropriate. *Prescribed treatment helps eliminate infection and meet the neonate's fluid and nutrient needs.*
- Discuss precipitating factors with family members *to help prevent recurrence.*
- PCC Instruct family members in preventive measures, such as dressing the neonate appropriately and providing adequate nutrition for the neonate's growth needs. If the family requires financial help, refer them to the appropriate social service agency. *These precautions may help protect the neonate from future cold stress episodes.*

Suggested NIC Interventions

Circulatory Precautions; Environmental Management; Fluid/Electrolyte Management; Hypothermia Treatment; Newborn Care; Skin Surveillance; Temperature Regulation

Evaluations for Expected Outcomes

- Neonate's temperature returns to normal range.
- Neonate exhibits warm, dry skin and capillary refill time within normal limits.
- Neonate has cardiovascular assessment findings within normal limits.
- Neonate doesn't develop complications of hypothermia.
- Neonate doesn't begin shivering.
- Neonate doesn't develop signs of hyperthermia related to radiant heat source.
- Neonate is successfully weaned from isolette or radiant warmer bed.
- Family members verbalize understanding of causes of hypothermia and preventive measures.
- Family members demonstrate proper axillary or inguinal temperature measurement technique.
- Family members demonstrate willingness to provide adequate home care for neonate.

Documentation

- Neonate's physical assessment findings, including cardiovascular status, temperature, and shivering
- Nursing interventions and neonate's response to them
- Family members' willingness and abilities to provide adequate home care
- Evaluations for expected outcomes

REFERENCES

Çağlar, S., Gözen, D., & İnce, Z. (2014). Heat loss prevention (help) after birth in preterm infants using vinyl isolation bag or polyethylene wrap. *Journal of Obstetric, Gynecologic & Neonatal Nursing, 43*(2), 216–223. doi:10.1111/1552-6909.12291

Fawcett, K. (2014). Preventing admission hypothermia in very low birth weight neonates. *Neonatal Network. 33*(3), 143–149.

Munday, J., Hines, S., Wallace, K., Chang, A. M., Gibbons, K., & Yates, P. (2014). A systematic review of the effectiveness of warming interventions for women undergoing cesarean section. *Worldviews on Evidence-Based Nursing, 11*(6), 383–393. doi:10.1111/wvn.12067

Vilinsky, A., & Sheridan, A. (2014). Hypothermia in the newborn: An exploration of its cause, effect, and prevention. *British Journal of Midwifery, 22*(8), 557–562.

RISK FOR HYPOTHERMIA

Definition

Vulnerable to a failure of thermoregulation that may result in a core body temperature below the normal diurnal range, which may compromise health

Assessment

- History of present illness
- Gestational age
- Prenatal and intrapartal history
- Presence of maternal risk factors, such as fever, diabetes mellitus, drug use, dystocia, and history of perinatal asphyxia
- Neurologic status, including level of consciousness (LOC) and sensory status
- Cardiovascular status, including core temperature, heart rate and rhythm, blood pressure, and capillary refill time

- Respiratory status, including rate, rhythm, and depth; breath sounds; and arterial blood gas values
- Integumentary status, including temperature, color (central vs. peripheral), and turgor
- Nutritional status, including dietary pattern, birth weight, current weight, and recent weight changes
- Fluid and electrolyte status, including intake and output, serum glucose and electrolyte levels, and urine specific gravity
- Psychosocial status, including behavior, parental stressors, parental coping skills, and financial resources

Risk Factors

- Alcohol consumption
- Damage to hypothalamus
- Economically disadvantaged
- Extremes of age
- Extremes of weight
- Heat transfer (e.g., conduction, convection, evaporation, radiation)
- Inactivity
- Insufficient caregiver knowledge of hypothermia prevention
- Insufficient clothing
- Insufficient supply of subcutaneous fat
- Low environmental temperature
- Malnutrition
- Pharmaceutical agent
- Radiation
- Trauma

Children and Adults: Accidental

- Mild hypothermia, core temperature approaching 35° C
- Moderate hypothermia, core temperature approaching 32° C
- Severe hypothermia, core temperature approaching 30° C

Children and Adults: Injured Patients

- Hypothermia, core temperature approaching 35° C
- Severe hypothermia, core temperature approaching 32° C

Neonates

- Decrease in metabolic rate
- Delay in breastfeeding
- Early bathing of newborn
- Grade 1 hypothermia, core temperature approaching 36.5° C
- Grade 2 hypothermia, core temperature approaching 36.0° C
- Grade 3 hypothermia, core temperature approaching 35.0° C
- Grade 4 hypothermia, core temperature approaching 34.0° C
- High-risk out-of-hospital birth
- Immature stratum corneum
- Increased body surface area- to-weight ratio
- Increase in oxygen demand
- Increase in pulmonary vascular resistance
- Ineffective vascular control
- Inefficient nonshivering thermogenesis
- Unplanned out-of-hospital birth

Expected Outcomes

- Neonate will exhibit body temperature within normal limits.
- Neonate will have warm, dry skin and capillary refill time within normal limits.
- Neonate's cardiovascular status will be within normal limits.
- Neonate won't develop complications of hypothermia.
- Neonate won't shiver.
- Family members will verbalize knowledge of how hypothermia develops and will state measures to prevent recurrent hypothermia.

- Family members will demonstrate ability to measure neonate's temperature accurately.
- Family members will demonstrate willingness to provide adequate home care for neonate.

Suggested NOC Outcomes

Neurological Status: Autonomic; Thermoregulation; Vital Signs; Risk Control: Hypothermia

Interventions and Rationales

- Monitor body temperature every 1 to 3 hours by axillary or inguinal route (avoid rectal measurement). Record temperature and route. *Monitoring body temperature helps to detect developing complications.* If using an electronic heat source, such as a radiant warmer, monitor the device's temperature reading hourly and compare it with the neonate's body temperature *to evaluate the effectiveness of interventions.*
- Monitor and record neurologic status every 1 to 4 hours. *Falling body temperature and slowed metabolic rate may cause decreased LOC.*
- Monitor and record vital signs every 1 to 4 hours. As ordered, initiate and maintain continuous electronic cardiorespiratory monitoring. *These measures help avert metabolic acidosis and respiratory arrest.*
- Provide supportive measures:
  - Maintain a neutral thermal environment—a narrow range of environmental temperatures that maintain a stable core temperature with minimal caloric and oxygen expenditure. Determination of a neutral thermal environment depends on the neonate's age and weight.
  - If indicated, place the neonate in an open crib. For mild hypothermia, dress the neonate with an undershirt, diaper, and knitted or stockinette cap and cover him with double blankets.
  - Avoid overheating the neonate.
  - Keep the diaper area dry.
  - Keep head covered.
  - Cover all metal or plastic surfaces that could come in contact with the neonate.
  - Maintain the room temperature between 75° F and 78° F (23.9° C and 25.6° C).
  - Perform all procedures under a radiant warmer, if possible. Postpone bathing the neonate.

  These measures protect the neonate from heat loss.
- Discuss precipitating factors with family members *to help prevent recurrence.*
- PCC Instruct family members in preventive measures, such as dressing the neonate appropriately and providing adequate nutrition for the neonate's growth needs. If the family requires financial help, refer them to the appropriate social service agency. *These precautions may help protect the neonate from future cold stress episodes.*

Suggested NIC Interventions

Comfort Level; Fluid Management; Hypothermia Treatment; Temperature Regulation; Vital Signs Monitoring

Evaluations for Expected Outcomes

- Neonate's temperature returns to normal range.
- Neonate exhibits warm, dry skin and capillary refill time within normal limits.

- Neonate has cardiovascular assessment findings within normal limits.
- Neonate doesn't develop complications of hypothermia.
- Neonate doesn't begin shivering.
- Family members verbalize understanding of causes of hypothermia and preventive measures.
- Family members demonstrate proper axillary or inguinal temperature measurement technique.
- Family members demonstrate willingness to provide adequate home care for neonate.

Documentation

- Neonate's physical assessment findings, including cardiovascular status, temperature, and shivering
- Nursing interventions and neonate's response to them
- Family members' willingness and abilities to provide adequate home care
- Evaluations for expected outcomes

REFERENCES

Çağlar, S., Gözen, D., & İnce, Z. (2014). Heat loss prevention (help) after birth in preterm infants using vinyl isolation bag or polyethylene wrap. *Journal of Obstetric, Gynecologic & Neonatal Nursing, 43*(2), 216–223. doi:10.1111/1552-6909.12291

Fawcett, K. (2014). Preventing admission hypothermia in very low birth weight neonates. *Neonatal Network, 33*(3), 143–149.

Munday, J., Hines, S., Wallace, K., Chang, A. M., Gibbons, K., & Yates, P. (2014). A systematic review of the effectiveness of warming interventions for women undergoing cesarean section. *Worldviews on Evidence-Based Nursing, 11*(6), 383–393. doi:10.1111/wvn.12067

Vilinsky, A., & Sheridan, A. (2014). Hypothermia in the newborn: An exploration of its cause, effect, and prevention. *British Journal of Midwifery, 22*(8), 557–562.

RISK FOR INFECTION

Definition

Vulnerable to invasion and multiplication of pathogenic organisms, which may compromise health

Assessment

- Gestational age
- Neonate's temperature and vital signs
- Labor and delivery record, including premature rupture of membranes, characteristics of amniotic fluid (odorous or foul-smelling), and maternal temperature
- Maternal infections (recent or current), maternal disease or infection during pregnancy, and maternal pathogens passed on during birth process
- Condition of umbilical cord and skin at base of cord, including redness, odor, and discharge
- Signs and symptoms of neonatal infection, including lethargy, poor weight gain, restlessness, jaundice, visible lesions, thrush, temperature elevations or unstable low temperature, hypoglycemia, altered feeding patterns, diarrhea, vomiting, and subtle color changes such as cyanosis, mottling, or grayish skin tones
- Signs of respiratory distress, including grunting, retractions, nasal flaring, and cyanosis
- Evidence of chronic intrauterine infections, including growth retardation, microcephaly, and hepatosplenomegaly

Risk Factors

- Chronic illness (e.g., diabetes mellitus)
- Inadequate vaccination
- Insufficient knowledge to avoid exposure to pathogens
- Invasive procedure
- Malnutrition
- Obesity

Inadequate Primary Defenses

- Alteration in peristalsis
- Alteration in pH of secretions
- Alteration in skin integrity
- Decrease in ciliary action
- Premature rupture of amniotic membrane
- Prolonged rupture of amniotic membrane
- Smoking
- Stasis of body fluids

Inadequate Secondary Defenses

- Decrease in hemoglobin
- Immunosuppression
- Leukopenia
- Suppressed inflammatory response (e.g., IL-6, CRP)
- Inadequate vaccination

Increased Environmental Exposure to Pathogens

- Exposure to disease outbreak

Expected Outcomes

- Neonate's vital signs will remain within normal range.
- Neonate will be alert and active.
- Neonate will remain free from signs and symptoms of infection.
- Neonate's umbilical cord will heal properly and remain free from infection.
- Family members will demonstrate good handwashing technique before handling neonate.

Suggested NOC Outcomes

Immune Status; Infection Severity; Infection Severity: Newborn

Interventions and Rationales

- Review the maternal chart and delivery record *to detect risk factors that predispose the neonate to infection.*
- Assess the neonate's gestational age. *Passive immunity of the neonate via the placenta increases significantly in the last trimester, making the premature neonate much more susceptible to infection.*
- S Follow sterile technique. Remove all rings, bracelets, and wristwatches before handling the neonate. Scrub your hands and arms with an antimicrobial preparation before entering the nursery and after contact with contaminated material. Wash your hands again after handling the neonate. Instruct the parents and siblings in handwashing techniques and procedures. *These measures help prevent the spread of pathogens.*
- Monitor all hospital personnel, parents, and visitors for potential infection *to prevent spreading infection to the neonate.*
- Organize the nursery. Make sure the aisles are 38 (1 m) wide and cribs are 189 (45.7 cm) apart. Keep individual supplies separate for each neonate. *These measures help prevent cross-contamination.*
- Provide cover gowns for non-nursing personnel who enter the nursery *to prevent the spread of pathogens.*
- Provide eye prophylaxis, as facility policy dictates, *to prevent ophthalmia neonatorum or gonococcal or chlamydia infections.*

- Perform umbilical cord care with each diaper change, as facility policy dictates, *to promote healing, remove urine and stools, and facilitate desiccation process.*
- Assess respirations, pulse, and blood pressure every 15 minutes for 1 hour, then every hour for 4 hours, then once per shift or more frequently, as indicated. Assess temperature every 4 hours for 24 hours, then every 8 hours, or as indicated. *Unstable vital signs, persistent elevations in temperature, or hypothermia may indicate neonatal infection.*
- Observe the neonate for signs and symptoms of infection. Notify the physician immediately if signs and symptoms of infection appear *to ensure rapid identification and early treatment.*
- Observe standard precautions. Wear gloves before the neonate's first bath and when in contact with blood and body secretions. *Following standard precautions prevents cross-contamination and transmission of pathogens, including human immunodeficiency virus.*
- PCC Encourage the mother to begin breast-feeding early. *Colostrum and breast milk contain high amounts of immunoglobulin (IgM) A, which provides passive immunity to the neonate and helps reduce infection.*
- As ordered, monitor laboratory studies, including white blood cell (WBC) count, serum levels of IgM, and blood cultures. Culture any lesions, pustules, or drainage. *A decreased WBC count commonly indicates infection in a neonate; elevated IgM levels indicate that an infectious process has occurred in utero. Cultures identify pathogens and help guide antibiotic therapy.*
- Administer topical, oral, and parenteral antibiotics, as ordered, *to eradicate pathogenic organisms.*
- Observe the circumcision site for color, healing, and presence of drainage. *A fresh, healing circumcision site is a port of entry for bacteria.*

Suggested NIC Interventions

Environmental Management; Infection Control; Infection Protection; Newborn Care; Surveillance; Vital Signs Monitoring

Evaluations for Expected Outcomes

- Neonate's vital signs remain within normal range.
- Neonate is alert and active.
- Neonate is free from signs and symptoms of infection.
- Neonate's umbilical cord is clean, dry, and healing.
- Family members demonstrate proper handwashing technique before handling neonate.

Documentation

- Vital signs
- Appearance of umbilical cord
- Date, time, and sites of cultures
- Feeding patterns and weight gain
- Bowel elimination patterns
- Condition of oral mucosa
- Skin color and rashes
- Activity pattern
- Interventions performed to reduce risk of infection
- Neonate's response to nursing interventions
- Evaluations for expected outcomes

REFERENCES

Ezeh, O. K., Agho, K. E., Dibley, M. J., Hall, J., & Page, A. N. (2014). Determinants of neonatal mortality in Nigeria: Evidence from the 2008 demographic and health survey. *BMC Public Health, 14*, 521. doi:10.1186/1471-2458-14-521

Ganchimeg, T., Ota, E., Morisaki, N., Laopaiboon, M., Lumbiganon, P., Zhang, J., . . . Mori, R. (2014). Pregnancy and childbirth outcomes among adolescent mothers: A world health organization multicountry study. *International Journal of Obstetrics and Gynaecology, 121*(Suppl 1), 40–48. doi:10.1111/1471-0528.12630

Imamoglu, E. Y., Gunay, M., Cilek, E. A., & Karatekin, G. (2014). Bilateral blepharoconjunctivitis as the presenting sign of disseminated herpes simplex 1 infection in a preterm neonate. *Ocular Immunology and Inflammation, 22*(4), 326–329. doi:10.3109/09273948.2013.807346

Netto, C. M., Whitten, M., & Shetty, N. (2015). Postpartum sepsis. *British Journal of Hospital Medicine, 76*(8), C118–C121. doi:10.12968/hmed.2015.76.8.C118

RISK FOR INFECTION

during the postpartum period

Definition

Vulnerable to invasion and multiplication of pathogenic organisms, which may compromise health

Assessment

- Laboratory studies, including white blood cell (WBC) and platelet count, clotting factors, hemoglobin level, hematocrit, serum albumin level, and cultures of blood, body fluid, sputum, urine, and wound drainage
- Labor and delivery record, including episiotomy; presence of invasive devices, such as IV and urinary catheters; and premature rupture of membranes
- Presence of medical conditions such as diabetes mellitus that may increase incidence of infection
- Signs and symptoms of infection, including pallor, fatigue, malaise, anorexia, chills, foul-smelling lochia, calf tenderness, elevated temperature, dysuria, marked abdominal tenderness, and tender, reddened breasts that are warm to the touch

Risk Factors

- Chronic illness (e.g., diabetes mellitus)
- Inadequate vaccination
- Insufficient knowledge to avoid exposure to pathogens
- Invasive procedure
- Malnutrition
- Obesity

Inadequate Primary Defenses

- Alteration in peristalsis
- Alteration in pH of secretions
- Alteration in skin integrity
- Decrease in ciliary action
- Premature rupture of amniotic membrane
- Prolonged rupture of amniotic membrane
- Smoking
- Stasis of body fluids

Inadequate Secondary Defenses

- Decrease in hemoglobin
- Immunosuppression
- Leukopenia
- Suppressed inflammatory response (e.g., IL-6, CRP)
- Inadequate vaccination

Increased Environmental Exposure to Pathogens

- Exposure to disease outbreak

Expected Outcomes

- Patient's vital signs will remain within normal range.
- Results of laboratory studies won't indicate infection.
- Patient's respiratory secretions and urine won't show evidence of infection.
- Patient's episiotomy or abdominal incision site will remain free from infection.
- Patient's IV sites won't become inflamed.
- Patient will maintain good personal hygiene.
- Patient will state risk factors that can lead to infection.
- Patient will remain free from signs and symptoms of infection.

Suggested NOC Outcomes

Immune Status; Infection Severity; Knowledge: Infection Control; Risk Detection; Wound Healing: Primary Intention

Interventions and Rationales

S
- Minimize the patient's risk of infection by:
  - washing your hands before and after providing care. *Handwashing is the single best way to avoid spreading pathogens.*
  - wearing gloves to maintain asepsis when providing direct care and when in contact with blood or body secretions. *Gloves reduce the possibility of transmitting disease.*
  - After delivery, monitor vital signs every 15 minutes for 1 hour, then every 4 hours for 24 hours, then every shift until discharge. Report abnormal readings. *Elevated temperature, pulse or respiratory rates, or blood pressure may indicate infection. A temperature greater than 100.4° F (38° C) on two consecutive readings after the first 24 hours postdelivery may indicate puerperal sepsis, urinary tract infection, endometritis, mastitis, or other infection.*
- Monitor the WBC count, as ordered, and promptly report abnormal values. *A total WBC count above 11,000/μL indicates increased production of leukocytes by bone marrow, usually in response to bacterial pathogens.*
- As ordered, culture urine, respiratory secretions, wound drainage, or blood *to identify pathogens and guide antibiotic therapy.*

PCC
- Instruct the patient in proper personal hygiene, such as use of a sitz bath and perineal irrigation bottle, handwashing, and breast care, *to reduce the risk of infection.* Explain to the patient that the most common site of localized postpartum infection is the episiotomy site. Tell the patient how to apply sanitary pads (front to back) and how to remove them (back to front). Tell her to wipe the perineum after elimination and to clean the perineum from front to back. *These measures decrease bacterial concentration and help prevent genitourinary infections.*

S
- Follow the facility's infection-control policy *to minimize the risk of nosocomial infection.*

S
- Use strict sterile technique when performing invasive procedures, such as urinary catheterization or IV line insertion, *to minimize the risk of introducing pathogens into the body.*
- Assess the IV site every 4 hours, noting the presence of redness or warmth. Change IV tubing and site every 72 hours, or as dictated by facility policy. *These measures keep pathogens from entering the body.*

PCC
- Instruct the postoperative patient to deep breathe and cough *to help remove secretions and prevent respiratory complications.*
- Ensure adequate nutritional intake. *A diet high in protein, iron, and vitamin C helps promote healing.*
- Assess the patient for generalized signs and symptoms of infection (pallor, fatigue, malaise, anorexia, and chills) every shift, and instruct her to report danger signs immediately. These include foul-smelling lochia, calf tenderness, elevated temperature, dysuria, marked abdominal tenderness, and tender, reddened breasts that feel warm to the touch. *Prompt detection of infection helps minimize complications.*

Suggested NIC Interventions

Allergy Management; Cesarean Section Care; Infection Control; Perineal Care; Postpartal Care

Evaluations for Expected Outcomes

- Patient's vital signs remain within normal limits.
- Patient's WBC count and differential remain within normal range, and cultures don't indicate any pathogens.
- Patient's respiratory secretions are clear and odorless, and urine is clear yellow, odorless, and sediment-free.
- Patient's episiotomy or abdominal incision site remains free from infection.
- Patient's IV sites don't become inflamed.
- Patient performs proper personal hygiene on a regular basis.
- Patient states risk factors that can lead to infection.
- Patient remains free from infection.

Documentation

- Vital signs
- Appearance of episiotomy or abdominal incision site
- Date, time, and sites of cultures
- Date, time, and sites of catheter insertions
- Appearance of invasive catheter and IV sites
- Patient teaching about infection control
- Interventions performed to reduce risk of infection
- Patient's response to nursing interventions
- Evaluations for expected outcomes

REFERENCES

Buchanan, J., & Beckmann, M. (2014). Postpartum voiding dysfunction: Identifying the risk factors. *The Australian & New Zealand Journal of Obstetrics & Gynaecology, 54*(1), 41–45. doi:10.1111/ajo.12130

Ganchimeg, T., Ota, E., Morisaki, N., Laopaiboon, M., Lumbiganon, P., Zhang, J., . . . Mori, R. (2014). Pregnancy and childbirth outcomes among adolescent mothers: A world health organization multicountry study. *BJOG: An International Journal of Obstetrics and Gynaecology, 121*(Suppl 1), 40–48. doi:10.1111/1471-0528.12630

Kamel, A., & Khaled, M. (2014). Episiotomy and obstetric perineal wound dehiscence: beyond soreness. *Journal of Obstetrics and Gynaecology, 34*(3), 215–217. doi:10.3109/01443615.2013.866080

RISK FOR INFECTION

during labor and delivery

Definition

Vulnerable to invasion and multiplication of pathogenic organisms, which may compromise health

Assessment

- Vital signs, including fetal heart rate
- Health history, including previous infections
- Rupture of membranes, including time of rupture and characteristics of amniotic fluid (amount, color [blood tinged or meconium stained], and odor)
- Laboratory studies, including white blood cell (WBC) and platelet count, clotting factors, hemoglobin level, hematocrit, serum albumin level, and cultures of blood or body fluid, sputum, urine, and wound drainage
- Signs and symptoms of chorioamnionitis, including maternal pulse rate over 160 beats/minute, malodorous amniotic fluid, increasing uterine tenderness, and fetal tachycardia

Risk Factors

- Chronic illness (e.g., diabetes mellitus)
- Inadequate vaccination
- Insufficient knowledge to avoid exposure to pathogens
- Invasive procedure
- Malnutrition
- Obesity

Inadequate Primary Defenses

- Alteration in peristalsis
- Alteration in pH of secretions
- Alteration in skin integrity
- Decrease in ciliary action
- Premature rupture of amniotic membrane
- Prolonged rupture of amniotic membrane
- Smoking
- Stasis of body fluids

Inadequate Secondary Defenses

- Decrease in hemoglobin
- Immunosuppression
- Leukopenia
- Suppressed inflammatory response (e.g., IL-6, CRP)
- Inadequate vaccination

Increased Environmental Exposure to Pathogens

- Exposure to disease outbreak

Expected Outcomes

- Patient will maintain good hygiene.
- Patient will remain free from infection.
- Patient's temperature will remain within normal range.

Suggested NOC Outcomes

Immune Status; Infection Severity; Risk Detection; Self-Care: Hygiene; Wound Healing: Primary Intention

Interventions and Rationales

- Monitor and record the patient's temperature every 4 hours before the membranes rupture and every 2 hours after they rupture. *Temperature elevations are an early sign of infection.*
- Use continuous fetal monitoring to assess the fetal heart rate and variability. Report rates over 160 beats/minute and variability under 3 to 5 beats/minute. *Fetal heart rates over 160 beats/minute and minimal variability may indicate maternal fever.*
- Wash your hands thoroughly, using proper technique, before and after providing care *to prevent the spread of infection.*
- Maintain standard precautions. Wear gloves if you might come into contact with the patient's blood and body secretions. *Standard precautions protect you and the patient from the transfer of micro-organisms.*
- Use strict sterile technique when suctioning the lower airway, applying scalp electrodes, or inserting urinary catheters, pressure catheters, or IV lines *to reduce the likelihood of nosocomial infections.*
- After spontaneous or artificial rupture of the membranes, assess the color, amount, and odor of the amniotic fluid and the presence of blood or meconium. *Alterations in the color, amount, and odor of the amniotic fluid may indicate infection. Meconium may indicate a predisposition to intrauterine infection and fetal distress.*
- After rupture of the membranes, minimize vaginal examinations and always use sterile gloves *to decrease the risk of chorioamnionitis or other uterine infection.*
- Maintain good patient hygiene. Clean the perineal area from front to back and keep the area dry *to reduce the risk of infection.*
- Carefully monitor intake and output *to assess for dehydration. Signs and symptoms of infection (tachycardia, dry mucous membranes, and poor skin turgor) may resemble those of dehydration.*

Suggested NIC Interventions

High-Risk Pregnancy Care; Infection Control; Infection Protection; Intrapartal Care: High-Risk Delivery; Postpartal Care

Evaluations for Expected Outcomes

- Patient maintains good hygiene.
- Patient remains free from infection, as evidenced by clear, odorless, sediment-free urine; WBC count within acceptable limits for labor and delivery (up to 20,000/μL); and cultures free from pathogens.
- Patient's temperature ranges from 97° F to 99° F (36.1° C to 37.2° C).

Documentation

- Maternal vital signs
- Fetal heart rate and variability
- Date, time, and sites of cultures
- Date, time, and sites of catheter insertions
- Appearance of all invasive catheter and tube sites and wounds
- Nursing interventions performed to reduce risk of infection
- Patient's response to nursing interventions
- Evaluations for expected outcomes

REFERENCES

Axelsson, D., & Blomberg, M. (2014). Prevalence of postpartum infections: a population-based observational study. *Acta Obstetricia et Gynecologica Scandinavica, 93*(10), 1065–1068. doi:10.1111/aogs.12455

Ganchimeg, T., Ota, E., Morisaki, N., Laopaiboon, M., Lumbiganon, P., Zhang, J., . . . Mori, R. (2014). Pregnancy and childbirth outcomes among adolescent mothers: A world health organization multicountry study. *International Journal of Obstetrics and Gynaecology, 121*(Suppl 1), 40–48. doi:10.1111/1471-0528.12630

Netto, C. M., Whitten, M., & Shetty, N. (2015). Postpartum sepsis. *British Journal of Hospital Medicine, 76*(8), C118-C121. doi:10.12968/hmed.2015.76.8.C118

Parriott, A. M., Brown, J. M., & Arah, O. A. (2014). Predischarge postpartum methicillin resistant Staphylococcus aureus infection and group B streptococcus carriage at the individual and hospital levels. *Infectious Diseases in Obstetrics and Gynecology, 2014*. doi:10.1155/2014/515646

RISK FOR INJURY

Definition

Vulnerable to physical damage due to environmental conditions interacting with the individual's adaptive and defense resources, which may compromise health

Assessment

- Ability of parents to care for neonate
- Apgar scores
- Developmental stage (neonate and parents or caregivers)
- Environment, including air temperature, water temperature, and stability of equipment
- Labor and delivery record
- Laboratory studies, including blood glucose and bilirubin levels, white blood cell count, clotting factors, platelet count, hemoglobin level, hematocrit, and maternal and neonatal blood types
- Neonatal health history, including traumatic delivery, blood dyscrasia, hypothermia, and hyperthermia
- Neurologic status (neonate and parents or caregivers)
- Prenatal history

Risk Factors

External

- Alteration in cognitive functioning
- Alteration in psychomotor functioning
- Compromised nutritional source (e.g., vitamins, food types)
- Exposure to pathogen
- Exposure to toxic chemical
- Immunization level within community
- Nosocomial agent
- Physical barrier (e.g., design, structure, arrangement of community, building, equipment)
- Unsafe mode of transport

Internal

- Abnormal blood profile
- Alteration in affective orientation
- Alteration in sensation (resulting from spinal cord injury, diabetes mellitus, etc.)
- Autoimmune dysfunction
- Effector dysfunction
- Extremes of age
- Immune dysfunction
- Impaired primary defense mechanisms (e.g., broken skin)
- Malnutrition
- Sensory integration dysfunction
- Tissue hypoxia

Expected Outcomes

- Neonate will have physical and safety needs met.
- Family members will provide safe environment for neonate after discharge.
- Family members will recognize and report dangerous or potentially dangerous situations.
- Neonate won't experience injury.

Suggested NOC Outcomes

Parenting: Infant/Toddler Physical Safety; Parenting: Psychosocial Safety; Risk Control; Safe Home Environment

Interventions and Rationales

- Assess family members' baseline knowledge of neonatal safety. Instruct them, as needed. *Education in safety techniques minimizes the risk of injury.* Consider which teaching methods (pamphlets, videotapes, or demonstrations) best suit each family member's individual learning style *to facilitate learning.*
- S Immediately report malfunctioning equipment to appropriate personnel for replacement or repair *to help prevent accidents.*
- Keep one hand 1 to 2 (2.5 to 5 cm) inches above the neonate when measuring weight *to prevent the neonate from accidentally slipping off the scale.*
- S When transporting neonates from the nursery, take one bassinet at a time, if possible, *to improve safety.*
- Discourage family members from walking in the hall while holding the neonate *to avoid falls caused by wet or slippery floors.*
- Discourage the mother from sleeping in bed with the neonate. *While sleeping, she may accidentally turn over onto, or lose her grip on, the neonate.*
- Monitor the neonate's skin color for signs of jaundice every shift. *Hyperbilirubinemia occurs in approximately 50% of neonates. Elevated bilirubin levels can lead to neurologic and developmental difficulties.*
- Test the water temperature before washing the neonate. The temperature shouldn't exceed 100° F (37.8° C). *A neonate's fragile skin can't tolerate high temperatures.*
- Don't allow ill staff members or visitors to approach the neonate *to prevent transfer of pathogens.*
- Assess the neonate's potential for injury based on prenatal and labor and delivery records. *Early detection and treatment can minimize injury from intrauterine or perinatal insults.*
- S Never leave neonates unattended in an unprotected area. *Neonates are totally dependent on others for their physical, emotional, and safety needs.*
- Monitor respiratory and neurologic status as well as laboratory test results. Promptly report abnormal findings *to ensure immediate intervention and prevent complications.*
- Avoid heat loss to the neonate from evaporation. *Cold stress leads to increased metabolic rate, which can result in oxygen consumption and hypoglycemia.*
- Review with family members the state regulations regarding car seats before discharge *to decrease the risk of automobile injury or fatality.*

Suggested NIC Interventions

Environmental Management; Parent Education: Infant; Risk Identification; Surveillance: Safety

Evaluations for Expected Outcomes

- Parents meet neonate's physical and safety needs.
- Family members express understanding of techniques to ensure neonate's safety, after discharge, and practice safety techniques during neonate's stay in hospital.
- Family members express understanding of potentially dangerous situations.
- Neonate doesn't experience injury.

Documentation

- Neonate's skin color
- Temperature of radiant warmer and presence of functioning temperature probe
- Laboratory results
- Observations of physical findings
- Observations or knowledge of unsafe practices
- Instructions given to family members and their responses
- Interventions performed to prevent injury
- Neonate's response to nursing interventions
- Evaluations for expected outcomes

REFERENCES

Axelsson, D., & Blomberg, M. (2014). Prevalence of postpartum infections: A population-based observational study. *Acta Obstetricia et Gynecologica Scandinavica, 93*(10), 1065–1068. doi:10.1111/aogs.12455

Ezeh, O. K., Agho, K. E., Dibley, M. J., Hall, J., & Page, A. N. (2014). Determinants of neonatal mortality in Nigeria: Evidence from the 2008 demographic and health survey. *BMC Public Health, 14*, 521. doi:10.1186/1471-2458-14-521

Imamoglu, E. Y., Gunay, M., Cilek, E. A., & Karatekin, G. (2014). Bilateral blepharoconjunctivitis as the presenting sign of disseminated herpes simplex 1 infection in a preterm neonate. *Ocular Immunology and Inflammation, 22*(4), 326–329. doi:10.3109/09273948.2013.807346

Ravisankar, S., Syed, S. S., Garg, P., & Higginson, J. (2014). Is cronobacter sakazakii infection possible in an exclusively breastfed premature neonate in the neonatal intensive care unit? *Journal of Perinatology, 34*(5), 408–409. doi:10.1038/jp.2014.14

RISK FOR INJURY

during labor

Definition

Vulnerable to physical damage due to environmental conditions interacting with the individual's adaptive and defense resources, which may compromise health

Assessment

- Previous pregnancies
- Prenatal history, including prenatal laboratory studies, pelvic measurements, allergies, weight gain, last menses, and estimated date of confinement
- Physical examination, including maternal vital signs, Leopold's maneuvers (to determine fetal position), palpation of uterus (to assess frequency, intensity, and duration of contractions), sterile vaginal examination (to assess ripeness of cervix [Bishop score]), presentation, estimation of maternal pelvis, and fetal heart rate

- Diagnostic studies, including ultrasound to determine gestational age and fetal size, and nonstress test or contraction stress test to assess fetal–placental function
- Laboratory studies, including complete blood count, blood type and Rh factor, platelets, Nitrazine test (to confirm rupture of membranes), and urine protein and glucose levels
- Contraindications to oxytocin stimulation, such as absolute cephalopelvic disproportion, fetal distress, grand multipara, overdistention of uterus from multiple gestation or polyhydramnios, vaginal bleeding, and unfavorable fetal presentation or position

Risk Factors

External

- Alteration in cognitive functioning
- Alteration in psychomotor functioning
- Compromised nutritional source (e.g., vitamins, food types)
- Exposure to pathogen
- Exposure to toxic chemical
- Immunization level within community
- Nosocomial agent
- Physical barrier (e.g., design, structure, arrangement of community, building, equipment)
- Unsafe mode of transport

Internal

- Abnormal blood profile
- Alteration in affective orientation
- Alteration in sensation (resulting from spinal cord injury, diabetes mellitus, etc.)
- Autoimmune dysfunction
- Effector dysfunction
- Extremes of age
- Immune dysfunction
- Impaired primary defense mechanisms (e.g., broken skin)
- Malnutrition
- Sensory integration dysfunction
- Tissue hypoxia

Expected Outcomes

- Patient will have uterine contractions every 2 to 3 minutes, with intensity of 40 to 60 mm Hg (by internal monitoring).
- Continuous fetal monitoring will show fetal heart rate maintains variability of 6 to 10 beats/minute, with reassuring pattern.
- Patient will achieve good labor pattern, and neonate will be delivered without complications.
- Medical personnel will monitor patient closely for adverse reactions to oxytocin stimulation and will initiate appropriate interventions.
- Patient will maintain fluid balance.
- Patient and fetus will maintain optimal well-being.

Suggested NOC Outcomes

Fetal Status: Intrapartum; Maternal Status: Intrapartum; Risk Detection

Interventions and Rationales

- Explain oxytocin protocol to the patient and her support person. Describe how oxytocin-induced contractions may peak more quickly and last longer than spontaneous contractions *to allay apprehension and encourage patient participation.*
- Before applying a fetal monitor or administering oxytocin, encourage the patient to void. Palpate the bladder every 2 hours for distention. *A full bladder causes discomfort, especially when equipment is placed on the patient's abdomen.*

- Monitor intake and output, and measure urine specific gravity. *Decreased output with increased specific gravity may indicate urine retention, which may impede fetal descent.*
- Place the patient in as comfortable a position as possible. Left lateral tilt relieves the pressure of a gravid uterus on the inferior vena cava and promotes blood flow to the placenta. *Correct positioning enhances patient comfort and may help you obtain a clearer fetal monitoring strip.*
- Apply the fetal monitor and obtain a 15- to 20-minute baseline strip *to ensure adequate assessment of fetal heart rate and contraction pattern.*
- Use an 18G or 20G catheter when starting a primary IV line *to prepare for possible emergency interventions, such as cesarean delivery or blood administration.*
- S Prepare oxytocin, as ordered. Add the drug to a dextrose 5% injection or normal saline solution (initially, 10 units to 1,000 mL of solution). Label the bottle with the patient's name, amount of oxytocin, date and time prepared, and your name. Note that a physician must be present in the facility during oxytocin infusion. *Strict procedure ensures uniform administration and accurate assessment of uterine response.*
- S Piggyback oxytocin solution to the primary IV line at the site most proximal to the patient. Use an IV infusion pump to control the flow rate. *Insertion at the most proximal site to the patient prevents bolus infusion if oxytocin is stopped and the flow rate of the primary IV solution is increased. The infusion pump guarantees exact dose administration.*
- Begin infusion at the rate of 0.5 to 1 mU/minute. Remain with the patient during the first 20 minutes. *Initiating oxytocin at this rate enables you to evaluate the patient's individual response to stimulation.*
- Increase the oxytocin infusion by increments of 1 to 2 mU/minute, as ordered, every 30 to 60 minutes until the desired contraction pattern is achieved and the cervix is dilated 5 to 6 cm. Monitor blood pressure before and after each increase in dosage. *Increasing oxytocin slowly avoids hyperstimulation, which can cause fetal distress and uterine hypoxia.*
- If you increase to an infusion rate of 20 mU/minute without the patient achieving the desired contraction pattern, notify the physician. *Increments above 20 mU/minute increase the risk of hyperstimulation and water intoxication.*
- Monitor maternal vital signs every 15 to 30 minutes, as indicated by facility policy, *to assess for oxytocin-induced hypertension.*
- Monitor the contractile pattern and fetal heart rate every 15 minutes. Assess contractions by palpation or intrauterine pressure catheter. At least every 30 minutes, document the heart rate, variability, and fetal monitor strip changes. *Assessment of the fetal heart rate and variability allows you to detect nonreassuring fetal heart patterns. Palpation of contractions or intrauterine catheter monitoring allows you to monitor uterine activity.*
- If the patient responds poorly to oxytocin infusion, take these steps:
  - Check the IV mixture.
  - Check the lines for patency.
  - Increase the oxytocin flow rate, according to facility policy.
  - Palpate the uterine fundus for quality, duration, and relaxation of contractions.

  Errors in oxytocin mixture and IV administration can cause poor uterine response. An unripe cervix or uterus will also diminish the desired response. If the patient's response doesn't improve, the infusion may have to be discontinued after 8 to 12 hours and restarted the next day.
- Observe for hypertonicity—contractions lasting longer than 90 seconds and occurring less than 2 minutes apart. When using an intrauterine pressure catheter, a reading greater than 75 mm Hg indicates hypertonicity. *Because hypertonicity is unpredictable, the patient must be monitored carefully.*

- If you detect hypertonicity, discontinue infusion immediately. Check maternal vital signs and notify the physician. Increase the flow rate of the primary IV solution, and position the patient on her left side. *These measures will help arrest hypertonicity.*
- Monitor continuously for loss of variability, late decelerations, or persistent bradycardia *to detect fetal distress. Fetal distress may result from impaired uteroplacental perfusion caused by increased tonicity of contractions.*
- If you detect signs of fetal distress, take these steps:
  - Discontinue oxytocin infusion *to minimize the risk to the fetus.*
  - Administer 8 to 12 L of oxygen via a tight rebreathing mask *to increase the oxygen supply to the fetus.*
  - Increase the flow rate of the primary IV line *to increase fluids.*
  - Reposition the patient on her left or opposite side *to increase placental blood flow.*
  - Notify the physician *to expedite medical evaluation of maternal and fetal status.*
  - Assess maternal vital signs *to monitor for early signs of distress.*
  - Perform or assist with a sterile vaginal examination *to rule out possibility of umbilical cord prolapse.*
  - Make sure the patient isn't left unattended *to promote safety.*
- Assess the patient's intake and output, and monitor the amount of oxytocin administered over the course of stimulation. Total fluid intake shouldn't exceed 125 mL/hour. *Over time, the antidiuretic effects of oxytocin combined with the administration of large volumes of electrolyte-free solutions can lead to water intoxication.*

Suggested NIC Interventions

Bleeding Precautions; Electronic Fetal Monitoring: Intrapartum; Environmental Management; Intrapartal Care: High-Risk Delivery; Labor Induction; Medication Administration

Evaluations for Expected Outcomes

- Patient has contractions every 2 to 3 minutes that last 30 to 60 seconds and are of moderate intensity with adequate resting tonus.
- Continuous fetal monitoring shows fetal heart rate maintains variability of 6 to 10 beats/minute, with reassuring pattern.
- Patient achieves good labor pattern and delivers neonate without complications.
- Medical personnel monitor patient closely for adverse reactions to oxytocin stimulation and initiate appropriate interventions.
- Patient maintains fluid balance.
- Patient and fetus maintain optimal well-being during labor and delivery.

Documentation

- Patient's vital signs on admission and every 15 to 30 minutes, according to facility policy
- Baseline assessment of uterine activity (frequency, intensity, interval, duration, and tonus) before oxytocin stimulation and every 30 minutes thereafter via continuous electronic fetal monitoring
- Assessment of fetal heart rate, including baseline rate, long-term variability, short-term variability (with internal monitoring), accelerations, and periodic changes
- Patient's physical and emotional response to induction or augmentation of labor or both
- Nursing interventions to reduce risk of injury to patient or fetus from oxytocin stimulation
- Patient's response to nursing interventions
- Evaluations for expected outcomes

REFERENCES

Aiken, C. E., Aiken, A. R., & Prentice, A. (2015). Influence of the duration of the second stage of labor on the likelihood of obstetric anal sphincter injury. *Birth: Issues in Perinatal Care, 42*(1), 86–93. doi:10.1111/birt.12137

Moore, J. E., Low, L. K., Titler, M. G., Dalton, V. K., & Sampselle, C. M. (2014). Moving toward patient-centered care: Women's decisions, perceptions, and experiences of the induction of labor process. *Birth: Issues in Perinatal Care, 41*(2), 138–146. doi:10.1111/birt.12080

Murtagh, M., & Folan, M. (2014). Women's experiences of induction of labour for post-date pregnancy. *British Journal of Midwifery, 22*(2), 105–110.

NEONATAL JAUNDICE

related to infant experiences of difficulty making the transition to extrauterine life

Definition

The yellow-orange tint of the neonate's skin and mucous membranes that occurs after 24 hours of life as a result of unconjugated bilirubin in the circulation

Assessment

- Infant weight gain patterns and trends
- Laboratory studies including bilirubin level. Maternal risk factors (Rh, ABO)
- Labor and delivery history
- Infant fluid and electrolyte status
- Infant bowel elimination, stool characteristics

Defining Characteristics

- Abnormal blood profile
- Bruised skin
- Yellow mucous membranes
- Yellow sclera
- Yellow-orange skin color

Expected Outcomes

- Neonate will establish effective feeding pattern (breast or bottle) that enhances stooling.
- Neonate will not experience injury as a result of increasing bilirubin levels.
- Neonate will receive bilirubin assessment and screening within first week of life to detect increasing levels of serum bilirubin.
- Neonate will receive appropriate therapy to enhance bilirubin excretion.
- Neonate will receive nursing assessment to determine risk for severity of jaundice.

Suggested NOC Outcomes

Bowel Elimination; Breastfeeding Establishment; Infant; Nutritional Status; Risk Control; Risk Detection

Interventions and Rationales

- Evaluate maternal and delivery history for risk factors for neonatal jaundice (Rh, ABO, G6PD deficiency, direct Coombs, prolonged labor, maternal viral illness, medications) *to anticipate which neonates are at highest risk for jaundice.*
- Collect and evaluate laboratory blood specimens as ordered or per unit protocol *to permit accurate and timely diagnosis and treatment of neonatal jaundice.*
- PCC Educate parents regarding newborn care at home in relation to appearance of jaundice in association with any of the following: no stool in 48 hours, lethargy with refusal to nurse or bottle-feed, less than 1 wet diaper in 12 hours, abnormal infant behavior. *Parent education is crucial for the time after the neonate is discharged from the hospital. Parents are the major decision makers concerning whether and when to bring the neonate back for medical and nursing assessments after being discharged from the hospital.*
- Provide caring support to the family if a breast-fed neonate must receive supplementation. *It can be upsetting and result in feelings of inadequacy to a breast-feeding mother for her neonate to require supplementation.*
- PCC Coordinate care and facilitate communication between family, nursing staff, pediatrician, and lactation specialist. *A multidisciplinary approach that includes the family enhances communication and improves outcomes.*

Suggested NIC Interventions

Attachment Promotion; Kangaroo Care; Newborn Monitoring; Vital Signs Monitoring; Infant Care; Breastfeeding Assistance; Bottle-Feeding; Teaching: Infant Nutrition; Capillary Blood Sample; Surveillance; Risk Identification: Childbearing Family; Bowel Management; Discharge Planning

Evaluations for Expected Outcomes

- An effective feeding pattern has been achieved for the neonate that enhanced stooling.
- Neonate did not experience any injury as a result of increased bilirubin levels.
- Bilirubin assessment and screening was completed within first week of life.
- Neonate received the appropriate therapy to enhance bilirubin excretion.

Documentation

- Neonate's feeding pattern
- Neonate will receive appropriate therapy to enhance bilirubin excretion
- Record of completed assessments
- Therapy used to promote bilirubin excretion
- Evaluations for expected outcomes

REFERENCES

Aydin, D., Karaca Ciftci, E., & Karatas, H. (2014). Identification of the traditional methods of newborn mothers regarding jaundice in Turkey. *Journal of Clinical Nursing, 23*(3/4), 524–530. doi:10.1111/jocn.12150

El-Radhi, A. S. (2015). Management of common neonatal problems. *British Journal of Nursing, 24*(5), 258–265. doi:10.12968/bjon.2015.24.5.258

Fonseca, M. J., Severo, M., Barros, H., & Santos, A. C. (2014). Determinants of weight changes during the first 96 hours of life in full-term newborns. *Birth: Issues in Perinatal Care, 41*(2), 160–168. doi:10.1111/birt.12087

Fullwood, D., & Sargent, S. (2014). Complications in acute liver failure: Managing hepatic encephalopathy and cerebral oedema. *Gastrointestinal Nursing, 12*(3), 27–34.

O'Brien, P. (2015). Delayed cord clamping: The new norm. *British Journal of Midwifery, 23*(5), 312.

RISK FOR NEONATAL JAUNDICE

Definition

Vulnerable to the yellow-orange tint of the neonate's skin and mucous membranes that occur after 24 hours of life as a result of unconjugated bilirubin in the circulation, which may compromise health

Assessment

- Infant weight gain patterns and trends
- Laboratory studies, including bilirubin level
- Maternal risk factors (e.g., Rh, ABO)
- Labor and delivery history
- Infant fluid and electrolyte status
- Infant bowel elimination, stool characteristics

Risk Factors

- Abnormal weight loss (>7 to 8% in breast-feeding newborn, 15% in non-breast-feeding newborn)
- Age <7 days
- Delay in meconium passage
- Feeding pattern not well established
- Infant experiences difficulty making the transition to extrauterine life
- Prematurity

Expected Outcomes

- Parents will identify factors that place infant at risk for neonatal jaundice.
- Parents will identify potential signs of neonatal jaundice in infant.
- Neonate will establish effective feeding pattern (breast or bottle) that enhances stooling.
- Neonate will not experience injury as a result of increasing bilirubin levels.
- Neonate will receive bilirubin assessment and screening within first week of life to detect increasing levels of serum bilirubin.

Suggested NOC Outcomes

Bowel Elimination; Breastfeeding Establishment; Infant; Nutritional Status; Risk Control; Risk Detection

Interventions and Rationales

- Review history of the mother and prior obstetrical and medical histories in determining risk factors leading to neonatal jaundice. *Utilizing the knowledge about the maternal factors and blood type incompatibilities that can lead to neonatal jaundice aids the provider team in preparations.*
- At birth, assess the neonate for gestational age. *Neonates less than 38 weeks are at higher risk for jaundice.*
- At birth, assess the neonate for birthing trauma such as excessive bruising. *Bruising is indicative of increased bleeding, which results in hemolysis and leading to increased bilirubin.*

- At birth, place the neonate to the breast for initial feeding. *This stimulates the production of milk, initiating the process to produce sufficient milk for the infant over the next days.*
- Inject vitamin K (phylloquinone) into the vastus lateralus muscle of the neonate as prescribed. *Neonates lack vitamin K and cannot produce sufficient amounts for several weeks; injecting vitamin K provides a primary chemical for the clotting factors.*
- Examine the skin and head of the neonate carefully to determine bruising or the presence of cephalohematoma. *Presence of bruising/hematoma indicates bleeding and increases the risk for jaundice as the red blood cells are reabsorbed.*
- Rely on laboratory analysis for total serum bilirubin (TSB) or calibrated transcutaneous bilirubin (TcB) graphed on the Bhutani nomogram. *Accurate clinical observations of the neonate's skin color for jaundice is difficult in varying lighting settings and varying skin tone pigmentation. Laboratory and calibrated cutaneous readings provide consistent accurate measures and are interpreted using the nomogram.*
- S Adhere to nursery protocol on time intervals to obtain readings/heel stick blood. *Clinical protocols are critical for assessment and treatment of hyperbilirubinemia since there are specific time-rate increase factors. This differentiates "normal physiologic" hyperbilirubinemia from more serious hemolytic forms.*
- If the neonate is less than 38 weeks, at 12 hours postpartum, obtain a heel stick blood sample for TSB; graph results to the Bhutani nomogram; continue every 12 hours per protocol or provider orders. *At- risk premature neonates have elevated TSB in comparison with 38-week neonates.*
- Maintain the nursery protocol on assessing vital signs, bilirubin, weight, intake, diaper output, and other parameters. *Close vigilance by the caregivers will inform the providers of progress in the neonate's health status and hydration status.*
- Institute the treatment plan—aggressive breast-feeding and/or phototherapy. *Sufficient breast milk intake by the neonate prevents dehydration and assists in the elimination of bilirubin; exposure to therapeutic photo light converts insoluble bilirubin to a water-soluble form that is easily eliminated.*
- Provide information to the mother/family unit of the identified factors that may lead to neonatal jaundice. *Understanding information and expectations reduces anxiety.*
- Breast-feeding 8 to 12 times a day (every 2 to 3 hours), beginning immediately at birth, with adequate amounts of milk, decreases the incidence of hyperbilirubinemia. *Understanding information and expectations allows the mother to participate in the care of her newborn.*
- PCC Provide detailed information to the family unit regarding the interventions to prevent bleeding and increased bilirubin, assessment findings, the lab values, and treatments for the neonate. *Understanding expectations improves confidence and reduces anxiety.*
- PCC Support the family when they receive the knowledge that risk factors exist. *Understanding information and expectations reduces anxiety and allows the family to prepare for their participation in the treatment plan.*
- PCC Encourage the mother to breast-feed her newborn. *This allows the mother to be the active agent intervening for her newborn by breast-feeding.*
- Support bonding of the neonate and mother/family unit if the neonate receives phototherapy. *Understanding information and expectations of how the neonate will appear during therapy reduces anxiety and reduces barriers to bonding.*
- PCC Refer to lactation consultant to manage breast-feeding and methods to enhance milk production. *Expertise and support provide the confidence to achieve success in breast-feeding.*
- Emphasize the importance of follow-up at discharge for any level of hyperbilirubinemia; adhere to the clinical protocols and clinical pathways. *Neonates are frequently discharged after 24 hours and need to have professional evaluation to ensure that the bilirubin levels follow a predicted decrease.*

Suggested NIC Interventions

Attachment Promotion; Kangaroo Care; Newborn Monitoring; Vital Signs Monitoring; Infant Care; Breastfeeding Assistance; Bottle-Feeding; Teaching: Infant Nutrition; Capillary Blood Sample; Surveillance; Risk Identification: Childbearing Family; Bowel Management; Discharge Planning

Evaluations for Expected Outcomes

- Parents identify risk factors for neonatal jaundice.
- Parents identify potential signs of neonatal jaundice.
- Neonate establishes effective feeding pattern.
- Neonate has no injuries related to elevated bilirubin.
- Neonate's bilirubin is within normal limits.

Documentation

- Results of risk assessment
- Parents' expression of knowledge of signs of neonatal jaundice
- Results of blood test, weight, urine, and stool
- Nursing interventions and mother's/infant's response to them
- Evaluations for expected outcomes

REFERENCES

El-Radhi, A. S. (2015). Management of common neonatal problems. *British Journal of Nursing, 24*(5), 258–265. doi:10.12968/bjon.2015.24.5.258

Fullwood, D., & Sargent, S. (2014). Complications in acute liver failure: Managing hepatic encephalopathy and cerebral oedema. *Gastrointestinal Nursing, 12*(3), 27–34.

O'Brien, P. (2015). Delayed cord clamping: The new norm. *British Journal of Midwifery, 23*(5), 312.

Snyder, S. R., Kivlehan, S. M., & Collopy, K. T. (2015). HELLP syndrome. *EMS World, 44*(6), 39–45.

DEFICIENT KNOWLEDGE

related to insufficient information about birthing process

Definition

Absence or deficiency of cognitive information related to a specific topic

Assessment

- Age
- Psychosocial status, including developmental stage, previous experience with childbearing, expectations of the birth process, interest in learning, and current level of knowledge about pregnancy, birth, and recovery
- Ability to learn, including cognitive domain, intellectual and conceptual skills, and attention span
- Support systems, including presence of support person and support person's interest in helping patient and ability to participate in doing so

Defining Characteristics

- Inaccurate follow-through of instruction
- Inaccurate performance on a test
- Inappropriate behavior (e.g., hysterical, hostile, agitated, apathetic)
- Insufficient knowledge

Expected Outcomes

- Patient will recognize that increased knowledge and skill will help her cope better with birth process.
- Patient will demonstrate understanding of what she's taught.
- Patient will demonstrate ability to perform skills needed for coping with labor.
- Patient will express realistic expectations about birth process.
- Patient's level of anxiety about giving birth will be realistic.
- Patient will express satisfaction with her increased knowledge.

Suggested NOC Outcomes

Concentration; Knowledge: Labor & Delivery; Knowledge: Pregnancy; Motivation

Interventions and Rationales

- Find a quiet, private environment for teaching *the patient and support person. Freed from distractions, the patient and support person will learn more effectively.*
- Establish a trusting relationship with the patient. Develop mutual goals for learning. *These measures will enhance learning.*
- PCC Select teaching strategies appropriate to the material and patient's learning style (lecture, discussion, demonstration, practice, or audiovisual materials). *Careful selection of teaching strategies will enable you to better meet the patient's needs.*
- PCC Teach information and skills needed for understanding and coping during birth *to decrease the patient's anxiety and increase her sense of competence.* Evaluate the patient's level of understanding and ability to use knowledge during the birth process.

Suggested NIC Interventions

Anticipatory Guidance; Childbirth Preparation; Learning Readiness Enhancement; Teaching: Individual

Evaluations for Expected Outcomes

- Patient expresses intention to put knowledge to use during labor.
- Patient describes birth process in her own words.
- Patient correctly performs labor skills.
- Patient expresses realistic expectations of labor.
- Patient responds to labor without undue anxiety, using breathing, relaxation, and position changes to cope.
- Patient voices satisfaction with newly acquired knowledge and skills.

Documentation

- Patient's current understanding about birth process
- Patient's expression of need for better understanding or skills

- Learning goals established in cooperation with patient
- Information and skills taught to patient
- Teaching method used
- Patient's response to teaching
- Patient's mastery of information, including demonstration of new skills
- Evaluations for expected outcomes

REFERENCES

Ferguson, T. D., Howell, T. L., & Parsons, L. C. (2014). The birth experience: Learning through clinical simulation. *International Journal of Childbirth Education, 29*(3), 66–72.

Hoang, S. (2014). Pregnancy and anxiety. *International Journal of Childbirth Education, 29*(1), 67–70.

Jacinto, G. A., Molina, O., & Kirven, J. (2015). Birth: A write of passage process. *International Journal of Childbirth Education, 30*(1), 38–41.

Lothian, J. A. (2014). Listen up: What we can learn from women's birth and postpartum experiences. *Journal of Perinatal Education, 23*(1), 3–5. doi:10.1891/1058-1243.23.1.3

DEFICIENT KNOWLEDGE

related to insufficient information about neonatal care

Definition

Absence or deficiency of cognitive information related to a specific topic

Assessment

- Psychosocial status, including age, learning ability (affective, cognitive, and psychomotor domains), decision-making ability, developmental stage, financial resources, health beliefs and attitudes, interest in learning, knowledge and skills regarding neonatal care, obstacles to learning, support systems (willingness and capability of others to help), and usual coping pattern
- Neurologic status, including level of consciousness, memory, mental status, and orientation

Defining Characteristics

- Inaccurate follow-through of instruction
- Inaccurate performance on a test
- Inappropriate behavior (e.g., hysterical, hostile, agitated, apathetic)
- Insufficient knowledge

Expected Outcomes

- Patient will express need to improve her understanding of neonatal care.
- Patient will set realistic learning goals for developing competence in caring for neonate.
- Patient will express understanding of neonatal care.
- Patient will demonstrate ability to care for neonate independently or with minimal assistance.
- Patient will identify specific learning goals and target dates for mastering new skills.
- Patient will express intention to adjust lifestyle to accommodate arrival of neonate.
- Patient or family member will contact community resources when necessary.
- Family members will take active role in caring for neonate.

Suggested NOC Outcomes

Concentration; Information Processing; Knowledge: Infant Care; Knowledge: Postpartum Maternal Health

Interventions and Rationales

- Establish an environment of mutual trust and respect *to enhance learning. Achieving rapport is especially important in light of the maternity patient's short length of stay.*
- Assess the patient's level of knowledge. Does she have other children? Has she had recent experience caring for a neonate? *Answering these questions will determine whether the patient requires the basic information or reinforcement of previous learning.*
- Negotiate with the patient to develop goals for learning. *Allowing the patient to participate in decision making enhances learning.*
- PCC Select teaching strategies appropriate for the patient's individual learning style, such as one-on-one discussion and demonstration, attending unit-based neonatal care class, or viewing audiovisual materials. *Choosing an approach that best serves the patient increases the chance for successful learning.*
- PCC Teach skills that the patient must incorporate into daily life *to ensure the relevance of the learning experience.* Have the patient give a return demonstration of each new skill, such as feeding, diapering, and bathing the neonate, *to increase the patient's comfort level and identify areas of misunderstanding.*
- Have the patient incorporate learned skills into her daily routine during the hospital stay. Encourage the patient to care for the neonate in the hospital and allow for rooming-in, if possible. *Practicing skills leads to proficiency.* Acknowledge positive efforts *to increase the patient's self-esteem.*
- Provide the patient with names and telephone numbers of resources (such as a local breast-feeding association or child welfare service) to contact with questions. *The patient may benefit from additional sources of support during her hospital stay as well as after discharge.*
- PCC Encourage family members to become involved in the care of the neonate *to promote family unity and bonding with the neonate.*

Suggested NIC Interventions

Childbirth Preparation; Counseling; Health Education; Learning Facilitation; Referral; Teaching: Infant Safety

Evaluations for Expected Outcomes

- Patient expresses need to improve her understanding of neonatal care.
- Patient sets realistic learning goals.
- Patient expresses understanding of neonatal care.
- Patient demonstrates ability to care for neonate, including comfortably holding and playing with neonate, bottle-feeding or breast-feeding and burping neonate at appropriate intervals, caring for circumcision (when applicable) and umbilical cord site, providing scalp care, and bathing and diapering neonate.
- Patient sets specific learning goals and target dates for mastering new skills.
- Patient adjusts lifestyle to accommodate arrival of neonate.

- Patient or family members express willingness to follow up on referrals to community resources.
- Family members demonstrate willingness to take active role in neonatal care.

Documentation

- Patient's current level of knowledge and skills
- Patient's expressions indicating her motivation to learn
- Patient's learning objectives
- Methods used to teach patient
- Teaching provided
- Skills demonstrated
- Patient's response to teaching
- Evaluations for expected outcomes

REFERENCES

Cleveland, L. M., & Bonugli, R. (2014). Experiences of mothers of infants with neonatal abstinence syndrome in the neonatal intensive care unit. *Journal of Obstetric, Gynecologic & Neonatal Nursing, 43*(3), 318–329. doi:10.1111/1552-6909.12306

Strand, H., Blomqvist, Y. T., Gradin, M., & Nyqvist, K. H. (2014). Kangaroo mother care in the neonatal intensive care unit: Staff attitudes and beliefs and opportunities for parents. *Acta Paediatrica, 103*(4), 373–378. doi:10.1111/apa.12527

Turner, M., Chur-Hansen, A., & Winefield, H. (2014). The neonatal nurses' view of their role in emotional support of parents and its complexities. *Journal of Clinical Nursing, 23*(21/22), 3156–3165. doi:10.1111/jocn.12558

DEFICIENT KNOWLEDGE

related to insufficient information about postpartum self-care

Definition

Absence or deficiency of cognitive information related to a specific topic

Assessment

- Psychosocial status, including age, learning ability (affective, cognitive, and psychomotor domains), decision-making ability, developmental stage, financial resources, health beliefs and attitudes, interest in learning, knowledge and skills regarding postpartum self-care, obstacles to learning, support systems (willingness and capability of others to help patient), and usual coping pattern
- Neurologic status, including level of consciousness, memory, mental status, and orientation
- Physical ability to perform self-care activities

Defining Characteristics

- Inaccurate follow-through of instruction
- Inaccurate performance on a test
- Inappropriate behavior (e.g., hysterical, hostile, agitated, apathetic)
- Insufficient knowledge

Expected Outcomes

- Patient will communicate desire to learn how to care for herself after delivery.
- Patient will establish realistic learning goals.
- Patient will verbalize or demonstrate understanding of what she has learned about self-care.
- Patient will incorporate newly learned skills into daily routine.
- Patient will make changes in postpartum routine, including seeking help from health care professional, if necessary.

Suggested NOC Outcomes

Knowledge: Health Resources; Knowledge: Postpartum Maternal Health

Interventions and Rationales

- Establish an environment of mutual trust and respect *to enhance the patient's learning. Establishing rapport is especially important in light of the maternity patient's short length of stay.*
- Assess the patient's level of understanding of postpartum self-care activities *to establish a baseline for learning and provide direction for goal development.*
- Negotiate with the patient target dates for mastering postpartum self-care skills. *Having the patient participate in decision making will promote learning.*
- PCC Select teaching strategies (discussion, demonstration, role playing, or audiovisual materials) best suited for the patient's individual learning style *to enhance learning.*
- PCC Teach skills that the patient must incorporate into her daily postpartum routine, including perineal care, use of a sitz bath, use of witch hazel compresses, application and removal of perineal pads, and breast care. *Relevant topics enhance the patient's motivation to learn.*
- Have the patient give a return demonstration of each new skill *to reinforce learning.*
- PCC Teach the patient about the process of involution *to help her understand postpartum occurrences.*
- PCC Teach the patient the importance of adequate nutrition and hydration *to ensure proper urinary and bowel elimination.*
- Discuss the importance of adequate rest *to promote emotional and physical stability.*
- Have the patient incorporate learned skills into her daily routine during hospitalization. Acknowledge her efforts. *Practicing learned skills will help the patient gain proficiency.*
- PCC Provide the patient with names and telephone numbers of appropriate resource people and community service agencies *to provide further resources to help with problem solving, both during the patient's stay and after discharge.*

Suggested NIC Interventions

Health Education; Learning Facilitation; Nutritional Counseling; Postpartal Care; Teaching: Prescribed Activity/Exercise

Evaluations for Expected Outcomes

- Patient expresses motivation to learn.
- Patient establishes realistic learning goals.

- Patient verbalizes or demonstrates understanding of what she has learned, including process of involution and deviations from normal that she should report, ability to use sitz bath, and knowledge of hemorrhoidal care.
- Patient incorporates skills into her daily routine, including performing breast and perineal care, resuming normal bowel and bladder elimination, and obtaining adequate rest and sleep.
- Patient states intention of making changes in daily routine and seeking help from health care professional, if necessary.

Documentation

- Patient's understanding of and skills in postpartum self-care (including insight into her own abilities)
- Patient's expressions that indicate her motivation to learn
- Learning objectives
- Methods used to teach patient
- Information imparted to patient
- Skills demonstrated to patient
- Patient's response to teaching
- Evaluations for expected outcomes

REFERENCES

Ehrenthal, D. B., Maiden, K., Rogers, S., & Ball, A. (2014). Postpartum healthcare after gestational diabetes and hypertension. *Journal of Women's Health, 23*(9), 760–764. doi:10.1089/jwh.2013.4688
Lothian, J. A. (2014). Listen up: What we can learn from women's birth and postpartum experiences. *Journal of Perinatal Education, 23*(1), 3–5. doi:10.1891/1058-1243.23.1.3
Moshki, M., Baloochi Beydokhti, T., & Cheravi, K. (2014). The effect of educational intervention on prevention of postpartum depression: An application of health locus of control. *Journal of Clinical Nursing, 23*(15/16), 2256–2263. doi:10.1111/jocn.12505
Suplee, P. D., Bloch, J. R., McKeever, A., Borucki, L. C., Dawley, K., & Kaufman, M. (2014). Focusing on maternal health beyond breast-feeding and depression during the first year postpartum. *Journal of Obstetric, Gynecologic & Neonatal Nursing, 43*(6), 782–791. doi:10.1111/1552-6909.12513

DEFICIENT KNOWLEDGE

related to insufficient knowledge about premature labor

Definition

Absence or deficiency of cognitive information related to a specific topic

Assessment

- Age
- Psychosocial status, including decision-making ability, developmental stage, financial resources, health beliefs and attitudes, interest in learning, knowledge and skills regarding pregnancy and birth process, learning ability (affective, cognitive, and psychomotor domains), obstacles to learning, previous experience with premature labor, support systems (willingness and ability of others to help patient), and usual coping pattern
- Neurologic status, including level of consciousness, memory, mental status, and orientation

Defining Characteristics

- Inaccurate follow-through of instruction
- Inaccurate performance on a test
- Inappropriate behavior (e.g., hysterical, hostile, agitated, apathetic)
- Insufficient knowledge

Expected Outcomes

- Patient will communicate desire to learn about premature labor and will set realistic learning goals.
- Patient will express understanding of causes, signs and symptoms, and management of premature labor.
- Patient will identify and immediately report danger signals during and after hospitalization.
- Patient will voice emotional response to premature labor.
- Patient will use available support systems.
- Patient will cope successfully with premature labor.
- Pregnancy will result in positive outcome.

Suggested NOC Outcomes

Communication: Receptive; Knowledge: Labor & Delivery; Knowledge: Pregnancy; Motivation

Interventions and Rationales

- Introduce yourself to the patient and support person, and orient them to their surroundings. Explain all procedures beforehand. *These measures reduce the patient's anxiety.*
- Establish an environment of mutual trust and respect *to calm the patient, decreasing uterine stimulation from stress, and to provide an atmosphere conducive to learning.*
- PCC Work with the patient to develop realistic learning goals. *Unrealistic goals will frustrate you and the patient. Failure to achieve goals may reduce the patient's interest in learning.*
- Select the teaching strategy most appropriate for the patient and support person *to enhance learning.*
- Assess the patient's understanding of pregnancy and premature labor *to establish a basis for a nursing care plan and help guide future interventions.*
- Explain the causes, signs and symptoms, and treatment of premature labor to the patient and support person *to prepare them to actively participate in care.* Avoid information overload. *Anxiety may limit the patient's ability to assimilate information.*
- Project a warm, caring attitude and convey a willingness to listen *to encourage the patient to ask questions and voice feelings.*
- Don't place unrealistic demands on the patient *to avoid exacerbating feelings of inadequacy and anxiety.*
- Remain with the patient for uninterrupted periods. Assure the patient and support person that they can rely on staff for emotional support *to ease anxiety and establish a therapeutic relationship.*
- PCC Include the patient in the decision-making process when possible *to give her a sense of participation and control.*

- Provide positive feedback to the patient *to strengthen her self-esteem.*
- PCC Provide the patient with information related to her health status and the condition of the fetus. Inform the support person as well. *Continued knowledge of maternal and fetal health status helps relieve anxiety.*
- PCC Teach the patient the danger signs to report immediately, such as contractions occurring every 10 minutes or less for 1 hour, fluid leaking from the vagina, or lack of or altered fetal movement. *Promptly identifying and reporting danger signs helps avoid premature labor.*
- If the patient is discharged to home before delivery, review discharge instructions. Emphasize taking prescribed medications; limiting activities, as instructed; and reporting danger signs. *If the patient understands her needs and limitations, she may be able to avoid a recurrence of premature labor.*

Suggested NIC Interventions

Childbirth Preparation; High-Risk Pregnancy Care; Teaching: Individual

Evaluations for Expected Outcomes

- Patient expresses desire to learn about premature labor and sets realistic learning goals.
- Patient identifies possible causes and signs and symptoms of premature labor and expresses understanding of methods of managing it.
- Patient promptly reports danger signs and receives appropriate interventions.
- Patient expresses emotional response to premature labor.
- Patient uses available support systems.
- Patient successfully copes with premature labor as demonstrated by verbal and nonverbal behaviors.
- Pregnancy results in positive outcome.

Documentation

- Patient's statements indicating her understanding of premature labor
- Patient's expressions indicating her motivation to learn
- Learning objectives
- Methods used to teach patient and support person
- Information discussed with patient and support person
- Patient's and support person's responses to teaching
- Maternal and fetal physical status
- Evaluations for expected outcomes

REFERENCES

Amis, D. (2014). Healthy birth practice #1: Let labor begin on its own. *Journal of Perinatal Education, 23*(4), 178–187. doi:10.1891/1058-1243.23.4.178

Baker, B. (2015). Evidence-based practice to improve outcomes for late preterm infants. *Journal of Obstetric, Gynecologic & Neonatal Nursing, 44*(1), 127–134. doi:10.1111/1552-6909.12533

Castrillio, S., Rankin, K., David, R., & Collins, J. (2014). Small-for-gestational age and preterm birth across generations: A population-based study of Illinois births. *Maternal & Child Health Journal, 18*(10), 2456–2464. doi:10.1007/s10995-014-1484-1

Gonçalves Vieira Fernandes, N., & Batoca Silva, E. M. (2015). Parents' experience during the hospitalisation of the preterm infant. *Revista de Enfermagem Referência, 4*(4), 107–115. doi:10.12707/RIV14032

DEFICIENT KNOWLEDGE

related to insufficient knowledge about self-care activities during pregnancy

Definition

Absence or deficiency of cognitive information related to a specific topic

Assessment

- Age
- Psychosocial status, including decision-making ability, developmental stage, financial resources, health beliefs and attitudes, interest in learning, knowledge and skills regarding pregnancy, learning ability (affective, cognitive, and psychomotor domains), obstacles to learning, previous obstetric history, support systems (willingness and ability of others to help patient), and usual coping pattern
- Neurologic status, including level of consciousness, memory, mental status, and orientation

Defining Characteristics

- Inaccurate follow-through of instruction
- Inaccurate performance on a test
- Inappropriate behavior (e.g., hysterical, hostile, agitated, apathetic)
- Insufficient knowledge

Expected Outcomes

- Patient will communicate need for more information about self-care and will set realistic learning goals.
- Patient will demonstrate understanding of material taught.
- Patient will demonstrate ability to perform new health-related behaviors she has learned.
- Patient will continue to practice appropriate health-related behaviors after pregnancy.

Suggested NOC Outcomes

Knowledge: Health Resources; Knowledge: Pregnancy

Interventions and Rationales

- Establish an environment of mutual trust and respect *to help the patient relax and be receptive to learning.*
- PCC Negotiate realistic learning goals with the patient. *Unrealistic goals will frustrate you and the patient. Failure to achieve goals may reduce the patient's interest in learning.*
- Using open-ended questions, assess the patient's knowledge of pregnancy-related health practices *to establish a basis for a nursing care plan and help guide future interventions.*
- PCC Adapt teaching strategies (discussion, demonstration, role playing, or use of audiovisual materials) to the patient's individual learning style. *Tailoring teaching and content to the patient's learning style helps enhance learning.*
- PCC Refer the patient to appropriate resource people, agencies, and organizations *to ensure comprehensive care.*

- Discuss appropriate dental care and instruct the patient to visit a dentist early in pregnancy. *Poor oral hygiene and caries may result from nausea, vomiting, heartburn, and gum hyperemia associated with pregnancy.*
- Review the possible effects of caffeine, alcohol, addictive drugs, and tobacco on the developing fetus *to help ensure fetal well-being.* Tell the patient that any substance she ingests during pregnancy can affect the fetus. Explain that alcohol may cause developmental anomalies; marijuana and tobacco may cause intrauterine growth retardation and prematurity; and cocaine may cause abruptio placentae in the mother, and prematurity, poor feeding patterns, irritability, neural tube defects, and increased respiratory and heart rates in the neonate.
- Urge the patient to consult her physician or nurse-midwife before taking any medications *to avoid possible teratogenic effects on the fetus.*
- Review exercise routines designed for pregnant women and, if appropriate, refer the patient to an organized exercise group. *A regular exercise program during pregnancy enhances well-being and helps improve muscle tone in preparation for childbirth.*
- Review dietary intake for 1 week and instruct the patient in proper nutrition during pregnancy. Explain to the patient that she needs an extra 300 calories each day, for a total of 2,100 to 2,400 calories/day. Refer the patient to a dietitian, if appropriate. *The patient needs more calories to maintain optimal use of protein, allow for fetal and maternal tissue synthesis, and meet increased basal metabolic needs.*
- Discourage the patient from wearing constrictive clothing and shoes or high-heeled shoes. *High-heeled shoes increase the likelihood of developing low back strain, backache, and poor balance. Constrictive clothing and shoes can alter venous circulation.*
- PCC Discuss exposure to possible sources of toxic chemicals or gases *to avoid possible teratogenic effects on the developing fetus.*
- Review the patient's daily routine at home and at work. *The patient may need to alter her routine during pregnancy. For example, if she holds a sedentary job, she should walk about periodically to increase circulation to her legs. If she stands for long periods, she may need to adopt a less physically demanding posture.*
- PCC Instruct the patient to contact a physician or nurse-midwife immediately if she experiences danger signs or symptoms, including severe vomiting, frequent and severe headaches, epigastric pain, vision disturbances, swelling of fingers or face, altered or absent fetal movements after quickening, signs of vaginal or urinary tract infection, unusual or severe abdominal pain, or fluid discharge from the vagina. *Prompt identification of danger signs reduces the risk of an atypical pregnancy.*

Suggested NIC Interventions

Energy Management; Health Education; Parenting Promotion; Teaching: Prescribed Activity/Exercise; Teaching: Prescribed Diet; Childbirth Preparation; Intrapartal Care; Prenatal Care

Evaluations for Expected Outcomes

- Patient communicates need for more information about self-care and establishes realistic learning goals.
- Patient demonstrates understanding of material taught, including importance of:
  - maintaining appropriate diet
  - following appropriate exercise regimen
  - limiting or stopping smoking (if applicable)
  - not consuming illicit drugs or alcohol

- checking with physician or nurse-midwife before taking any medication
- limiting caffeine intake
- obtaining sufficient rest
- avoiding areas that may contain toxic chemicals or gases
- not wearing constrictive clothing and shoes or high-heeled shoes
- reporting danger signals to physician or nurse-midwife
- visiting dentist early in pregnancy
- taking prenatal vitamins as prescribed.

- Patient demonstrates ability to perform health-related behaviors she has learned during pregnancy.
- Patient continues to practice appropriate health-related behaviors after pregnancy.

Documentation

- Patient's knowledge of self-care activities during pregnancy
- Expressions indicating patient's motivation to learn
- Learning objectives
- Teaching methods
- Subject matter discussed in teaching session
- Record of dietary intake for 1 week
- Demonstration and return demonstration of skills
- Written and audiovisual materials given to patient
- Patient's response to teaching
- Evaluations for expected outcomes

REFERENCES

Bonura, K. B. (2016). Guest editor—Prenatal exercise as self-care: A gentle approach for childbirth educators. *International Journal of Childbirth Education, 31*(1), 7.

Chang, S., Chen, K., Lin, M., Lin, H., Huang, L., & Lin, W. (2014). A repeated measures study of changes in health-related quality of life during pregnancy and the relationship with obstetric factors. *Journal of Advanced Nursing, 70*(10), 2245–2256. doi:10.1111/jan.12374

Kolu, P., Raitanen, J., & Luoto, R. (2014). Physical activity and health-related quality of life during pregnancy: A secondary analysis of a cluster-randomised trial. *Maternal & Child Health Journal, 18*(9), 2098–2105. doi:10.1007/s10995-014-1457-4

Leppänen, M., Aittasalo, M., Raitanen, J., Kinnunen, T., Kujala, U., & Luoto, R. (2014). Physical activity during pregnancy: Predictors of change, perceived support and barriers among women at increased risk of gestational diabetes. *Maternal & Child Health Journal, 18*(9), 2158–2166. doi:10.1007/s10995-014-1464-5

RISK FOR DISTURBED MATERNAL–FETAL DYAD

Definition

Vulnerable to disruption of the symbiotic maternal–fetal dyad as a result of comorbid or pregnancy-related conditions, which may compromise health

Assessment

- Patient's understanding of health condition and treatment plan, past participation in health care planning, and decision making
- Patient's recognition and realization of potential growth, health, and autonomy
- Support systems, expressed concerns regarding maternal role

- Family status, including roles of family members
- Cultural status, including affiliation with racial, ethnic, or religious groups

Risk Factors

- Alteration in glucose metabolism (e.g., diabetes mellitus, steroid use)
- Compromised fetal oxygen transport (due to anemia, asthma, cardiac disease, hypertension, seizures, premature labor, hemorrhage, etc.)
- Inadequate prenatal care
- Pregnancy complication (e.g., premature rupture of membranes, placenta previa/abruption, multiple gestation)
- Presence of abuse (e.g., physical, psychological, sexual)
- Substance abuse
- Treatment regimen

Expected Outcomes

- Patient will be compliant with recommendations for self-care activities to minimize prenatal complications and optimize maternal/fetal health.
- Patient will verbalize fears and uncertainty related to prenatal conditions.
- Patient will actively involve significant other/support systems with pregnancy expectations and plan of care.
- Patient will demonstrate the "maternal tasks of pregnancy" culminating in an unconditional acceptance of the fetus before delivery.

Suggested NOC Outcomes

Prenatal Health Behavior; Knowledge: Pregnancy; Role Performance; Family Integrity

Interventions and Rationales

- Assess physical condition, psychosocial well-being, and cultural beliefs at each prenatal visit *to be able to counsel and/or refer as needed.*
- PCC Encourage support/involvement of significant other(s) during course of pregnancy *to enhance maternal role adaptation.*
- Incorporate the cultural beliefs, rites, and rituals of the childbearing family into the plan of care *to foster feelings of normalcy with pregnancy.*
- PCC Educate patient/significant other on role transition and maternal tasks of pregnancy *to provide anticipatory guidance on expected psychosocial changes.*
- PCC Teach trimester-specific risk/danger signs and emphasize importance of self-monitoring *to empower the patient and reduce potential for adverse fetal effects.*
- PCC Encourage patient to express disappointments/concerns related to relationships, physical condition, and fetal well-being *to promote therapeutic communication.*
- PCC Refer to community resources as needed (e.g., prenatal classes, psychological counseling, pastoral care, social services) *to facilitate appropriate role adaptation.*

Suggested NIC Interventions

Anticipatory Guidance; Childbirth Preparation; Coping Enhancement; Role Enhancement

Evaluations for Expected Outcomes

- Patient's physical and psychosocial well-being remained stable.
- Patient's maternal role adaptation was enhanced by support from significant other.
- Patient's cultural beliefs regarding childbearing were incorporated into the plan of care.
- Patient understood the trimester-specific risks and dangers and the importance of self-monitoring.
- Patient was able to express concerns related to relationships, physical condition, and fetal well-being.
- Patient was aware of appropriate resources to use to help with role adaptation.

Documentation

- Patient's prenatal record of physical and psychosocial condition
- Plan of care, including cultural beliefs related to childbearing
- Patient's understanding of trimester-specific risks and dangers and self-monitoring abilities
- Evaluations for expected outcomes

REFERENCES

Baker, B. (2015). Evidence-based practice to improve outcomes for late preterm infants. *Journal of Obstetric, Gynecologic & Neonatal Nursing, 44*(1), 127–134. doi:10.1111/1552-6909.12533

Dietz, P., Bombard, J., Mulready-Ward, C., Gauthier, J., Sackoff, J., Brozicevic, P., . . . Taylor, A. (2014). Validation of self-reported maternal and infant health indicators in the pregnancy risk assessment monitoring system. *Maternal & Child Health Journal, 18*(10), 2489–2498. doi:10.1007/s10995-014-1487-y

Folger, A. (2014). Maternal chlamydia trachomatis infections and preterm birth: The impact of early detection and eradication during pregnancy. *Maternal & Child Health Journal, 18*(8), 1795–1802. doi:10.1007/s10995-013-1423-6

Krans, E., Moloci, N., Housey, M., & Davis, M. (2014). Impact of psychosocial risk factors on prenatal care delivery: A national provider survey. *Maternal & Child Health Journal, 18*(10), 2362–2370. doi:10.1007/s10995-014-1476-1

IMBALANCED NUTRITION: LESS THAN BODY REQUIREMENTS

related to inability to ingest food

Definition

Intake of nutrients insufficient to meet metabolic needs

Assessment

- Gestational age
- Perinatal history
- Apgar score
- Suck and swallow reflex, including intactness of lips and palate
- Gastrointestinal assessment, including vomiting and regurgitation, stool characteristics (color, amount, consistency, and frequency), inspection of abdomen, auscultation of bowel sounds, palpation for masses, and percussion for tympany or dullness
- Nutritional status, including intake and output, current weight, weight change since delivery, skin turgor, urine characteristics (frequency and amount), signs of dehydration, and feedings (type, amount, and frequency)

- Laboratory studies, including urine glucose levels, urine bilirubin levels, and urine specific gravity
- Maternal assessment, including anesthetic used during labor and delivery, parity, knowledge level, and breast-feeding (condition of nipples and positioning of neonate)

Defining Characteristics

- Abdominal cramping
- Abdominal pain
- Alteration in taste sensation
- Body weight 20% or more below ideal weight range
- Capillary fragility
- Diarrhea
- Excessive hair loss
- Food aversion
- Food intake less than recommended daily allowance
- Hyperactive bowel sounds
- Insufficient information
- Insufficient interest in food
- Insufficient muscle tone
- Misinformation
- Misperception
- Pale mucous membranes
- Perceived inability to ingest food
- Satiety immediately upon ingesting food
- Sore buccal cavity
- Weakness of muscles required for mastication
- Weakness of muscles required for swallowing
- Weight loss with adequate food intake

Expected Outcomes

- Mother will demonstrate effective feeding techniques.
- Neonate won't lose more than 10% of birth weight.
- Neonate will retain entire feeding without vomiting or regurgitating.
- Neonate will ingest 130 to 200 oz/kg and 95 to 145 calories/kg/day.
- Neonate will establish effective suck and swallow reflexes, allowing for adequate nutritional intake.
- Neonate will maintain good (elastic) skin turgor, moist mucous membranes, urine specific gravity between 1.005 and 1.015, and flat, soft fontanels.
- Infant will gain at least 1 oz (28.4 g) each day for first 6 months after birth.

Suggested NOC Outcomes

Nutritional Status; Nutritional Status: Food & Fluid Intake; Nutritional Status: Nutrient Intake; Weight: Body Mass

Interventions and Rationales

- Obtain the neonate's weight at the same time each day, using the same scale, *to ensure early recognition of excessive weight loss.*
- If bottle-feeding, record the amount ingested at each feeding. If breast-feeding, record the number of minutes the neonate nurses at each feeding as well as ingestion of any supplement *to aid in early recognition of inadequate caloric and fluid intake.*
- Assess the parents' knowledge of feeding techniques. As needed, teach the parents how much and how often to feed the neonate, how to prepare formula, how to position the neonate during and after feeding, and how to burp the neonate. *Early detection of knowledge deficits and appropriate instruction help eliminate misconceptions.*
- Regularly assess the neonate's sucking pattern. Try to correct ineffective sucking patterns *to help eliminate ongoing difficulties.*

- Provide a preemie nipple or breast shell, as appropriate. *The preemie nipple's larger hole and softer texture make it easier for the neonate to obtain formula. A breast shell helps draw out an inverted nipple.*
- Make sure the neonate's tongue is properly positioned under the nipple *to enable the neonate to suck adequately.*
- Make sure the neonate is awake before feeding. Unwrap the blanket and tap the soles of the feet. *A tightly wrapped, drowsy neonate is less likely to be interested in feeding. The neonate must be fully awake and stimulated to suck effectively.*
- Record the number of stools and amount of urine voided each shift. *Decreased amounts of concentrated urine may indicate dehydration; an altered bowel elimination pattern may indicate decreased food intake.*
- Monitor the neonate for signs of dehydration, such as poor (inelastic) skin turgor, dry mucous membranes, decreased or concentrated urine, and sunken fontanels and eyeballs, *to establish the need for immediate medical intervention.*
- Assess the neonate for neurologic or other physical causes of ineffective sucking *to identify the need for more extensive evaluation.*
- Assess the need for gavage feeding. *The neonate may temporarily require an alternative means of obtaining adequate fluids and calories.*

Suggested NIC Interventions

Bottle-Feeding; Bowel Management; Fluid Monitoring; Nutrition Management; Teaching: Prescribed Diet; Weight Management

Evaluations for Expected Outcomes

- Mother demonstrates effective feeding techniques.
- Neonate returns to birth weight by 10 days after delivery.
- Neonate retains entire feeding.
- Neonate ingests 130 to 200 oz/kg and 95 to 145 calories/kg each day.
- Neonate establishes effective suck and swallow reflexes.
- Neonate maintains good skin turgor, moist mucous membranes, urine specific gravity between 1.005 and 1.015, and flat, soft fontanels.
- Infant gains at least 1 oz each day for first 6 months after birth.

Documentation

- Frequency, amount, and type of fluid ingested
- Incidence of vomiting and regurgitation
- Effectiveness of suck reflex
- Neonate's daily weight
- Parent's knowledge, level of caregiving, and bonding with neonate
- Frequency of bowel elimination and urination
- Signs of dehydration
- Nursing interventions and neonate's response
- Use of special nipple (such as preemie nipple)
- Results of laboratory studies
- Presence of physical or neurologic impairment
- Evaluations for expected outcomes

REFERENCES

Coleman Smith, V. (2016). The importance of infant nutrition. *International Journal of Childbirth Education, 31*(1), 32–34.

Martino, K., Wagner, M., Froh, E. B., Hanlon, A. L., & Spatz, D. L. (2015). Postdischarge breastfeeding outcomes of infants with complex anomalies that require surgery. *Journal of Obstetric, Gynecologic & Neonatal Nursing, 44*(3), 450–457. doi:10.1111/1552-6909.12568

Radzyminski, S. (2016). Mother's beliefs, attitudes, and decision making related to infant feeding choices. *Journal of Perinatal Education, 25*(1), 18–28. doi:10.1891/1058-1243.25.1.18

ACUTE PAIN

related to physical injury agent (e.g., abscess, amputation, burn, cut, heavy lifting, operative procedure, trauma, overtraining); physiologic changes of pregnancy

Definition

An unpleasant sensory and emotional experience associated with actual or potential tissue damage, or described in terms of such damage (International Association for the Study of Pain); sudden or slow onset of any intensity from mild to severe with an anticipated or predictable end

Assessment

- Characteristics of pain, including location, quality, intensity on a scale of 1 to 10, temporal factors, and sources of relief
- Physiologic variables, such as age and pain tolerance
- Psychological variables, such as body image, personality, previous experience with pain, anxiety, and secondary gain from symptoms
- Sociocultural variables, such as cognitive style, culture or ethnicity, and attitude and values
- Environmental variables, such as setting and time
- Understanding of pregnancy and birth process

Defining Characteristics

- Appetite change
- Change in physiologic parameter (e.g., blood pressure, heart rate, respiratory rate, oxygen saturation, and end-tidal CO_2)
- Diaphoresis
- Distraction behavior
- Evidence of pain using standardized pain behavior checklist for those unable to communicate verbally (e.g., Neonatal Infant Pain Scale, Pain Assessment Checklist for Seniors with Limited Ability to Communicate)
- Expressive behavior (e.g., restlessness, crying, vigilance)
- Facial expression of pain (e.g., eyes lack luster, beaten look, fixed or scattered movement, grimace)
- Guarding behavior
- Hopelessness
- Narrowed focus (e.g., time perception, thought processes, interaction with people and environment)
- Positioning to ease pain

- Protective behavior
- Proxy report of pain behavior/activity changes (e.g., family member, caregiver)
- Pupil dilation
- Self-focused
- Self-report of intensity using standardized pain scale (e.g., Wong-Baker FACES scale, visual analog scale, numeric rating scale)
- Self-report of pain characteristics using standardized pain instrument (e.g., McGill Pain Questionnaire, Brief Pain Inventory)

Expected Outcomes

- Patient will identify characteristics of pain.
- Patient will articulate factors that intensify pain and will modify behavior accordingly.
- Patient will carry out appropriate interventions for pain relief.

Suggested NOC Outcomes

Client Satisfaction: Symptom Control; Comfort Level; Nausea and Vomiting Severity; Pain Control; Pain Level

Interventions and Rationales

- Provide care for the patient experiencing nausea and vomiting:
  - Assess and document the extent of nausea and vomiting *to create a database for nursing interventions and patient teaching.*
  - Reassure the patient that nausea will usually subside by the fourth month of pregnancy *to reduce the patient's anxiety level and enhance compliance with nursing interventions.*
  - PCC Instruct the patient to eat dry, unsalted crackers before rising in the morning *to prevent nausea resulting from an empty stomach.*
  - Tell the patient to avoid greasy or spicy foods. Spicy foods irritate the stomach. *Fats with meals depress gastric motility and digestive enzyme secretion and slow intestinal peristalsis. These effects may lead to gastroesophageal reflux.*
  - Tell the patient to avoid cooking odors that predispose her to nausea and to use an electric fan while cooking *to help avoid nausea. Air circulation dilutes odors.*
  - Advise the patient to eat six small meals per day instead of three large ones *to avoid overloading the stomach.*
  - Advise the patient to eat foods high in carbohydrates. *Such foods are easier to digest.*
  - Tell the patient to take iron pills and vitamins after meals *to avoid irritating the stomach.*
  - Advise the patient to take frequent walks outdoors. *Walking in fresh air reduces nausea and helps reinforce a positive outlook.*
  - Tell the patient to separate food and fluid intake by ½ hour. *Drinking excessive fluids with meals distends stomach, predisposing patient to nausea. Taking fluids between meals also prevents dehydration.*
  - Advise the patient to avoid very cold fluids and foods at mealtimes. *Cold fluids and foods may cause nausea and abdominal cramping.*
  - Caution the patient to consult a physician before taking over-the-counter medications to treat nausea and vomiting *to avoid harmful effects on fetus.*

- Provide care for the patient experiencing urinary frequency:
  - Assess the patient for frequency and dysuria *to rule out a possible urinary tract infection (UTI).*
  - Reassure the patient that urinary frequency is normal in the early and late stages of pregnancy because the enlarging uterus places pressure on the bladder. *Reassurance may reduce the patient's confusion and anxiety.*
  - Tell the patient to avoid drinking large amounts of liquids within 2 to 3 hours of bedtime *to prevent frequent nocturnal urination and sleep loss.*
  - PCC Instruct the patient to ingest the required amount of liquids early in the day *to reduce the need for evening liquids.*
  - PCC Instruct the patient to void when the urge occurs *to prevent bladder distention and urinary stasis, which may predispose patient to UTI.*
  - PCC Teach the patient signs and symptoms of UTI. Urge her to report signs and symptoms promptly. *Early detection of UTI allows early treatment and helps prevent complications, such as pyelonephritis and premature labor.*
- Provide care for the patient experiencing breast fullness and tingling:
  - Assess the patient's breast discomfort *to obtain a database for further interventions.*
  - Assure the patient that breast changes and discomfort are natural. Tell her that fullness will last the entire pregnancy but that tenderness will resolve after the first trimester. *Reassurance decreases the patient's anxiety level and promotes compliance.*
  - Advise the patient to wear a supportive bra with wide, adjustable straps and smooth lining *to decrease irritation and provide support for enlarging breasts.*
  - PCC Instruct the patient to avoid tight bras and clothing that may confine breasts. *Pressure increases tenderness, tingling sensations, and discomfort.*
  - PCC Teach the patient the anatomy and physiology of breast changes during pregnancy. If indicated, begin preparation for breast-feeding at the end of the third trimester *to enhance breast-feeding experience.*
- Provide care for the pregnant patient who develops a headache:
  - Assess the type and location of the headache and associated signs and symptoms. *Assessment provides information for selection of interventions and clues to the patient's discomfort. The presence of associated factors, such as proteinuria, weight gain, edema, elevated blood pressure, and hyperreflexia, may indicate the occurrence of gestational hypertension.*
  - Advise the patient to sleep 8 hours each night and to nap or rest for 2 hours in the afternoon *to alleviate fatigue.*
  - Advise the patient to drink 6 to 8 glasses (1,500 to 2,000 mL) of fluid/day to prevent or alleviate a headache resulting from dehydration. *Increasing fluids may eliminate the headache by increasing vascular space and dilating cerebral veins.*
  - PCC Instruct the patient to apply cool, wet compresses to the forehead and back of the neck and to massage the neck, shoulders, face, and scalp. *Cool compresses may eliminate headaches resulting from emotional tension and spasms of sternocleidomastoid muscles of the neck and back.*
  - PCC Instruct the patient to take two acetaminophen tablets every 4 to 6 hours, as ordered. Tell her to avoid aspirin because of its anticoagulant action. Remind her to consult a physician before taking over-the-counter medications. *Acetaminophen effectively relieves minor headaches of pregnancy.*
- Provide care to the patient experiencing heartburn:
- Assess the patient's nutritional habits *to obtain clues to the patient's discomfort and information for selection of interventions.*
- Reassure the patient that normal pregnancy changes can cause heartburn *to decrease anxiety and increase compliance with nursing interventions.*

- Advise the patient to eliminate greasy and spicy foods from her diet and to avoid fats. *Such foods decrease stomach motility and increase the secretion of stomach acids and gastric acidity.*
- PCC Instruct the patient to reduce fluid intake with meals. *Liquids tend to inhibit gastric juices.*
- PCC Instruct the patient to avoid very cold foods. *Very cold foods promote gastric reflux.*
- PCC Instruct the patient to drink cultured milk, such as buttermilk, rather than regular whole milk. *Cultured milk has less fat than regular milk.*
- PCC Instruct the patient in good posture. *Good posture gives the patient's stomach more room to function.*
- PCC Instruct the patient to take small, frequent meals *to avoid overloading the stomach* and to remain upright for 3 to 4 hours after each meal *to decrease the possibility of reflux.*
- Advise the patient to use antacids that are low in sodium *to reduce the risk of tissue edema.* Tell her to take antacids that contain both aluminum and magnesium (such as Maalox and Riopan). *Aluminum-based antacids (such as Amphojel) may cause constipation. Magnesium-based antacids (such as Milk of Magnesia) have laxative effects. Aluminum–magnesium combinations tend to balance these effects.* Tell the patient to avoid antacids that contain sodium bicarbonate *to prevent hypokalemia, metabolic alkalosis, and hypernatremia.*

• Provide care for the patient with round ligament pain:
- Assess the onset and site of round ligament discomfort and associated uterine activity *to rule out the possibility of premature labor activity.*
- Reassure the patient that round ligament pain is normal during pregnancy and results from the stretching of ligaments that support the expanding uterus. *Reassurance will decrease anxiety and promote cooperation.*
- PCC Instruct the patient to avoid sudden jerky movement, to rise slowly from recumbent positions, and to avoid excessive exercise, standing, or walking. *Sudden, jerky movements or twisting of the torso pulls on round ligaments, causing unilateral or bilateral pain. Excessive exercise, standing, or walking can also strain abdominal muscles.*

• Provide care to the patient who experiences backache:
- Assess the patient's posture, lifting techniques, and footwear *to pinpoint causes of pain.*
- PCC Instruct the patient to wear low-heeled shoes, maintain good posture, and hold her shoulders back *to increase spinal curvature, which may reduce backache.*
- PCC Instruct the patient in proper body mechanics *to help her avoid stress to her lower back.*
- Tell the patient to rest in a recumbent position or with her legs bent and elevated on a bed or chair *to relieve strain on the lower back.*
- PCC Instruct the patient to perform moderate daily exercise *to tone and maintain muscle strength in the lower back.*
- Discuss the benefits of massaging and applying warm, moist heat to the lower back. *These measures will help relax and soothe tight muscles.*

• Provide care for the patient with hemorrhoids:
- Assess the patient's diet for fiber, fluids, and iron intake *to plan an appropriate diet that will enhance bowel function.*
- Assess prepregnancy bowel habits and history of hemorrhoids *to provide a database for planning interventions.*
- PCC Instruct the patient to avoid constipation by increasing intake of dietary fiber, bran cereals, and fluids. She should also drink warm water when she arises in the morning. *Avoiding constipation helps prevent straining at stool and lessens the risk of*

hemorrhoids. Dietary fiber, bran cereals, and fluids increase intestinal peristalsis and facilitate bowel function.
  - Encourage the patient to take sitz baths and to use witch hazel and Epsom salt compresses. *Warm sitz baths cause tissue dilation, increased blood flow, and healing. Witch hazel pads (such as Tucks) and Epsom salt compresses reduce tissue swelling.*
  - According to the physician's recommendation, encourage the use of analgesic ointments and topical preparations *to reduce pain.*
  - Administer stool softeners, as ordered, *to allow normal evacuation without straining.*
- Provide care for the pregnant patient with varicosities:
  - Assess for the degree of pain, family history, level of exercise, extent of varicosities, and history of varicosities before pregnancy. *Assessing pain helps rule out thrombophlebitis. Assessing the extent of varicosities and the patient's level of exercise helps plan for nursing interventions.*
  - Reassure the patient about the cause and usual duration of her discomfort *to decrease anxiety and promote compliance.*
  - Tell the patient to rest in a recumbent position, with her legs elevated above body level, twice per day *to promote venous return and avoid stagnation and pooling of venous blood.*
  - PCC Instruct the patient to put on supportive stockings before arising in the morning and to raise her legs when putting them on. *Supportive stockings promote venous return and increase comfort.*
  - Tell the patient to avoid garters and tight knee-high stockings and not to cross her legs *to reduce the risk of venous pooling and thrombus formation.*
  - Advise the patient to perform regular exercise, take frequent walks, and avoid sitting for long periods *to increase blood flow and retard stasis and pooling.*
- Provide care for the patient suffering from leg cramps:
  - Assess the patient's diet for excessive soft drink intake or inadequate dairy protein. *Inadequate dairy protein or excessive intake of soft drinks, which contain large amounts of phosphorus, can disrupt the body's calcium–phosphorus ratio, thereby leading to leg cramps.*
  - Reassure the patient that leg cramps are normal during pregnancy *to reduce anxiety and promote compliance.*
  - Tell the patient to consult with a physician about supplementing milk intake with aluminum hydroxide (Amphojel). *Taken with milk, aluminum hydroxide helps remove dietary phosphorus from the intestinal tract.*
  - PCC Instruct the patient to elevate her legs periodically and to avoid lying prone with toes pointed. *Lying prone with toes pointed predisposes the patient to blood vessel occlusion and subsequent cramping.*
  - Tell the patient to exercise and use good body mechanics to prevent leg cramping *by increasing general circulation.*
  - Advise the patient to take warm baths at bedtime *to relax muscle fibers and increase blood flow circulation to the muscles.*
  - If cramping occurs, tell the patient to straighten the affected leg and dorsiflex the foot. *These measures pull contracted muscle taut, thus relieving a cramp caused by contraction.*
  - Caution the patient not to rub the affected calf *to avoid risk of dislodging undetected thrombus.*
- Provide care for the patient who experiences Braxton Hicks contractions:
  - Assess the patient for frequency, strength, and regularity of contractions *to rule out preterm or true labor.*
  - Reassure the patient that Braxton Hicks contractions are normal in pregnancy *to reduce anxiety.*

PCC

- Instruct the patient to walk. *Walking may cause Braxton Hicks contractions to cease and can help distinguish them from true labor.*
- Advise the patient to assume a left lateral position when at rest *to increase blood flow to the uterus, which may decrease the intensity and frequency of contractions.*

Suggested NIC Interventions

Anxiety Reduction; Coping Enhancement; Environmental Management; Pain Management; Teaching: Individual

Evaluations for Expected Outcomes

- Patient identifies characteristics of pain.
- Patient lists factors that intensify pain and modifies behavior accordingly.
- Patient carries out appropriate interventions for pain relief.

Documentation

- Patient's description of pain and expression of feelings about pain
- Observations about patient's physical, psychological, and sociocultural responses to pain
- Comfort measures and medications provided to reduce pain
- Effectiveness of pain relief interventions
- Patient teaching about pain and pain relief
- Additional nursing interventions performed to assist patient with pain control
- Evaluations for expected outcomes

REFERENCES

Amorin-Woods, L. G., Beck, R. W., Parkin-Smith, G. F., Lougheed, J., & Bremner, A. P. (2014). Adherence to clinical practice guidelines among three primary contact professions: A best evidence synthesis of the literature for the management of acute and subacute low back pain. *Journal of the Canadian Chiropractic Association, 58*(3), 220–237.

Fitzgerald, K. (2015). Sixteen-year-old female with acute abdominal pain: A case report. *Integrative Medicine: A Clinician's Journal, 14*(6), 26–29.

Kwan, W. S., & Li, W. W. (2014). Effect of ear acupressure on acute postpartum perineal pain: A randomised controlled study. *Journal of Clinical Nursing, 23*(7/8), 1153–1164. doi:10.1111/jocn.12281

Sanders, R., & Lamb, K. (2014). An exploration of the benefits and drawbacks of intrapartum pain management strategies. *British Journal of Midwifery, 22*(9), 642–649.

ACUTE PAIN

related to physical injury agent (e.g., abscess, amputation, burn, cut, heavy lifting, operative procedure, trauma, overtraining); physiologic response to labor

Definition

An unpleasant sensory and emotional experience associated with actual or potential tissue damage, or described in terms of such damage (International Association for the Study of Pain); sudden or slow onset of any intensity from mild to severe with an anticipated or predictable end

Assessment

- Descriptive characteristics of pain, including location, quality, intensity on scale of 1 to 10, temporal factors, and sources of relief
- Physiologic variables, including age and pain tolerance
- Psychological variables, including body image, personality, previous experience with pain, anxiety, and secondary gain from symptoms
- Sociocultural variables, including cognitive style, culture or ethnicity, and attitude and values
- Environmental variables, including setting and time
- Understanding and expectations of labor and delivery

Defining Characteristics

- Appetite change
- Change in physiological parameter (e.g., blood pressure, heart rate, respiratory rate, oxygen saturation, and end-tidal CO_2)
- Diaphoresis
- Distraction behavior
- Evidence of pain using standardized pain behavior checklist for those unable to communicate verbally (e.g., Neonatal Infant Pain Scale, Pain Assessment Checklist for Seniors with Limited Ability to Communicate)
- Expressive behavior (e.g., restlessness, crying, vigilance)
- Facial expression of pain (e.g., eyes lack luster, beaten look, fixed or scattered movement, grimace)
- Guarding behavior
- Hopelessness
- Narrowed focus (e.g., time perception, thought processes, interaction with people and environment)
- Positioning to ease pain
- Protective behavior
- Proxy report of pain behavior/activity changes (e.g., family member, caregiver)
- Pupil dilation
- Self-focused
- Self-report of intensity using standardized pain scale (e.g., Wong-Baker FACES scale, visual analog scale, numeric rating scale)
- Self-report of pain characteristics using standardized pain instrument (e.g., McGill Pain Questionnaire, Brief Pain Inventory)

Expected Outcomes

- Patient will identify characteristics of pain and will describe factors that intensify it.
- Patient will modify behavior to decrease pain.
- Patient will express decrease in intensity of discomfort.
- Patient will experience satisfaction with her performance during labor and delivery.

Suggested NOC Outcomes

Client Satisfaction: Symptom Control; Comfort Level; Pain Control; Pain Level

Interventions and Rationales

- Orient the patient on admission to the labor and delivery suite. Show the patient her room and explain the operations of her bed and call bell. Explain admission protocol and the labor process. *These measures will allay the patient's initial anxiety.*
- Assess the patient's knowledge of the labor process and her current anxiety level *to plan supportive strategies.*
- PCC Explain available analgesics and anesthesia to the patient and support person. *Awareness that medications are available reduces anxiety.*
- PCC Encourage the support person to remain with the patient in labor. *A woman in labor will respond more readily to supportive measures offered by a familiar, caring person.*
- PCC Instruct the patient and support person in techniques to decrease the discomfort of labor:
  - Discuss techniques of conscious relaxation. *During labor, relaxation enables the patient to use coping techniques.*
  - Tell the patient to concentrate on an internal or external focal point. *A focal point allows controlled thoughts while breathing.*
  - Instruct the patient in basic deep chest breathing, which is similar to normal breathing but slower and deeper. *Deep chest breathing creates a sense of relaxation during contractions.*
  - Instruct the patient in shallow chest breathing. Tell her to take slow, panting-like breaths. *Slow breathing avoids hyperventilation. Shallow chest breathing lifts the diaphragm from the uterus during contractions, decreasing the intensity of contractions.*
  - Instruct the patient in effleurage. *This technique stimulates large- diameter sensory nerve fibers and interferes with the transmission of pain impulses to the brain.*
- In early labor, provide the patient with diversional activities, such as watching television, *to decrease anxiety.*
- As labor progresses, modify the environment to reduce distractions (close door, turn off television, and close curtains). *These measures help the patient to concentrate during the active phase of labor.*
- Apply sacral pressure to the patient, if needed, *to decrease back pain.*
- Help the patient change positions and use pillows *to make herself more comfortable.* Make sure all body parts are supported, with joints slightly flexed. *Frequent position changes reduce stiffness, prevent pressure sores, and promote comfort.*
- Assess the bladder for distention and encourage the patient to void every 2 hours. *A distended bladder increases the patient's discomfort during contractions and interferes with fetal descent.*
- Provide frequent mouth care. According to facility protocol, provide ice chips, water-based jelly, or a wet 4″ × 4″ gauze swab for dry lips *to relieve dry mouth and lips caused by breathing techniques and nothing-by-mouth status.*
- Apply a cool, damp cloth to the patient's forehead *to relieve diaphoresis.*
- Change the patient's gown and bed linens, as needed. *Diaphoresis and vaginal discharge can dampen the gown and bed and cause discomfort.*
- Encourage the patient to rest and relax between contractions *to decrease fatigue. Fatigue worsens pain perception and decreases the patient's ability to cope with contractions.*
- Discuss with the patient and support person which pain medications are available if alternative pain control methods prove inadequate. *The patient may need prescribed analgesics to cope with the labor process.*

Suggested NIC Interventions

Calming Technique; Medication Management; Pain Management; Simple Massage; Support System Enhancement

Evaluations for Expected Outcomes

- Patient identifies characteristics of pain and describes factors that intensify it.
- Patient modifies behavior to decrease pain, including using breathing techniques, asking for analgesia, when needed, and assuming more comfortable position.
- Patient reports decrease in intensity of discomfort.
- Patient expresses satisfaction with her performance during childbirth.

Documentation

- Patient's childbirth preparation and plans for giving birth
- Patient's description of pain
- Observation of patient's response to labor
- Nursing interventions to decrease discomfort
- Patient's response to nursing interventions
- Evaluations for expected outcomes

REFERENCES

Ondeck, M. (2014). Healthy birth practice #2: Walk, move around, and change positions throughout labor. *Journal of Perinatal Education, 23*(4), 188–193. doi:10.1891/1058-1243.23.4.188

Shirvani, M. A., & Ganji, Z. (2014). The influence of cold pack on labour pain relief and birth outcomes: A randomised controlled trial. *Journal of Clinical Nursing, 23*(17/18), 2473–2480. doi:10.1111/jocn.12413

Steel, A., Adams, J., Sibbritt, D., Broom, A., Frawley, J., & Gallois, C. (2014). The influence of complementary and alternative medicine use in pregnancy on labor pain management choices: Results from a nationally representative sample of 1,835 women. *Journal of Alternative & Complementary Medicine, 20*(2), 87–97. doi:10.1089/acm.2013.0171

Sullivan, D. H., & McGuiness, C. (2015). Natural labor pain management. *International Journal of Childbirth Education, 30*(2), 20–25.

ACUTE PAIN

related to physical injury agent (e.g., abscess, amputation, burn, cut, heavy lifting, operative procedure, trauma, overtraining); postpartum physiologic changes

Definition

An unpleasant sensory and emotional experience associated with actual or potential tissue damage, or described in terms of such damage (International Association for the Study of Pain); sudden or slow onset of any intensity from mild to severe with an anticipated or predictable end

Assessment

- Descriptive characteristics of pain, including location, quality, intensity on scale of 1 to 10, temporal factors, and sources of relief
- Physiologic variables, such as age and pain tolerance
- Psychological variables, such as body image, personality, previous experience with pain, anxiety, and secondary gain from symptoms
- Sociocultural variables, including cognitive style, culture or ethnicity, attitude and values, and birth order
- Environmental variables, such as setting and time

- Physical factors, including perineal pain, sulcus tears, hemorrhoids, hematomas, uterine discomfort, breast fullness and engorgement, nipple soreness or cracking, and episiotomy (type, extension, redness, edema, ecchymosis, discharge, and approximation)

Defining Characteristics

- Appetite change
- Change in physiologic parameter (e.g., blood pressure, heart rate, respiratory rate, oxygen saturation, and end-tidal CO_2)
- Diaphoresis
- Distraction behavior
- Evidence of pain using standardized pain behavior checklist for those unable to communicate verbally (e.g., Neonatal Infant Pain Scale, Pain Assessment Checklist for Seniors with Limited Ability to Communicate)
- Expressive behavior (e.g., restlessness, crying, vigilance)
- Facial expression of pain (e.g., eyes lack luster, beaten look, fixed or scattered movement, grimace)
- Guarding behavior
- Hopelessness
- Narrowed focus (e.g., time perception, thought processes, interaction with people and environment)
- Positioning to ease pain
- Protective behavior
- Proxy report of pain behavior/activity changes (e.g., family member, caregiver)
- Pupil dilation
- Self-focused
- Self-report of intensity using standardized pain scale (e.g., Wong-Baker FACES scale, visual analog scale, numeric rating scale)
- Self-report of pain characteristics using standardized pain instrument (e.g., McGill Pain Questionnaire, Brief Pain Inventory)

Expected Outcomes

- Patient will identify characteristics of pain and will describe factors that intensify it.
- Patient will understand and carry out appropriate interventions for pain relief.
- Patient will express comfort and relief from pain.

Suggested NOC Outcomes

Client Satisfaction: Symptom Control; Comfort Level; Pain Control; Pain Level

Interventions and Rationales

- Assess the patient's pain symptoms *to obtain information and plan appropriate nursing interventions.*
- As ordered, administer pain medications *to provide pain relief.*
- Discuss with the patient the reasons for her discomfort and its expected duration *to decrease anxiety and increase compliance.*
- Examine the episiotomy site for redness, edema, ecchymosis, drainage, and approximation *to detect trauma to perineal tissues or developing complications.*

- Inspect the rectum for hemorrhoids. Provide instruction on hemorrhoidal care, as appropriate. Tell the patient to apply ice for 20 minutes every 4 hours, apply a witch hazel compress, and use sitz baths. *Hemorrhoidal care will help decrease patient discomfort. Ice aids in the regression of hemorrhoids and vulval irritation by promoting localized vasoconstriction.*
- Apply ice packs to the episiotomy site for the first 24 hours *to increase vasoconstriction and reduce edema and discomfort.*
- Encourage the use of sitz baths. Baths should be cool to cold for the first day and warm (100° F to 105° F [37.8° to 40.6° C]) thereafter. The patient should take sitz baths three or four times per day, with each lasting about 20 minutes. *Sitz baths with cold water decrease edema and promote comfort. After 24 hours, moist heat increases circulation to the perineum, reduces edema, promotes healing, and enhances oxygenation and nutrition of tissues.*
- As ordered, teach the patient how to use sprays, creams, and ointments for the perineal area. *These products penetrate sensory nerve endings, providing a depressant effect on peripheral nerves, thereby reducing the response to sensory stimulation. Astringents, such as witch hazel, shrink tissues and reduce swelling.*
- Assess for uterine tenderness and the presence and frequency of after-birth pains every hour for first 24 hours, then every shift, as indicated. *In the first 12 hours after birth, uterine contractions are strong and regular. Factors that may intensify contractions include multiparity, breast-feeding, and oxytocin administration.*
- Encourage the patient to tighten the buttocks before sitting and to sit on a flat, padded surface. She should avoid foam donuts or soft pillows. *Tightening gluteal muscles before sitting reduces stress and direct pressure on the perineum. Because foam donuts separate the buttocks, they may decrease venous blood flow to the affected area, thereby increasing discomfort.*
- Inspect breast and nipple tissue for engorgement or cracked nipples *to ensure selection of appropriate nursing interventions.*
- PCC Encourage the breast-feeding mother to wear a supportive bra *to increase comfort* and to position the neonate properly during feedings. She shouldn't use the same position every time. *This will help prevent sore nipples.*
- If the breast-feeding patient is engorged, instruct her to use warm compresses or take a warm shower before breast-feeding and to breast-feed more often *to relieve discomfort. Warm compresses and showers help stimulate the flow of milk and may help relieve stasis and engorgement.*
- If the breast-feeding mother's nipples become sore, instruct her to air-dry the nipples for 20 to 30 minutes after feedings *to help toughen the nipples* and to apply breast creams, as ordered, *to soften the nipples and relieve irritation.* If only one nipple is sore or cracked, instruct her to offer the nontender nipple first for several feedings *to reduce potential trauma on the sore nipple.*
- Tell the non-breast-feeding patient to wear a tight supportive bra or breast binder and apply ice packs, as needed, *to prevent or reduce lactation.*
- Assess for bladder distention. Implement measures to facilitate voiding, and provide appropriate patient teaching. *Bladder fullness can cause discomfort.*
- After epidural or spinal anesthesia, assess the patient for spinal headache. Pain is primarily located behind the eyes but may radiate to the temples and occipital area. The supine position decreases pain; sitting or standing increases pain. Don't give pain medications before a medical evaluation of the source of the headache. Increase oral fluids, and notify the physician or anesthesiologist, as indicated. *Epidural or spinal anesthesia may lead to leakage of cerebrospinal fluid (CSF) and subsequent headache. Increasing oral fluids helps to compensate for the loss of CSF.*
- After a cesarean delivery, provide an abdominal pillow and teach the patient to splint the incision site when moving or coughing *to provide support for the abdominal muscles.*

Suggested NIC Interventions

Distraction; Heat/Cold Application; Pain Management; Presence; Simple Relaxation Therapy; Sleep Enhancement

Evaluations for Expected Outcomes

- Patient identifies characteristics of pain and describes factors that intensify it.
- Patient understands and carries out appropriate interventions for pain relief, including taking sitz baths and prescribed medications.
- Patient expresses comfort and relief from pain.

Documentation

- Patient's description of physical pain, pain relief, and feelings about pain
- Nurse's observations about patient's physical, psychological, and sociocultural responses to pain
- Comfort measures and medications provided to reduce pain
- Effectiveness of pain relief interventions
- Information provided to patient about pain and pain relief
- Additional nursing interventions performed to help patient control pain
- Evaluations for expected outcomes

REFERENCES

Chin, E. G., Vincent, C., & Wilkie, D. (2014). A comprehensive description of postpartum pain after cesarean delivery. *Journal of Obstetric, Gynecologic & Neonatal Nursing, 43*(6), 729–741. doi:10.1111/1552-6909.12483

Kwan, W. S., & Li, W. W. (2014). Effect of ear acupressure on acute postpartum perineal pain: A randomised controlled study. *Journal of Clinical Nursing, 23*(7/8), 1153–1164. doi:10.1111/jocn.12281

Power, T., Jackson, D., Carter, B., & Weaver, R. (2015). Misunderstood as mothers: Women's stories of being hospitalized for illness in the postpartum period. *Journal of Advanced Nursing, 71*(2), 370–380. doi:10.1111/jan.12515

LABOR PAIN

related to cervical dilation; fetal expulsion

Definition

Sensory and emotional experience that varies from pleasant to unpleasant, associated with labor and childbirth

Assessment

- Characteristics of pain, including intensity on 0 to 10 scale, location, quality, duration, and alleviating factors
- Behavioral response to pain
- Assessment of vital signs
- Understanding and expectations of labor and delivery

Defining Characteristics

- Alteration in blood pressure
- Alteration in heart rate
- Alteration in muscle tension
- Alteration in neuroendocrine functioning
- Alteration in respiratory rate
- Alteration in sleep pattern
- Alteration in urinary functioning
- Decrease in appetite
- Diaphoresis
- Distraction behavior
- Expressive behavior
- Facial expression of pain (e.g., eyes lack luster, beaten look, fixed or scattered movement, grimace)
- Increase in appetite
- Narrowed focus
- Nausea
- Pain
- Perineal pressure
- Positioning to ease pain
- Protective behavior
- Pupil dilation
- Self-focused
- Uterine contraction
- Vomiting

Expected Outcomes

- Patient will identify characteristics of pain and will describe factors that intensify it.
- Patient will modify behavior to decrease pain.
- Patient will express decrease in intensity of discomfort.
- Patient will experience satisfaction with her pain control during labor and delivery.

Suggested NOC Outcomes

Anxiety Level; Client Satisfaction: Pain Control; Comfort Status; Comfort Status: Physical; Nausea & Vomiting Severity; Vital Signs

Interventions and Rationales

- Orient the patient to the labor and delivery suite upon admission. *This helps alleviate the patient's initial anxiety.*
- Assess the patient's knowledge of the labor and delivery process and her current anxiety level *to plan supportive strategies.*
- Explain available analgesics and anesthesia to patient and support person. *Awareness of available medications will reduce anxiety.*
- PCC Explain available nonpharmacologic pain reductions strategies available to patient and support person. *Awareness of available methods will reduce anxiety.*
- PCC Encourage the support person to stay with the patient in labor *as a woman in labor will respond more readily to supportive measures offered by a familiar caring person.*
- Assist the patient and the support person in techniques to decrease the discomfort of labor:
  - Conscious relaxation. *During labor, relaxation enables the patient to use coping techniques.*
  - Concentration on an internal or external focal point. *A focal point allows controlled thoughts while breathing.*
  - Slow, deep chest breathing. *Deep chest breathing creates a sense of relaxation during contractions.*
  - Shallow chest breathing: slow panting like breaths. *Slow breathing avoids hyperventilation. Shallow chest breathing lifts the diaphragm from the uterus during contractions, decreasing the intensity of the contractions.*

- Effleurage. *This technique stimulated large- diameter sensory nerve fibers and interferes with the transmission of pain impulses to the brain.*
- In the first stage of labor, provide the patient with diversional activities *to decrease anxiety.*
- As labor progresses, modify the environment to reduce distractions (close the door, turn off television, and close curtains). *These measures help the patient concentrate during the active phase of labor.*
- If needed, apply sacral pressure to the patient, *to decrease back pain.*
- Assist the patient with position changes and use pillows to make her more comfortable. Assure all body parts are supported and joints are slightly flexed. *Frequent position changes promotes comfort, prevents stiffness, and prevents pressure ulcers.*
- Assess for bladder distention and encourage patient to void every 2 hours. *A distended bladder increases discomfort during contractions.*
- Provide frequent mouth care *to relieve dry mouth and lips caused by breathing techniques.*
- Apply a cool damp cloth to the patient's forehead *to relieve diaphoresis.*
- Change the patient's gown and linens as needed *to ease discomfort caused by diaphoresis or vaginal discharge.*
- Encourage patient to rest and relax between contractions to decrease fatigue. *Fatigue worsens pain perception and decreases the patient's ability to cope with contractions.*

Suggested NIC Interventions

Energy Management; Environmental Management: Comfort; Guided Imagery; Massage; Medication Administration; Music Therapy; Positioning; Relaxation Therapy; Vital Signs Monitoring

Evaluations for Expected Outcomes

- Patient identifies characteristics of pain and describes factors that intensify it.
- Patient modifies behavior to decrease pain, including using breathing techniques, asking for analgesia, when needed, and assuming more comfortable position.
- Patient reports decrease in intensity of discomfort.
- Patient expresses satisfaction with her pain control during childbirth.

Documentation

- Patient's childbirth preparation and plans for pain control while giving birth
- Patient's description of pain
- Observation of patient's response to labor
- Nursing interventions to decrease discomfort
- Patient's response to nursing interventions
- Evaluations for expected outcomes

REFERENCES

Garthus-Niegel, S., Knoph, C., Soest, T., Nielsen, C. S., & Eberhard-Gran, M. (2014). The role of labor pain and overall birth experience in the development of posttraumatic stress symptoms: A longitudinal cohort study. *Birth: Issues in Perinatal Care, 41*(1), 108–115. doi:10.1111/birt.12093

Sanders, R., & Lamb, K. (2014). An exploration of the benefits and drawbacks of intrapartum pain management strategies. *British Journal of Midwifery, 22*(9), 642–649.

Sullivan, D. H., & McGuiness, C. (2015). Natural labor pain management. *International Journal of Childbirth Education, 30*(2), 20–25.

IMPAIRED PARENTING

related to insufficient knowledge about child health maintenance; insufficient knowledge about parenting skills; insufficient response to infant cues

Definition

Inability of the primary caretaker to create, maintain, or regain an environment that promotes the optimum growth and development of the child

Assessment

- Parental status, including age and maturity, apprehension, parental role models during childhood, knowledge of child care and normal growth and development, previous bonding history, available support systems, coping mechanisms, and feelings about pregnancy and neonate
- Family status, including age, sex, status, and developmental stage of other children and parents' relationship with each other and with other children
- Mother's medical condition
- Neonatal status, including medical condition, separation from parents, and presence of medical equipment
- Psychosocial status, including financial stressors and work demands

Defining Characteristics

Infant or Child

- Behavior disorder (e.g., attention deficit, oppositional defiant)
- Delay in cognitive development
- Diminished separation anxiety
- Failure to thrive
- Frequent accidents
- Frequent illness
- History of abuse (e.g., physical, psychological, sexual)
- History of trauma (e.g., physical, psychological, sexual)
- Impaired social functioning
- Insufficient attachment behavior
- Low academic performance
- Runaway

Parental

- Abandonment
- Decrease in ability to manage child
- Decrease in cuddling
- Deficient parent–child interaction
- Frustration with child
- History of childhood abuse (e.g., physical psychological, sexual)
- Hostility
- Inadequate child health maintenance
- Inappropriate care-taking skills
- Inappropriate child-care arrangements
- Inappropriate stimulation (e.g., visual, tactile, auditory)
- Inconsistent behavior management
- Inconsistent care
- Inflexibility in meeting needs of child
- Neglects needs of child
- Perceived inability to meet child's needs
- Perceived role inadequacy
- Punitive
- Rejection of child
- Speaks negatively about child
- Unsafe home environment

Expected Outcomes

- Parents will establish contact with neonate.
- Parents will communicate feelings and anxieties about neonate's condition and their parenting skills.

- Parents will express willingness to care for neonate and will demonstrate competent parenting skills.
- Parents will demonstrate knowledge of neonate's developmental needs.
- Parents will become involved in planning and providing neonate's care.
- Parents will use available support systems to assist with care of neonate.

Suggested NOC Outcomes

Family Coping; Knowledge: Infant Care; Parent–Infant Attachment; Parenting Performance

Interventions and Rationales

- Before the parents' first visit to the neonatal intensive care unit (NICU), explain the appearance of the neonate and the presence of supportive devices *to prepare the parents for sights and sounds that may otherwise upset them.*
- PCC Encourage the mother to visit the NICU. Assess whether the mother can physically go, and offer assistance, if necessary. *The mother may hesitate to ask for help or may be unsure of her physical surroundings.*
- Provide the parents with a picture of the neonate *to help them accept the reality of the birth.*
- If the neonate must be transferred to another facility, arrange for the parents to meet the transfer team and visit with the neonate beforehand. *Seeing the neonate and meeting the transfer team will increase the parents' feelings of involvement and help them come to terms with the neonate's condition.*
- PCC Encourage the father or other family member to visit the neonate soon after admittance to the NICU or transfer to another facility, especially if the mother can't visit. *Firsthand reports from a family member about the neonate's condition and physical surroundings will help allay fears of the rest of the family.*
- Assess the parents' level of understanding of the neonate's condition and their expectations *to clear up misunderstandings, allow for prompt intervention, and promote realistic planning.*
- PCC Encourage the parents to express their anxieties related to the neonate's condition and their parenting skills *to identify and clarify misconceptions.*
- Make sure the parents are informed of the neonate's ongoing condition *to help decrease their anxiety and help them plan for the future.*
- PCC Encourage the parents to touch and talk to the neonate and call the neonate by name. Reassure them that touching the infant won't cause any harm. *This will stimulate bonding between the parents and the infant.*
- Allow time for the parents to care for the neonate within the secure environment of the hospital. Provide positive feedback for the parents' efforts to care for the neonate *to increase the parents' self-confidence.*
- Provide the parents with the NICU telephone number and encourage phone calls at any time *to make information about the neonate readily available.*
- PCC Refer the parents to social services, as needed, *to help ensure comprehensive care.*
- Encourage the parents to bring in personal items for the neonate, such as small stuffed animals or pictures of family members, *to encourage emotional bonding with the neonate.*

Suggested NIC Interventions

Attachment Promotion; Environmental Management: Attachment Process; Family Integrity Promotion; Infant Care; Parent Education: Infant

Evaluations for Expected Outcomes

- Parents initiate regular contact with neonate.
- Parents voice their anxieties about neonate's condition and their ability to provide care.
- Parents express willingness to meet neonate's basic needs and, if appropriate, special care needs, and display appropriate caregiving and attachment behaviors, including providing appropriate verbal, tactile, and auditory stimulation for neonate.
- Parents demonstrate knowledge of neonate's developmental needs.
- Parents take part in planning and providing neonate's care.
- Parents express awareness of and willingness to contact available sources of support.

Documentation

- Observations of parents' behavior
- Parents' statements concerning neonate
- Information provided to parents and their level of understanding
- Parents' interactions with neonate
- Parents' willingness to meet neonate's physical and emotional needs
- Consultations with health care team members
- Parents' and neonate's responses to nursing interventions
- Evaluations for expected outcomes

REFERENCES

Rossman, B., Greene, M. M., & Meier, P. P. (2015). The role of peer support in the development of maternal identity for 'NICU moms'. *Journal of Obstetric, Gynecologic & Neonatal Nursing, 44*(1), 3–16. doi:10.1111/1552-6909.12527

Samra, H. A., McGrath, J. M., Fischer, S., Schumacher, B., Dutcher, J., & Hansen, J. (2015). The NICU parent risk evaluation and engagement model and instrument (PREEMI) for neonates in intensive care units. *Journal of Obstetric, Gynecologic & Neonatal Nursing, 44*(1), 114–126. doi:10.1111/1552-6909.12535

Shao-Hui, S., Ying-Li, L., Hayter, M., & Ruey-Hsia, W. (2014). Efficacy of swaddling and heel warming on pain response to heel stick in neonates: A randomised control trial. *Journal of Clinical Nursing, 23*(21/22), 3107–3114. doi:10.1111/jocn.12549

Wuytack, F., Curtis, E., & Begley, C. (2015). Experiences of first-time mothers with persistent pelvic girdle pain after childbirth: Descriptive qualitative study. *Physical Therapy, 95*(10), 1354–1364. doi:10.2522/ptj.20150088

READINESS FOR ENHANCED PARENTING

Definition

A pattern of providing an environment for children or other dependent person(s) to nurture growth and development, which can be strengthened

Assessment

- Parental status that includes parents' age and maturity, parental role models during childhood, role satisfaction, adjustment to parental role, ability to relate appropriately to various age levels of children, willingness to adjust to various age needs, social support available, education needs of parent, present parenting skills, coping mechanisms, knowledge of child care and growth and development, discipline methods utilized, bonding and attachment issues

- Family status, including relationship of parents to each other, relationship of parents to children and to other dependent person(s), sibling relationships, spirituality, community involvement, age-appropriate safety issues, nutritional status, health care practices
- Psychosocial status including financial, single parent or dual parent family, educational level, employment, environment, stressors, affection and concern, consistency and reliability of parenting techniques

Defining Characteristics

- Children express desire to enhance home environment
- Expresses desire to enhance parenting
- Parent expresses desire to enhance emotional support of children
- Parent expresses desire to enhance support of other dependent person

Expected Outcomes

- Parents will express satisfaction in role of parent.
- Parents will express confidence in ability to parent.
- Home will exhibit signs of safe and functional environment.
- Child care or dependent persons care routines will be adequate.
- Children and dependent persons will appear nutritionally healthy.
- Family will appear to be physically healthy.
- Family will express belief in a higher spiritual power.
- Family will express enjoying spending time together.
- Parents will demonstrate consistency and effectiveness related to discipline.
- Family will express confidence in social and community resources available related to family needs.

Suggested NOC Outcomes

Parent–Infant Attachment; Parenting: Psychosocial Safety

Interventions and Rationales

- Discuss with the parents their perceptions and philosophy related to the role of parents in a family. *Verbalizing perceptions and beliefs provides an opportunity to clarify the parents' thinking.*
- PCC Offer the parents an opportunity to express their doubts or convictions about the adequacy of their parenting skills. *An open and receptive attitude provides an atmosphere for increased trust and enhanced learning.*
- PCC Support family efforts as they adapt to the ever-changing issues of family needs. *Recognition of and appreciation for one's efforts enhances motivation to continue to improve skills.*
- S Observe the home environment and discuss the issues of safety and cleanliness, if needed. *Family members need to have privacy and a sense of personal space as well as an environment that's free from environmental hazards, both chemical and physical.*
- Request that the parents describe a typical day with normal routines related to family dynamics and functioning. *This provides a concrete example for reflection of family functioning.*
- Discuss the food likes and dislikes of the family. *Parents need to be aware of nutritional preferences in order to increase family compliance for change.*

- Review the elements of a well-balanced diet for the various age groups represented in the family. *Different ages and developmental levels have different nutritional needs.*
- Discuss health care beliefs and practices with regard to the health maintenance of all family members. *Knowledge of sound health care practices enhances the well-being of family members.*
- Explore the family's value system as well as their spiritual beliefs and practices. *Spirituality and values provide a basis for ethical and moral reasoning and an enhanced meaning to life.*
- Encourage the family to "play" together. *Laughter and joy increase enjoyment and bonding as well as growth in the family unit.*
- Praise the family for traditions and activities that they do together. *Sharing meaningful activities increases loyalty, security, and a sense of belonging for family members.*
- PCC Engage the parents in a discussion of discipline practices and offer suggestions to enhance their present skills. *Discipline needs to be consistent, loving, and have reasonable guidelines. Children want and need limits so as to feel secure and safe.*
- PCC Explore the parents' perception of social support and community resources available to the family. *Social support and community resources provide guidance and positive reinforcement for parenting techniques and are a source of assistance and strength when families are experiencing stress.*

Suggested NIC Interventions

Developmental Enhancement: Child; Family Integrity Promotion: Childbearing Family; Family Involvement Promotion

Evaluations for Expected Outcomes

- Parents state enjoyment and satisfaction in the role of parent.
- Parents relate a positive sense of self and confidence in their ability to parent.
- Home environment is clean and free from chemical and physical hazards.
- Family functions in a structured and goal-oriented direction.
- Family members express participating in regular health and dental checkups.
- Family members express belief in a higher power and participation in their spiritual community.
- Family members look forward to family traditions, especially those related to holidays and vacations, and to spending time together as a family at school and community activities.
- Children are provided with consistent structure and guidelines; they express awareness of family rules and belief that those rules are fair.
- Family utilizes various social support venues as well as community resources to meet the needs of the family and individual family members.

Documentation

- Parents' feelings and concerns about parenting
- Discipline methods described by parents
- Interventions to assist family with identifying nutritional needs of various age groups
- Health care teaching for family with different age groups
- Parents' perception of social and community support and resources
- Evaluations for expected outcomes

REFERENCES

Collins, C., Duncanson, K., & Burrows, T. (2014). A systematic review investigating associations between parenting style and child feeding behaviours. *Journal of Human Nutrition & Dietetics, 27*(6), 557–568. doi:10.1111/jhn.12192

Seay, A., Freysteinson, W. M., & McFarlane, J. (2014). Positive parenting. *Nursing Forum, 49*(3), 200–208. doi:10.1111/nuf.12093

Wright, D. (2015). Supporting transitions to parenthood: Bonding with a baby that has down's syndrome. *Midwifery Matters, 2015* (147), 9–12.

RISK FOR SITUATIONAL LOW SELF-ESTEEM

Definition

Vulnerable to developing a negative perception of self-worth in response to a current situation, which may compromise health

Assessment

- Availability of support
- Patient's and support person's perception of labor and delivery
- Patient history, including past labor and delivery experience, ethnic and cultural background, and usual pattern of coping with stress
- Physiologic and behavioral changes during labor and delivery

Risk Factors

- Alteration in body image
- Alteration in social role
- Behavior inconsistent with values
- Decrease in control over environment
- Developmental transition
- Functional impairment
- History of abandonment
- History of abuse (e.g., physical, psychological, sexual)
- History of loss
- History of neglect
- History of rejection
- Inadequate recognition
- Pattern of failure
- Pattern of helplessness
- Physical illness
- Unrealistic self-expectations

Expected Outcomes

- Patient will express feelings about labor and delivery.
- Patient will set realistic goals for her behavior during labor and delivery.
- Patient will receive adequate emotional and physical support during labor and delivery.
- Patient will project positive self-concept through behavioral and verbal expression.

Suggested NOC Outcomes

Coping; Psychosocial Adjustment: Life Change; Self-Esteem

Interventions and Rationales

PCC
- Encourage the patient and support person to articulate their expectations of the labor and delivery experience *to identify and correct misconceptions early in the couple's experience.*

- Provide ongoing, positive feedback about the patient's behavior *to clear up misconceptions and increase feelings of self-esteem.*
- Emphasize realistic goals for behavior during labor and delivery. *Placing unrealistic demands on the patient can lead to feelings of inadequacy and poor self-esteem.*
- PCC Encourage the support person to express feelings about labor and delivery. *The patient may misunderstand how the support person viewed her behavior during labor.*
- PCC Encourage the patient to take active role in self-care activities after delivery *to reinforce the patient's ability to care for herself and increase self-esteem.*

Suggested NIC Interventions

Active Listening; Coping Enhancement; Emotional Support; Self-Esteem Enhancement

Evaluations for Expected Outcomes

- Patient expresses feelings about labor and delivery.
- Patient expresses realistic understanding of what to expect from her own behavior during labor and delivery.
- Patient expresses satisfaction with emotional and physical support received during labor and delivery.
- Patient's behavior and remarks reflect positive self-image.

Documentation

- Patient's behaviors and expressions that indicate low self-esteem
- Nurse's perceptions of patient's readiness for decision making
- Nursing interventions to improve patient's self-concept
- Patient's response to nursing interventions
- Patient's willingness to perform self-care activities
- Patient's expressions of well-being
- Evaluations for expected outcomes

REFERENCES

Gottesman, C. (2014). Stress relief at your finger tips for labor, delivery, and afterward. *International Journal of Childbirth Education, 29*(4), 28–31.

Kennell, J., & McGrath, S. (2005). Starting the process of mother–infant bonding. *Acta Paediatrica, 94*(6), 775–777.

Rossignol, M., Chaillet, N., Boughrassa, F., & Moutquin, J. (2014). Interrelations between four antepartum obstetric interventions and cesarean delivery in women at low risk: A systematic review and modeling of the cascade of interventions. *Birth: Issues in Perinatal Care, 41*(1), 70–78. doi:10.1111/birt.12088

Wiklund, I., Edman, G., & Andolf, E. (2007). Cesarean section on maternal request: Reasons for the request, self-estimated health, expectations, experience of birth and signs of depression among first-time mothers. *Acta Obstetricia et Gynecologica Scandinavica, 86*(4), 451–456.

IMPAIRED SKIN INTEGRITY

related to mechanical factor (e.g., shearing forces, pressure, physical immobility)

Definition

Altered epidermis and/or dermis

Assessment

- Age
- Vital signs
- Integumentary status, including color, elasticity, hygiene, lesions, moisture, quantity and distribution of hair, sensation, temperature, texture, and turgor
- Musculoskeletal status, including area affected by anesthetic procedure, joint mobility, muscle strength and mass, paralysis, and range of motion
- Health history, including past skin problems, trauma, surgery, chronic debilitating disease, and immobility
- Nutritional status, including appetite, dietary intake, hydration, present weight, and change from normal
- Laboratory studies, including hemoglobin levels, hematocrit, and serum albumin levels
- Psychosocial status, including coping patterns, family or significant other, mental status, occupation, self-concept, and body image
- Knowledge, including patient's current understanding of her physical condition and physical, mental, and emotional readiness to learn
- Presence of medical condition that may interfere with healing
- Extent of interruption in skin integrity because of delivery

Defining Characteristics

- Alteration in skin integrity
- Foreign matter piercing skin

Expected Outcomes

- Patient will demonstrate understanding of self-care activities.
- Patient will perform skin care routine.
- Patient will identify possible danger signs and report them immediately to physician.
- Patient will regain skin integrity.
- Patient's episiotomy or abdominal incision will heal without infection.
- Patient and partner will express feelings about possible change in body image.

Suggested NOC Outcomes

Tissue Integrity: Skin & Mucous Membranes; Wound Healing: Primary Intention

Interventions and Rationales

- Inspect the incision every shift using the REEDA (redness, edema, ecchymosis, discharge, and approximation) method. Document findings. *Frequent assessments can detect signs and symptoms of possible infection.*
- Perform the prescribed treatment regimen. Monitor progress and report favorable and adverse responses. *Periodic cleaning decreases bacterial concentrations, thus aiding the healing process. Monitoring response to treatment can help identify a possible need for alternative interventions.*
- PCC Instruct and assist the patient with general hygiene, including handwashing and toileting practices. *Proper handwashing is the most effective method of disease prevention. Bacteria from hands can easily contaminate other areas.*

PCC • Instruct and assist the patient in the use of sitz baths (three to four times daily) and perineal irrigation bottle (after each elimination). *Sitz baths aid the healing process by increasing circulation to the perineum and decreasing edema. Perineal irrigation bottles maintain cleanliness, thus decreasing bacterial concentration.*

PCC • Teach the patient how to apply and remove a maternity perineal pad. Tell her to apply a clean pad from front to back and to remove a soiled pad from back to front *to decrease the risk of contaminating the vaginal area with stools.*

PCC • Maintain infection control standards *to help minimize the risk of nosocomial infections.*

- Provide a splinting pillow for the patient with an abdominal incision. *Splinting provides support to the area, minimizing discomfort and encouraging the patient to move and cough.*
- Help the patient assume a comfortable position *to minimize the incidence of pain-induced immobility.*
- Inform the patient of the purpose of self-care practices *to increase compliance.*

PCC • Encourage the patient and partner to discuss the impact of impaired skin integrity. The patient's self-esteem may be lowered because of a scar from the abdominal incision. The patient or partner may be concerned about the effect the episiotomy will have on sexual relations. *Open communication increases understanding between partners.*

PCC • Instruct the patient and partner in the possible danger signs and symptoms that should be reported to the physician immediately. These include:
  - temperature above 100.4° F (38° C) on two consecutive readings
  - incisional drainage
  - increased discomfort at the episiotomy or incision site
  - reddened or warm skin surrounding the episiotomy or incision site

  Prompt reporting of danger signs and symptoms may help prevent major complications.

Suggested NIC Interventions

Cesarean Section Care; Incision Site Care; Perineal Care; Skin Surveillance

Evaluations for Expected Outcomes

- Patient demonstrates correct self-care practices.
- Patient performs skin care routine.
- Patient identifies possible danger signs and reports them immediately to physician.
- Patient regains skin integrity.
- Patient's episiotomy or abdominal incision site shows no redness, edema, ecchymosis, or discharge, and edges are approximated.
- Patient and partner communicate feelings about possibly altered body image or sexuality.

Documentation

- Patient's concerns about change in skin integrity
- Patient's willingness and ability to perform self-care practices
- Observations of episiotomy or abdominal incision site and response to treatment regimen
- Presence and type of skin closure method
- Instructions regarding treatment regimen and patient's understanding of instructions
- Prescribed treatment
- Interventions to provide supportive care
- Patient's response to nursing interventions
- Self-care practices performed by patient
- Evaluations for expected outcomes

REFERENCES

Gizzo, S., Andrisani, A., Noventa, M., Di Gangi, S., Quaranta, M., Cosmi, E., . . . Ambrosini, G. (2015). Caesarean section: Could different transverse abdominal incision techniques influence postpartum pain and subsequent quality of life? A systematic review. *Plos One, 10*(2), e0114190. doi:10.1371/journal.pone.0114190

Kamel, A., & Khaled, M. (2014). Episiotomy and obstetric perineal wound dehiscence: Beyond soreness. *Journal of Obstetrics and Gynaecology, 34*(3), 215–217. doi:10.3109/01443615.2013.866080

Melo, I., Katz, L., Coutinho, I., & Amorim, M. M. (2014). Selective episiotomy vs. implementation of a non- episiotomy protocol: A randomized clinical trial. *Reproductive Health,* 1166. doi:10.1186/1742-4755-11-66

RISK FOR SUDDEN INFANT DEATH SYNDROME

Definition

Vulnerable to unpredicted death of an infant

Assessment

- Age, sex, weight, ethnic background
- Perinatal history (gestational age, Apgar score, birth weight, birth order)
- Maternal history (age, socioeconomic status, level of education, parenting experience; smoking, alcohol, and drug history)
- Cardiovascular status (pulse, blood pressure, heart sounds)
- Respiratory status (respiratory rate, quality, depth, breath sounds)
- Neurologic status (alertness, reflexes—especially gag, suck, swallow, response to touch)
- Sleep routines (position, mattress, sleepwear, room temperature, co-bedding)
- Feeding routines (breast- or bottle-fed, ease of feeding, spitting up)

Risk Factors

Modifiable

- Delay in prenatal care
- Exposure to smoke
- Infant overheating
- Infant overwrapping
- Infant placed in prone position to sleep
- Infant placed in side-lying position to sleep
- Insufficient prenatal care
- Soft underlayment (e.g., loose items placed near infant)

Potentially Modifiable

- Low birth weight
- Prematurity
- Young maternal age

Nonmodifiable

- Age 2 to 4 months
- Ethnicity (e.g., African-American or Native American)
- Male gender
- Season of the year (i.e., winter and fall)

Expected Outcomes

- Parents will be receptive to teaching and guidance.
- Parents will verbalize understanding of risk factors and provide all precautions possible to prevent disorder.
- Infant will be placed in proper position on back with head of crib slightly elevated.

- Infant will be able to move extremities and head freely without restriction or without becoming tangled in loose bedding or articles.
- Infant will sleep alone in appropriate crib on firm sleep surface.
- Infant's body temperature will remain within normal limits.
- Infant will be monitored with apnea monitor during sleep.
- Parents state that they feel prepared and have the ability to handle emergencies utilizing CPR techniques and 911 services.
- Parents will handle the stress of knowing they have a high-risk infant with appropriate coping skills.

Suggested NOC Outcomes

Risk Control; Risk Detection

Interventions and Rationales

- PCC Educate the family about the risk factors of SIDS *so that they'll be aware of the current practices to reduce risk and prevent its occurrence.*
- S Position the infant on the back when placed in the crib. *Incidence of SIDS is higher among infants placed prone.*
- Make sure the infant's head is slightly elevated *to decrease abdominal pressure on the diaphragm and allow better expansion of the lungs.*
- PCC Teach the parents to avoid having loose blankets, toys, or other articles in the crib *to decrease the risk of accidental suffocation.*
- S Make sure the infant lies on a firm surface so that the infant doesn't sink into the mattress, mattress cover, or blanket *to decrease the risk of suffocation.*
- Avoid overheating the room and wrapping the infant's body in heavy blankets. *Overheating the infant increases the body's demand for oxygen.*
- Encourage the mother to breast-feed the infant *because this is associated with a lower incidence of SIDS.*
- S When an apnea monitor is ordered for the high-risk infant, teach the parents how to correctly apply the apparatus and leads and ensure that alarms are set correctly. The machine will sound an alarm if the respiratory rate or heart rate falls below a predetermined level (typically specified by the physician). *The benefit of the monitor can only be achieved if it's utilized appropriately.*
- S Instruct the parents in the correct application of CPR *to reduce anxiety and promote confidence in technique.*
- Assess the level of anxiety in the parents and family members routinely and provide suggestions for coping mechanisms *to assist the family in dealing with the period of vulnerability for the infant.*
- PCC Make appropriate referrals for community health nursing and home visits *to allow an opportunity to assess the home situation, care provided, and coping level of the family.*

Suggested NIC Interventions

Anticipatory Guidance; Anxiety Reduction; Caregiver Support; Coping-Enhancement; Emotional Support; Environmental Management: Safety; Family Integrity Promotion: Childbearing Family; Infant Care; Learning Facilitation; Parent Education: Childrearing Family; Positioning; Risk Identification: Childbearing Family; Teaching: Infant Safety

Evaluations for Expected Outcomes

- Parents listen and cooperate with patient teaching.
- Parents readily participate in education regarding SIDS risk factors and management.
- Parents utilize appropriate positioning of infant in crib.
- Infant moves freely without entanglement or suffocation in crib during sleep.
- Parents allow infant to sleep alone on firm surface.
- Infant's temperature remains within normal limits.
- Apnea monitor is utilized correctly.
- Parents utilize CPR and activate emergency services appropriately.
- Family members recognize need for heightened coping skills to deal with stress of high-risk infant.

Documentation

- Information given to parents regarding SIDS, positioning the infant, and sleeping arrangements
- Infant's temperature
- Demonstration of apnea monitor
- Attendance at CPR class
- Evaluations for expected outcomes

REFERENCES

Ball, H. L. (2015). Empowering families to make informed choices about sleep safety. *British Journal of Midwifery, 23*(3), 164–165.

Bartlow, K. L. (2016). Nurses' knowledge and adherence to sudden infant death syndrome prevention guidelines. *Pediatric Nursing, 42*(1), 7–13.

Brännström, I. (2014). Speaking discourses and silent lips: Women and gender-based portraits in sudden infant death publications. *Journal of Clinical Nursing, 23*(7/8), 1120–1132. doi:10.1111/jocn.12288

INEFFECTIVE THERMOREGULATION

related to extremes of age

Definition

Temperature fluctuation between hypothermia and hyperthermia

Assessment

- Gestational age
- Weight in relation to gestational age
- Neurologic status, including level of consciousness and motor and sensory status
- Cardiovascular status, including blood pressure, capillary refill time, electrocardiogram results, heart rate and rhythm, pulses (apical and peripheral), and temperature
- Respiratory status, including arterial blood gas measurements, breath sounds, and rate, depth, and character of respirations
- Integumentary status, including color, temperature, and turgor
- Fluid and electrolyte status, including blood urea nitrogen levels, intake and output, serum electrolyte levels, and urine specific gravity

- Laboratory studies, including clotting factors, hemoglobin levels, hematocrit, and platelet and white blood cell counts
- Environmental factors that contribute to heat loss, including radiation (loss of heat to objects not in direct contact with neonate), conduction (loss of heat through direct contact with cooler objects), convection (loss of heat from body surface to cooler surrounding air), and evaporation (changing of liquid to vapor)
- Coexisting conditions and diagnoses
- Maternal sedation before delivery

Defining Characteristics

- Cyanotic nail beds
- Fluctuations in body temperature above or below normal range
- Flushed skin
- Hypertension
- Increase in body temperature above normal range
- Increase in respiratory rate
- Mild shivering
- Moderate pallor
- Piloerection
- Reduction in body temperature below normal range
- Seizures
- Skin cool to touch
- Skin warm to touch
- Slow capillary refill
- Tachycardia

Expected Outcomes

- Neonate will maintain body temperature at normal levels.
- Neonate will have warm, dry skin.
- Neonate will maintain heart rate, respiratory rate, and blood pressure within normal range.
- Neonate won't exhibit signs of compromised neurologic status.
- Staff members will take steps to maintain neonate's body temperature at normal level.
- Parents will recognize and avoid possible sources of heat loss.
- Parents will express understanding of neonate's thermoregulatory disturbance and thermoregulation.

Suggested NOC Outcomes

Hydration; Newborn Adaptation; Thermoregulation: Newborn

Interventions and Rationales

- Monitor the neonate's body temperature after delivery *to obtain a baseline.* According to facility protocol, continue routine monitoring of the neonate's body temperature until discharge *to determine the need for intervention and the effectiveness of therapy. Timely intervention prevents complications related to prolonged cold stress.*
- Monitor and record the heart rate, respiratory rate, and blood pressure after delivery and routinely thereafter until discharge *to help ensure prompt diagnosis and treatment of conditions that may affect thermoregulation.*
- Monitor the results of laboratory studies for indications of sepsis or of metabolic or respiratory disorders. *Difficulty maintaining normal body temperature may indicate an underlying disorder. Conditions resulting from cold stress may further interfere with effective thermoregulation. For example, hypoxia, central nervous system trauma, and hypoglycemia may impair the neonate's ability to maintain normal body temperature.*

- Place the neonate under a radiant warmer device, with a temperature probe. When temperature is stable, transfer a healthy neonate to a regular open crib. Transfer a sick neonate to a servo-controlled open warmer bed or incubator. *These measures will help minimize oxygen consumption and metabolic rate, cause sweat gland activity to cease, and maintain deep body temperature at appropriate level.*
- Closely monitor the neonate's temperature and compare it with the temperature of the warming device. Be aware of potential hazards:
  - Make sure the temperature probe doesn't become detached from the neonate's skin *to prevent hyperthermia. Overheating increases the metabolic rate and, subsequently, oxygen consumption and may lead to apneic spells, particularly in a premature neonate.*
  - Don't place the temperature probe between the neonate and the mattress. *This can result in a falsely high reading, causing the warming device to decrease heat output, thus leading to hypothermia.*
  - Maintain an accurate record of environmental and core temperatures. Observe for variations in heater output. *Consistent variations in heater output may be symptomatic of sepsis.*
  - Monitor the neonate for signs of dehydration, including inelastic skin turgor, increased urine specific gravity, and dry mucous membranes. *Warming devices may contribute to insensible water loss.*
- Provide fluids based on the neonate's age, size, and condition. Monitor intake and output, and administer parenteral fluids, as ordered. *The neonate may need an increase in fluids to compensate for water loss caused by an increase in metabolic rate.*
- Maintain the environmental temperature at a comfortable setting. Take these steps:
  - Dry the neonate thoroughly after delivery.
  - Provide a bath only when the neonate's temperature is stable. After the bath, return the neonate to an incubator or warmer device until the neonate's temperature returns to the normal range.
  - Monitor the nursery temperature and humidity.
  - Provide heated, nebulized oxygen, when ordered.
  - Use an overhead warmer during procedures and extensive examinations.
  - Keep the incubator or radiant warmer away from windows and cold walls.
  - Ensure that linen and clothing are clean and dry.
  - Warm your hands before performing examinations and procedures.
  - Warm the examination table and instruments, such as scales and stethoscope, when possible, before exposure to the neonate.

  Maintaining the temperature of the external environment reduces the effects of heat loss from the body surface to the environment.
- PCC Teach family members about:
  - signs and symptoms of altered body temperature, such as cool extremities
  - factors in the home that contribute to neonatal heat loss and ways to minimize heat loss
  - signs of prolonged heat loss, including poor weight gain
  - the importance of contacting a health care provider when problems related to temperature regulation arise

  Careful teaching allows family members to take an active role in maintaining the neonate's health.

Suggested NIC Interventions

Environmental Management; Fluid Monitoring; Newborn Care; Newborn Monitoring; Temperature Regulation

Evaluations for Expected Outcomes

- Neonate's temperature is stable at 96.8° F to 98.6° F (36° C to 37° C) within 4 hours of birth.
- Neonate has warm, dry skin.
- Neonate maintains heart rate, respiratory rate, and blood pressure within normal limits.
- Neonate exhibits no signs of compromised neurologic status.
- Staff members keep neonate in neutral thermal environment throughout hospitalization.
- Parents minimize or eliminate potential for heat loss in home environment and incorporate precautions against ineffective thermoregulation into routine care of neonate.
- Parents express understanding of neonate's thermoregulatory disturbance and thermoregulation.

Documentation

- Physical findings
- Intake and output
- Laboratory results
- Vital signs, including blood pressure
- Environmental temperature
- Teaching provided to parents regarding thermoregulation
- Parents' expressions indicating understanding of problems related to thermoregulation
- Nursing interventions
- Neonate's response to interventions
- Evaluations for expected outcomes

REFERENCES

Nimbalkar, S. M., Patel, V. K., Patel, D. V., Nimbalkar, A. S., Sethi, A., & Phatak, A. (2014). Effect of early skin-to-skin contact following normal delivery on incidence of hypothermia in neonates more than 1800 g: Randomized control trial. *Journal of Perinatology: Official Journal of the California Perinatal Association, 34*(5), 364–368. doi:10.1038/jp.2014.15

Park, H., Choi, B. S., Lee, S. J., Son, I., Seol, I., & Lee, H. J. (2014). Practical application of kangaroo mother care in preterm infants: Clinical characteristics and safety of kangaroo mother care. *Journal of Perinatal Medicine, 42*(2), 239–245. doi:10.1515/jpm-2013-0066

Teodoro, J. S., Zouhar, P., Flachs, P., Bardova, K., Janovska, P., Gomes, A. P., . . . Kopecký, J. (2014). Enhancement of brown fat thermogenesis using chenodeoxycholic acid in mice. *International Journal of Obesity, 38*(8), 1027–1034. doi:10.1038/ijo.2013.230

IMPAIRED URINARY ELIMINATION

related to sensory impairment during labor

Definition

Dysfunction in urine elimination

Assessment

- Vital signs
- History of sensory or neuromuscular impairment, urinary tract trauma, surgery, or infection

- Genitourinary status, including palpation of bladder, voiding pattern, urine characteristics, and presence of pain or discomfort
- Labor and delivery, including anesthesia (regional or local) and oxytocin induction or augmentation
- Fluid and electrolyte status, including skin turgor, intake and output, urine specific gravity, and inspection of mucous membranes
- Neuromuscular status, including ability to perceive bladder fullness

Defining Characteristics

- Dysuria
- Frequent voiding
- Hesitancy
- Nocturia
- Urinary incontinence
- Urinary retention
- Urinary urgency

Expected Outcomes

- Patient's vital signs will remain within normal limits.
- Patient will empty bladder regularly, as confirmed by abdominal palpation.
- Patient's intake and output will remain approximately equivalent.
- Patient's urinary function will remain normal and free from complications.

Suggested NOC Outcomes

Urinary Continence; Urinary Elimination

Interventions and Rationales

- Review the patient's intake and output before and during labor. Note the color, amount, concentration, and urine specific gravity. *Decreased output may indicate dehydration, hemorrhage, gestational hypertension, and excessive oxytocin stimulation. Urine specific gravity reflects the kidneys' ability to concentrate urine and the patient's hydration status.*
- Assess for dehydration (poor skin turgor; flushed, dry skin; confusion; dry mucous membranes; fever; and rapid, thready pulse). *Dehydration leads to decreased circulatory blood volume and decreased urine output.*
- Palpate the abdomen above the symphysis pubis every 2 hours *to detect bladder distention and the degree of fullness.*
- Encourage the patient to void every 2 hours *to promote optimum bladder tone, prevent distention, and assist in promoting fetal descent.*
- To facilitate voiding, help the patient relax by:
  - having her sit in an upright position. Assist her to the bathroom, if appropriate. *An upright or squatting position promotes contraction of the pelvis and intra-abdominal muscles, thereby assisting in sphincter control and bladder contraction.*
  - providing privacy *to promote relaxation.*
  - pouring warm water over the perineum *to stimulate the urge to void.*
  - providing an audible sound of slow-running water. *This technique helps many patients void through power of suggestion.*

- As ordered, catheterize the patient if she can't void independently. *An overdistended bladder can cause atony and impede fetal descent or can become traumatized by the presenting part of the fetus during delivery.*

Suggested NIC Interventions

Prompted Voiding; Urinary Catheterization; Urinary Elimination Management

Evaluations for Expected Outcomes

- Patient's vital signs remain within normal range.
- Patient empties her bladder adequately at least every 2 hours.
- Patient's intake approximately equals output.
- Patient's urinary function remains normal and free from complications.

Documentation

- Intake and output
- Vital signs
- Results of bladder assessment
- Nursing interventions performed to promote voiding
- Patient's response to nursing interventions
- Evaluations for expected outcomes

REFERENCES

Buchanan, J., & Beckmann, M. (2014). Postpartum voiding dysfunction: Identifying the risk factors. *The Australian & New Zealand Journal of Obstetrics & Gynaecology, 54*(1), 41–45. doi:10.1111/ajo.12130

Pifarotti, P., Gargasole, C., Folcini, C., Gattei, U., Nieddu, E., Sofi, G., . . . Meschia, M. (2014). Acute postpartum urinary retention: Analysis of risk factors, a case-control study. *Archives of Gynecology and Obstetrics, 289*(6), 1249–1253. doi:10.1007/s00404-014-3144-5

Reilly, E. C., Freeman, R. M., Waterfield, M. R., Waterfield, A. E., Steggles, P., & Pedlar, F. (2014). Prevention of postpartum stress incontinence in primigravidae with increased bladder neck mobility: A randomised controlled trial of antenatal pelvic floor exercises. *International Journal of Obstetrics and Gynaecology, 121*(Suppl 7), 758–766. doi:10.1111/1471-0528.13213

PART V

Geriatric Health

APPLYING EVIDENCE-BASED PRACTICE

The Question

Does coffee consumption prevent memory disturbance in Alzheimer's patients?

Evidenced-Based Resources

Alzheimer's Association. (2016). 2016 Alzheimer's disease fact and figures. Retrieved from http://www.alz.org/documents_custom/2016-Facts-and-Figures-Fact-Sheet.pdf

Carman, A. J., Dacks, P. A., Lane, R. F., Shineman, D. W., & Fillit, H. M. (2014). Current evidence for the use of coffee and caffeine to prevent age-related cognitive decline and Alzheimer's disease. *Journal of Nutrition, Health & Aging*, *18*(4), 383–392. doi:10.1007/s12603-014-0021-7

National Institute on Aging. (2015, May.). Alzheimer's disease fact sheet. Retrieved March 1, 2016 from https://www.nia.nih.gov/alzheimers/publication/alzheimers-disease-fact-sheet

Panza, F., Solfrizzi, V., Barulli, M., Bonfiglio, C., Guerra, V., Osella, A., . . . Logroscino, G. (2015). Coffee, tea, and caffeine consumption and prevention of late-life cognitive decline and dementia: A systematic review. *Journal of Nutrition, Health & Aging*, *19*(3), 313–328. doi:10.1007/s12603-014-0563-8

Sugiyama, K., Tomata, Y., Kaiho, Y., Honkura, K., Sugawara, Y., & Tsuji, I. (2016). Association between coffee consumption and incident risk of disabling dementia in elderly Japanese: The Ohsaki cohort 2006 Study. *Journal of Alzheimer's Disease*, *50*(2), 491–500. doi:10.3233/JAD-150693

Evaluating the Evidence

Dementia and chronic confusion are not a normal part of aging. Alzheimer's disease (AD) is the most common form of dementia. AD attacks the brain, creating problems related to memory, thinking, and behavior. Symptoms usually develop gradually and get worse over time. As the disease progresses, it interferes with activities of daily living and the ability to perform tasks. There is no cure for AD but there are treatments to delay disease progression (Alzheimer's Association, 2016; National Institute on Aging, 2015). Considerable research has been conducted worldwide to find a cure. A focus of research today is prevention of AD.

Caffeine is a known stimulant that increases alertness and improves cognitive function. Because coffee is one of the most popular beverages in the world and contains caffeine, coffee consumption has become the subject of much AD prevention research. Panza et al. (2014) completed a systematic review of the literature that explored caffeine consumption and prevention of late-life cognitive decline and dementia. After review of 28 studies, Panza et al. (2014) concluded that the risk of cognitive decline and dementia related to AD may be decreased by consuming moderate amounts of coffee, tea, or caffeine.

A study conducted by Sugiyama et al. (2016) examined the association between coffee consumption and the risk of dementia in elderly Japanese. The study population consisted of over 31,000 residents aged 65 or older living in Ohsaki City, Miyagi Prefecture, and northeastern Japan. Data was collected about health habits, history of disease, and dietary habits including coffee consumption frequency. A significant association between coffee consumption and lower dementia incidence was observed.

Carmen, Dacks, Lane, Shineman, and Fillit (2014) examined random controlled trials that attempted to determine if caffeine or coffee protects against age-related cognitive decline. Evidence suggested that coffee consumption in midlife may decrease the risk of dementia in certain individuals. Carmen et al. (2014) conclude that potential health benefits of coffee and caffeine consumption outweigh any health risks as a low-cost strategy to prevent dementia.

Applying the Results and Making a Decision

AD attacks nearly half of Americans aged 85 and older and, along with other dementias, triples health care costs for those aged 65 and older (Alzheimer Association, 2016). There have been numerous research studies to suggest that caffeine/coffee could be an effective therapeutic agent against AD. These studies open up the possibility that dietary interventions could modify the risk of dementia/AD.

Reevaluating Process and Identifying Areas for Improvement

Nurses should continue to care for Alzheimer patients according to present standards. However, the results of the studies might have important implications in the prevention or delaying the onset of dementia and AD. Evidence suggests that moderate consumption of coffee is the best dietary option for long-term protection against AD and memory loss.

INTRODUCTION

Improvements in health care are enabling adults to live longer and as a result, the incidence of chronic disease has increased. Health promotion and disease prevention have become a priority for older adults. Nurses and other health care providers are challenged with meeting the unique needs of the geriatric patient. This section focuses on caring for adults aged 65 and older. The selected nursing diagnoses and associated care plans in this section relate to meeting the needs of geriatric patients.

Holistic geriatric care involves not only helping the patient cope with the effects of aging and chronic illness but also supporting efforts to maintain self-reliance and autonomy. Your assessment should include the patient's psychosocial functioning as well as physiologic status. When planning care, consider factors such as the amount and quality of contact with family and friends, the opportunity to perform meaningful life roles, access to transportation, and available financial resources. These factors have a tremendous influence on an older adult's well-being.

Because older adults now lead longer and more productive lives, geriatric care is increasingly focused on health promotion. Your interventions may include encouraging the patient to make lifestyle changes such as seeking and maintaining social support, moving to a more healthful environment, exercising, and eating properly.

If the patient becomes ill, your task may be to help restore optimal functioning. If recovery is unlikely, your task may be to foster adjustment and acceptance of the health condition and help the patient receive necessary assistance.

Always keep in mind that interventions must be tailored to the patient's unique needs. Although aging is common to all, each person ages differently. Factors that influence aging include genetics, culture, nutrition, environment, stress, and lifestyle. Planning care to meet the patient's distinctive needs demonstrates respect for the patient's rich life experiences.

RISK FOR ACTIVITY INTOLERANCE

Definition

Vulnerable to experiencing insufficient physiological or psychological energy to endure or complete required or desired daily activities, which may compromise health

Assessment

- Usual activity level, including self-care (dressing, feeding self, toileting), transfer, walking, stair climbing, and aids for ambulation
- Pain
- Cardiovascular status, including blood pressure, heart rate and rhythm (at rest and with activity), skin temperature and color, edema, and chest pain or discomfort
- Respiratory status, including arterial blood gas results, auscultation of breath sounds, and rate, rhythm, depth, and pattern of respiration at rest and with activity
- Musculoskeletal status, including range of motion and muscle size, strength, tone, and functional mobility grades as follows:
  0 = completely independent
  1 = requires use of equipment or device
  2 = requires help, supervision, or teaching from another person
  3 = requires help from another person and equipment or device
  4 = dependent; doesn't participate in activity
- Laboratory studies, including complete blood count

- Environmental factors, including safety hazards
- History of chronic illnesses (cardiopulmonary, cardiovascular, musculoskeletal, and neuromuscular)
- Sensory deficits, including hearing, vision, and tactile
- Psychosocial status, including cognitive and mental status, mood, affect, behavior, family support, and coping style
- Economic status
- Medication history, including use of prescription and over-the-counter medications

Risk Factors

- Circulatory problems
- History of previous intolerance
- Inexperience with an activity
- Physical deconditioning
- Respiratory condition

Expected Outcomes

- Patient's pulse, respirations, and blood pressure will remain within established parameters.
- Patient will use assistive devices, as needed, to carry out activities.
- Patient will modify activities to adjust to decreased activity tolerance.
- Patient will seek help in performing activities of daily living (ADLs), as needed.
- Patient will demonstrate willingness to perform activities needed to follow prescribed care plan.
- Patient will verbalize acceptance of decreased activity level.
- Patient will experience less discomfort when ambulating, transferring, or performing other activities.
- Patient will state plan to use support services.

Suggested NOC Outcomes

Activity Tolerance; Endurance; Energy Conservation; Self-Care: Activities of Daily Living (ADLs); Self-Care: Instrumental Activities of Daily Living (IADLs)

Interventions and Rationales

- Establish realistic goals for improving the patient's activity level, taking into account the patient's physical limitations and energy level *to help improve the patient's quality of life. Keep in mind that in some older patients with chronic conditions, even minimal improvements in activity level are noteworthy.*
- S Demonstrate the use of assistive devices, such as a cane or walker, shopping cart on wheels, or trapeze, *to teach methods of conserving energy and maintaining independence.*
- Establish progressive goals to increase ambulation, for example:
  - ambulate 20 feet (6.1 m) three times/day for 1 week
  - ambulate 40 feet (12.2 m) three times/day for 1 week
  - ambulate 60 feet (18.3 m) three times/day for 1 week

  Older patients may tire easily; therefore, the activity level should be increased gradually.
- Monitor vital signs before and after ambulation *to detect cardiovascular insufficiency.*

- PCC Provide encouragement if the patient achieves even small improvements in activity level *to help restore self-confidence.*
- PCC Coordinate the activities of the interdisciplinary team when developing an activity regimen for the patient. For example, the physician can prescribe treatment for the medical condition, a physical therapist can design an exercise program, a dietitian can devise a nutrition plan, and a social worker can locate community resources, such as Meals on Wheels or home health care services. *All of these measures address the patient's physical and psychosocial needs.*
- PCC Refer a depressed patient to a mental health practitioner *to address the psychosocial problems that may be causing impairment in activity.*
- Encourage the patient to express feelings about the decreased energy levels that may accompany advanced age *to enhance acceptance.*
- PCC Teach the patient about good nutrition and the importance of getting adequate rest *to improve poor health practices.*
- Monitor the patient's medication regimen regularly *to identify drugs that may cause gait, posture, or ambulatory problems.*
- Help the patient identify activities that are personally meaningful and develop a realistic plan to incorporate meaningful activities into the daily routine *to heighten satisfaction with energy expenditure.*
- PCC Encourage the patient to take part in exercise and social activities, as tolerated, *to increase stamina and decrease social isolation.*
- S Modify the environment *to maximize independent activity.* For example, place the bed on the first floor of the home with easy access to the bathroom and instruct the patient to obtain and use energy-saving devices, such as an elevated toilet seat, trapeze bar on the bed, and a chair with arms and a seat that raises the patient to standing position, *to promote independence.*
- Perform periodic health assessments and monitor for complaints of weakness or fatigue *to assess whether acute illness or exacerbation of chronic condition is causing activity intolerance.*
- PCC Refer the patient to a home health care agency for follow-up care. Encourage the patient to interview and select home health care personnel *to foster the patient's sense of independence.*

Suggested NIC Interventions

Energy Management; Exercise Promotion; Home Maintenance Assistance; Nutrition Management; Self-Care Assistance

Evaluations for Expected Outcomes

- Patient's pulse, respirations, and blood pressure are within established parameters.
- Patient uses assistive devices to carry out activities.
- Patient demonstrates necessary skills for modifying activity level to adjust to activity intolerance.
- Patient requests help to complete ADLs, as needed.
- Patient demonstrates willingness to perform activities needed to follow care plan, including maintaining balanced diet, getting adequate rest, and participating in modified exercise program.
- Patient's verbal statements indicate that the patient is learning to accept decreased energy level and to come to terms with the fact that the patient may not regain former level of activity.

- Patient reports experiencing less discomfort and pain when ambulating, transferring, and performing ADLs.
- Patient states that acceptance of support services won't damage self-esteem or alter independent living efforts.

Documentation

- Observations of patient's activity level, both deficits and improvements
- Patient's compliance with treatment regimen and response to multidisciplinary approach
- Teaching provided to patient and family members and their responses
- Modification of home or facility environment to ease patient's activity level
- Evaluations for expected outcomes

REFERENCES

Casaburi, R., & Duvall, K. (2014). Improving early-stage diagnosis and management of COPD in primary care. *Postgraduate Medicine, 126*(4), 141–154. doi:10.3810/pgm.2014.07.2792

Elbehairy, A. F., Ciavaglia, C. E., Webb, K. A., Guenette, J. A., Jensen, D., Mourad, S. M., . . . O'Donnell, D. E. (2015). Pulmonary gas exchange abnormalities in mild chronic obstructive pulmonary disease. Implications for dyspnea and exercise intolerance. *American Journal of Respiratory & Critical Care Medicine, 191*(12), 1384–1394. doi:10.1164/rccm.201501-0157OC

Kongoji, K., Yoneyama, K., Koyama, K., Mitarai, T., Kamijima, R., Kida, K., . . . Akashi, Y. J. (2014). Early defects identified by computed tomography angiography are associated with left ventricular dysfunction and exercise intolerance following acute myocardial infarction. *Japanese Journal of Radiology, 32*(10), 585–591. doi:10.1007/s11604-014-0344-7

Yates, B. C., Norman, J., Meza, J., Stanek Krogstrand, K., Harrington, S., Shurmur, S., . . . Schumacher, K. (2015). Effects of partners together in health intervention on physical activity and healthy eating behaviors. *Journal of Cardiovascular Nursing, 30*(2), 109–120. doi:10.1097/JCN.0000000000000127

DISTURBED BODY IMAGE

related to psychosocial factors

Definition

Confusion in mental picture of one's physical self

Assessment

- Sensory acuity, including vision and hearing
- Skin changes, including discoloration (e.g., age spots), thinning, sagging, dryness associated with diminished sebaceous gland production, and wrinkling associated with diminished underlying connective structures
- Hair, including thinning and loss of color
- Musculature, including diminished muscle mass, alterations in body shape, and sagging skin
- Mental status, including denial, depression, discouragement, fear, and grief
- Activity level, including activities of daily living and physical exercise

Defining Characteristics

- Absence of body part
- Alteration in body function

- Alteration in body structure
- Alteration in view of one's body (e.g., appearance, structure, function)
- Avoids looking at one's body
- Avoids touching one's body
- Behavior of acknowledging one's body
- Behavior of monitoring one's body
- Change in ability to estimate spatial relationship of body to environment
- Change in lifestyle
- Change in social involvement
- Depersonalization of body part by use of impersonal pronouns
- Emphasis on remaining strengths
- Extension of body boundary (e.g., includes external object)
- Fear of reaction by others
- Focus on past appearance
- Focus on past function
- Heightened achievement
- Hiding of body part
- Negative feeling about body
- Nonverbal response to change in body (e.g., appearance, structure, function)
- Overexposure of body part
- Perceptions that reflect an altered view of one's body appearance
- Personalization of body part by name
- Personalization of loss by name
- Preoccupation with change
- Preoccupation with loss
- Refusal to acknowledge change
- Trauma to nonfunctioning body part

Expected Outcomes

- Patient will alter skin care routine to reflect age-related changes and will use cosmetics appropriately.
- Patient will identify physical changes caused by aging without disparaging comments.
- Patient will identify at least one positive aspect of aging.
- Patient will use vision and hearing aids appropriately.
- Patient will dress appropriately with regard to safety, comfort, and personal taste.
- Patient will clean and style hair appropriately, without excessive coloring.
- Patient will demonstrate increased flexibility and willingness to consider lifestyle changes.
- Patient will participate in at least one social activity or group regularly.
- Patient will exercise and engage in other physical activities at level consistent with desire, ability, and safety.

Suggested NOC Outcomes

Body Image; Grief Resolution; Self-Esteem

Interventions and Rationales

- Encourage the patient to express feelings about the physical changes associated with aging. *Active listening conveys a caring and accepting attitude.*

PCC
- Provide information on appropriate self-care activities, such as:
  - maintaining a proper diet
  - bathing less frequently
  - using skin lotions to combat dryness
  - exercising appropriately to maintain muscle mass, bone strength, and cardiorespiratory health
  - avoiding fractures related to osteoporosis.

  Providing accurate self-care information helps the patient establish realistic goals.
- Encourage the patient to consider new grooming styles or to seek advice from a barber or cosmetologist on "updating" hair and makeup styles. *Attractive, tasteful grooming may help the older patient achieve a sense of control over the aging process.*

PCC
- Provide the patient with referrals for corrective eyewear and hearing aids *to address sensory deficits.*
- Provide the patient with positive role models. For example, offer to share literature that emphasizes the accomplishments, capabilities, and contributions of older adults *to promote a positive self-image and a more positive view of the elderly population.*
- During conversations with the patient, focus on the patient's strengths and what the patient can do; emphasize the positive aspects of aging *to increase the patient's self-esteem.*

PCC
- Encourage the patient to engage in social activities with people from all age groups *to increase opportunities for human interaction, positive feedback, and development of new interests.*

Suggested NIC Interventions

Active Listening; Body Image Enhancement; Counseling; Grief Work Facilitation; Self-Esteem Enhancement

Evaluations for Expected Outcomes

- Patient has clean, well-cared-for skin and uses cosmetics appropriately.
- Patient identifies age-related physical changes and comments on them positively.
- Patient identifies at least one personal advantage to growing older and one aspect of own life or personality that's better than it was 10 years ago.
- Patient uses vision and hearing aids comfortably.
- Patient dresses appropriately.
- Patient's hair appears clean and well- groomed.
- Patient demonstrates increased flexibility and willingness to consider lifestyle changes.
- Patient participates in at least one social activity or group regularly.
- Patient engages in regular, appropriate exercise or activity.

Documentation

- Patient's statements about appearance, ability, and age
- Mental status assessment (baseline and ongoing)
- Physical assessment
- Interventions directed toward improving patient's body image
- Patient's response to nursing interventions
- Evaluations for expected outcomes

REFERENCES

A systematic review of interventions on body image and disordered eating outcomes among women in midlife. (2016). *International Journal of Eating Disorders, 49*(1), 5–18. doi:10.1002/eat.22480

Breast cancer and body image as a prognostic factor of depression: A case study in México City. (2015). *Nutricion Hospitalaria, 31*(1), 371–379. doi:10.3305/nh.2015.31.1.7863

Rhoten, B. A., Deng, J., Dietrich, M. S., Murphy, B., & Ridner, S. H. (2014). Body image and depressive symptoms in patients with head and neck cancer: An important relationship. *Supportive Care in Cancer, 22*(11), 3053–3060. doi:10.1007/s00520-014-2312-2

Taylor, C. (2015). Body image concerns after colorectal cancer surgery. *British Journal of Nursing, 24*, S8–S14.

RISK FOR IMBALANCED BODY TEMPERATURE

Definition

Vulnerable to failure to maintain body temperature within normal parameters, which may compromise health

Assessment

- Age
- History of present illness
- Medical history, especially endocrine or nervous system illness
- Environmental temperature
- Medication history
- Neurologic status, including level of consciousness, knowledge level, and sensory, motor, and mental status
- Cardiovascular status, including heart rate and rhythm, blood pressure, pulses, capillary refill time, and electrocardiogram results
- Respiratory status, including breath sounds, arterial blood gas results, and respiratory rate, depth, and character
- Integumentary status, including temperature, color, and turgor
- Gastrointestinal status, including evidence of enema or laxative abuse, inspection of abdomen, and auscultation of bowel sounds
- Support systems, including family, friends, volunteer organizations, and clergy

Risk Factors

- Acute brain injury
- Alteration in metabolic rate
- Condition affecting temperature regulation
- Decreased sweat response
- Dehydration
- Extremes of age
- Extremes of environmental temperature
- Extremes of weight
- Inactivity
- Inappropriate clothing for environmental temperature
- Increase in oxygen demand
- Increased body surface area- to- weight ratio
- Inefficient nonshivering thermogenesis
- Insufficient supply of subcutaneous fat
- Pharmaceutical agent
- Sedation

- Sepsis
- Vigorous activity

Expected Outcomes

- Patient's body temperature will remain normal.
- Patient's skin will remain warm and dry.
- Patient will state feelings of comfort.
- Patient won't exhibit signs of hypothermia or hyperthermia.
- Patient or family member will identify warning signs of hypothermia and hyperthermia.
- Patient or family member will express understanding of factors that cause hypothermia and hyperthermia.
- Patient or family member will describe ways to prevent imbalanced body temperature.

Suggested NOC Outcomes

Risk Control; Risk Detection; Thermoregulation

Interventions and Rationales

- Monitor the patient's body temperature every 8 hours or more frequently, as indicated, *to ensure the temperature doesn't vary more than 1° F from average normal (98.6° F [37° C] oral).* If it does, monitor it more frequently.
- Assess the patient's knowledge and lifestyle before teaching about hypothermia and hyperthermia *to gear the teaching plan to the patient's needs.*
- Using large black type, provide the patient with a list of the signs and symptoms of imbalanced body temperature:
  - *Hypothermia:* shallow respirations; slow, weak pulse; decreased body temperature; low blood pressure; and pallor
  - *Hyperthermia:* shivering, shaking chill; feeling hot; extreme thirst; elevated body temperature; and high blood pressure.

  Listing the signs and symptoms helps the patient learn and identify warning signals of imbalanced body temperature. Large black type is easier for the older patient to read.
- Encourage the patient to remain active when in a cool environment *to keep warm and maintain normal metabolism.*
- Explain to the patient or family member why the patient needs warm clothing in cool climates, even indoors. Suggest socks, nonslip house shoes, and leg warmers *to provide warmth to vulnerable lower extremities, where vascular changes may cause decreased temperature sensation.*
- PCC Instruct the patient or family member to label home thermostats with large numbers and to use black or bright contrasting colors to indicate appropriate temperature settings. *Easy-to-read labels will help the patient maintain room temperature.*
- PCC Teach the patient or family member about the dangers of too much direct sunlight on warm days *to prevent overheating in an older patient with faulty thermoreceptors.*
- Discuss appropriate clothing for warm and cool climates. Suggest wearing clothes in layers, which can be removed or added, as needed, *to accommodate an increased susceptibility to temperature variations caused by aging vasculature.*
- Suggest that a friend, family member, or volunteer from a local community organization visit the patient daily *to help ensure the patient's safety.*

Suggested NIC Interventions

Environmental Management; Temperature Regulation; Vital Signs Monitoring

Evaluations for Expected Outcomes

- Patient's body temperature remains within normal limits.
- Patient's skin remains warm and dry.
- Patient reports absence of pain.
- Patient doesn't exhibit or report signs or symptoms of hypothermia or hyperthermia.
- Patient or family member identifies warning signs of hypothermia and hyperthermia.
- Patient or family member correctly identifies factors that may cause hypothermia or hyperthermia.
- Patient or family member describes changes to lifestyle that will prevent recurrence of imbalanced body temperature.

Documentation

- Patient's or family member's perception of problem, including reports of excessive cold or heat
- Patient's temperature
- Observations of risk factors for imbalanced body temperature
- Instructions regarding preventive measures
- Patient's or family member's statements of understanding of instructions
- Evaluations for expected outcomes

REFERENCES

Baillot, M., & Hue, O. (2015). Hydration and thermoregulation during a half-ironman performed in tropical climate. *Journal of Sports Science & Medicine*, *14*(2), 263–268.

Erdling, A., & Johansson, A. (2015). Core temperature—The intraoperative difference between esophageal versus nasopharyngeal temperatures and the impact of prewarming, age, and weight: A randomized clinical trial. *AANA Journal*, *83*(2), 99–105.

Sloane, P. D., Kistler, C., Mitchell, C. M., Beeber, A. S., Bertrand, R. M., Edwards, A. S., . . . Zimmerman, S. (2014). Role of body temperature in diagnosing bacterial infection in nursing home residents. *Journal of the American Geriatrics Society*, *62*(1), 135–140. doi:10.1111/jgs.12596

DECREASED CARDIAC OUTPUT

related to reduced myocardial perfusion

Definition

Inadequate blood pumped by the heart to meet the metabolic demands of the body

Assessment

- Mental status, especially sudden mental deterioration accompanied by confusion, agitation, and restlessness
- Cardiovascular status, including history of arrhythmias and syncope; skin color, temperature, and turgor; jugular vein distention; hepatojugular reflux; heart rate

and rhythm; heart sounds; blood pressure; peripheral pulses; electrocardiogram (ECG),echocardiogram, and phonocardiogram results; serum digoxin level; and aspartate aminotransferase, lactate dehydrogenase, and creatine kinase isoenzyme levels
- Respiratory status, including respiratory rate and depth, breath sounds, chest X-ray, and arterial blood gas results
- Renal status, including weight, intake and output, urine specific gravity, and serum electrolyte levels

Defining Characteristics

Altered Heart Rate/Rhythm

- Bradycardia
- ECG change (e.g., arrhythmia, conduction abnormality, ischemia)
- Heart palpitations
- Tachycardia

Altered Preload

- Decrease in central venous pressure (CVP)
- Decrease in pulmonary artery wedge pressure (PAWP)
- Edema
- Fatigue
- Heart murmur
- Increase in CVP
- Increase in PAWP
- Jugular vein distension
- Weight gain

Altered Afterload

- Abnormal skin color (e.g., pale, dusky, cyanosis)
- Alteration in blood pressure
- Clammy skin
- Decrease in peripheral pulses
- Decrease in pulmonary vascular resistance (PVR)
- Decrease in systemic vascular resistance (SVR)
- Dyspnea
- Increase in PVR
- Increase in SVR
- Oliguria
- Prolonged capillary refill

Altered Contractility

- Adventitious breath sounds
- Coughing
- Decrease in cardiac index
- Decrease in ejection fraction
- Decrease in left ventricular stroke work index
- Decrease in stroke volume index
- Orthopnea
- Paroxysmal nocturnal dyspnea
- Presence of S3 heart sound
- Presence of S4 heart sound

Behavioral/Emotional

- Anxiety
- Restlessness

Expected Outcomes

- Patient won't experience tachypnea, restlessness, anxiety, dyspnea, confusion, fainting, dizzy spells, light-headedness, nausea, fatigue, or weakness.
- Patient will tolerate exercise and activities at usual level, taking into account any cardiac damage.
- Patient will maintain respiratory status within established parameters.
- Patient's cardiac status will stabilize, with no evidence of arrhythmias.
- Patient and family members will understand and comply with prescribed therapeutic regimen.

Suggested NOC Outcomes

Cardiac Disease Self-Management; Cardiac Pump Effectiveness; Circulation Status; Vital Signs

Interventions and Rationales

- Administer medications, as ordered; monitor intake and output; and observe for adverse reactions. *In older patients, decreased renal and liver function may lead to rapid development of toxicity.*
- Monitor for dyspnea or breathlessness every 2 to 4 hours, and report changes from baseline. *Older patients with silent or painless myocardial infarction frequently develop dyspnea related to left-sided heart failure.*
- Monitor mental status every 2 to 4 hours and report deviations from baseline. *Dizziness, confusion, light-headedness, and restlessness may indicate decreased cerebral blood flow caused by slow carotid sinus reflex.*
- S Administer diuretics cautiously to the patient. Monitor closely for cardiac overload by taking frequent vital signs and documenting intake and output accurately. Report signs and symptoms of cardiac overload, such as elevated CVP, fluid intake above output, and increased pulmonary artery pressure. *When fluid in the lungs and lower extremities is mobilized and returns to circulation, it may overtax the patient's weakened myocardium.*
- Assess apical and radial pulses every 2 to 4 hours and report deviations from the baseline *to monitor for arrhythmias, impending cardiac arrest, hypertension, or shock.*
- Administer oxygen to the patient, as ordered, especially after the patient eats or during increased activity, *to increase oxygenation of the brain and heart.*
- Make sure the patient gets adequate rest and doesn't exceed activity tolerance level *to ease dyspnea, decrease oxygen demand on myocardium, and prevent hydrostatic pneumonia, venous thrombosis, and cardiovascular deconditioning.*
- PCC Teach the patient or family member the symptoms of possible cardiac problems:
  - dizziness
  - indigestion
  - nausea
  - retrosternal pain
  - shortness of breath
  - unusual fatigue and weakness

  showing the symptoms of decreased cardiac functioning gives the patient a sense of greater control over the situation and encourages compliance with the treatment plan.
- Reduce stressful elements, such as excessive noise or light in the patient's environment, *to help decrease anxiety and restlessness, which may lead to arrhythmias.*
- Encourage the patient to increase fluid intake and dietary fiber and to take natural stool softeners *to avoid Valsalva's maneuver during defecation, which can increase heart rate and blood pressure, cause reflex bradycardia, and decrease cardiac output.*

Suggested NIC Interventions

Cardiac Care; Cardiac Precautions; Hemodynamic Regulation; Vital Signs Monitoring

Evaluations for Expected Outcomes

- Patient experiences fewer dyspneic episodes, with no syncope or dizzy spells.
- Patient returns to normal activity and exercise levels, taking into account the extent of cardiac damage.
- Patient maintains normal respiratory status.
- Physical examination reveals no evidence of arrhythmias.
- Patient and family members understand and comply with prescribed therapeutic regimen.

Documentation

- Patient's chief complaint
- Signs or symptoms of decreased cardiac output
- Therapeutic interventions and patient's response
- Activity and exercise tolerance
- Diet and sleep patterns
- Teaching provided to patient and family member
- Evaluations for expected outcomes

REFERENCES

Caitlin, B. J., Lewis, K. B., Nichols, N., & Parsons, L. M. (2015). Advance care planning and the role of the cardiovascular nurse. *Canadian Journal of Cardiovascular Nursing, 25*(3), 5–9.
McLaughlin, D., Hoy, L., & Glackin, M. (2015). Heart failure nurse specialist crisis interventions and avoided hospital admissions. *British Journal of Cardiac Nursing, 10*(7), 326–333.
Unverzagt, S., Oemler, M., Braun, K., & Klement, A. (2014). Strategies for guideline implementation in primary care focusing on patients with cardiovascular disease: A systematic review. *Family Practice, 31*(3), 247–266. doi:10.1093/fampra/cmt080

RISK FOR IMPAIRED CARDIOVASCULAR FUNCTION

Definition

Vulnerable to internal or external causes that can damage one or more vital organs and the circulatory system itself

Assessment

- 12 lead electrocardiogram
- Activity level
- Blood pressure
- Body weight
- Lab values (HDL, LDL, total cholesterol levels, triglycerides, HgA1C, BNP)
- Pulse assessment, including rate, rhythm, amplitude, sounds
- Skin assessment, including color, temperature, pain, pallor, clubbing of fingers, presence of ulcers
- Urine output

Risk Factors

- Age ≥65 years
- Diabetes mellitus
- Dyslipidemia
- Family history of cardiovascular disease
- History of cardiovascular disease
- Hypertension
- Insufficient knowledge of modifiable risk factors
- Obesity
- Pharmaceutical agent
- Sedentary lifestyle
- Smoking

Expected Outcomes

- Patient will have no damage to cardiovascular system or one or more other major organs.
- Patient will have improved myocardial contractility/systemic perfusion.

Suggested NOC Outcomes

Cardiac Pump Effectiveness; Circulation Status; Tissue Perfusion: Peripheral; Vital Signs

Interventions and Rationales

- Administer diuretics as ordered. *When used in conjunction with low sodium diet and restriction of fluids, can lead to clinical improvement.*
- Administer vasodilators as ordered. *Can increase cardiac output*
- PCC Educate about testing such as cardiac stress test, echocardiography, CT, MRI, cardiac catheterization, etc. *Testing may be needed to determine possible damage to one or more vital organs.*
- PCC Educate importance of rest periods during activity. *Adequate rest is needed to improve efficiency of cardiac contractility and oxygen consumption.*
- Educate on lifestyle changes such as low salt diet, no smoking, exercise, etc. *Education will decrease risk.*
- Elevate legs. *Decreases venous stasis*
- Provide passive range of motion exercises. *Decreases venous stasis*

Suggested NIC Interventions

Cardiac Precautions; Circulatory Precautions; Fluid Management; Homodynamic Regulation; Vital Signs Monitoring

Evaluations for Expected Outcomes

- Patient will have no damage to cardiovascular system or one or more other major organs.
- Patient will have improved myocardial contractility/systemic perfusion.
- Improved myocardial function

Documentation

- Cardiovascular assessment
- Intake and output
- Medication administration
- Skin assessment
- Vital signs
- Weight

REFERENCES

Centers for Disease Control and Prevention. (n.d.). *Preventing heart disease: Healthy living habits.* Retrieved from http://www.cdc.gov/heartdisease/healthy_living.htm

Unverzagt, S., Oemler, M., Braun, K., & Klement, A. (2014). Strategies for guideline implementation in primary care focusing on patients with cardiovascular disease: A systematic review. *Family Practice, 31*(3), 247–266. doi:10.1093/fampra/cmt080

Wang, W., Zhang, H., Lopez, V., Wu, V. X., Poo, D. C., & Kowitlawakul, Y. (2015). Improving awareness, knowledge, and heart-related lifestyle of coronary heart disease among working population through a mHealth programme: Study protocol. *Journal of Advanced Nursing, 71*(9), 2200–2207. doi:10.1111/jan.12668

CONSTIPATION

related to diet, fluid intake, activity level, and personal bowel habits

Definition

Decrease in normal frequency of defecation accompanied by difficult or incomplete passage of stool and/or passage of excessively hard, dry stool

Assessment

- History of bowel disorder or surgery
- Gastrointestinal (GI) status, including nausea and vomiting, usual bowel habits, tenesmus, distention, flatulence, laxative or enema use, and medications
- Oral status, including inspection of oral cavity (gums, tongue, and dentition), pain or discomfort, and salivation
- Activity status, including type, duration, and frequency of exercise; lifestyle; and access to toilet facilities during work and leisure
- Nutritional status, including appetite, dietary intake, amount and type of dietary fiber, fluid intake, food likes and dislikes, meal pattern, access to food supply and storage facilities, access to shopping and transportation, and financial resources available for food
- Drug history, including use of constipating agents (such as aluminum-based antacids, anticholinergics, antidepressants, iron supplements, laxatives, and opioids) and history of laxative abuse

Defining Characteristics

- Abdominal pain
- Abdominal tenderness with palpable muscle resistance

- Abdominal tenderness without palpable muscle resistance
- Anorexia
- Atypical presentations in older adults (e.g., changes in mental status, urinary incontinence, unexplained falls, elevated body temperature)
- Borborygmi
- Bright red blood with stool
- Change in bowel pattern
- Decrease in stool frequency
- Decrease in stool volume
- Distended abdomen
- Fatigue
- Hard, formed stool
- Headache
- Hyperactive bowel sounds
- Hypoactive bowel sounds
- Inability to defecate
- Increase in intra-abdominal pressure
- Indigestion
- Liquid stool
- Pain with defecation
- Palpable abdominal mass
- Palpable rectal mass
- Percussed abdominal dullness
- Rectal fullness
- Rectal pressure
- Severe flatus
- Soft, paste-like stool in rectum
- Straining with defecation
- Vomiting

Expected Outcomes

- Patient will participate in the development of bowel program.
- Patient will report urge to defecate, as appropriate.
- Patient will increase fluid and fiber intake.
- Patient will report easy and complete evacuation of stools.
- Patient will increase activity level.
- Patient will have elimination pattern within normal limits.
- Patient will describe changes in personal habits that will help maintain normal elimination.

Suggested NOC Outcomes

Bowel Elimination; Hydration; Symptom Control

Interventions and Rationales

- Monitor the frequency and characteristics of the patient's stools. *Careful monitoring forms the basis of an effective treatment plan.*

- Monitor and record the patient's fluid intake and output. *Inadequate fluid intake contributes to dry feces and constipation. Monitoring fluid balance ensures adequate fluid intake and promotes elimination.*
- Provide privacy for elimination *to promote physiologic functioning.*
- Encourage the patient to use a bedside commode or walk to toilet facilities. Avoid the use of a bedpan *because such use may inhibit normal positioning for evacuation, thereby exacerbating constipation.*
- PCC Work with the patient to plan and implement an individualized bowel regimen *to establish a regular elimination schedule.*
- Emphasize to the patient the importance of responding to the urge to defecate. Be alert for any mental status changes that may impair the patient's ability to recognize or attend to the need to defecate or to report the need to the caregiver. *A timely response to the urge to defecate is necessary to maintain normal physiologic functioning and to avoid pressure and discomfort in the lower GI tract.*
- PCC Teach the patient to locate public restrooms and to wear easily removable clothing on outings *to promote normal bowel functioning.*
- PCC Teach the patient to massage the abdomen once per day. Show the patient how to locate and gently massage along the transverse and descending colon. *In the older patient, the neural centers in the lower intestinal wall may be impaired, making it more difficult for the body to evacuate feces. Massage may help stimulate peristalsis and the urge to defecate.*
- If abdominal pressure is inadequate to complete defecation, encourage the patient to perform a rocking motion of the upper body *to aid in elimination.*
- Plan and implement an exercise routine, such as walking, leg raising, abdominal muscle strengthening, and Kegel exercises. *Exercise promotes the abdominal and pelvic muscle tone necessary for normal elimination.*
- Encourage the intake of high-fiber foods. *Many older patients have reduced intestinal muscle tone and decreased strength in abdominal muscles, resulting in slower peristalsis, dry feces, and decreased ability to exert pressure for evacuation. High-fiber foods supply bulk for normal elimination and improve intestinal muscle tone.*
- Unless contraindicated, encourage fluid intake of 6 to 8 glasses (1,420 to 1,900 mL) daily *to maintain normal metabolic processes and prevent excessive reabsorption of fluid from GI contents.*
- PCC Teach the patient the sensible use of laxatives and enemas *to avoid laxative dependency. Overuse of laxatives and enemas may cause fluid and electrolyte loss and damage to intestinal mucosa.*
- Help the patient understand the diet modification plan. If appropriate, have the patient consult with a dietitian *to encourage compliance with the prescribed diet.*

Suggested NIC Interventions

Bowel Management; Constipation/Impaction Management; Exercise Promotion; Fluid Management; Nutrition Management

Evaluations for Expected Outcomes

- Patient participates in planning and implementing bowel program.
- Patient reports urge to defecate, as appropriate.
- Patient's daily diet includes high-fiber foods and adequate fluids.
- Patient reports easy and complete evacuation of stools.
- Patient increases activity level.

- Patient achieves routine bowel function without excessive use of laxatives, enemas, straining, or discomfort.
- Patient makes adaptations to lifestyle to ensure maintenance of bowel function.

Documentation

- Patient's expressions of concern regarding constipation, dietary changes, laxative use, and bowel pattern
- Physical findings
- Intake and output
- Observations of diet, characteristics of stool, and activity level
- Teaching provided and patient's response
- Patient's expressions indicating understanding of bowel program
- Evaluations for expected outcomes

REFERENCES

Bardsley, A. (2015). Approaches to managing chronic constipation in older people within the community setting. *British Journal of Community Nursing, 20*(9), 444–450. doi:10.12968/bjcn.2015.20.9.444

Holroyd, S. (2015). How can community nurses manage chronic constipation? *Journal of Community Nursing, 29*(5), 74–82.

Lee, A. (2015). Combating the causes of constipation. *Nursing & Residential Care, 17*(6), 327–331.

INEFFECTIVE COPING

related to inability to solve problems or adapt to demands of daily living

Definition

Inability to form a valid appraisal of the stressors, inadequate choices of practiced responses, and/or inability to use available resources

Assessment

- Age
- Lifestyle changes necessitated by disease or illness
- Role changes caused by retirement, relocation, or death of spouse, family members, or friends
- Changes associated with normal aging, such as decreased vision, hearing, and physical endurance
- Perceived coping ability
- Usual coping mechanisms
- Support systems, including family, friends, and religious and community organizations

Defining Characteristics

- Alteration in concentration
- Alteration in sleep pattern
- Change in communication pattern
- Destructive behavior toward others
- Destructive behavior toward self

- Difficulty organizing information
- Fatigue
- Frequent illness
- Inability to ask for help
- Inability to attend to information
- Inability to deal with a situation
- Inability to meet basic needs
- Inability to meet role expectation
- Ineffective coping strategies
- Insufficient access of social support
- Insufficient goal-directed behavior
- Insufficient problem resolution
- Insufficient problem-solving skills
- Risk-taking behavior
- Substance abuse

Expected Outcomes

- Patient will verbalize increased ability to cope.
- Patient will expand support network to meet social and emotional needs.
- Patient will locate and use appropriate resources for help in problem solving.
- Patient will report increased ability to meet demands of daily living.
- Patient will make changes to environment to ensure enhanced coping or move into long-term care facility, as needed.

Suggested NOC Outcomes

Coping; Decision-Making; Impulse Self-Control; Information Processing; Social Interaction Skills

Interventions and Rationales

- PCC Refer the patient to social service agencies, such as geriatric assessment centers, adult day-care programs, and home health care agencies, as appropriate, *to expand the patient's support network and to help in coping with physical, psychosocial, and economic stressors.*
- PCC Assist the patient in becoming involved with informal community programs, such as volunteer, foster grandparent, or religious groups, *to provide peer and social contact and decrease the patient's loneliness and isolation.*
- Encourage the patient to reminisce about the past *to help the patient recall past challenges and successful coping strategies.*
- PCC Provide the patient with information about the aging process, methods of coping with stress, and techniques used by other older adults to meet the demands of daily living *to assist the patient in implementing coping strategies.*
- If the patient must enter a long-term care facility or undergo lengthy home-based convalescence, help the patient put the situation in perspective. Explain to the patient that extreme stress can overwhelm anyone, even well-adapted individuals with strong support systems. When stress becomes overwhelming, rehabilitation in a secure environment may be the best option. Entering a long-term care facility isn't "the beginning of the end," as many people think, but rather an additional mechanism for ensuring optimal recovery. *Taking time to provide a carefully worded explanation may help the patient come to terms with the situation.*

- If the patient requires treatment in a long-term care facility, provide the least restrictive environment possible *to reduce the patient's fear and anxiety, help the patient to retain a sense of control, and encourage the patient to use own abilities to the maximum.*
- PCC Discuss with the patient the possibility of making lifestyle changes, such as moving closer to relatives, moving to a retirement community, or hiring someone to help with housework, *to improve ability to cope.*

Suggested NIC Interventions

Coping Enhancement; Decision-Making Support; Emotional Support; Environmental Management; Impulse Control Training; Support System Enhancement

Evaluations for Expected Outcomes

- Patient verbalizes an increased ability to cope.
- Patient reports success in developing support network to meet social and emotional needs.
- Patient contacts resources to help with problem solving.
- Patient reports increased ability to meet demands of daily living.
- Patient identifies lifestyle changes that will improve own ability to cope or states understanding and accepting the need to move to long-term care facility or retirement community.

Documentation

- Patient's expression of feelings about present life situation and difficulty coping
- Formal and informal sources of support identified by patient or family members
- Observations of patient's behavior in response to stressful situations
- Teaching provided and patient's response
- Use of outside support services
- Evaluations for expected outcomes

REFERENCES

Jacobs, N. L., Dehue, F., Völlink, T., & Lechner, L. (2014). Determinants of adolescents' ineffective and improved coping with cyberbullying: A Delphi study. *Journal of Adolescence, 37*(4), 373–385. doi:10.1016/j.adolescence.2014.02.011

Meredith, P. J., Rappel, G., Strong, J., & Bailey, K. J. (2015). Sensory sensitivity and strategies for coping with pain. *American Journal of Occupational Therapy, 69*(4), 1–10. doi:10.5014/ajot.2015.014621

Regier, N. G., & Parmelee, P. A. (2015). The stability of coping strategies in older adults with osteoarthritis and the ability of these strategies to predict changes in depression, disability, and pain. *Aging & Mental Health, 19*(12), 1113–1122. doi:10.1080/13607863.2014.1003286

COMPROMISED FAMILY COPING

related to caring for dependent, aging family member

Definition

A usually supportive primary person (family member, significant other, or close friend) provides insufficient, ineffective, or compromised support, comfort, assistance, or encouragement that may be needed by the client to manage or master adaptive tasks related to his or her health challenge

Assessment

- Patient status, including age, medical history, self-concept, physical disabilities or limitations, present living arrangements, and role in family
- Family assessment, including communication style, family coping style, perceptions of the aging process (myths versus realities), health problems of other members, financial status, support systems, and additional stressors
- Patient's current health crisis (emotional or physical)

Defining Characteristics

- Assistive behaviors by support person produce unsatisfactory results
- Client complaint about support person's response to health problem
- Client concern about support person's response to health problem
- Limitation in communication between support person and client
- Protective behavior by support person incongruent with client's abilities
- Protective behavior by support person incongruent with client's need for autonomy
- Support person reports inadequate understanding that interferes with effective behaviors
- Support person reports insufficient knowledge that interferes with effective behaviors
- Support person reports preoccupation with own reaction to client's need
- Support person withdraws from client

Expected Outcomes

- Family members will assume responsibilities formerly held by patient, as appropriate.
- Family members will express feelings about responsibilities in caring for an older relative.
- Patient and family members will express understanding of maturational and developmental issues that contributed to crisis.
- Patient and family members will identify and make use of appropriate community services.
- Family members will demonstrate improved capacity to plan care for older relative.
- Patient and family members will express satisfaction with their improved ability to cope with current crisis.

Suggested NOC Outcomes

Caregiver Emotional Health; Caregiver–Patient Relationship; Caregiver Stressors; Family Coping; Family Normalization

Interventions and Rationales

- Identify the primary caregiver in the family and assess the roles of other family members *to establish family hierarchy and plan interventions.*
- PCC Educate the patient and family members about the aging process. Discuss how changes in the patient have affected the family *to assess the needs of the patient and family members.*
- Avoid becoming involved in a power struggle among family members. *The patient may no longer be able to fulfill the family role, and the sudden shift in roles may lead to a power struggle among family members. The patient or family members may try to manipulate you as part of this power struggle. Maintaining a neutral, objective approach will help family members adjust to role changes.*

- PCC As appropriate, arrange and conduct a conference for family members; include the patient when possible. *Long-established communication patterns may interfere with family members' ability to resolve conflicts and make decisions. Your presence may help family members express feelings, identify needs and resources, and develop healthier ways of interacting.*
- Encourage family members to express their feelings about caring for the older family member. *A nonjudgmental attitude promotes effective communication.*
- PCC Encourage family members to identify strengths and weaknesses in the family system. Help them explore values, beliefs, perceived changes, and actual role changes related to the older patient's altered physical or emotional condition *to enhance insight.*
- PCC Assist the patient and family members in developing short-term and long-term goals and contingency plans *to increase a sense of control and direction for the future.*
- PCC Help the patient and family members identify appropriate community services, such as adult day care, respite care, and geriatric outreach services, *to provide access to additional sources of support.*
- Suggest using a care manager to help with the ongoing coordination of the patient's needs. Help the family identify a care manager they can relate to. *A care manager may help simplify decision making and limit family conflict.*
- PCC Help family members explore coping strategies used effectively during past crises and discuss how to apply these strategies to the present situation *to make family members aware of their demonstrated ability to adapt to change.*
- PCC Provide emotional support for the primary caregiver. *The family member who takes on the most responsibility for the patient has the double burden of caring for an older adult and adjusting to a new role in the family.*
- Maintain a nonjudgmental attitude while working with family members. Some families may hesitate to accept outside help. Other families may be unwilling to make even small sacrifices to care for an older relative. Remember that if family members haven't been supportive or close to the patient before, you're unlikely to change their attitudes. *A nonjudgmental outlook benefits the patient and family members. Learning to accept your limitations will help you avoid burnout.*
- Remain supportive and understanding if the patient or family members are reluctant to use needed community resources, such as adult day care, respite care, and home health care services. *An older patient may feel that using outside resources means sacrificing independence; family members may feel that asking for help indicates lack of caring.*

Suggested NIC Interventions

Caregiver Support; Coping Enhancement; Family Involvement Promotion; Respite Care

Evaluations for Expected Outcomes

- Family members assume responsibilities formerly held by patient, as appropriate.
- Patient and family members share feelings about current crisis.
- Patient and family members express understanding of maturational and developmental issues that led to crisis.
- Patient and family members acknowledge need for outside help to cope with crisis and identify and contact community resources.
- Family members demonstrate improved capacity for short-term and long-term planning.
- Patient and family members express satisfaction with their improved ability to cope with current crisis.

Documentation

- Patient's and family members' understanding of aging process and current health crisis
- Observations of patient's and family members' reactions to crisis
- Family members' willingness to become involved in patient care
- Nursing interventions
- Teaching provided
- Patient's and family members' responses to interventions and instructions
- Referrals to community agencies
- Evaluations for expected outcomes

REFERENCES

del-Pino-Casado, R., Pérez-Cruz, M., & Frías-Osuna, A. (2014). Coping, subjective burden, and anxiety among family caregivers of older dependents. *Journal of Clinical Nursing, 23*(23/24), 3335–3344. doi:10.1111/jocn.12561

Santos de Araújo Dantas, M., Amador Silva, D., Ataíde Melo de Pinho, T., Barros Torquato, I. M., Dantas de Assis, W., & dos Santos, S. R. (2015). Family coping strategies for leukemia diagnosis: Social and religious aspects. *Journal of Nursing UFPE, 9*(1), 137–142. doi:10.5205/reuol.6817-60679-1-ED.0901201519

Washington, K. T., & Rakes, C. R. (2015). Coping responses among hospice family caregivers: A confirmatory factor analysis. *Journal of Pain & Symptom Management, 50*(6), 867–873. doi:10.1016/j.jpainsymman.2015.07.002

INEFFECTIVE DENIAL

related to fear or anxiety about aging

Definition

Conscious or unconscious attempt to disavow knowledge or meaning of an event to reduce anxiety and/or fear, leading to the detriment of health

Assessment

- Age
- Appearance
- Activity patterns, including sudden interest or participation in activities that may be dangerous
- Self-concept, including self-esteem, body image, and perception of self in life continuum
- Coping behaviors
- Mental status, including affect, communication, memory, mood, orientation, perception, abstract thinking, judgment, and insight

Defining Characteristics

- Delay in seeking health care
- Denies fear of death
- Denies fear of invalidism
- Displaces fear of impact of the condition

- Displaces source of symptoms
- Does not admit impact of disease on life
- Does not perceive relevance of danger
- Does not perceive relevance of symptoms
- Inappropriate affect
- Minimizes symptoms
- Refusal of health care
- Use of dismissive gestures when speaking of distressing event
- Use of dismissive comments when speaking of distressing event
- Use of treatment not advised by health care professional

Expected Outcomes

- Patient will discuss aging process and impact on ability to participate in hobbies and other activities.
- Patient will express interest in age-appropriate community activities.
- Patient will set aside time for reminiscing as part of daily routine.
- Patient will express a more positive view of growing older.
- Patient will adapt activities to avoid unnecessary physical stress on body.

Suggested NOC Outcomes

Acceptance: Health Status; Anxiety Self-Control; Fear Self-Control

Interventions and Rationales

- Discuss the challenge of being an older adult in today's youth-oriented society *for encouraging the patient to express own feelings and helping the patient in recognizing not having to accept society's prejudices about aging.*
- PCC Discuss with the patient and family members the changes that normally occur as part of the aging process *to correct misconceptions.*
- Discuss how to adapt activities and hobbies to accommodate the physical changes that occur with aging *to avoid excess physical stress.*
- Discuss the advantages of growing older, such as having more time to pursue hobbies and other interests, *to help the patient develop a positive view of aging.*
- Emphasize various activities that the patient can continue to do well *to enhance self-esteem.*
- Encourage the patient to set aside time for reminiscing as part of daily routine. *Reminiscing helps the patient to affirm the past and promotes self-esteem.*
- PCC Provide information about senior volunteer groups and part-time work or volunteer opportunities *to help the patient maintain physical and mental functioning and promote social interaction.*
- Invite an active member of a senior citizens club, social group, senior sports league, or advocacy group to visit the patient *to provide a positive role model.*

Suggested NIC Interventions

Coping Enhancement; Health Education; Self-Awareness Enhancement

Evaluations for Expected Outcomes

- Patient expresses positive and negative feelings about aging.
- Patient states intention to engage in age-appropriate community activity.
- Patient expresses willingness to set aside time for reminiscing.
- Patient expresses a more positive view of growing older.
- Patient adapts activities to avoid unnecessary physical stress on body.

Documentation

- Evidence of patient's difficulty adjusting to the aging process
- Nursing interventions
- Referrals provided
- Patient's response to nursing interventions
- Patient's statements that indicate a more positive attitude toward growing older
- Evaluations for expected outcomes

REFERENCES

Kaldy, J. (2014). Denial: When it helps, when it hurts. *Caring for the Ages, 15*(10), 1–7.
Paris, J. J., Cummings, B. M., & Moore, M. P. (2014). "Brain death," "dead," and parental denial. *Cambridge Quarterly of Healthcare Ethics, 23*(4), 371–382. doi:10.1017/S0963180114000048
Williams, A. R., Olfson, M., & Galanter, M. (2015). Assessing and improving clinical insight among patients "in denial". *JAMA Psychiatry, 72*(4), 303–304. doi:10.1001/jamapsychiatry.2014.2684

RISK FOR FALLS

Definition

Vulnerable to increased susceptibility to falling, which may cause physical harm and compromise health

Assessment

- Psychosocial status, including age, developmental stage, learning ability, decision-making ability, health beliefs and attitudes, interest in learning, knowledge and skills regarding current health problem, obstacles to learning, financial resources, support systems, and usual coping pattern
- Neurologic status, including level of consciousness, memory, mental status, and orientation
- Physical impairment or limitation, recent joint replacement, other surgery or illness
- Environmental hazards such as throw rugs, carpet edges, stairways, slippery floors, tubs and showers, unsteady handrails

Risk Factors

Adult

- Age ≥65 years
- History of falls
- Living alone
- Lower limb prosthesis
- Use of assistive device (e.g., walker, cane, wheelchair)

Child

- Absence of stairway gate
- Absence of window guard
- Age ≤2 years
- Inadequate supervision
- Insufficient automobile restraints
- Male gender when <1 year of age

Cognitive

- Alteration in cognitive functioning

Environment

- Cluttered environment
- Exposure to unsafe weather-related condition (e.g., wet floors, ice)
- Insufficient lighting
- Insufficient antislip material in bathroom
- Unfamiliar setting
- Use of restraints
- Use of throw rugs

Pharmaceutical Agents

- Alcohol consumption
- Pharmaceutical agent

Physiologic

- Acute illness
- Alteration in blood glucose level
- Anemia
- Arthritis
- Condition affecting the foot
- Decrease in lower extremity strength
- Diarrhea
- Difficulty with gait
- Faintness when extending neck
- Faintness when turning neck
- Hearing impairment
- Impaired balance
- Impaired mobility
- Incontinence
- Neoplasm
- Neuropathy
- Orthostatic hypotension
- Postoperative recovery period
- Proprioceptive deficit
- Sleeplessness
- Urinary urgency
- Vascular disease
- Visual impairment

Expected Outcomes

- Patient and family will identify the factors that increase potential for falls.
- Patient and family will assist in identifying and applying safety measures to prevent injury.
- Patient and family will make necessary physical changes in the environment to ensure increased safety.
- Patient and family will develop strategies to maintain safety.
- Patient will optimize activities of daily living within sensorimotor limitations.

Suggested NOC Outcomes

Fall Prevention Behavior; Falls Occurrence; Mobility; Risk Control; Knowledge: Fall Prevention; Coordinated Movement; Safe Home Environment

Interventions and Rationales

- S Identify factors that may cause or contribute to injury from a fall *in order to enhance the patient, family, caregiver awareness of the risks.*
- S Improve environmental safety factors as needed. *Doing frequent assessments of the patient's environment is necessary to make sure new risks have not occurred.*
- S Spend time orienting the patient and the family to the patient's environment. Assess the patient's ability to use call bell or other safety emergency system. Remove anything from the environment that will increase the risk of falls; for example, throw rugs, cords, furniture blocking the patient's path to the bathroom, etc. *The patient's immediate environment must be reviewed frequently to prevent unnecessary falls.*
- PCC Teach the patient and family about the need for safe illumination. Advise the patient to wear sunglasses when outside *to reduce the glare.* Suggest the use of contrasting colors in household furnishings *to enable the patient to distinguish difference in things when walking and sitting.*
- For patients with hearing loss, encourage the use of a hearing aid *to minimize hearing deficit.*
- PCC Teach the patient with unstable gait the proper use of assistive devices. Many patients never learn to use canes, crutches, etc. properly, *to decrease the potential for falling.*
- S Review medications with the patient and family. Help the patient understand which medications put the patient at greater risk for falls. Knowing the risk may help the patient take more care in moving about. It may also call for reviewing with the primary care physician. *Two or more medications taken by a patient put the patient at higher risk. Many medications taken by the elderly can cause dizziness, sleepiness, lowered blood pressure, and confusion. Without sufficient instructions, the patient may be at a higher risk for falls.*
- S Provide additional patient education for household safety. Refer patient to appropriate resources (such as police, fire, home health nurses) for safety education. There is interest in the community for educating the elderly in the area of fall prevention. *Many hospitalizations of elderly people because of trauma are caused by falls.*

Suggested NIC Interventions

Fall Prevention; Environmental Management: Safety; Risk Identification; Medication Management; Exercise Therapy: Balance

Evaluation for Expected Outcomes

- Patient and family are able to point out things in the environment that put them at risk.
- Patient and family members assist in making the changes necessary to promote fall prevention.
- Patient demonstrates the ability to move about without falling.
- Patient identifies resources in the community to help the patient with ongoing fall prevention.

Documentation

- Statements by the patient and family about potential for injury as a result of sensory or motor deficits
- Interventions to reduce risk of fall by the patient
- Information about sources of risk to the patient
- Patient response to implementation of preventive measures
- Evaluation of expected outcomes

REFERENCES

Godlock, G. (2016). Implementation of an evidence-based patient safety team to prevent falls in inpatient medical units. *Medsurg Nursing*, *25*(1), 17–23.

Leone, R. M., & Adams, R. J. (2016). Safety standards: Implementing fall prevention interventions and sustaining lower fall rates by promoting the culture of safety on an inpatient rehabilitation unit. *Rehabilitation Nursing*, *41*(1), 26–32. doi:10.1002/rnj.250

Tomita, M. R., Saharan, S., Rajendran, S., Nochajski, S. M., & Schweitzer, J. A. (2014). Psychometrics of the home safety self-assessment tool (HSSAT) to prevent falls in community-dwelling older adults. *American Journal of Occupational Therapy*, *68*(6), 711–718. doi:10.5014/ajot.2014.010801

FRAIL ELDERLY SYNDROME

Definition

Dynamic state of unstable equilibrium that affects the older individual experiencing deterioration in one or more domain of health (physical, functional, psychological, or social) and leads to increased susceptibility to adverse health effects, in particular disability

Assessment

- Ability to complete activities of daily living
- Cognitive level
- Level of physical activity
- Nutritional status
- Oxygenation status
- Presence of depression
- Self-report of exhaustion
- Slowness
- Weakness
- Weight

Defining Characteristics

- Activity intolerance
- Bathing self-care deficit
- Decreased cardiac output
- Dressing self-care deficit
- Fatigue
- Feeding self-care deficit

- Hopelessness
- Imbalanced nutrition: Less than body requirements
- Impaired physical mobility
- Impaired walking
- Social isolation
- Toileting self-care deficit

Expected Outcomes

- Patient will have improved physical function.
- Patient will have improved psychological function.
- Patient will have improved social function.

Suggested NOC Outcomes

Physical Aging; Psychosocial Adjustment: Life Change; Client Satisfaction: Functional Assistance

Interventions and Rationales

- S Conduct environmental assessment. *Can identify risks for falls and ability to manage care outside the hospital.*
- PCC Educate on importance of regular exercise. *Can improve mobility, improve gait, decrease incidence of falls, increase muscle strength.*
- PCC Implement interdisciplinary treatment plan. *Can improve physical and psychological function, improve patient satisfaction, decrease need for hospitalization.*
- Provide antidepressants as ordered. *Delay of treatment may accelerate decline of patient status.*
- Provide appetite stimulating medications as ordered. *May increase appetite.*
- Provide patient with ample time to complete activities of daily living (ADLs). *Can increase ability to complete ADLs.*
- Provide physical and occupational therapy as needed. *Can improve functional impairment.*
- Provide socialization opportunities. *Isolation can exacerbate depression.*
- Provide stimulating activities. *Keeps cognitive mind engaged.*
- Provide supplemental nutritional drinks. *Can provide extra calories and energy intake.*

Suggested NIC Interventions

Physical Exercise; Strength Training; Balance Training

Evaluations for Expected Outcomes

- Patient has no deterioration of physical function.
- Patient has no deterioration of psychological function.
- Patient has no deterioration of social function.

Documentation

- Ability to complete ADLs
- Body weight

- Cognitive level
- Mental status
- Mobility status
- Vital signs

REFERENCES

Chen, X., Mao, G., & Leng, S. X. (2014). Frailty syndrome: An overview. *Clinical Interventions in Aging, 9*, 433–441. doi: 10.2147/CIA.S45300

Lenardt, M. H., Hammerschmidt Kolb Carneiro, N., Albino, J., & Hautsch Willig, M. (2014). Quality of life of frail elderly users of the primary care. *Acta Paulista De Enfermagem, 27*(5), 399–404. doi:10.1590/1982-0194201400067

Palace, A. J., & Flood-Sukhdeo, J. (2014). The frailty syndrome. *Today's Geriatric Medicine, 7*(1), 18.

RISK FOR FRAIL ELDERLY SYNDROME

Definition

Vulnerable to a dynamic state of unstable equilibrium that affects the older individual experiencing deterioration in one or more domain of health (physical, functional, psychological, or social) and leads to increased susceptibility to adverse health effects, in particular disability

Assessment

- Ability to complete activities of daily living (ADLs)
- Cognitive level
- Fall risk
- Level of physical activity
- Muscle strength
- Nutritional status
- Oxygenation status
- Presence of depression
- Self-report of exhaustion
- Slowness
- Weakness
- Weight

Risk Factors

- Activity intolerance
- Age >70 years
- Alteration in cognitive functioning
- Altered clotting process (e.g., Factor VII, D-dimers)
- Anorexia
- Anxiety
- Average daily physical activity is less than recommended for gender and age
- Chronic illness
- Constricted life space
- Decrease in energy
- Decrease in muscle strength
- Decrease in serum 25-hydroxyvitamin D concentration
- Depression

- Economically disadvantaged
- Endocrine regulatory dysfunction (e.g., glucose intolerance, increase I 1GF-1, androgen, DHEA, and cortisol)
- Ethnicity other than Caucasian
- Exhaustion
- Fear of falling
- Female gender
- History of falls
- Immobility
- Impaired balance
- Impaired mobility
- Insufficient social support
- Living alone
- Low educational level
- Malnutrition
- Muscle weakness
- Obesity
- Prolonged hospitalization
- Sadness
- Sarcopenia
- Sarcopenic obesity
- Sedentary lifestyle
- Sensory deficit (e.g., visual, hearing)
- Social isolation
- Social vulnerability (e.g., disempowerment, decreased life control)
- Suppressed inflammatory response (e.g., II-6, CRP)
- Unintentional loss of 25% of body weight over one year
- Unintentional weight loss >10 lb (>4.5 kg) in one year
- Walking 15 feet requires >6 seconds (4 m >5 seconds)

Expected Outcomes

- Patient will not experience deterioration in physical domain.
- Patient will not experience deterioration in functional domain.
- Patient will not experience deterioration in psychological domain.
- Patient will not experience deterioration in social domain.
- Patient will not be susceptible to adverse health effects.

Suggested NOC Outcomes

Physical Aging; Psychosocial Adjustment: Life Change; Client Satisfaction: Functional Assistance

Interventions and Rationales

- S Conduct environmental assessment. *Can identify risks for falls and ability to manage care outside the hospital.*
- PCC Educate on importance of regular exercise. *Can improve mobility, improve gait, decrease incidence of falls, increase muscle strength.*
- PCC Implement interdisciplinary treatment plan. *Can improve physical and psychological function, improve patient satisfaction, decrease need for hospitalization.*
- Provide patient with ample time to complete ADLs. *Can increase ability to complete ADLs.*

- Provide physical and occupational therapy as needed. *Can improve functional impairment.*
- Provide socialization opportunities. *Isolation can exacerbate depression.*
- Provide stimulating activities. *Keeps cognitive mind engaged.*
- Provide supplemental nutritional drinks. *Can provide extra calories and energy intake.*

Suggested NIC Interventions

Physical Exercise; Strength Training; Balance Training

Evaluations for Expected Outcomes

- Patient has no deterioration in physical domain.
- Patient has no deterioration in psychological domain.
- Patient has no deterioration in functional domain.
- Patient has no deterioration in social domain.
- Patient is not susceptible to adverse health effects.

Documentation

- Ability to complete ADLs
- Body weight
- Cognitive level
- Fall risk
- Mental status
- Mobility status
- Vital signs

REFERENCES

Chen, X., Mao, G., & Leng, S. X. (2014). Frailty syndrome: An overview. *Clinical Interventions in Aging, 9,* 433–441. doi: 10.2147/CIA.S45300

Lenardt, M. H., Hammerschmidt Kolb Carneiro, N., Albino, J., & Hautsch Willig, M. (2014). Quality of life of frail elderly users of the primary care. *Acta Paulista De Enfermagem, 27*(5), 399–404. doi:10.1590/1982-0194201400067

Palace, A. J., & Flood-Sukhdeo, J. (2014). The frailty syndrome. *Today's Geriatric Medicine, 7*(1), 18.

IMPAIRED GAS EXCHANGE

related to carbon dioxide retention or excess mucus production

Definition

Excess or deficit in oxygenation and/or carbon dioxide elimination at the alveolar-capillary membrane

Assessment

- Age
- Gender
- Smoking history

- Occupational or environmental risk factors, such as exposure to asbestos, smog, and pollutants
- Respiratory status, including history of respiratory disorders, breath sounds, sputum characteristics, accessory muscle use, cyanosis, and arterial blood gas (ABG) levels
- Cardiovascular status, including skin color and temperature, heart rate and rhythm, heart sounds, blood pressure, hemoglobin levels, hematocrit, red and white blood cell and platelet counts, prothrombin and partial thromboplastin times, and serum iron concentrations
- Psychosocial status, including mental status, knowledge level, lifestyle, and support systems
- Activity status, including ability to perform activities of daily living (ADLs)

Defining Characteristics

- Abnormal arterial blood gases
- Abnormal arterial pH
- Abnormal breathing pattern (e.g., rate, rhythm, depth)
- Abnormal skin color (e.g., pale, dusky, cyanosis)
- Confusion
- Cyanosis
- Decrease in carbon dioxide
- Diaphoresis
- Dyspnea
- Headache upon awakening
- Hypercapnia
- Hypoxemia
- Hypoxia
- Irritability
- Nasal flaring
- Restlessness
- Somnolence
- Tachycardia
- Vision disturbance

Expected Outcomes

- Patient will exercise and perform ADLs without experiencing dyspnea or excessive fatigue.
- Patient will maintain adequate fluid intake.
- Patient will maintain adequate ventilation and have clear breath sounds on auscultation.
- Patient or family members will state understanding of causes for impaired gas exchange and behaviors to prevent it.

Suggested NOC Outcomes

Fluid and Electrolyte Balance; Respiratory Status: Gas Exchange; Tissue Perfusion: Pulmonary; Vital Signs

Interventions and Rationales

- Establish baseline values for respiratory assessment *to distinguish age-related changes that may mimic disease states from disease. Older adults take shorter breaths. This decreases maximum breathing capacity, vital capacity, residual volume, and functional capacity.*

- Auscultate lungs every 4 hours, taking into account anatomic changes that may occur in older patients, such as kyphosis, deviated trachea, and dowager's hump, *to detect abnormal breath sounds. Report abnormalities.*
- Administer and monitor oxygen therapy, as ordered, *to enhance oxygenation and detect signs of decompensation. Older patients have a high incidence of chronic cardiac and chronic pulmonary disorders. Detecting early changes in condition allows for early intervention.*
- PCC Teach the patient relaxation techniques and ask for a return demonstration. *Using relaxation techniques may help reduce tissue oxygen demand.*
- Incorporate the patient's past experiences into the teaching plan when conveying information about disease, medications, and lifestyle changes. *Information becomes more meaningful when related to previous experiences.*
- PCC Help the patient schedule ADLs to allow for rest periods. *The older patient has more fibrous, less elastic alveoli that contain fewer functional capillaries, which decrease exertional capacity. The patient needs rest periods to conserve respiratory effort.*
- PCC Help the patient identify positions that maximize ventilatory capacity, such as leaning over the bedside table when sitting or using a large wedge pillow under the shoulders. *In an older patient, accessory muscles of the pharynx and larynx may atrophy, making it necessary for the patient to assume breathing positions that maximize ventilation, perfusion, and thoracic expansion.*
- Encourage adequate fluid intake. *Older adults may have a diminished sense of thirst, which may lead to dry mucous membranes. Dry mucous membranes, in turn, may impede removal of secretions and promote respiratory infection. Consuming adequate fluids helps to liquefy secretions, reducing the energy required to mobilize them.* Record intake and output *to monitor fluid status.*
- Perform bronchial hygiene, such as positioning, coughing, deep breathing, percussion, postural drainage, and suctioning, *to promote and maintain a patent airway.*
- S Evaluate the home environment and recommend changes, such as moving the patient's bedroom to the first floor, *to reduce exertion.*

Suggested NIC Interventions

Acid-Base Management; Hemodynamic Regulation; Oxygen Therapy; Vital Signs Monitoring

Evaluations for Expected Outcomes

- Patient performs exercise and ADLs with minimum fatigue and increased endurance.
- Patient maintains adequate fluid intake.
- Patient maintains adequate ventilation and has clear breath sounds on auscultation.
- Patient or family members state understanding of causes for impaired gas exchange and behaviors to prevent it.

Documentation

- Patient's complaints of dyspnea or fatigue
- Observations of patient's condition
- Patient's response to nursing interventions
- Teaching provided and patient's response

- Patient's expressions indicating understanding of care plan
- Evaluations for expected outcomes

REFERENCES

Casaburi, R., & Duvall, K. (2014). Improving early-stage diagnosis and management of COPD in primary care. *Postgraduate Medicine, 126*(4), 141–154. doi:10.3810/pgm.2014.07.2792
Fratantoro, M. (2014). Reducing and preventing COPD readmissions. *RT: The Journal for Respiratory Care Practitioners, 27*(5), 4.
Linden, A., & Butterworth, S. W. (2014). A comprehensive hospital-based intervention to reduce readmissions for chronically ill patients: A randomized controlled trial. *American Journal of Managed Care, 20*(10), 783–792.

GRIEVING

related to perceived potential loss of life

Definition

A normal complex process that includes emotional, physical, spiritual, social, and intellectual responses and behaviors by which individuals, families, and communities incorporate an actual, anticipated, or perceived loss into their daily lives

Assessment

- Age
- Developmental stage
- Presence of living will, durable power of attorney for health care, and other advance directives
- History of chronic illness or terminal diagnosis
- Mental status, including level of consciousness and orientation
- Emotional status, including evidence of anger, apathy, depression, or hostility
- Support systems, including family members, significant other, friends, and clergy
- Spiritual practices, including religious affiliation and use of spiritual support systems
- Customs and beliefs related to illness, death, and suffering

Defining Characteristics

- Alterations in activity level
- Alteration in dream pattern
- Alteration in immune functioning
- Alteration in neuroendocrine functioning
- Alteration in sleep pattern
- Anger
- Blaming
- Despair
- Detachment
- Disorganization
- Finding meaning in a loss
- Guilt about feeling relieved
- Maintaining a connection to the deceased
- Pain

- Panic behavior
- Personal growth
- Psychological distress
- Suffering

Expected Outcomes

- Patient will express and accept feelings about anticipated death.
- Patient will progress through stages of grieving process in own way.
- Patient will practice religious rituals and use other coping mechanisms appropriate to end of life.
- Family members or significant other will participate in providing supportive care and comfort to patient.

Suggested NOC Outcomes

Coping; Family Coping; Grief Resolution; Psychosocial Adjustment: Life Change

Interventions and Rationales

- Provide time for the patient to express feelings about death or terminal illness. *Active listening helps the patient lessen feelings of loneliness and isolation.* Don't approach the patient with a busy, hurried attitude, *which can block communication.*
- Establish a relationship that encourages the patient to express concerns about death. *Basic nursing care combined with genuine interest in the patient fosters trust and understanding.*
- Guide the patient in life review. Encourage the patient to write or tape record own life history as a lasting gift to family members. *Life review allows the patient to survey events from the past and give them meaningful interpretation.*
- PCC Involve an interdisciplinary team (psychologist, nurse, patient, nutritionist, physician, physical therapist, and chaplain) in providing care for a dying patient. *Each team member offers unique expertise for meeting the dying patient's needs.*
- PCC Encourage family members to become involved in the care of the dying patient. Communicate with the patient and family members honestly and compassionately. *Giving family members a role in patient care helps relieve anxiety and lessen feelings of regret and guilt. Honest communication is important because family members need an opportunity to acknowledge their loss and say farewell.*
- Demonstrate acceptance of the patient's response to own anticipated death, whatever that response may be: crying, sadness, anger, fear, or denial. *Each patient responds to dying in own way. Helping the patient express feelings freely will enhance the patient's ability to cope.*
- Help the patient progress through the psychological stages associated with anticipated death, including shock and denial, anger, bargaining, depression, and acceptance, *to help you anticipate the dying patient's psychological needs. Keep in mind, however, that not all dying patients go through each stage.*
- Support the patient's spiritual coping behaviors. For example, arrange for the patient to have objects that provide spiritual comfort (such as a Bible, prayer shawl, Menorah, Shofar, misbaha, pictures, statues, or rosary beads) at the bedside. *Even patients for whom religious practice hasn't been a dominant part of life may turn to religion when confronted by death or serious illness.*

- Inform the patient about hospice services. Hospice services emphasize symptomatic relief and caring, with the aim of improving patient and family comfort until death occurs, instead of prolonging life for its own sake. *Hospice care is an appropriate alternative for a patient with an incurable illness.*
- PCC Provide referrals for home health care assistance if the patient will be cared for at home *to support the patient's decision to remain at home.*

Suggested NIC Interventions

Anticipatory Guidance; Coping Enhancement; Family Support; Grief Work Facilitation

Evaluations for Expected Outcomes

- Patient expresses and accepts feelings brought about by anticipated death.
- Patient progresses through stages of grieving in own way.
- Patient participates in religious rituals and uses other appropriate coping mechanisms.
- Patient receives adequate support during end of life from family members, friends, and members of health care team.

Documentation

- Patient's verbal expressions indicating feelings about anticipated death
- Observations of emotional responses, such as crying, anger, and withdrawal
- Interventions to help patient cope with anticipated death
- Patient's requests for assistance in achieving spiritual comfort (spiritual objects and visits from minister, priest, or rabbi)
- Patient's response to interventions
- Evaluations for expected outcomes

REFERENCES

Miller, E. T. (2015). The grieving process: A necessary step toward healing. *Rehabilitation Nursing, 40*(4), 207–208. doi:10.1002/rnj.220

Raitio, K., Kaunonen, M., & Aho, A. L. (2015). Evaluating a bereavement follow-up intervention for grieving mothers after the death of a child. *Scandinavian Journal of Caring Sciences, 29*(3), 510–520. doi:10.1111/scs.12183

Waller, A., Turon, H., Mansfield, E., Clark, K., Hobden, B., & Sanson-Fisher, R. (2016). Assisting the bereaved: A systematic review of the evidence for grief counselling. *Palliative Medicine, 30*(2), 132–148. doi:10.1177/0269216315588728

IMPAIRED HOME MAINTENANCE

related to impaired cognitive, emotional, or psychomotor functioning

Definition

Inability to independently maintain a safe growth-promoting immediate environment

Assessment

- Age
- Gender

- Home environment
- Financial resources
- Patient's psychosocial status, including perception of reality, communication patterns, role responsibilities, degree of awareness and concern, history of psychiatric-related illness, support systems, and cognitive, memory, and motor abilities
- Caregiver's psychosocial status, including stressors, support systems, and understanding of patient's care requirements

Defining Characteristics

- Difficulty maintaining a comfortable environment
- Excessive family responsibilities
- Financial crisis (e.g., debt, insufficient finances)
- Insufficient clothing
- Insufficient cooking equipment
- Insufficient equipment for maintaining home
- Insufficient linen
- Pattern of disease caused by unhygienic conditions
- Pattern of infection caused by unhygienic conditions
- Request for assistance with home maintenance
- Unsanitary environment

Expected Outcomes

- Patient and caregiver will express concern about poor home maintenance and verbalize plans to correct health and safety hazards in the home.
- Patient and caregiver will identify community organizations that can help ease transition from hospital to home or long-term care facility.
- Patient and caregiver will develop schedule for doing household tasks.

Suggested NOC Outcomes

Family Functioning; Role Performance; Self-Care: Instrumental Activities of Daily Living (IADLs)

Interventions and Rationales

- Help the patient and caregiver identify the strengths and weaknesses in current home maintenance practices *to provide a focus for interventions.*
- Discuss with the patient and caregiver obstacles to meeting home maintenance needs *to provide the basis for a program to meet health and safety requirements.*
- Determine the patient's ability and motivation to achieve a higher level of home maintenance. *Self-motivation is necessary to ensure change.*
- PCC Help the patient and caregiver explore community resources, such as Meals On Wheels, senior centers, home health care agencies, homemaker services, cleaning services, self-help groups, religious programs, and retired senior volunteer programs, *to ease the transition from hospital to home.*
- Allow the caregiver to express feelings about having responsibility for the patient's health care regimen and household upkeep. When appropriate, discuss opportunities for the caregiver to assign responsibility to other family members or make use of community resources. Encourage the caregiver to ask questions, seek help, and make decisions

to enhance communication and help the caregiver and family members form realistic expectations.

S
- Conduct a home visit or evaluate the patient's description of own home *to assess safety needs and make recommendations for structural alterations. For example, the patient may benefit from installing ramps, enlarging doorways, or moving a second-floor bedroom to the first-floor family room.*
- Discuss alternative housing opportunities with the patient and caregiver, such as moving the patient to a life-care community, *to provide necessary information to make appropriate decisions regarding the patient's future.*

S
- Based on assessment of the patient's health and home environment, determine the need for assistive devices, including:
  - hearing aids
  - handheld or table-stand magnifying glasses
  - hospital bed
  - large-print items
  - telephones for hearing impaired
  - telephone dial covers with large numbers
  - telephones with programmed dialing
  - wheelchair
  - amplifiers for phone receivers
  - clocks that chime or recite time
  - canes
  - walkers
  - handrails
  - safety bars for toilet and bath
  - automatic chair lifts
  - commode chairs
  - shower chairs
  - orthotics

  Using assistive devices helps the patient remain independent and improves self-confidence and self-esteem.
- Help the patient develop written daily and weekly schedules for performing household tasks *to provide structure and consistency and set standards for measuring progress.*

PCC
- Involve the patient in the decision-making process by providing a choice of where, when, and how to carry out appropriate home maintenance activities *to increase the patient's feelings of independence and self-esteem.*
- If the patient can't perform certain tasks without assistance, teach the caregiver or others how to provide help *to ensure the patient's needs are met.*

Suggested NIC Interventions

Environmental Management; Family Integrity Promotion; Home Maintenance Assistance; Role Enhancement

Evaluations for Expected Outcomes

- Patient and caregiver express understanding of changes needed to promote maximum health and safety in home.
- Patient and caregiver list community resources to assist with home maintenance deficits.
- Patient and caregiver establish and follow daily and weekly schedules for home maintenance activities.

Documentation

- Patient's perception of problems in home maintenance
- Observations regarding magnitude of home maintenance deficits
- Interventions to alleviate home maintenance deficits
- Responses of caregiver and others asked to assist patient with home maintenance
- Evaluations for expected outcomes

REFERENCES

Jang, M., & Lee, Y. (2015). The effects of an education program on home renovation for fall prevention of Korean older people. *Educational Gerontology, 41*(9), 653–669. doi:10.1080/03601277.2015.1033219

Kelly, A. J., Fausset, C. B., Rogers, W., & Fisk, A. D. (2014). Responding to home maintenance challenge scenarios: The role of selection, optimization, and compensation in aging-in-place. *Journal of Applied Gerontology, 33*(8), 1018–1042. doi:10.1177/0733464812456631

Smith, L. P., Shu Wen, N., & Popkin, B. M. (2014). Resistant to the recession: Low-income adults' maintenance of cooking and away-from-home eating behaviors during times of economic turbulence. *American Journal of Public Health, 104*(5), 840–846. doi:10.2105/AJPH.2013.301677

RISK FOR PERIOPERATIVE HYPOTHERMIA

Definition

Vulnerable to an inadvertent drop in core body temperature below 36° C/96.8° F occurring one hour before to 24 hours after surgery, which may compromise health

Assessment

- Body weight
- Environment temperature
- Patient temperature
- Patient's thermal comfort level
- Skin assessment

Risk Factors

- American Society of Anesthesiologists (ASA) Physical Status classification score >I
- Cardiovascular complications
- Combined regional and general anesthesia
- Diabetic neuropathy
- Heat transfer (e.g., high volume of unwarmed infusion, unwarmed irrigation >20 L)
- Low body weight
- Low environmental temperature
- Low preoperative temperature (<36° C/96.8° F)
- Surgical procedure

Expected Outcomes

- Patient will maintain normothermia before surgery.
- Patient will maintain normothermia during surgery.
- Patient will maintain normothermia after surgery.

Suggested NOC Outcomes

Neurological Status: Autonomic; Thermoregulation; Vital Signs; Risk Control: Hypothermia

Interventions and Rationales

- Implement passive warming measures such as cotton blankets, surgical drapes, plastic sheeting, and reflective blankets during the intraoperative period. *Decreases risk of subsequent hypothermia.*
- Increase ambient temperature to between 20° C and 25° C. *Ambient temperature can reduce risk of heat loss through convection.*
- Measure patient's temperature 1 to 2 hours before start of anesthesia and either continuously or every 15 minutes during surgery, and every hour post-surgery. *Monitor for higher risk for hypothermia*
- Prewarm IV infusions. *May reduce the risk of subsequent hypothermia*
- Prewarm patient 20 to 30 minutes before surgery. *Counteracts decline in temperature*

Suggested NIC Interventions

Comfort Level; Fluid Management; Hypothermia Treatment; Temperature Regulation; Vital Signs Monitoring

Evaluations for Expected Outcomes

- Patient expresses thermal comfort level
- Patient maintains normothermic body temperature.

Documentation

- Environmental temperature
- Use of passive warming measures
- Vital signs

REFERENCES

Putnam, K. (2015). New resource for preventing perioperative hypothermia. *AORN Journal, 102*(2), P7–P9. doi:10.1016/S0001-2092(15)00617-1

Singh, A. (2014). Strategies for the management and avoidance of hypothermia in the perioperative environment. *Journal of Perioperative Practice, 24*(4), 75–78.

Torossian, A., Bräuer, A., Höcker, J., Bein, B., Wulf, H., & Horn, E.-P. (2015). Preventing inadvertent perioperative hypothermia. *Deutsches Ärzteblatt International, 112*(10), 166–172. doi:10.3238/arztebl.2015.0166

STRESS URINARY INCONTINENCE

Definition

Sudden leakage of urine with activities that increase intra-abdominal pressure

Assessment

- History of incontinence symptoms, including onset and pattern
- Physical observations, including personal and perineal hygiene and complete bladder assessment
- Genitourinary status, including pain or discomfort, urinalysis, urine specific gravity, use of urinary assistive devices, voiding pattern, and cystometrogram results
- Fluid and electrolyte status, including intake and output, mucous membranes, postvoiding residual volume, skin turgor, and serum electrolyte, blood urea nitrogen, and creatinine levels
- Mental status, including cognition and affect
- Mobility status
- Emotional status, including evidence of social withdrawal
- Current medication regimen

Defining Characteristics

- Involuntary leakage of small volume of urine (e.g., with coughing, laughing, sneezing, on exertion)
- Involuntary leakage of small volume of urine in the absence of detrusor contraction
- Involuntary leakage of small volume of urine in the absence of overdistended bladder

Expected Outcomes

- Patient will understand causes of stress incontinence.
- Patient will establish plan compatible with lifestyle to manage symptoms.
- Patient will resume normal social activities.
- Patient will maintain continence with the aid of incontinence pads or frequent toileting.
- Patient will perform Kegel exercises.

Suggested NOC Outcomes

Knowledge: Treatment Regimen; Tissue Integrity: Skin/Mucous Membranes; Urinary Continence; Urinary Elimination

Interventions and Rationales

- Discuss stress incontinence and associated social stigma with the patient in a nonjudgmental manner. Tell the patient that many people experience incontinence. *The patient may be reluctant to discuss incontinence, which can have a negative effect on self-image. A nonjudgmental approach may help ease embarrassment and encourage open discussion of the problem.*
- PCC Assist the patient in obtaining appropriate evaluation and care for the underlying causes of stress incontinence *to ensure prompt diagnosis and treatment.*
- Review the current medication regimen for drugs that can contribute to stress incontinence, including diuretics, central nervous system depressants, and anticholinergics. Discuss with the physician the possibility of changing medications or the medication schedule *to relieve symptoms.*
- Develop an individualized toileting schedule, increasing intervals by 30 minutes until the patient achieves a 2- to 3-hour pattern. *Bladder retraining may help alleviate symptoms.*

PCC
- Teach the patient to do Kegel exercises to strengthen pelvic floor muscles. Instruct the patient to tighten the muscles of the pelvic floor to stop the flow of urine while urinating and then to release the muscles to restart the flow *to strengthen the urinary sphincter muscle and restore control.*
- Discuss the benefits and costs of adult incontinence pads with the patient. *Pads, although costly, are nonintrusive, easy to manage, and easily removed.*
- Encourage the patient to take short trips outside the home when symptoms are under control *to enhance the patient's confidence and reduce social embarrassment.*
- When mobility is a problem, help the patient obtain a bedside commode *to reduce the need for adult incontinence pads, which can adversely affect the patient's self-image.*

Suggested NIC Interventions

Pelvic Muscle Exercise; Urinary Elimination Management; Urinary Incontinence Care

Evaluations for Expected Outcomes

- Patient expresses, without embarrassment, understanding of causes of stress incontinence.
- Patient manages symptoms successfully.
- Patient begins to resume social activity.
- Patient maintains continence with aid of incontinence pads or frequent toileting.
- Patient performs Kegel exercises.

Documentation

- Patient's symptoms of stress incontinence, including onset and pattern
- Patient teaching, including Kegel exercises, use of incontinence pads, and other control strategies
- Patient's response to nursing interventions
- Evaluations for expected outcomes

REFERENCES

Knarr, J., Musil, C., Warner, C., Kless, J. R., & Long, J. (2014). Female stress urinary incontinence: An evidence-based, case study approach. *Urologic Nursing*, *34*(3), 143–151. doi:10.7257/1053-816X.2014.34.3.143

Ng, S. F., Lok, M. K., Pang, S. M., & Wun, Y. T. (2014). Stress urinary incontinence in younger women in primary care: Prevalence and opportunistic intervention. *Journal of Women's Health*, *23*(1), 65–68. doi:10.1089/jwh.2013.4382

Shin, D. C., Shin, S. H., Lee, M. M., Lee, K. J., & Song, C. H. (2016). Pelvic floor muscle training for urinary incontinence in female stroke patients: A randomized, controlled and blinded trial. *Clinical Rehabilitation*, *30*(3), 259–267. doi:10.1177/0269215515578695

RISK FOR URGE URINARY INCONTINENCE

Definition

Vulnerable to involuntary passage of urine occurring soon after a strong sensation of urgency to void, which may compromise health

Assessment

- Age and gender
- Vital signs

- Drug history
- History of illness that may cause neuromuscular dysfunction, including stroke, spinal cord injury, head injury, urinary tract disease, and infection
- Genitourinary status, including pain or discomfort, urinalysis, urine specific gravity, use of urinary assistive devices, voiding pattern, and cystometrogram results
- Fluid and electrolyte status, including intake and output, mucous membranes, postvoiding residual volume, skin turgor, and serum electrolyte, blood urea nitrogen, and creatinine levels
- Neuromuscular status, including ambulation ability, cognitive status, sensory ability, and degree of neuromuscular function
- Sexuality status, including patient's or partner's expressions of concern
- Psychosocial status, including coping skills, self-concept, stressors (finances, family, job), patient's and family members' perceptions of health problem, and patient's motivation to meet self-care needs

Risk Factors

- Alcohol consumption
- Atrophis urethritis
- Atrophic vaginitis
- Detrusor hyperactivity with impaired bladder contractility
- Fecal impaction
- Impaired bladder contractility
- Ineffective toileting habits
- Involuntary sphincter relaxation
- Small bladder capacity
- Treatment regimen

Expected Outcomes

- Patient will state possibility of anticipating when episodes of incontinence are likely to occur.
- Patient will state understanding of potential causes of urge incontinence and its treatment.
- Patient will avoid complications of urge incontinence or such complications will be minimized.
- Patient will discuss potential effects of urologic dysfunction on self and family members.
- Patient or family members will demonstrate skill in managing incontinence.
- Patient and family members will identify community resources to help them cope with alterations in urinary status.

Suggested NOC Outcomes

Knowledge: Treatment Regimen; Urinary Continence; Urinary Elimination

Interventions and Rationales

- Observe the patient's voiding pattern and document intake and output *to ensure correct fluid replacement therapy and provide information about the patient's ability to void adequately.*

- Determine the patient's premorbid elimination status *to ensure that interventions are realistic and based on the patient's health status and goals.*
- PCC Use an interdisciplinary approach to management of incontinence. Incorporate recommendations from a urologist, urology nurse specialist, other health care providers, and the patient. Monitor progress and report the patient's response to interventions. *An interdisciplinary approach helps to ensure that the patient receives adequate care. Encouraging patient participation on the team will help foster motivation.*
- Assess the patient's ability to sense and communicate elimination needs *to maximize self-care.*
- Make sure the patient's toilet environment is warm, clean, and free from odor *to promote continence.*
- Place a commode beside the bed if impaired mobility is an issue. *A bedside commode requires less energy expenditure than using a bedpan or ambulating to a bathroom.*
- Keep the bed and commode at same level *to facilitate easy access.*
- Provide good lighting from bed to bathroom *to reduce confusion and risk of falls.*
- S Remove all obstacles between bed and bathroom *to reduce risk of falls.*
- Unless contraindicated, provide 2.5 to 3 L of fluid daily *to moisten mucous membranes and ensure adequate hydration.* Space out fluid intake through the day and limit it to 150 mL after supper *to reduce the need to void at night.*
- Have the patient wear easily removed articles of clothing (a gown instead of pajamas, Velcro fasteners instead of buttons or zippers) *to facilitate the removal of clothing and foster independence.*
- Instruct the patient to stop and take a deep breath if experiencing an intense urge to urinate before reaching a bathroom. *Anxiety and rushing may increase bladder contraction.*
- Have the patient keep a diary recording episodes of incontinence. Use the information from the diary as a basis for planning interventions. Possible bladder training interventions may include voiding every 2 hours, avoiding high fluid intake, maintaining proper hygiene, or notifying a health care professional if urge incontinence occurs frequently. *Individualized interventions help promote self-care, foster motivation, and avoid incontinence.*
- PCC Incorporate the patient's suggestions for managing incontinent episodes into a care plan *to foster motivation.*
- Encourage the patient to express feelings regarding incontinence *to provide emotional support and identify areas for further patient teaching.*
- PCC Explain urge incontinence to the patient and family members, especially preventive measures and potential underlying causes, *to foster compliance.*
- Note if the patient expresses concern about the effect of incontinence on sexuality. If appropriate, refer him to a sex therapist *to promote sexual health.*
- PCC Refer the patient and family members to community resources such as support groups, as appropriate, *to help ensure continuity of care.*

Suggested NIC Interventions

Fluid Monitoring; Urinary Elimination Management; Urinary Habit Training; Urinary Incontinence Care

Evaluations for Expected Outcomes

- Patient states the possibility of anticipating when episodes of incontinence are likely to occur.
- Patient states understanding of potential causes of urge incontinence and its treatment.

- Patient avoids complications of urge incontinence or complications are minimized.
- Patient discusses potential effects of urologic dysfunction on self and family members.
- Patient or family members demonstrate skill in managing incontinence.
- Patient and family members identify community resources to help them cope with alterations in urinary status.

Documentation

- Patient's urologic status
- Episodes of urge incontinence
- Nursing interventions and patient's response
- Instruction given to patient and family and their responses
- Demonstrated ability to meet self-care needs
- Patient's expression of concern about potential changes in urologic status and its impact on body image and lifestyle
- Patient's statements indicating motivation to meet self-care needs
- Evaluations for expected outcomes

REFERENCES

Amano, T., Earle, C., Imao, T., & Takemae, K. (2016). Are urge incontinence and aging risk factors of erectile dysfunction in patients with male lower urinary tract symptoms? *Aging Male*, *19*(1), 54–57. doi:10.3109/13685538.2015.1103219

Tenfelde, S., & Janusek, L. W. (2014). Yoga: A biobehavioral approach to reduce symptom distress in women with urge urinary incontinence. *Journal of Alternative & Complementary Medicine*, *20*(10), 737–742. doi:10.1089/acm.2013.0308

Testa, A. (2015). Understanding urinary incontinence in adults. *Urologic Nursing*, *35*(2), 82–86. doi:10.7257/1053-816X.2015.35.2.82

RISK FOR INJURY

Definition

Vulnerable to physical damage due to environmental conditions interacting with the individual's adaptive and defensive resources, which may compromise health

Assessment

- Age
- Gender
- Patient's health status, including presence of acute or chronic illness and changes or deterioration in mental or physical functioning
- Family status, including communication patterns and presence or absence of extended family
- Family members' willingness and ability to provide physical and emotional support to patient
- Evidence of physical abuse, including malnutrition, imprint of hand or fingers, marks from restraints, and unexplained bruises, burns, welts, cuts, dislocations, or abrasions
- Evidence of emotional abuse, including observation or reports of insults, ridicule, or humiliation
- Evidence of financial abuse, including unexplained changes in bank accounts and transfer of funds to caregivers

- Evidence of neglect, including inappropriate clothing, unsanitary living conditions, inadequate food supplies, lack of medication, and absence of needed eyeglasses, hearing aids, cane, or walker

Risk Factors

External

- Alteration in cognitive functioning
- Alteration in psychomotor functioning
- Compromised nutritional source (e.g., vitamins, food types)
- Exposure to pathogen
- Exposure to toxic chemical
- Immunization level within community
- Nosocomial agent
- Physical barrier (e.g., design, structure, arrangement of community, building, equipment)
- Unsafe mode of transport

Internal

- Abnormal blood profile
- Alteration in affective orientation
- Alteration in sensation (resulting from spinal cord injury, diabetes mellitus, etc.)
- Autoimmune dysfunction
- Effector dysfunction
- Extremes of age
- Immune dysfunction
- Impaired primary defense mechanisms (e.g., broken skin)
- Malnutrition
- Sensory integration dysfunction
- Tissue hypoxia

Expected Outcomes

- Patient will remain free from injury and will state that incidents of abuse no longer occur.
- Patient will express understanding of right to be free from abuse.
- Patient will report increased social contact outside family.
- Patient will establish "buddy system," whereby the patient and friend visit or telephone each other at regularly scheduled intervals.
- Patient will maintain control over mail, telephone, and other personal effects.
- Caregiver will state intention to contact respite care services, support groups, and other community resources.
- Caregiver will report increased ability to cope with responsibilities of caring for older family member.
- Patient and caregiver will report improved communication patterns.

Suggested NOC Outcomes

Risk Control; Safe Home Environment

Interventions and Rationales

- Monitor the patient closely at each visit for evidence of physical or mental abuse or neglect. Observe for bruises or abrasions, body odor, or a dirty, unkempt appearance *to ensure safety and well-being.* Question the patient privately about findings *to encourage trust and promote open communication.*
- PCC Encourage the patient to discuss incidents of abuse or threats of abuse. Be willing to listen and be careful to convey a nonjudgmental attitude. *Older patients may be reluctant to discuss abuse or threats of abuse because of the fear of retaliation, embarrassment, or reluctance to report family members to authorities. By communicating that you care and are willing to listen, you may help the patient overcome these barriers.*
- PCC Teach the patient about the right to be free from abuse. Discuss the responsibility of law enforcement agencies to investigate incidents of abuse. Provide a list of social service agencies that can provide counseling *to empower the patient to resist or prevent episodes of abuse.*
- Encourage the patient to maintain the use of a personal telephone and open own mail *to promote a sense of control and self-worth and maintain contact with people outside the home.*
- PCC Encourage the patient to participate in community activities, such as religious groups and senior volunteer organizations, *to establish social contacts and develop a strong support network.*
- Suggest the use of Meals on Wheels or a community geriatric outreach for the homebound patient *to prevent isolation and provide respite for the family caregiver.*
- PCC Encourage friends to visit the patient at home. Suggest that the patient and a friend develop a "buddy system," whereby each takes turns telephoning or visiting the other at regular intervals *to provide social contact, respite for the caregiver, and an additional safeguard against abuse.*
- If appropriate, encourage the patient and family members to periodically hold conferences. Help the patient and family members identify productive topics for discussion, such as strategies for dealing with the patient's self-care deficits or scheduling respite care, *to foster open communication, defuse tension, and develop solutions to practical problems of caring for an older family member.*
- PCC Inform the caregiver about state and county services for the elderly, respite services, adult day care, support groups for children of aging parents, and other community resources *to enhance the caregiver's ability to cope and thereby diminish the likelihood of abuse.*
- S Report actual or suspected elder abuse to local authorities and provide follow-up or emergency care, if needed. *Nearly every state has laws mandating that suspected elder abuse be reported to authorities.*

Suggested NIC Interventions

Abuse Protection Support; Environmental Management: Violence Prevention; Family Mobilization; Risk Identification; Surveillance: Safety

Evaluations for Expected Outcomes

- Patient doesn't exhibit injuries and states that incidents of abuse have stopped.
- Patient expresses understanding of right to be protected from abuse.
- Patient reports satisfaction with ability to maintain or increase social contacts outside family.
- Patient establishes "buddy system" with friend outside home.

- Patient maintains control over mail, telephone, and other personal effects.
- Caregiver regularly attends community support group and contacts appropriate social service agencies and other sources of support.
- Caregiver reports increased ability to cope with responsibilities of caring for older family member.
- Patient and caregiver report improved communication.

Documentation

- Evidence of emotional, physical, or financial neglect or abuse
- Patient's statements that indicate risk of abuse
- Caregiver's statements indicating feelings about caring for older family member
- Caregiver's statements indicating willingness to attend support groups or use community resources
- Patient's and caregiver's expressed understanding of teaching provided by nurse
- Patient's response to nursing interventions
- Evaluations for expected outcomes

REFERENCES

Murphy, M. P., Carmine, H., & Kolakowsky-Hayner, S. (2014). Modifiable and nonmodifiable risk factors for falls after traumatic brain injury: An exploratory investigation with implications for medication use. *Rehabilitation Nursing*, *39*(3), 113–122. doi:10.1002/rnj.89

Sherwood, G., & Zomorodi, M. (2014). A new mindset for quality and safety: The QSEN competencies redefine nurses' roles in practice. *Nephrology Nursing Journal*, *41*(1), 15–72.

Ulrich, B., & Kear, T. (2014). Patient safety and patient safety culture: Foundations of excellent health care delivery. *Nephrology Nursing Journal*, *41*(5), 447–457.

DEFICIENT KNOWLEDGE (SPECIFY)

related to insufficient information

Definition

Absence or deficiency of cognitive information related to a specific topic

Assessment

- Current knowledge level
- Interest and motivation to learn
- Preferred learning style
- Comprehension ability and reading level
- Other factors that may affect learning, such as cultural influences; religious practices and beliefs; sensory, cognitive, or physical impairment; support systems; economic status; and feelings of anger, depression, or hopelessness

Defining Characteristics

- Inaccurate follow-through of instruction
- Inaccurate performance on a test
- Inappropriate behavior (e.g., hysterical, hostile, agitated, apathetic)
- Insufficient knowledge

Expected Outcomes

- Patient will express understanding of disease process, medication regimen, and treatment plan.
- Patient will make informed choices when addressing health care problems and self-care deficits.
- Patient will demonstrate ability to effectively implement chosen health care strategy.

Suggested NOC Outcomes

Knowledge: Disease Process; Knowledge: Medication; Knowledge: Treatment Procedure(s)

Interventions and Rationales

- Consider the older patient's life experiences when developing a teaching plan. *New information is easier to assimilate if it's built on existing knowledge.*
- Provide a quiet, calm environment for learning *to enable the patient to process information without distraction from background noise or stress.*
- Limit the length of each teaching session *to avoid information overload.*
- Ask if the patient wants to learn new or additional information. If not, discuss why. *Open discussion helps identify barriers to learning and determines if these barriers may be eliminated. Discussion also promotes acceptance of the patient's right to choose own level of participation.*
- Encourage the patient to use memory aids, such as preset alarms on a watch, a calendar for noting scheduled appointments, and a small notepad for recording questions or symptoms, *to help compensate for memory lapses.*
- PCC Write instructions in large letters, using black ink or contrasting colors. *Older patients see black best and may have difficulty distinguishing pastels or monochromatic color schemes.*
- PCC Modify your teaching style to accommodate normal aging changes:
  - Face the patient when speaking.
  - Use a well-modulated voice.
  - Allow ample time for teaching sessions.

  Understanding normal age-related changes enhances teaching effectiveness.
- Set aside time during each session for answering questions and clarifying information. An older patient may need affirmation that the knowledge the patient possesses is current and correct. Discussion may also stimulate an exchange of ideas and further learning.
- PCC Encourage the patient to join a support group, such as a club for stroke survivors or a support group for cancer patients, to reinforce education and promote contact with others in the same situation.
- PCC Involve the caregiver in teaching sessions, when appropriate, to reinforce information and ensure continuity of care at home.

Suggested NIC Interventions

Family Support; Health System Guidance; Support Group; Teaching: Disease Process; Teaching: Prescribed Medication; Teaching: Procedure/Treatment

Evaluations for Expected Outcomes

- Patient expresses increased understanding of disease process, medication regimen, and treatment plan, describing at least three basic concepts relevant to disease process and its impact on activities of daily living (ADLs).
- Patient states at least four strategies to improve self-care and expresses understanding of how chosen strategies will provide relief from disease process and improve own ability to perform ADLs.
- Patient demonstrates ongoing ability to implement chosen health care strategies.

Documentation

- Patient's verbal statements and behavior that indicate deficient knowledge
- Teaching provided and patient's or caregiver's response, including questions and comments made during teaching sessions
- Patient's description of chosen intervention strategies
- Patient's statements and behaviors that indicate implementation of strategies
- Evaluations for expected outcomes

REFERENCES

Fujii, M., Ishizuka, S., & Sasaki, H. (2015). Small group teaching in a psychiatric hospital for dementia patients. *Geriatrics & Gerontology International*, *15*(2), 239–240. doi:10.1111/ggi.12370

Goldschmidt, J., & Song, H. (2015). Active engagement: Teaching cooking skills to young adults with autism. *Journal of Nutrition Education & Behavior*, *47*(4), S29. doi:10.1016/j.jneb.2015.04.078

Meuris, K., Maes, B., & Zink, I. (2015). Teaching adults with intellectual disability manual signs through their support staff: A key word signing program. *American Journal of Speech-Language Pathology*, *24*(3), 545–560. doi:10.1044/2015_AJSLP-14-0062

IMPAIRED BED MOBILITY

related to neuromuscular impairment

Definition

Limitation of independent movement from one bed position to another

Assessment

- Age and gender
- Vital signs
- History of neuromuscular disorder or dysfunction
- Drug history
- Musculoskeletal status, including coordination, muscle size and strength, muscle tone, range of motion (ROM), and functional mobility as follows:
  0 = completely independent
  1 = requires use of equipment or device
  2 = requires help, supervision, or teaching from another person
  3 = requires help from another person and equipment or device
  4 = dependent; doesn't participate in activity
- Neurologic status, including level of consciousness, motor ability, and sensory ability

Defining Characteristics

- Impaired ability to move between long sitting and supine positions
- Impaired ability to move between prone and supine positions
- Impaired ability to move between sitting and supine positions
- Impaired ability to reposition self in bed
- Impaired ability to turn from side to side

Expected Outcomes

- Patient won't exhibit complications associated with impaired bed mobility, such as altered skin integrity, contractures, venous stasis, thrombus formation, depression, altered health maintenance, and falls.
- Patient will maintain or improve muscle strength and joint ROM.
- Patient will achieve highest level of bed mobility possible (independence, independence with device, verbalization of needs for assistance with bed mobility, requires assistance of one person, requires assistance of two people).
- Patient will maintain safety while in bed.
- Patient will demonstrate ability to use equipment or devices to assist with moving about in bed safely.
- Patient will adapt to alteration in ability to move about in bed.
- Patient will participate in social, physical, and occupational activities to the extent possible.

Suggested NOC Outcomes

Body Positioning: Self-Initiated; Immobility Consequences: Physiological; Immobility Consequences: Psychocognitive Mobility

Interventions and Rationales

- Perform ROM exercises to affected joints, unless contraindicated, at least once per shift. Progress from passive to active ROM, as tolerated, *to prevent joint contractures and muscle atrophy.*
- Assist the patient in maintaining anatomically correct and functional body positioning. Encourage repositioning every 2 hours while in bed. Establish a turning schedule for immobile patients. *Proper positioning relieves pressure, thereby preventing skin breakdown, and helps prevent fluid accumulation in dependent extremities.*
- Identify the patient's level of independence using the functional mobility scale. Communicate your findings to staff *to provide continuity of care and preserve the documented level of independence.*
- Monitor and record daily evidence of complications related to impaired bed mobility (contractures, venous stasis, skin breakdown, thrombus formation, depression, altered health maintenance or self-care skills, falls). *Patients with neuromuscular dysfunction are at risk for complications.*
- Perform prescribed medical regimen to manage or prevent complications (e.g., administer prophylactic heparin for venous stasis) *to promote the patient's health and well-being.*
- Assess the patient's skin every 2 hours *to maintain skin integrity.*
- Help the patient move about in bed. Encourage progressive mobility up to the limits imposed by the patient's condition *to maintain muscle tone, prevent complications associated with immobility, and promote self-care.*

- PCC Refer the patient to a physical therapist for development of a program to improve bed mobility *to assist with rehabilitation of musculoskeletal deficits.*
- PCC Refer the patient to an occupational therapist for development of a program to maximize self-care *to promote restoration of self-care skills.*
- PCC Encourage the patient to participate in physical and occupational therapy sessions. Incorporate equipment, devices, and techniques used by therapists into your care. Request written instructions from the patient's therapists to use as a reference *to help ensure continuity of care and reinforce learned skills.*
- If you're uncertain about your ability to move the patient, request help from colleagues *to maintain safety.*
- PCC Instruct the patient and family members in techniques to improve bed mobility and ways to prevent complications *to help prepare the patient and family members for discharge.*
- Demonstrate the patient's bed mobility regimen and note the date. Have the patient and family members perform a return demonstration *to ensure continuity of care and use of proper technique.*
- PCC Assist the patient in identifying and contacting resources for social and spiritual support *to promote the patient's reintegration into the community and help him maintain psychosocial health.*

Suggested NIC Interventions

Bed Rest Care; Body Mechanics Promotion; Circulatory Precautions; Exercise Promotion: Strength Training; Exercise Therapy: Joint Mobility; Fall Prevention; Positioning; Skin Surveillance

Evaluations for Expected Outcomes

- Patient doesn't exhibit complications associated with impaired bed mobility, such as altered skin integrity, contractures, venous stasis, thrombus formation, depression, altered health maintenance, and falls.
- Patient maintains or improves muscle strength and joint ROM.
- Patient achieves highest level of bed mobility possible (independence, independence with device, verbalization of needs for assistance with bed mobility, requires assistance of one person, requires assistance of two people).
- Patient maintains safety while in bed.
- Patient demonstrates ability to use equipment or devices to assist with moving about in bed safely.
- Patient adapts to alteration in ability to move about in bed.
- Patient participates in social, physical, and occupational activities to the greatest extent possible.

Documentation

- Patient's bed mobility status
- Presence of complications
- Referrals for physical or occupational therapy
- Response to program to improve or restore bed mobility
- Patient's statements regarding the loss of bed mobility skills and goals for improving bed mobility
- Teaching provided to patient and family members
- Patient's and family members' demonstrated skill in carrying out bed mobility program
- Evaluations for expected outcomes

REFERENCES

Janssens, J., Malfroid, K., Nyffeler, T., Bohlhalter, S., & Vanbellingen, T. (2014). Application of LSVT BIG intervention to address gait, balance, bed mobility, and dexterity in people with Parkinson's disease: A case series. *Physical Therapy*, *94*(7), 1014–1023. doi:10.2522/ptj.20130232

Lindemann, U., van Oosten, L., Evers, J., Becker, C., van Dieen, J. H., & van Lummel, R. C. (2014). Effect of bed height and use of hands on trunk angular velocity during the sit-to-stand transfer. *Ergonomics*, *57*(10), 1536–1540. doi:10.1080/00140139.2014.933889

Wysocki, A., Thomas, K. S., & Mor, V. (2015). Functional improvement among short-stay nursing home residents in the MDS 3.0. *Journal of the American Medical Directors Association*, *16*(6), 470–474. doi:10.1016/j.jamda.2014.11.018

IMPAIRED WHEELCHAIR MOBILITY

related to neuromuscular impairment

Definition

Limitation of independent operation of wheelchair within environment

Assessment

- Age and gender
- Vital signs
- History of neuromuscular disorder or dysfunction
- Drug history
- Musculoskeletal status, including coordination, gait, muscle size and strength, muscle tone, range of motion (ROM), and functional mobility as follows:
  0 = completely independent
  1 = requires use of equipment or device
  2 = requires help, supervision, or teaching from another person
  3 = requires help from another person and equipment or device
  4 = dependent; doesn't participate in activity
- Neurologic status, including level of consciousness, motor ability, and sensory ability
- Characteristics of patient's wheelchair (e.g., whether standard or motorized) and adequacy of wheelchair for meeting patient's needs (right size, appropriate safety features, and easy for patient to operate)
- Endurance (length of time patient can operate wheelchair before becoming fatigued)

Defining Characteristics

- Impaired ability to operate power wheelchair on a decline
- Impaired ability to operate power wheelchair on an incline
- Impaired ability to operate power wheelchair on curbs
- Impaired ability to operate power wheelchair on even surface
- Impaired ability to operate power wheelchair on uneven surface
- Impaired ability to operate wheelchair on a decline
- Impaired ability to operate wheelchair on an incline
- Impaired ability to operate wheelchair on curbs
- Impaired ability to operate wheelchair on even surface
- Impaired ability to operate wheelchair on uneven surface

Expected Outcomes

- Patient won't exhibit complications associated with impaired wheelchair mobility, such as skin breakdown, contractures, venous stasis, thrombus formation, depression, alteration in health maintenance, and falls.
- Patient will maintain or improve muscle strength and joint ROM.
- Patient will achieve highest level of independence possible with regard to wheelchair use.
- Patient will express feelings regarding alteration in ability to use wheelchair.
- Patient will maintain safety when using wheelchair.
- Patient will adapt to alteration in ability.
- Patient will participate in social and occupational activities to the greatest extent possible.
- Patient will demonstrate understanding of techniques to improve wheelchair mobility.

Suggested NOC Outcomes

Ambulation: Wheelchair; Balance; Immobility Consequences: Physiological; Immobility Consequences: Psychocognitive; Mobility

Interventions and Rationales

- Perform ROM exercises for affected joints, unless contraindicated, at least once per shift. Progress from passive to active ROM, as tolerated, *to prevent joint contractures and muscle atrophy.*
- Make sure the patient maintains anatomically correct and functional body positioning while in the wheelchair *to promote comfort.* Explain to the patient where vulnerable pressure points are and teach the patient to shift and reposition own weight *to prevent skin breakdown.*
- S Assess whether the patient's wheelchair is adequate to meet the patient's needs *to help maintain mobility and independence.* Consider the following:
  - Is the seat the right size? It should be wide and deep enough to support the patient's thighs and allow the patient to sit comfortably. It should be low enough so that the patient's feet touch the floor but high enough to allow easy transfer from bed to chair. The chair's back should be tall enough to support the patient's upper body.
  - Is the chair easy for the patient to operate when weak? If the patient has little or no arm strength, the patient may need a motorized wheelchair.
  - Is the chair safe? All wheelchairs have safety features, such as brakes that lock the wheels, but some safety features can be modified to meet the patient's needs. For example, seat belts can be attached at the waist, hips, or chest.
- S Identify the patient's level of independence using the functional mobility scale. Communicate findings to staff *to promote continuity of care and preserve the documented level of independence.*
- Monitor and record daily evidence of complications related to impaired wheelchair mobility (contractures, venous stasis, skin breakdown, thrombus formation, depression, and alteration in health maintenance or self-care skills). *Patients with neuromuscular dysfunction are at risk for complications.*
- PCC Encourage the patient to operate the wheelchair independently to the limits imposed by the patient's condition *to maintain muscle tone, prevent complications of immobility, and promote independence in self-care and health maintenance skills.*
- PCC Refer the patient to a physical therapist for development of a program to enhance wheelchair mobility *to assist with rehabilitation of musculoskeletal deficits.*

PCC
- Encourage attendance at physical therapy sessions and reinforce prescribed activities on the unit by using equipment, devices, and techniques used in the therapy session. Request a written copy of the patient's rehabilitation program to use as a reference *to maintain continuity of care and promote patient safety.*
- Assess the patient's skin on return to bed and request a wheelchair cushion, if necessary, *to maintain the patient's skin integrity.*

S
- Demonstrate techniques to promote wheelchair mobility to the patient and family members, and note the date *to help prepare the patient for discharge and maintain safety.* For example, teach the patient and family members how to perform wheelchair push-ups. If the patient can move the arms, have the patient grip the arms of the chair and push down hard with hands and arms to try to raise the body off the seat. Have the patient and family members perform a return demonstration *to ensure continuity of care and use of proper technique.*

PCC
- Assist in identifying resources for helping the patient maintain the highest level of mobility, such as a community stroke program, sports associations for people with disabilities, or the National Multiple Sclerosis Society, *to promote the patient's reintegration into the community.*

Suggested NIC Interventions

Exercise Promotion: Strength Training; Exercise Therapy: Balance; Exercise Therapy: Muscle Control; Mutual Goal Setting; Positioning: Wheelchair

Evaluations for Expected Outcomes

- Patient doesn't exhibit complications associated with impaired wheelchair mobility, such as skin breakdown, contractures, venous stasis, thrombus formation, depression, alteration in health maintenance, and falls.
- Patient maintains or improves muscle strength and joint ROM.
- Patient achieves highest level of independence possible with regard to wheelchair use.
- Patient expresses feelings regarding alteration in ability to use wheelchair.
- Patient maintains safety when using wheelchair.
- Patient adapts to alteration in ability.
- Patient participates in social and occupational activities to the greatest extent possible.
- Patient demonstrates understanding of techniques to improve wheelchair mobility.

Documentation

- Observations of changes in patient's mobility status and related complications
- Patient's expression of concern about loss of wheelchair mobility
- Patient's goals for future regarding mobility status
- Teaching provided to patient
- Patient's return demonstration of skills in carrying out wheelchair mobility program
- Patient's response to nursing interventions
- Evaluations for expected outcomes

REFERENCES

Best, K. L., Routhier, F., & Miller, W. C. (2015). A description of manual wheelchair skills training: current practices in Canadian rehabilitation centers. *Disability & Rehabilitation: Assistive Technology*, *10*(5), 393–400. doi:10.3109/17483107.2014.907367

Sakakibara, B. M., Miller, W. C., Eng, J. J., Backman, C. L., & Routhier, F. (2014). Influences of wheelchair-related efficacy on life-space mobility in adults who use a wheelchair and live in the community. *Physical Therapy*, *94*(11), 1604–1613. doi:10.2522/ptj.20140113
Slavens, B. A., Schnorenberg, A. J., Aurit, C. M., Graf, A., Krzak, J. J., Reiners, K., . . . Harris, G. F. (2015). Evaluation of pediatric manual wheelchair mobility using advanced biomechanical methods. *Biomed Research International*, *2015*, 1–11. doi:10.1155/2015/634768

RISK FOR IMPAIRED ORAL MUCOUS MEMBRANE

Definition

Vulnerable to injury to the lips, soft tissues, buccal cavity, and/or oropharynx, which may compromise health

Assessment

- Fluid intake
- Nutritional status
- Oral mucosa
- Ill-fitting dentures
- Ability to swallow
- Pain level
- Ability to provide oral hygiene

Risk Factors

- Alcohol consumption
- Allergy
- Alteration in cognitive functioning
- Autoimmune disease
- Autosomal disorder
- Barrier to dental care
- Barrier to oral self-care
- Behavior disorder (e.g., attention deficit, oppositional defiant)
- Chemotherapy
- Decrease in hormone level in women
- Economically disadvantaged
- Immunodeficiency
- Immunosuppression
- Inadequate nutrition
- Infection
- Insufficient knowledge of oral hygiene
- Insufficient oral hygiene
- Mechanical factor (e.g., orthodontic appliance, device for ventilation or food, ill-fitting dentures)
- Radiation therapy
- Smoking
- Stressors
- Surgical procedure
- Syndrome (e.g., Sjögren's)
- Trauma

Expected Outcomes

- Patient will have pink, moist, and intact oral mucosa.
- Patient will have no reports of oral dryness and pain.

Suggested NOC Outcomes

Hydration; Immune Status; Knowledge: Health Promotion; Nutritional Status; Self-Care: Oral Hygiene

Interventions and Rationales

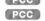

- Assist with oral care before meals, after meals and snacks. *Good oral care can decrease risk for impaired oral mucosa.*
- Avoid serving hot, cold, spicy, fried, or citrus foods. *Can damage oral mucosa.*
- PCC Educate about regular dental checkups. *Can ensure health of teeth and gums.*
- PCC Educate to breathe through nose and not mouth. *Mouth breathing can further dry the oral mucosa.*
- Encourage 2,500 to 3,000 ml of oral intake daily unless contraindicated. *Adequate fluid intake will help prevent dehydration and dryness of mouth.*
- Encourage patient to not smoke or use tobacco. *Smoking dries the mucosa and tobacco is an irritant to the oral mucosa.*
- Lubricate lips. *Prevents cracking and irritation.*
- Rinse mouth every 2 hours if unable to take fluid by mouth or presence of drainage or lesions. *Prevents dryness.*
- Suction mouth as needed. *Can reduce risk of developing infection.*
- Use tap water or saline to provide oral care. *Use of alcohol-based products or hydrogen peroxide will dry and damage the mouth.*

Suggested NIC Interventions

Fluid Management; Nutrition Management; Oral Health Maintenance; Oral Health Promotion

Evaluations for Expected Outcomes

- Patient does not have impaired oral mucosa.
- Patient does not report any oral dryness or pain.

Documentation

- Ability to provide oral hygiene
- Evaluations for expected outcomes
- Intake and output
- Nutritional status
- Oral mucosa assessment
- Pain level

REFERENCES

Dahm, T. S., Bruhn, A., & LeMaster, M. (2015). Oral care in the long-term care of older patients: How can the dental hygienist meet the need? *Journal of Dental Hygiene*, *89*(4), 229–237.

Eilers, J., Harris, D., Henry, K., & Johnson, L. A. (2014). Evidence-based interventions for cancer treatment-related mucositis: Putting evidence into practice. *Clinical Journal of Oncology Nursing, 18*, 80–96. doi:10.1188/14.CJON.S3.80-96
Özden, D., Türk, G., Düger, C., Güler, E. K., Tok, F., & Gülsoy, Z. (2014). Effects of oral care solutions on mucous membrane integrity and bacterial colonization. *Nursing in Critical Care, 19*(2), 78–86. doi:10.1111/nicc.12057

READINESS FOR ENHANCED NUTRITION

Definition

A pattern of nutrient intake, which can be strengthened

Assessment

- Biologic factors, including age, gender, and height, weight, and body mass index
- Psychological factors, including self-esteem, history of depression, and attitudes toward food and eating
- Sociocultural factors, including moral or health concerns about food and eating, financial status, and cultural background and influences of same in food choices
- Environmental factors, including ability to read and understand food labels, percentage of meals that are takeout, fast food, or eaten in restaurants, and cost of food in a particular geographical area

Defining Characteristics

- Expresses desire to enhance nutrition

Expected Outcomes

- Patient will articulate present understanding of factors that enable and hinder enhanced nutritional status.
- Patient will evaluate each of the barriers to enhancing nutritional status.
- Patient will articulate the personal value of practicing positive behaviors.
- Patient will plan modifications of environment, which will reinforce change in eating habits.
- Patient will express positive feelings about self.

Suggested NOC Outcomes

Knowledge: Diet; Nutritional Status; Nutritional Status: Biochemical Measures

Interventions and Rationales

- PCC Provide the patient with materials that are intellectually and culturally appropriate for enhancing nutritional knowledge. *It's important to engage the patient in information gathering before beginning to develop a plan to change behavior.*
- Help the patient list the internal and external barriers to improving nutritional status. *Lack of understanding of the patient's individual barriers, such as unclear goals, lack of skill, or lack of motivation will prevent change from occurring.*
- PCC Have the patient make a list of the positive outcomes of changing the behaviors, such as wearing smaller size clothing, feeling better about being with others who are health

conscious, enjoying feelings of physical and emotional well-being. *Positive reinforcers make the changes more appealing to effect.*

PCC • Teach the patient to read food labels, to plan meals using a standard method such as the Food Guide Pyramid (American Dietetic Association), and to shop for and stock the refrigerator and pantry with smart food choices. *New behaviors require practice in a practical sense for the kind of reinforcement that will produce the desired change.*

PCC • Encourage the patient to join or form some type of group *to help maintain the motivation to continue new behaviors.*

Suggested NIC Interventions

Nutrition Management; Nutritional Monitoring; Nutritional Counseling; Teaching: Prescribed Diet

Evaluations for Expected Outcomes

- Patient articulates present understanding of factors that enable and hinder enhanced nutritional status.
- Patient evaluates each of the barriers to enhancing nutritional status.
- Patient articulates the personal value of practicing positive behaviors.
- Patient plans modifications of environment, which will reinforce change in eating habits.
- Patient expresses positive feelings about self.

Documentation

- Weight changes
- Patient's expressed attitudes toward food and eating
- Patient's expressed feelings about weight, body image, and emotional status
- Patient's participation in a group
- Patient's response to nursing interventions
- Evaluations for expected outcomes

REFERENCES

Better nutrition when cooking for one. (2016). *Harvard Health Letter, 41*(4), 5.

Kamphuis, C. M., de Bekker-Grob, E. W., & van Lenthe, F. J. (2015). Factors affecting food choices of older adults from high and low socioeconomic groups: A discrete choice experiment. *American Journal of Clinical Nutrition, 101*(4), 768–774. doi:10.3945/ajcn.114.096776

Sobow, T. (2014). Healthy cognitive aging with a healthier diet and better nutrition? *European Journal of Clinical Nutrition, 68*(11), 1177–1178. doi:10.1038/ejcn.2014.179

RISK FOR POISONING

Definition

Vulnerable to accidental exposure to, or ingestion of, drugs or dangerous products in sufficient doses, which may compromise health

Assessment

- Age
- Gender

- Drug history, including use of prescription and over-the-counter medications
- Use of alcoholic beverages
- Health history, including evidence of hepatic or renal impairment
- Nutritional status, including weight changes, protein intake, and fluid status
- Psychosocial history, including activity level, knowledge level, financial status, mental status, and living arrangements
- Laboratory studies, including toxicology screening; serum digoxin, serum electrolyte, blood urea nitrogen, serum creatinine, and bilirubin levels; liver enzymes, such as aspartate aminotransferase, alanine aminotransferase, and alkaline phosphatase; and total serum protein and albumin to globulin ratio

Risk Factors

External

- Access to dangerous product
- Access to illicit drugs potentially contaminated by poisonous additives
- Access to large supply of pharmaceutical agents in house
- Access to pharmaceutical agent

Internal

- Alteration in cognitive functioning
- Emotional disturbance
- Inadequate precautions against poisoning
- Insufficient knowledge of pharmacologic agents
- Insufficient knowledge of poisoning prevention
- Occupational setting without adequate safeguards
- Reduced vision

Expected Outcomes

- Patient will express understanding of medication regimen.
- Patient won't experience episodes of toxicity.
- Patient's medical condition will remain under control.
- Patient will take only prescribed medications in correct quantities at correct times.

Suggested NOC Outcomes

Personal Safety Behavior; Safe Home Environment

Interventions and Rationales

- PCC Instruct the patient or family member in the drug regimen, including the reasons for taking drugs, safety precautions, and how to monitor the effectiveness of drugs, *to increase compliance.*
- S Regularly review and document the patient's medication regimen *to monitor medication use, assess whether certain medications should be discontinued, and monitor for drug interactions.*
- PCC Instruct the patient or family member to store drugs in secure area away from the bedside *to prevent accidental ingestion. Many older patients keep medications at their bedside to decrease the need to arise during the night.*

S
- If color-coding medications, use only bright, contrasting colors. *Older patients can't distinguish pastel colors well.*
- Help the patient or family member identify behaviors that contribute to the risk of toxicity, such as obtaining prescriptions from various health care providers or using different pharmacies, *to raise awareness of potential hazards.*
- Encourage the patient or family member to retain a primary physician who coordinates care. *Older patients with multiple health problems may receive care from various providers who are unaware of each other's treatment plans and medication regimens.*

PCC
- Provide instructions for the use of medications, including quantity, frequency, and number of doses, *to enhance understanding of the medication regimen and increase compliance.* Make sure the instructions are clearly written in black or blue ink. *Older patients can read black or blue ink more easily.*

S
- Make sure all medication labels are inscribed in large print and include dosage instructions *to avoid medication errors.*
- Help the patient maintain an accurate and effective system for following the medication regimen, such as a check-off calendar system or separate pill boxes labeled for each day of the week, *to reduce errors.* Encourage the patient to work with a pharmacist when developing this system.
- Monitor the patient's urine and serum toxicity levels, when indicated, *to reduce the risk of toxicity. Age-related changes in body function may lead to decreased renal, liver, and GI clearance of drugs, increasing the patient's risk of toxicity. Also, various drugs commonly used by the older patient increase the risk of toxicity from drug interactions.*

PCC
- Discuss with the physician the possibility of using alternative drugs, such as long-acting preparations or drugs that require only one dose per day, *to simplify the drug regimen and thereby decrease the risk of toxicity.*

Suggested NIC Interventions

Environmental Management: Safety; Health Education; Risk Identification; Substance Use Prevention

Evaluation for Expected Outcomes

- Patient expresses understanding of medication regimen.
- Patient doesn't experience episodes of toxicity.
- Patient's existing medical condition remains under control.
- Patient takes only prescribed drugs in correct quantities at correct times.

Documentation

- Evidence of patient's or family member's lack of understanding of or poor compliance with medication regimen
- Additional factors that increase patient's risk of drug toxicity
- Physical findings
- Instructions provided about safe drug practices
- Patient's or family member's response to instructions
- Patient's response to nursing interventions
- Evaluations for expected outcomes

REFERENCES

Marcus, D. M., & Grollman, A. P. (2016). Toxicity of botanical medicines: An overlooked global health problem. *American Journal of Public Health*, *106*(1), 16–17.

Morris, D. S., & Fiala, S. C. (2015). Online electronic cigarette retailers can do more to prevent accidental poisonings. *Tobacco Control*, *24*(4), 415–416. doi:10.1136/tobaccocontrol-2014-051779
Wong, C., Lin, Y., Hong, L., Chen, T., Ma, H., Hsu, Y., . . . Wu, M. (2016). Increased long-term risk of dementia in patients with carbon monoxide poisoning: A population-based study. *Medicine*, *95*(3), 1–5. doi:10.1097/MD.0000000000002549

POWERLESSNESS

Definition

The lived experience of lack of control over a situation, including a perception that one's actions do not significantly affect an outcome

Assessment

- Environmental factors, such as institutional setting
- Impact of therapeutic regimens on lifestyle, including use of cane or walker, changes in diet, and medication regimen
- Economic status, including retirement income, medical expenses such as ongoing home care or placement in nursing home, and Medicare or other insurance coverage
- Emotional status, including recent loss of spouse and history of dependence on others
- Physical impairments, including arthritic conditions, loss of limb use, diminished vision, and lengthy or chronic illness

Defining Characteristics

- Alienation
- Dependency
- Depression
- Doubt about role performance
- Frustration about inability to perform previous activities
- Inadequate participation in care
- Insufficient sense of control
- Shame

Expected Outcomes

- Patient will identify aspects of life still under patient's control.
- Patient will help develop schedule for self-care activities.
- Patient will participate in decisions about own care and lifestyle.
- Patient will express more realistic expectations and increased satisfaction with current situation.

Suggested NOC Outcomes

Depression Self-Control; Family Participation in Professional Care; Health Beliefs; Health Beliefs: Perceived Resources

Interventions and Rationales

- Guide the patient through a life review. Encourage the patient to reflect on past achievements *to foster a sense of satisfaction and promote acceptance of current status.*
- PCC Help the patient establish realistic expectations and goals. *Having realistic expectations helps prevent failures, which might exacerbate feelings of powerlessness.*
- Help the patient identify the aspects of own life that are still under control. For example, offer the patient a chance to request changes to the arrangement of the furniture in the patient's room. Recognize the patient's right to express feelings. *Empowering the older patient in any way possible may prevent feelings of powerlessness from becoming overwhelming.*
- PCC Encourage the patient to make choices in scheduling his daily routine, including personal hygiene, dressing and grooming, meals, and physical therapy. Emphasize that the patient, not staff members, has the authority to make scheduling decisions. *This helps the patient reassert control.*
- Ask the patient open-ended questions rather than questions that the patient can answer with "yes" or "no." *Open-ended questions encourage the patient to assert own opinions and thereby regain a feeling of control.*
- Encourage staff members to express interest in the patient's progress and set aside time to listen attentively to the patient *to acknowledge and reinforce own efforts to regain control.*
- PCC Encourage the patient to take an active role in choosing among social and recreational activities *to enhance the patient's lifestyle and further diminish feelings of powerlessness.*

Suggested NIC Interventions

Decision-Making Support; Family Involvement Promotion; Financial Resource Assistance; Health System Guidance; Self-Esteem Enhancement; Values Clarification

Evaluations for Expected Outcomes

- Patient identifies aspects of life still under own control and describes actions that can be taken to improve or modify the routine.
- Patient displays an appropriate sense of responsibility in scheduling self-care activities.
- Patient takes part in decisions about own care and lifestyle.
- Patient expresses more realistic expectations and increased satisfaction with current situation.

Documentation

- Patient's verbal and behavioral expressions of powerlessness
- Patient's level of involvement in self-care activities
- Patient's level of participation in therapeutic and social milieu
- Patient's response to nursing interventions
- Patient's statements indicating increased feelings of control
- Evaluations for expected outcomes

REFERENCES

Sheridan, N. F., Kenealy, T. W., Kidd, J. D., Schmidt-Busby, J. G., Hand, J. E., Raphael, D. L., . . . Rea, H. H. (2015). Patients' engagement in primary care: Powerlessness and compounding jeopardy. A qualitative study. *Health Expectations*, *18*(1), 32–43. doi:10.1111/hex.12006

Taylor, H. (2014). Promoting a patient's right to autonomy: Implications for primary health care practitioners. Part 1. *Primary Health Care, 24*(2), 36–41.
Uy, V., May, S. G., Tietbohl, C., & Frosch, D. L. (2014). Barriers and facilitators to routine distribution of patient decision support interventions: A preliminary study in community-based primary care settings. *Health Expectations, 17*(3), 353–364. doi:10.1111/j.1369-7625.2011.00760.x

RISK FOR RELOCATION STRESS SYNDROME

Definition

Vulnerable to physiological and/or psychosocial disturbance following transfer from one environment to another that may compromise health

Assessment

- Consideration of transfer or relocation
- Nature of possible relocation
- Physical and mental status of patient, including health condition, cognitive functioning, and functional abilities
- Financial resources
- Support systems, including family, friends, and health care workers
- Resources available to help prepare for relocation
- Conditions in original environment versus conditions in new environment
- Coping and problem-solving abilities, including educational level, past experiences with relocation, and participation in recreational activities or hobbies

Risk Factors

- Compromised health status
- Deficient mental competence
- History of loss
- Ineffective coping strategies
- Insufficient predeparture counseling
- Insufficient support system
- Move from one environment to another
- Powerlessness
- Significant environmental change
- Unpredictability of experience

Expected Outcomes

- Patient will request information about new environment.
- Patient will participate in decision making regarding relocation.
- Patient will communicate understanding of need for relocation.
- Patient will take steps to prepare for relocation along with family members or partner.
- Patient will express satisfaction with adjustment to new environment.

Suggested NOC Outcomes

Loneliness Severity; Psychosocial Adjustment: Life Change; Quality of Life; Stress Level

Interventions and Rationales

- Assess the patient's needs for additional health care services before relocation *to ensure that the patient receives appropriate care in the new environment.*
- PCC If possible, include the patient in the decision-making process regarding potential location, dates, and circumstances of relocation *to promote a feeling of participation in choices, which will allow a feeling of control.*
- If possible, allow the patient and family members to visit the new location and provide introductions to the new staff. *The more familiar the environment, the less stress the patient will experience during relocation.*
- PCC Educate family members about relocation stress syndrome and its potential effects *to encourage family members to provide needed emotional support throughout the transition period.*
- Help the patient and family members prepare for relocation. Conduct group discussions, provide pictures of setting, and communicate any information that will ease transition *to help the patient with the new environment.*
- Encourage the patient to express emotions associated with relocation *to provide an opportunity to correct misconceptions, answer questions, and reduce anxiety.*
- PCC Communicate all aspects of the patient's discharge plan to appropriate staff members at the new location *to ensure continuity of care.*
- Reassure the patient that family members and friends know the new location and will continue to visit *to reduce feelings of abandonment and anxiety.*

Suggested NIC Interventions

Active Listening; Coping Enhancement; Self-Responsibility Facilitation; Spiritual Support

Evaluations for Expected Outcomes

- Patient requests information about new environment.
- Patient expresses understanding of relocation process.
- Patient and family members complete preparations for relocation.
- Patient makes use of available resources to smooth transition to new environment.
- Patient expresses feelings associated with adjustment to new environment.

Documentation

- Evidence of patient's emotional distress over relocation
- Patient's needs in preparing for relocation
- Available resources and support systems
- Intervention to prepare patient and family members for relocation and patient's and family members' responses
- Discharge plan instructions communicated to new staff
- Evaluations for expected outcomes

REFERENCES

McGrath, P. (2015). Findings on family issues during relocation for hematology care. *Oncology Nursing Forum*, *42*, E250–E256. doi:10.1188/15.ONF.E250-E256

Oh, H., Lee, S., Kim, J., Lee, E., Min, H., Cho, O., & Seo, W. (2015). Clinical validity of a relocation stress scale for the families of patients transferred from intensive care units. *Journal of Clinical Nursing*, *24*(13/14), 1805–1814. doi:10.1111/jocn.12778

Yueh-Ying, Y., Shu-Ming, C., Chien-Lin, K., & Hsin-Ju, L. (2014). Exploring relocation stress and diabetes control in the elderly residents of long-term care facilities. *Journal of Nursing*, *61*(6), 57–65. doi:10.6224/JN.61.6.57

INEFFECTIVE ROLE PERFORMANCE

Definition

A pattern of behavior and self-expression that does not match the environmental context, norms, and expectations

Assessment

- Age
- Gender
- Patient's perception of social, vocational, and family roles
- Neurologic status, including level of consciousness, memory, mental status, orientation, and cognitive and perceptual functioning
- Physical disabilities or limitations
- Coping behaviors
- Developmental status, including evaluation of age-appropriate task resolution, such as accepting changes in mental and physical capacities, relinquishing past roles, creating new social relationships, substituting new activities and interests for those that can no longer be pursued, and revising goals, values, and self-concept to accommodate lifestyle changes
- Family status, including roles of family members, effect of illness on patient's family, and family members' understanding of patient's illness
- Family members' perceptions of patient's ability to perform social, vocational, and family roles

Defining Characteristics

- Alteration in role perception
- Anxiety
- Change in capacity to resume role
- Change in others' perception of role
- Change in self-perception of role
- Change in usual pattern of responsibility
- Depression
- Discrimination
- Domestic violence
- Harassment
- Inappropriate development expectations
- Ineffective adaptation to change
- Ineffective coping strategies
- Ineffective role performance
- Insufficient confidence
- Insufficient external support for role enactment
- Insufficient knowledge of role requirements
- Insufficient motivation
- Insufficient opportunity for role enactment
- Insufficient self-management
- Insufficient skills
- Pessimism
- Powerlessness
- Role ambivalence

- Role conflict
- Role confusion
- Role denial
- Role dissatisfaction
- Role strain
- System conflict
- Uncertainty

Expected Outcomes

- Patient will express feelings about limitations imposed by aging.
- Patient will discuss plans to reevaluate social, family, and vocational roles and adapt them to present physical and mental status.
- Family members will express willingness to take over responsibilities previously performed by patient.
- Patient will continue to perform usual social, family, and vocational roles to the extent possible.
- Family members will express willingness to provide emotional support as patient adjusts to ineffective role performance.

Suggested NOC Outcomes

Caregiver Lifestyle Disruption; Coping; Role Performance

Interventions and Rationales

- Discuss with the patient factors that make it difficult to fulfill the patient's usual vocational role. For example, has the patient recently been forced to retire? How does the patient cope with free time? How does the patient feel about no longer being the family breadwinner? *Discussion helps the patient gain insight and rationally define problems and potential solutions.*
- PCC Help the patient develop an activity program and explore ways the patient can contribute to society, such as participation in a senior volunteer program, *to help restore the patient's sense of purpose.*
- Discuss factors that make it difficult for the patient to fulfill usual social roles. For example, have many of the patient's close friends died? Is it difficult for the patient to obtain transportation to social events? *This will help the patient identify the causes of diminished social interaction.*
- PCC Investigate support groups, senior citizen centers, and other community resources *to help the patient find new outlets for forming social relationships.*
- PCC Discuss with family members ways they can help the patient cope with ineffective role performance, such as visiting frequently, providing emotional support, and requesting the patient's input in family decisions, *to help maintain the patient's self-esteem.*
- Encourage the patient to fulfill life roles within the constraints imposed by aging *to maintain a sense of purpose and preserve a connection with others.*
- Encourage family members to express feelings about the patient's ineffective role performance. Discuss alternate ways for family members to partially or fully assume roles formerly performed by the patient *to enhance family coping.*
- PCC Provide the patient and family members with information about developmental tasks that the patient must perform to master the process of aging. These may include accepting changes in mental and physical capacities, relinquishing past roles, creating new social

relationships, substituting new activities and interests for those that patient can no longer pursue, and revising goals, values, and self-concept to accommodate lifestyle changes. *Helping the patient and family members understand that these tasks are a normal part of the aging process may enhance coping.*

Suggested NIC Interventions

Anticipatory Guidance; Coping Enhancement; Counseling; Mood Management; Role Enhancement

Evaluations for Expected Outcomes

- Patient expresses feelings about limitations imposed by aging.
- Patient describes plans to adapt to role changes related to aging and chronic illness.
- Family members express willingness to take on responsibilities formerly held by patient.
- Patient continues to fulfill family, social, and vocational responsibilities to the extent possible.
- Family members express willingness to provide emotional support for patient as he adjusts to ineffective role performance.

Documentation

- Patient's expression of feelings and concerns associated with ineffective role performance
- Nursing interventions to help patient understand and accept changes in role performance
- Patient's response to nursing interventions
- Statements by family members indicating their attitude toward patient's ineffective role performance
- Referrals to support services for patient and family members
- Evaluations for expected outcomes

REFERENCES

Cavalcanti, B. C., Marques, D. R., Guimarães, F. J., de Oliveira Mangueira, S., da Silva Frazão, I., & Perrelli, J. A. (2014). "Ineffective role performance" nursing diagnosis in postpartum women: A descriptive study. *Online Brazilian Journal of Nursing, 13*(2), 246–254.

Chen, Y., Shaffer, M., Westman, M., Chen, S., Lazarova, M., & Reiche, S. (2014). Family role performance: Scale development and validation. *Applied Psychology: An International Review, 63*(1), 190–218. doi:10.1111/apps.12005

Watkins, S. L., Lounsbury, P. A., & Fleming-Castaldy, R. P. (2016). The self-assessment of role performance and activities of daily living abilities (SARA™): Development and clinical utility of a client-centered screening tool and outcome measure. *Occupational Therapy in Health Care, 30*(1), 42–57. doi:10.3109/07380577.2015.1050621

RISK FOR SELF-DIRECTED VIOLENCE

Definition

Vulnerable to behaviors in which an individual demonstrates that he or she can be physically, emotionally, and/or sexually harmful to self

Assessment

- Age 45 or older
- Gender
- Race
- Religion
- Marital status (widowed, divorced, married, or single)
- Life situation, including isolation (living alone or in urban area) and recent retirement, unemployment, or move to new area
- Mental health history, including coping behaviors, statements of low self-esteem, family dynamics, and communication patterns
- Recent stressors, including divorce, death of spouse, and relocation
- Mental status, including orientation, level of consciousness, and thought processes
- Support systems

Risk Factors

- Age ≥45 years
- Age 15 to 19 years
- Behavioral cues (e.g., writing forlorn love notes, directing angry messages at a significant other who has rejected the person, giving away personal items, taking out a large life insurance policy)
- Conflict about sexual orientation
- Conflict in interpersonal relationship(s)
- Employment concern (e.g., unemployed, recent job loss/failure)
- Engaged in autoerotic sexual acts
- History of multiple suicide attempts
- Insufficient personal resources (e.g., achievement, insight, affect unavailable and poorly controlled)
- Marital status (e.g., single, widowed, divorced)
- Mental health issue (e.g., depression, psychosis, personality disorder, substance abuse)
- Occupation (e.g., executive, administrator/owner of business, professional, semiskilled worker)
- Pattern of difficulties in family background (e.g., chaotic or conflictual, history of suicide)
- Physical health issue
- Psychological disorder
- Social isolation
- Suicidal ideation
- Suicidal plan
- Verbal cues (e.g., talking about death, "better off without me," asking about lethal dosage of medication)

Expected Outcomes

- Patient won't harm self and will remain in safe environment.
- Patient will discuss sadness, despair, and other feelings.
- Patient will discuss events that led up to current crisis.
- Patient will acknowledge suicidal thoughts.
- Patient will receive referral to mental health professional.
- Patient will express improved self-concept.
- Patient will report decreased desire to kill self.
- Patient will discuss appropriate coping skills to avoid future suicidal episodes.

Suggested NOC Outcomes

Impulse Self-Control; Self-Mutilation Restraint; Suicide Self-Restraint

Interventions and Rationales

- Be aware of key facts about suicide in older patients:
  - Suicide among older adults is a serious problem. Those with the highest risk of suicide are at least 85 years old, depressed, with high self-esteem and a need to control life.
  - The suicide rate for older adult men is seven times that for older women.
  - Most suicides by older patients are planned and aren't just gestures or threats; even frail nursing home residents can find strength to carry out suicide, if sufficiently determined.

  Awareness of suicide risks may help prevent attempts.
- S Remove items from the patient's surroundings that could be used in a suicide attempt *to ensure the patient's safety.*
- Set aside time for listening to the patient *to communicate that you care.*
- Approach the patient with understanding and concern *to alleviate angry or embarrassed feelings related to emotional breakdown or a previous unsuccessful suicide attempt.*
- Communicate a nonjudgmental attitude *to build trust and rapport.*
- Assess the patient for signs and symptoms of depression, such as a persistent depressed mood, diminished interest in daily activities, sleep disturbances, inappropriate guilt, loss of energy, poor concentration, changes in appetite, psychomotor retardation or agitation, and a passive wish for death. *Elderly patients are at increased risk for depression. Depression increases in frequency and intensity with advancing age. Factors that contribute to an increase in depression include changes in neurotransmitter levels, multiple losses, diminished health, and decreased resources. Depression may also occur in the early stages of dementia.*
- Discuss the problems that led the patient to this episode of depression. *Talking about specific events may help the patient achieve catharsis and develop appropriate coping skills.* Events that may contribute to depression in older patients include recent major loss, experience of rejection by or isolation from family or friends, recent disability, loss of partner, loss of sexual function, and loss of social, family, or occupational role.
- Recognize the patient's feelings of inadequacy and take steps to bolster self-esteem. Encourage the patient to participate in a life review, revisit places where significant past events took place, put together a scrapbook, research family genealogy, or attend family, class, or church reunions. *These activities help the patient experience emotions, which ultimately promotes improved self-esteem.*
- Avoid comparing the patient with others *to reduce stereotyping and foster individuality.*
- Support the patient but don't give false reassurances that everything will work out. Let the patient know that, although no easy answer exists, help is available and you'll help find alternative solutions *to ease despair.*
- S Supervise the administration of prescribed medications. Be aware of drug actions and adverse effects and make sure that the patient doesn't hoard medications *to ensure the patient won't harm self, even inadvertently.*
- Decrease environmental stimuli, when necessary, and provide a safe outlet that allows patient to release emotions and anger. Review situations that cause stress for the patient and help the patient develop plans for dealing with them. *These measures will help the patient cope better with depression.*

- Assess for signs of suicidal thinking that warrant further investigation, such as sudden hoarding of medications, giving away possessions, sudden interest in guns, and despondent remarks, *to determine if the patient is at risk for suicide.*
- PCC Ask the patient directly, "Have you thought about killing yourself?" If so, ask, "What do you plan to do?" *to assess for suicidal ideation.*
- If you suspect that the patient is at risk for suicide, refer the patient to a mental health professional for immediate evaluation *to ensure safety.*
- PCC Educate the patient or family member in the use of prescribed antidepressants. Explain that geriatric doses differ from those for younger patients. *Knowledge of medications and careful monitoring help guard against adverse effects.*
- PCC Help the patient identify community resources *to obtain continued therapy and support after hospitalization.*
- PCC Encourage family members to talk with one another and develop improved coping strategies *to foster enhanced family functioning.*

Suggested NIC Interventions

Environmental Management: Violence Prevention; Impulse Control Training; Suicide Prevention

Evaluations for Expected Outcomes

- Patient doesn't harm self and the patient's environment is safe, with items that could be used in suicide attempt removed.
- Patient expresses feelings and thoughts in way that promotes healing process.
- Patient discusses events that led up to current crisis.
- Patient acknowledges suicidal thoughts.
- Patient receives referral to mental health professional.
- Patient states feeling better about self.
- Patient states experiencing fewer suicidal thoughts.
- Patient expresses understanding the importance of increased social support and improved coping skills in avoiding future suicidal episodes.

Documentation

- Patient's exact description of suicidal thoughts and recent suicide attempt
- Observations of patient's behavior
- Interventions to prevent suicide
- Patient's response to therapy
- Evaluations for expected outcomes

REFERENCES

Ho, R. M., Ho, E. L., Tai, B. C., Ng, W. Y., & Chia, B. H. (2014). Elderly suicide with and without a history of suicidal behavior: Implications for suicide prevention and management. *Archives of Suicide Research*, *18*(4), 363–375. doi:10.1080/13811118.2013.826153

Shah, A., & Zarate-Escudero, S. (2014). Can some aspects of the epidemiology of elderly suicides be applied to dementia. *International Psychogeriatrics*, *26*(2), 185–191. doi:10.1017/S1041610213001026

Wright, P. P., & Thorpe, C. W. (2016). Triple threat among the elderly: Depression, suicide risk, and handguns. *Journal of Emergency Nursing*, *42*(1), 14–18. doi:10.1016/j.jen.2015.01.0100

SITUATIONAL LOW SELF-ESTEEM

related to alteration in social role; functional impairment

Definition

Development of a negative perception of self-worth in response to a current situation

Assessment

- Changes in physical appearance, including wrinkles, sagging skin, gray hair, aging spots, scoliosis, dowager's hump, and increased truncal fat
- Changes in social status, including recent retirement (forced or voluntary)
- Changes in sleep patterns, including trouble falling asleep, frequent awakenings, and restless sleep
- Family status, including recent loss of spouse or significant other
- Reason for current hospitalization
- Medical history, including chronic illnesses
- Mental status, including evidence of depression, hopelessness, discouragement, preoccupation with body functions, and unrealistic fear of developing serious disease

Defining Characteristics

- Helplessness
- Indecisive behavior
- Nonassertive behavior
- Purposelessness
- Self-negating verbalizations
- Situation challenge to self-worth
- Underestimates ability to deal with situation

Expected Outcomes

- Patient will participate in care.
- Patient will maintain eye contact and initiate conversations.
- Patient will maintain upright and open posture.
- Patient's body language and speech content will be congruent.
- Patient will talk about impact of changes caused by chronic illness or aging on lifestyle.
- Patient will express (verbally or through behavior) increased acceptance of changes caused by chronic illness or aging.
- Patient will express increased self-esteem.

Suggested NOC Outcomes

Decision-Making; Grief Resolution; Psychosocial Adjustment: Life Change; Self-Esteem

Interventions and Rationales

- Ask permission to enter the patient's personal space, including areas around the bed, bedside tables, and closet. *As the patient's self-esteem decreases, the significance of personal space increases. Asking permission provides the patient with a sense of control and raises self-esteem.*

- Encourage the patient to wear own pajamas or gowns and robes *to contribute to positive self-identity.*
- Arrange the patient's personal items on the bedside stand so that they're in easy reach *to maintain the patient's independence.*
- Incorporate appropriate exercise activities into the patient's daily care *to enhance strength, endurance, and coordination, and improve self-esteem.*
- Encourage the patient to reminisce *to focus the patient's attention on past accomplishments.*
- If the patient has limited mobility, install an over-the-bed trapeze *to promote independence.*
- Incorporate tactile stimulation into daily activities through techniques such as back rubs, foot massages, and touching of the hand or arm. *Frequent touching enhances the patient's sense of self-worth.*
- PCC Encourage the patient to express feelings about chronic illness or aging and fears about loss of independence and ability to participate in work and leisure activities. *This allows the patient to gain insight and to rationally define problems and possible solutions.*
- PCC Provide information about appropriate support groups and encourage interacting with individuals who have successfully adapted to illness or limitations *to increase the patient's coping skills.*

Suggested NIC Interventions

Coping Enhancement; Decision-Making Support; Grief Work Facilitation; Self-Esteem Enhancement

Evaluations for Expected Outcomes

- Patient carries out activities of daily living while in hospital.
- Patient maintains eye contact and initiates conversations.
- Patient maintains upright and open posture.
- Patient's body language and speech are congruent.
- Patient states at least two ways that chronic illness or aging will affect the patient's lifestyle.
- Patient discusses feelings about aging, chronic illness, loss of independence, and diminished ability to participate in work and leisure activities.
- At least once per day, patient makes statements reflecting greater self-esteem.

Documentation

- Patient's expressions that indicate lowered self-esteem
- Mental status assessment (baseline and ongoing)
- Interventions to improve patient's self-esteem
- Patient's response to nursing interventions
- Evaluations for expected outcomes

REFERENCES

La Mela, C., Maglietta, M., Caini, S., Casu, G. P., Lucarelli, S., Mori, S., & Ruggiero, G. M. (2015). Perfectionism, weight and shape concerns, and low self-esteem: Testing a model to predict bulimic symptoms. *Eating Behaviors*, *19*, 155–158. doi:10.1016/j.eatbeh.2015.09.002

Noser, A., & Zeigler-Hill, V. (2014). Investing in the ideal: Does objectified body consciousness mediate the association between appearance contingent self-worth and appearance self-esteem in women? *Body Image*, *11*(2), 119–125. doi:10.1016/j.bodyim.2013.11.006
Garofalo, C., Holden, C. J., Zeigler-Hill, V., & Velotti, P. (2016). Understanding the connection between self-esteem and aggression: The mediating role of emotion dysregulation. *Aggressive Behavior*, *42*(1), 3–15. doi:10.1002/ab.21601

INEFFECTIVE SEXUALITY PATTERN

Definition

Expressions of concern regarding own sexuality

Assessment

- Changes in female reproductive organs related to aging
- History of hormone replacement therapy (postmenopause or postoophorectomy), including estrogen, progesterone, or both
- Relationship with spouse or significant other
- Psychosocial status, including self-perception, ability to cope with aging process, usual sexual activity pattern, and social interaction patterns
- Chronic illnesses
- Impaired mobility
- Perceived changes in sexual activity resulting from surgery or illness

Defining Characteristics

- Alteration in relationship with significant other
- Alteration in sexual activity
- Alteration in sexual behavior
- Change in sexual role
- Difficulty with sexual activity
- Difficulty with sexual behavior
- Value conflict

Expected Outcomes

- Patient will express feelings about sexuality and self-concept.
- Patient will discuss options for maintaining intimacy throughout life span.
- Patient will express understanding of normal physiologic changes in reproductive organs that occur with aging.
- Patient will express understanding of options to relieve discomfort associated with menopause or hysterectomy.

Suggested NOC Outcomes

Body Image; Role Performance; Sexual Identity

Interventions and Rationales

PCC
- Provide information about hysterectomy and menopause. *After menopause or hysterectomy, older women may need reassurance that sexual activity can still be enjoyable.*

PCC
- Teach the patient about the impact of normal physiologic changes caused by aging on sexuality. For example, the vagina becomes smaller and less elastic, vaginal walls become thin and smooth, and external genitalia may become softer. Also, vaginal lubrication may take longer. Patient may also have abdominal pain or bladder irritability during intercourse. *Explaining how aging affects sexuality may help the patient accept these physiologic changes.*
- Encourage the patient to express feelings about sexuality *to reassure the patient that you're willing to discuss her concerns.*
- Discuss other options for intimacy, such as hugging, touching, and closeness, *to reaffirm the patient's identity as a sexual being.*

PCC
- Provide information about alternative techniques and adaptations that can assist sexual satisfaction *to encourage the patient to explore and accept her sexuality.* Topics may include the use of lubricants, Kegel exercises (for vaginal muscle tone), self-stimulation, and alternative sexual positions and activities.
- Discuss the impact that a chronic illness or adverse drug reactions can have on the patient's sexuality *to explore ways of eliminating barriers to sexual enjoyment.* Discuss with the physician the possibility of providing alternative medications.

PCC
- Teach the patient the benefits and risks associated with hormone replacement therapy, including:
  - reduced postmenopausal osteoporosis
  - increased risk of endometrial cancer (with estrogen therapy alone)
  - presence of monthly menses with combined estrogen and progestin therapy
  - increased risk of breast cancer.

  Education helps the patient make the most informed decision possible.
- Discuss psychosocial issues that may affect the patient's sexuality, such as financial concerns about remarriage or a family member's objections to her relationship with a male companion, *to help the patient focus on specific concerns and avoid misunderstandings.*

PCC
- If the patient lives in a long-term care facility or life-care community, encourage her to participate in social activities *to enhance opportunities for sexual expression.*

Suggested NIC Interventions

Body Image Enhancement; Self-Awareness Enhancement; Self-Esteem Enhancement

Evaluations for Expected Outcomes

- Patient discusses feelings related to sexuality and self-concept.
- Patient discusses options for maintaining intimacy throughout life.
- Patient describes physiologic changes in reproductive organs that occur with aging.
- Patient describes options to relieve discomfort associated with menopause or hysterectomy, including risks and benefits of hormone replacement therapy.

Documentation

- Patient's expression of feelings about sexuality and aging
- Teaching provided and patient's response
- Patient's behavioral response to care
- Patient's expression of improved ability to achieve sexual enjoyment and intimacy
- Evaluations for expected outcomes

REFERENCES

Erden, S., & Kaya, H. (2015). Sexual dysfunction and anxiety levels of type 2 male diabetics. *Applied Nursing Research*, *28*(3), 239–243. doi:10.1016/j.apnr.2015.04.014

Perz, J., Ussher, J. M., & Gilbert, E. (2014). Feeling well and talking about sex: Psychosocial predictors of sexual functioning after cancer. *BMC Cancer*, *14*(1), 228–228. doi:10.1186/1471-2407-14-228

Villaamil, F. (2014). Shared embarrassment: (Not) Talking about sex in HIV-related doctor–patient encounters. *Medical Anthropology*, *33*(4), 335–350. doi:10.1080/01459740.2013.826215

RISK FOR IMPAIRED SKIN INTEGRITY

Definition

Vulnerable to alteration in epidermis and/or dermis, which may compromise health

Assessment

- Age
- Physical examination, including inspection of lower limbs, testing for sensation in lower limbs, palpation of peripheral pulses, and presence of edema
- Integumentary status, including color, elasticity, hygiene, lesions, moisture, quantity and distribution of hair, sensation, temperature and blood pressure, texture, turgor, and condition of nails
- Psychosocial status, including coping patterns, lifestyle, presence of family members or significant other, mental status, self-concept, and body image
- Mobility status, including activity level, joint range of motion, contractures, muscle mass, and tone
- Mental status
- Evidence of incontinence
- Recent changes in medication regimen
- History of skin problems, including pressure ulcers, dermatitis, and trauma
- Ability to perform skin care regimen

Risk Factors

External

- Chemical injury agent (e.g., burn, capsaicin, methylene chloride, mustard agent)
- Excretions
- Extremes of age
- Humidity
- Hyperthermia
- Hypothermia
- Mechanical factor (e.g., shearing forces, pressure, physical immobility)
- Moisture
- Radiation therapy
- Secretions

Internal

- Alteration in metabolism
- Alteration in pigmentation
- Alteration in sensation (resulting from spinal cord injury, diabetes mellitus, etc.)
- Alteration in skin turgor
- Hormonal change
- Immunodeficiency
- Impaired circulation
- Inadequate nutrition
- Pharmaceutical agent
- Pressure over bony prominence
- Psychogenetic factor

Expected Outcomes

- Patient will maintain intact skin.
- Patient or caregiver will describe normal aging changes in skin and risk factors for disturbance in skin integrity.
- Patient or caregiver will implement strategies to prevent skin breakdown and will carry out skin care regimen.

Suggested NOC Outcomes

Immobility Consequences: Physiological; Tissue Integrity: Skin & Mucous Membranes

Interventions and Rationales

- PCC Educate the patient or caregiver about changes to skin caused by aging *to motivate the patient or caregiver to implement a skin care regimen. Physiologic changes associated with aging increase the risk of skin breakdown. For example, older patients, especially those immobilized with chronic health problems, are at high risk for pressure ulcers. Physiologic changes also leave older patients vulnerable to problems associated with dry skin.*
- Help the patient obtain appropriate evaluation and treatment of the underlying skin condition *to promote healing and minimize complications.*
- Help the patient or caregiver implement a pressure-relief movement and massage program *to prevent pressure ulcers.* The patient should change position at least every 2 hours. *Frequent turnings and massage promote adequate tissue perfusion and prevent necrosis.*
- Use preventive skin care devices as needed, such as a foam mattress, alternating pressure mattress, sheepskin, pillows, or padding, *to avoid discomfort and skin breakdown. These measures don't replace the need for turning.*
- PCC Teach the patient about the need for good nutrition, including the importance of meeting caloric requirements and benefits of adequate vitamin and protein intake. *Good nutrition helps maintain adequate tissue nourishment, perfusion, and oxygenation.*
- Help the patient or caregiver develop and implement a daily routine of skin inspection and care. Discuss the need to maintain good personal hygiene; use nonirritating (nonalkaline) soap; pat rather than rub skin dry; inspect skin regularly; avoid prolonged exposure to water, sun, cold, and wind; and recognize and report signs of skin breakdown (redness, blisters, and discoloration). *A daily program of skin inspection and maintenance will protect the older patient's skin integrity.*
- Encourage the patient or caregiver to seek immediate attention if skin injury or trauma occurs *to help prevent further injury and conditions that may require extensive treatment.*
- Monitor wounds or incisions for infection and follow a prescribed treatment regimen *to prevent infection, which may delay healing.*

Suggested NIC Interventions

Bed Rest Care; Circulatory Precautions; Pressure Management; Skin Surveillance

Evaluations for Expected Outcomes

- Patient's skin remains intact.
- Patient or caregiver describes skin changes that result from aging and lists risk factors for impaired skin integrity.
- Patient or caregiver implements daily program of skin inspection and care, including frequent turning and movement.

Documentation

- Observations of patient's skin
- Presence of risk factors for impaired skin integrity
- Patient teaching provided and patient's response
- Patient's response to nursing interventions
- Evaluations for expected outcomes

REFERENCES

Cowdell, F., & Garrett, D. (2014). Older people and skin: Challenging perceptions. *British Journal of Nursing*, *23*, S4–S8.

Cowdell, F., & Radley, K. (2014). What do we know about skin-hygiene care for patients with bariatric needs? Implications for nursing practice. *Journal of Advanced Nursing*, *70*(3), 543–552. doi:10.1111/jan.12208

Yamaguti, W. P., Moderno, E. V., Yamashita, S. Y., Gomes, T. C., Maida, A. V., Kondo, C. S., . . . de Brito, C. M. (2014). Treatment-related risk factors for development of skin breakdown in subjects with acute respiratory failure undergoing noninvasive ventilation or CPAP. *Respiratory Care*, *59*(10), 1530–1536. doi:10.4187/respcare.02942

SOCIAL ISOLATION

Definition

Aloneness experienced by the individual and perceived as imposed by others and as a negative or threatening state

Assessment

- Age
- Psychosocial status, including support systems, financial resources, coping and problem-solving ability, cultural background, and activities or hobbies
- Health status, including vision or hearing deficits, chronic illness, incontinence, and pain
- Self-care abilities, including knowledge and use of adaptive equipment and supplies, and technical and mechanical skills
- Living conditions, including home environment, site of activities and resources, and transportation
- Mental status, including behavior, mood, and affect
- Musculoskeletal status, including coordination, functional ability, gait, range of motion, presence of tremor or paralysis, and muscle tone, size, and strength

Defining Characteristics

- Absence of support system
- Aloneness imposed by others
- Cultural incongruence
- Desire to be alone
- Developmental delay
- Developmentally inappropriate interests
- Disabling condition
- Feeling different from others
- Flat affect
- History of rejection
- Hostility
- Illness
- Inability to meet expectations of others
- Insecurity in public
- Meaningless actions
- Member of a subculture
- Poor eye contact
- Preoccupation with own thoughts
- Purposelessness
- Repetitive actions
- Sad affect
- Values incongruent with cultural norms
- Withdrawn

Expected Outcomes

- Patient will express feelings associated with social isolation.
- Patient will seek assistance or information from staff to overcome social isolation.
- Patient will make use of community resources.
- Patient will describe increased number of social contacts.
- Patient will express satisfaction with level of social contacts.

Suggested NOC Outcomes

Leisure Participation; Loneliness Severity; Mood Equilibrium; Social Interaction Skills

Interventions and Rationales

- Assign a primary nurse or case manager to the patient *to provide consistency and promote trust.*
- Discuss with the patient causes and contributing factors of social isolation. Find out what factors the patient believes interfere most with the ability to develop relationships with others *to determine the patient's wants and needs.*
- Determine if the patient is willing to make changes in lifestyle or daily routine to increase contact with others. *The patient needs to have motivation for nursing interventions to succeed.*
- If appropriate, address physical limitations that interfere with the patient's ability to form social relationships. For example, if the patient has a hearing deficit, make a referral to an audiologist for a hearing aid; if the patient has a mobility impairment, make a referral to

a physical therapist for an exercise program or for recommendations for assistive devices. *The patient may need physical limitations addressed before the patient can overcome social isolation.*

- Assess the influence of the home environment on the patient's social life. For example, is the patient afraid to go outside because of a high crime rate in the neighborhood? If so, consider investigating options, such as a retirement community or residential care facility, which might offer better social opportunities. *The patient may not be aware of alternative living options.*
- PCC Investigate activity groups, support groups, senior citizens centers, health education programs, and other community resources *to develop an activity program for the patient.*
- Investigate the availability and cost of public transportation. Familiarize the patient with the route to planned activities. *The patient must overcome barriers to transportation to gain access to the outside world.*
- PCC Involve the patient in planning activities that will enhance the patient's social life and assist the patient in identifying resources *to individualize care planning and reduce feelings of dependency and helplessness.*

Suggested NIC Interventions

Behavior Modification: Social Skills; Mood Management; Socialization Enhancement

Evaluations for Expected Outcomes

- Patient expresses feelings associated with social isolation.
- Patient expresses desire to overcome social isolation and seeks help from staff to increase participation in social activities.
- Patient makes use of resources, such as social services, senior citizens centers, American Association of Retired Persons, and religious organizations.
- Patient indicates that social contacts have increased and feelings of social isolation have diminished.
- Patient expresses satisfaction with level of social contacts.

Documentation

- Factors that have caused or contributed to patient's social isolation
- Patient's statements indicating dissatisfaction with social situation
- Community resources identified for patient
- Planning done by patient, family member, primary nurse, and case manager
- Patient's use of community resources
- Evaluations for expected outcomes

REFERENCES

Medvene, L. J., Nilsen, K. M., Smith, R., Ofei-Dodoo, S., DiLollo, A., Webster, N., . . . Nance, A. (2016). Social networks and links to isolation and loneliness among elderly HCBS clients. *Aging & Mental Health*, *20*(5), 485–493. doi:10.1080/13607863.2015.1021751

Pettigrew, S., Donovan, R., Boldy, D., & Newton, R. (2014). Older people's perceived causes of and strategies for dealing with social isolation. *Aging & Mental Health*, *18*(7), 914–920. doi:10.1080/13607863.2014.899970

Price, B. (2015). Approaches to counter loneliness and social isolation. *Nursing Older People*, *27*(7), 31–39.

READINESS FOR ENHANCED SPIRITUAL WELL-BEING

Definition

A pattern of experiencing and integrating meaning and purpose in life through connectedness with self, others, art, music, literature, nature, and/or a power greater than oneself, which can be strengthened

Assessment

- Spiritual status, including personal religious habit; religious or church affiliation; perceptions of faith, life, death, and suffering; support network; embarrassment at practicing religious rituals; beliefs opposed by family members, peers, and health care providers; conflicts with belief system
- Health history, including medical conditions that change body image, chronic or terminal illness, debilitating disease
- Psychological status, including reactions to illness and disability; change in appetite, energy level, motivation, personal hygiene, self-image, sleep, and sex drive; alcohol or drug abuse; moodiness; recent divorce, job loss, losses through separation or death; personality traits, maladaptive behaviors; relationships with peers, group involvement, life events in childhood, family pressure; recreational activities; quality of authority relationships, peer relationships; situational crisis; occupation changes; dating and marital history
- Brief Psychiatric Rating Scale, Hamilton Depression Rating Scale, and others, as needed
- Self-care status, including neurologic, musculoskeletal, sensory or psychological impairment, ability to carry out activities and adapt
- Family status, including marital status; communication, methods of conflict resolution; ability of family to meet physical, social, and emotional needs of its members; socioeconomic factors; family health history; evidence of abuse
- Nutritional status, including height, weight, and any special dietary habits
- Sleep pattern status, including hours of sleep, energy level before and after sleep, rest and relaxation patterns; difficulty falling asleep, nocturnal awakening, early morning awakening, hypersomnia, insomnia, sleep pattern reversal; sleep EEG; dyssomnia, parasomnia, unipolar depression, bipolar disorder, sleep apnea

Defining Characteristics

Connections to Self

- Expresses desire to enhance acceptance
- Expresses desire to enhance coping
- Expresses desire to enhance courage
- Expresses desire to enhance hope
- Expresses desire to enhance joy
- Expresses desire to enhance love
- Expresses desire to enhance meaning in life
- Expresses desire to enhance meditative practice
- Expresses desire to enhance purpose in life
- Expresses desire to enhance satisfaction with philosophy of life
- Expresses desire to enhance self-forgiveness
- Expresses desire to enhance serenity (e.g., peace)
- Expresses desire to enhance surrender

Connections with Others

- Expresses desire to enhance forgiveness from others
- Expresses desire to enhance interaction with significant other
- Expresses desire to enhance interaction with spiritual leaders
- Expresses desire to enhance service to others

Connections with Art, Music, Literature, and Nature

- Expresses desire to enhance creative energy (e.g., writing, poetry, music)
- Expresses desire to enhance spiritual reading
- Expresses desire to enhance time outdoors
- Expresses desire to enhance mystical experiences
- Expresses desire to enhance participation in religious activity
- Expresses desire to enhance prayerfulness
- Expresses desire to enhance reverence

Expected Outcomes

- Patient will discuss spiritual conflicts.
- Patient will be provided with opportunity to meet with chosen religious authority.
- Patient will be supported in the efforts to pursue enhanced spiritual well-being.
- Patient will pursue religious or spiritual practices to the extent that the patient feels comfortable.
- Patient will describe plan to continue to enhance spiritual well-being.
- Patient will receive referrals for continued support.

Suggested NOC Outcomes

Hope; Quality of Life; Spiritual Health

Interventions and Rationales

- Monitor the patient for potential signs of spiritual distress that might harm the patient's well-being (altered self-care, sleep pattern disturbance, and change in exercise and eating habits) *to plan appropriate interventions.*
- Assess the significance of spirituality in the patient's life and in coping with illness. Note whether the patient participates in religious rituals, observes religious practices (such as prayer, meditation, or dietary restrictions), or wishes to discuss spiritual beliefs. Keep an open view of what constitutes spirituality. *Before the nurse can intervene in spiritual matters, she must determine if spirituality is significant for the patient.*
- Ask the patient if illness has affected the spiritual outlook and tell the patient you're willing to help in addressing spiritual issues, if the patient wishes, *to reduce isolation and help bring issues related to spiritual distress out into the open.*
- PCC Ask if the patient wishes to discuss spiritual concerns with a chosen religious authority *to allow access to expert spiritual care resources.*
- Encourage the patient to pursue spiritual questions. Reassure the patient that spiritual concerns are valid and that by strengthening spirituality, the patient can enhance overall well-being *to demonstrate acceptance.*
- PCC Provide the patient with resources for coping with spiritual distress (such as referrals to religious or spiritual organizations or books on prayer and meditation) *to enhance the opportunity to attend to spiritual needs.* Make sure the resources selected are

appropriate with regard to the patient's religious affiliation and spiritual beliefs *to demonstrate respect for own beliefs and values.* If you lack knowledge about the patient's beliefs and practices, consult the patient's chosen religious authority *to best meet the patient's needs.*

- Help the patient arrange travel to a place selected for prayer, reflection, or contemplation. Use resources such as church-affiliated vans or volunteer escorts *to enhance the patient's contact with outside sources of support.*
- Demonstrate to the patient that you're willing to discuss issues related to spirituality, such as the patient's view of God, how illness has affected the patient's religious beliefs, or how hospital stays affect the patient's spiritual practices, *to bring spiritual issues into the open.* Keep an open mind when listening. Keep the conversation focused on the patient's spiritual values and the role they play in recovering from illness and coping with changes in body image *to ensure that interaction between the nurse and the patient remains therapeutic.*
- Discuss with the patient the importance of maintaining a healthy diet, getting regular exercise and sleep, and maintaining healthy interaction with family members and friends. *A patient in spiritual distress may neglect day-to-day well-being.*
- Praise the patient for taking time to attend to spiritual needs and encourage the patient to continue to develop spirituality after leaving the health care setting *to provide continued encouragement.*
- PCC Provide the patient with referrals to appropriate religious groups, spiritually centered organizations, and social service organizations *to help provide additional support and to ensure continuity of care.*
- Consider resources such as parish nurses, home-visiting services, and computer networks *to help provide continued opportunity for spiritual development and to ensure continuity of care.*

Suggested NIC Interventions

Active Listening; Emotional Support; Hope Instillation; Presence; Spiritual Growth Facilitation; Spiritual Support

Evaluations for Expected Outcomes

- Patient becomes comfortable discussing spiritual conflicts.
- Patient is visited by a religious representative of choice.
- Patient is supported in efforts to pursue enhanced spiritual well-being.
- Patient takes the initiative to pursue desire for active religious participation.
- Patient openly discusses effects of illness on own beliefs and other spiritual issues.
- Patient develops a plan for continued involvement in religious activity.
- Patient accepts referrals for continued religious growth.

Documentation

- Statements about spiritual conflicts
- Visits with chosen religious authority
- Engagement in religious or spiritual practices
- Suggested religious resources outside of hospital
- Statements about ability to cope with changes in body image as a result of illness, to maintain spiritual values in face of long-term or chronic illness, and to pursue spiritual practices during hospital stays

- Eating patterns, exercise schedules, and sleep patterns
- Stated plans to continue to enhance spiritual well-being
- Evaluations for expected outcomes

REFERENCES

Adib-Hajbaghery, M., & Faraji, M. (2015). Comparison of happiness and spiritual well-being among the community dwelling elderly and those who lived in sanitariums. *International Journal of Community Based Nursing & Midwifery*, *3*(3), 216–226.

Ali, J., Marhemat, F., Sara, J., & Hamid, H. (2015). The relationship between spiritual well-being and quality of life among elderly people. *Holistic Nursing Practice*, *29*(3), 128–135. doi:10.1097/HNP.0000000000000081

Elham, H., Hazrati, M., Momennasab, M., & Sareh, K. (2015). The effect of need-based spiritual/religious intervention on spiritual well-being and anxiety of elderly people. *Holistic Nursing Practice*, *29*(3), 136–143. doi:10.1097/HNP.0000000000000083

IMPAIRED VERBAL COMMUNICATION

related to physiologic or psychosocial changes

Definition

Decreased, delayed, or absent ability to receive, process, transmit, and/or use a system of symbols

Assessment

- History of neurologic disease
- Speech characteristics, including pattern (rate of speech, phrase length, effort, fluency, prosody, repetition, and information content), vocabulary, level of comprehension, and presence of aphasia (Broca's, Wernicke's, transcortical, receptive, or global) or dysarthria
- Ability to use alternative forms of communication (eye blinks, gestures, pictures, nods, or written notes)
- Auditory status, including use of hearing aid, history of hearing deficits, and presence of cerumen
- Vision status, including use of eyeglasses, history of vision deficits, visual acuity (near and distant), and visual fields
- Neurologic status, including level of consciousness, orientation, cognition, memory (recent and remote), insight, judgment, cranial nerves (IX, X, XII), primitive reflexes (snout, suck, and palm-chin), and results of diagnostic studies (arteriogram, EEG, and computed tomography and magnetic resonance imaging scans)
- Psychosocial status, including family, friends, other support system; recent relocation; recent losses; and efforts to express sadness, frustration, anxiety, or other emotions associated with verbal communication impairment
- Medication status, including use of prescription and over-the-counter medications

Defining Characteristics

- Absence of eye contact
- Difficulty comprehending communication
- Difficulty expressing thoughts verbally (e.g., aphasia, dysphasia, apraxia, dyslexia)
- Difficulty forming sentences
- Difficulty forming words (e.g., aphonia, dyslalia, dysarthria)

- Difficulty in selective attending
- Difficulty in use of body expressions
- Difficulty in use of facial expressions
- Difficulty maintaining communication
- Difficulty speaking
- Difficulty verbalizing
- Disoriented to person
- Disoriented to place
- Disoriented to time
- Does not speak
- Dyspnea
- Inability to speak
- Inability to speak language of caregiver
- Inability to use body expressions
- Inappropriate verbalization
- Partial visual deficit
- Refusal to speak
- Slurred speech
- Stuttering
- Total visual deficit

Expected Outcomes

- Patient will improve communication skills to the extent possible.
- Patient will attend sessions with speech therapist.
- Visitors and staff members will demonstrate appropriate respect when speaking with patient.
- Patient will communicate needs without excessive frustration.
- Patient will take steps to decrease isolation from friends and family members.
- Patient or family member will identify and contact appropriate support services.
- Patient will indicate through gestures, behavior, writing, or speaking that the patient is coming to terms with impaired ability to communicate.

Suggested NOC Outcomes

Communication; Communication: Expressive; Communication: Receptive

Interventions and Rationales

- When initiating communication, face the patient, maintain eye contact, speak slowly, and enunciate clearly *to make it easier for the patient to receive and process your message.*
- S Take steps to enhance communication while providing care:
  - Communicate one idea at a time.
  - Use "yes" and "no" questions.
  - Avoid abstract thoughts and controversial topics.
  - Use plain, everyday vocabulary.
  - Allow longer response time.
  - Guess at the meaning of incorrect words.
  - Reduce distractions.
  - Eliminate unnecessary noise.
  - Encourage the patient to use gestures or other alternative means of communication.

  Facilitating communication efforts will help decrease the patient's frustration.

- If the patient's communication problems are exacerbated by hearing deficits, use appropriate techniques to overcome hearing problems:
  - Minimize glare in the patient's room *to make it easier for the patient to read your lips.*
  - Check for the proper use of adaptive hearing devices. If the patient wears a hearing aid, make sure the battery is working and the hearing aid is placed correctly *to enhance hearing ability.*
  - Use paper and a pencil if hearing is severely impaired *to provide alternative means of communication.*
- If the patient doesn't follow your conversation, rephrase ideas using simpler wording *to overcome differences in language or culture that may block communication.*
- Don't rush the patient when struggling to express own thoughts. Demonstrate tact and willingness to listen. Even if you can't understand the patient, let the patient know you accept the patient's efforts to communicate and you empathize with patient's frustration. *A patient with impaired verbal communication experiences isolation, despair, and frustration. Demonstrating compassion and fostering a therapeutic relationship is the most important step for improving communication.*
- Avoid conversing with the patient when the patient is tired. *The patient's attention span may deteriorate when fatigued, thereby making efforts to communicate even more frustrating.*
- PCC Encourage the patient to engage in social activities, such as attending therapy sessions and eating with other patients at group tables, *to reduce feelings of isolation.*
- If appropriate, help the patient reintegrate into family life. *Impaired speech may affect the patient's role in the family. Providing an opportunity to reintegrate the patient into family life, through family gatherings, may diminish loneliness and anxiety.*
- Encourage the patient to reminisce. Use photographs, gestures, and visits from family members and friends to stimulate the patient's desire for self-expression. *Recalling meaningful experiences may motivate the patient to try to communicate and may enhance feelings of self-worth.*
- PCC Encourage family members and colleagues to use speech appropriate for adults when talking to the patient and not to talk about the patient within range of hearing *to convey respect.*
- PCC Obtain a referral to a speech therapist. Educate family members and colleagues about the methods prescribed by the therapist to enhance communication *to ensure continuity of care.*
- PCC Refer the patient and family members to appropriate community resources, such as a club for stroke survivors or support group for relatives of Alzheimer's patients, *to help them cope with communication impairment after discharge.*

Suggested NIC Interventions

Active Listening; Communication Enhancement: Speech Deficit; Presence; Touch

Evaluations for Expected Outcomes

- Patient improves communication skills to the extent possible.
- Patient attends sessions with speech therapist ___ times/week.
- Visitors and staff demonstrate appropriate respect when speaking with patient by using adult speech and not talking about the patient within the patient's hearing range.
- Patient communicates needs, using gestures, behavior, writing, or speech, without excessive frustration.

- Patient takes steps to decrease isolation from friends and family members.
- Patient or family member identifies and contacts appropriate support services.
- Patient indicates coming to terms with own impaired ability to communicate.

Documentation

- Observations of impaired speaking ability, use of communication aids, and expressions of frustration
- Interventions implemented to decrease barriers to effective communication
- Patient's efforts to communicate using gestures, behavior, writing, and speech
- Patient teaching and patient's response
- Referrals to speech therapist and other support services
- Evaluations for expected outcomes

REFERENCES

Cheba, M., Żuralska, R., & Skrzypek-Czerko, M. (2014). Difficulties related to the communication with the patient with aphasia according to the nursing staff. *Journal of Neurological & Neurosurgical Nursing, 3*(2), 75–80. doi:10.15225/PNN.2014.3.2.4

Dark, J., & Sander, R. (2014). An overview of communication, movement, and perception difficulties after stroke. *Nursing Older People, 26*(5), 32–37. doi:10.7748/nop.26.5.32.e567

Johnson, M., & Feng, L. (2014). Communication difficulty and relevant interventions in mild cognitive impairment: Implications for neuroplasticity. *Topics in Geriatric Rehabilitation, 30*(1), 18–34. doi:10.1097/TGR.0000000000000001

PART VI

Psychiatric and Mental Health

APPLYING EVIDENCE-BASED PRACTICE

The Question

Do middle and high school suicide awareness programs decrease adolescent suicide attempts?

Evidence-Based Resources

American Academy of Pediatrics. (n.d.). *Teen suicide statistics*. Retrieved from https://www.healthychildren.org/English/health-issues/conditions/emotional-problems/Pages/Teen-Suicide-Statistics.aspx

Brent, D. A., & Brown, C. H. (2015). Effectiveness of school-based suicide prevention programmes. *Lancet*, *385*(9977), 1489–1491. doi:10.1016/S0140-6736(14)61586-5

Centers for Disease Control and Prevention. (2015). *Suicide facts at a glance*. Retrieved from http://www.cdc.gov/violenceprevention/pdf/suicide-datasheet-a.pdf

Kim, S. M., Baek, J. H., Han, D. H., Lee, Y. S., & Yurgelun-Todd, D. A. (2015). Psychosocial–environmental risk factors for suicide attempts in adolescents with suicidal ideation: Findings from a sample of 73,238 adolescents. *Suicide & Life-Threatening Behavior*, *45*(4), 477–487. doi:10.1111/sltb.12143

Meril, M., & Vineetha, J. (2015). Effectiveness of School Based Teaching Programme (SBTP) for teachers regarding 'Prevention of Suicide among Students' in selected schools, Mangalore. *International Journal of Nursing Education*, *7*(1), 292–294. doi:10.5958/0974-9357.2015.00058.6

Schilling, E. A., Lawless, M., Buchanan, L., & Aseltine R. H., Jr. (2014). 'Signs of suicide' shows promise as a middle school suicide prevention program. *Suicide & Life-Threatening Behavior*, *44*(6), 653–667. doi:10.1111/sltb.12097

Schmidt, R. C., Iachini, A. L., George, M., Koller, J., & Weist, M. (2015). Integrating a suicide prevention program into a school mental health system: A case example from a rural school district. *Children & Schools*, *37*(1), 18–26.

Walrath, C., Godoy Garraza, L., Reid, H., Goldston, D. B., & McKeon, R. (2015). Research and practice. Impact of the Garrett Lee Smith youth suicide prevention program on suicide mortality. *American Journal of Public Health*, *105*(5), 986–993. doi:10.2105/AJPH.2014.302496

Evaluating the Evidence

The adolescent years can be a highly stressful period filled with uncertainty, mood swings, depression, and anxiety. Adolescents may be victims of abuse, face problems with family or friends, have difficulty at school, have a substance abuse problem, or struggle with sexual identity (American Academy of Pediatrics, n.d.; Kim, Baer, Han, Lee, & Yurgelun-Todd, 2015). Adolescents who are overwhelmed by emotional turmoil and psychological stress may have underdeveloped coping skills, leaving them vulnerable to making poor decisions and having poor impulse control. In 2013, 17% of U. S. students in grades 9 through 12 seriously considered attempting suicide. Suicide is the third leading cause of death among 10 to 14 year olds and the second leading cause of death for 15 to 34 year olds (Centers for Disease Control and Prevention, 2015).

Because adolescents attend school for a considerable portion of time, school-based programs are ideal to reach large populations of students (Meril & Vineetha, 2015). Schilling, Lawless, Buchanan, and Aseltine (2014) examined the effectiveness of the Signs of Suicide (SOS) program on fifth through eighth grade students from eight middle schools. The SOS program lesson plans include how to recognize depression, how to recognize the signs and symptoms of possible suicide, and how to approach someone for help. Comparison of student pre- and post-tests indicated a decrease in suicidal ideation and increased knowledge of depression and suicide.

A rural school district in Maryland was the focus of a study conducted to measure the effectiveness of a mental health and suicide awareness program (Schmidt, Iachini, George, Koller, & Weist, 2015). Students (n = 5,949) in grades 6 through 12 participated in a 4-year program designed to increase knowledge of suicide risk, suicide ideation, and how to ask for help. Students completed questionnaires throughout the 4 years to measure program effectiveness. At the end of the study period, data indicated a decrease in student suicidal thoughts.

Community-based mental health and suicide prevention programs have had successful results. Walrath, Garraza, Reid, Goldston, and McKeon (2015) examined the effectiveness of a community-based Garrett Lee Smith (GLS) youth suicide prevention program on suicide mortality across 466 counties in the United States. The GLS program is a comprehensive program that includes suicide screening, life skills development, helplines and hotlines, and gatekeeper training. Gatekeepers are individuals who have contact with large numbers of adolescents on a regular basis; teachers, public school staff, physicians, etc. Gatekeepers learn the warning signs of suicide and are trained to identify individuals at risk. In counties where the GLS program was implemented, evaluation of data after 1 year indicated significantly lower suicide rates of 10 to 24 year olds.

Applying the Results and Making a Decision

Recognizing suicidal behavior is only one part of intervention programs aimed to reduce the number of adolescents who attempt suicide. Programs that teach coping skills, screen for depression and anxiety, and teach how to seek help are the most effective (Brent & Brown, 2015). Intervention programs should empower students by giving them tools to deal with adversity and stress. Reaching the greatest numbers of adolescents can be accomplished in schools, making schools the ideal vehicle for suicide prevention and mental health awareness programs.

Reevaluating Process and Identifying Areas for Improvement

Suicide, a leading cause of death for adolescents, can be prevented. Providing mental health support programs in schools is a proactive intervention that supports healthy development. Current interventions must be updated to improve the future mental health of adolescents. Student programs should include educational components for suicide behavior awareness, how to recognize depression in themselves and others, and how to seek out help. Providing education to teachers and school personnel can improve identification of students at risk. Because school-based suicide prevention programs may help to decrease the number of students who consider and/or attempt suicide, all schools should include mental health and suicide prevention programs in their curriculum.

INTRODUCTION

All nurses have a responsibility to respond to the psychological as well as the physical needs of patients. Caring for patients with psychiatric disorders and psychological health problems requires empathy and expert observation, assessment, and therapeutic communication skills. This section focuses on providing care to patients with diverse needs related to mental health and well-being.

Patients with psychiatric disorders require well-organized care; however, in addition to maintaining medication schedules and regulating daily routine, nurses must also establish and maintain a therapeutic relationship. The nurse–patient relationship should foster trust and encourage open communication, which allows the nurse to interpret patient needs and concerns. Because the social stigma that often accompanies mental illness can be difficult for the patient to overcome, the nurse should maintain a nonjudgmental attitude throughout care.

In addition to psychiatric disorders, nurses provide comprehensive care to patients who are affected by substance abuse, domestic violence, sexual abuse, and related issues. When responding to patients in distress, care should be provided in a nonthreatening manner. The nurse acts as patient advocate by providing emotional support and may coordinate support groups and refer patients to crisis centers.

As more patients cope with anxiety and depression that may accompany chronic disease, nurses are called to provide holistic care that encompasses the mind, body, and spirit. The nursing diagnoses and associated care plans in this section will assist you in planning care to meet the psychological needs of your patients.

ANXIETY

related to situational crisis

Definition

Vague, uneasy feeling of discomfort or dread accompanied by an autonomic response (the source is often nonspecific or unknown to the individual); a feeling of apprehension caused by anticipation of danger. It is an alerting sign that warns of impending danger and enables the individual to take measures to deal with that threat

Assessment

- History of panic symptoms (choking feeling in throat, hyperventilation, light-headedness, dizziness, and other physical signs and symptoms of anxiety)
- Psychological status, including patient's explanation of problem, onset, duration, precipitating events, past and present coping (note use of repression and denial and escape–avoidance behaviors), insight (note patient's understanding of irrationality of fears),

motivation to change, anxiety level (+1, +2, +3, +4), secondary gains (what kind and from whom), current stressors, results of mental status examination (note expression of anxiety in terms of personal fears, concentration, judgment, affect, and impulse control, as well as all other aspects of mental status), and personal abilities, talents, and strengths
- Sociologic status, including support systems, hobbies, interests, work history, family makeup, family roles (evidence of harmony or disharmony), family coping mechanisms, evidence of reinforcement of problem by family, and lifestyle (how this reinforces irrational fears)
- Medication history, including response, effectiveness, and adverse effects

Defining Characteristics

Behavioral

- Decrease in productivity
- Extraneous movement
- Fidgeting
- Glancing about
- Hypervigilance
- Insomnia
- Poor eye contact
- Restlessness
- Scanning behavior
- Worried about change in life event

Affective

- Anguish
- Apprehensiveness
- Distress
- Fear
- Feeling of inadequacy
- Helplessness
- Increase in wariness
- Irritability
- Jitteriness
- Overexcitement
- Rattled
- Regretful
- Self-focused
- Uncertainty
- Worried

Physiologic

- Facial tension
- Hand tremors
- Increase in perspiration
- Increase in tension
- Shakiness
- Trembling
- Voice quivering

Sympathetic

- Alteration in respiratory pattern
- Anorexia
- Brisk reflexes
- Cardiovascular excitation
- Diarrhea
- Dry mouth
- Facial flushing
- Twitching
- Weakness
- Heart palpitations
- Increase in blood pressure
- Increase in heart rate
- Increase in respiratory rate
- Pupil dilation
- Superficial vasoconstriction

Parasympathetic

- Abdominal pain
- Alteration in sleep pattern
- Decrease in heart rate
- Decreased blood pressure

- Diarrhea
- Faintness
- Fatigue
- Nausea
- Tingling in extremities
- Urinary frequency
- Urinary hesitancy
- Urinary urgency

Cognitive

- Alteration in attention
- Alteration in concentration
- Awareness of physiologic symptoms
- Blocking of thoughts
- Confusion
- Decrease in perceptual field
- Diminished ability to learn
- Diminished ability to problem-solve
- Fear
- Forgetfulness
- Preoccupation
- Rumination
- Tendency to blame others

Expected Outcomes

- Patient will experience reduced anxiety by identifying precipitating situations.
- Patient will connect life events to occurrence of anxiety.
- Patient will identify current stressors.
- Patient will set limits and compromises on behavior when ready.
- Patient will develop effective coping behaviors.
- Patient will maintain autonomy and independence without disabling fears or use of phobic behavior.

Suggested NOC Outcomes

Aggression Self-Control; Anxiety Level; Anxiety Self-Control; Concentration; Coping; Impulse Self-Control; Psychosocial Adjustment: Life Change

Interventions and Rationales

- Identify your feelings toward the patient *to keep your feelings from interfering with treatment.*
- Accept the patient as is. *Forcing the patient to change before the patient is ready causes panic.*
- Explore factors that precipitate phobic reactions and anxiety. *This is important for understanding the patient's behavioral dynamics.*
- Reassure the patient about being safe. *The patient may perceive being at risk, which may increase the patient's level of anxiety.*
- Support the patient with desensitization techniques *to help overcome the patient's problem.*
- Give the patient a chance to ventilate own feelings. *This reduces the patient's tendency to suppress or repress bottled-up feelings, which may continue to affect behavior even though the patient may be unaware of them.*
- PCC Teach relaxation techniques (breathing exercises, progressive muscle relaxation, guided imagery, meditation) *to counteract the fight-or-flight response.*
- Help the patient set limits and compromises on behavior when ready, and allow the patient to be afraid. *Fear is a feeling, neither right nor wrong.*
- Give the patient facts about fear and anxiety and their consequences *to reduce anxiety and encourage the patient to help manage the problem.*

- Encourage the patient not to run away when afraid *to help the patient learn that fear can be faced and managed.*
- PCC Help the patient develop own techniques for dealing with fears *to establish alternatives to escape or avoidance behaviors.*

Suggested NIC Interventions

Anger Control Assistance; Anxiety Reduction; Calming Technique; Coping Enhancement; Impulse Control Training; Presence; Progressive Muscle Relaxation; Meditation Facilitation

Evaluations for Expected Outcomes

- Patient identifies precipitating situations and demonstrates fewer physical symptoms of anxiety, improved concentration, and reduced preoccupation with fears.
- Patient discusses possible relationship between anxiety and past and present experiences.
- Patient lists stressors.
- Patient limits phobic behavior when ready.
- Patient participates in desensitization therapy and learns to better manage stress, health, and responsibilities.
- Patient makes decisions, shows greater independence, and decreases behaviors that limit spontaneous activity.

Documentation

- Observation of subjective and objective data
- Interventions to reduce anxiety and increase coping
- Patient's response to interventions
- Evaluations for expected outcomes

REFERENCES

Charon, R., & Charon, C. (2014). Management of dental fear, anxiety and phobia. *Dental Nursing, 10*(7), 378–383.

Garcia-Lopez, L. J., Sáez-Castillo, A. J., Beidel, D., & La Greca, A. M. (2015). Brief measures to screen for social anxiety in adolescents. *Journal of Developmental & Behavioral Pediatrics, 36*(8), 562–568. doi:10.1097/DBP.0000000000000213

Heatherington, L., Harrington, N. T., Harrington, J., Niemeyer, K. F., Weinberg, S. C., & Friedlander, M. L. (2014). Applying group cognitive behavioral therapy for anxiety disorders in community settings: Retention, outcome, and clinical considerations. *Journal of Cognitive Psychotherapy, 28*(2), 117–133. doi:10.1891/0889-8391.28.2.117

INEFFECTIVE COPING

related to inadequate opportunity to prepare for stressor; uncertainty

Definition

Inability to form a valid appraisal of the stressors, inadequate choices of practiced responses, and/or inability to use available resources

Assessment

- Patient's perception of present health problem or crisis
- Usual problem-solving techniques/behaviors used to cope with life problems
- Physical or emotional impairment
- Occupation
- Diversional activities
- Financial resources
- Support systems, including family members, friends, and clergy
- Reaction of family members to patient's crisis

Defining Characteristics

- Alteration in concentration
- Alteration in sleep pattern
- Change in communication pattern
- Destructive behavior toward others
- Destructive behavior toward self
- Difficulty organizing information
- Fatigue
- Frequent illness
- Inability to ask for help
- Inability to attend to information
- Inability to deal with a situation
- Inability to meet basic needs
- Inability to meet role expectation
- Ineffective coping strategies
- Insufficient access of social support
- Insufficient goal-directed behavior
- Insufficient problem resolution
- Insufficient problem-solving skills
- Risk-taking behavior
- Substance abuse

Expected Outcomes

- Patient will express understanding of the relationship between emotional state and behavior.
- Patient will become actively involved in planning own care.
- Patient will reduce use of manipulative behavior to gratify needs.
- Patient will accept responsibility for behavior.
- Patient will identify effective and ineffective coping techniques.
- Patient will use available support systems, such as family, friends, and psychotherapist, to develop and maintain effective coping skills.

Suggested NOC Outcomes

Aggression Self-Control; Coping; Decision-Making; Impulse Self-Control; Social Interaction Skills

Interventions and Rationales

- If possible, assign a primary nurse to the patient *to provide continuity of care and promote development of a therapeutic relationship.*
- PCC Spend consistent, uninterrupted time with the patient. Encourage open expression of feelings. *An open environment will help the patient ventilate intense emotion. Through discussion, you can help the patient understand the personal meaning attached to recent events and foster a realistic assessment of the situation.*
- As the patient becomes able to express feelings more openly, discuss the relationship between feelings and behavior. *To change, the patient must understand this relationship.*
- Discourage dependent behavior by assisting the patient only when necessary. Provide positive reinforcement for independent behavior *to enhance self-esteem, encourage repetition of desired behavior, and promote effective coping.*
- PCC Encourage the patient to make decisions about care *to reduce feelings of helplessness and enhance the patient's sense of mastery over the current situation.*
- Set limits on manipulative behavior. Provide the patient with clear expectations for behavior, and describe the consequences if limits are violated. *If the patient can't curb inappropriate behavior, consistent limit-setting imposes external controls.*
- Recognize that manipulative behaviors reduce the patient's sense of insecurity by increasing feelings of power. *Understanding the patient's motivation may help you deal better with manipulative behavior.*
- Help the patient recognize and accept responsibility for own actions. Discourage the patient from unfairly placing blame on others. *Developing a sense of responsibility is necessary before change can occur.*
- Help the patient recognize and feel good about positive personal qualities and accomplishments. Provide rewards to reinforce acceptable coping behaviors. *As self-esteem increases, the patient will feel less need to manipulate others.*
- Help the patient analyze the current situation and evaluate the effectiveness of coping strategies *to foster an objective outlook.*
- Praise the patient for identifying and using effective coping techniques *to reinforce appropriate behavior.*
- Suggest alternatives to ineffective behaviors identified by the patient. Encourage the patient to determine what new behaviors can be effectively incorporated into the lifestyle. *Fostering patient participation in care promotes feelings of independence.*
- PCC Encourage the patient to use support systems, such as a psychotherapist, family, and friends, *to maintain effective coping skills.*

Suggested NIC Interventions

Anger Control Assistance; Coping Enhancement; Decision-Making Support; Environmental Management: Violence Prevention; Impulse Control Training; Support System Enhancement

Evaluations for Expected Outcomes

- Patient describes emotions triggered by illness or personal crisis and usual coping behaviors.
- Patient works with primary nurses to plan care.
- Patient describes two instances in which needs were met through direct communication.
- Patient describes one difficult interpersonal situation that was solved by identifying the problem, choosing alternative ways to communicate, and taking action.
- Patient identifies two effective and two ineffective coping behaviors.
- Patient enlists support and assistance from family and friends.

Documentation

- Patient's perception of present situation
- Emotions expressed by patient
- Observations of patient's behaviors
- Interventions performed to help patient develop coping skills
- Patient's response to nursing interventions
- Evaluations for expected outcomes

REFERENCES

Jacobs, N. L., Dehue, F., Völlink, T., & Lechner, L. (2014). Determinants of adolescents' ineffective and improved coping with cyberbullying: A Delphi study. *Journal of Adolescence, 37*(4), 373–385. doi:10.1016/j.adolescence.2014.02.011

Meredith, P. J., Rappel, G., Strong, J., & Bailey, K. J. (2015). Sensory sensitivity and strategies for coping with pain. *American Journal of Occupational Therapy, 69*(4), 1–10. doi:10.5014/ajot.2015.014621

Regier, N. G., & Parmelee, P. A. (2015). The stability of coping strategies in older adults with osteoarthritis and the ability of these strategies to predict changes in depression, disability, and pain. *Aging & Mental Health, 19*(12), 1113–1122. doi:10.1080/13607863.2014.1003286

IMPAIRED EMANCIPATED DECISION MAKING

related to decrease in understanding of all available health care options; limited decision-making experience

Definition

A process of choosing a health care decision that does not include personal knowledge and/or consideration of social norms, or does not occur in a flexible environment, resulting in decisional dissatisfaction

Assessment

- Levels of consciousness and orientation
- Age
- Stage of development
- Presence of cognitive impairment
- Level of education
- Language fluency

Defining Characteristics

- Delay in enacting chosen health care option
- Distress when listening to other's opinion
- Excessive concern about what others think is the best decision
- Feeling constrained in describing own opinion
- Inability to choose a health care option that best fits current lifestyle
- Inability to describe how option will fit into current lifestyle
- Limited verbalization about health care option in other's presence

Expected Outcomes

- The patient will demonstrate consideration of how available health care choices fit with their values, beliefs, preferences, and lifestyle.
- The patient will express consideration of their own values, beliefs, and preferences, independent of those of others in considering the available health care options.

- The patient will verbalize opinion freely.
- The patient will make a health care choice.
- The patient will verbalize satisfaction with health care choice based on the available options.

Suggested NOC Outcomes

Decision-Making; Information Processing; Participation in Health Care Decisions

Interventions and Rationales

- Engage the patient in the therapeutic relationship. Demonstrate an attitude of respect, patience, and acceptance. *Persons who feel cared for, understood, and respected in health care situations are better motivated to collaboratively participate in their care.*
- PCC Continually assess for readiness to make a health care choice *to promote timely decision making.*
- PCC Ensure privacy for one-to-one interaction between patient and nurse. *The patient's status in relationships with family/loved ones may inhibit frank discussion in their presence.*
- PCC Ensure that communications and information provided are at a level consistent with the patient's cognitive abilities *to ensure understanding.*
- Avoid limiting choices based on health care provider preference, values, or beliefs and avoid encouraging one choice over another. *The health care team is accountable to the patient to provide appropriate information on all available options and to promote autonomous decision making.*
- Explore with the patient the meaning of experience of making a health care decision. Ask what meanings the current health care situation and having to make a health care decision have for the patient. *The health care need and necessity to make a health care decision may represent a crisis for the patient. Understanding the patient's experience of this can direct the identification of other necessary assessments and interventions.*
- Discuss the patient's emotional experience of needing to make a health care choice. *The patient may feel anger, fear, anxiety, pressured, or overwhelmed by the need to choose or the choices offered.*
- Validate the patient's experience, and ask permission to discuss the patient's thoughts and feelings about own choices. Identify any anxiety or fear related to making a decision. *Fear and anxiety can lead to anger, feeling pressured or overwhelmed, procrastination, and/or excessive seeing of reassurance or opinions from others.*
- If fear or anxiety is present, validate the patient's experience *to promote self-esteem, strengthen the therapeutic relationship, and promote autonomous decision making.*
- S Provide clarifying information about choices, if needed. *Misinterpretations of information may lead to difficulty making a decision.*
- PCC Refer to professional support to address anxious distorted thoughts, if needed. *Counseling may be required to assist the patient to work through distorted thoughts and determine own best course of action.*
- Share with the patient observation of distress when hearing other's opinion. Ask the patient to share thoughts that are leading to distress. *Sharing thoughts that lead to distress regarding others' opinions may reveal relationship barriers to decision making. Indecision may arise from dissonance between the patient's own values, beliefs, and preferences and*

those of loved ones or health care providers. Validate those thoughts. *Validation of the patient's distressing thoughts promotes self-esteem, builds the therapeutic relationship, and promotes autonomous decision making.*

- If needed, clarify perceptions of health care team decisional preference. *The patient may feel pressured to make an unwanted choice by a perceived power differential within the therapeutic relationship.*
- PCC Engage the patient to use a problem-solving framework to identify and to evaluate the possible available choices. Ask the patient to list the advantages and drawbacks to each choice, as well as personal values, goals, and preferences related to each choice. Encourage the patient to identify personal and social barriers to enacting any of the choices. Then ask the patient to rate the suitability of each choice based on appraisal of each one. *Use of a problem-solving framework in consideration of health care choices encourages the patient to consider health care options from the context of own experience, and to identify own best choices given the patient's life situation.*

Suggested NIC Interventions

Active Listening; Assertiveness Training; Decision-Making Support; Learning Facilitation; Mutual Goal Setting

Evaluations for Expected Outcomes

- The patient states how available health care choices fit with their values, beliefs, preferences, and lifestyle.
- The patient expresses own values, beliefs, and preferences in making the health care decision, comparing and contrasting how they differ from loved ones.
- The patient does not perceive pressure to choose or preference of a choice by the health care team.
- The patient freely verbalizes own opinion.
- The patient chooses health care option and expresses satisfaction with own choice based on the options available.

Documentation

- Assessment findings
- Health teaching regarding the patient's health need and available health care choices
- Patient verbatim statements regarding perceptions of health care situation and available choices
- Patient verbatim statements regarding own emotional experience of making a health care decision, related interventions undertaken, and patient response
- Observations of patient distress when hearing others' opinions, related interventions enacted, and patient response
- Use of problem-solving framework and patient response to same

REFERENCES

Kramer-Roy, D. (2015). Using participatory and creative methods to facilitate emancipatory research with people facing multiple disadvantage: A role for health and care professionals. *Disability and Society, 30*(8), 1207–1224.

Olesen, M. L., Graungaard, A. H., & Husted, G. R. (2015). Deciding treatment for miscarriage—Experiences of women and health care professionals. *Scandinavian Journal of Caring Sciences, 29*(2), 386–394.

Welzel, C., & Delhey, J. (2015). Generalizing trust: The benign force of emancipation. *Journal of Cross-Cultural Psychology, 46*(7), 875–896.
Wittmann-Price, R. A., & Price, S. W. (2014). Development and revision of the Wittmann-Price emancipated decision-making scale. *Journal or Nursing Measurement, 22*(3), 361–367.

READINESS FOR ENHANCED EMANCIPATED DECISION MAKING

related to decrease in understanding of all available health care options; limited decision-making experience

Definition

A process of choosing a health care decision that includes personal knowledge and/or consideration of social norms, which can be strengthened

Assessment

- Levels of consciousness and orientation
- Age
- Stage of development
- Presence of cognitive impairment
- Level of education
- Language fluency

Defining Characteristics

- Expresses desire to enhance ability to choose health care options that best fit current lifestyle
- Expresses desire to enhance ability to enact chosen health care option
- Expresses desire to enhance ability to understand all available health care options
- Expresses desire to enhance ability to verbalize own opinion with constraint
- Expresses desire to enhance comfort to verbalize health care options in the presence of others
- Expresses desire to enhance confidence in decision making
- Expresses desire to enhance confidence to discuss health care options openly
- Expresses desire to enhance decision making
- Expresses desire to enhance privacy to discuss health care options

Expected Outcomes

- The patient will engage with the nurse to meet needs for privacy
- The patient will openly seek information, and verbalize that the patient's information needs are met
- The patient will assertively communicate own opinions regarding own health care choices
- The patient will self-select a health care choice that meets the patient's lifestyle needs and reflects the patient's values, beliefs, and preferences
- The patient will verbalize satisfaction with own health care decision given the available choices

Suggested NOC Outcomes

Decision-Making; Information Processing; Participation in Health Care Decisions

Interventions and Rationales

- PCC Collaborate with the patient to determine strategies to meet the patient's needs for privacy. *To promote self-care, self-esteem, and decision making.*
- PCC Provide information proactively in anticipation of the patient's needs, as well as upon request by the patient. Encourage the patient to ask questions and provide meaningful answers to them. *To promote psychological readiness to make a decision, self-esteem, and confidence in knowledge.*
- Avoid the use of technical terms when at all possible; explain the meaning of technical terms when they must be used in communication with or in the presence of the patient. *To prevent a perceived power differential, which can be a barrier to patient understanding and self-esteem, and impede the therapeutic relationship.*
- PCC Ensure that communications and information provided are at a level consistent with the patient's cognitive abilities *to ensure understanding.*
- Promote self-esteem through active listening, validation of concerns, knowledge and feelings, conveyance of respect for the patient's values, beliefs, and preferences. *To promote psychological readiness to make a decision, and to strengthen the therapeutic relationship.*
- Use active listening to identify and reflect back to the patient the opinions of choices available to the patient. *To promote autonomous consideration of options by the patient and confidence in own opinions.*
- Ask the patient to verbalize what lifestyle, social, and other factors the patient needs to consider in making a decision, and how these would impact or be impacted by the health care choices available to the patient. *To promote consideration of the context of the patient's decision making.*
- Ask the patient about strategies used in the past to make decisions. Validate the patient's past choices in strategies. Engage the patient in realistic appraisal of the applicability of past strategies to current situation. *To identify and draw on personal experiences and strengths in decision making.*
- PCC Teach the patient about the utility of problem-solving frameworks to assist in decision making. As desired, ask the patient to use a problem-solving framework to identify and to evaluate the possible choices available. Ask the patient to list the advantages and drawbacks to each choice, as well as personal values, goals and preferences related to each choice. Encourage the patient to identify personal and social barriers to enacting any of the choices. Then ask the patient to rate the suitability of each choice based on the patient's appraisal of each one. *Use of a problem-solving framework in consideration of health care choices encourages the patient to consider health care options from the context of own experience, and to identify own best choices given the patient's life situation.*
- As needed, assist the patient to practice assertive expression of opinions. Encourage the patient to communicate in a way that is authentic, and simultaneously respectful of own feelings, values, beliefs, and wishes, as well as those of others. *Assertive expression of opinions promotes self-esteem within and after interpersonal interactions.*
- Role playing assertive expression of opinions may be helpful to prepare the patient to do so in real-life situations. *Role play can be an effective strategy toward the development of skill mastery.*

Suggested NIC Interventions

Active Listening; Assertiveness Training; Decision-Making Support; Learning Facilitation; Mutual Goal Setting

Evaluations for Expected Outcomes

- The patient collaborates on meeting own needs for privacy
- The patient openly seeks information.
- The patient verbalizes having sufficient information to make own health care decision.
- The patient communicates own opinions regarding health care choices while remaining respectful of those of others.
- The patient self-selects a health care choice that meets the patient's lifestyle needs and reflects the patient's values, beliefs, and preferences
- The patient verbalizes satisfaction with health care decision given the available choices

Documentation

- Assessment findings
- Patient engagement in planning and enacting interventions to ensure privacy; interventions taken to ensure privacy.
- Information sought and health teaching provided, including patient response.
- Past decision-making strategies used and patient's verbatim perceptions of utility for application in current situation.
- Patient's verbatim opinions of the available health care choices.
- Patient response to education regarding problem-solving framework, and as appropriate, the patient's use of it in the current situation.
- Patient-identified factors in making own health care decision.
- As applicable, patient engagement in practice of assertive expression of opinions.
- Decision made by patient.
- Patient verbalizations regarding satisfaction with choices and own decision.

REFERENCES

Kayser, J. W., Cossette, S., & Alderson, M. (2014). Autonomy-supportive intervention: An evolutionary concept analysis. *Journal of Advanced Nursing, 70*(6), 1254–1266.

Linehan, M. (2014). *DBT skills training manual* (2nd ed.). New York: Guilford Press.

Olesen, M. L., Graungaard, A. H., & Husted, G. R. (2015). Deciding treatment for miscarriage—Experiences of women and health care professionals. *Scandinavian Journal of Caring Sciences, 29*(2), 386–394.

Welzel, C., & Delhey, J. (2015). Generalizing trust: The benign force of emancipation. *Journal of Cross-Cultural Psychology, 46*(7), 875–896.

RISK FOR IMPAIRED EMANCIPATED DECISION MAKING

related to insufficient information regarding health care options; insufficient self-confidence in decision making

Definition

Vulnerable to a process of choosing a health care decision that does not include personal knowledge and/or consideration of social norms, or does not occur in a flexible environment, resulting in decisional dissatisfaction

Assessment

- Levels of consciousness and orientation
- Age

- Stage of development
- Presence of cognitive impairment
- Level of education
- Language fluency

Risk Factors

- Inadequate time to discuss health care options
- Insufficient confidence to openly discuss health care options
- Insufficient privacy to openly discuss health care options
- Limited decision-making experience
- Traditional hierarchical family
- Traditional hierarchical health care systems

Expected Outcomes

- The patient will verbalize own opinion freely
- The patient will verbalize own values, beliefs, and preferences
- The patient will identify any disparities between self and others' values, beliefs, and preferences
- The patient's information needs will be met
- The patient will make an autonomous health care choice

Suggested NOC Outcomes

Decision-Making; Information Processing; Participation in Health Care Decisions

Interventions and Rationales

- PCC Engage the patient in the therapeutic relationship. Demonstrate an attitude of respect, patience, and acceptance. *Persons who feel cared for, understood, and respected in health care situations are better motivated to collaboratively participate in own care.*
- PCC Ensure privacy for one-to-one interaction between patient and nurse. *The patient's status in relationships with family/loved ones may inhibit frank discussion in their presence.* If necessary, move the interaction, modify the environment, or remove others to ensure privacy.
- Avoid limiting choices based on health care provider preference, values, or beliefs and avoid encouraging one choice over another. *The health care team is accountable to the patient to provide appropriate information on all available options and to promote autonomous decision making.*
- PCC Ensure that communications and information provided are at a level consistent with the patient's cognitive abilities *to ensure understanding.*
- Ask the patient about understanding of the patient's health care need and the available choices. *To identify any misperceptions.*
- Validate the patient's understanding *to promote self-esteem, confidence in knowledge, and strengthen the therapeutic relationship.*
- Accept the patient's personal knowledge as relevant to the decision-making process. Discourage the patient from discounting personal knowledge and deferring to others' knowledge *to promote self-empowerment, confidence, and self-esteem.*
- PCC Provide education as needed in an accepting, nonjudgmental, supportive manner. Avoid taking a stance of correcting the patient; rather build on the patient's knowledge and understanding *to build knowledge capacity while preserving self-esteem.*
- Respectfully inquire as to the patient's cultural background, including gender roles, generational roles, and social expectations. *The patient is the best source of knowledge of own particular culture.*

- Encourage the patient to explore any cultural considerations in health care decision making, and to share what it is like for the patient to include those considerations. *Negative or conflicting emotions, or indecision may arise in the patient due to incongruence between the patient's cultural values and beliefs and personal values, beliefs, and preferences.*
- Explore with the patient the meaning of experiencing making a health care decision. Ask what meaning the current health care situation and having to make a health care decision has for the patient. *The health care need and necessity to make a health care decision may represent a crisis for the patient. Understanding the patient's experience of this can direct the identification of other necessary assessments and interventions.*
- Ask the patient about strategies used in the past to make decisions. Validate the patient's past choices in strategies. Reinforce independent strategies. *To identify and draw on personal experiences and strengths in decision making.*
- If past experience in decision making is limited, engage the patient to use a problem-solving framework to identify and to evaluate the possible available choices. Ask the patient to list the advantages and drawbacks to each choice, as well as personal values, goals, and preferences related to each choice. Encourage the patient to identify personal and social barriers to enacting any of the choices. Then ask the patient to rate the suitability of each choice based on appraisal of each one. *Use of a problem-solving framework in consideration of health care choices encourages the patient to consider health care options from the context of own experience, and to identify own best choices given the patient's life situation.*

Suggested NIC Interventions

Active Listening; Assertiveness Training; Decision-Making Support; Learning Facilitation; Mutual Goal Setting

Evaluations for Expected Outcomes

- The patient freely verbalizes personal opinions about the available health care choices
- The patient verbalizes how health care choices align with personal values, beliefs, and preferences
- The patient identifies conflicts between own choice and others' values, beliefs, and preferences
- The patient verbalizes feeling informed about own choices
- The patient makes an autonomous health care choice
- The patient verbalizes satisfaction with own health care choice given the available options

Documentation

- Assessment findings
- Interventions taken to ensure privacy, and patient and loved ones response
- Patient verbatim statements regarding the patient's understanding and perceptions of own health care choices, own cultural identification and norms, and the meaning the patient makes of own health concern and the need to make a health care decision. Related interventions undertaken and patient response.
- Past decision-making strategies used and utility for application in current situation
- Health teaching regarding health care choices, including patient response
- Any use of a problem-solving framework and patient response to same
- Patient's decision made and verbatim statements regarding the patient's satisfaction with it given the choices available

REFERENCES

Kramer-Roy, D. (2015). Using participatory and creative methods to facilitate emancipatory research with people facing multiple disadvantage: A role for health and care professionals. *Disability and Society, 30*(8), 1207–1224.

Olesen, M. L., Graungaard, A. H., & Husted, G. R. (2015). Deciding treatment for miscarriage—Experiences of women and health care professionals. *Scandinavian Journal of Caring Sciences, 29*(2), 386–394.

Papastavrou, E., Efstathiou, G., Tsangari, H., Karlou, C., Patiraki, E., Jarosova, D., ... Suhonen, R. (2016). Patients' decisional control over care: A cross-national comparison from both the patients' and nurses' points of view. *Scandinavian Journal of Caring Sciences, 30*(1), 26–36.

Welzel, C., & Delhey, J. (2015). Generalizing trust: The benign force of emancipation. *Journal of Cross-Cultural Psychology, 46*(7), 875–896.

Wittmann-Price, R., & Price, S. (2014). Development and revision of the Wittmann-Price emancipated decision-making scale. *Journal or Nursing Measurement, 22*(3), 361–367.

LABILE EMOTIONAL CONTROL

related to brain injury; emotional disturbance; stressors

Definition

Uncontrollable outbursts of exaggerated and involuntary emotional expression

Assessment

- Physiologic status, including patterns of nutrition, pain, elimination, activity, and rest
- Developmental delay or disability
- History of or current neurologic disease and/or traumatic brain injury
- History of or current exposure to trauma involving own or a loved one's death or the threat of death, serious injury, or sexual violence
- History of or current mental illness, including ADHD, mood, anxiety, eating, somatoform, autism spectrum, or borderline personality disorders
- History of impulse control disorder
- Mental status exam, including appearance, affect, mood, sensorium, cognition, motor (i.e., speech, movements, gait), thought process, thought content, perceptual disturbance)
- Childhood experience of parental responsiveness to emotional and psychological needs
- Substance use, including alcohol, street drugs, and prescription medications used differently than as prescribed, and patient's perceived benefits of substance use
- Usual pattern of emotional response. For areas of distress intolerance, specific types of stressors, frequency, and maladaptive response(s)
- Presence of rumination on stressors, or a typical pattern of rumination on stressors
- Patient's perception of health situation
- Patient's perception of own exaggerated and involuntary emotional expression

Defining Characteristics

- Absence of eye contact
- Difficulty in use of facial expressions
- Embarrassment regarding emotional expression
- Excessive crying without feeling sadness
- Excessive laughing without feeling happiness

- Expression of emotion incongruent with triggering factor
- Involuntary crying
- Involuntary laughing
- Tearfulness
- Uncontrollable crying
- Uncontrollable laughing
- Withdrawal from occupational situation
- Withdrawal from social situation

Expected Outcomes

- Patient will identify the personal and social impacts of emotional outbursts, and own goals for managing/limiting outbursts.
- Patient will discuss bodily, cognitive, and situational experiences correlating with periods of emotional outbursts.
- Patient will practice strategies to promote emotional control.
- Patient will express positive self-esteem.

Suggested NOC Outcomes

Aggression Control; Anxiety Control; Coping; Impulse Control; Self-Esteem; Self-Mutilation Restraint; Social Interaction Skills

Interventions and Rationales

- PCC Do not attempt to teach new skills/information while the patient is in the midst of an intense emotional outburst *as the patient's cognitive capacity may be reduced at this time.*
- PCC Teach new skills when the patient is calm. *Emotional outbursts physiologically are time-limited.*
- S PCC During the outburst, use a calm tone and communicate in short, direct, specific statements. Expect that the patient may need extra time to process information and that instructions may need to be repeated *as diminished cognitive capacity may impact processing of information.*
- When the outburst has ended, ensure that the patient's immediate physiologic needs (i.e., rest, nutrition, hydration, elimination) are addressed prior to engaging in interventions to reduce and prevent future outbursts. *Basic physiologic needs must be met for the patient to be able to engage therapeutically.*
- PCC Teach the patient about the social impact of the patient's emotional outbursts (as needed). Ask the patient to identify at least one person, besides self, who has been impacted by emotional outbursts. Ask the patient to identify at least one way the patient has been impacted socially, and one way the patient has been impacted occupationally (i.e., work, school) by outbursts *to promote insight and stimulate motivation to engage in strategies to limit outbursts.*
- Use nonjudgmental, matter-of-fact language *to promote self-esteem.*
- Engage the patient in discussion of how life would be different if the patient had better control over emotional outbursts *to foster motivation and engagement in care.*
- Ask the patient to decide at least one reason why the patient wants to better control emotional expression *to foster motivation and engagement in interventions, and to promote self-efficacy.*

- PCC Teach the patient to practice awareness of bodily sensations *to help learn the early signs of emotional arousal.*
- Assist the patient to make linkages between bodily sensations and emotional state. Teach strategies to decrease physiologic arousal *to help the patient to limit unwanted emotional outbursts.*
- Assist the patient to identify environmental and situational triggers to physiologic arousal, and engage the patient to create a plan to limit physiologic arousal *to promote self-efficacy in proactive management of emotional outbursts.*
- Promote self-esteem. Emphasize therapeutic gains made by the patient and encourage nonjudgmental, realistic appraisal of therapeutic challenges. *Higher self-esteem promotes cognitive self-regulatory capacity.*
- Assist the patient to identify and practice strategies to manage distressing/exciting situations and strong emotions. Use vicarious learning or role play exercises to practice plan of response to limit emotional outbursts. *Practice of strategies in a safe and controlled environment develops skills in strategies and builds confidence to apply strategies in triggering situations.*
- PCC Involve the patient in own care. Provide options and solicit feedback on the patient's experience of care. *Partnering with the patient promotes self-efficacy and self-esteem, and strengthens the therapeutic alliance.*
- Solicit the patient's thoughts and experience of bodily sensations during care. Reinforce and support use of adaptive coping strategies to limit emotional outbursts. *To help the patient further develop awareness of signs and triggers, and to promote use of strategies to limit/prevent outbursts.*
- Communicate continuous nonjudgmental acceptance of the patient through verbal and meta-communication. *To strengthen the therapeutic alliance, promote self-esteem.*
- Provide the patient with specific, simple, step-by-step information on what to expect in care *to reduce/prevent emotional arousal, communicate respect, and engage patient in care.*
- Chunk information according to immediate care requirements, and provide updates as each stage of care ensues. *Chunking information decreases cognitive stress and promotes retention.*
- PCC Assist the patient with referral to specialized resources in Mindfulness, Dialectical Behavior Therapy, and/or Cognitive Behavioral Therapy, as indicated, in consultation with the interdisciplinary care team. *Mindfulness improves attention and body awareness, and promotes cognitive control and attentional capability in situations of high emotion. Mindfulness, Dialectical Behavioral Therapy, and Cognitive Behavior Therapy each have applications for improving cognitive control and emotional dysregulation.*

Suggested NIC Interventions

Anger Control Assistance; Anxiety Reduction; Cognitive Restructuring; Coping Enhancement; Impulse Control Training; Support Group

Evaluations for Expected Outcomes

- The patient discusses experience of own emotional outbursts, and identifies ways they have affected the patient. Also, there is discussion on ways emotional outbursts have impacted the patient socially, including the effects on other people, relationships, social, and occupational opportunities. The patient identifies reasons to work toward better control of emotional expression.

- The patient identifies bodily sensations/changes, thoughts, and situations antecedent to emotional outbursts. The patient notes any trends in antecedents.
- The patient practices strategies to notice own physiologic, cognitive and emotional states, and practices strategies to decrease physiologic and emotional arousal.
- The patient identifies achievements inherent in decision to engage in interventions to limit emotional outbursts, setting goals, skills learned, skills practiced, and positive gains made in treatment.

Documentation

- Food and fluid intake, assessment of pain (if present), bowel and bladder activity, sleep patterns, activity, and exercise
- Relevant medical, developmental, and psychiatric history
- History of trauma
- Substance use, (if applicable) the patient's reasons for using, and relationship of substance use to emotional outbursts
- Patient, family, and nurse's observations of emotional outbursts, antecedents, impacts of and responses to outbursts
- Interventions implemented to limit uncontrolled emotional outbursts, including patient engagement and response
- Evaluations for expected outcomes
- Referrals to other services

REFERENCES

Grecucci, A., Pappaianni, E., Siugzdaite, R., Theuninck, A., & Job, R. (2015). Mindful emotion regulation: Exploring the neurocognitive mechanisms behind mindfulness. *BioMed Research International,* 1–9.

Linehan, M. (2014). *DBT skills training manual* (2nd ed.). New York: Guilford Press.

Sullivan-Bolyai, S., Johnson, K., Cullen, K., Hamm, T., Bisordi, J., Blaney, K., … Melkus, G. (2014). Tried and true: Self-regulation theory as a guiding framework for teaching parents diabetes education using human patient simulation. *Advances in Nursing Science, 37*(4), 340–349.

Thomson, K., Burnham Riosa, P., & Weiss, J. (2015). Brief report of preliminary outcomes of an emotion regulation intervention for children with autism spectrum disorder. *Journal of Autism and Developmental Disorders, 45*(11), 3487–3495.

Zawadzki, M. J. (2015). Rumination is independently associated with poor psychological health: Comparing emotion regulation strategies. *Psychology & Health, 30*(10), 1146–1163. doi:10.1080/08870446.2015.1026904

DYSFUNCTIONAL FAMILY PROCESSES

related to family history of substance abuse; substance abuse

Definition

Psychosocial, spiritual, and physiological functions of the family unit are chronically disorganized, which leads to conflict, denial of problems, resistance to change, ineffective problem solving, and a series of self-perpetuating crises

Assessment

- Family status, including alcoholic family member's ability to function in occupational and family roles, ability of other family members to function in their roles, family conflicts, financial status, and rituals during holidays and family celebrations

- Coping patterns, including type and number of changes family has recently experienced, usual response to stress, ability to adapt to change, and use of support systems
- Family health history, including medication use, mental illness, stress-related illnesses, history of alcohol or drug abuse, and evidence of emotional, physical, or sexual abuse of spouse or children
- Parental status, including age, marital status, number and ages of dependent children, and knowledge of normal child behavior
- Drinking pattern, including continuous or binge drinking, periods of abstinence and relapse, use of other substances, symptoms of withdrawal, and past drinking patterns and treatment
- Psychological status, including self-image and self-esteem, functional ability, independence level, and problem-solving and decision-making skills
- Spiritual status, including affiliation with a religious group and religious practices

Defining Characteristics

Behavioral

- Agitation
- Alteration in concentration
- Blaming
- Broken promises
- Chaos
- Complicated grieving
- Conflict avoidance
- Contradictory communication pattern
- Controlling communication pattern
- Criticizing
- Decrease in physical comfort
- Denial of problems
- Dependency
- Difficulty having fun
- Difficulty with intimate relationship
- Difficulty with life cycle transition
- Disturbances in academic performance in children
- Enabling substance use pattern
- Escalating conflict
- Failure to accomplish developmental tasks transitions
- Harsh self-judgment
- Immaturity
- Inability to accept a wide range of feelings
- Inability to accept help
- Inability to adapt to change
- Inability to deal constructively with traumatic experiences
- Inability to express a wide range of feelings
- Inability to meet emotional needs of its members
- Inability to meet the security needs of its members
- Inability to meet spiritual needs of its members
- Inability to receive help appropriately
- Inappropriate anger expression
- Insufficient knowledge about substance abuse

- Insufficient problem-solving skills
- Lying
- Manipulation
- Nicotine addiction
- Orientation favors tension relief rather than goals
- Paradoxical communication pattern
- Power struggles
- Rationalization
- Refusal to get help
- Seeking of affirmation
- Seeking of approval
- Self-blame
- Social isolation
- Special occasions centered on substance use
- Stress-related physical illnesses
- Substance abuse
- Unreliable behavior
- Verbal abuse of children
- Verbal abuse of parent
- Verbal abuse of partner

Feelings

- Abandonment
- Anger
- Anxiety
- Confuses love and pity
- Confusion
- Depression
- Dissatisfaction
- Embarrassment
- Emotional isolation
- Emotionally controlled by others
- Failure
- Fear
- Feeling different from others
- Feeling misunderstood
- Feeling unloved
- Guilt
- Hopelessness
- Hostility
- Hurt
- Insecurity
- Lingering resentment
- Loneliness
- Loss
- Loss of identity
- Low self-esteem
- Mistrust
- Moodiness
- Powerlessness
- Rejection

- Repressed emotions
- Shame
- Surgical procedure
- Taking responsibility for substance abuser's behavior
- Tension
- Unhappiness
- Vulnerability
- Worthlessness

Roles and Relationships

- Change in role function
- Chronic family problems
- Closed communication system
- Conflict between partners
- Deterioration in family relationships
- Diminished ability of family members to relate to each other for mutual growth and maturation
- Disrupted family rituals
- Disrupted family roles
- Disturbance in family dynamics
- Economically disadvantaged
- Family denial
- Inconsistent parenting
- Ineffective communication with partner
- Insufficient cohesiveness
- Insufficient family respect for autonomy of its members
- Insufficient family respect for individuality of its members
- Insufficient relationship skills
- Intimacy dysfunction
- Neglect of obligation to family member
- Pattern of rejection
- Perceived insufficient parental support
- Triangulating family

Expected Outcomes

- Family members will acknowledge that there's a problem with alcoholism within the family.
- Alcoholic family member will sign a contract stating that the person agrees to abstain from alcohol.
- Family members will sign contracts stating that they won't engage in abusive behavior.
- Family members will communicate their needs using "I" statements.
- Parents will take steps to reassert appropriate boundaries with children and resume parental responsibilities.
- Family members will discuss problems in an open, safe environment.
- Family members will acknowledge their strengths and their progress in resolving problems.
- Number and intensity of family crises will diminish.
- Family members will state their plans to continue to seek counseling and attend appropriate support group meetings.

Suggested NOC Outcomes

Family Coping; Family Functioning; Family Normalization; Role Performance; Substance Addiction Consequences

Interventions and Rationales

- Encourage family members to acknowledge that alcoholism is a problem within the family *to break through family denial.* Encourage individual family members to take responsibility for their problems. *Problems can't be addressed until family members take responsibility for them.*
- Inform the alcoholic family member that the person will have to address alcoholism before progress can be made in rebuilding family relations. Tell the person that abstinence with the help of a support group such as Alcoholics Anonymous is the only proven effective treatment for alcoholism *to establish abstinence as basis for treatment.*
- Ask the alcoholic family member to sign a contract stating the person will abstain from alcohol *to help the person take responsibility for own behavior.*
- S Help family members evaluate the consequences of abusive and violent behavior. Inform them that any suspected abuse will be reported. Ask family members to sign contracts stating they won't abuse each other *to help ensure the safety of family members.*
- PCC Teach family members to communicate their needs assertively. Encourage family members to use "I" statements to express feelings, for example, "I'm mad because you didn't show up for the school play like you promised," *to help family members get in touch with and talk about their feelings.*
- Discuss with the parents their ideas and beliefs regarding parental authority. Ask if they feel they have abdicated authority. Work with the parents to develop steps to reassert parental authority *to reestablish appropriate boundaries and relieve children of the need to assume parental roles.*
- Provide an opportunity for family members to discuss conflicts in an open, safe atmosphere *to decrease anxiety and help family members develop confidence in their ability to resolve problems.*
- PCC Assist family members in identifying their strengths and their progress in addressing problems *to build self-esteem.*
- PCC Encourage family members to continue to seek counseling *to enhance interpersonal skills and strengthen the family unit.*
- PCC Encourage family members to participate in Al-Anon or Alateen *to foster recovery.*

Suggested NIC Interventions

Coping Enhancement; Family Process Maintenance; Family Support; Substance Use Prevention; Substance Use Treatment

Evaluations for Expected Outcomes

- Family members acknowledge that alcoholism is a problem in the family.
- Alcoholic family member signs a contract stating that the person agrees to abstain from alcohol.
- Family members sign contracts stating that they won't engage in abusive behavior.
- Family members communicate their needs using "I" statements.
- Parents take steps to reassert appropriate boundaries with children and to resume parental responsibilities.

- Family members discuss problems in an open, safe environment.
- Family members acknowledge their strengths and the progress they have made in resolving problems.
- Number and intensity of family crises diminish.
- Family members state their plans to continue to seek counseling and attend appropriate support groups.

Documentation

- Family's reactions to and experience with alcoholism
- Interventions to assist family and family's response to them
- Referrals to community agencies
- Evaluations for expected outcomes

REFERENCES

Harrison, R., Lawton, R., Perlo, J., Gardner, P., Armitage, G., & Shapiro, J. (2015). Emotion and coping in the aftermath of medical error: A cross-country exploration. *Journal of Patient Safety, 11*(2), 29–35.

Montero-Marin, J., Prado-Abril, J., Piva Demarzo, M. M., Gascon, S., & García-Campayo, J. (2014). Coping with stress and types of burnout: Explanatory power of different coping strategies. *PLoS One*, *9*(2), e89090. doi:10.1371/journal.pone.0089090

Nijjar, R., Ellenbogen, M., & Hodgins, S. (2014). Personality, coping, risky behavior, and mental disorders in the offspring of parents with bipolar disorder: A comprehensive psychosocial assessment. *Journal of Affective Disorders, 166*, 315–324.

INTERRUPTED FAMILY PROCESSES

related to power shift among family members; shift in family roles

Definition

Change in family relationships and/or functioning

Assessment

- Family status, including marital status, family's developmental stage, family roles, family rules, communication patterns, family goals, and socioeconomic status
- Family health history, including history of mental illness, stress-related illnesses, history of substance abuse, and sexual abuse of spouse or children
- Parental status, including ages of dependent children and knowledge of normal child behavior
- Psychological status, including self-image and self-esteem, functional ability, independence level, and problem-solving and decision-making skills

Defining Characteristics

- Alteration in availability for affective responsiveness
- Alteration in family conflict resolution
- Alteration in family satisfaction
- Alteration in intimacy
- Alteration in participation for problem solving
- Change in communication pattern
- Change in somatization

- Change in stress-reduction behavior
- Change in expressions of conflict with community resources
- Change in expressions of isolation from community resources
- Change in participation for decision making
- Change in available emotional support
- Decrease in mutual support
- Ineffective task completion
- Power alliance change
- Ritual change

Expected Outcomes

- Family members won't experience verbal, physical, emotional, or sexual abuse.
- Family members will communicate clearly, honestly, consistently, and directly.
- Family members will establish clearly defined roles and equitable responsibilities.
- Family members will express understanding of rules and expectations.
- Family members will report that methods of solving problems and resolving conflicts have improved.
- Family members will report a decrease in the number and intensity of family crises.
- Family members will seek ongoing treatment.

Suggested NOC Outcomes

Family Coping; Family Functioning; Family Normalization; Social Interaction Skills; Substance Addiction Consequences

Interventions and Rationales

- Meet with family members *to establish levels of authority and responsibility in the family.*
- In family meeting, arrange seating so adults present a unified front *to reinforce their function as a decision-making unit.*
- Hold adults accountable for their alcohol or substance abuse and have them sign a "Use Contract" *to decrease denial, increase trust, and promote change.*
- S Assist family to set limits on abusive behaviors and have them sign "Abuse Contracts" *to foster feelings of safety and trust.*
- PCC Teach family to communicate clearly and honestly to increase their ability *to express thoughts and feelings in a positive way.*
- Encourage family members to evaluate communication patterns periodically *to reinforce benefits of effective communication skills.*
- PCC Refer to outside agencies, if needed, *to ensure continuing support.*

Suggested NIC Interventions

Coping Enhancement; Family Integrity Promotion; Family Process Maintenance; Family Support; Normalization Promotion; Substance Use Prevention; Substance Use Treatment

Evaluations for Expected Outcomes

- Family members don't experience any type of abuse.
- Family members report that family communication is clear, honest, and respectful.
- Family members describe clearly defined roles and responsibilities.

- Family members demonstrate understanding of roles and responsibilities.
- Family members identify problems and work together to solve them.
- Family members report fewer family crises.
- Family members recognize the need for professional assistance.

Documentation

- Problems and conflicts described by family members
- Behavioral contracts signed by family members
- Changes in roles and responsibilities and information about how these changes were negotiated
- Evidence of changes in family communication patterns
- Family's response to nursing interventions
- Evaluations for expected outcomes

REFERENCES

Feldman, R. (2014). When maternity doesn't matter: Dispersing pregnant women seeking asylum. *British Journal of Midwifery, 22*(1), 23–28.

Gazmararian, J., Elon, L., Yang, B., Graham, M., & Parker, R. (2014). Text4baby program: An opportunity to reach underserved pregnant and postpartum women? *Maternal & Child Health Journal, 18*(1), 223–232. doi:10.1007/s10995-013-1258-1

Webb, M. S., Passmore, D., Cline, G., & Maguire, D. (2014). Ethical issues related to caring for low birth weight infants. *Nursing Ethics, 21*(6), 731–741. doi:10.1177/0969733013513919

Zani, A. V., Pamplona Tonete, V. L., & de Lima Parada, C. G. (2014). Maternal representations about the provision of care to newborns at risk: A collective discourse. *Online Brazilian Journal of Nursing, 13*(3), 321–331.

HOPELESSNESS

related to chronic stress

Definition

Subjective state in which an individual sees limited or no alternatives or personal choices available and is unable to mobilize energy on own behalf

Assessment

- Family status, including family composition, level of education of family members, parents' occupation, child's grade level, ability of family to meet child's physical and emotional needs, coping patterns, and evidence of abuse
- Psychological status, including changes in appetite, energy level, motivation, and personal hygiene
- Sleep pattern
- Social status, including quality of relationships, degree of trust in others, level of self-esteem, and ability to function in social or academic roles

Defining Characteristics

- Alteration in sleep pattern
- Decrease in affect

- Decrease in appetite
- Decrease in initiative
- Decrease in response to stimuli
- Decrease in verbalization
- Despondent verbal cues (e.g., "I can't," sighing)
- Inadequate involvement in care
- Passivity
- Poor eye contact
- Shrugging in response to speaker
- Turning away from speaker

Expected Outcomes

- Child won't harm self while in hospital.
- Child will complete activities of daily living (ADLs) with assistance.
- Child will identify feelings and seek help when they're overwhelming.
- Child will identify ways to deal with stress at home and school.
- Child will begin making positive statements about self and others.

Suggested NOC Outcomes

Decision-Making; Depression Self-Control; Hope; Mood Equilibrium; Psychomotor Energy; Quality of Life

Interventions and Rationales

- Assign a small, consistent number of caregivers *to allow for the development of a trusting relationship between the child and the caregiver.*
- S Provide a safe environment *to maintain the child's safety.*
- Spend time each shift with the child. Allow the child to play in lieu of talking. *Playing is a form of communication for children.*
- Encourage the child to perform self-care activities to the extent possible and praise the smallest efforts *to enhance self-esteem and reduce feelings of hopelessness.*
- PCC Help the child make contact with other children *to reduce feelings of hopelessness.*
- Have family members bring toys, pictures, and other personal belongings *to reduce the child's stress.*
- PCC Teach the child, parents, and teachers about interventions that increase self-esteem *so that the child continues to receive support after discharge.*

Suggested NIC Interventions

Energy Management; Family Support; Hope Instillation; Mood Management

Evaluations for Expected Outcomes

- Child remains safe and unharmed.
- Child completes ADLs.
- Child asks for help when unable to cope with feelings.
- Child demonstrates positive methods of dealing with stress.
- Child attempts to make positive statements about self and others.

Documentation

- Observations of child's behavior
- Child's participation in self-care activities
- Child's expressions during play therapy
- Nursing interventions that stabilize mood and maintain safety
- Child's response to nursing interventions
- Evaluations for expected outcomes

REFERENCES

Boles, J. (2015). Bearing bad news: Supporting patients and families through difficult conversations. *Pediatric Nursing*, *41*(6), 306–308.

MacPhee, D., Lunkenheimer, E., & Rigges, N. (2015). Resilience as a regulation of family process. *Family Relations*, *64*(1), 153–175.

Svavarsdottir, E. K., Sigurdardottir, A. O., Konradsdottir, E., Stefansdottir, A., Sveinbjarnardottir, E. K., Ketilsdottir, A., ... Guðmundsdottir, H. (2015). The process of translating family nursing knowledge into clinical practice. *Journal of Nursing Scholarship*, *47*(1), 5–15. doi:10.1111/jnu.12108

INEFFECTIVE IMPULSE CONTROL

Definition

A pattern of performing rapid, unplanned reactions to internal or external stimuli without regard for the negative consequences of these reactions to the impulsive individual or to others

Assessment

- History or current presence of stress reactions in response to internal or external forces expressed by such physical findings as choking sensation, hyperventilation, dizziness, increased heart rate and/or blood pressure, perspiration, pupillary dilation, polyuria, and elevated blood glucose, cholesterol, and free fatty acid levels
- History or current presence of stress reactions in response to internal or external forces expressed by such behavioral cues as insomnia, restlessness, "scattered" thoughts, disorganized speech, restlessness, irritability, and altered concentration
- Physical stressors, including extreme heat or cold, malnutrition, disease, infection, and pain
- Psychological stressors, including fear, sense of failure, change in company or home location, success, holiday, vacation, or promotion
- Level of stress, positive coping mechanisms, realistic thought patterns, behaviors, or energy level
- Medication history, including use of drugs, caffeine, tobacco, or alcohol, which stimulate the sympathetic nervous system
- Sleep patterns or changes in daily activities that could be perceived as stressful, including too many or too few activities
- Sociologic factors, including job satisfaction, presence of support systems, family coping mechanisms, or hobbies

Defining Characteristics

- Acting without thinking
- Asking personal questions despite discomfort of others

- Gambling addiction
- Inability to save money or regulate finances
- Inappropriate sharing of personal details
- Irritability
- Overly familiar with strangers
- Sensation seeking
- Sexual promiscuity
- Temper outburst
- Violent behavior

Expected Outcomes

- Patient will identify triggers that lead to self-destructive actions.
- Patient will identify appropriate coping mechanisms to prevent self-harm and minimize engaging in impulsive behaviors.
- Patient will identify strategies that will aid in maintaining positive relationships.
- Patient will report to staff any thoughts of harming self or others.
- Patient will work with staff in planning ongoing treatment.

Suggested NOC Outcomes

Aggression Control; Anxiety Control; Coping; Impulse Control; Self-Esteem; Self-Mutilation Restraint; Social Interaction Skills

Interventions and Rationales

- S Assess the patient for thoughts of suicide, homicide, or self-mutilation. *Findings may require immediate safety precautions and psychological support.*
- Assess for history of previous or current medical conditions and any pharmacologic side effects that may be contributing to current symptoms, *as brain trauma, organic brain disorders, or medications can present with impulse control symptoms.*
- Decrease environmental stimuli if the patient is feeling unsafe. *A quiet and nonstimulating environment will assist in decreasing level of anxiety.*
- PCC Assist the patient in identifying stressors that lead to inappropriate or harmful impulsive behaviors, *as the patient is usually unaware of impulsive behaviors and will require assistance in identifying them.*
- PCC Encourage the patient to attend milieu therapies. *Milieu therapies will offer the patient an opportunity to share feelings and learn/practice new coping and social skills with peers.*
- PCC Educate the patient regarding cognitive therapies that can be used *to reinforce appropriate coping and social skills.*
- Dedicate quality time to the patient in a therapeutic and consistent manner *in order to help the patient feel safe and allow an open and trusting relationship to develop.*
- PCC Refer the patient for treatment, which may include but is not limited to medication management, individual therapy sessions, peer support groups, and crisis center contacts *to ensure continuation of treatment.*

Suggested NIC Interventions

Anger Control Assistance; Anxiety Reduction; Cognitive Restructuring; Coping Enhancement; Impulse Control Training; Support Group

Evaluations for Expected Outcomes

- Patient shows no physical or mental signs of self-destructive actions.
- Patient uses appropriate coping mechanisms.
- Patient can manage own impulsive behavior.
- Patient reports no harm to self or others.
- Patient states plan for continuing therapy.

Documentation

- Results of assessment for suicidal ideation, thoughts of homicide, or self-mutilation
- Response to decreased environmental stimuli
- Milieu therapies attended and response to treatment
- Response to nursing interventions
- External agencies suggested
- Evaluations for expected outcomes

REFERENCES

Bancos, I., Nannenga, M. R., Bostwick, J. M., Silber, M. H., Erickson, D., & Nippoldt, T. B. (2014). Impulse control disorders in patients with dopamine agonist-treated prolactinomas and nonfunctioning pituitary adenomas: A case-control study. *Clinical Endocrinology*, *80*(6), 863–868. doi:10.1111/cen.12375

Cicolini, G., Simonetti, V., Comparcini, D., Galli, F., Luisa, D. L., Mercanti, R., & Sepede, G. (2014). Impulsivity in inpatient substance abusers: An exploratory study. *Journal of Clinical Nursing*, *23*(5/6), 896–899. doi:10.1111/jocn.12373

Hayes, D. J., Jupp, B., Sawiak, S. J., Merlo, E., Caprioli, D., & Dalley, J. W. (2014). Brain γ-aminobutyric acid: A neglected role in impulsivity. *European Journal of Neuroscience*, *39*(11), 1921–1932. doi:10.1111/ejn.12485

RISK FOR INJURY

Definition

Vulnerable to physical damage due to environmental conditions interacting with the individual's adaptive and defense resources, which may compromise health

Assessment

- Age
- Health history, including accidents, falls, exposure to environmental hazards, marks from restraints, and unexplained bruising
- Evidence of neglect, including inappropriate clothing, unsanitary living conditions, inadequate food supplies, lack of medication, and absence of needed eyeglasses, hearing aid, cane, or walker
- Family status, including caregiver relationship to patient; time and resources available for caregiving; willingness and ability to meet patient's physical, social, and psychological needs; feelings of frustration; and history of abuse of any family member

Risk Factors

External

- Alteration in cognitive functioning
- Alteration in psychomotor functioning

- Compromised nutritional source (e.g., vitamins, food types)
- Exposure to pathogen
- Exposure to toxic chemical
- Immunization level within community
- Nosocomial agent
- Physical barrier (e.g., design, structure, arrangement of community, building, equipment)
- Unsafe mode of transport

Internal

- Abnormal blood profile
- Alteration in affective orientation
- Alteration in sensation (resulting from spinal cord injury, diabetes mellitus, etc.)
- Autoimmune dysfunction
- Effector dysfunction
- Extremes of age
- Immune dysfunction
- Impaired primary defense mechanisms (e.g., broken skin)
- Malnutrition
- Sensory integration dysfunction
- Tissue hypoxia

Expected Outcomes

- Patient will remain free from injury.
- Patient will state that no incidents of abuse occur.
- Patient will maintain control of mail, telephone, and other personal effects.
- Caregiver will state intention to contact respite care services and support groups.
- Patient and caregiver will report improved communication patterns.

Suggested NOC Outcomes

Abuse Protection; Falls Occurrence; Personal Safety Behavior; Risk Control; Safe Home Environment

Interventions and Rationales

- S Monitor the patient closely for signs of physical or mental abuse or neglect (bruises, abrasions, body odor, and unkempt appearance) *to ensure the patient's safety and well-being.*
- S Encourage the patient to discuss abuse or threats of abuse. Be willing to listen, and be careful to convey a nonjudgmental attitude. *The patient may hesitate to talk openly for fear of retaliation.*
- Report actual or suspected abuse to local authorities. *Every state has an agency that investigates and makes decisions about how a patient can best be protected from further abuse. Nurses are mandatory reporters of suspected abuse.*
- PCC Encourage the patient to answer own telephone and open own mail. *This gives the patient a sense of control and self-worth.*
- PCC Inform the patient and caregiver about state and county services for elderly people, respite services, adult day care, and support groups for children of aging parents *to enhance the caregiver's ability to cope.*

Suggested NIC Interventions

Environmental Management: Safety; Incident Reporting; Risk Identification; Surveillance: Safety

Evaluations for Expected Outcomes

- Patient shows no physical or mental signs of abuse.
- Patient reaffirms there has been no abuse.
- Patient can manage own mail and telephone messages.
- Caregiver contacts community agencies that offer assistance.
- Patient and family demonstrate improved communication.

Documentation

- Evidence of abuse
- Comments by patient that indicate abuse
- Reports made to state agencies
- Changes in caregiver–patient relationship
- External agencies contacted by caregiver
- Changes occurring as a result of using outside resources
- Evaluations for expected outcomes

REFERENCES

Carney, A. (2015). Indicators of abuse in the elderly ICU patient. *Critical Care Nursing Quarterly, 38*(3), 293–297.

Martins, H., Assunção, L., Caldas, I., & Magalhães, T. (2014). Victims of intimate partner violence. The physician's intervention in the Portuguese National Health Service. *Journal of Family Violence, 29*(3), 315–322. doi:10.1007/s10896-014-9586-5

Mercado, R. C., Wiltsey-Stirman, S., & Iverson, K. M. (2015). Impact of childhood abuse on physical and mental health status and health care utilization among female veterans. *Military Medicine, 180*(10), 1065–1074. doi:10.7205/MILMED-D-14-00719

DEFICIENT KNOWLEDGE

related to insufficient information

Definition

Absence or deficiency of cognitive information related to a specific topic

Assessment

- Age
- Developmental stage
- Educational level
- Ethnic group
- Religion
- Beliefs, values, and attitudes about health and illness
- Family status, including marital status, family roles, and family communication patterns

- Mental status, including level of consciousness, thought and speech, mood and affect, orientation, memory, capacity to read and write, and judgment
- Legal status, including patient's authority to give consent, presence of a legal guardian, and nature of treatment

Defining Characteristics

- Inaccurate follow-through of instruction
- Inaccurate performance on a test
- Inappropriate behavior (e.g., hysterical, hostile, agitated, apathetic)
- Insufficient knowledge

Expected Outcomes

- Patient will describe treatment and name the person who will perform it.
- Patient will express awareness of right to refuse treatment.

Suggested NOC Outcomes

Knowledge: Health Resources; Knowledge: Illness Care

Interventions and Rationales

- Ask the patient to describe understanding of the procedure to be performed *to determine how much the patient can assimilate.*
- S Answer questions in terms the patient can understand. If the patient can't understand, refer the patient to the physician *to ensure the patient's right to informed consent is protected.*
- If the patient can't understand, make sure the patient's legal guardian understands the procedure and the reason for doing it. *The nurse can be held liable if informed consent isn't obtained.*
- PCC If treatment is ongoing, continue to educate the patient about care and legal rights *to ensure continuity of care.*

Suggested NIC Interventions

Health Care Information Exchange; Health System Guidance; Teaching: Individual

Evaluations for Expected Outcomes

- Patient explains treatment accurately.
- Patient states understanding of legitimate right to refuse treatment.

Documentation

- Patient's or guardian's understanding of treatment
- Actions taken to ensure informed consent
- Signed consent (or refusal to sign)
- Evaluations for expected outcomes

REFERENCES

Ejaredar, M., & Hagen, B. (2014). I was told it restarts your brain: Knowledge, power, and women's experiences of ECT. *Journal of Mental Health*, *23*(1), 31–37. doi:10.3109/09638237.2013.841870

Griffith, R. (2015). Understanding the code: Acting in a patient's best interests. *British Journal of Community Nursing*, *20*(9), 458–461.
Nunes, S. T., Rego, G., & Nunes, R. (2016). Right or duty of information. *Nursing Ethics*, *23*(1), 36–47. doi:10.1177/0969733014557116

IMPAIRED MOOD REGULATION

related to anxiety; chronic illness; pain

Definition

A mental state characterized by shifts in mood or affect and which is comprised of a constellation of affective, cognitive, somatic, and/or physiological manifestations varying from mild to severe

Assessment

- Vital signs
- Weight
- Presence of mental illness, medical illness, infectious disease, acquired brain injury, or developmental delay or disability.
- Presence of, and if any the characteristics of, a relationship between mood state and therapeutic, accidental, or recreational substance use (i.e., medication, toxins, illicit/misused drugs/medication)
- Mental status exam, including appearance, affect, mood, sensorium, cognition, motor (i.e., speech, movements, gait), thought process, thought content, perceptual disturbance)
- Nutritional, hydration, and elimination status
- Patterns of activity and rest
- Suicidal ideation—current, recent, past
- Thoughts or history of self-harm without suicidal intent
- Presence/absence of hope, plans for the future
- Risk of any disinhibited behavior (i.e., personal, social, sexual, financial, legal, safety)
- Developmental stage

Defining Characteristics

- Changes in verbal behavior
- Disinhibition
- Dysphoria
- Excessive guilt
- Excessive self-awareness
- Excessive self-blame
- Flight of thoughts
- Hopelessness
- Impaired concentration
- Influenced self-esteem
- Irritability
- Psychomotor agitation
- Psychomotor retardation
- Sad affect
- Withdrawal

Expected Outcomes

- The patient will not engage in self-harm and suicidal behavior.
- The patient will not engage in risky behavior.
- The patient will have a balanced pattern of activity and rest.
- The patient's food and fluid intake will meet the patient's physiologic needs.

- The patient will participate in psychoeducation.
- The patient will verbalize a realistic understanding of the meaning of own symptoms.
- The patient will identify own goals for care.
- The patient will collaborate with the nurse to create a wellness recovery plan that includes goals and positive plans for the future.
- The patient will verbalize having hope for future.
- The patient will demonstrate awareness of distorted thoughts, if present, and will identify alternative balanced thought(s).
- The patient will complete activities of daily living.

Suggested NOC Outcomes

Anxiety Level; Coping; Depression Level; Impulse; Self-Control; Quality of Life; Stress Level

Interventions and Rationales

S
- Initiate suicide and/or self-harm precautions as necessary *to ensure the patient remains safe from suicide and self-harm.*

S
- Initiate precautions to reduce risks, if any, related to disinhibition. *Patient insight into risks and potential consequences of disinhibited behavior may be limited or absent.* The disinhibited patient may require increased observation and/or frequent redirection to avoid risky behavior.
- If indicated, support measures to resolve effects of substance action or substance withdrawal *to promote safe elimination of substance from the body and prevent complications of substance action or withdrawal.*
- Ensure dietary and fluid intake to meet physiologic needs *to prevent dehydration, electrolyte imbalances, muscles loss, unhealthy weight change, elimination changes, complications of hypoglycemia. Persons with mood disturbances may not meet diet and hydration needs. Persons with mood disturbance may manifest hyper- or hypoactivity.*
- Encourage and support appropriate levels of rest and activity (according to the patient's physiologic needs and capabilities) *to prevent complications of inactivity (e.g., skin break down, deep vein thrombosis, muscle atrophy, constipation, etc.) as well as to prevent complications of excessive activity (e.g., exhaustion, injury, electrolyte imbalances, exertional rhabdomyolysis).*

PCC
- Use short, simple phrases to convey instructions or questions. Permit ample time for the patient to respond, and expect to at times need to repeat instructions or questions. Tasks may need to be presented to the patient for completion one step at a time, and in small, simple steps. *Impaired concentration, psychomotor agitation, psychomotor retardation, or flight of ideas may inhibit processing of information and capability to remain on task.*
- Convey a nonjudgmental, supportive attitude and do not take personally any irritable statements/responses. Use effective therapeutic communication skills to avoid power struggles. *Maintenance of a therapeutic nurse–patient relationship is a key nursing responsibility.*
- Provide assistance, cues, or reminders, as needed, for the completion of activities of daily living (ADLs) *as impaired concentration, flight of ideas, psychomotor agitation, or psychomotor retardation may restrict independent skill or follow through on ADLs.*

PCC
- Assist the patient to access psychoeducation resources appropriate to the patient's clinical situation *to promote understanding of etiology of the patient's mood symptoms, promote engagement in care, and build self-efficacy in symptom recognition and management.*

PCC
- Engage the patient to develop and enact a wellness recovery plan in own care, which includes positive goals for the future *to promote hope and engagement in self-care.*
- Assist the patient to evaluate the efficacy of the patient's strategies to meet goals. Emphasize gains made toward recovery goals, and assist in problem solving new solutions for strategies attempted but ineffective to meet goals. *To promote self-esteem, self-efficacy, development of problem-solving skills.*
- Assist the patient with excessive guilt, excessive self-blame, or excessive self-awareness to counter distorted thinking through the Best Friend Technique. *Excessive guilt, self-blame, or excessive self-awareness can be linked to cognitive distortions. Cognitive distortions are negative thoughts that do not truly reflect reality.*
- Ask the patient to identify the specific thoughts the patient has about self that link to feelings of guilt or blame, or excessive awareness of self, and then to identify what a caring and realistic best friend would tell about the patient's distorted thought. *Cognitive Behavioral Therapy (CBT) strategies, such as the Best Friend Technique, can help the patient to become aware of the emotionally charged, distorted thoughts and to consider an alternative, more neutral, less emotionally charged thought.*

PCC
- Assist the patient with referral to specialty psychotherapy resources, as indicated by the patient's presentation and as determined by the clinical team. *Psychotherapies, such as CBT, Interpersonal and Social Rhythm Therapy (IPSRT), Acceptance and Commitment Therapy (ACT), and Interpersonal Psychotherapy, have indications for use in persons with mood disturbances.*

Suggested NIC Interventions

Anxiety Reduction; Coping Enhancement; Emotional Support; Improved Quality of Life; Improved Well-Being; Mood Management

Evaluations for Expected Outcomes

- The patient remains safe from self-harm and suicidal behavior.
- The patient refrains from risky behavior.
- The patient engages in a balanced pattern of activity and rest.
- The patient's food and fluid intake meet the patient's physiologic needs.
- The patient participates in psychoeducation and verbalizes a realistic understanding of the meaning of the patient's symptoms and goals in care.
- The patient participates in creating own wellness recovery plan.
- The patient verbalizes hope and plans for future.
- The patient demonstrates awareness of distorted thinking, if present, and identifies alternative balanced thought(s).
- The patient completes ADLs.

Documentation

- Risk assessments
- Mental status exam findings
- Observations of patient behavior and activity level
- Patient verbatim statements regarding own experience(s) of hopelessness, excessive guilt, excessive self-awareness, excessive self-blame
- Interventions implemented, including patient engagement and response
- Content of wellness recovery plan

- Relevant medical, developmental, and psychiatric history
- Referrals to other services
- Evaluations for expected outcomes

REFERENCES

Fountoulakis, K. N. (2015). *Bipolar disorder: An evidence-based guide to manic depression*. Berlin: Springer-Verlag.

Furman, J. (2015). When exercise causes exertional rhabdomyolysis. *Journal of the American Academy of Physician Assistants, 28*(4), 38–43.

Greenberger, D., & Padesky, C. A. (2016). *Mind over mood: Change how you feel by changing the way you think* (2nd ed.). New York Guilford Press.

Videbeck, S. L. (2014). *Psychiatric-mental health nursing*. Philadelphia, PA: Lippincott Williams & Wilkins.

Yatham, L. N., Kennedy, S. H., Parikh, S. V., Schaffer, A., Beaulieu, S., Alda, M., … Berk, M. (2013). Canadian Network for Mood and Anxiety Treatments (CANMAT) and International Society for Bipolar Disorders (ISBD) collaborative update of CANMAT guidelines for the management of patients with bipolar disorder: Update 2013. *Bipolar Disorders, 15*, 1–44.

RISK FOR OTHER DIRECTED VIOLENCE

Definition

Vulnerable to behaviors in which an individual demonstrates that he or she can be physically, emotionally, and/or sexually harmful to others

Assessment

- Age
- Gender
- Recent stressors and coping strategies
- Patient history, including health history, substance abuse history (type and effects on mental status), and previous episodes of violence (circumstances, behavior, arrests)
- Reactions of family members to episodes of violence
- Mental status examination (with emphasis on insight and judgment)
- Physical findings, including neurologic examination
- Laboratory studies, including electroencephalography, toxicology screening, and blood chemistry

Risk Factors

- Access to weapon
- Alteration in cognitive functioning
- Cruelty to animals
- Fire-setting
- History of childhood abuse (e.g., physical, psychological, sexual)
- History of substance abuse
- History of witnessing family violence
- Impulsiveness
- Motor vehicle offense (e.g., traffic violations, use of a motor vehicle to release anger)
- Negative body language (e.g., rigid posture, clenching of fists/jaw, hyperactivity, pacing, threatening stances)
- Neurologic impairment (e.g., positive EEG, head trauma, seizure disorders)
- Pathologic intoxication

- Pattern of indirect violence (e.g., tearing objects off walls, urinating/defecating on floor, stamping feet, temper tantrum, throwing objects, breaking a window, slamming doors, sexual advances)
- Pattern of other-directed violence (e.g., hitting/kicking/spitting/scratching others, throwing objects/biting someone, attempted rape, rape, sexual molestation, urinating/defecating on a person)
- Pattern of threatening violence (e.g., verbal threats against property/people, social threats, cursing, threatening notes/gestures, sexual threats)
- Pattern of violent antisocial behavior (e.g., stealing, insistent borrowing, insistent demands for privileges, insistent interrupting, refusal to eat/take medication, ignoring instructions)
- Perinatal complication
- Prenatal complications
- Psychotic disorder
- Suicidal behavior

Expected Outcomes

- Patient will maintain control over anger.
- Patient will successfully rechannel hostility into socially acceptable behaviors.
- Patient will discuss angry feelings and will verbalize ways to tolerate frustration appropriately.
- Patient will express need for long-term treatment by appropriate professional.

Suggested NOC Outcomes

Abuse Cessation; Abusive Behavior Self-Restraint; Aggression Self-Control; Impulse Self-Control

Interventions and Rationales

- Maintain a low level of stimuli in the patient's environment *to avoid increasing agitation and provoking violent behavior.*
- S Remove all objects from the environment that the patient could use to injure others *to provide for the patient's safety and protect potential victims of violence.*
- Instruct staff members to maintain and convey a calm attitude toward the patient. *Anxiety is contagious and can be transferred to the patient. A calm attitude reinforces a feeling of safety.*
- Explain in a firm, calm voice that you'll help the patient remain in control. *Communicating willingness to help the patient maintain self-control encourages the patient to take control of own behavior.*
- Set limits on the patient's behavior *to reinforce the expectation that the patient will act in a responsible, controlled manner.*
- Express understanding of the patient's feelings and encourage open discussion *to provide support, reassurance, and positive reinforcement for desirable behaviors.*
- Administer prescribed medications to help the patient control aggressive behavior and remain calm. Monitor for effectiveness. *When used appropriately, medications commonly remove the need for physical restraint.*
- PCC Explain the medication program to the patient *to promote compliance* and make sure the patient takes medications, as prescribed, *to help keep the patient calm.*
- According to facility policy, restrain or seclude the patient, as necessary, *to prevent serious injury to self or others.* Use seclusion or restraint only after less restrictive

measures have failed. Both measures require a physician's order as well as accurate documentation.

- Establish a daily routine of strenuous exercise, and encourage the patient to adhere to it. *Exercise provides an alternative way to handle frustration.*
- Encourage the patient to gradually begin discussing hostile feelings *to help develop more appropriate ways of dealing with hostility.*
- PCC Refer the patient for appropriate long-term treatment; for example, to a drug or alcohol rehabilitation center, psychiatrist, or psychologist. *The patient may require help from specialized professionals or agencies.*

Suggested NIC Interventions

Anger Control Assistance; Behavior Management; Environmental Management: Violence Prevention; Impulse Control Training

Evaluations for Expected Outcomes

- Patient behaves in nonaggressive manner.
- Patient rechannels hostility by participating in strenuous physical exercise on daily basis.
- Patient states what precipitates anger and describes consequences of failing to control it.
- Patient expresses need for ongoing treatment.

Documentation

- Patient behaviors that indicate escalating agitation
- Other observations about patient's verbal and nonverbal behavior
- Factors that precipitate acts of violence
- Nursing interventions performed to reduce or prevent violent behavior
- Nursing interventions performed to ensure safety of other patients and staff members
- Patient's response to nursing interventions
- Referrals to specialized professionals and agencies
- Evaluations for expected outcomes

REFERENCES

Berends, L., Ferris, J., & Laslett, A. (2014). On the nature of harms reported by those identifying a problematic drinker in the family, an exploratory study. *Journal of Family Violence*, *29*(2), 197–204. doi:10.1007/s10896-013-9570-5

Cha, S., & Masho, S. (2014). Discussions about intimate partner violence during prenatal care in the United States: The role of race/ethnicity and insurance status. *Maternal & Child Health Journal*, *18*(6), 1413–1422. doi:10.1007/s10995-013-1381-z

Davis, C., Landon, D., & Brothers, K. (2015). Safety alert: Protecting yourself and others from violence. *Nursing*, *45*(1), 55–59.

DISTURBED PERSONAL IDENTITY

related to low self-esteem

Definition

Inability to maintain an integrated and complete perception of self

Assessment

- Choices of vocation, sexual orientation, religious orientation, and friendships
- Ability to defend choices regarding long-range goals, to recognize alternatives, and to appreciate consequences
- Comfort level with decisions made about long-range goals
- Degree of anxiety or depression about long-range goals
- Loss of interest or social isolation from usual activities or friends
- Level of irritability about long-range goals
- Sleep difficulties
- Changes in eating habits
- Rape trauma
- Family status, including method of dealing with general conflicts, level of patient's communication with parents, handling of negotiations regarding restriction of freedom, degree of patient's separation from family, tolerance of patient's expressed opinions, reaction of parents to patient's long-range goals, and age-appropriateness of dating, curfew regulation, and money responsibilities
- Family and cultural standards related to separation issues

Defining Characteristics

- Alteration in body image
- Confusion about cultural values
- Confusion about goals
- Confusion about ideological values
- Delusional description of self
- Feeling of emptiness
- Feeling of strangeness
- Fluctuating feelings about self
- Gender confusion
- Inability to distinguish between internal and external stimuli
- Inconsistent behavior
- Ineffective coping strategies
- Ineffective relationships
- Ineffective role performance

Expected Outcomes

- Patient will establish trusting relationship with caregiver.
- Patient's issues will be discussed.
- Family's issues will be discussed.
- Patient will establish a firm, positive sense of self and personal identity.
- Patient will choose long-range goals using problem-solving techniques and will be comfortable with choices.
- Family will accept patient's choices of long-range goals.

Suggested NOC Outcomes

Distorted Thought Self-Control; Identity; Personal Well-Being; Self-Esteem

Interventions and Rationales

- Assess the patient alone, without family, *to gather baseline data and begin a therapeutic relationship.*
- PCC Explain your role as a patient advocate; negotiate rules of interaction, including confidentiality and depth and breadth of discussion *to establish your role as a resource for the patient rather than as the family's agent.*
- Explore personal identity issues distressing to the patient *to isolate issues into smaller, more solvable units.*
- Help the patient identify own values, beliefs, hopes, dreams, skills, and interests. *The patient's deficits may lie in a lack of self-exploration, problem-solving methods used, or separation issues with parents.*
- Integrate personal identity issues into decisions and choices *to help the patient develop skill in problem-solving methods.*
- Help the patient identify the likely consequences of each choice. *Discussion and explanation aid problem-solving skills.*
- Promote choices with the most likelihood of success. *Specific instructions can help the patient gain problem-solving ability and maturity.*
- Encourage family conferences to explore potential reactions to the patient's choices, and promote support for the patient's independent decision making. *Meetings can help the patient and family members identify problems and find better ways to interact. Meetings also allow the patient and family members to ventilate true feelings in a safe environment.*
- PCC Encourage peer support groups *to explore and share personal identity experiences. Adolescents and young adults commonly accept support from peers more readily than from older adults.*
- PCC Promote outpatient counseling and family meetings, as appropriate, to reinforce progress. *Establishing outpatient support systems can reduce regression.*
- Listen to the patient's personal values and beliefs, but remain nonjudgmental, even if the patient's values and beliefs differ from your own. *Remaining nonjudgmental, but attentive, shows your support.*

Suggested NIC Interventions

Delusion Management; Environmental Management: Violence Prevention; Hallucination Management; Reality Orientation

Evaluations for Expected Outcomes

- Patient openly discusses concerns with caregiver.
- Patient describes personal identity struggles.
- Family members discuss their reactions to patient's personal identity choices.
- Patient describes values, beliefs, skills, and interests in a positive way.
- Patient identifies choices and possible alternatives, postulates consequences, and makes decisions about long-range goals.
- Family members accept patient's choices of long-range goals.

Documentation

- Assessment of patient's initial issues and problem-solving ability, including family's reactions, as well as assessment of level of separation achieved by patient

- Patient's level of emotional distress and changes in sleep and eating, initially and as hospitalization continues
- Patient's progress in problem solving and making choices
- Patient–family interactions and content of family meetings
- Patient's interaction in peer-group meetings
- Outpatient resources identified and suggested to patient and family members
- Evaluations for expected outcomes

REFERENCES

Brand, B. L., Loewenstein, R. J., & Spiegel, D. (2014). Dispelling myths about dissociative identity disorder treatment: An empirically based approach. *Psychiatry: Interpersonal & Biological Processes*, 77(2), 169–189. doi:10.1521/psyc.2014.77.2.169

Kamen, C. S., Smith-Stoner, M., Heckler, C. E., Flannery, M., & Margolies, L. (2015). Social support, self-rated health, and lesbian, gay, bisexual, and transgender identity disclosure to cancer care providers. *Oncology Nursing Forum*, 42(1), 44–51. doi:10.1188/15.ONF.44-51

Li, Y., Ho, C., & Wang, H. (2016). Demoralization in cancer patients and related factors in Taiwan. *Cancer Nursing*. doi:10.1097/NCC.0000000000000352

DISTURBED PERSONAL IDENTITY

related to psychiatric disorders

Definition

Inability to maintain an integrated and complete perception of self

Assessment

- Degree of anxiety or depression about self-perception
- Family status, including method of dealing with general conflicts
- Changes in sleep or eating patterns
- Cultural status and standards

Defining Characteristics

- Alteration in body image
- Confusion about cultural values
- Confusion about goals
- Confusion about ideological values
- Delusional description of self
- Feeling of emptiness
- Feeling of strangeness
- Fluctuating feelings about self
- Gender confusion
- Inability to distinguish between internal and external stimuli
- Inconsistent behavior
- Ineffective coping strategies
- Ineffective relationships
- Ineffective role performance

Expected Outcomes

- Patient will contract for safety.
- Patient will identify internal versus external stimuli.
- Patient will maintain adequate nutritional intake.
- Patient will identify personal goals and realistic steps toward those goals.
- Patient will compile a list of resources to call when needed.
- Patient will remain free of substance abuse.
- Patient will secure a safe place to live.

Suggested NOC Outcomes

Coping; Self-esteem; Impulse Self Control; Distorted Thought Self Control

Interventions and Rationales

- S Safety-assess for suicidal/homicidal ideation, self-induced cuts or burns. Assess for self-induced vomiting or restricting of food. Thorough mental status exam. *Individuals struggling with identity issues are at an increased safety risk.*
- S Contract with patient for safety. Schedule meeting with client to process feeling and experiences. *Demonstrating care and compassion for the client allows the patient to feel safe and promotes healing.*
- Instruct client to write about feelings in a journal and to list coping strategies. *Journaling can help a client maintain self-control and may increase insight.*
- Accept the client in own struggle. Reinforce taking healthy risks and appropriate expression of feelings. *Appropriate expression of feelings enhances self-esteem and promotes resiliency.*
- PCC Refer patients to mental health services for medication and symptom management. *Disturbed personal identity may require ongoing mental health care.*

Suggested NIC Interventions

Environmental Management: Safety; Self-Esteem Enhancement; Coping Enhancement; Role Enhancement; Journaling

Evaluations for Expected Outcomes

- Patient expresses freedom from harming self or others.
- Patient does not engage in substance abuse.
- Patient maintains adequate nutritional status.
- Patient shares personal goals and realistic strategies for achievement.
- Patient secures a safe place to live.
- Patient develops list of resources in time of need.

Documentation

- Patient's contract for safety
- Patient's planned health promotion behaviors
- Patient's understanding of available resources if needed
- Evaluations for expected outcomes

REFERENCES

Brand, B. L., Loewenstein, R. J., & Spiegel, D. (2014). Dispelling myths about dissociative identity disorder treatment: An empirically based approach. *Psychiatry: Interpersonal & Biological Processes*, *77*(2), 169–189. doi:10.1521/psyc.2014.77.2.169

Kamen, C. S., Smith-Stoner, M., Heckler, C. E., Flannery, M., & Margolies, L. (2015). Social support, self-rated health, and lesbian, gay, bisexual, and transgender identity disclosure to cancer care providers. *Oncology Nursing Forum*, *42*(1), 44–51. doi:10.1188/15.ONF.44-51

Li, Y., Ho, C., & Wang, H. (2016). Demoralization in cancer patients and related factors in Taiwan. *Cancer Nursing*. doi:10.1097/NCC.0000000000000352

RISK FOR DISTURBED PERSONAL IDENTITY

Definition

Vulnerable to the inability to maintain an integrated and complete perception of self, which may compromise health

Assessment

- Choices of vocation, sexual orientation, religious orientation, and friendships
- Ability to defend choices regarding long-range goals, to recognize alternatives, and to appreciate consequences
- Comfort level with decisions made about long-range goals
- Degree of anxiety or depression about long-range goals
- Loss of interest in or social isolation from usual activities or friends
- Level of irritability about long-range goals
- Sleep difficulties
- Changes in eating habits
- Family status, including method of dealing with general conflicts, level of patient's communication with family members/others, handling of negotiations regarding restriction of freedom, degree of patient's separation from family, tolerance of patient's expressed opinions, reaction to patient's long-range goals, and age-appropriateness of dating, curfew regulation, and money responsibilities
- Family and cultural standards

Risk Factors

- Alteration in social role
- Cult indoctrination
- Cultural incongruence
- Developmental transition
- Discrimination
- Dissociative identity disorder
- Dysfunctional family processes
- Exposure to toxic chemical
- Low self-esteem
- Manic states
- Organic brain disorder
- Perceived prejudice
- Pharmaceutical agent
- Psychiatric disorder
- Situational crisis
- Stages of growth

Expected Outcomes

- Patient will actively participate in milieu therapies.
- Patient will maintain safety and report any thoughts of suicide to staff.

- Patient will perform relaxation techniques during periods of stress.
- Patient will verbalize understanding of the need for long-term therapy.

Suggested NOC Outcomes

Anxiety Control; Coping; Depression Level; Distorted Thought Control; Impulse Control; Self-Esteem; Substance Addiction Consequences

Interventions and Rationales

- S Assess patient for thoughts of suicide *as patient may require immediate safety precautions and psychological support.*
- Assess for history of previous or current medical conditions, substance abuse, and any pharmacologic side effects. *Brain trauma, organic brain disorders, substance abuse, or medication side effects can present with similar symptoms.*
- PCC Work with patient to identify triggers that provoke anxiety. *The patient may not remember or be aware of the events that trigger the patient's symptoms and will need assistance in identifying them.*
- Provide patient with emotional support and reassurance of safety during episodes of dissociation *as the symptoms the patient is experiencing can be disturbing and anxiety provoking in and of themselves.*
- Reorient patient as necessary *in order to reduce anxiety related to confusion.*
- PCC Educate patient on positive coping mechanisms such as cognitive therapies and relaxation techniques, and assist the patient in applying these techniques. *Assisting the patient with relaxation therapies during times of anxiety decreases anxiety and helps assure the patient of the efficacy of these coping mechanisms.*
- Dedicate quality time to the patient in a therapeutic and consistent manner *in order to help the patient feel safe, allow time for open expression of feelings, and develop a trusting relationship.*
- PCC Refer patient for long-term therapy and educate patient regarding the length of treatment. *Patient may not be aware that long-term treatment may be necessary.*
- PCC Refer patient to support groups in the community *as this will help the patient to realize that he/she is not alone and because these groups provide further anxiety prevention strategies and support.*

Suggested NIC Interventions

Anxiety Reduction; Coping Enhancement; Decision-Making Support; Risk Identification; Self-Esteem Enhancement; Substance Use Prevention; Suicide Prevention; Relaxation Therapy

Evaluations for Expected Outcomes

- Patient participates in milieu therapy.
- Patient expresses no thoughts of suicide.
- Patient uses appropriate stress management techniques.
- Patient verbalizes need for long-term therapy.

Documentation

- Results of assessment for suicidal ideation

- Assessment of health history and use/reaction to medications
- Patient's responses to therapeutic actions
- Patient–family interactions and content of family meetings
- Cognitive therapies and relaxation techniques used
- Outpatient resources identified and suggested to patient
- Evaluations for expected outcomes

REFERENCES

Brand, B. L., Loewenstein, R. J., & Spiegel, D. (2014). Dispelling myths about dissociative identity disorder treatment: An empirically based approach. *Psychiatry: Interpersonal & Biological Processes*, *77*(2), 169–189. doi:10.1521/psyc.2014.77.2.169

Fraser, G. (2014). The diagnosis and treatment of dissociative identity disorder: A case study and contemporary perspective. *Canadian Journal of Psychiatry*, *59*(2), 115–116.

Jacobson, L., Fox, J., Bell, H., Zeligman, M., & Graham, J. (2015). Survivors with dissociative identity disorder: Perspectives on the counseling process. *Journal of Mental Health Counseling*, *37*(4), 308–322. doi:10.17744/mehc.31.4.03

POSTTRAUMA SYNDROME

related to history of criminal victimization

Definition

Sustained maladaptive response to a traumatic, overwhelming event

Assessment

- History and circumstances of assault
- Patient's perception of event
- Physical injuries sustained, including cardiopulmonary, genitourinary, integumentary, and musculoskeletal
- Neurologic status
- Emotional reactions, including grief reaction and changes in self-concept and sleep pattern
- Cognitive reactions, including concentration, memory, and orientation
- Behavioral reactions, including coping patterns and social interactions
- Available support systems

Defining Characteristics

- Aggression
- Alienation
- Alteration in concentration
- Alteration in mood
- Anger
- Anxiety
- Avoidance behaviors
- Compulsive behavior
- Denial
- Depression
- Dissociative amnesia
- Enuresis
- Exaggerated startle response
- Fear Flashbacks
- Gastrointestinal irritation
- Grieving
- Guilt
- Headache
- Heart palpitations
- History of detachment
- Hopelessness
- Horror

- Hypervigilence
- Intrusive dreams
- Intrusive thoughts
- Irritability
- Neurosensory irritability
- Nightmares
- Panic attacks
- Rage
- Reports feeling numb
- Repression
- Shame
- Substance abuse

Expected Outcomes

- Patient will recover from physical injuries to the extent possible.
- Patient will express feelings of anger, blame, fear, and guilt. Patient will spend less time recriminating himself.
- Patient will express feelings of physical safety.
- Patient will use effective coping mechanisms to reduce fear.
- Patient will mobilize support systems and professional resources, as needed.
- Patient will reestablish and maintain adaptive interpersonal relationships.

Suggested NOC Outcomes

Abuse Recovery: Emotional; Abuse Recovery: Sexual; Coping; Fear Self-Control

Interventions and Rationales

- Follow the medical regimen to manage physical injuries. *This reduces anxiety as the patient perceives the body's ability to recover from injury.*
- Provide the patient with psychological support:
  - Visit frequently *to decrease the patient's fear of being left alone and to encourage a trusting relationship.*
  - Be available to listen *to express empathy with the patient's feelings.*
  - Accept the patient's feelings and behaviors *to reassure the patient that they're appropriate and valid.*
  - Reassure the patient of safety, and take appropriate measures to ensure it. *The patient's feelings of safety are compromised by fear of repeated assaults.*
- Avoid care-related activities and environmental stimuli (loud noises, bright lights, abrupt entrances to room, painful procedures or treatments) that may intensify symptoms. *The patient's traumatic experience may be intensified by misinterpreting procedures or environmental factors as repeated assaults.*
- Monitor mental status, reorienting the patient to surroundings and interpreting reality as often as necessary, *to alleviate psychic numbing, a characteristic symptom of assault.*
- Instruct the patient in at least one fear-reducing behavior, such as seeking support from others when frightened, *to help the patient gain a sense of mastery over the current situation.*
- Support family members:
  - Provide time for them to express their feelings.
  - Help them understand the phases of crisis and the patient's reactions to them.

  These measures help reduce anxiety.
- PCC Offer referrals to community or professional resources, including clergy, mental health professionals, social services, and support groups, *to help the patient regain a sense of universality, decrease isolation, share fears, and deal constructively with feelings.*
- Recognize that the patient's culture may affect response to assault; remain supportive and nonjudgmental *to show you support and accept the patient's response.*

Suggested NIC Interventions

Coping Enhancement; Counseling; Rape-Trauma Treatment; Security Enhancement; Support System Enhancement

Evaluations for Expected Outcomes

- Patient recovers from injuries to the extent possible and resumes normal or near-normal activities of daily living.
- Patient expresses feelings of anger, blame, fear, and guilt. Patient spends less time recriminating self.
- Patient reports feeling safe.
- Patient demonstrates at least one fear-reducing behavior during times of panic (specify).
- Patient uses available support groups or mental health crisis center.
- Patient interacts socially with others.

Documentation

- Patient's perception of event
- Observations of patient's verbal and nonverbal behaviors
- Observations of patient's interaction with others
- Patient's response to nursing interventions
- Referrals to other support systems
- Evaluations for expected outcomes

REFERENCES

Anderson, K. M., Renner, L. M., & Bloom, T. S. (2014). Rural women's strategic responses to intimate partner violence. *Health Care for Women International*, *35*(4), 423–441. doi:10.1080/07399332.2013.815757

Saindon, C., Rheingold, A. A., Baddeley, J., Wallace, M. M., Brown, C., & Rynearson, E. K. (2014). Restorative retelling for violent loss: An open clinical trial. *Death Studies*, *38*(4), 251–258. doi:10.1080/07481187.2013.783654

Stoddard, S., Varela, J., & Zimmerman, M. (2015). Future expectations, attitude toward violence, and bullying perception during early adolescence: A mediation evaluation. *Nursing Research, 64*(6), 422–433.

Sutherland, M. A., Fontenot, H. B., & Fantasia, H. C. (2014). Beyond assessment: Examining providers' responses to disclosures of violence. *Journal of the American Association of Nurse Practitioners*, *26*(10), 567–573. doi:10.1002/2327-6924.12101

POSTTRAUMA SYNDROME

related to history of abuse (e.g., physical, psychological, sexual)

Definition

Sustained, maladaptive response to a traumatic, overwhelming event

Assessment

- Age
- Gender
- Education level

- Customs and rituals, especially pertaining to sexuality
- Family roles, rules, and subsystems
- Evidence of physical, sexual, or emotional abuse within family
- Ability of family members to protect children and correctly judge situations as being safe or unsafe
- Family history of alcoholism, substance abuse, or incarceration of family members

Defining Characteristics

- Aggression
- Alienation
- Alteration in concentration
- Alteration in mood
- Anger
- Anxiety
- Avoidance behaviors
- Compulsive behavior
- Denial
- Depression
- Dissociative amnesia
- Enuresis
- Exaggerated startle response
- Fear Flashbacks
- Gastrointestinal irritation
- Grieving
- Guilt
- Headache
- Heart palpitations
- History of detachment
- Hopelessness
- Horror
- Hypervigilence
- Intrusive dreams
- Intrusive thoughts
- Irritability
- Neurosensory irritability
- Nightmares
- Panic attacks
- Rage
- Reports feeling numb
- Repression
- Shame
- Substance abuse

Expected Outcomes

- Child won't harm self or others.
- Child will agree to maintain personal safety.
- Child will begin expressing feelings in words.
- Child will describe steps to take to maintain safety.
- Child will express awareness of placement after discharge (home, foster care, group home, day treatment program).

Suggested NOC Outcomes

Abuse Cessation; Abuse Recovery: Sexual; Anxiety Level; Coping; Fear Self-Control; Self-Mutilation Restraint

Interventions and Rationales

- Inform members of the treatment team and appropriate community agencies that the child may be victim of incest. *You have a responsibility to ensure the child's safety after discharge.*
- S Observe the child for changes in mood or behavior and for statements of intention to harm self. *Children who have recently disclosed sexual abuse have a high rate of suicide.*
- S Ask the child to agree to verbal and written safety contracts stating the child won't harm self *to provide the child with a tangible reminder of how to cope with crises.*

- If the child wants to talk about the traumatic event, actively listen *to reassure that what the child tells you is important.*
- Praise the child for participating in one-on-one therapy sessions *to enhance participation and sense of self-worth.*
- Help the child identify adults who can be trusted, such as a school counselor, clergy person, or school nurse, *to help prevent further episodes of incest.*
- PCC Make appropriate referrals to mental health professionals and social service agencies *to ensure the child's safety in the community.*

Suggested NIC Interventions

Behavior Management: Self-Harm; Coping Enhancement; Counseling; Mutual Goal Setting; Patient Contracting; Security Enhancement

Evaluations for Expected Outcomes

- Child doesn't harm self or others.
- Child enters into a contract to refrain from injuring self or others.
- Child finds positive ways of expressing feelings.
- Child follows steps defined in the plan to maintain safety.
- Child cooperates in looking at a positive living environment after discharge.

Documentation

- Written or verbal safety contract
- Exact quotes of child if any disclosures are made regarding incest
- Child's behavior with peers, staff, and family during visits
- Responses to nursing interventions
- Evaluations for expected outcomes

REFERENCES

Morrill, M. (2014). Sibling sexual abuse: An exploratory study of long-term consequences for self-esteem and counseling considerations. *Journal of Family Violence*, *29*(2), 205–213. doi:10.1007/s10896-013-9571-4

Nowakowski, E., & Mattern, K. (2014). An exploratory study of the characteristics that prevent youth from completing a family violence diversion program. *Journal of Family Violence*, *29*(2), 143–149. doi:10.1007/s10896-013-9572-3

Symes, L., Maddoux, J., McFarlane, J., Nava, A., & Gilroy, H. (2014). Physical and sexual intimate partner violence, women's health and children's behavioural functioning: Entry analysis of a seven-year prospective study. *Journal of Clinical Nursing*, *23*(19/20), 2909–2918. doi:10.1111/jocn.12542

POWERLESSNESS

related to insufficient interpersonal interactions

Definition

The lived experience of lack of control over a situation, including a perception that one's actions do not significantly affect an outcome

Assessment

- Age
- Gender
- Level of education
- Occupation
- Ethnic group
- Family status, including marital status; developmental stage; socioeconomic status; support systems; history of physical, sexual, or emotional support; and family health history
- Beliefs, values, and attitudes about health and illness
- History of substance abuse
- Description of physical, sexual, or emotional abuse

Defining Characteristics

- Alienation
- Dependency
- Depression
- Doubt about role performance
- Frustration about inability to perform previous activities
- Inadequate participation in care
- Insufficient sense of control
- Shame

Expected Outcomes

- Patient will identify feelings of powerlessness.
- Patient will identify risks to personal safety.
- Patient will make decisions related to care.
- Patient will identify life situations over which the patient has no control.
- Patient will develop a plan to take control of life.

Suggested NOC Outcomes

Depression Self-Control; Health Beliefs: Perceived Control; Health Beliefs: Perceived Resources

Interventions and Rationales

- S Evaluate the patient's potential for harm. *Ensuring the patient's safety is your primary responsibility.*
- Discuss the patient's abusive relationship. Help the patient identify feelings of powerlessness and the circumstances that lead to such situations *to help the patient recognize things that threaten loss of control.*
- Contact social services *to ensure the patient receives legal and financial support, as needed.*
- Assist the patient to take responsibility for making decisions about self-care by setting care goals and making an activity schedule *to increase feelings of control over life.*
- Help the patient recognize situations in which determination and control over life is exhibited *to reinforce past successes and develop a foundation for establishing future goals.*
- PCC Refer the patient to a shelter *to ensure continued safety after discharge.*

Suggested NIC Interventions

Decision-Making Support; Financial Resource Assistance; Patient Rights Protection; Referral; Self-Responsibility Facilitation

Evaluations for Expected Outcomes

- Patient discusses feelings of powerlessness.
- Patient describes circumstances in which safety is threatened.
- Patient makes decisions in relation to care.
- Patient understands situations in life over which the patient has no control.
- Patient develops plan that will help take control of own life.

Documentation

- Observations of patient's behavior
- Visits and phone calls from abusive spouse
- Patient's plan for her future
- Patient's response to nursing interventions
- Referrals to specialized professionals and support groups
- Evaluations for expected outcomes

REFERENCES

Dudgeon, A. (2014). Intimate partner violence in rural U.S. areas: What every nurse should know. *American Journal of Nursing, 114*(5), 26–35.

Jaspaert, E., & Vervaeke, G. (2014). Exploring the indirect effect of preference discrepancy on intimate partner violence. *Journal of Family Violence, 29*(8), 829–837. doi:10.1007/s10896-014-9636-z

Symes, L., Maddoux, J., McFarlane, J., Nava, A., & Gilroy, H. (2014). Physical and sexual intimate partner violence, women's health and children's behavioural functioning: Entry analysis of a seven-year prospective study. *Journal of Clinical Nursing, 23*(19/20), 2909–2918. doi:10.1111/jocn.12542

RAPE-TRAUMA SYNDROME

Definition

Sustained maladaptive response to a forced, violent, sexual penetration against the victim's will and consent

Assessment

- History and circumstances of traumatic event
- Physical injuries sustained, including genitourinary, integumentary, musculoskeletal, and neurologic
- Emotional reactions, including grief reaction, changes in self-concept, and spiritual distress
- Support systems available to patient, including clergy, family members, and friends
- Problem-solving techniques usually employed by patient

Defining Characteristics

- Aggression
- Agitation
- Alteration in sleep pattern
- Anger

- Anxiety
- Change in relationship(s)
- Confusion
- Denial
- Dependency
- Depression
- Disorganization
- Dissociative identity disorder
- Embarrassment
- Fear
- Guilt
- Helplessness
- History of suicide attempt
- Humiliation
- Hyperalertness
- Impaired decision making
- Low self-esteem
- Mood swings
- Muscle spasm
- Muscle tension
- Nightmares
- Paranoia
- Perceived vulnerability
- Phobias
- Physical trauma
- Self-blame
- Sexual dysfunction
- Shame
- Shock
- Substance abuse
- Thoughts of revenge

Expected Outcomes

- Patient will recover from physical injuries to fullest extent possible.
- Patient will express feelings and fears.
- Patient will use support systems.

Suggested NOC Outcomes

Abuse Protection; Abuse Recovery: Emotional; Coping

Interventions and Rationales

- Explain the assessment procedures to the patient *to reduce the level of fear associated with data gathering after a rape.*
- Follow the medical regimen to manage physical injuries caused by the traumatic event. *This is the first step in meeting the patient's hierarchy of needs and depends on the extent of the patient's other injuries and the intensity of the psychological response.*
- Follow the facility's protocol regarding legal responsibilities. Be aware of the potential legal issues of rape and of the role nurses may play as witnesses in legal proceedings. *These steps will help protect the patient's legal rights.*
- Provide emotional support:
  - Be available to listen. *Active listening allows an empathetic response to the patient's feelings while being aware of one's own thoughts and behaviors.*
  - Accept the patient's feelings *to let her know her feelings are valid and acceptable.*
  - Approach the patient in a warm, caring manner *to cultivate her trust and cooperation.*
  - Provide privacy during the physical examination and interviewing process. *To protect the patient's rights, no information should be released without prior consent.*
  - Assure the patient of her safety, and take all necessary measures to ensure it. *This reduces the patient's fears of repeated assault.*
- Support the patient's family members in their reactions to the traumatic event:
  - Provide time for them to express their feelings and concerns.
  - Help them understand the patient's reactions.

  Giving them time to talk and providing accurate information helps them support their loved one.

PCC • Offer referral to other support persons or groups, such as clergy, a crisis center, mental health professionals, rape counselors, and Women Organized Against Rape. *This will help the patient express her feelings and develop coping skills.*

Suggested NIC Interventions

Abuse Protection Support; Anxiety Reduction; Crisis Intervention; Rape-Trauma Treatment; Self-Esteem Enhancement

Evaluations for Expected Outcomes

- Patient recovers from physical injuries.
- Patient expresses feelings common to rape victims, such as anger, blame, humiliation, and fear of disease or pregnancy.
- Patient contacts local mental health, rape counseling, or crisis center.

Documentation

- Patient's expressions of feelings about herself and traumatic event
- Physical findings and treatment
- Observations of family's interaction with patient
- Referrals to support persons
- Patient's response to nursing interventions
- Evaluations for expected outcomes

REFERENCES

Burns, B., Grindlay, K., Holt, K., Manski, R., & Grossman, D. (2014). Military sexual trauma among U.S. servicewomen during deployment: A qualitative study. *American Journal of Public Health*, *104*(2), 345–349. doi:10.2105/AJPH.2013.301576

Coyle, C. T., Shuping, M. W., Speckhard, A., & Brightup, J. E. (2015). The relationship of abortion and violence against women: Violence prevention strategies and research needs. *Issues in Law & Medicine*, *30*(2), 111–127.

Özcan, N. K., Boyacıoğlu, N. E., Enginkaya, S., Dinç, H., & Bilgin, H. (2014). Reproductive health in women with serious mental illnesses. *Journal of Clinical Nursing*, *23*(9/10), 1283–1291. doi:10.1111/jocn.12332

INEFFECTIVE RELATIONSHIP

Definition

A pattern of mutual partnership that is insufficient to provide for each other's needs

Assessment

- Coping status, including method of dealing with general conflicts, level of patient's communication with family and others; handling of negotiations regarding restriction of freedom, degree of patient's separation from family, tolerance of patient's expressed opinions, reaction to patient's long-range goals; and age-appropriateness of dating, curfew regulation, and money responsibilities
- Family and cultural standards

- Family status, including family composition; responsibilities assumed in caring for family members (including patient); and ability of family to meet their physical, social, emotional, and economic needs
- Individual's past response to crises, including stress management and communication patterns to express anger, affection, and confrontation
- Sociological factors, including job satisfaction, presence of support systems, or hobbies

Defining Characteristics

- Delay in meeting of developmental goals appropriate for family life cycle stage
- Dissatisfaction with complementary relationship between partners
- Dissatisfaction with emotional need fulfillment between partners
- Dissatisfaction with idea sharing between partners
- Dissatisfaction with information sharing between partners
- Dissatisfaction with physical need fulfillment between partners
- Inadequate understanding of partner's compromised functioning (e.g., physical psychological, social)
- Insufficient balance in autonomy between partners
- Insufficient balance in collaboration between partners
- Insufficient mutual respect between partners
- Insufficient mutual support in daily activities between partners
- Partner not identified as support person
- Unsatisfying communication with partner

Expected Outcomes

- Patient will actively participate in activities that build cohesion with partner/family.
- Patient will express understanding of role as an individual, partner, and/ or member of the family.
- Patient will identify negative behaviors that contribute to the dysfunction of the patient's relationship(s) and a desire to change them.
- Patient will verbalize positive aspects of own relationship(s).

Suggested NOC Outcomes

Abusive Behavior Self-Control; Coping; Family Functioning; Role Performance; Psychosocial Adjustment: Social Support; Substance Addiction Consequences

Interventions and Rationales

- Assess the patient and involve family and other health care providers as appropriate, *as they can provide additional information and/or perspectives that the patient may not be aware of.*
- Assess the patient and family for signs of addiction or abuse, *as both can contribute negatively to the physiologic and psychological status of the patient and partner/family and the status of their relationship.*
- Assist the patient with cognitive therapies that develop positive coping skills to help build self-esteem, *as this fosters self-confidence and a positive attitude toward personal relationships.*
- PCC Educate the patient and partner/family regarding importance of everyone following through with the treatment plan, *as joint participation is necessary to facilitate a successful outcome.*

- Provide a safe environment and assist the patient and partner/family in communicating openly regarding positive aspects of their relationship *in order to help facilitate positive interaction.*
- PCC • Work with the patient and partner/family to set up a treatment plan. *Encouraging the patient to work with partner/family helps to create cohesiveness and mutual support in implementing the treatment plan.*
- PCC • Work with outside agencies/programs if abuse or addiction is a factor *in order to ensure patient and partner/family safety.*

Suggested NIC Interventions

Anxiety Reduction; Abuse Protection Support; Coping Enhancement; Complex Relationship Building; Family Support; Role Enhancement; Sexual Counseling; Substance Use Treatment; Support Group

Evaluations for Expected Outcomes

- Patient participates in activities.
- Patient identifies negative behaviors and states plans for their resolution.
- Patient verbalizes positive aspects of relationships.

Documentation

- Assessment of patient's relationships and evidence of addiction or drug abuse
- Patient's progress in problem solving and making choices
- Patient–family interactions and content of family meetings
- Patient's response to interventions
- Outpatient resources identified and suggested to patient and family members
- Evaluations for expected outcomes

REFERENCES

Coy, J. S., & Miller, M. M. (2014). Intimate partners who struggle with formal commitments: Attachment styles, major challenges, and clinical implications. *American Journal of Family Therapy, 42*(3), 232–242. doi:10.1080/01926187.2013.808138

Grant, M. (2014). Resolving communication challenges in the intensive care unit. *AACN Advanced Critical Care, 26*(2), 123–130. doi:10.1097/NCI.0000000000000076

Snelling, P. C. (2015). Who can blame who for what and how in responsibility for health? *Nursing Philosophy, 16*(1), 3–18. doi:10.1111/nup.12061

RISK FOR INEFFECTIVE RELATIONSHIP

Definition

Vulnerable to developing a pattern that is insufficient for providing a mutual partnership to provide for each other's needs

Assessment

- Coping status, including method of dealing with general conflicts, level of patient's communication with family and others; handling of negotiations regarding restriction of freedom, degree of patient's separation from family; tolerance of patient's expressed opinions,

reaction to patient's long-range goals; and age-appropriateness of dating, curfew regulation, and money responsibilities
- Family and cultural standards
- Family status, including family composition; responsibilities assumed in caring for family members (including patient); and ability of family to meet their physical, social, emotional, and economic needs
- Individual's past response to crises, including stress management and communication patterns to express anger, affection, and confrontation
- Sociological factors, including job satisfaction, presence of support systems, or hobbies

Risk Factors

- Alteration in cognitive functioning in one partner
- Developmental crisis
- History of domestic violence
- Incarceration of one partner
- Ineffective communication skills
- Stressor
- Substance abuse
- Unrealistic expectations

Expected Outcomes

- Patient will actively participate in activities that help build cohesion with partner/family.
- Patient will express understanding of own role as an individual, a partner, and/or member of the family.
- Patient will identify healthy coping mechanisms that will support the patient as an individual, a partner, and/or family member.
- Patient will verbalize desire to work with partner/family in developing healthy communication skills.

Suggested NOC Outcomes

Family Functioning; Family Integrity; Role Performance; Psychosocial Adjustment; Life Change; Social Interaction Skills; Social Support

Interventions and Rationales

- Assess the patient and partner/family, *since the partner/family can provide additional information/perspectives that the patient may not be aware of.*
- Assess support system and availability. *The partner may travel frequently and immediate family may not live in proximity to the patient, which can cause emotional strain.*
- Assist the patient and partner/family to identify positive activities that they can participate in together *to help build cohesion.*
- Assist the patient with cognitive therapies and stress reduction techniques. *Positive coping skills can help foster self-confidence and a positive attitude and positive behaviors toward personal relationships.*
- PCC Educate the patient and partner/family regarding the need for family treatment, *as the partner/family is also affected by the status of the relationship, and only together can they begin to repair the relationship.*

- Provide a safe environment and assist the patient and partner/family in communicating openly *in order to help facilitate a positive interaction.*
- PCC Work with the patient and partner/family to ensure that the treatment plan is sensitive to their cultural practices and developmental needs *in order to help build unity and confidence in their ability to follow-through with the treatment plan.*

Suggested NIC Interventions

Anxiety Reduction; Abuse Protection Support; Complex Relationship Building; Family Support; Role Enhancement; Sexual Counseling; Substance Use Treatment; Support Group

Evaluations for Expected Outcomes

- Patient participates in activities.
- Patient verbalizes accurate knowledge of role in family.
- Patient states effective coping strategies.
- Patient and family demonstrate improved communication.

Documentation

- Assessment of family dynamics
- Cognitive therapies and stress reduction techniques used
- Referrals to family treatment modalities
- Changes in relationship
- External agencies contacted by patient
- Evaluations for expected outcomes

REFERENCES

Harvey, P., & Ahmann, E. (2016). Validation: A family-centered communication skill. *Nephrology Nursing Journal, 43*(1), 61–66.
Laursen, J. (2015). Spouses needs for professional support: The spouses' perspective on communication. *MEDSURG Nursing, 24*(5), 325–362.
Snelling, P. C. (2015). Who can blame who for what and how in responsibility for health? *Nursing Philosophy, 16*(1), 3–18. doi:10.1111/nup.12061

IMPAIRED RESILIENCE

related to psychological disorder

Definition

Decreased ability to sustain a pattern of positive responses to an adverse situation or crisis

Assessment

- Patient's perception of problem, coping mechanisms, problem-solving ability, decision-making competencies, relationships, family system
- Health history, history of chronic illness
- Activity status, nutritional status, sleep patterns
- Cultural status, including affiliation with racial, ethnic, or religious groups

Defining Characteristics

- Decrease interest in academic activities
- Decrease interest in vocational activities
- Depression
- Guilt
- Impaired health status
- Ineffective coping strategies
- Low self-esteem
- Renewed elevation of distress
- Shame
- Social isolation

Expected Outcomes

- Patient will remain free from harming self or others.
- Patient will avoid abusing substances.
- Patient will identify personal strengths.
- Patient will engage in activities that promote health.
- Patient will identify strategies that have been successful in previous times of stress.

Suggested NOC Outcomes

Role Performance; Effective/Enhanced Resilience; Knowledge: Health Behavior

Interventions and Rationales

- Explore with the patient what maladaptive behaviors the patient is exhibiting due to impaired individual resilience. *The patient must take ownership of behaviors before change can take place.*
- PCC Assist the patient in making a list of strengths and resources with contact information and the parameters for contacting those resources. *Planning for needs decreases anxiety and increases self-care.*
- Instruct the patient to engage in positive health behaviors. *Adequate sleep, nutritional intake, and activity improve decision making.*
- Encourage the patient to wait to make life-changing decisions until the current crisis is over. *Decision making is impaired during times of crisis.*
- PCC Refer patients to mental health resources in the event of maladaptive coping or safety risk. *Individuals with impaired individual resilience face an increased risk of physical and mental illness.*

Suggested NIC Interventions

Anxiety Reduction; Coping Enhancement; Decision-Making Support; Spiritual Support

Evaluations for Expected Outcomes

- Patient expresses freedom from harming self or others.
- Patient does not engage in substance abuse.
- Patient identifies at least three personal strengths that lead to increased resilience.
- Patient shares strategies that were successful during other stressful periods.
- Patient states activities that will promote health.

Documentation

- Patient's expressions of feelings regarding current crisis
- Patient's planned health promotion behaviors

- Patient's understanding of available resources if needed
- Evaluations for expected outcomes

REFERENCES

Baker, A. Z., & Procter, N. G. (2014). Losses related to everyday occupations for adults affected by mental illness. *Scandinavian Journal of Occupational Therapy*, *21*(4), 287–294. doi:10.3109/11038128.2014.894571

Laursen, J. (2015). Spouses needs for professional support: The spouses' perspective on communication. *MEDSURG Nursing*, *24*(5), 325–362.

Zalonis, R., & Slota, M. (2014). The use of palliative care to promote autonomy in decision making. *Clinical Journal of Oncology Nursing*, *18*(6), 707–711. doi:10.1188/14.CJON.707-711

RISK FOR IMPAIRED RESILIENCE

Definition

Vulnerable to decreased ability to sustain a pattern of positive response to an adverse situation or crisis, which may compromise health

Assessment

- Patient perception of problem, coping mechanisms, problem-solving ability, decision-making competencies, relationships, family system
- Health history, history of chronic illness
- Activity status, nutritional status, sleep patterns
- Cultural status, including affiliation with racial, ethnic, or religious groups

Risk Factors

- Chronicity of existing crisis
- Multiple coexisting adverse situations
- New crisis (e.g., unplanned pregnancy, loss of housing, death of family member)

Expected Outcomes

- Patient will identify available support systems to maintain resilience.
- Patient will identify healthy coping strategies.
- Patient will verbalize belief in self to withstand current situation.
- Patient will engage in activities that promote health.
- Patient will identify strategies that have been helpful in previous times of stress.

Suggested NOC Outcomes

Role Performance; Effective/Enhanced Resilience

Interventions and Rationales

- Evaluate previous mechanisms of effective coping in difficult situations. *Assimilating current situation to previous successes enhances resilience.*
- Assist the patient in making a list of strengths and resources. Be knowledgeable of cultural aspects of resilience. *Cultural relevance is critical to all aspects of patient care.*

- Instruct the patient to engage in positive self-talk: "I can handle this"; "I will accomplish one thing today and celebrate it." *A positive outlook increases endorphins and enhances self-efficacy.*
- Encourage the patient to maintain activities of health promotion, including adequate sleep, nutritious eating, and activity. *Maintaining adequate self-care enhances resilience.*
- PCC Refer patients to mental health resources in the event of maladaptive coping or safety risk. *Risk of compromised resilience may lead to actual compromised resilience.*

Suggested NIC Interventions

Anxiety Reduction; Coping Enhancement; Decision-Making Support; Spiritual Support

Evaluations for Expected Outcomes

- Patient acknowledges previous strategies of effective coping in difficult situations.
- Patient makes list of strengths and resources, including cultural considerations.
- Patient engages in positive self-talk.
- Patient engages in positive health promotion activities.

Documentation

- Patient's acknowledgment of effective strategies
- Patient's list of strengths and resources
- Patient's identified health promotion activities
- Evaluations for expected outcomes

REFERENCES

Baker, A. Z., & Procter, N. G. (2014). Losses related to everyday occupations for adults affected by mental illness. *Scandinavian Journal of Occupational Therapy*, *21*(4), 287–294. doi:10.3109/11038128.2014.894571

Laursen, J. (2015). Spouses needs for professional support: The spouses' perspective on communication. *MEDSURG Nursing*, *24*(5), 325–362.

Zalonis, R., & Slota, M. (2014). The use of palliative care to promote autonomy in decision making. *Clinical Journal of Oncology Nursing*, *18*(6), 707–711. doi:10.1188/14.CJON.707-711

CAREGIVER ROLE STRAIN

related to unpredictability of care situation

Definition

Difficulty in performing the family/significant other caregiver role

Assessment

- Caregiver's age, sex, level of education, occupation, and marital status
- Caregiver's physical and mental status, including chronic health problems, self-care abilities and limitations, and level of cognitive function
- Patient's physical and mental status, including history of psychiatric illness, self-care limitations, and level of cognitive function

- Support systems, including financial resources, family members and friends, community services, health-related services such as geriatric or psychiatric day care, and religious affiliation
- Cultural, ethnic, and religious background of family
- Family roles, coping patterns, family alliances, goals, and values

Defining Characteristics

Caregiving Activities

- Apprehensiveness about future ability to provide care
- Apprehensiveness about future health of care receiver
- Apprehensiveness about potential institutionalization of care receiver
- Apprehensiveness about well-being of care receiver if unable to provide care
- Difficulty completing required tasks
- Difficulty performing required tasks
- Dysfunctional change to caregiving activities
- Preoccupation with care routine

Caregiver Health Status: Physiologic

- Cardiovascular disease
- Diabetes mellitus
- Fatigue
- Gastrointestinal distress
- Headache
- Hypertension
- Rash
- Weight change

Caregiver Health Status: Emotional

- Alteration in sleep pattern
- Anger
- Depression
- Emotional vacillation
- Frustration
- Impatience
- Ineffective coping strategies
- Insufficient time to meet personal needs
- Nervousness
- Somatization
- Stressors

Caregiver Health Status: Socioeconomic

- Change in leisure activities
- Low work productivity
- Refusal of career advancement
- Social isolation

Caregiver–Care Receiver Relationship

- Difficulty watching care receiver with illness
- Grieving of changes in relationship with care receiver
- Uncertainty about changes in relationship with care receiver

Family Processes

- Concern about family member(s)
- Family conflict

Expected Outcomes

- Family members will discuss how patient's illness has altered established roles and responsibilities within family.
- Family members will assign responsibilities to prevent too much from falling on one individual's shoulders.

- Family members will establish limits on patient's behavior and will work together to uphold them.
- Family members will refrain from using destructive coping mechanisms, such as substance abuse and physical or mental abuse of care recipient.
- Family members will make use of outside support systems, such as community resources, religious organizations, and day hospitals.
- Family members will recognize need for professional assistance.

Suggested NOC Outcomes

Caregiver Emotional Health; Caregiver Lifestyle Disruption; Caregiver Well-Being; Family Coping; Family Support During Treatment; Role Performance

Interventions and Rationales

- Assist family members to clarify needs, set individual goals, and develop plans to meet them. *This will instill in each person a sense of empowerment and control over life.*
- Encourage discussion among family members about role changes and added responsibilities that have occurred as a result of the patient's health status *to establish open and honest communication among family members.*
- Encourage discussion of the family's past experience with crises, comparing them with the present situation *to help the family see they have survived difficulties together and encourage them to seek viable solutions.*
- Encourage family members to retain involvement with social and religious networks *to avoid feelings of isolation and abandonment.*
- PCC Refer the family to appropriate professional services *to ensure their needs are being met. Caregiver support groups may provide the family with helpful strategies that have worked for others facing the same problems.*

Suggested NIC Interventions

Caregiver Support; Coping Enhancement; Respite Care; Role Enhancement; Teaching: Individual

Evaluations for Expected Outcomes

- Family members adjust to changes in roles and responsibilities.
- Family members share responsibilities of caregiving equally.
- Patient behaves within limits set by caregiver.
- Family members don't exhibit signs of stress.
- Family members use community resources, as needed.
- Family members attend support groups or seek other forms of professional assistance.

Documentation

- Family members' beliefs and attitudes about patient's illness
- Role adjustment and flexibility of family members
- Coping patterns
- Patient's behavior
- Goals articulated by family members
- Use of support systems

- Referrals for professional help
- Patient's and family members' responses to nursing interventions
- Evaluations for expected outcomes

REFERENCES

del-Pino-Casado, R., Pérez-Cruz, M., & Frías-Osuna, A. (2014). Coping, subjective burden and anxiety among family caregivers of older dependents. *Journal of Clinical Nursing*, *23*(23/24), 3335–3344.

Litzelman, K., Skinner, H. G., Gangnon, R. E., Nieto, F. J., Malecki, K., & Witt, W. P. (2014). Role of global stress in the health-related quality of life of caregivers: Evidence from the survey of the health of Wisconsin. *Quality of Life Research: An International Journal of Quality of Life Aspects of Treatment, Care and Rehabilitation*, *23*(5), 1569–1578. doi:10.1007/s11136-013-0598-z

Zeleníková, R., Kozáková, R., & Jarošová, D. (2014). Clinical validation of the nursing diagnosis caregiver role strain in the Czech Republic. *International Journal of Nursing Knowledge*, *25*(2), 80–84. doi:10.1111/2047-3095.12020

RISK FOR CHRONIC LOW SELF-ESTEEM

Definition

Vulnerable to longstanding negative self-evaluating/feelings about self or self-capabilities, which may compromise health

Assessment

- Reason for hospitalization or outpatient treatment
- Age
- Gender
- Developmental stage
- Family system, including marital status, role in family, and sibling position
- Perception of health problem
- Past experience with health care system
- Mental status, including abstract thinking, affect, communication, general appearance, judgment or insight, memory, mood, orientation, perception, and thinking process
- Belief system, including norms, religion, and values
- Social interaction pattern
- Social and occupational history
- Perception of self (past and present), including body image, coping mechanisms, problem-solving ability, and self-worth
- Past experience with crisis
- Past history of treatment for psychosocial disturbance, including hospitalization, medication, psychotherapy, and suicidal ideation, plans, and attempts
- Neurovegetative signs, including ability to experience pleasure, appetite, energy level, and sleep

Risk Factors

- Cultural incongruence
- Exposure to traumatic situation
- Inadequate affection received
- Inadequate group membership
- Inadequate respect from others
- Ineffective coping with loss
- Insufficient feeling of belonging
- Psychiatric disorder

- Repeated failures
- Repeated negative reinforcement
- Spiritual incongruence

Expected Outcomes

- Patient will attend milieu therapies and interact with peers.
- Patient will use cognitive therapies to modify negative thoughts about self.
- Patient will maintain safety and report any thoughts of self-harm to staff.
- Patient will report decrease in feelings of anger, fear, guilt, and self-doubt.
- Patient will verbalize positive self-characteristics and accomplishments.

Suggested NOC Outcomes

Anxiety Control; Body Image; Coping; Depression Level; Mood Equilibrium; Risk Control; Self-Esteem; Social Interaction Skills

Interventions and Rationales

- Assess the patient's mental status per unit protocols. *Recurring assessments will aid in identifying interventions, expected outcomes, and allow for modifications based on the patient's progress.*
- Obtain thorough history upon admission *in order to determine if patient past history has additional risk factors for low self-esteem.*
- Assist the patient in applying cognitive therapies and positive self-talk *in order to identify and modify negative actions and thoughts that lead to feelings of anger, fear, guilt, and self-doubt.*
- PCC Work with the patient to set a daily schedule that promotes self-care and attendance at milieu therapies, and give sincere praise when the patient follows through. *Independence and positive feedback from peers and staff will aid in developing self-confidence and increasing self-esteem.*
- PCC Educate the patient on the importance of being assertive and reinforce by having the patient state particular needs or preferences for the day, *as this will help build independence, self-confidence, and decrease fear of rejection.*
- PCC Educate the patient regarding the importance of setting realistic treatment goals *in order to continue to build self-confidence and self-esteem.*
- PCC Educate the patient regarding resources available in the community, such as support groups, and *their positive impact on building self-esteem.*
- Dedicate quality time to the patient in a therapeutic and consistent manner *in order to help the patient feel safe, allow time for open expression of feelings, and allow for the development of a trusting relationship.*
- PCC Work together with the patient to develop a treatment plan and schedule appointments. *This will help to build the patient's independence, confidence, social skills, and self-esteem.*

Suggested NIC Interventions

Anxiety Reduction; Body Image Enhancement; Cognitive Restructuring; Coping Enhancement; Self-Esteem Enhancement; Support Group

Evaluations for Expected Outcomes

- Patient attends milieu therapy.
- Patient interacts with peers.

- Patient uses cognitive therapies.
- Patient expresses reduction in anger, fear, self-doubt, and guilt.
- Patient expresses positive thoughts about self.

Documentation

- Mental status assessment
- Cognitive therapies used
- Treatment goals set and results achieved
- Responses to interventions
- External agencies suggested
- Changes occurring as a result of using outside resources
- Evaluations for expected outcomes

REFERENCES

Baker, A. Z., & Procter, N. G. (2014). Losses related to everyday occupations for adults affected by mental illness. *Scandinavian Journal of Occupational Therapy*, *21*(4), 287–294. doi:10.3109/11038128.2014.894571

Kitzinger, C., & Kitzinger, J. (2014). Grief, anger and despair in relatives of severely brain injured patients: Responding without pathologising. *Clinical Rehabilitation*, *28*(7), 627–631. doi:10.1177/0269215514527844

Zalonis, R., & Slota, M. (2014). The use of palliative care to promote autonomy in decision making. *Clinical Journal of Oncology Nursing*, *18*(6), 707–711. doi:10.1188/14.CJON.707-711

SELF-MUTILATION

Definition

Deliberate self-injurious behavior causing tissue damage with the intent of causing nonfatal injury to attain relief of tension

Assessment

- Age
- Gender
- Developmental history
- Current stress level and coping behaviors
- Mental status, including judgment, thought content, and mood
- Family history, including abusive behavior
- Previous episodes of self-mutilation or suicide attempts
- Substance abuse history
- Social history, including sexual activity and aggression within peer group

Defining Characteristics

- Abrading
- Biting
- Constricting a body part
- Cuts on body
- Hitting
- Ingestion of harmful substances
- Inhalation of harmful substance
- Insertion of object into body orifice
- Picking at wound
- Scratches on body
- Self-inflicted burn
- Severing of a body part

Expected Outcomes

- Patient will refrain from harming self while in the hospital.
- Patient will express an increased sense of security.
- Patient will report being able to cope better with disorganization, aggressive impulses, anxiety, and hallucinations.
- Patient will verbalize absence of or fewer dissociative states.
- Patient will participate in therapeutic milieu.
- Patient will describe community resources that can provide assistance when the patient feels out of control.

Suggested NOC Outcomes

Impulse Self-Control; Risk Control; Self-Mutilation Restraint

Interventions and Rationales

- Assess behavioral responses; coping strategies; number and types of stressors; social factors; and spiritual beliefs. *Assessment information will assist in identifying appropriate goal and interventions.*
- Move patient to a quiet room *to reduce stimuli if the patient is in a dissociative state.*
- S Remove all dangerous objects from patient's room *to prevent injury.* Place patient under observation *to provide protection and increase the patient's sense of security.*
- Administer psychotropic medications, as prescribed, *to reduce tension, impulse behavior, hallucinations, and panic.*
- PCC Teach patient's coping strategies to family members. *Family members and friends can help patient practice adaptive methods of coping with self-destructive feelings.*
- Have patient and family members practice role playing *to increase the confidence in the patient's ability to handle difficult situations.*
- PCC Teach self-healing techniques to both patient and family such as meditation, guided imagery, yoga, and prayer. Teach patient how to incorporate the use of self-healing techniques in carrying out usual daily activities. *These techniques can reduce the anxiety that comes from attempting to cope with disease.*
- PCC Teach additional skills that enhance coping and relaxation strategies for the patient and family (i.e., meditation, guided imagery, yoga, exercise). *Self-healing gives the patient a better sense of control over regaining independence.*
- Limit the number of staff who interact with patient *to provide continuity of care and enhance a sense of security.*
- If patient is participating in a therapeutic milieu, discuss the patient's risk of self-harm with community members *to provide patient with enhanced protection and psychological support.*
- S If patient causes harm to self, provide care in a calm, nonjudgmental manner. Encourage discussion of feelings that caused self-mutilation *to help patient connect self-destructive behavior to feelings that preceded it, and provide an opportunity to explore alternative ways of dealing with negative feelings.*
- Accept patient's feelings of powerlessness as normal. *This indicates respect for the patient and enhances feelings of self-respect.*
- Encourage patient to take an active role in self-care *to promote a sense of control.*
- Organize frequent staff meetings *to ensure patient care is consistent with current behavior.*
- PCC Organize family conferences to allow opportunities for the family to discuss their particular frustrations and hopes in relation to the patient's current situation. *Family*

conferences can help the patient and family members ventilate true feelings in a safe environment.

Suggested NIC Interventions

Area Restriction; Behavior Management; Self-Harm; Environmental Management; Impulse Control; Coping Behaviors; Guided Imagery; Meditation Facilitation

Evaluations for Expected Outcomes

- Patient keeps terms of verbal contract that the patient won't harm self.
- Patient expresses increased sense of security.
- Patient describes coping skills that help in dealing better with disorganization, aggressive impulses, anxiety, and hallucinations.
- Patient experiences fewer or no dissociative states.
- Patient participates in therapeutic milieu.
- Patient tells staff member about suicidal thoughts.

Documentation

- Nursing interventions performed and patient's response to them
- Verbal contracts between patient and nurse
- Patient's responses to medication and behavior modification program
- Revisions to treatment plan
- Drawing of self-inflicted injuries
- Evidence of suicidal ideation
- Evaluations for expected outcomes

REFERENCES

Klonsky, E. D., Victor, S. E., & Saffer, B. Y. (2014). Nonsuicidal self-injury: What we know, and what we need to know. *Canadian Journal of Psychiatry*, *59*(11), 565–568.

Larkin, C., Corcoran, P., Perry, I., & Arensman, E. (2014). Severity of hospital-treated self-cutting and risk of future self-harm: A national registry study. *Journal of Mental Health*, *23*(3), 115–119. doi:10.3109/09638237.2013.841867

Morales, Y. M., & Guarnero, P. A. (2014). Non-suicidal self-injury among adult males in a correctional setting. *Issues in Mental Health Nursing*, *35*(8), 628–634. doi:10.3109/01612840.2014.927943

RISK FOR SELF-MUTILATION

Definition

Vulnerable to deliberate self-injurious behavior causing tissue damage with the intent of causing nonfatal injury to attain relief of tension

Assessment

- Age
- Gender
- Developmental history
- Current stress level and coping behaviors
- Mental status, including judgment, thought content, and mood

- Family history, including abusive behavior
- Previous episodes of self-mutilation or suicide attempts
- Substance abuse history
- Social history, including sexual activity and aggression within peer group

Risk Factors

- Adolescence
- Alteration in body image
- Autism
- Battered child
- Borderline personality disorder
- Character disorder
- Childhood illness
- Childhood surgery
- Depersonalization
- Developmental delay
- Dissociation
- Disturbance in interpersonal relationships
- Eating disorder
- Emotional disorder
- Family divorce
- Family history of self-destructive behavior
- Family substance abuse
- Feeling threatened with loss of significant relationship
- History of childhood abuse (e.g., physical, psychological, sexual)
- History of self-directed violence
- Impaired self-esteem
- Impulsiveness
- Inability to express tension verbally
- Incarceration
- Ineffective coping strategies
- Irresistible urge for self-directed violence
- Isolation from peers
- Living in nontraditional setting (e.g., foster group, or institutional care)
- Loss of control over problem-solving situation
- Loss of significant relationship(s)
- Low self-esteem
- Mounting tension that is intolerable
- Negative feelings (e.g., depression, rejection, self-hatred, separation anxiety, guilt, depersonalization)
- Pattern of inability to plan solutions
- Pattern of inability to see long-term consequences
- Peers who self-mutilate
- Perfectionism
- Psychotic disorder
- Requires rapid stress reduction
- Sexual identity crisis
- Substance abuse
- Use of manipulation to obtain nurturing relationship with others
- Violence between parental figures

Expected Outcomes

- Patient won't harm self while in facility.
- Patient will express increased sense of security.
- Patient will report being able to cope better with disorganization, aggressive impulses, anxiety, and hallucinations.
- Patient will experience fewer or no dissociative states.
- Patient will participate in therapeutic milieu.
- Patient will report suicidal thoughts to staff members.

Suggested NOC Outcomes

Abuse Recovery Status; Anxiety Level; Impulse Self-Control; Risk Control; Self-Mutilation Restraint

Interventions and Rationales

- Limit the number of staff members interacting with the patient *to provide continuity of care and increase the patient's sense of security.*
- Have staff members make frequent, short contacts with the patient *to reassure the patient without stifling independence.*
- **S** Remove all dangerous objects from the patient's environment *to promote safety.*
- **S** Make short-term verbal contracts with the patient on not harming self *to make the patient aware about being ultimately responsible for own safety and that the patient can guarantee it.*
- Administer psychotropic medications, as ordered, *to reduce tension, impulsive behavior, hallucinations, and panic.*
- If the patient enters a dissociative state or hallucinates, move the patient to a quiet room with reduced stimuli. If restraint is needed, remain with the patient and provide reassurance *to calm and orient the patient to reality.*
- As ordered, place the patient under observation *to provide protection and increase the patient's sense of security*. If hospitalized, the patient can be "zoned" or asked to remain in areas within sight of staff members.
- If the patient is participating in a therapeutic milieu, discuss the patient's risk of self-harm with community members *to provide enhanced protection and psychological support.*
- **S** If the patient harms self, care for injuries in a calm, nonjudgmental manner. Encourage the patient to talk about the feelings that prompted self-mutilation. *Discussion may help the patient connect self-destructive behavior to the feelings that preceded it and allow exploration of alternative ways of dealing with negative thoughts and feelings.*
- If self-destructive acts persist, consider developing a behavior modification program, in which the patient is rewarded with benefits (personal attention, material items) for demonstrating self-control *to reinforce self-control.*
- **S** Ask the patient directly whether the patient is thinking of suicide and, if so, what is the plan. *A self-destructive patient may become suicidal and may require additional precautions.*
- **PCC** Hold frequent treatment team meetings *to ensure consistent care that's appropriate to the patient's current behavior.*

Suggested NIC Interventions

Area Restriction; Behavior Management: Self-Harm; Environmental Management: Violence Prevention; Impulse Control Training; Limit Setting

Evaluations for Expected Outcomes

- Patient keeps terms of verbal contract on not harming self.
- Patient expresses increased sense of security.
- Patient describes coping skills that help in dealing better with disorganization, aggressive impulses, anxiety, and hallucinations.
- Patient experiences fewer or no dissociative states.
- Patient participates in therapeutic milieu.
- Patient tells staff member about suicidal thoughts.

Documentation

- Nursing interventions performed and patient's response to them
- Verbal contracts between patient and nurse
- Patient's responses to medication and behavior modification program
- Revisions to treatment plan
- Drawing of self-inflicted injuries
- Evidence of suicidal ideation
- Evaluations for expected outcomes

REFERENCES

Klonsky, E. D., Victor, S. E., & Saffer, B. Y. (2014). Nonsuicidal self-injury: What we know, and what we need to know. *Canadian Journal of Psychiatry*, *59*(11), 565–568.

Larkin, C., Corcoran, P., Perry, I., & Arensman, E. (2014). Severity of hospital-treated self-cutting and risk of future self-harm: A national registry study. *Journal of Mental Health*, *23*(3), 115–119. doi:10.3109/09638237.2013.841867

Morales, Y. M., & Guarnero, P. A. (2014). Non-suicidal self-injury among adult males in a correctional setting. *Issues in Mental Health Nursing*, *35*(8), 628–634. doi:10.3109/01612840.2014.927943

SEXUAL DYSFUNCTION

related to alteration in body function (due to anomaly, disease, medication, pregnancy, radiation, surgery, trauma, etc.)

Definition

A state in which an individual experiences a change in sexual function during the sexual response phases of desire, excitation, and/or orgasm, which is viewed as unsatisfying, unrewarding, or inadequate

Assessment

- Comprehensive sexual history, including attitude toward sex, sexual preference, sexual responsiveness of partner, previous sexual response patterns, and sexual desire, enjoyment, and performance
- Psychological factors, including self-esteem, body image, guilt, symptoms of depression, and suicidal ideation
- Support systems, including family, friends, and clergy
- Attitude of spouse or significant other
- Sociocultural factors, including educational level, socioeconomic status, ethnic group, and religious beliefs and practices

- Physiologic factors, including medication history (response, effectiveness, and adverse reactions), current medication regimen (including tricyclic antidepressants or monoamine oxidase [MAO] inhibitors), and substance abuse history (type and effect on mental status)
- Coping and problem-solving ability and ability to concentrate

Defining Characteristics

- Alteration in sexual activity
- Alteration in sexual excitation
- Alteration in sexual satisfaction
- Change in interest toward others
- Change in self-interest
- Change in sexual role
- Decrease in sexual desire
- Perceived sexual limitation
- Seeks confirmation of desirability
- Undesired change in sexual function

Expected Outcomes

- Patient will acknowledge depressive episode and problem in sexual function.
- Patient will voice feelings about decreases in sexual desire.
- Patient will identify ways to enhance pleasure and improve interpersonal communication with partner.
- Patient will regain sexual desire with recovery from depression.
- Patient will accept referral for sex therapy, if necessary.

Suggested NOC Outcomes

Body Image; Fear Level; Self-Esteem; Sexual Functioning

Interventions and Rationales

- Initiate a trusting therapeutic relationship with the patient. Make the purpose, nature, and parameters of this relationship clear *to help the patient feel secure and develop trust.*
- PCC Educate the patient and family members about the nature of depression, its treatment, and its effect on sexual desire. *Understanding the link between depression and sexual desire may diminish feelings of guilt and worthlessness and help raise self-esteem.*
- Allow the patient to express feelings openly in a nonthreatening, nonjudgmental atmosphere *to foster communication and help the patient cope with unresolved issues.* Offer feedback *to validate the patient's feelings and promote self-esteem.*
- PCC Include the patient and partner in planning care and interventions *to enhance a feeling of control for both partners.*
- Reinforce compliance with the treatment plan for depression. *Even though tricyclic antidepressants and MAO inhibitors may diminish sexual desire, the patient needs to comply to resolve depression.*
- Discuss with the patient and partner alternative expressions of affection to enhance their relationship during treatment *to help the couple preserve intimacy during a temporary loss of libido.*
- PCC Refer the patient for sex counseling or therapy if low sexual desire persists after the resolution of depression. *Sexual desire should return to its usual level after successful treatment for depression. If it doesn't, the patient should receive professional therapy.*

Suggested NIC Interventions

Self-Awareness Enhancement; Self-Responsibility Facilitation; Sexual Counseling; Teaching: Sexuality

Evaluations for Expected Outcomes

- Patient describes depressive episode, treatment plan, and effects on sexual desire.
- Patient expresses concerns to staff and family members.
- Patient identifies at least three activities to enhance pleasure and communication with partner.
- Patient reports return of sexual fantasies and desire for sexual activity.
- Patient communicates willingness to follow through with referral for sex therapy.

Documentation

- Patient's perceptions and concerns
- Observation of patient's behavior, depressive symptoms, and suicidal risk
- Interventions to assist patient and family members
- Patient's and partner's responses to nursing interventions
- Evaluations for expected outcomes

REFERENCES

Bostock-Cox, B. (2015). Long term conditions, medication and sexual health. *Practice Nurse*, *45*(11), 22–25.
Kaya Erten, Z., Zincir, H., Özkan, F., Selçuk, A., & Elmali, F. (2014). Sexual lives of women with diabetes mellitus (type 2) and impact of culture on solution for problems related to sexual life. *Journal of Clinical Nursing*, *23*(7/8), 995–1004. doi:10.1111/jocn.12273
Mola, J. R. (2015). Erectile dysfunction in the older adult male. *Urologic Nursing*, *35*(2), 87–93. doi:10.7257/1053-816X.2015.35.2.87

SEXUAL DYSFUNCTION

related to misinformation about sexual function

Definition

A state in which an individual experiences a change in sexual function during the sexual response phase of desire, excitation, and/or orgasm, which is viewed as unsatisfying, unrewarding, or inadequate

Assessment

- History of behaviors indicating excessive elation, such as hypersexuality, intrusiveness, grandiose thoughts, looseness of association, flight of ideas, extreme levels of energy, lack of sleep, lack of proper nutrition, poor judgment, elevated mood, expansiveness, pressured and rapid speech, and strained interpersonal relationships
- History of psychiatric illness, including personality disorders exemplified by lack of impulse control
- Sexual history, including attitude toward sex, previous sexual patterns, sexual preference, sexual response of partners, and appropriateness of sexual behavior
- Sociocultural factors, including educational level, socioeconomic status, and ethnic group
- Patient's perception of sexual behaviors and practices
- Partner's perception of patient's sexual behaviors
- Coping and problem-solving abilities

- Health history, including medication history (response, effectiveness, and adverse reactions), use of psychosis-inducing drugs (such as phencyclidine and amphetamines), use of disinhibiting drugs (such as alcohol, amphetamines, and cocaine), and other substance abuse (type and effect on mental status)

Defining Characteristics

- Alteration in sexual activity
- Alteration in sexual excitation
- Alteration in sexual satisfaction
- Change in interest toward others
- Change in self-interest
- Change in sexual role
- Decrease in sexual desire
- Perceived sexual limitation
- Seeks confirmation of desirability
- Undesired change in sexual function

Expected Outcomes

- Patient will meet sexual needs in socially appropriate manner.
- Patient will reduce or eliminate sexual behaviors that may harm self or others.
- Patient will learn how to recognize indicators of impending episodes of hypersexuality and how to prevent such episodes from occurring.
- Patient will state plan to participate in recommended therapy.

Suggested NOC Outcomes

Anxiety Level; Self-Esteem; Sexual Functioning; Sexual Identity

Interventions and Rationales

- Help the patient recognize potentially harmful sexual behavior. Set limits on high-risk sexual behavior. *Indiscriminate, impulsive sexual behavior can lead to unwanted pregnancy, sexually transmitted diseases, and physical and emotional trauma.*
- Encourage the patient to express sexual urges in socially acceptable ways (including masturbation in a private setting) *to help the patient discover positive methods of relieving sexual tension.*
- Discuss with the patient hypersexual behaviors and feelings associated with hypersexuality *to promote insight into behavior.*
- PCC Refer the patient to a medical and psychiatric specialist or sex therapist, if needed. *Indiscriminate and impulsive hypersexuality usually indicates a physical or psychiatric illness that requires further evaluation and treatment by an appropriate professional.*

Suggested NIC Interventions

Behavior Management: Sexual; Energy Management; Sexual Counseling

Evaluations for Expected Outcomes

- Patient states desire to express sexual drive in socially acceptable manner.
- Patient reports sexual relationships that aren't harmful to self or others.
- Patient develops increased understanding of hypersexual urges and the ability to cope with intense sexual desire.
- Patient expresses willingness to participate in psychiatric care or sex therapy, if needed.

Documentation

- Patient's perception of sexual behaviors and level of sexual activities
- Patient's statements about sexual behaviors
- Observations of patient's behavior, including inappropriate sexual expression
- Interventions to help patient set limits on hypersexuality
- Patient's response to nursing interventions
- Evaluations for expected outcomes

REFERENCES

Bostock-Cox, B. (2015). Long term conditions, medication and sexual health. *Practice Nurse, 45*(11), 22–25.

Kolbe, N., Kugler, C., Schnepp, W., & Jaarsma, T. (2016). A silent phenomenon: Results from a convergent parallel mixed method study. Sexual counseling in patients with heart failure. *Journal of Cardiovascular Nursing, 31*(1), 53–61.

Saunamäki, N., & Engström, M. (2014). Registered nurses' reflections on discussing sexuality with patients: Responsibilities, doubts and fears. *Journal of Clinical Nursing, 23*(3/4), 531–540. doi:10.1111/jocn.12155

SOCIAL ISOLATION

related to inability to engage in satisfying personal relationships

Definition

Aloneness experienced by the individual and perceived as imposed by others and as a negative or threatening state

Assessment

- Age
- Gender
- Level of education
- Ethnic group
- Family status, including marital status, family roles, ability of family to meet patient's physical and emotional needs, and communication style
- Coping patterns
- Evidence of physical, sexual, or emotional abuse
- Mental status, including motor activity, thought and speech, mood and affect, perceptions, orientation, memory, general information, attention span, abstraction, and judgment

Defining Characteristics

- Absence of support system
- Aloneness imposed by others
- Cultural incongruence
- Desire to be alone
- Developmental delay
- Developmentally inappropriate interest
- Disabling condition
- Feeling different from others
- Flat affect
- History of rejection
- Hostility
- Illness
- Inability to meet expectations of others
- Insecurity in public
- Meaningless actions
- Member of a subculture

- Poor eye contact
- Preoccupation with own thoughts
- Purposelessness
- Repetitive actions
- Sad affect
- Values incongruent with cultural norms
- Withdrawn

Expected Outcomes

- Patient will articulate feelings of isolation.
- Patient will agree to spend time daily talking to others.
- Patient will express comfort in talking to others.
- Patient will plan to continue social interactions with family and friends after discharge.

Suggested NOC Outcomes

Family Social Climate; Loneliness Severity; Personal Well-Being; Social Interaction Skills; Social Involvement; Social Support

Interventions and Rationales

- Spend time with the patient each shift *to establish a trusting relationship.*
- Encourage the patient to articulate feelings. Listen nonjudgmentally *to let the patient know that the patient's ideas are valued.*
- Demonstrate eye contact, appropriate physical boundaries, and other socially appropriate behavior *to provide a model for the patient.*
- Encourage the patient to begin relating to others through participation in unit activities *to help the patient practice newly acquired social skills.*
- Encourage the patient to increase level of social contact gradually *to avoid becoming overwhelmed.*
- PCC Help the patient locate community resources and support groups *to decrease isolation and provide support.*

Suggested NIC Interventions

Caregiver Support; Family Integrity Promotion; Mood Management; Socialization Enhancement

Evaluations for Expected Outcomes

- Patient discusses difficulty interacting with others.
- Patient is observed communicating with others.
- Patient appears to communicate with increasing ease.
- Patient has developed a personal plan for continued ease in communicating with others.

Documentation

- Patient's comments about own interpersonal problems
- Patient's expression of feeling alone
- Patient's participation in group activities
- Resources provided to patient for ongoing care
- Evaluations for expected outcomes

REFERENCES

Cantrell, K. A., & Boles, J. (2015). The children's corner: Perspectives on supportive care. Bridging isolation for youth with chronic conditions: Are we thinking virtually? *Pediatric Nursing*, *41*(5), 254–256.

Hagan, R., Manktelow, R., Taylor, B. J., & Mallett, J. (2014). Reducing loneliness amongst older people: A systematic search and narrative review. *Aging & Mental Health*, *18*(6), 683–693. doi:10.1080/13607863.2013.875122

McCarthy, A. (2015). Summer camp for children and adolescents with chronic conditions. *Pediatric Nursing*, *41*(5), 245–250.

SOCIAL ISOLATION

related to insufficient personal resources (e.g., poor achievement, poor insight, affect unavailable and poorly controlled)

Definition

Aloneness experienced by the individual and perceived as imposed by others as a negative or threatening state

Assessment

- Reason for hospitalization (physiologic or psychiatric)
- Support systems, including clergy, family members, and friends
- Diversional interests
- Attitudes of family members toward patient in this situation
- Financial resources
- Occupation
- Level of education and intelligence
- Coping and problem-solving ability
- Self-esteem

Defining Characteristics

- Absence of support system
- Aloneness imposed by others
- Cultural incongruence
- Desire to be alone
- Developmental delay
- Developmentally inappropriate interest
- Disabling condition
- Feeling different from others
- Flat affect
- History of rejection
- Hostility
- Illness
- Inability to meet expectations of others
- Insecurity in public
- Meaningless actions
- Member of a subculture
- Poor eye contact
- Preoccupation with own thoughts
- Purposelessness
- Repetitive actions
- Sad affect
- Values incongruent with cultural norms
- Withdrawn

Expected Outcomes

- Patient will interact positively with caregivers.
- Patient will express feelings about lack of supportive relationships.
- Patient will express desire to be involved with others.

- Patient will express desire to improve self and current condition; for example, by obtaining further education or learning how to better manage finances.
- Patient will use available resources (social services, home health care, psychology services, self-improvement classes) to establish realistic plan for future.
- Patient will state plan to participate in social activity.

Suggested NOC Outcomes

Client Satisfaction: Communication; Mood Equilibrium; Personal Well-Being; Social Involvement; Social Support

Interventions and Rationales

- Assign the same caregivers to the patient *to promote a trusting relationship with staff members. Consistent care promotes the patient's ability to communicate openly.*
- Assign a primary nurse to coordinate the patient's care. *This reduces the potential for fragmented nursing interventions.*
- Plan a 15-minute period each shift to sit with the patient. If the patient doesn't wish to talk, remain silent. *Active listening communicates concern, allows time to collect thoughts, and encourages the patient to initiate interaction.*
- PCC Involve the patient in planning care and have the patient participate in self-care continuously *to provide structure, reduce feelings of helplessness, and foster independent action.*
- Discuss the patient's living accommodations and lifestyle outside the facility to *help you understand the patient and facilitate discharge planning.*
- PCC Refer the patient to social services for follow-up, if necessary, *to ensure a comprehensive approach to care.*
- PCC Help the patient identify social outlets (peer group, associations, group activity) *to draw the patient's attention to specific data and promote goal-directed interaction.*

Suggested NIC Interventions

Coping Enhancement; Family Support; Referral; Socialization Enhancement; Support System Enhancement

Evaluations for Expected Outcomes

- Patient seeks information from and expresses feelings to caregivers.
- Patient acknowledges concern about absence of supportive relationships.
- Patient expresses desire to develop meaningful relationships.
- Patient states at least two methods of achieving personal growth and improving current situation.
- Patient identifies and contacts social service agencies.
- Patient states plan to participate in social activities.

Documentation

- Patient's perceptions of current situation
- Patient's expressions of plans for future
- Observations of patient's behavior
- Planning done by patient with nurse, physician, social worker, and others

- Patient's response to nursing interventions
- Evaluations for expected outcomes

REFERENCES

Cantrell, K. A., & Boles, J. (2015). The children's corner: Perspectives on supportive care. Bridging isolation for youth with chronic conditions: Are we thinking virtually? *Pediatric Nursing*, *41*(5), 254–256.

Hagan, R., Manktelow, R., Taylor, B. J., & Mallett, J. (2014). Reducing loneliness amongst older people: A systematic search and narrative review. *Aging & Mental Health*, *18*(6), 683–693. doi:10.1080/13607863.2013.875122

McCarthy, A. (2015). Summer camp for children and adolescents with chronic conditions. *Pediatric Nursing*, *41*(5), 245–250.

CHRONIC SORROW

related to chronic disability (e.g., physical, mental); chronic illness

Definition

Cyclical, recurring, and potentially progressive pattern of pervasive sadness experienced (by a parent, caregiver individual with chronic illness or disability) in response to continual loss, throughout the trajectory of an illness or disability

Assessment

- Age and sex
- History of recent loss
- Patient's usual pattern of coping with loss, including cultural, intellectual, and emotional responses
- Expressed feelings of loss of control over current situation
- Behavioral manifestations of grieving, including their intensity
- Somatic problems associated with grieving, including changes in appetite, sleep patterns, activity level, and libido
- Lifestyle changes related to illness (mobility restrictions, risk of complications, and medication regimen)
- Psychosocial status, including religious beliefs and practices, personal philosophy, educational background, and effect of altered health status on social life
- Physical and social environment
- Sources of support, including family members, friends, and clergy

Defining Characteristics

- Feelings that interfere with well-being (e.g., personal, social)
- Overwhelming negative feelings
- Sadness (e.g., periodic, recurrent)

Expected Outcomes

- Patient will identify losses associated with changes in health status.
- Patient will express feelings about changes in health status.
- Patient will seek assistance in dealing with emotions related to loss.

- Patient will begin to develop healthy coping mechanisms such as open expression of grief.
- Patient will seek out support from family, friends, clergy, or others when necessary.
- Patient will begin to plan for discharge and for future.
- Patient will express realistic expectations with regard to health status.

Suggested NOC Outcomes

Acceptance: Health Status; Depression Self-Control; Hope; Mood Equilibrium

Interventions and Rationales

- Spend at least 15 minutes each shift with the patient to focus on expression of feelings. Encourage the patient to express thoughts and feelings openly. *Dysfunctional grieving may result from the inability to freely express feelings.*
- Communicate to the patient that feelings of anger are acceptable, but place limits on destructive behavior. *Inability to identify anger as normal response to loss may cause the patient to express aggression inappropriately.*
- Help the patient focus realistically on changes in health status because of loss *to help the patient plan for the future.*
- PCC Encourage the patient to reach out to people who can offer support, such as family, friends, and clergy, *to increase emotional strength.*
- Encourage the patient and family members to reminisce. *Engaging in life review promotes a peaceful atmosphere and helps in understanding the meaning of loss in relation to health and life.*
- Inform the patient and family members about additional sources of support within the facility or community *to facilitate adaptive responses to loss and encourage community integration.*
- PCC Encourage the patient to take an active part in setting goals for health care *to facilitate independence and enhance self-esteem.*
- Help the patient and family set realistic goals for discharge and the future *to help the patient place the loss in perspective and move on to new opportunities and relationships.*
- Encourage the patient to be as independent as possible in self-care activities *to enhance self-esteem and promote optimal functioning.*
- PCC Refer the patient to a psychologist, psychiatrist, or social worker as appropriate. *Restoring emotional health may require assistance from a mental health professional.*

Suggested NIC Interventions

Coping Enhancement; Decision-Making Support; Emotional Support; Hope Instillation; Mood Management; Spiritual Support; Support Group

Evaluations for Expected Outcomes

- Patient identifies losses associated with changes in health status.
- Patient expresses feelings about changes in health status.
- Patient seeks assistance in dealing with emotions related to loss.
- Patient begins to develop healthy coping mechanisms such as open expression of grief.
- Patient seeks out support from family, friends, clergy, or others when necessary.
- Patient begins to plan for discharge and for future.
- Patient expresses realistic expectations with regard to health status.

Documentation

- Patient's statements regarding loss
- Patient's behavioral response to loss, including interactions with family members and staff
- Nursing interventions to help patient overcome chronic sorrow
- Patient's response to nursing interventions
- Patient's statements indicating understanding that grief is normal
- Patient's statements regarding goals for discharge and future
- Referrals to a mental health professional
- Evaluations for expected outcomes

REFERENCES

Bjorgvinsdottir, K., & Halldorsdottir, S. (2014). Silent, invisible and unacknowledged: Experiences of young caregivers of single parents diagnosed with multiple sclerosis. *Scandinavian Journal of Caring Sciences*, *28*(1), 38–48. doi:10.1111/scs.12030

Knight, C. C., Dailey, K. D., & Currie, E. R. (2015). An introduction to unexpected grief for pre-licensure nursing students: A simulation and interprofessional expert panel regarding fetal demise. *Nursing Education Perspectives*, *36*(6), 414–416.

Monaro, S., Stewart, G., & Gullick, J. (2014). A 'lost life': Coming to terms with haemodialysis. *Journal of Clinical Nursing*, *23*(21/22), 3262–3273. doi:10.1111/jocn.12577

RISK FOR SUICIDE

Definition

Vulnerable to self-inflicted, life-threatening injury

Assessment

- Age
- Gender
- Medical history
- Patient's life situation
- Recent stressors and coping behaviors
- Available support systems
- History of suicide attempts, including aggressiveness of suicide attempts, lethality of suicide attempts, and number of prior suicide attempts
- History of substance abuse (type and effects on mental status)
- Reaction of family members
- Safety hazards
- Mental status, including abstract thinking, affect, content of thought, general information, insight, judgment, mood, orientation, recent and remote memory, and thought processes

Risk Factors

Behavioral

- Changing a will
- Giving away possessions
- History of suicide attempt
- Impulsiveness

- Making a will
- Marked change in attitude
- Marked change in behavior
- Marked change in school performance
- Purchase of a gun
- Stockpiling medication
- Sudden euphoric recovery from a major depression

Demographic

- Age (e.g., elderly people, young adult males, adolescents)
- Divorced status
- Ethnicity (e.g., white, Native American)
- Male gender
- Widowed

Physical

- Chronic pain
- Physical illness
- Terminal illness

Psychological

- Family history of suicide
- Guilt
- History of childhood abuse (e.g., physical, psychological, sexual)
- Homosexual youth
- Psychiatric disorder
- Substance abuse

Situational

- Access to weapon
- Adolescents living in nontraditional settings (e.g., juvenile detention center, prison, half-way house, group home)
- Economically disadvantaged
- Institutionalization
- Living alone
- Loss of autonomy
- Loss of independence
- Relocation
- Retired

Social

- Cluster suicides
- Disciplinary problems
- Disruptive family life
- Grieving
- Helplessness
- Hopelessness
- Insufficient social support
- Legal difficulty
- Loneliness
- Loss of important relationship
- Social isolation

Verbal

- Reports desire to die
- Threat of killing self

Expected Outcomes

- Patient's environment will be free from potential suicide weapons.
- Patient will recover from suicidal episode.
- Patient will discuss feelings that precipitated suicide attempt.
- Patient will consult mental health professional.
- Patient will describe available resources for crisis prevention and management.
- Patient will voice improvement in self-worth.

Suggested NOC Outcomes

Impulse Self-Control; Self-Mutilation Restraint; Suicide Self-Restraint

Interventions and Rationales

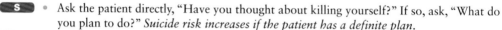

- **S** Ask the patient directly, "Have you thought about killing yourself?" If so, ask, "What do you plan to do?" *Suicide risk increases if the patient has a definite plan.*
- **S** Initiate appropriate safety protocols by removing from the patient's environment anything that could be used to inflict further self-injury (razor blades, belts, glass objects, pills) *to help ensure the patient's safety.*
- **S** Make a short-term contract with the patient on not harming self during a specific period. Continue negotiating until no evidence of suicidal ideation exists. *A contract gets the subject of suicide out in the open, places some responsibility for safety on the patient, and conveys acceptance of the patient as a worthwhile person.*
- Supervise the administration of prescribed medications. *Medications may be appropriate alternative to verbal interventions.* Be aware of drug actions and adverse effects. Make sure that the patient doesn't hoard medications.
- Provide supervision (one-on-one observation when possible) for the patient based on facility policy *to ensure compliance with legal requirements to protect the patient and to reassure the patient of staff concern.*
- Use a warm, caring, nonjudgmental manner *to show unconditional positive regard.*
- Listen carefully to the patient and don't challenge the patient *to communicate care and support.*
- Demonstrate understanding, but don't reinforce denial of the current situation *because denial can mask the roots of suicidal feelings.*
- **PCC** Make appropriate referrals to mental health professionals *to help the patient work through suicidal feelings and develop healthier alternatives.*
- Help the patient set a goal for obtaining long-term psychiatric care. *Ambivalence about psychiatric care or refusal to consult with a therapist marks the suicidal patient's lack of insight and use of denial.*
- **PCC** Provide the patient with telephone numbers and other information about crisis centers, hot lines, and counselors. *Alternatives may ease anxiety about the perceived threat of long-term psychotherapy.*

Suggested NIC Interventions

Behavior Management: Self-Harm; Environmental Management: Violence Prevention; Impulse Control Training; Suicide Prevention

Evaluations for Expected Outcomes

- Patient won't harm self in hospital.

- In aftermath of initial suicide attempt, patient makes commitment not to act on suicidal thoughts.
- Patient states reasons for suicide attempt.
- Patient contacts mental health professional.
- Patient identifies crisis prevention resources, such as hotline phone number, local crisis center, and name of therapist.
- Patient expresses positive feelings about self.

Documentation

- Patient's comments about suicide attempt and current feelings about it
- Observations of patient's behavior
- Interventions to reduce or prevent self-destructive behavior
- Patient's observable response to interventions
- Evaluations for expected outcomes

REFERENCES

Greenlee, K., & Hyde, P. S. (2014). Suicide and depression in older adults: Greater awareness can prevent tragedy. *Generations*, *38*(3), 23–26.

Procter, N., & Ferguson, M. (2015). Are there warning signs for suicide? *Australian Nursing & Midwifery Journal*, *23*(5), 31.

Xu, G., & Li, N. (2014). A comparison study on mental health status between suicide survivors and survivors of accidental deaths in rural China. *Journal of Psychiatric & Mental Health Nursing*, *21*(10), 859–865. doi:10.1111/jpm.12147

IMPAIRED VERBAL COMMUNICATION

related to psychological condition (e.g., brain tumor, decreased circulation to brain, weakened musculoskeletal system)

Definition

Decreased, delayed, or absent ability to receive, process, transmit, and/or use a system of symbols

Assessment

- Neurologic status, including history of neurologic disorders, mental status (orientation, level of consciousness, mood or behavior, knowledge and intelligence, vocabulary, and memory), and speech (pattern, language, level of comprehension and expression, and ability to use other forms of communication, such as gestures, pictures, and drawings)
- Psychological status, including history of mental or psychiatric disorders, history of alcohol or psychoactive drug use, stressors, phobias, and coping strategies

Defining Characteristics

- Absence of eye contact
- Difficulty comprehending communication
- Difficulty expressing thoughts verbally (e.g., aphasia, dysphasia, apraxia, dyslexia)
- Difficulty forming sentences
- Difficulty forming words (e.g., aphonia, dyslalia, dysarthria)
- Difficulty in selective attending
- Difficulty in use of body expressions

- Difficulty in use of facial expressions
- Difficulty maintaining communication
- Difficulty speaking
- Difficulty verbalizing
- Disoriented to person
- Disoriented to place
- Disoriented to time
- Does not speak
- Dyspnea
- Inability to speak
- Inability to speak language of caregiver
- Inability to use body expressions
- Inappropriate verbalization
- Partial visual deficit
- Refusal to speak
- Slurred speech
- Stuttering
- Total visual deficit

Expected Outcomes

- Patient will communicate needs and desires to staff, family, or friends.
- Staff members will meet patient's needs.
- Patient will incur no injury or harm.
- Patient's communication ability will return to baseline level.
- Patient will explain relationship of causative factors, such as alcohol, to inability to communicate effectively.
- Patient will begin to make plans to use self-help groups and other resources to improve psychological status.

Suggested NOC Outcomes

Communication; Communication: Expressive; Communication: Receptive

Interventions and Rationales

- Observe the patient closely *to anticipate the patient's needs* (e.g., restlessness may indicate a need to urinate).
- Minimize environmental stimuli and maintain a quiet, nonthreatening environment *to reduce anxiety.*
- S Introduce yourself, and explain procedures in simple terms. Encourage consistent use of the same terms for common objects. *Treating the patient as normal may enhance responsiveness.*
- Encourage communication attempts and allow the patient time to say or write words in response *to decrease frustration.*
- Assess the patient's communication status daily and record. Match communication needs to interventions: For disorientation, use reality orientation techniques; for a manic state, reduce environmental stimuli and talk softly and calmly; for alcohol withdrawal syndrome, reassure the patient, don't reinforce the presence of hallucinations, and provide a quiet environment; for stuttering, use rhythm or song. *Each patient needs communication status interventions tailored to the patient's situation.*

- Determine the patient's past interests and habits from family members and discuss them with the patient *to stimulate nonthreatening two-way conversation.*
- S Maintain a safe environment by using side rails, soft restraints, and other safety measures according to established policies *to protect the patient.*
- PCC Refer the patient to a psychiatric liaison nurse, social services, community agencies, and self-help groups such as Alcoholics Anonymous. *Resolution of communication problems may require long-term follow-up.*

Suggested NIC Interventions

Active Listening; Anxiety Reduction; Decision-Making Support; Environmental Management; Presence; Referral

Evaluations for Expected Outcomes

- Patient consistently communicates needs to staff, family, or friends.
- Staff members meet patient's basic needs.
- Patient doesn't show signs of neglect (weight loss, dehydration, constipation) or evidence of falls (bruises, contusions, cuts).
- Patient demonstrates return to baseline communication level by stating name, place, and time.
- Patient describes relationship between causative factors and impaired communication.
- Patient expresses intent to attend self-help groups and identifies resources appropriate to resolving underlying psychological problem.

Documentation

- Patient's concern with the level of communication
- Observations of patient's needs, communication attempts, orientation, and safety measures
- Interventions carried out to promote communication
- Contributing factors to poor communication and plans to improve psychological status
- Patient's response to nursing interventions
- Evaluations for expected outcomes

REFERENCES

Bird, J., & Parente, R. (2014). Recognition of nonverbal communication of emotion after traumatic brain injury. *Neurorehabilitation*, *34*(1), 39–43. doi:10.3233/NRE-131006

Lavelle, M., Dimic, S., Wildgrube, C., McCabe, R., & Priebe, S. (2015). Non-verbal communication in meetings of psychiatrists and patients with schizophrenia. *Acta Psychiatrica Scandinavica*, *131*(3), 197–205. doi:10.1111/acps.12319

Maul, K. K., Conner, P. S., Kempler, D., Radvanski, C., & Goral, M. (2014). Using informative verbal exchanges to promote verb retrieval in nonfluent aphasia. *American Journal of Speech-Language Pathology/American Speech-Language-Hearing Association*, *23*(3), 407–420. doi:10.1044/2014_AJSLP-13-0004

PART VII

Community-Based Health

APPLYING EVIDENCE-BASED PRACTICE

The Question

Should residents of multiunit housing (e.g., apartments, condominiums, town homes) be allowed to smoke in their residence?

Evidence-Based Resources

American Lung Association. (n.d.). Is secondhand smoke infiltrating your apartment or condominium? Retrieved March 18, 2016, from http://www.lung.org/assets/documents/tobacco/secondhand-smoke-infiltrating.pdf

Azagba, S. (2015). Effect of smoke-free patio policy of restaurants and bars on exposure to secondhand smoke. *Preventive Medicine*, *76*, 74–78. doi:10.1016/j.ypmed.2015.04.012

Fischer, F., & Kraemer, A. (2015). Meta-analysis of the association between secondhand smoke exposure and ischaemic heart diseases, COPD and stroke. *BMC Public Health*, *15*, 1–18. doi:10.1186/s12889-015-2489-4

Russo, E. T., Hulse, T. E., Adamkiewicz, G., Levy, D. E., Bethune, L., Kane, J., . . . Shah, S. N. (2015). Comparison of indoor air quality in smoke-permitted and smoke-free multiunit housing: Findings from the Boston Housing Authority. *Nicotine & Tobacco Research*, *17*(3), 316–322. doi:10.1093/ntr/ntu146

Stooke, V. D. (2014). Sharing the air, the legal and ethical considerations of extending tobacco legislation to include multiunit dwellings in Alberta. *Public Health Nursing*, *31*(1), 60–68. doi:10.1111/phn.12068

U.S. Department of Health and Human Services. (2006). *The health consequences of involuntary exposure to tobacco smoke: A report of the surgeon general*. Atlanta, GA: U.S. Department of Health and Human Services, Centers for Disease Control and Prevention, Coordinating Center for Health Promotion, National Center for Chronic Disease Prevention and Health Promotion, Office on Smoking and Health. Retrieved from http://www.surgeongeneral.gov/library/reports/secondhandsmoke/fullreport.pdf

Evaluating the Evidence

The dangers of smoking are well documented. Likewise, secondhand smoke exposure places individuals at risk for serious health problems. Secondhand smoke causes more than 41,000 deaths/year and worsens many health conditions, including respiratory infections, heart disease, stroke, cancer, and asthma (American Lung Association, n.d.). Evidence shows that the relative risk between second hand smoke and ischemic heart disease, chronic obstructive pulmonary disease, and stroke is substantial (Fischer & Kraemer, 2015). Children are especially vulnerable to secondhand smoke with infants and children under 18 months of age experiencing between 150,000 and 300,000 respiratory tract infections a year (American Lung Association, n.d.).

Those living in multiple unit housing (e.g., apartments, condominiums, duplexes, row houses, town homes) can be at increased risk of secondhand smoke exposure. Close proximity to a smoking neighbor increases smoke transfer between residences through air ventilation systems, cracks in walls or floors, around plumbing, and spaces under doors (Stooke, 2014). The U.S. Surgeon General states there is no safe level of exposure to second hand smoke and that the only complete protection is to eliminate smoking in indoor areas (U.S. Department of Health and Human Services, 2006).

To examine smoke transfer between residences, Russo et al. (2015) recorded smoking activity, airborne nicotine amounts, and fine particulate matter amounts in five Boston multiunit housing buildings. The 32 sample residences were comparable in size; residents of 15 units were smokers, residents of 11 units were nonsmokers, and 6 units were vacant. Measurable increases in particulate matter were recorded in nonsmoking residences directly adjacent to smoking residences. An examination of the data revealed that while particulate matter in smoking residences dramatically peaked and declined, the pattern of measurable particulate matter in unoccupied residences tended to increase slowly and remain in the residence for extended periods of time.

In many cities in the United States, smoking in public venues is prohibited indoors; however, many restaurants and bars permit smoking in open areas outside, such as patios. A common misconception is that because patrons smoke outside, the exposure to second hand smoke is reduced. Azagba (2015) examined data from the 2005 to 2012 Canadian Tobacco Use Monitoring Survey. Analysis of 89,743 surveys provided insight about self-reported exposure to secondhand smoke. Data indicated that secondhand smoke exposure was significantly reduced for indoor patrons at venues where smoking was prohibited both indoors and outdoors compared to venues where smoking was allowed in patio areas.

Applying the Results and Making a Decision

Secondhand smoke exposure continues to be a health and safety focus. Evidence proves that exposure to secondhand smoke causes serious health problems. Currently in the United States, there is no federal statute or regulation to protect nonsmokers from secondhand smoke in multiunit dwellings. Because people spend more time in their homes than anywhere else, eliminating smoking in multiunit housing can significantly contribute to the health and well-being of those residents. Providing a safe living environment for those in multiunit housing should be a priority for health care providers.

Reevaluating Process and Identifying Areas for Improvement

Health promotion and illness prevention is a major focus in health care today. Smoke-free policies will benefit all residents of multiunit housing by improving air quality and reducing the risk for serious health problems. Nurses advocate for the health and wellness of communities by raising public awareness of the dangers of secondhand smoke. Providing education to the community as well as residents of multiunit housing will promote policy change. Nurses should be proactive in encouraging health promotion programs in local communities.

INTRODUCTION

Evolving health care trends require nurses to be prepared to provide care in a variety of settings. Inpatient hospital acute care has become shorter in duration, increasing the need for home-based care or care in alternative settings. More and more patients are treated in nontraditional settings, including hospice, home health, geriatric centers, ambulatory care centers, schools, homeless shelters, faith communities, and prisons just to name a few. The care plans in this section focus on community-based health care to help you meet the needs of individuals, families, and communities while in nontraditional settings.

Home health nurses provide care to patients with complex chronic illnesses, acute conditions, and postoperative care needs. When planning interventions in the home care setting, the nurse should encourage patient and family participation. Participating in planning care fosters knowledge that motivates patients and families to take responsibility for health.

Providing care to communities requires creativity and flexibility. In addition to educating communities through health and wellness programs, your role may include helping individuals access health information from a variety of sources. The community health nurse must be knowledgeable of resources on the internet and through community service agencies. Community members may require help sorting through the vast amount of information available to them.

Planning care in the community requires specialized assessment, communication, collaboration, cultural competence, management skill, and leadership abilities. Developing therapeutic relationships with community members builds trust and fosters communication. Through teaching efforts, you may have the opportunity to improve the lives of individual patients and enhance the well-being of an entire community.

CONTAMINATION

Definition

Exposure to environmental contaminants in doses sufficient to cause adverse health effects

Assessment

- Community demographics, including age and sex distribution, education and income levels, and ethnic, racial, and religious groups
- Community health status, including prevalence of health problems in community, environmental pollutants, pesticide usage, biologic or radiation hazards, availability of health care services, community members' use of health care services, and beliefs, values, and attitudes about health and illness
- Living conditions, including number of occupants, sanitation, and ventilation
- Occupation and work history

Defining Characteristics

Pesticides

- Dermatologic effects of pesticide exposure
- Gastrointestinal (GI) effects of pesticide exposure
- Neurologic effects of pesticide exposure
- Pulmonary effects of pesticide exposure
- Renal effects of pesticide exposure

Chemicals

- Dermatologic effects of chemical exposure
- GI effects of chemical exposure
- Immunologic effects of chemical exposure
- Neurologic effects of chemical exposure
- Pulmonary effects of chemical exposure
- Renal effects of chemical exposure

Biological

- Dermatologic effects of biologic exposure
- GI effects of biologic exposure
- Neurologic effects of biologic exposure
- Pulmonary effects of biological exposure
- Renal effects of biological exposure

Pollution

- Neurologic effects of pollution exposure
- Pulmonary effects of pollution exposure

Waste

- Dermatologic effects of waste exposure
- GI effects of waste exposure
- Hepatic effects of waste exposure
- Pulmonary effects of waste exposure

Radiation

- Exposure to radioactive material
- Genetic effects of radiation exposure
- Immunologic effects of radiation exposure
- Neurologic effects of radiation exposure
- Oncologic effect of radiation

Suggested NOC Outcomes

Anxiety Level; Community Health Status; Fear Level; Community Disaster Readiness

Expected Outcomes

- Community members will have minimized health effects associated with contamination.
- Community members will utilize health surveillance data system to monitor for contamination incidents.
- Community members will utilize disaster plan to evacuate and triage affected members.
- Community members will minimize exposure to contaminants.

Interventions and Rationales

- Triage, stabilize, transport, and treat affected community members. *Accurate triage and early treatment provide the best chance of survival to affected persons.*
- Monitor individuals for therapeutic effects, side effects, and compliance with post-exposure drug therapy. *Drug therapy may extend over a long period of time and will require monitoring for compliance as well as therapeutic and side effects.*
- Help individuals cope with contamination incident; use groups that have survived terrorist attacks as useful resource for victims *to aid in support; those with experience can share reactions and useful coping mechanisms.*
- Help individuals deal with feelings of fear, vulnerability, and grief *to minimize risk of traumatic stress.*
- S Decontaminate persons, clothing, and equipment using approved procedure. Victims may first require decontamination before entering health facility *to receive care in order to prevent the spread of contamination.*
- S Use appropriate isolation precautions, including universal, airborne, droplet, and contact isolation. *Proper use of isolation precautions prevents cross-contamination.*

PCC
- Provide accurate information on risks involved, preventive measures, and use of antibiotics and vaccines *to enhance the use of protective measures.*
- Encourage individuals to talk to others about their fears. *Interventions aimed at supporting an individual's coping can help the person deal with feelings of fear, helplessness, and loss of control that are normal reactions in a crisis situation.*

PCC
- Collaborate with other agencies (local health department, emergency medical services, state and federal agencies). *Communication and collaboration among agencies increase ability to handle crises efficiently and correctly.*

Suggested NIC Interventions

Anxiety Reduction; Crisis Intervention; Environmental Management; Infection Control; Health Education; Triage

Evaluations for Expected Outcomes

- There is no evidence of contamination.
- Health surveillance data negative for contamination.
- Community participates in disaster planning efforts.
- Community's exposure to contaminants is minimized.

Documentation

- Results of health surveillance data
- Evaluation of simulated disaster plans
- Evaluations for expected outcomes

REFERENCES

Hoover, E., Renauld, M., Edelstein, M. R., & Brown, P. (2015). Social science collaboration with environmental health. *Environmental Health Perspectives*, *123*(11), 1100–1106. doi:10.1289/ehp.1409283

Hore, P., Ahmed, M., Nagin, D., & Clark, N. (2014). Intervention model for contaminated consumer products: A multifaceted tool for protecting public health. *American Journal of Public Health*, *104*(8), 1377–1383. doi:10.2105/AJPH.2014.301912

Jackson Allen, P. (2015). Primary care approaches. Climate change: It's our problem. *Pediatric Nursing*, *41*(1), 42–46.

Jianghong, L., & Lewis, G. (2014). Environmental toxicity and poor cognitive outcomes in children and adults. *Journal of Environmental Health*, *76*(6), 130–138.

RISK FOR CONTAMINATION

Definition

Vulnerable to exposure to environmental contaminants, which may compromise health

Assessment

- Community demographics, including age and sex distribution, education and income levels, and ethnic, racial, and religious groups
- Community health status, including prevalence of health problems in community, environmental pollutants, pesticide usage, biologic or radiation hazards, availability of health care services, community members' use of health care services, and beliefs, values, and attitudes about health and illness
- Living conditions, including number of occupants, sanitation, and ventilation
- Occupation and work history

Risk Factors

External

- Carpeted flooring
- Chemical contamination of food
- Chemical contamination of water
- Economically disadvantaged
- Exposure to areas with high contaminant level
- Exposure to atmospheric pollutants
- Exposure to bioterrorism
- Exposure to disaster (natural or man-made)
- Exposure to radiation
- Flaking, peeling surface in presence of young children (e.g., paint, plaster)
- Inadequate breakdown of contaminant
- Inadequate household hygiene practices
- Inadequate municipal services (e.g., trash removal, sewage treatment facilities)
- Inadequate personal hygiene practices
- Inadequate protective clothing
- Inappropriate use of protective clothing
- Playing where environmental contaminants are used
- Unprotected exposure to chemical (e.g., chromium, lead)
- Use of environmental contaminant in the home
- Use of noxious material in insufficiently ventilated area (e.g., lacquer, paint)
- Use of noxious material without effective protection (e.g., lacquer, paint)

Internal

- Concomitant exposure
- Developmental characteristics of children
- Extremes of age
- Female gender
- Gestational age during exposure
- Inadequate nutrition
- Preexisting disease
- Pregnancy
- Previous exposure to contaminant
- Smoking

Expected Outcomes

- Community will remain free from adverse effects of contamination.
- Community will utilize health surveillance data system to monitor for contamination incidents.
- Community will participate in mass casualty and disaster readiness drills.
- Community will remain free from contamination-related health effects.
- Community will have minimal exposure to contaminants.

Suggested NOC Outcomes

Community Disaster Readiness; Community Health Status; Health Beliefs: Perceived Threat; Knowledge: Health Behavior; Knowledge: Health Resources; Risk Control

Interventions and Rationales

- Monitor individuals for therapeutic effects, side effects, and compliance with post-exposure drug therapy. *Drug therapy may extend over a long period of time and will require monitoring for compliance as well as therapeutic and side effects.*
- S Conduct surveillance for environmental contamination; notify agencies authorized to protect the environment of contaminants in the area. *Early surveillance and detection are critical components of preparation.*
- S Assist individuals in relocating to safer environment *to decrease their risk of contamination.*
- S Modify environment to minimize risk. *Modification of the environment will decrease the risk of actual contamination.*

S
- Implement decontamination of persons, clothing, and equipment by using approved procedure. Victims may first require decontamination before entering health facility *to receive care in order to prevent the spread of contamination.*

S
- Use appropriate isolation precautions: universal, airborne, droplet, and contact isolation. *Proper use of isolation precautions prevents cross-contamination by contaminating agent.*

PCC
- Provide accurate information on risks involved, preventive measures, use of antibiotics and *vaccines to reduce anxiety and increase compliance.*
- Assist community members with feelings of fear and vulnerability. *Interventions aimed at supporting an individual's coping help the person deal with feelings of fear, helplessness, and loss of control that are normal reactions in a crisis situation.*
- In conjunction with other healthcare providers, schedule mass casualty and disaster readiness drills. *Practice in handling contamination occurrences will decrease the risk of exposure during actual contamination events.*

Suggested NIC Interventions

Bioterrorism Preparedness; Communicable Disease Management; Community; Community Disaster Preparedness; Environmental Management: Safety; Environmental Risk Protection; Health Education; Health Policy Monitoring; Health Screening; Immunization/Vaccination Management; Risk Identification; Surveillance: Safety

Evaluations for Expected Outcomes

- No evidence of contamination.
- Health surveillance data negative for contamination.
- Community participates in disaster planning efforts.
- Community exposure to contaminants is minimized.

Documentation

- Results of health surveillance data
- Evaluation of simulated disaster plans
- Evaluations for expected outcomes

REFERENCES

Chalupka, S. (2014). Climate change and health. *American Journal of Nursing, 114*(8), 67–69.

Fowler, S., & Schnall, J. (2014). TOXNET: Information on toxicology and environmental health. *American Journal of Nursing, 114*(2), 61–63.

Hore, P., Ahmed, M., Nagin, D., & Clark, N. (2014). Intervention model for contaminated consumer products: A multifaceted tool for protecting public health. *American Journal of Public Health, 104*(8), 1377–1383. doi:10.2105/AJPH.2014.301912

INEFFECTIVE COMMUNITY COPING

related to insufficient community resources (e.g., respite, recreation, social support)

Definition

A pattern of community activities for adaptation and problem solving that is unsatisfactory for meeting the demands or needs of the community

Assessment

- Community demographics, including age and sex distribution, education and income levels, and ethnic, racial, and religious groups
- Family status, including family composition (percentage of single-parent families in community), responsibilities assumed by teenagers in caring for siblings, and ability of families to meet their physical, social, emotional, and economic needs
- Community health status, including prevalence of health problems in community, attitudes toward sex and sexuality, availability of health care services, community members' use of health care services, and beliefs, values, and attitudes about health and illness
- Education system, including availability of sex education in schools, availability of programs to help pregnant teens complete their education, and willingness of parents to allow children to participate
- Political system, including government officials' support for or opposition to sex education
- Attitude of religious groups toward sex and sexuality and religious groups' influence on educators
- Transportation availability to clinics and other social services and recreation opportunities for adolescents
- Welfare and health care system and reliance of teen mothers on welfare for support

Defining Characteristics

- Community does not meet expectation of its members
- Deficient community participation
- Elevated community illness rate
- Excessive community conflict
- Excessive stress
- High incidence of community problems (e.g., homicides, vandalism, terrorism, robbery, abuse, unemployment, poverty, militancy, mental illness)
- Perceived community powerlessness
- Perceived community vulnerability

Expected Outcomes

- Community members will express desire to develop improved communication among community members.
- Community members will express need for plan to improve community functioning.
- Community members express desire to develop and implement plans to strengthen community resources.
- Community members will express willingness to participate in problem-solving strategies.
- Community members will evaluate success of plan in meeting goals and objectives and will continue to revise it, as necessary.

Suggested NOC Outcomes

Community Competence; Community Health Status; Risk Control

Interventions and Rationales

- Work with the community to assess and develop needed programs *to provide community members with information about risks, problems, and complications of community needs.*

- Work closely with community to assess strengths and weaknesses of community functioning *to assess their needs and provide care.*
- Implement an outreach and health promotion program *to raise community members' awareness of community problems.* Consider these steps:
  - Work with teachers, school psychologists, counselors, school nurses, students, and the parent–teacher association *to determine the needs among the child and adolescent population.*
  - Encourage local youth groups, religious organizations, and social service organizations to feature guest speakers on community issues at their meetings. *Speakers with expertise in the area of community dynamics are able to provide information that help community members build stronger resources.*
  - Contact representatives of local corporations *to ask for funding for educational programs.*
  - Help community members establish work groups for organization and collaboration. *Organizing community teams will foster problem solving.*
  - Provide education on community issues and problems. *Access to information allows for greater problem solving.*
- Encourage community members to establish work groups or a task force *to develop and implement needed programs within the community.*
- Work with community members to evaluate the effectiveness of the programs and assist with modifying programs, as needed, *to ensure the program's effectiveness and promote use of the program as a model for preventive health.*
- Collect statistical data as needed *to help evaluate the effectiveness of programs.*

Suggested NIC Interventions

Community Health Development; Health Education; Health Screening; Program Development; Consultation; Family Planning: Contraception; Referral

Evaluations for Expected Outcomes

- Community members have improved communication among community members.
- Community members develop plan to improve community functioning.
- Community members develop and implement plan to strengthen community resources.
- Community members participate in problem-solving strategies.
- Community members evaluate success of plan and revise it, as needed.

Documentation

- Community perception of problem
- Statistics that support existence of problem
- Community resources that already exist to alleviate problem
- Future plans to deal with problem
- Evaluations for expected outcomes

REFERENCES

Chabot, M. J., Navarro, S., Swann, D., Darney, P., & Thiel de Bocanegra, H. (2014). Association of access to publicly funded family planning services with adolescent birthrates in California counties. *American Journal of Public Health*, *104*(Suppl 1), e1–e6. doi:10.2105/AJPH.2013.301454

Freed, P., & SmithBattle, L. (2016). Promoting teen mother's mental health. *American Journal of Maternal Child Nursing*, *41*(2), 84–89.

Kirven, J. (2014). Maintaining their future after teen pregnancy: Strategies for staying physically and mentally fit. *International Journal of Childbirth Education*, *29*(1), 57–61.
Smyth, S., & Anderson, G. (2014). Family nurse partnership: Meeting the needs of teenage mothers. *British Journal of Midwifery*, *22*(12), 870–875.

FEAR

related to innate response to stimuli (e.g., sudden noise, height)

Definition

Response to perceived threat that is consciously recognized as a danger

Assessment

- Patient's age and sex
- Developmental status, including cognitive, psychosexual, and psychosocial stages; cognitive and motor capabilities; and communication and socialization skills
- Temperature, pulse rate, blood pressure, respiratory rate, and skin color and temperature
- Health history, especially past or present bruises, burns, fractures, dislocations, and other injuries
- Changes in behavior, eating or sleeping habits, and ability to concentrate
- Parental status, including parents' age and maturity level, marital status, stability of parental relationship, educational levels, financial needs and resources, employment status, developmental state of family, parents' knowledge of normal growth and development, relationship with child, understanding of child's fear, past responses to crises, and coping mechanisms

Defining Characteristics

- Apprehensiveness
- Decrease in self-assurance
- Excitedness
- Feeling of dread
- Feeling of fear
- Feeling of panic
- Feeling of terror
- Feeling of alarm
- Increase in blood pressure
- Increase in tension
- Jitteriness
- Muscle tension
- Nausea
- Pallor
- Pupil dilation
- Vomiting

Cognitive

- Decrease in learning ability
- Decrease in problem-solving ability
- Decrease in productivity
- Identifies object of fear
- Stimulus believed to be a threat

Behaviors

- Attack behaviors
- Avoidance behaviors
- Focus narrowed to the source of fear
- Impulsiveness
- Increase in alertness

Physiologic

- Anorexia
- Change in physiologic response (e.g., blood pressure, heart rate, respiratory rate, oxygen saturation, and end-title CO_2)
- Diarrhea
- Dry mouth
- Dyspnea
- Fatigue
- Increase in perspiration
- Increase in respiratory rate

Expected Outcomes

- Child will identify sources of fear.
- Child will exhibit marked decrease in physiologic and behavioral manifestations of fear and will report feeling safe and comfortable.
- Child will experience no further injury or abuse.
- Child will attend school regularly, participate actively in activities, and develop positive relationships with peers, teachers, and school nurse.
- If removed from home, child will grieve loss of parents.
- Parents will acknowledge abuse and will do everything possible to protect child.
- Parents will seek individual and group support.
- Parents will receive counseling for problems that might lead to abuse, such as dysfunction in family and lack of food, shelter, or medical care.

Suggested NOC Outcomes

Anxiety Self-Control; Comfort Level; Coping; Fear Self-Control

Interventions and Rationales

- Observe the child for signs of possible abuse, and elicit as much information as possible from the child about the injuries. *Discrepancies between physical evidence and reported history may be important signs of possible child abuse.* Report the case to a social service agency as soon as possible.
- Spend as much time as possible establishing rapport with the child. Communicate at the child's eye level. Speak in a soft, reassuring voice. *Establishing rapport encourages the child to express feelings and provides comfort.*
- Help the child identify sources of fear *to enable the child to put emotions into perspective.*
- During your discussion with the child, be careful not to condemn the parents in any way for their actions. *Listening nonjudgmentally helps to maintain a therapeutic relationship.*
- Refrain from asking the child too many questions. *Excessive questioning may upset the child and make it more difficult for professionals who will investigate the incident formally.*
- Emphasize that the child has done nothing wrong *to prevent feelings of guilt that may interfere with the child's ability to communicate about the problem.*
- Reassure that no one is permitted to hurt the child. Tell the child about the right to refuse to let anyone touch in a way that makes the child uncomfortable. *Accurate information dispels misconceptions that exacerbate the child's fear.*
- S Report suspected abuse to the appropriate social service agency as soon as the problem is discovered. *In many states, failure to report abuse constitutes a crime.*
- Evaluate whether to tell the parents that you're reporting suspected abuse. *The child might be in danger if the parents know they're being reported. Protecting the child is the first priority.*
- Be available if the child wishes to talk about interactions with outside social service agencies or ways in which life has changed. *Having someone the child trusts will enhance the child's ability to cope.*

Suggested NIC Interventions

Anxiety Reduction; Coping Enhancement; Security Enhancement; Therapeutic Play

Evaluations for Expected Outcomes

- Child discusses sources of fear.
- Child exhibits marked decrease in physiologic and behavioral manifestations of fear and reports feeling safe and comfortable.
- Child experiences no further injury or abuse.
- Child attends school regularly, participates in school activities and support groups, and reports improved relationships with peers and adults.
- If removed from home, child grieves loss of parents.
- Parents acknowledge abuse and do everything possible to protect child.
- Parents seek individual and group support.
- Parents receive counseling for problems that might lead to abuse.

Documentation

- Child's verbal and behavioral expressions of fear
- Physical manifestations of fear
- Communication with parents
- Details of report to social service agency
- Child's and parents' responses to nursing interventions
- Evaluations for expected outcomes

REFERENCES

Chieng, Y. S., Chan, W. S., Klainin-Yobas, P., & He, H. (2014). Perioperative anxiety and postoperative pain in children and adolescents undergoing elective surgical procedures: A quantitative systematic review. *Journal of Advanced Nursing*, *70*(2), 243–255. doi:10.1111/jan.12205

Copanitsanou, P., & Valkeapää, K. (2014). Effects of education of pediatric patients undergoing elective surgical procedures on their anxiety—A systematic review. *Journal of Clinical Nursing*, *23*(7/8), 940–954. doi:10.1111/jocn.12187

Jolly, A. A. (2015). Handle with care: Top ten tips a nurse should know before caring for a hospitalized child with autism spectrum disorder. *Pediatric Nursing*, *41*(1), 11–22.

GRIEVING

related to anticipatory loss of significant object (e.g., possession, job, status)

Definition

A normal complex process that includes emotional, physical, spiritual, social, and intellectual responses and behaviors by which individuals, families, and communities incorporate an actual, anticipated, or perceived loss into their daily lives

Assessment

- Patient's status, including present condition, estimated life expectancy, and recent treatments and interventions
- Pain control and management, including patient's wishes and the family's expectations
- Patient's and family's status, including events leading to decision to use hospice services, family's cultural and religious beliefs, family members' understanding of hospice care, and family support, including family dynamics, family's special needs, and family member in charge

- Concepts of death, dying, and loss, including willingness of patient and family to discuss terminal illness, willingness to make plans, anger expressed by family members, communication patterns among family members and with health care professionals, awareness of processes and events leading up to death, understanding of what occurs at moment of death, and ethical, financial, and social decisions faced by family members
- Advance directives, including presence of living will
- Involvement with community resources such as religious or support group

Defining Characteristics

- Alteration in activity level
- Alteration in dream pattern
- Alteration in immune functioning
- Alteration in neuroendocrine functioning
- Alteration in sleep pattern
- Anger
- Blaming
- Despair
- Detachment
- Disorganization
- Finding meaning in a loss
- Guilt about feeling relieved
- Maintaining a connection to the deceased
- Pain
- Panic behavior
- Personal growth
- Psychological distress
- Suffering

Expected Outcomes

- Patient will report no pain, show no sign of infection, and be as comfortable as possible.
- Patient will express own needs.
- Patient will grieve own loss of life.
- Patient will communicate with family and other members of support network.
- Patient will receive care from family or friends.
- Patient will remain as independent as possible for as long as possible.
- Patient will talk openly about illness and impending death.
- Patient will receive support through stages of dying.
- Patient will die with dignity.

Suggested NOC Outcomes

Coping; Dignified Life Closure; Family Coping; Family Social Climate; Hope; Grief Resolution; Spiritual Health

Interventions and Rationales

- On each hospice visit, conduct a thorough physical assessment, monitor the patient's vital signs, and note signs of complications or impending death. *Assessment provides information needed to modify the care plan.*
- Assess the patient's and family members' psychosocial status *to determine the need for continued support.*
- Answer all questions honestly *to support the patient's and family members' right to know.*

PCC
- Help the patient understand the grieving process and accept the feelings the patient experiences as normal. Discuss and help the patient progress through the psychological stages of anticipated death: shock and denial, anger, bargaining, depression, and acceptance. *Knowing these stages will help you and family members anticipate the patient's needs. Remember that not all patients go through each stage.*

- Guide the patient in reviewing own life. Encourage the patient to write or tape own life history as a lasting gift to family members *to help the patient give events from the past meaningful interpretation.*
- PCC Encourage the patient to make simple decisions related to own care *to give the patient a sense of functional ability and control.*
- Express acceptance of the patient's response to own anticipated death, whatever that response: crying, sadness, anger, fear, or denial. *Each patient responds to dying in own way. Helping the patient express feelings freely enhances coping.*
- PCC Teach the patient and family members about pain control, comfort measures, diet, medications, hydration, palliative care, skin care, and how to respond to complications or a serious change in the patient's condition. *Knowledge of how to meet the basic needs of the terminally ill enhances the patient's and family members' feeling of control.*
- Perform skilled care related to indwelling urinary catheters, I.V. therapy, medications, supplemental oxygen, and other treatments prescribed by the physician *to fulfill professional nursing responsibilities.*
- Evaluate the needs of the patient and caregiver for additional resources that hospice can provide. *Commonly, the family may be able to use social, financial, religious, or volunteer services.* Be aware that they may hesitate to ask about such services.
- Support the patient's spiritual coping behaviors. For example, arrange for the patient to have at the bedside objects that provide spiritual comfort, such as a bible, prayer shawl, pictures, statues, rosary beads, or other items. *Even nonobservant individuals commonly turn to religion when confronted by death.*
- PCC Recommend that the family call the American Cancer Society at 1-800-ACS-2345 and request publication *Caring for the Patient with Cancer at Home. This guide for patients and families is a good quick reference for caring for terminally ill patients. The information is also appropriate for patients with terminal illnesses other than cancer.*
- PCC If grief counseling is available, refer family members to this service. Also, provide support to family members after the patient's death *to prevent feelings of being abandoned by the hospice staff.*

Suggested NIC Interventions

Anticipatory Guidance; Coping Enhancement; Family Support; Grief Work Facilitation; Referral

Evaluations for Expected Outcomes

- Patient reports no pain, shows no signs of infection, and indicates state of relative comfort.
- Patient expresses own needs.
- Patient grieves own loss of life.
- Patient communicates with family members and other members of support network.
- Patient receives care from family or friends.
- Patient remains as independent as possible for as long as possible.
- Patient talks openly about impending death and accepts death peacefully.
- Patient receives support through stages of dying.
- Patient dies with dignity.

Documentation

- Assessment of patient's physical and emotional status
- Patient's and family members' adaptation to situation

- Interventions to meet patient's needs
- Patient's response to nursing interventions
- Referrals to community agencies
- Evaluations for expected outcomes

REFERENCES

Clipsham, L., Islam, Z., & Faull, C. (2015). Experiences of hospice inpatient nurses in supporting children before the death of a parent. *International Journal of Palliative Nursing*, *21*(9), 453–459. doi:10.12968/ijpn.2015.21.9.453

Holdsworth, L. M. (2015). Bereaved carers' accounts of the end of life and the role of care providers in a 'good death': A qualitative study. *Palliative Medicine*, *29*(9), 834–841. doi:10.1177/0269216315584865

Mullen, J. E., Reynolds, M. R., & Larson, J. S. (2015). Caring for pediatric patients' families at the child's end of life. *Critical Care Nurse*, *35*(6), 46–56. doi:10.4037/ccn2015614

DEFICIENT COMMUNITY HEALTH

Definition

Presence of one or more health problems or factors that deter wellness or increase the risk of health problems experienced by an aggregate

Assessment

- Community demographics, including age and sex distribution, ethnic and racial groups, education, and income levels
- Prevalence of health problems in community, availability of health care services, and use of health care services
- Psychosocial status of community members, including cognitive abilities, access to transportation, physical disabilities, communication problems, environmental factors, financial resources, support systems, and beliefs and practices regarding health

Defining Characteristics

- Health problem experienced by aggregates or populations
- Program unavailable to eliminate health problem(s) of an aggregate or population
- Program unavailable to enhance wellness of an aggregate or population
- Program unavailable to prevent health problem(s) of an aggregate or population
- Program unavailable to reduce health problem(s) of an aggregate or population
- Risk of hospitalization experienced by aggregates or population
- Risk of physiologic states experienced by aggregates or population
- Risk of psychological states experienced by aggregates or population

Expected Outcomes

- Community members will conduct a formal comprehensive survey assessing the parameters of the community that impact its health.
- Community members will develop a plan to secure professional, governmental, social, and financial/economic resources that sustain a community's health.
- Community members will develop processes that enable individuals, organizations, and agencies to work together to accomplish the community's health goals.
- Community members will implement systems that meet the community's health needs.

Suggested NOC Outcomes

Health-Promoting Behavior; Health-Seeking Behavior; Knowledge: Health Behavior; Knowledge: Health Resources; Community Health Status

Interventions and Rationales

- Select a qualified leader/coordinator to establish and direct community resources to assess the health care needs of the residents. *A leader is necessary to coordinate the efforts of individuals working to improve the structures supporting community health.*
- Communicate widely and through multiple media outlets the need for participation in surveys and assessments to determine deficiencies in community health. *Understanding proposed actions and expectations reduces anxiety and suspicion; it increases cooperation among the community residents.*
- Assess the community demographics. *An understanding of who has health needs to be addressed provides efficiency and effectiveness in delivering care.*
- Evaluate the prevalence of health problems and risk behaviors. *Understanding the medical conditions and nursing needs are essential components of providing professional services to meet the community's needs.*
- Establish the scope of need and the reality of resources available to meet the needs. *Integrating the knowledge gained about the community deficit enables the community leaders to identify scope of need, scope of work, and means to accomplish it.*
- Create opportunities for community resources to begin services to the community residents in need. *Volunteers and concerned individuals can provide local services to meet the needs of "their neighbors" and promote goodwill.*
- Foster relationships at all levels (local, regional, and national) that secure resources to enable policy, funding, and actions plans that correct deficiencies in community health. *In communities of any size, working together for common goals creates synergy and moves the agenda forward.*
- Plan for resident (community) centered, safe, equitable, effective, efficient, quality, and timely delivery of health care. *These aims from the Institute for Medicine provide guidance in the outcomes desired for the community health care delivery.*
- PCC Teach the community members about their roles in self-care, disease management, and community care. *This facilitates autonomy to improve health and promote community-centered care.*
- PCC Educate students about their responsibilities, self-care, health maintenance, and health protection. *Positive health habits, positive self-esteem, disease avoidance, pregnancy avoidance, and successful completion of high school coupled with plans for a vocation or higher education reduces the current and future burden on the community's health.*
- Support and encourage the community as it moves forward. *Barriers and challenges to initiatives may develop and can be surmounted with professional guidance.*
- Encourage groups, agencies, and residents to find common ground and goals to work on together to identify solutions to meet the needs of the community. *In finding common ground, a commitment to the group process and the outcomes goal evolve into a solution.*
- Solicit a cadre of individuals with expertise to enhance the assessment, planning, and implementation phases of the community health plan. *Advanced knowledge of the community health assessment and promotion process enables local leaders and residents to move steadily toward positive health outcomes*

PCC
- Engage local educators and community leaders to provide insight and recommendations for implementing the health plan. *Local experts can be translational leaders in bringing the right residents forward to benefit from the ideas and resources made available through the community health initiatives.*

Suggested NIC Interventions

Community Health Development; Program Development; Environmental Management: Community; Health Screening; Community Disease Management

Evaluations for Expected Outcomes

- Community members complete health surveys and assessments.
- Community members develop health care plan.
- Community members participate in health care planning, implementation, and evaluation.
- Community resources are adequate to meet health care needs.

Documentation

- Results of surveys and assessments done
- Minutes of meetings held
- Public relations announcements
- Educational materials produced
- Evaluations for expected outcomes

REFERENCES

Best, S. (2015). Innovating in rural health in Wales: Applied findings from the practitioner's perspective. *British Journal of Community Nursing*, *20*(11), 559–563. doi:10.12968/bjcn.2015.20.11.559

Mohammad, Y., Jan, R., McIntyre, H., Lakhani, A., Anwar, S., & Levi, A. J. (2015). Community midwives' workplace experiences: A case study from a resource-poor country. *British Journal of Midwifery*, *23*(12), 886–893. doi:10.12968/bjom.2015.23.12.886

Turner, C. (2015). Mobile working: Positively engaging community nurses. *British Journal of Community Nursing*, *20*(3), 134–138.

INEFFECTIVE HEALTH MAINTENANCE

related to insufficient resources (e.g., financial, social, knowledge)

Definition

Inability to identify, manage, and/or seek out help to maintain health

Assessment

- Community demographics, including age and sex distribution, ethnic and racial groups, education, and income levels
- Prevalence of health problems in community, availability of health care services, and use of health care services

- Psychosocial status of community members, including cognitive abilities, access to transportation, physical disabilities, communication problems, environmental factors, financial resources, support systems, and beliefs and practices regarding health

Defining Characteristics

- Absence of adaptive behaviors to environmental changes
- Absence of interest in improving health behaviors
- Inability to take responsibility for meeting basic health practices
- Insufficient knowledge about basic health practices
- Insufficient social support
- Pattern of lack of health-seeking behavior

Expected Outcomes

- Community members will express desire to learn about available resources.
- Community members will identify local resources and how to access them.
- Community members will contact community agencies.
- Community organizations will develop resource information guides for their members and will promote increased access to needed resources.

Suggested NOC Outcomes

Health-Promoting Behavior; Health-Seeking Behavior; Knowledge: Health Behavior; Knowledge: Health Resources

Interventions and Rationales

- Assess factors that hinder community members' learning about neighborhood resources in order *to identify areas where education may bring about change.*
- PCC Assist members to learn about community and resources available to them, such as the American Heart Association, Agency on Aging, American Cancer Society, Meals On Wheels, and Alzheimer's support group, *to help empower community members.*
- Plan specific programs to familiarize members of community organizations with neighborhood resources. For example, have an agency spokesperson attend senior citizen lunch meetings to distribute program materials, *to enhance acceptance and reach more people.*
- PCC Help community members identify specific neighborhood resources they need. For example, a senior citizen group may need nutrition support services, whereas young families may need information about immunizations and child safety. *Targeting resources that meet specific health needs increases chances that they 'll be used.*
- Assist community organizations—such as neighborhood civic associations, religious groups, or social clubs—develop a manual describing health care resources available to group members *to provide an ongoing resource and help community members become self-sufficient.*
- Ask members of community organizations to evaluate community resources. Discuss ways in which organizations may become politically active in requesting needed services. *When members are aware of resources, evaluation may help point out the need for changes.*

Suggested NIC Interventions

Health Education; Health System Guidance; Self-Responsibility Facilitation; Support System Enhancement

Evaluations for Expected Outcomes

- Community members express lack of familiarity with neighborhood resources and desire to learn about them.
- Community members seek out and obtain information about neighborhood resources.
- Community members contact appropriate neighborhood resources.
- Community organizations develop resource information guides for their members and promote increased access to needed resources.

Documentation

- Perception of problem as expressed by community members
- Response of community members to presentations by agency spokespeople
- Evaluation of neighborhood resources
- Evaluations for expected outcomes

REFERENCES

Best, S. (2015). Innovating in rural health in Wales: Applied findings from the practitioner's perspective. *British Journal of Community Nursing*, *20*(11), 559–563. doi:10.12968/bjcn.2015.20.11.559

Cross, S. L., Suharwardy, S. H., Bodavula, P., Schechtman, K., Overton, E. T., Onen, N. F., & Lane, M. A. (2014). Improving cervical cancer screening rates in an urban HIV clinic. *AIDS Care*, *26*(9), 1186–1193. doi:10.1080/09540121.2014.894610

Smith, L. P., Shu Wen, N., & Popkin, B. M. (2014). Resistant to the recession: Low-income adults' maintenance of cooking and away-from-home eating behaviors during times of economic turbulence. *American Journal of Public Health*, *104*(5), 840–846. doi:10.2105/AJPH.2013.301677

RISK FOR INFECTION

Definition

Vulnerable to invasion and multiplication of pathogenic organisms, which may compromise health

Assessment

- Patient's health status, including age, weight, reason for home infusion therapy, vital signs, nutritional status, and motor skills
- Health history, including drug allergies, substance abuse, chronic metabolic or systemic disease, and recent or present respiratory, urinary, or oral infection
- Current medical treatments, including radiation therapy, chemotherapy, antibiotic or antifungal therapy, steroid treatment, and anticoagulant, thrombolytic, or immunosuppressive therapy
- Mental status, including level of consciousness, orientation, judgment, and affect
- Caregiver's physical and mental status, including chronic health problems, self-care abilities, mobility limitations, and level of cognitive function
- Home environment, including structural barriers, availability of soap and water for hand washing, clean preparation area, access to telephone, and need for special equipment
- Financial status, including insurance coverage and understanding of co-payments and out-of-pocket expenses

Risk Factors

- Chronic illness (e.g., diabetes mellitus)
- Inadequate vaccination
- Insufficient knowledge to avoid exposure to pathogens
- Invasive procedure
- Malnutrition
- Obesity

Inadequate Primary Defenses

- Alteration in peristalsis
- Alteration in pH of secretions
- Alteration in skin integrity
- Decrease in ciliary action
- Premature rupture of amniotic membrane
- Prolonged rupture of amniotic membrane
- Smoking
- Stasis of body fluids

Inadequate Secondary Defenses

- Decrease in hemoglobin
- Immunosuppression
- Leukopenia
- Suppressed inflammatory response (e.g., IL-6, CRP)
- Inadequate vaccination

Increased Environmental Exposure to Pathogens

- Exposure to disease outbreak

Expected Outcomes

- Patient or caregiver will demonstrate ability to administer drugs and fluids, as prescribed.
- Patient or caregiver will demonstrate ability to prevent infection from home infusion therapy.
- Patient or caregiver will monitor site and general condition of patient for complications (redness or tenderness at insertion site, swelling, burning, cool skin, decreased flow rate, blood backup in line, pain along vein, general discomfort, fever, chills, malaise, and respiratory distress) and will report complications immediately.
- Patient or caregiver will exhibit capability and comfort in carrying out all necessary procedures.

Suggested NOC Outcomes

Risk Control; Risk Detection; Safe Home Environment; Knowledge: Infection Control

Interventions and Rationales

- During the initial visit, approach care in a systematic and organized fashion. Have available written materials, checklists, supplies, equipment, and other items. Conduct teaching sessions in a quiet place where you, the patient, and the caregiver will be undisturbed. *An organized approach may reduce anxiety and help the patient and caregiver perceive the responsibility as series of well-defined tasks.*
- PCC Use verbal and written instructions, demonstrate each step, and have the patient and caregiver perform return demonstrations. *Some patients and caregivers may have difficulty learning new skills and require repeated reinforcement.*
- Make sure that the patient and caregiver understand the purpose of treatment, and enlist their participation throughout the course of therapy. *Understanding the treatment and its goals helps the home care patient assume a greater role in administering, monitoring, and maintaining therapy.*
- Provide emotional support and encouragement *to decrease the patient's and caregiver's anxiety regarding home infusion therapy.*
- Provide all necessary supplies, including solution, sterile I.V. tubing, pole and infusion pump, intake and output record, and dressings. Explain how to get additional

supplies and help the patient and caregiver make these arrangements *to promote independence.*

S • Stress the need to use sterile technique *to reduce the risk of infection at the access site.*
S • Emphasize the importance of following safety precautions when disposing of used supplies *to protect caregivers and the patient from injury.*
- Tell the patient to protect the catheter from coming into contact with granular or lint-producing surfaces. *Airborne particles and surface contaminants can cause localized infection.*

PCC • Teach the patient to change the site dressing, as ordered (usually every 2 or 3 days), or whenever it becomes wet, soiled, or nonocclusive *to reduce the risk of infection.*
PCC • Teach the patient and family members drug names, treatment protocols, administration procedures, potential adverse effects and drug toxicity, and signs, indicating the need to call a physician or nurse immediately *to reinforce the need to be precise in drug administration.*
PCC • Teach the patient and caregiver how to manage complications related to improper catheter placement and fluid administration. These may include redness, tenderness, swelling, heat, or fluid leakage at site; streaking or pain along the vein; a decreased flow rate or blood backflow in tubing; and fever, chills, malaise, or shortness of breath. *Detecting complications as early as possible may prevent more serious consequences.*

Suggested NIC Interventions

Environmental Management; Health System Guidance; Infection Protection; Venous Access Device (VAD) Maintenance; Infection Control

Evaluations for Expected Outcomes

- Patient receives drugs and fluids, as prescribed.
- Patient remains free from infection associated with home infusion therapy.
- Patient or caregiver detects and immediately reports complications associated with home infusion therapy.
- Patient or caregiver exhibits capability and comfort in carrying out all necessary procedures.

Documentation

- Explanation and demonstration of each procedure and return demonstration by patient (documented on comprehensive teaching checklist)
- Times of care measures, especially dressing, tubing, and solution changes
- Observations of patient's condition, complications, and subsequent treatments
- Evidence of patient's and caregiver's learning
- Evaluations for expected outcomes

REFERENCES

Holmdahl, S., Sävenstedt, S., & Imoni, R. (2014). Parenteral nutrition in home-based palliative care: Swedish district nurses experiences. *Scandinavian Journal of Caring Sciences*, *28*(1), 89–96. doi:10.1111/scs.12038

Lyons, M., & Phalen, A. (2014). A randomized controlled comparison of flushing protocols in home care patients with peripherally inserted central catheters. *Journal of Infusion Nursing*, *35*(1), 52–64.

Meyer, B. (2014). Broadening infusion specialization as an adjunct to organizational sustainability. *Journal of Infusion Nursing*, *37*(1), 44–54.

DEFICIENT KNOWLEDGE

related to insufficient knowledge of resources

The Americans with Disabilities Act

Definition

Absence or deficiency of cognitive information related to a specific topic

Assessment

- Psychosocial status, including age, learning ability (affective, cognitive, and psychomotor domains), decision-making ability, developmental stage, financial resources, health beliefs and attitudes, interest in learning, knowledge and skill regarding current health problem, obstacles to learning, support systems, and usual coping pattern
- Neurologic status, including level of consciousness, memory, mental status, and orientation
- Musculoskeletal status, including coordination, gait, muscle size and strength, muscle tone, range of motion, and functional mobility as follows:
  0 = completely independent
  1 = requires use of equipment or device
  2 = requires help, supervision, or teaching from another person
  3 = requires help from another person and equipment or device
  4 = dependent; doesn't participate in activity

Defining Characteristics

- Inaccurate follow-through of instruction
- Inaccurate performance on a test
- Inappropriate behavior (e.g., hysterical, hostile, agitated, apathetic)
- Insufficient knowledge

Expected Outcomes

- Patient will express need for information about rights of individuals with disabilities.
- Patient will state understanding of rights as disabled person under Americans with Disabilities Act (ADA).
- Patient will state intention to seek adaptations to work environment or other accommodations as a consequence of learning about ADA.

Suggested NOC Outcomes

Knowledge: Health Behavior; Knowledge: Health Resources

Interventions and Rationales

- Establish an environment of mutual trust and respect *to enhance learning.*
- Listen to the patient's concerns about coping with a disability in society. *As a community health nurse, you should be concerned not only with the patient's physiologic well-being but also with the patient's ability to function to maximum potential in the community.*

- Discuss with the patient about the feeling of being fully informed about own rights under law. Ask whether the patient is aware of laws that protect the rights of disabled people. *Open, direct discussion will establish the need for information.*
- Inform the patient about ADA *to enhance the patient's understanding of own legal rights.* Tell the patient Congress passed this law in 1990. Explain that many important rights of disabled people, defined as anyone "with a physical or mental impairment that substantially limits one or more major life activities," are set out in the law.
- PCC Teach the patient about own rights under ADA. Explain that ADA:
  - provides for equal employment opportunities for people with disabilities. Explain that the law doesn't mandate for quotas, affirmative action, preferential treatment, or guarantee of job.
  - states that employers must make work-related accommodation for a qualified person with a disability.
  - prohibits discrimination against a qualified person with a disability by a department or agency of any state or local government.
  - requires that programs and services of all state and local governments be readily accessible to and usable by individuals with disabilities.
  - provides for access to public accommodations and services; for example, widening or enlarging doors, removing architectural and communication barriers, or providing alternative arrangements if accommodation isn't possible. This provision affects hotels, theaters, shopping centers, professional offices, pharmacies, banks, schools, health centers, and other establishments.
  - provides for access to telecommunications for people with hearing and speech impairments.

  Discussion of specific provisions of law may help patient to reevaluate past experiences and alert the patient to the possibility of taking appropriate action to assert own rights.
- If the patient requests more information, refer the patient to resources available from the library or Internet *to help increase the patient's knowledge about issues related to disability.* For example, tell the patient to read *Complying with the Americans with Disabilities Act: A Guidebook for Management and People with Disabilities* by Don Fersh and Peter W. Thomas, Esq., published by Greenwood Publishing Group; or to contact Job Accommodation Center at http://askjan.org/media/index.htm.

Suggested NIC Interventions

Health Care Information Exchange; Health Education; Health System Guidance

Evaluations for Expected Outcomes

- Patient expresses desire to obtain information about ADA.
- Patient demonstrates initiative in searching for information about ADA and develops realistic understanding of rights under ADA.
- Patient identifies specific changes the patient will seek in response to information about ADA, such as accommodation to disabilities by employer.

Documentation

- Patient's statements of desire for information related to disability
- Patient's stated goals of learning more about rights of disabled under law
- Methods used to teach patient
- Patient's statements indicating enhanced understanding of ADA
- Evaluations for expected outcomes

REFERENCES

25th Anniversary of the Americans with Disabilities Act—July 2015. (cover story). (2015). *MMWR: Morbidity & Mortality Weekly Report*, *64*(29), 777.

Douglas, M. D., Dawes, D. E., Holden, K. B., & Mack, D. (2015). Missed policy opportunities to advance health equity by recording demographic data in electronic health records. *American Journal of Public Health*, *105*, S380–S388. doi:10.2105/AJPH.2014.302384

Stoelzle, H., & Sames, K. (2014). Disabilities act compliance of fitness facilities in an American metropolitan area. *International Journal of Therapy & Rehabilitation*, *21*(4), 169–174.

U.S. Department of Justice Civil Rights Division. (n.d.). *Information and technical assistance of the Americans with disabilities act*. Retrieved from http://www.ada.gov/

DEFICIENT KNOWLEDGE

related to insufficient information

Definition

Absence or deficiency of cognitive information related to a specific topic

Assessment

- Psychosocial status, including age, developmental stage, learning ability, decision-making ability, health beliefs and attitudes, interest in learning, knowledge and skills regarding current health problem, obstacles to learning, financial resources, support systems, and usual coping pattern
- Neurologic status, including level of consciousness, memory, mental status, and orientation

Defining Characteristics

- Inaccurate follow-through of instruction
- Inaccurate performance on a test
- Inappropriate behavior (e.g., hysterical, hostile, agitated, apathetic)
- Insufficient knowledge

Expected Outcomes

- Patient will keep insurance card, written material about plan requirements, and name and phone numbers of primary care physician and managed care plan readily available.
- Patient will express understanding of how to use managed care plan, discuss benefits of managed care, and describe role of primary care physician.
- Patient will demonstrate understanding of co-payments, deductibles, and other financial issues and will explain how to get additional information, when needed.
- Patient will schedule preventive screening appointments to which the patient is entitled.

Suggested NOC Outcomes

Knowledge: Health Behavior; Knowledge: Health Resources; Knowledge: Illness Care

Interventions and Rationales

- Allow the patient time to identify frustrations about managed care. *Managed care concepts are complex and difficult to understand. Providing the patient with an opportunity to express current understanding of managed care may allow you to identify misperceptions. The patient may view managed care as a mechanism for denying the patient's choice of physicians, hospitals, and other health care options.*
- Provide a simple explanation of managed care and its benefits. Point out the advantages and disadvantages of managed care to the health consumer. Explain the difference between an HMO and a PPO in simple terms:
  - HMO stands for Health Maintenance Organization. There are four different HMO models. A staff-model HMO employs physicians who care for enrollees. In network, group practice, and individual practice association models, the HMO contracts directly with physicians, either individually or in groups, to provide care to their enrollees.
  - PPO stands for Preferred Provider Organization. This is a slightly more flexible type of plan. It's less restrictive than an HMO but has many built-in safeguards. In this case, the managed care organization contracts with a group of selected or preferred providers for its members. These physicians then agree to accept whatever reimbursement the PPO determines is fair.

  Understanding the structure of managed care may help patients who are accustomed to fee-for-service plans adjust to a new system.
- Review the highlights of the patient's plan. Explain the importance of keeping the insurance card and phone numbers for the plan handy at all times. *A better understanding of how to use the plan will enhance the patient's opportunity to obtain needed health care.*
- Explore the patient's understanding of the primary care physician's role. Stress the importance of always going through a primary care physician to meet health care needs. *Understanding the primary care physician's role is the key to using a managed care plan successfully.*
- Determine what screening examinations are covered under the plan and how often they're allowed. Screening examinations may include routine physical examinations, mammograms, prostate-specific antigen screening, eye examinations, and other procedures. *Accessing these benefits may allow for the diagnosis of major illnesses at an earlier stage.*
- Have the patient incorporate learned material into a plan that defines how to use a managed care plan for specific medical problems, how and when to obtain referrals, and whom to contact for billing problems. *Developing a plan allows the patient to use new information and receive feedback.*
- Urge the patient to ask questions *to clarify the need for further information and allow you to evaluate the patient's understanding.*

Suggested NIC Interventions

Health Education; Health System Guidance; Learning Facilitation; Teaching: Disease Process

Evaluations for Expected Outcomes

- Patient carries insurance card and keeps essential phone numbers readily available for self or caregivers.
- Patient expresses understanding of how to use managed care plan, discusses benefits of plan, and describes role of primary care physician.

- Patient demonstrates understanding of co-payments, deductibles, and other financial issues, and explains how to get additional information, when needed.
- Patient schedules preventive screening appointments.

Documentation

- Information provided to patient
- Patient's response to teaching
- Appointments made by patient as a result of teaching
- Evaluations for expected outcomes

REFERENCES

Ely, L. T. (2015). Nurse-managed clinics: Barriers and benefits toward financial sustainability when integrating primary care and mental health. *Nursing Economics*, *33*(4), 193–203.
Howard, S. W., Bernell, S. L., Yoon, J., Luck, J., & Ranit, C. M. (2015). Point–counterpoint. Oregon's experiment in health care delivery and payment reform: Coordinated care organizations replacing managed care. *Journal of Health Politics, Policy & Law*, *40*(1), 245–255.
Quinn, K. (2015). The 8 basic payment methods in health care. *Annals of Internal Medicine*, *163*(4), 300–306. doi:10.7326/M14-2784

IMBALANCED NUTRITION: LESS THAN BODY REQUIREMENTS

related to economically disadvantaged

Definition

Intake of nutrients insufficient to meet metabolic needs

Assessment

Adult

- Age, sex, height, and weight
- Nutritional history, hereditary influences, usual daily intake, meal preparation habits, and use of alcohol or drugs
- Cultural influences, including education level, occupation, nationality, or ethnic group; beliefs, values, and attitudes about health and illness; and health practices and customs

Child

- Parents' educational level and knowledge of child development
- Home environment and financial resources
- Child's capabilities, including communication skills, motor skills, cognitive abilities, and socialization skills

Defining Characteristics

- Abdominal cramping
- Abdominal pain
- Alteration in taste sensation
- Body weight 20% or more below ideal weight range
- Capillary fragility
- Diarrhea
- Excessive hair loss
- Food aversion

- Food intake less than recommended daily allowance
- Hyperactive bowel sounds
- Insufficient information
- Insufficient interest in food
- Insufficient muscle tone
- Misinformation
- Misperception
- Pale mucous membranes
- Perceived inability to ingest food
- Satiety immediately upon ingesting food
- Sore buccal cavity
- Weakness of muscles required for mastication
- Weakness of muscles required for swallowing
- Weight loss with adequate food intake

Expected Outcomes

- Patient will describe reasons for not obtaining adequate nutrition.
- Patient will state food preferences.
- Patient will consume adequate calories daily. Specify ______ calories
- Patient will gain a specified amount of weight weekly. Specify _____ lb/week
- Patient will eat independently without constant encouragement.
- Patient will use community resources to improve nutritional status as needed.

Suggested NOC Outcomes

Nutritional Status; Nutritional Status: Nutrient Intake; Weight Control

Interventions and Rationales

Adult

- Identify patients who don't have resources to eat properly or who neglect nutritional needs. *Nurses working in community settings frequently encounter patients whose nutritional needs aren't met. Nursing responsibilities include identifying these individuals and intervening on their behalf.*
- Encourage the patient to discuss reasons for not eating *to assess the cause of the problem and develop a care plan.*
- Determine the patient's food preferences, and attempt to obtain preferred foods. Offer foods that appeal to the senses *to enhance the patient's appetite.*
- Suggest the patient eats high-protein, high-calorie foods *to prevent body protein breakdown and provide caloric energy.*
- If the patient is eligible for food stamps, help the patient obtain them and teach the patient how to use them *to buy foods that provide well-balanced meals.*
- Depending on the patient's resources, help locate soup kitchens for the homeless, senior centers that serve meals for a nominal fee, Meals On Wheels, or similar programs *to promote access to appropriate community resources.*

Child

- Assess the child for evidence of balanced nutrition patterns. Stress to the parents the importance of good nutrition *to reinforce to the child and parents the value of good nutrition in relation to growth and development.*
- Encourage the child to take advantage of a school breakfast program *to begin the school day with adequate nutrients.*
- Determine the child's food preferences *to use as a basis for teaching the child and parents.*
- PCC Teach the child and parents about required daily nutrients. Stress the need for the parents to supervise the child's meals. *Parental support helps the child develop good eating habits.*

PCC • If you work in a school, confer with teachers to develop stimulating lessons on nutrition. *Working together, teachers and school nurses can reinforce lessons about nutrition.*
- Document cases of undernourished children and noncompliant parents. If necessary, refer the family to an appropriate social service agency. *Cases in which parents can't or won't cooperate on the child's behalf may require further intervention.*

Suggested NIC Interventions

Eating Disorders Management; Nutrition Management; Nutritional Counseling; Weight Gain Assistance

Evaluations for Expected Outcomes

- Patient describes reasons for not obtaining adequate nutrition.
- Patient states food preferences.
- Patient consumes adequate calories daily.
- Patient gains a specified amount of weight weekly.
- Patient eats independently without constant encouragement.
- Patient uses community resources as needed.

Documentation

- Patient's weight
- Daily intake
- Teaching provided
- Referrals
- Patient's response to nursing interventions
- Evaluations for expected outcomes

REFERENCES

Nordén, J., Grönberg, A. M., Bosaeus, I., Forslund, H. B., Hulthén, L., Rothenberg, E., . . . Slinde, F. (2015). Nutrition impact symptoms and body composition in patients with COPD. *European Journal of Clinical Nutrition*, *69*(2), 256–261. doi:10.1038/ejcn.2014.76

Rocks, T., Pelly, F., & Wilkinson, P. (2014). Nutritional management of anorexia nervosa in children and adolescent inpatients: The current practice of Australian dietitians. *Nutrition & Dietetics*, *71*(2), 100–107. doi:10.1111/1747-0080.12058

Tuval-Mashiach, R., Hasson-Ohayon, I., & Ilan, A. (2014). Attacks on linking: Stressors and identity challenges for mothers of daughters with long lasting anorexia nervosa. *Psychology & Health*, *29*(6), 613–631. doi:10.1080/08870446.2013.879135

RISK FOR POISONING

Definition

Vulnerable to accidental exposure to, or ingestion of, drugs or dangerous products in sufficient doses, which may compromise health

Assessment

- Age and gender
- Results of test for blood lead concentration

- Sources of lead in child's environment, such as living in or frequently visiting older building, living in area with heavy traffic, or living near lead smelter
- Occupations and hobbies of family members that include use of lead
- Cultural use of folk remedies that contain lead
- History of pica, such as biting nails or sucking on pencils or other items
- Nutritional deficiencies, such as inadequate amounts of protein, iron, calcium, and zinc
- Mental status, including ability to concentrate and mental acuity
- History of developmental delays
- Behavior such as irritability, restlessness, and hyperactivity

Risk Factors

External

- Access to dangerous product
- Access to illicit drugs potentially contaminated by poisonous additives
- Access to large supply of pharmaceutical agents in house
- Access to pharmaceutical agent

Internal

- Alteration in cognitive functioning
- Emotional disturbance
- Inadequate precautions against poisoning
- Insufficient knowledge of pharmacologic agents
- Insufficient knowledge of poisoning prevention
- Occupational setting without adequate safeguards
- Reduced vision

Expected Outcomes

- Laboratory tests will indicate blood lead concentration less than 9 mcg/dL.
- Patient will have no signs or symptoms of elevated blood lead levels.
- Environmental factors for lead poisoning in home will be eliminated as much as possible.
- Parents and teachers will demonstrate understanding of safety guidelines and will promote them at home and in school.
- Children will practice safety measures to prevent lead poisoning.

Suggested NOC Outcomes

Personal Safety Behavior; Physical Injury Severity; Safe Home Environment

Interventions and Rationales

- Assess the patient for anemia, distractibility, hearing impairment, hyperactivity, impulsivity, and mild intellectual deficit *to detect low-dose lead poisoning. Blindness, coma, seizures, mental retardation, or paralysis may indicate high-dose poisoning.*
- If there's any indication that a child needs blood level tested, request an order to have a test performed. *Early intervention reduces levels and prevents more serious complications. When children are registered for preschool, kindergarten, or first grade, their blood should be tested for elevated lead levels. All children under age 6, or as state regulations dictate, should be tested for elevated blood lead levels.*

- In cases of elevated blood levels, communicate with the child's primary physician to determine what actions must be taken. *Nursing responsibilities include following up when the child's health may be jeopardized.*
- PCC Set up educational programs for children, parents, and teachers about the dangers of lead poisoning. Tailor the sessions to the appropriate educational level. *Education is the first defense against lead poisoning.* Make sure parents understand these critical concepts:
  - Before eating, carefully wash hands with hot soapy water. *Dirt and dust on hands may contain lead that may be ingested while eating.*
  - Teach children to keep hands, toys, and all other objects out of their mouth *because they contain dirt.* Wash pacifiers and other items meant to be put into the mouth (especially if the item falls on the floor or other dirty surface).
  - Provide children with a healthful, balanced diet to ensure that they receive adequate amounts of iron, protein, calcium, and zinc. Be sure to provide fresh fruits, vegetables, whole grains, and meat. *Eating regularly is important because lead is absorbed more quickly on an empty stomach.*
  - Allow water to run for 2 minutes before using for drinking, cooking, or making formula *to decrease amount of lead in water.* This is especially important in areas where lead content of water is high.
  - Don't store food in open cans, and be cautious about using cookware and ceramic dishes that may contain lead or may have been fired incorrectly. *These can be insidious sources of lead.*
- Assess whether the child or family members use folk remedies. *Various cultures use folk remedies that contain large quantities of lead. For example, Mexican azarcon and greta (both nearly 100% lead) and Asian* pay-loo-ah *are used as remedies for diarrhea and vomiting.* Suggest alternative remedies to these highly toxic compounds.
- PCC Teach parents to be alert for stomach aches, irritability, and headaches. *These may be early signs of higher-than-normal lead levels.*

Suggested NIC Interventions

Environmental Management: Safety; Health Education; Home Maintenance Assistance; Surveillance: Safety

Evaluations for Expected Outcomes

- Screening results show normal blood lead levels.
- Patient doesn't have signs and symptoms of elevated blood lead levels.
- Environmental factors for lead poisoning in home are eliminated.
- Parents and teachers promote safety guidelines at home and in school.
- Children practice safety measures to prevent lead poisoning.

Documentation

- Blood lead levels
- Physical and behavioral manifestations of elevated blood lead levels
- Referrals to physician for treatment and follow-up visits
- Teaching provided
- Response to nursing interventions
- Evaluations for expected outcomes

REFERENCES

Hanna-Attisha, M., LaChance, J., Casey Sadler, R., & Champney Schnepp, A. (2016). Elevated blood lead levels in children associated with the flint drinking water crisis: A spatial analysis of risk and public health response. *American Journal of Public Health*, *106*(2), 283–290. doi:10.2105/AJPH.2015.303003

Rogers, M. L., Lucht, J. A., Sylvaria, A. J., Cigna, J., Vanderslice, R., & Vivier, P. M. (2014). Primary prevention of lead poisoning: Protecting children from unsafe housing. *American Journal of Public Health*, *104*(8), e119–e124. doi:10.2105/AJPH.2014.301908

Schnur, J., & John, R. M. (2014). Childhood lead poisoning and the new centers for disease control and prevention guidelines for lead exposure. *Journal of the American Association of Nurse Practitioners*, *26*(5), 238–247. doi:10.1002/2327-6924.12112

RISK FOR CAREGIVER ROLE STRAIN

Definition

Vulnerable to difficulty in performing the family/significant other caregiver role, which may compromise health

Assessment

- Caregiver's age, gender, and general health
- Cultural status, including level of education, occupation, nationality, area of residence (rural, suburban, or urban), beliefs and attitudes about Alzheimer's disease, and race, ethnicity, and religion
- Family status, including caregiver's relationship to patient, roles, rules, communication skills, family subsystems, support network, ability of family members to meet caregiver's and patient's physical and emotional needs, social and economic factors, coping patterns, and evidence of abuse
- Caregiver's psychological status, including quality of relationship with patient, sense of self-worth, hobbies, recreational activities, and recent life changes
- Patient's self-care status, including functional ability and ability to perform activities of daily living (ADLs)
- Caregiver's spiritual status, including religious affiliation, religious practices, and attitudes about life, death, suffering, and faith

Risk Factors

- Alteration in cognitive functioning in care receiver
- Care receiver discharges home with significant needs
- Care receiver exhibits bizarre behavior
- Care receiver exhibits deviant behavior
- Caregiver health impairment
- Caregiver isolation
- Caregiver not developmentally ready for caregiver role
- Caregiver's competing role commitments
- Caregiving task complexity
- Codependency
- Congenital disorder
- Developmental delay
- Developmental delay of caregiver
- Excessive caregiving activities
- Exposure to violence
- Extended duration of caregiving required
- Family isolation
- Female caregiver
- Illness severity of care receiver
- Inadequate physical environment for providing care
- Ineffective caregiver coping pattern

- Ineffective family adaptation
- Inexperience with caregiving
- Instability in care receiver's health
- Insufficient caregiver recreation
- Insufficient respite for caregiver
- Partner as caregiver
- Pattern of family dysfunction prior to the caregiving situation
- Pattern of ineffective relationship between caregiver and care receiver
- Prematurity
- Presence of abuse (e.g., physical, psychological, sexual)
- Psychological disorder in caregiver
- Psychological disorder in care receiver
- Stressors
- Substance abuse
- Unpredictability of illness trajectory

Expected Outcomes

- Caregiver will realistically describe current obligations and challenges that lie ahead.
- Caregiver will distinguish obligations she must fulfill from those that she can control or limit.
- In conjunction with nurse, caregiver will develop care plan for patient and demonstrate ability to follow care plan.
- Caregiver will exhibit positive sense of self-worth.
- Caregiver will describe emotional response to caring for patient.
- Caregiver will express less role strain.
- Caregiver will describe help available from informal and formal support systems in community and will take steps to obtain help.

Suggested NOC Outcomes

Caregiver Emotional Health; Caregiver Performance: Direct Care; Caregiver Home Care Readiness; Caregiver Physical Health; Caregiving Endurance Potential; Caregiver Well-Being

Interventions and Rationales

- Assess the caregiver's stress level. Several tools allow such assessment, including one in the book *Alzheimer's: A Caregiver's Guide and Sourcebook* by Howard Gruetzner. *Pinpointing specific areas of stress will enable the nurse to assist the caregiver more precisely in developing a "stress relief" plan.*
- Describe the five stages of Alzheimer's disease to the caregiver (early and late confusional states and early, middle, and late dementia). Discuss the characteristics of each stage and ways to respond to the behavioral problems of each stage. *Understanding the progressive nature of the disease will help the caregiver cope and adapt to each new stage.*
- PCC Help the caregiver develop a realistic care plan that considers the patient's abilities and limitations. The plan will require modification as the patient decompensates. *A plan provides consistency for both the caregiver and the patient.*
- Instruct the caregiver to encourage the patient to participate in social and self-care activities, such as bathing, dressing, dining out with friends, and playing cards, to the greatest extent possible. *Allowing the patient to become dependent too soon increases the caregiver's stress.*
- Facilitate a family meeting to help the primary caregiver seek assistance from other family members. *The caregiver may feel guilty about asking for help. A nurse's presence may lend support and validity to the request for assistance and decrease the caregiver's feelings of guilt and embarrassment.*

- Support the caregiver and family members as they adjust to the degenerative nature of the disease. Be aware that over time the stress associated with caring for the patient increases. *Providing ongoing support will help family members avoid physical and emotional problems associated with stress.*
- PCC Identify community resources that may offer the caregiver relief from constant supervision of the patient. Examples of resources include home health nursing assistants, respite care, and adult day care. *Caregivers can use outside resources to provide care for the patient while the caregiver tends to her own needs.*
- PCC Help the caregiver contact informal sources of support, such as religious groups, extended family, and community volunteers, *for support and relief.*
- S If the patient is taking drug therapy for Alzheimer's disease, ensure that the caregiver understands dosages, adverse effects, and signs and symptoms to report to the physician. *Patients receiving drug therapy for Alzheimer's disease require careful monitoring.*
- Encourage the caregiver to accept help from a care manager, *who can coordinate the patient's care.*
- PCC Encourage the caregiver to attend an Alzheimer's support group *for an opportunity to interact with people who share similar experiences.*
- PCC Refer the caregiver to the Alzheimer's Association *so the caregiver can be aware of current advances in treatment.*

Suggested NIC Interventions

Caregiver Support; Coping Enhancement; Decision-Making Support; Family Involvement Promotion; Respite Care; Referral

Evaluations for Expected Outcomes

- Caregiver develops realistic assessment of situation.
- Caregiver distinguishes obligations that must be fulfilled from those the caregiver can control or limit.
- Caregiver develops care plan for patient and demonstrates ability to carry out the plan.
- Caregiver exhibits positive sense of self-worth.
- Caregiver describes emotional response to caring for patient.
- Caregiver expresses less role strain.
- Caregiver describes and accepts help from informal and formal support systems and resources.

Documentation

- Caregiver's comments related to:
  - Fatigue
  - Family members' reactions to caregiver's experience
  - Feelings about patient's behavior
  - Financial concerns
  - Contact with friends or feelings of isolation
  - Attendance at support group meetings
  - Feelings of self-worth
- Contacts made in community on behalf of caregiver
- Evaluations for expected outcomes

REFERENCES

del-Pino-Casado, R., Pérez-Cruz, M., & Frías-Osuna, A. (2014). Coping, subjective burden and anxiety among family caregivers of older dependents. *Journal of Clinical Nursing*, *23*(23/24), 3335–3344. doi:10.1111/jocn.12561

Smith-Johnson, B., Davis, B. L., Burns, D., Montgomery, A. J., & McGee, Z. T. (2015). African American wives and perceived stressful experiences: Providing care for stroke survivor spouses. *ABNF Journal*, *26*(2), 39–42.

Zeleníková, R., Kozáková, R., & Jarošová, D. (2014). Clinical validation of the nursing diagnosis caregiver role strain in the Czech Republic. *International Journal of Nursing Knowledge*, *25*(2), 80–84. doi:10.1111/2047-3095.12020

READINESS FOR ENHANCED SPIRITUAL WELL-BEING

related to parish nursing

Definition

A pattern of experiencing and integrating meaning and purpose in life through connectedness with self, others, art, music, literature, nature, and/or a power greater than oneself, which can be strengthened

Assessment

- Spiritual status, including personal religious habits; religious or church affiliation; perceptions of life, faith, death, and suffering; support network; embarrassment at practicing religious rituals; opposition to beliefs by family, peers, or health care providers; and conflicts with belief system
- Health history, including medical conditions that change body image, chronic or terminal illness, and debilitating disease
- Psychological status, including reactions to illness and disability, job loss, loss through separation or death, relationships with peers, and change in appetite, energy level, motivation, personal hygiene, self-image, and sleep habits
- Self-care status, including neurologic, musculoskeletal, sensory, or psychological impairment and ability to carry out activities and adapt
- Family status, including marital status, communication skills and methods of conflict resolution, cultural factors that affect health practices, socioeconomic factors, family goals, family health history, ability of family to meet physical, social, and emotional needs

Defining Characteristics

Connections to Self

- Expresses desire to enhance acceptance
- Expresses desire to enhance coping
- Expresses desire to enhance courage
- Expresses desire to enhance hope
- Expresses desire to enhance joy
- Expresses desire to enhance love
- Expresses desire to enhance meaning in life
- Expresses desire to enhance meditative practice
- Expresses desire to enhance purpose in life

- Expresses desire to enhance satisfaction with philosophy of life
- Expresses desire to enhance self-forgiveness
- Expresses desire to enhance serenity (e.g., peace)
- Expresses desire to enhance surrender

Connections with Others

- Expresses desire to enhance forgiveness from others
- Expresses desire to enhance interaction with significant other
- Expresses desire to enhance interaction with spiritual leaders
- Expresses desire to enhance service to others

Connections with Art, Music, Literature, and Nature

- Expresses desire to enhance creative energy (e.g., writing, poetry, music)
- Expresses desire to enhance spiritual reading
- Expresses desire to enhance time outdoors
- Expresses desire to enhance mystical experiences
- Expresses desire to enhance participation in religious activity
- Expresses desire to enhance prayerfulness
- Expresses desire to enhance reverence

Expected Outcomes

- Patient will discuss spiritual concerns.
- Patient will meet with appropriate religious figure.
- Patient will openly discuss effect of illness on beliefs and other spiritual issues.
- Patient will receive referrals for continued support.
- Patient will receive support in an effort to pursue enhanced spiritual well-being.

Suggested NOC Outcomes

Dignified Life Closure; Hope; Quality of Life; Spiritual Health

Interventions and Rationales

- Assess the patient's desire for spiritual intervention as part of care *to promote physical, emotional, and spiritual health.*
- Listen attentively to the patient's concerns *to ascertain the impact of spirituality on the patient's life.*
- Encourage patient to discuss health concerns or other circumstances that affect spiritual outlook. Discuss spirituality if patient wishes to do so. *This reduces the patient's feeling of isolation and allows for open discussion of spiritual distress.*
- Discuss ways in which the patient believes the community can provide support. *Learning how the patient defines own expectations will help you assess the feasibility of meeting expectations.*
- Help the patient determine a mechanism for soliciting support from the community, such as placing a request for assistance in a religiously affiliated bulletin or requesting a visit from a member of the clergy. *The patient may know the type of support that is needed but may not know how to go about getting it.*
- Demonstrate to the patient that you're willing to discuss issues related to spirituality or to pray with the patient. Keep an open mind. Keep the conversation focused on the patient's spiritual values *to maintain the therapeutic value of interaction between patient and nurse.*

PCC
- Provide information about other community resources that might benefit the patient and family members *to help provide continuity of care.*

Suggested NIC Interventions

Spiritual Growth Facilitation; Spiritual Support; Values Clarification; Referral

Evaluations for Expected Outcomes

- Patient discusses spiritual concerns.
- Patient receives opportunity to meet with clergy member.
- Patient openly discusses effects of illness on beliefs and other spiritual issues.
- Patient receives referrals for continued support.
- Patient recognizes and verbalizes support given to own efforts to pursue enhanced spiritual well-being.

Documentation

- Spiritual needs as defined by patient and nurse
- Interventions initiated by nurse
- Referrals to outside agencies
- Patient's statements about spiritual well-being
- Evaluations for expected outcomes

REFERENCES

Taylor, E. J., Park, C. G., & Pfeiffer, J. B. (2014). Nurse religiosity and spiritual care. *Journal of Advanced Nursing*, *70*(11), 2612–2621. doi:10.1111/jan.12446

Wordsworth, H., Moore, R., & Woodhouse, D. (2016). Parish nursing: A unique resource for community and district nurses. *British Journal of Community Nursing*, *21*(2), 66–74. doi:10.12968/bjcn.2016.21.2.66

Yilmaz, M., & Gurler, H. (2014). The efficacy of integrating spirituality into undergraduate nursing curricula. *Nursing Ethics*, *21*(8), 929–945. doi:10.1177/0969733014521096

IMPAIRED SPONTANEOUS VENTILATION

related to home ventilation therapy

Definition

Decreased energy reserves resulting in an inability to maintain independent breathing that is adequate to support life

Assessment

- Age and sex
- Health history, including previous respiratory problems, neurologic or neuromuscular disease, and recent hospitalization
- Respiratory status, including rate and depth of respiration, chest excursion and symmetry, presence of cyanosis, use of accessory muscles for respiration, effectiveness of cough, suctioning demands, and sputum characteristics
- Neuromuscular strength and endurance

- Mental and emotional status, including cognitive state and ability to follow directions
- Functional status, including ability to perform ADLs
- Family status, including usual coping patterns, family roles, communication patterns, financial resources, effect of patient's illness on family, and beliefs and attitudes about health, illness, death, and other issues
- Home environment, including electrical safety, availability of hot water, house layout, lighting, and fire hazards
- Knowledge of safety precautions

Defining Characteristics

- Alteration in metabolism
- Apprehensiveness
- Decrease in arterial oxygen saturation
- Decrease in cooperation
- Decrease in partial pressure of oxygen
- Decrease in tidal volume
- Dyspnea
- Increase in accessory muscle use
- Increase in heart rate
- Increase in partial pressure of carbon dioxide
- Restlessness

Expected Outcomes

- Patient will exhibit clear breath sounds.
- Patient won't exhibit signs of respiratory distress or infection.
- Patient will incorporate mechanical ventilation into ADLs and family life.
- Patient will demonstrate adequate use of communication aids.
- Patient will remain free from complications.
- Caregiver will demonstrate ease in using equipment and procedures to keep patient comfortable and free from infection.
- Caregiver will implement and maintain safety measures for using oxygen in home.

Suggested NOC Outcomes

Respiratory Status: Gas Exchange; Respiratory Status: Ventilation; Vital Signs

Interventions and Rationales

- Ascertain what the patient and family members know about home ventilation therapy *to determine what the patient needs to learn. Building on current knowledge enhances learning.*
- PCC Teach the patient and family members the setup, use, and care of all parts of the equipment *to promote independence and decrease anxiety.*
- S Explain the meanings of ventilator alarms and what to do if alarms sound *to help reduce anxiety and minimize complications.*
- Explain how to get help in case of emergency *to decrease the potential for injury.*
- PCC Emphasize the importance of the patient's involvement in family activities, even though the patient is on mechanical ventilation, *to increase the patient's sense of well-being.*
- S Emphasize to family members that the patient needs to be attended to at all times *to ensure ongoing care.*
- PCC Demonstrate to family members how to clean and disinfect equipment *to ensure that the patient doesn't develop an infection.*
- PCC Teach home oxygen safety *to avoid fire or injury to the patient and family members.*

- Inform the patient and family members about signs and symptoms of complications, such as atelectasis, fluid overload, respiratory infection, and tension pneumothorax. Encourage immediate reporting of complications *to ensure early intervention for respiratory distress.*

Suggested NIC Interventions

Airway Management; Mechanical Ventilation; Respiratory Monitoring; Vital Signs Monitoring

Evaluations for Expected Outcomes

- Patient has clear breath sounds.
- Patient doesn't exhibit respiratory distress or infection.
- Patient incorporates mechanical ventilation into daily life.
- Patient demonstrates use of communication aids.
- Patient remains free from complications.
- Caregiver demonstrates ease in using equipment and procedures to keep patient comfortable and free from infection.
- Caregiver implements and maintains safety measures for using oxygen in home.

Documentation

- Assessment results, such as vital signs and breath sounds
- Checks of ventilator settings, alarms, and backup equipment
- Arterial blood gas analysis results
- Patient's response to respiratory treatment
- Patient's response to nursing interventions
- Patient teaching and patient's and family members' responses to teaching
- Evaluations for expected outcomes

REFERENCES

Laakso, K., Markström, A., Havstam, C., Idvall, M., & Hartelius, L. (2014). Communicating with individuals receiving home mechanical ventilation: The experiences of key communication partners. *Disability & Rehabilitation*, *36*(11–13), 875–883. doi:10.3109/09638288.2013.822572

Manhas, K. P., & Mitchell, I. (2015). (Dis)-Trust in transitioning ventilator-dependent children from hospital to homecare. *Nursing Ethics*, *22*(8), 913–927. doi:10.1177/0969733014551598

Warlan, H., & Howland, L. (2015). Posttraumatic stress syndrome associated with stays in the intensive care unit: Importance of nurses' involvement. *Critical Care Nurse*, *35*(3), 44–54. doi:10.4037/ccn2015758

PART VIII

Wellness

APPLYING EVIDENCE-BASED PRACTICE

The Question

Do physical activity programs in the community preserve mobility in older adults who are in poor health?

Evidence-Based Resources

Administration on Aging. (n.d.). *Aging statistics*. Retrieved March 30, 2016, from http://www.aoa.acl.gov/aging_statistics/index.aspx

Bethancourt, H. J., Rosenberg, D. E., Beatty, T., & Arterburn, D. E. (2014). Barriers to and facilitators of physical activity program use among older adults. *Clinical Medicine & Research*, *12*(1/2), 10–20. doi:10.3121/cmr.2013.1171

Centers for Disease Control and Prevention. (2015). *The benefits of physical activity*. Retrieved from http://www.cdc.gov/physicalactivity/basics/pa-health/

Pahor, M., Guralnik, J. M., Ambrosius, W. T., Blair, S., Bonds, D. E., Church, T. S., . . . Williamson, J. D. (2014). Effect of structured physical activity on prevention of major mobility disability in older adults: The LIFE study randomized clinical trial. *Journal of the American Medical Association*, *311*(23), 2387–2396. doi:10.1001/jama.2014.5616

Yang, H., Chen, K., Chen, M., Wu, H., Chang, W., Wang, Y., & Huang, H. (2015). Applying the transtheoretical model to promote functional fitness of community older adults participating in elastic band exercises. *Journal of Advanced Nursing*, *71*(10), 2338–2349. doi:10.1111/jan.12705

Yao, L., Foley, K. T., Kolanowski, A. M., & Smith, B. A. (2014). Proto Tai Chi: In search of a promising group exercise for the frail elderly. *Geriatric Nursing*, *35*(2 Suppl), S21–S26. doi:10.1016/j.gerinurse.2014.02.021

Evaluating the Evidence

The population of adults aged 65 and older is expected to grow to about 98 million by 2060 (Administration on Aging, n.d.). Health promotion that preserves independence and functioning in later years is of great value to older adults. Regular exercise has many health benefits for all ages, but is especially important for older adults to maintain function and ability to perform everyday activities (Centers for Disease Control and Prevention, 2015). Older adults who lose mobility are at greater risk of disability, morbidity, and mortality (Pahor et al., 2014).

Community programs may help to fill the gap of physical fitness needs. Pahor et al. (2014) studied the effects of regular physical activity versus health education on mobility disability over a 2-year period. Education is an important component of health programs; however, Pahor et al. (2014) found that persistent mobility disability was significantly reduced in participants of a structured physical activity program as compared to a health education only program.

A small convenience sample of 24 older adults participated in a study to investigate the effectiveness of group Tai Chi (Yao, Foley, Kolanowski, & Smith, 2014). Tai Chi incorporates physical, motivational, and behavioral elements. The exercise program consisted of 2 days/week at a community center and 3 to 4 days/week at home. Engagement in the program was high with 22 participants attending all scheduled classes. No injuries, falls, or adverse events occurred during exercise. Participants rated the overall program as helpful, fun, and easy to learn.

The Senior Elastic Band (SEB) exercise program addresses common health problems of older adults. The SEB exercise program is well suited for older adults because the only equipment required is one elastic band, the exercises are easy to learn, and the program can be undertaken at home. Yang et al. (2015) completed a 6-month study to investigate the effectiveness of SEB exercise on functional fitness of participants from six senior activity centers. Exercises were performed for 40 minutes, three times a week for 6 months. Participants had significant improvement in fitness and endurance performance at 3- and 6-month evaluations.

Traditional exercise programs may not provide the motivation, instruction, or practice in developing the skills needed for behavior change toward an independent regimen of physical activity. Programs for older adults must be enjoyable, easy to perform, and safe. Factors to consider when developing an exercise program for older adults are physical and mental health, individual preference, physical environment, level of guidance needed, and program characteristics (Bethancourt, Rosenberg, Beatty, & Arterburn, 2014).

Applying the Results and Making a Decision

Evidence suggests that all individuals, including older adults, who participate in regular physical exercise have improved mobility. The most successful and beneficial exercise programs provide participants with consistent moderate activity that does not over stress the body. Participants often lose motivation when programs are too rigid or do not provide a sense of community. Organized programs that are supported by the community yield the most positive results.

Reevaluating Process and Identifying Areas for Improvement

Health promotion and wellness programs should focus on maintaining long-term physical, cognitive, and emotional well-being. Physical activity is important in developing a healthier lifestyle. Community support and organized group exercise programs foster improved health and increased mobility.

INTRODUCTION

For decades, nurses have promoted health in an illness-oriented model of health care. Today, a holistic model of care is encouraged. Care that embraces the whole person with a holistic philosophy optimizes functioning and wellness. This section focuses on assisting individuals, families, and communities to optimize health and wellness by developing care plans that promote healthier lifestyles and emphasize the interconnectedness of body, mind, and spirit.

The focus on holism and wellness has sparked a great deal of interest on the part of health consumers. Complementary and alternative modalities, in addition to traditional medical therapy, are gaining popularity in meeting physiologic, psychological, and spiritual needs. Holistic nursing practice facilitates the healing process and enhances overall wellness.

Wellness plans begin with your assessment. You will want to know about the individual's current health status and past health problems. Encourage the patient to identify areas of strengths and weaknesses of their health. Together with the patient, determine what areas of wellness the patient is most motivated to improve. Your individualized plan of care will focus on those areas.

Establish outcomes the patient expects to achieve. Encourage development of plans that include health goals, appropriate activity levels, diet preferences, and rewards for milestones completed. Because achieving wellness is a process, break the process into outcomes that the individual, family, or community can achieve and measure. Guide the patient in exploring a variety of activities and/or programs that will provide motivation toward meeting chosen goals. Help the patient in developing a plan that is practical and attainable.

While many healthy individuals or groups desire to enhance their levels of wellness, developing wellness plans for patients with chronic diseases may improve functioning and decrease frequent hospitalizations. Older adults may be interested in improving health to control risk factors for problems such as falls. Individuals with physical or mental disabilities, such as limitations in sight, hearing, mobility, intellect, or emotion, will benefit from optimizing the capabilities they possess.

By working together with each patient in your care, you can develop plans that will promote a higher state of wellness.

READINESS FOR ENHANCED CHILDBEARING PROCESS

Definition

A pattern of preparing for and maintaining a healthy pregnancy, childbirth process, and care of the newborn for ensuring well-being, which can be strengthened

Assessment

- Patient's understanding of health problem and treatment plan
- Patient's health status, support systems, expressed concerns regarding childbirth process

Defining Characteristics

During Pregnancy

- Expresses desire to enhance knowledge of childbearing process
- Expresses desire to enhance management of unpleasant pregnancy symptoms

- Expresses desire to enhance prenatal lifestyle (e.g., elimination, exercise, nutrition, personal hygiene, sleep)
- Expresses desire to enhance preparation for newborn

During Labor and Delivery

- Expresses desire to enhance lifestyle appropriate for stage of labor (e.g., elimination, exercise, nutrition, personal hygiene, sleep)
- Expresses desire to enhance proactivity during labor and delivery

After Birth

- Expresses desire to enhance attachment behavior
- Expresses desire to enhance baby care techniques
- Expresses desire to enhance baby feeding techniques
- Expresses desire to enhance breast care
- Expresses desire to enhance safety for the baby
- Expresses desire to enhance postpartum lifestyle (e.g., elimination, exercise, nutrition, personal hygiene, sleep)
- Expresses desire to enhance use of support system

Expected Outcomes

- Patient/childbearing family will demonstrate willingness to maintain/modify lifestyle for optimal prenatal health.
- Patient will convey confidence and knowledge of pregnancy, the labor and delivery process, and newborn care.
- Patient will express appropriate self-control and readily cooperate with recommendations of the health care team during labor and delivery.
- After delivery, parent–newborn attachment will be evident.
- Newborn's physical, social, and nutritional needs will be met.

Suggested NOC Outcomes

Prenatal Health Behavior; Knowledge: Pregnancy; Knowledge: Labor & Delivery; Knowledge: Newborn Care; Parent–Infant Attachment

Interventions and Rationales

- Assess baseline knowledge of prenatal self-care, labor and delivery process, and newborn care *to identify and resolve knowledge deficits.*
- PCC Provide written literature on prenatal wellness, labor and delivery expectations, and newborn care. *Providing written materials allows adequate time to synthesize and understand new information.*
- PCC Teach self-care for common prenatal discomforts *to promote patient autonomy.*
- PCC Teach the childbearing family labor and delivery process, and newborn care. *Understanding expectations improves confidence and reduces anxiety.*
- PCC Assist the childbearing family with development of a birth plan. *This allows childbearing family to participate in managing the birth experience and promotes communication with the health care team.*
- PCC Encourage and support the childbearing family throughout the course of the pregnancy *to improve self-confidence and promote compliance with health recommendations.*

PCC • Refer to Certified Childbirth Educator for classes on prenatal care, labor and delivery (to include cesarean birth), breastfeeding, and newborn care. *Advanced knowledge of the childbearing process promotes empowerment and positive maternal outcomes.*

Suggested NIC Interventions

Anticipatory Guidance; Prenatal Care; Childbirth Preparation; Emotional Support; Parent Education: Infant

Evaluations for Expected Outcomes

- Childbearing family shows willingness to maintain/modify lifestyle for optimal prenatal health.
- Patient conveys confidence related to the labor and delivery process and newborn care.
- Patient accepts recommendations of the health care team during labor and delivery.
- Newborn's physical, social, and nutritional needs are met.

Documentation

- Patient and family statement of lifestyle changes if needed
- Patient's understanding of the labor and delivery process
- Referrals to Certified Childbirth Educator
- Evaluations for expected outcomes

REFERENCES

Daniels, M., & Wedler, J. A. (2015). Enhancing childbirth education through technology. *International Journal of Childbirth Education*, *30*(3), 28–32.
Frazer, C., Hussey, L., Bosch, E., & Squire, M. (2015). Pregnancy apps: A closer look at the implications for childbirth educators. *International Journal of Childbirth Education*, *30*(3), 12–16.
McCants, B. M., & Greiner, J. R. (2016). Prebirth education and childbirth decision making. *International Journal of Childbirth Education*, *31*(1), 24–27.

READINESS FOR ENHANCED COMFORT

Definition

A pattern of ease, relief, and transcendence in physical, psychospiritual, environmental, and/or social dimensions, which can be strengthened

Assessment

- Patient's perception of current state of comfort
- Patient's responsibility for actions taken to maintain a state of comfort
- Support systems, including family members, friends, and clergy
- Attitude of contentment
- Reliance on health care system to resolve complaints

Defining Characteristics

- Expresses desire to enhance comfort
- Expresses desire to enhance feeling of contentment

- Expresses desire to enhance relaxation
- Expresses desire to enhance resolution of complaints

Expected Outcomes

- Patient will express positive perception of nursing assistance to perform activities that promote comfort.
- Patient will experience physical and psychological ease.
- Patient will develop plans to optimize level of comfort.
- Patient will report an increase in relaxation.

Suggested NOC Outcomes

Client Satisfaction; Comfort Level; Comfortable Death; Hope; Personal Autonomy; Personal Well-Being; Quality of Life

Interventions and Rationales

- Assess the patient's satisfaction with the amount of assistance the nurse is currently offering *to determine whether the patient perceives self as performing own physical, psychosocial, and spiritual activities at a level that's comfortable for the patient.*
- PCC Assist the patient in developing plan for increasing comfort *to maximize the patient's level of contentment and rest.*
- Implement a program to promote resolution of complaints *to prevent or alleviate the patient's stress or discomfort.*
- PCC Involve staff, family, and community in promoting the patient's comfort *to include all resources that can contribute to the patient's comfort and well-being.*
- PCC Teach the patient methods of deep breathing, meditation, and guided imagery *in order to reduce anxiety and promote enhanced comfort.*
- Provide pharmacologic relief when ordered to relieve symptoms related to discomfort. *Making the patient comfortable helps the patient cooperate in a more positive way with treatment.*

Suggested NIC Interventions

Coping Enhancement; Emotional Support; Environmental Management: Comfort; Touch

Evaluations for Expected Outcomes

- Patient expresses positive perception of nursing assistance with activities that promote comfort.
- Patient reports feelings of encouragement, acceptance, and reassurance during times of stress.
- Patient develops plan to adapt to perceived stressors, changes, and interferences with a state of comfort.
- Patient expresses an increase in relaxation and level of comfort.

Documentation

- Patient's perception of level of comfort
- Patient's plan for increasing comfort

- Community resources that exist to increase patient comfort
- Future plans to address comfort and contentment
- Evaluations for expected outcomes

REFERENCES

de Azevedo Ponte, K. M., & de Fátima da Silva, L. (2015). Comfort as a result of nursing care: An integrative review. *Revista de Pesquisa: Cuidado é Fundamental*, 7(2), 2603–2614. doi:10.9789/2175-5361.2015.v7i2.2603-2614

Serrano, B., Baños, R. M., & Botella, C. (2016). Virtual reality and stimulation of touch and smell for inducing relaxation: A randomized controlled trial. *Computers in Human Behavior*, *55*, 1–8. doi:10.1016/j.chb.2015.08.007

Slatyer, S., Williams, A. M., & Michael, R. (2015). Seeking empowerment to comfort patients in severe pain: A grounded theory study of the nurse's perspective. *International Journal of Nursing Studies*, *52*(1), 229–239. doi:10.1016/j.ijnurstu.2014.06.010

READINESS FOR ENHANCED COMMUNICATION

related to wellness diagnosis

Definition

A pattern of exchanging information and ideas with others, which can be strengthened

Assessment

- Gender and age as variables in communication patterns
- Developmental history of communication patterns and practices
- Effect of stress on communication
- Family history of communication patterns
- Cultural and religious communication patterns
- Knowledge of difference between passive, aggressive, and assertive patterns of communication

Defining Characteristics

- Expresses desire to enhance communication

Expected Outcomes

- Patient will express message clearly as evidenced by feedback that receiver understood the message.
- Patient will express an increased sense of confidence in communicating thoughts and feelings to nurse, family, health care teams, and any kind of reference groups in which an individual participates (e.g., friends, school groups, community groups, faith groups, etc.) throughout the life span and the continuum of care.
- Patient will report enhanced ability to respond assertively to individuals who relate with passive or aggressive communication styles.
- Patient will report feelings of confidence in social encounters because of enhanced communication skills.
- Patient will gain practice in applying enhanced communication techniques with individuals, family, and groups.

- Patient communication will be enhanced by nonverbal means, such as use of electronic mail and Internet connections, pictures, and drawings.
- Patient will use enhanced communication skills to negotiate and advocate for self with health care providers and in conflict situations.

Suggested NOC Outcomes

Communication: Expressive; Communication: Receptive; Health-Seeking Behaviors

Interventions and Rationales

- Establish a clear purpose for interaction. *This provides the patient with goals and a time frame for interaction.*
- Provide environment that diminishes physical space between nurse and patient to eliminate barriers to communications such as noise and lack of privacy. *Reducing barriers to communication nonverbally communicates to patient that nurse wants to be involved with patient.*
- Use verbal and nonverbal communication patterns that integrate warmth, genuineness, empathy, and respect to facilitate patient empowerment and relationship building. *Therapeutic nurse–patient relationship building increases patient's feeling of security. The nurse modeling caring behaviors encourages patient to incorporate the same attitudes.*
- Provide support through active listening, appropriate periods of silence, reflection of feelings, and paraphrasing and summarizing comments. *Active listening techniques encourage increased patient participation in communication.*
- Incorporate questions that are open-ended, and start with such words as "what," "how," and "could," rather than "why." *Open-ended, nonthreatening questioning encourages patient to discuss issues of concern and improve communication skills.*
- Refrain from interrupting, changing subject, revealing too much personal information about self, or responding too quickly to questions during interactions. *Skillful role modeling of positive communication skills keeps focus on patient.*
- Encourage patient verbally and nonverbally to explore strategies to enhance self-advocacy communication skills with health care providers. *Self-advocacy communication skills can guide patient toward autonomy, confidence, and independence.*
- Avoid critical, overprotective, or over-controlling communication patterns when working with patient. *Positive communication patterns reflect respect and facilitate development of patient trust and relationship building.*
- Include role playing as a teaching strategy to model methods of enhanced verbal and nonverbal communication skills. *Role playing of verbal and nonverbal communication methods in a nonthreatening, safe environment can enhance communication skills.*
- Explore and discuss thoughts and feelings regarding any overuse of negative cognitions and expressions on the part of the patient by suggesting strategies such as rubber band on wrist to snap every time negative expressions start. *Exploration and discussion of negative cognitions may provide an opportunity to explore alternative ways of dealing with negative thoughts and feelings.*
- PCC Teach theory of assertive behavior, and role play assertive communication approaches. *Assertiveness training can decrease passive or aggressive communication patterns.*
- Listen for themes presented during nurse–patient interactions *because themes can provide areas of focus for patient discussions with caregiver.*
- Schedule frequent treatment team meetings regarding communication skill development with patient. *Team meetings with patient can ensure continuity of care and the*

development of communication patterns, facilitating patient's coping with health and illness.

PCC
- Communicate a plan to patient regarding mutual decision making (partnering) toward goals and direction of future encounters *to reinforce patient's role within the relationship.*
- Consider factors such as age, gender, culture, religion, and spirituality in communicating with patient *to facilitate the provision of holistic and individual care.*
- Communicate use of positive self-talk to patient *to enhance confidence in communication.*

Suggested NIC Interventions

Active Listening; Animal-Assisted Therapy; Anticipatory Guidance; Art Therapy; Assertiveness Training; Behavioral Modification: Social Skills; Complex Relationship Building; Music Therapy; Socialization Enhancement

Evaluations for Expected Outcomes

- Patient expresses message clearly as evidenced by feedback that receiver understood the message.
- Patient expresses satisfaction with feedback received from caregivers and others.
- Patient reports that nurse and other health care team members provide an increased sense of security through verbal and nonverbal communication.
- Patient reports less anxiety and guilt and more control in providing assertive responses when relating to individuals with passive or aggressive communication styles.
- Patient expresses belief that nurse uses interactions that convey respect, warmth, empathy, and genuineness that can result in enhanced communication skill building.
- Patient discloses feelings of confidence and increased life quality related to enhanced communication skills with family, groups, health care team, and confrontational persons.
- Patient describes enhanced ability to advocate for self in coping with chronic and acute illness.
- Patient reports successful negotiations within health care milieu.

Documentation

- Efforts made by nurse to provide didactic information on communication theory and to role model enhanced communication skills, such as assertiveness training
- Patient's response to didactic discussions and strategies, such as role playing and interactive videos
- Nursing interventions regarding coaching and supporting patient progress toward enhanced communication patterns
- Patient's expressed thoughts and feelings about personal progress toward enhanced communication responses
- Revisions to treatment plan
- Evaluations for expected outcomes

REFERENCES

Clochesy, J. M., Dolansky, M. A., Hickman, R. L., Jr., Gittner, L. S., & Hickman, R. J. (2015). Enhancing communication between patients and healthcare providers: SBAR3. *Journal of Health & Human Services Administration*, *38*(2), 237–252.

Liermann, K., & Norton, C. (2016). Enhancing family communication: Examining the impact of a therapeutic wilderness program for struggling teens and parents. *Contemporary Family Therapy: An International Journal*, *38*(1), 14–22. doi:10.1007/s10591-015-9371-5

Weis, J., Zoffmann, V., & Egerod, I. (2015). Enhancing person-centered communication in NICU: A comparative thematic analysis. *Nursing in Critical Care*, *20*(6), 287–298. doi:10.1111/nicc.12062

READINESS FOR ENHANCED COPING

Definition

A pattern of cognitive and behavioral efforts to manage demands related to well-being, which can be strengthened

Assessment

- Age
- Usual coping mechanisms
- Perceived coping ability
- Role responsibilities
- Social support
- Spiritual resources

Defining Characteristics

- Awareness of possible environmental change
- Expresses desire to enhance knowledge of stress management strategies
- Expresses desire to enhance management of stressors
- Expresses desire to enhance social support
- Expresses desire to enhance use of emotion-oriented strategies
- Expresses desire to enhance use of problem-oriented strategies
- Expresses desire to enhance use of spiritual resource

Expected Outcomes

- Patient will identify major issues that require ongoing enhancement of coping strategies.
- Patient will express feelings associated with present coping strategies.
- Patient will demonstrate readiness to develop enhanced strategies.
- Patient will identify support persons and activities that will assist in goal attainment.

Suggested NOC Outcomes

Coping; Quality of Life

Interventions and Rationales

- Establish a trusting relationship with the patient. *Building trust will allow the patient to be more open.*
- Begin discussions at the patient's level of comfort. *If the patient wants to discuss feelings, it won't benefit the patient or nurse to begin presenting strategies that require logical reasoning.*
- Determine from listening to the patient options that might be attractive to the patient in reaching new goals for coping; for example, support group, spiritual direction, and journaling. *The patient will strive to enhance coping skills using those opportunities to which the patient feels best suited.*
- Arrange to meet with the patient regularly to assist in helping the patient focus on goals and evaluate progress. *Recognizing even small attempts at successful coping encourages the patient to increase own efforts.*

Suggested NIC Interventions

Active Listening; Coping Enhancement

Evaluations for Expected Outcomes

- Patient has successfully articulated major areas where enhanced coping strategies are needed.
- Patient expresses feelings associated with current coping strategies.
- Patient demonstrates readiness to develop enhanced strategies.
- Patient identifies the person(s) perceived as being able to support therapeutically in the patient's efforts.
- Patient identifies with group support or attends class or session to learn more about coping.

Documentation

- Patient's assessment of coping skills
- Patient's goals for enhanced coping
- Actions taken by patient to cope from situation to situation
- Patient's response to nursing interventions
- Evaluations for expected outcomes

REFERENCES

Akiko, K., Ashby, J., Jess, A., Chernenko, A., Tabler, J., Ha Ngoc, T., . . . Reel, J. J. (2015). Stress, coping strategies, and depression—Uninsured primary care patients. *American Journal of Health Behavior*, *39*(6), 742–750. doi:10.5993/AJHB.39.6.1

Campion, M., & Levita, L. (2014). Enhancing positive affect and divergent thinking abilities: Play some music and dance. *Journal of Positive Psychology*, *9*(2), 137–145. doi:10.1080/17439760.2013.848376

Serlachius, A., Pulkki-Råback, L., Elovainio, M., Hintsanen, M., Mikkilä, V., Laitinen, T. T., . . . Keltikangas-Järvinen, L. (2015). Is dispositional optimism or dispositional pessimism predictive of ideal cardiovascular health? The Young Finns Study. *Psychology & Health*, *30*(10), 1221–1239. doi:10.1080/08870446.2015.1041394

READINESS FOR ENHANCED COMMUNITY COPING

related to immunization

Definition

A pattern of community activities for adaptation and problem solving for meeting the demands or needs of the community, which can be strengthened

Assessment

- Community demographics, including age and gender distribution, ethnic groups, racial groups, religious groups, and education and income levels
- Community health status, including availability of health care services, use of health care services, prevalence of childhood illnesses in the community, epidemiologic statistics, and beliefs, values, and attitudes about health and illness
- Education system, including educational level of adult population and state law or school system's requirements for immunization before school attendance
- Religious institutions and their support for, or objections to, immunization
- Social services, including availability of clinics and other social services, access to health care, welfare system, and parents' dependence on welfare for support

Defining Characteristics

- Expresses desire to enhance availability of community recreation programs
- Expresses desire to enhance availability of community relaxation programs
- Expresses desire to enhance communication among community members
- Expresses desire to enhance communication between aggregates and larger community
- Expresses desire to enhance community planning for predictable stressors
- Expresses desire to enhance community resources for managing stressors
- Expresses desire to enhance community responsibility for stress management
- Expresses desire to enhance problem solving for identified issue

Expected Outcomes

- Community members will express understanding of problems associated with failure to immunize population and will recognize need for plan to reduce number of children and adults who aren't immunized.
- Community members will establish plan to increase rate of immunization and ensure adequate protection from communicable diseases.
- Community members will work to reduce spread of communicable diseases and increase rate of immunization within community.
- Community members will evaluate established plans for ensuring that all children become immunized and will make changes to plans as needed.

Suggested NOC Outcomes

Community Competence; Community Health Status; Community Health Status: Immunity; Community Risk Control: Communicable Disease

Interventions and Rationales

- PCC Work with community members to pinpoint potential problems associated with inadequate immunization of the population *to ensure adequate protection against communicable diseases.* Consider taking these steps:
  - Identify new members of the community, such as immigrants and refugees, *to help reach parents who need information about immunization.*
  - Identify parents who don't follow through with the required series of immunizations *to protect children from incomplete immunization.*
- Encourage community members to implement a program to disseminate information about problems associated with inadequate immunization *to educate residents and promote the community's established immunization program.*
- PCC Provide extensive education about communicable diseases and the importance of immunizations *to empower community residents and help decrease the risk of communicable diseases.*
- S Encourage health departments, clinics, and practitioners' offices to provide information on the recommended childhood immunization schedule to the public *to foster education about immunization.*
- S Contact the parents of children who aren't immunized in person or by handwritten note. Make it clear that your purpose in promoting immunization is to protect their child from illness *to build parents' trust in immunization programs.*
- PCC Provide immunization information in the parents' first language *to overcome a lack of understanding caused by language barriers.*

PCC
- Develop a list of referrals for the parents of children who aren't immunized. Include information on low-cost health insurance, city health centers, and well-baby clinics *to encourage compliance.*

S
- Coordinate with local nursing schools, health department nurses, and other interested nursing groups to provide the necessary number of professionals to deliver adequate immunizations *to reduce the risk of communicable disease.*
- Conduct a follow-up survey on immunization rates *to measure the effectiveness of educational efforts.*
- Collect statistical data from community sources, such as health department and schools, *to continue to identify children who haven't been immunized.*

Suggested NIC Interventions

Communicable Disease Management; Community Health Development; Health Education; Health Policy Monitoring; Immunization/Vaccination Management

Evaluations for Expected Outcomes

- Community members understand risks of failing to immunize population and recognize need for plan.
- Community members put forth plan to meet community's immunization needs, which contains definite actions yet allows for modifications.
- Community members implement plan to reduce spread of communicable diseases and increase rate of immunization.
- Community members evaluate plan and make changes, as needed, to help solve problems and further the goal of meeting community's immunization needs.

Documentation

- Evidence of need for immunization program
- Statistical data documenting problem
- Written plan to resolve problem
- Efforts made to disseminate written information to community
- Evaluations for expected outcomes

REFERENCES

Craig, S. L., Betancourt, I., & Muskat, B. (2015). Thinking big, supporting families, and enabling coping: The value of social work in patient- and family-centered health care. *Social Work in Health Care*, *54*(5), 422–443. doi:10.1080/00981389.2015.1017074

Kimhi, S. (2016). Levels of resilience: Associations among individual, community, and national resilience. *Journal of Health Psychology*, *21*(2), 164–170. doi:10.1177/1359105314524009

Reifsnider, E., Bishop, S. L., An, K., Mendias, E., Welker-Hood, K., Moramarco, M. W., & Davila, Y. R. (2014). We stop for no storm: Coping with an environmental disaster and public health research. *Public Health Nursing*, *31*(6), 500–507. doi:10.1111/phn.12160

READINESS FOR ENHANCED FAMILY COPING

Definition

A pattern of management of adaptive tasks by primary person (family member, significant other, or close friend) involved with the client's health change, which can be strengthened

Assessment

- Family process, including normal pattern of interaction among family members, family's understanding and knowledge of patient's present condition, support systems available (financial, social, and spiritual), family's past response to crises (coping patterns), and communication patterns used to express anger, affection, and confrontation
- Patient's illness, including progression and severity of illness, patient's perception of health problem, and problem-solving techniques used by patient to cope with life problems

Defining Characteristics

- Expresses desire to acknowledge growth impact of crisis
- Expresses desire to choose experiences that optimize wellness
- Expresses desire to enhance connection with others who have experienced a similar situation
- Expresses desire to enhance enrichment of lifestyle
- Expresses desire to enhance health promotion

Expected Outcomes

- Family members will discuss impact of patient's illness and feelings about it.
- Family members will participate in treatment plan.
- Family members will establish a visiting routine beneficial to patient and themselves.
- Family members will demonstrate care needed to maintain patient's health status.
- Family members will identify and use available support systems.

Suggested NOC Outcomes

Family Coping; Family Normalization; Family Participation in Professional Care

Interventions and Rationales

- Allow time for family members to discuss impact of the patient's illness and their feelings. Encourage expression of feelings *to allow family members to realistically adjust to the patient's problems.*
- PCC Encourage family conferences; help family members identify key issues and select support services, if needed, *to develop sense of shared responsibility and feelings of safety, adequacy, and comfort.*
- Help the patient and family establish a visiting routine that won't tax the patient's or family's resources. Use the patient's daily routine to aid in planning—for example, no visiting during treatments or during periods of uninterrupted sleep. *Involving family members reassures the patient of their care and reduces family's fear and anxiety.*
- Reinforce family members' efforts to care for the patient *to let them know they're doing their best and to ease adaptation and grieving process.*
- Demonstrate care procedures, and encourage participation in treatment and planning decisions (such as selecting times for pulmonary toilet for the patient with cystic fibrosis). *Meeting others' needs promotes self-esteem.*
- PCC Provide family members with clear, concise information about the patient's condition. Be aware of what they have been told, and help them interpret information. *This information will help alleviate their concerns.*

- Ensure privacy for the patient and family during visits *to foster open communication.*
- Help family support the patient's independence. Encourage attendance at therapy sessions, and allow the patient to demonstrate new skills and abilities. *Independence helps the patient reach maximum functional level.*
- Provide emotional support to family by being available to answer questions. *Attentive listening conveys empathy, recognition, and respect for a person.*
- PCC Inform family of community resources and support groups available to assist in managing the patient's illness and providing emotional or financial support to caretakers, such as Easter Seals Association, Visiting Nurse Association, and Meals On Wheels. *Community resources may help the patient develop potential, independence, and self-reliance.*

Suggested NIC Interventions

Caregiver Support; Family Involvement Promotion; Health Education; Self-Modification Assistance

Evaluations for Expected Outcomes

- Family members acknowledge their feelings about patient's illness.
- Family members spend adequate time with patient and seek to participate in care.
- Family members establish a visiting routine beneficial to patient and themselves.
- Family members display competence in caring for patient through return demonstration and provide adequate level of care to maintain patient's health.
- Family members make contact with support resources available in their community.

Documentation

- Family's response to patient's illness
- Family's current understanding of patient's illness
- Observations about family's interaction with patient and acceptance of current situation
- Evaluations for expected outcomes

REFERENCES

Bademli, K., & Duman, Z. Ç. (2014). Effects of a family-to-family support program on the mental health and coping strategies of caregivers of adults with mental illness: A randomized controlled study. *Archives of Psychiatric Nursing*, *28*(6), 392–398. doi:10.1016/j.apnu.2014.08.011

Bradshaw, S., Shumway, S. T., Wang, E. W., Harris, K. S., Smith, D. B., & Austin-Robillard, H. (2015). Hope, readiness, and coping in family recovery from addiction. *Journal of Groups in Addiction & Recovery*, *10*(4), 313–336. doi:10.1080/1556035X.2015.1099125

Rossetto, K. R. (2015). Developing conceptual definitions and theoretical models of coping in military families during deployment. *Journal of Family Communication*, *15*(3), 249–268. doi:10.1080/15267431.2015.1043737

READINESS FOR ENHANCED DECISION MAKING

Definition

A pattern of choosing a course of action for meeting short- and long-term health-related goals, which can be strengthened

Assessment

- Patient's perception of own ability to make decisions
- Patient's expression of desire to align decisions with personal values and goals
- Patient's expression of desire to improve congruence between decisions and sociocultural values and goals
- Patient's desire to evaluate the efficacy of own decisions
- Patient's need for reliable information on which to base own decisions

Defining Characteristics

- Expresses desire to enhance congruency of decisions with sociocultural goals
- Expresses desire to enhance congruency of decisions with sociocultural values
- Expresses desire to enhance congruency of decisions with goals
- Expresses desire to enhance congruency of decisions with values
- Expresses desire to enhance decision making
- Expresses desire to enhance risk–benefit analysis of decisions
- Expresses desire to enhance understanding of choices for decision making
- Expresses desire to enhance understanding of the meaning of choices
- Expresses desire to enhance use of reliable evidence for decisions

Expected Outcomes

- Patient will express desire to make effective decisions to meet short- and long-term goals.
- Patient will share decision-making goals and concerns.
- Patient will discuss measures used to evaluate quality of decisions made.
- Patient will make decisions that promote maximal physical, mental, social, and psychological well-being.
- Patient will involve family, community, friends, and clergy in health care decisions.

Suggested NOC Outcomes

Decision-Making; Participation in Health Care Decisions; Self-Care: Instrumental Activities of Daily Living (IADLs)

Interventions and Rationales

- Assess the patient's ability to make decisions that affect the patient's well-being *to determine the patient's level of ability to participate in health care decisions.*
- PCC Work with the patient to enhance the patient's decision-making capabilities *to promote personal actions of a competent individual to exercise governance in life decisions.*
- Provide the patient with decision-making support *to enhance self-care and well-being of the patient and family.*
- Assist the patient with decisions that involve family, community, friends, and clergy *to provide opportunities for shared decision making and enhanced support for the patient.*

Suggested NIC Interventions

Decision-Making Support; Health System Guidance; Self-Responsibility Facilitation

Evaluations for Expected Outcomes

- Patient expresses desire to make effective decisions to meet short- and long-term goals.
- Patient shares decision-making goals and concerns.
- Patient discusses measures used to evaluate the quality of decisions made.
- Patient makes decisions that promote maximal physical, mental, social, and psychological well-being.
- Patient involves family, community, friends, and clergy in health care decisions.

Documentation

- Patient's perception of decision-making abilities
- Patient's involvement of family, community, friends, and clergy in decision making
- Future plans to make decisions that improve physical, mental, social, and psychological well-being
- Evaluations for expected outcomes

REFERENCES

Ali, S. F., & Muhammad, M. P. (2014). Patient preference regarding their role in clinical decision-making process: A systematic review. *International Journal of Nursing Education*, *6*(2), 192–195. doi:10.5958/0974-9357.2014.00632.1

Stacey, D., & Légaré, F. (2015). Engaging patients using an interprofessional approach to shared decision making. *Canadian Oncology Nursing Journal*, *25*(4), 455–461.

Tuominen, L., Leino-Kilpi, H., & Suhonen, R. (2016). Older people's experiences of their free will in nursing homes. *Nursing Ethics*, *23*(1), 22–35. doi:10.1177/0969733014557119

READINESS FOR ENHANCED FLUID BALANCE

Definition

A pattern of equilibrium between the fluid volume and chemical composition of body fluids, which can be strengthened

Assessment

- Cardiovascular status, including pulse and blood pressure, capillary filling, and electrocardiogram (ECG) results
- Gastrointestinal (GI) status, including types and amounts of fluid and food intake; maintenance of stable weight; and recent episodes of acute, limited GI disturbance with intestinal loss of fluid (vomiting or diarrhea)
- Fluid and electrolyte status, including skin turgor; mucous membranes (lips) for moistness or cracks; temperature and color of skin; absence or presence of diaphoresis; and presence of dependent edema or fingerprint edema
- Renal–urinary status, including normal pattern and amount of voiding and evidence of straw-colored urine
- Respiratory status, including rate and depth of respirations through nasal passages; cough; and auscultation of lungs for fine crackles
- Neurologic status, including level of consciousness and mental status
- Skeletal muscles, including normal tone and strength and absence of cramping
- Laboratory studies, including serum electrolyte, plasma glucose, and blood urea nitrogen (BUN) levels; plasma osmolarity; hemoglobin (Hb) level and hematocrit (HCT); and urine analysis that includes specific gravity and glucose

Defining Characteristics

- Expresses desire to enhance fluid balance

Expected Outcomes

- Patient's vital signs will remain stable and within normal ranges; ECG shows no abnormality in rhythm.
- Patient's skin temperature, moistness, turgor, and color will be normal.
- Patient's mucous membranes will be moist and noncracked.
- Patient's weight will remain stable.
- Patient's fluid volume intake will remain adequate; patient will experience thirst satiety.
- Patient will produce adequate urine volume (approximately equal to fluid intake) of light to straw-colored urine.
- Patient's urine-specific gravity will remain between 1.015 and 1.025.
- Patient's plasma and serum values for electrolytes, osmolarity, glucose, BUN, HCT, and Hb will be within normal ranges.
- Patient will be alert and responsive to demands of living and react appropriately to reflex needs such as thirst; patient's muscle reflexes, strength, and tone will be normal.
- Patient will express understanding of factors that contribute to normal fluid and electrolyte balance.
- Patient will adhere to prescribed therapies to manage coexisting disease processes such as diabetes mellitus, heart failure, renal insufficiency, and thyroid excess or deficiency, which interfere with electrolyte and osmolar homeostasis.

Suggested NOC Outcomes

Fluid Balance; Hydration; Nutritional Status: Food & Fluid Intake; Tissue Integrity: Skin & Mucous Membranes; Tissue Perfusion: Abdominal Organs; Vital Signs

Interventions and Rationales

- Explain and reinforce to the patient the need to drink 1.5 to 2 L fluids daily, divided equally throughout the day. *Although daily intake should be between 2.5 and 3.5 L daily, food liberates about 1 L of fluid and, in the process of food oxidation, cells liberate up to 0.4 L of water.*
- Encourage the patient to select healthy, appropriate beverages such as drinking plenty of water; other beverages, such as soda, should be consumed in moderation. *Many beverages, including carbonated soft drinks and fruit juices, have a high sugar content and increase the osmolar content of the body, causing a greater thirst and an increased load on the renal system and diuresis. Beverages with caffeine cause diuresis and may cause an increased fluid loss. Patient should carefully select and judiciously use beverages and sports drinks that claim to replenish electrolytes. Alcoholic beverages are discouraged during hot weather because these can cause fluid and electrolyte disturbances through excess diuresis.*
- PCC Educate the patient on how to read and interpret labels on beverage and food containers. For example, humans require 0.5 g (500 mg) of sodium/day; typical intake is 5 to 6 g daily. *Reducing the amount of sodium reduces the amount of fluid volume in the vascular system, thus controlling thirst and blood pressure. Individuals with treatment*

plans that include nutritional therapy should be encouraged to adhere to prescribed restrictions.

- PCC Teach the patient about adequate water intake during demanding daily events, such as increased exercise or high environmental temperatures. *During extreme exercise conditions, unmeasured fluid losses through diaphoresis and lung evaporation can be significant (1,200 to 2,000 mL). Advise the patient to hydrate well before (750 mL), during (250 mL every 15 minutes of activity), and after (500 mL) exercise events. To prevent dehydration, gauge fluid need on urine color and amount. It should remain light to straw-colored and normal in volume.*
- PCC Educate the patient on signs and symptoms of dehydration (dry mouth and mucous membranes), light-headedness (blood pressure and vital sign changes), and scant urine output (glycosuria and polyuria). *By recognizing onset of dehydration, one can avoid severe complications.*
- PCC Educate the patient on signs and symptoms of over hydration and fluid retention, such as scant urine output, cough, increased weight gain, dependent edema, and jugular vein distention. *By recognizing onset of overhydration or fluid retention, one can avoid severe complications.*

Suggested NIC Interventions

Electrolyte Management; Fluid/Electrolyte Management; Fluid Management; Fluid Monitoring

Evaluations for Expected Outcomes

- Patient's vital signs, skin temperature and turgor, and ECG are within normal range.
- Patient maintains fluid volume equilibrium with normal electrolyte and osmolar balance.
- Patient responds to natural thirst mechanism and drinks 1,400 to 1,800 mL daily.
- Patient manages nutrient intake to reduce sodium intake toward daily requirement and maintains serum sodium between 135 and 145 mEq/L.
- Patient manages food and nutrient intake and treatment plan (if applicable) to maintain plasma glucose level below 120 mg/dL.
- Patient maintains plasma osmolality between 280 and 295 mOsm/kg.
- Patient doesn't experience weight gain or loss related to fluid gain or loss.

Documentation

- Patient's weight and weight changes over time
- Vital signs; capillary filling
- Daily intake and types of fluids
- Daily urine output; characteristics of urine (color, concentration, odor)
- Thirst and patient's ability to satisfy thirst
- Skin turgor; moist or dry mucous membranes
- Laboratory electrolyte results, if available
- Evaluations for expected outcomes

REFERENCES

Maughan, R. J., Watson, P., Cordery, P. A., Walsh, N. P., Oliver, S. J., Dolci, A., . . . Galloway, S. R. (2016). A randomized trial to assess the potential of different beverages to affect hydration status: Development of a beverage hydration index. *American Journal of Clinical Nutrition*, *103*(3), 717–723. doi:10.3945/ajcn.115.114769

Perry, C. S., 3rd, Rapinett, G., Glaser, N. S., & Ghetti, S. (2015). Hydration status moderates the effects of drinking water on children's cognitive performance. *Appetite*, *95*, 520–527. doi:10.1016/j.appet.2015.08.006

Phillips, S. M., Sykes, D., & Gibson, N. (2014). Hydration status and fluid balance of elite European youth soccer players during consecutive training sessions. *Journal of Sports Science & Medicine*, *13*(4), 817–822.

READINESS FOR ENHANCED HOPE

Definition

A pattern of expectations and desires for mobilizing energy on one's own behalf, which can be strengthened

Assessment

- Patient's perception of ability to set personal goals
- Patient's expression of desire to build on possibilities for the future
- Patient's ability to align desires and expectations
- Patient's expression of hope regarding health situation
- Patient's desire to maintain and enhance relationships with others
- Patient's problem-solving approach to health situation
- Patient's expressed need for increased spiritual connection

Defining Characteristics

- Expresses desire to enhance ability to set achievable goals
- Expresses desire to enhance belief in possibilities
- Expresses desire to enhance congruency of expectation with goal
- Expresses desire to enhance connectedness with others
- Expresses desire to enhance hope
- Expresses desire to enhance problem solving to meet goal
- Expresses desire to enhance sense of meaning to life
- Expresses desire to enhance spirituality

Expected Outcomes

- Patient will express desire for positive health outcomes.
- Patient will share personal goals to increase autonomy and personal satisfaction.
- Patient will discuss measures to increase quality of life.
- Patient will develop plan to promote maximal physical, mental, social, and psychological abilities.
- Patient will share strategies to live a meaningful life.
- Patient will express awareness of the need for developing and maintaining a positive attitude of hope.
- Patient will state plan for own role enhancement.
- Patient will share need for emotional support.
- Patient will maintain a sense of humor and positive sense of self.
- Patient will seek spiritual support as needed.

Suggested NOC Outcomes

Hope; Personal Well-Being; Quality of Life; Will to Live

Interventions and Rationales

- Assist the patient in adapting to disability *to promote acceptance and understanding of physical condition, thereby improving management of therapeutic regimen.*
- S Assess the patient's adaptation to current health status; *baseline assessment is needed to develop care plan.*
- Implement a plan to build on the patient's optimal role performance; *establish a plan with the patient that promotes clear mutual expectations.*
- PCC Facilitate opportunities for spiritual nourishment and growth *to address the patient's holistic needs for maximal therapeutic environment.*
- Assist the patient to build and maintain meaningful interpersonal relationships *to maintain highest level of well-being.*
- Discuss the issue of hope with the patient's family. Encourage the patient to allow including the family in your discussions about hope. *It is important to understand what the differences and similarities are in their expectations*

Suggested NIC Interventions

Emotional Support; Hope Instillation; Self-Esteem Enhancement; Spiritual Growth Facilitation; Support Systems

Evaluations for Expected Outcomes

- Patient expresses desire for positive health outcomes.
- Patient shares personal goals to increase autonomy and personal satisfaction.
- Patient discusses measures utilized to increase quality of life.
- Patient develops a plan to promote maximal physical, mental, social, and psychological abilities.
- Patient shares own strategies for living a meaningful life.
- Patient demonstrates awareness of the need for developing and maintaining a positive attitude of hope.
- Patient states plan for own role enhancement.
- Patient shares the need for emotional support.
- Patient maintains a sense of humor and positive sense of self.
- Patient seeks spiritual support as needed.

Documentation

- Patient's assessment of situation and hopeful resolution of problems
- Community resources to support patient's positive outcomes
- Future plans to maximize patient's preferred outcomes
- Evaluations for expected outcomes

REFERENCES

Paley, J. (2014). Hope, positive illusions, and palliative rehabilitation. *Progress in Palliative Care*, 22(6), 358–362. doi:10.1179/1743291X14Y.0000000084

Waynor, W. R., & Gill, K. J. (2015). The role of hope in predicting supported employment success. *Journal of Rehabilitation, 81*(2), 26–31.
Yarcheski, A., & Mahon, N. E. (2016). Meta-analyses of predictors of hope in adolescents. *Western Journal of Nursing Research, 38*(3), 345–368. doi:10.1177/0193945914559545

READINESS FOR ENHANCED KNOWLEDGE

Definition

A pattern of cognitive information related to a specific topic, or its acquisition, which can be strengthened

Assessment

- Age and gender
- Developmental state
- Mental status
- Health problems, restrictions, and limitations
- Roles in family and community
- Socioeconomic factors
- Cultural background

Defining Characteristics

- Expresses a desire to enhance learning

Expected Outcomes

- Patient will identify new sources for enhancing knowledge in the topic of interest.
- Patient will make use of all relevant resources to enhance knowledge.
- Patient will ask questions where new information needs clarification.
- Patient will begin practicing new behaviors gleaned from enhanced knowledge.

Suggested NOC Outcomes

Knowledge: Health Promotion

Interventions and Rationales

- Determine exactly what the patient knows and to what level the patient wishes to and can enhance knowledge and understanding. *This information will assist the nurse in planning with the patient.*
- PCC Provide books and videos that will help the patient's quest for enhanced knowledge. *Supplying some materials directly may motivate the patient to want to search further.*
- PCC Direct the patient to use other sources for information, such as libraries, Internet, or professional organizations. *An independent search results in the patient developing confidence in own ability to go much deeper into the area of interest.*
- PCC Be available to answer questions and correct misconceptions for the patient *in order to enhance the effectiveness of what the patient is learning.*
- Provide feedback to the patient for incorporating new knowledge into lifestyle. *This reinforces behaviors resulting from enhanced knowledge.*

Suggested NIC Interventions

Learning Facilitation; Learning Readiness Enhancement

Evaluations for Expected Outcomes

- Patient expresses motivation for enhanced knowledge.
- Patient uses various resources to achieve success.
- Patient questions things that aren't clearly understood.
- Patient practices skills derived from enhanced knowledge.

Documentation

- Patient's current level of knowledge and skill
- Patient's expressions of motivation to enhance knowledge
- Resources used to enhance knowledge
- Patient's response to learning resources
- Evaluations for expected outcomes

REFERENCES

Bannister, S. L., Hanson, J. L., Maloney, C. G., & Dudas, R. A. (2015). Practical framework for fostering a positive learning environment. *Pediatrics*, *136*(1), 6–9. doi:10.1542/peds.2015–1314
Hume, K., & Tomsik, E. (2014). Enhancing patient education and medication reconciliation strategies to reduce readmission rates. *Hospital Pharmacy*, *49*(2), 112–114. doi:10.1310/hpj4902-112
Price, B. (2015). Helping patients to learn about self-management. *Nursing Standard*, *30*(2), 51–60. doi:10.7748/ns.30.2.51.e10145

READINESS FOR ENHANCED POWER

Definition

A pattern of participating knowingly in change for well-being, which can be strengthened

Assessment

- Patient's perception of present state of power
- Patient's perception of ability to enhance power
- Support systems, including family members, friends, clergy
- Patient's ability to identify choices
- Patient's readiness for change to occur
- Reliance on health care system to resolve complaints or assume power

Defining Characteristics

- Expresses desire to enhance awareness of possible changes
- Expresses desire to enhance identification of choices that can be made for change
- Expresses desire to enhance independence with actions for change
- Expresses desire to enhance involvement in change
- Expresses desire to enhance knowledge for participation in change
- Expresses desire to enhance participation in choices for daily living

- Expresses desire to enhance participation in choices for health
- Expresses desire to enhance power

Expected Outcomes

- Patient will express perceived control in influencing health outcomes.
- Patient will participate in choices that enhance his care and well-being.
- Patient will develop a plan for adjusting to significant life changes.

Suggested NOC Outcomes

Family Resiliency; Health Beliefs: Perceived Control; Personal Autonomy; Psychosocial Adjustment: Life Change

Interventions and Rationales

- Assess the patient's understanding of need for changes to improve well-being; *knowledge increases power in independent decisions for change.*
- Assess the patient's participation in choices to be made *to enhance care and well-being.*
- Assist the patient in acquiring knowledge necessary for positive decision making. *Making positive decisions that produce benefits will reinforce health-seeking behaviors.*
- Help the patient to involve family, community, clergy, and friends with changes to the care plan *to increase the patient's perceived control to affect maximal self-care outcomes.*
- PCC Work with the patient to help develop a plan that takes into account the resources identified as being helpful to the patient in attaining an optimal level of self-care. *This will help the patient maintain control of own decision making about health while using the input of others whom the patient trusts.*

Suggested NIC Interventions

Assertiveness Training; Coping Enhancement; Self-Modification Assistance; Self-Responsibility Facilitation

Evaluations for Expected Outcomes

- Patient expresses understanding of the need for changes to improve well-being.
- Patient participates in choices that enhance own care and well-being.
- Patient develops a plan for adjusting to significant life changes.

Documentation

- Patient's understanding of needed changes for own care and well-being
- Patient's choices that enhance own care and well-being
- Patient's knowledge to make ongoing changes to own care and well-being
- Evaluations for expected outcomes

REFERENCES

Irving, P. (2015). Self-empowerment in later life as a response to ageism. *Generations*, *39*(1), 72–77.

Mazzoni, D., Cicognani, E., Laghi, M., Sgarlato, V., & Mosconi, G. (2014). Patients' direction, empowerment, and quality of life in hemodialysis. *Psychology, Health & Medicine*, *19*(5), 552–558. doi:10.1080/13548506.2013.855316

Stoffel, V. (2015). Engagement, exploration, empowerment. *American Journal of Occupational Therapy*, *69*(6), 1–8. doi:10.5014/ajot.2015.696002

READINESS FOR ENHANCED RELATIONSHIP

Definition

A pattern of mutual partnership to provide for each other's needs, which can be strengthened

Assessment

- Sexual status, including usual patterns of sexuality
- Patient's health status, support systems, expressed concerns regarding relationship
- Communication patterns

Defining Characteristics

- Expresses desire to enhance autonomy between partners
- Expresses desire to enhance collaboration between partners
- Expresses desire to enhance communication between partners
- Expresses desire to enhance emotional need fulfillment for each partner
- Expresses desire to enhance mutual respect between each partner
- Expresses desire to enhance satisfaction with complementary relationship between partners
- Expresses desire to enhance satisfaction with emotional need fulfillment for each partner
- Expresses desire to enhance satisfaction with idea sharing between partners
- Expresses desire to enhance satisfaction with information sharing between partners
- Expresses desire to enhance satisfaction with physical need fulfillment for each partner
- Expresses desire to enhance understanding of partner's functional deficit (e.g., physical, psychological, social)

Expected Outcomes

- Patient will communicate effectively with partner and family members.
- Patient will articulate ways to mutually meet physical and emotional needs of partner and self.
- Patient will participate in appropriate counseling (premarital, preconceptual, sexual) as needed.
- Patient will verbalize that relationships are characterized by well-balanced autonomy and self-efficacy.

Suggested NOC Outcomes

Family Functioning; Role Performance; Sexual Functioning; Social Interaction Skills

Interventions and Rationales

- Assess communication techniques and effectiveness of couple and family *to be able to counsel and/or refer appropriately as needed.*
- Suggest that the patient and partner/family members attend counseling sessions as appropriate for their life cycle stage. *Patients may need permission from a health care professional in order to feel comfortable seeking relationship assistance.*

PCC • Teach the patient and family members normal family life cycle stages *so that they can better understand what is normal and are able to anticipate challenges.*
- Encourage the patient and family members to share information and ideas *in order to enhance communication.*

PCC • Refer as needed to colleagues in other disciplines such as social workers or counselors *to facilitate enhanced communication.*

Suggested NIC Interventions

Family Integrity Promotion; Family Support; Preconceptual Counseling; Sexual Counseling; Socialization Enhancement; Support System Enhancement

Evaluations for Expected Outcomes

- Patient communicates effectively with partner and family.
- Patient states ways to meet physical and emotional needs of partner and self.
- Patient actively participates in recommended counseling.

Documentation

- Patient's statement of improved communication with partner/family members
- Patient's participation in recommended counseling
- Referrals to other disciplines
- Evaluations for expected outcomes

REFERENCES

Fortune-Britt, A. G., Nieuwsma, J. A., Gierisch, J. M., Datta, S. K., Stolldorf, D. P., Cantrell, W. C., . . . Jackson, G. L. (2015). Evaluating the implementation and sustainability of a program for enhancing veterans' intimate relationships. *Military Medicine*, *180*(6), 676–683. doi:10.7205/MILMED-D-14-00336

Kemp, D. (2016). Improving mental health through social support: Building positive and empowering relationships. *Mental Health Nursing*, *36*(1), 21.

Lundy, B. L., & Drouin, M. (2016). From social anxiety to interpersonal connectedness: Relationship building within face-to-face, phone, and instant messaging mediums. *Computers in Human Behavior*, *54*, 271–277. doi:10.1016/j.chb.2015.08.004

READINESS FOR ENHANCED RESILIENCE

Definition

A pattern of positive responses to an adverse situation or crisis, which can be strengthened

Assessment

- Patient's perception of situation, coping mechanisms, problem-solving ability, decision-making competencies, relationships, family system

Defining Characteristics

- Demonstrates positive outlook
- Exposure to crisis
- Expresses desire to enhance available resources
- Expresses desire to enhance communication skills
- Expresses desire to enhance environmental safety
- Expresses desire to enhance goal setting
- Expresses desire to enhance involvement in activities
- Expresses desire to enhance own responsibility for action
- Expresses desire to enhance progress toward goal
- Expresses desire to enhance relationship with others
- Expresses desire to enhance resilience
- Expresses desire to enhance self-esteem
- Expresses desire to enhance sense of control
- Expresses desire to enhance support system
- Expresses desire to enhance use of conflict management strategies
- Expresses desire to enhance use of coping skills
- Expresses desire to enhance use of resource

Expected Outcomes

- Patient will acknowledge readiness for enhanced resilience.
- Patient will verbalize the feelings of resilience.
- Patient will identify impact of resilience on growth.

Suggested NOC Outcomes

Enhanced Self-Esteem; Enhanced Personal Potential; Knowledge: Health Behavior

Interventions and Rationales

- Explore with the patient the process and growth in mastering a situation or crisis that enhanced the patient's resilience. *Mastery of responses in crisis situations can generalize to future situations.*
- Listen therapeutically to the patient's self-exploration and mastery. *Active listening is the key to the therapeutic alliance and accurate assessment.*
- Instruct the patient to journal experiences for future reflection. *Journaling is a therapeutic tool for self-exploration and expansion.*
- Guide the patient to review life goals that might now be attainable. *Personal potential is maximized in an environment of resilience.*
- Encourage the patient to assist others or get involved to enrich the lives of others. *Humans benefit from shared positive experiences.*

Suggested NIC Interventions

Coping Enhancement; Enhanced Human Potential

Evaluations for Expected Outcomes

- Patient acknowledges readiness for enhanced resilience.
- Patient verbalizes the feelings of resilience.
- Patient identifies the impact of resilience toward growth.

Documentation

- Patient's acknowledgement of readiness for increased resilience
- Patient's statements regarding the impact of resilience on personal growth

- Patient's feelings of resilience
- Evaluations for expected outcomes

REFERENCES

Ellis, L., Gergen, J., Wohlgemuth, L., & Nolan, M. T. (2016). Empowering the "cheerer": Role of surgical intensive care unit nurses in enhancing family resilience. *American Journal of Critical Care*, *25*(1), 39–45. doi:10.4037/ajcc2016926

Ottmann, G., & Maragoudaki, M. (2015). Fostering resilience later in life: A narrative approach involving people facing disabling circumstances, carers and members of minority groups. *Ageing & Society*, *35*(10), 2071–2099. doi:10.1017/S0144686X14000828

Wong, P. S., Fong, K. W., & Lam, T. L. (2015). Enhancing the resilience of parents of adults with intellectual disabilities through volunteering: An exploratory study. *Journal of Policy & Practice in Intellectual Disabilities*, *12*(1), 20–26. doi:10.1111/jppi.12101

READINESS FOR ENHANCED SELF-CARE

Definition

A pattern of performing activities for oneself to meet health-related goals, which can be strengthened

Assessment

- Patient's perception of adequacy of self-care
- Family responsibilities assumed in caring for patient
- Patient's attitude toward use of health care services
- Patient's use of family, friends, and clergy support systems
- Health history, including self-care abilities, disabilities, or deformities
- Patient's reliance on community for health and welfare support

Defining Characteristics

- Expresses desire to enhance independence with health
- Expresses desire to enhance independence with life
- Expresses desire to enhance independence with personal development
- Expresses desire to enhance independence with well-being
- Expresses desire to enhance knowledge of self-care strategies
- Expresses desire to enhance self-care

Expected Outcomes

- Patient will demonstrate positive decision making toward maximizing potential for self-care.
- Patient will express satisfaction with independence in assuming responsibility for planning self-care
- Patient will involve staff, family, and community in developing strategies for self-care.

Suggested NOC Outcomes

Adherence Behavior; Client Satisfaction: Functional Assistance; Discharge Readiness: Independent Living; Health Beliefs: Perceived Ability to Perform

Interventions and Rationales

- Assess the patient's satisfaction with level of self-care *in order to support general well-being.*
- PCC Assist the patient to develop plan to promote autonomous decision making *to increase patient's responsibility for facilitating care.*
- Support the patient's implementation of a program to sustain health-seeking behavior *to promote patient autonomy in self-care.*
- Promote health team, family, and community efforts to participate in the patient's self-care initiatives *to promote satisfactory mutual goal setting and group efforts.*
- PCC Encourage the patient and family to participate in support networks that promote patient's independence, where possible, *to promote patient and family resilience.*
- PCC Develop a referral list for community resources *to promote the patient's enhanced self-care.*

Suggested NIC Interventions

Mutual Goal Setting; Resiliency Promotion; Self-Responsibility Facilitation

Evaluations for Expected Outcomes

- Patient expresses awareness of need to maintain independence in health management.
- Patient develops and maintains a plan for enhanced self-care.
- Patient involves staff, family, and community in developing strategies for self-care.

Documentation

- Patient's perception of readiness for enhancing self-care
- Family, friends, community, and clergy resources available to promote patient's independence
- Future plans to maintain and enhance independence in self-care
- Evaluations for expected outcomes

REFERENCES

Lamers, S. M., Bohlmeijer, E. T., Korte, J., & Westerhof, G. J. (2015). The efficacy of life-review as online-guided self-help for adults: A randomized trial. *Journals of Gerontology Series B: Psychological Sciences & Social Sciences*, *70*(1), 24–34. doi:10.1093/geronb/gbu030

Vargas Chaves, S., & Fernández Chaves, J. J. (2014). Effectiveness of nursing home care in improving self-care of older persons. *Enfermería Actual en Costa Rica*, (27), 1–11. doi:10.15517/revenf.v0i27.16059

Vaughan Dickson, V., D'Eramo Melkus, G., Dorsen, C., Katz, S., & Riegel, B. (2015). Improving heart failure self-care through a community-based skill-building intervention. *Journal of Cardiovascular Nursing*, *30*(4 Suppl 1), S14–S24. doi:10.1097/JCN.0000000000000161

READINESS FOR ENHANCED SELF-CONCEPT

Definition

A pattern of perceptions or ideas about the self, which can be strengthened

Assessment

- Age
- Gender
- Developmental stage
- Health problems
- Past experience with health care system
- Mental status
- Belief system (norms, values, religion)
- Social interaction patterns
- Family system
- Perception of self (past and present), including body image, coping mechanisms, problem-solving ability, and self-worth

Defining Characteristics

- Acceptance of limitations
- Acceptance of strengths
- Actions congruent with verbal expressions
- Confidence in abilities
- Expresses desire to enhance role performance
- Expresses desire to enhance self-concept
- Satisfaction with body image
- Satisfaction with personal identity
- Satisfaction with sense of worth
- Satisfaction with thoughts about self

Expected Outcomes

- Patient will articulate long- and short-term goals.
- Patient will express motivation necessary to achieve goals.
- Patient will develop realistic plan to achieve stated goals.
- Patient will practice self-management strategies needed to be successful.
- Patient will evaluate progress and modify behavior as needed.

Suggested NOC Outcomes

Body Image; Neglect Recovery; Personal Autonomy; Self-Esteem

Interventions and Rationales

- PCC Provide the patient with materials and resources on health-related issues that affect this individual's attitude. *Knowledge will enhance or inhibit patient's motivation or resolve.*
- Answer questions related to written material *so the patient is adequately prepared to establish realistic goals.*
- PCC Assist the patient in writing long- and short-term goals. *These goals can serve as tools for self-evaluation as new behaviors are being practiced.*
- Have the patient list one or two realistic, practical behaviors that will facilitate achieving goals. *The more positive the behaviors are, the greater the chance the patient has of being successful.*
- PCC Assist the patient to determine positive rewards for successful behavioral changes. *Reinforcement is needed for new behavior to continue.*

Suggested NIC Interventions

Hope Instillation; Self-Awareness Enhancement; Self-Responsibility Facilitation

Evaluations for Expected Outcomes

- Patient has realistic goals and workable plan for change.
- Patient responds positively to changes in self-concept.
- Patient demonstrates interest in evaluating progress.
- Patient shows a willingness to modify plan to continue reaching goals.

Documentation

- Patient's expressions of self-concept
- Patient's adherence to plan
- Modifications to plan
- Patient's response to nursing interventions
- Evaluations for expected outcomes

REFERENCES

Düring, C., & Jessop, D. C. (2015). The moderating impact of self-esteem on self-affirmation effects. *British Journal of Health Psychology*, *20*(2), 274–289. doi:10.1111/bjhp.12097

Searle, L. (2014). Surviving girlhood: Building positive relationships, attitudes, and self-esteem to prevent teenage girl bullying. *Child & Adolescent Mental Health*, *19*(2), 159. doi:10.1111/camh.12061_2

Yeung, J. C., & Lun, V. M. (2016). When self-help materials help: Examining the effects of self-discrepancy and modes of delivery of positive self-statements. *Journal of Positive Psychology*, *11*(2), 163–172. doi:10.1080/17439760.2015.1037862

READINESS FOR ENHANCED SLEEP

Definition

A pattern of natural, periodic suspension of relative consciousness to provide rest and sustain a desired lifestyle, which can be strengthened

Assessment

- Age
- Daytime activity and work patterns
- Cognitive status
- Possible precipitating factors
- Daytime consequences of sleeplessness
- Underlying conditions or medications
- Situational daily stressors
- Overall quality and duration of sleep
- Sleep environment
- Exposure to bright lights, exercise, and social interaction
- Recent changes in health status or lifestyle
- Dietary and drug history, including ingestion of caffeine or other stimulants, nicotine, alcohol, sedatives, hypnotics, and fluid intake

Defining Characteristics

- Expresses desire to enhance sleep

Expected Outcomes

- Patient will identify factors that enhance readiness for sleep.
- Patient will demonstrate readiness for enhanced sleep through the use of appropriate sleep hygiene measures.
- Patient's amount of sleep and rapid eye movement (REM) sleep will be congruent with developmental needs.
- Patient will express feeling rested after sleep.
- Institutional policies and staff behaviors will reflect measures to enhance readiness for sleep.

Suggested NOC Outcomes

Anxiety Level; Rest; Sleep

Interventions and Rationales

- Ask patient to keep a log of sleep and wake times, number of awakenings, total time asleep, quality of sleep, and any precipitating factors that may influence sleep *to determine sleep efficiency.*
- PCC Educate patient about normal age-related changes to sleep and strategies to improve sleep that are specific to patient's health status, lifestyle, and environment *to decrease anxiety about sleeplessness.*
- Make a behavioral modification plan based on the assessment of condition, patient history, and precipitating factors *to enhance compliance.*
- PCC Provide education about sleep *to dispel myths about sleep requirements and faulty strategies.*
- Increase exposure to light, exercise, and social interaction as synchronizers *to help rematch the circadian rhythms with normal day and night cycles.*
- Provide an environment conducive to relaxation, including low level of stimuli, dimmed lights, silence, and comfortable furniture, *to maximize sleep response.*
- Develop interventions within the facility that address quality sleep; for example, scheduling procedures and care activities *to avoid unnecessary awakenings*; modifying environmental factors *to promote a quiet, warm, relaxed sleep setting*; addressing lifestyle changes, such as having a roommate and the unfamiliarity of relocation; and orienting older adults to facility's setting *to enhance the ability to sleep.*
- Implement environmental strategies that cause people to lower their voices and thereby reduce noise; for example, closing the patient's door, placing phones on low volume, speaking at lower volumes, and dimming lights *to reduce extraneous sounds.*
- Instruct the patient to avoid dietary substances and drugs that may influence sleep, including ingestion of caffeine or other stimulants, nicotine, alcohol, sedatives, hypnotics, and fluid intake *to enhance the ability to sleep.*
- Provide warm, light snacks containing protein at bedtime and small amounts of liquids *to promote a sense of comfort.*
- Provide a cup of water close to the bed *to avoid a dry mouth and facilitate returning to sleep after awakening.*
- Advise the patient to avoid strenuous exercise at least 2 hours before bedtime *to enhance the ability to sleep.*
- PCC Teach the patient to relax before going to bed with reading, music, meditation, or other comforting and soothing activity *to enhance the ability to sleep.*
- PCC Educate the patient about sleep hygiene measures: to use the bedroom and bed only for sleep (or sexual activity), and to avoid other activities in the bedroom, such as watching television, reading, and eating, *to enhance the ability to sleep.*

Suggested NIC Interventions

Energy Management; Environmental Management; Environmental Management: Comfort; Progressive Muscle Relaxation; Sleep Enhancement

Evaluations for Expected Outcomes

- Patient identifies factors that enhance readiness for sleep.
- Patient demonstrates readiness for enhanced sleep through the use of appropriate sleep hygiene measures.

- Patient's amount of sleep and REM sleep is congruent with developmental needs.
- Patient expresses feeling rested after sleep.
- Institutional policies and staff behaviors reflect measures to enhance readiness for sleep.

Documentation

- Patient's sleep history
- Patient's plan for behavioral modification
- Observations of sleep hygiene behaviors
- Nursing interventions to enhance sleep readiness
- Patient's response to nursing interventions
- Evaluations for expected outcomes

REFERENCES

Halpern, J., Cohen, M., Kennedy, G., Reece, J., Cahan, C., & Baharav, A. (2014). Yoga for improving sleep quality and quality of life for older adults. *Alternative Therapies in Health & Medicine*, *20*(3), 37–46.

Hwang, E., & Shin, S. (2015). The effects of aromatherapy on sleep improvement: A systematic literature review and meta-analysis. *Journal of Alternative & Complementary Medicine*, *21*(2), 61–68. doi:10.1089/acm.2014.0113

Wu, W., Kwong, E., Lan, X., & Jiang, X. (2015). The effect of a meditative movement intervention on quality of sleep in the elderly: A systematic review and meta-analysis. *Journal of Alternative & Complementary Medicine*, *21*(9), 509–519. doi:10.1089/acm.2014.0251

READINESS FOR ENHANCED SPIRITUAL WELL-BEING

Definition

A pattern of experiencing and integrating meaning and purpose in life through connectedness with self, others, art, music, literature, nature, and/or a power greater than oneself, which can be strengthened

Assessment

- Spiritual status, including personal religious habits, religious or church affiliation, embarrassment at practicing religious rituals, and opposition to beliefs by family, peers, and health care providers
- Health history, including medical conditions that change body image, chronic or terminal illness, and debilitating disease
- Psychological status, including reactions to illness and disability; change in appetite, energy level, motivation, personal hygiene, self-image, sleep, and sex drive; alcohol or drug abuse; moodiness; recent divorce, job loss, or losses through separation or death; personality traits; and relationships with peers
- Self-care status, including neurologic, musculoskeletal, sensory, or psychological impairment and ability to carry out activities and adapt
- Family status, including marital status and communication patterns
- Nutritional status, including malabsorption or nutritional deficiencies, obesity, anorexia, bulimia, weight loss or gain, nausea, vomiting, fainting, constipation, diarrhea, pallor, irritability, cravings, food hoarding, and alteration in personal habits such as exercise, drug and alcohol use, and use of laxatives
- Sleep pattern status, including hours of sleep, energy level before and after sleep, difficulty falling asleep, nocturnal awakening, early morning awakening, hypersomnia, insomnia, and sleep pattern reversal

Defining Characteristics

Connections to Self

- Expresses desire to enhance acceptance
- Expresses desire to enhance coping
- Expresses desire to enhance courage
- Expresses desire to enhance hope
- Expresses desire to enhance joy
- Expresses desire to enhance love
- Expresses desire to enhance meaning in life
- Expresses desire to enhance meditative practice
- Expresses desire to enhance purpose in life
- Expresses desire to enhance satisfaction with philosophy of life
- Expresses desire to enhance self-forgiveness
- Expresses desire to enhance serenity (e.g., peace)
- Expresses desire to enhance surrender

Connections with Others

- Expresses desire to enhance forgiveness from others
- Expresses desire to enhance interaction with significant other
- Expresses desire to enhance interaction with spiritual leaders
- Expresses desire to enhance service to others

Connections with Art, Music, Literature, and Nature

- Expresses desire to enhance creative energy (e.g., writing, poetry, music)
- Expresses desire to enhance spiritual reading
- Expresses desire to enhance time outdoors
- Expresses desire to enhance mystical experiences
- Expresses desire to enhance participation in religious activity
- Expresses desire to enhance prayerfulness
- Expresses desire to enhance reverence

Expected Outcomes

- Patient will discuss spiritual conflicts.
- Patient will have opportunity to meet with chosen religious figure.
- Patient will receive support in efforts to pursue enhanced spiritual well-being.
- Patient will pursue religious or spiritual practices to the extent the patient feels comfortable.
- Patient will openly discuss effects of illness on own beliefs and other spiritual issues.
- Patient will describe plan to continue to enhance spiritual well-being.
- Patient will receive referrals for continued support.

Suggested NOC Outcomes

Hope; Quality of Life; Spiritual Health

Interventions and Rationales

- Monitor for potential signs of spiritual distress that might harm the patient's well-being (altered self-care, sleep pattern disturbance, and change in exercise and eating habits) *to plan appropriate interventions.*
- Assess the significance of spirituality in the patient's life and ability to cope with illness. Note whether the patient participates in religious rituals, observes religious practices (prayer, meditation, and dietary restrictions), or wishes to discuss spiritual beliefs. Keep an open view of what constitutes spirituality. *Before you can intervene in spiritual matters, you must determine the significance of spirituality for the patient.*

- Ask the patient whether illness has affected the patient's spiritual outlook, and tell the patient you're willing to help address spiritual issues if the patient wishes *to reduce isolation and help bring issues related to spiritual distress out into the open.*
- Ask whether the patient wishes to discuss spiritual concerns with a religious figure *to allow access to expert spiritual care resources.*
- Encourage the patient to pursue spiritual questions. Reassure the patient that spiritual concerns are valid and that by strengthening spirituality, the patient can enhance overall well-being *to demonstrate acceptance.*
- PCC Provide the patient with resources for coping with spiritual distress (referrals to religious or spiritual organizations and books on prayer and meditation) *to enhance the opportunity to attend to spiritual needs.* Make sure the patient receives materials appropriate to own religious affiliation and spiritual beliefs *to demonstrate respect for personal beliefs and values.* If you lack knowledge about the patient's beliefs and practices, consult a religious figure *to best meet the patient's needs.*
- Help the patient arrange travel to a place selected for prayer, reflection, or contemplation. Use resources such as church-affiliated vans or volunteer escorts *to enhance the patient's contact with outside sources of support.*
- Demonstrate to the patient that you're willing to discuss issues related to spirituality, such as the patient's view of God, how illness has affected the patient's religious beliefs, and how hospital stays affect the patient's spiritual practices *to bring spiritual issues into the open.* Keep an open mind when listening. Keep conversation focused on the patient's spiritual values and the role they play in recovering from illness and coping with changes in body image *to ensure that interaction between you and the patient remains therapeutic.*
- Discuss with the patient the importance of maintaining a healthful diet, getting regular exercise and sleep, and maintaining healthy interaction with family and friends. *A patient in spiritual distress may neglect day-to-day well-being.*
- Praise the patient for taking time to attend to own spiritual needs, and encourage the patient to continue to develop spirituality after leaving the facility *to provide continued encouragement.*
- PCC Provide the patient with referrals to appropriate religious groups, spiritually centered organizations, and social service organizations. Consider resources such as parish nurses, home-visiting services, and computer networks *to help provide a continued opportunity for spiritual development and to ensure continuity of care.*

Suggested NIC Interventions

Coping Enhancement; Self-Awareness Enhancement; Spiritual Growth Facilitation; Spiritual Support; Values Clarification

Evaluations for Expected Outcomes

- Patient discusses spiritual conflicts.
- Patient has opportunity to meet with chosen religious figure.
- Patient recognizes and expresses support received in own efforts to pursue enhanced spiritual well-being.
- Patient pursues religious or spiritual practices to the extent the patient feels comfortable.
- Patient discusses effects of illness on own beliefs and other spiritual issues openly.
- Patient describes plan to continue to enhance spiritual well-being.
- Patient identifies religious resources offered outside facility or agency.

Documentation

- Statements about spiritual conflicts
- Visits with religious representative
- Engagement in religious or spiritual practices
- Religious resources suggested outside facility or agency
- Statements about ability to cope with changes in body image as a result of illness, to maintain spiritual values in the face of long-term or chronic illness, and to pursue spiritual practices during hospital stays
- Eating patterns, exercise schedules, and sleep patterns
- Stated plans to continue to enhance spiritual well-being
- Evaluations for expected outcomes

REFERENCES

Kidwell, M. D. (2014). Music therapy and spirituality: How can I keep from singing? *Music Therapy Perspectives*, *32*(2), 129–135. doi:10.1093/mtp/miu023

Scott, H. (2016). The importance of spirituality for people living with dementia. *Nursing Standard*, *30*(25), 41–50.

Taylor, E. J., Park, C. G., & Pfeiffer, J. B. (2014). Nurse religiosity and spiritual care. *Journal of Advanced Nursing*, *70*(11), 2612–2621. doi:10.1111/jan.12446

Appendix A

A Selected Nursing Diagnoses by Medical Diagnosis

Abnormal rupture of membranes
- Deficient fluid volume
- Fear
- Hyperthermia
- Impaired resilience
- Readiness for enhanced childbearing process
- Risk for bleeding
- Risk for disturbance of maternal–fetal dyad
- Risk for imbalanced fluid volume
- Risk for infection
- Risk for shock

Abortion
- Anxiety
- Complicated grieving
- Ineffective coping
- Hopelessness
- Impaired resilience
- Moral distress
- Readiness for enhanced coping
- Readiness for enhanced decision making
- Risk for bleeding
- Risk for complicated grieving
- Risk for infection
- Risk for interruption of maternal–fetal dyad
- Readiness for enhanced resilience
- Risk for impaired resilience
- Risk for shock
- Situational low self-esteem

Abruptio placentae
- Acute pain
- Anxiety
- Risk for bleeding
- Complicated grieving
- Readiness for enhanced hope
- Risk for shock

Acoustic neuroma
- Chronic pain
- Disturbed sensory perception (auditory)
- Nausea
- Imbalanced nutrition: Less than body requirements
- Impaired skin integrity
- Ineffective breathing pattern
- Ineffective tissue cerebral perfusion
- Insomnia
- Readiness for enhanced knowledge
- Risk for deficient fluid volume
- Risk for electrolyte imbalance
- Risk for interruption of maternal–fetal dyad

Acquired immunodeficiency syndrome
- Caregiver role strain
- Chronic confusion
- Death anxiety
- Decisional conflict
- Defensive coping
- Deficient community health
- Grieving
- Hopelessness
- Impaired resilience
- Impaired memory
- Ineffective community coping
- Ineffective denial
- Ineffective protection
- Ineffective health management
- Ineffective sexuality patterns
- Ineffective therapeutic regimen management
- Moral distress
- Powerlessness
- Readiness for enhanced communication
- Readiness for enhanced emancipated decision making
- Readiness for enhanced resilience
- Readiness for enhanced self-care
- Risk for caregiver role strain
- Risk for complicated grieving
- Risk for compromised human dignity
- Risk for contamination
- Risk for delayed surgical recovery
- Risk for impaired oral mucous membrane

- Risk for infection
- Risk for loneliness
- Risk-prone health behavior
- Social isolation

Acute pancreatitis

- Acute pain
- Deficient knowledge (specify)
- Impaired comfort
- Insomnia
- Nausea
- Readiness for enhanced coping
- Risk for dysfunctional gastrointestinal motility
- Risk for electrolyte imbalance
- Risk for imbalanced fluid volume
- Risk for impaired liver function
- Risk for unstable glucose level
- Risk-prone health behavior

Acute renal failure

- Death anxiety
- Decreased cardiac output
- Deficient fluid volume
- Disturbed thought processes
- Dressing or grooming self-care deficit
- Excess fluid volume
- Fear
- Impaired physical mobility
- Impaired skin integrity
- Ineffective tissue perfusion (renal)
- Interrupted family processes
- Readiness for enhanced spiritual well-being
- Risk for acute confusion
- Risk for complicated grieving
- Risk for electrolyte imbalance
- Risk for imbalanced fluid volume
- Risk for ineffective renal perfusion
- Risk for infection
- Risk-prone health behavior
- Sexual dysfunction
- Disturbed sleep pattern
- Sleep deprivation
- Spiritual distress

Acute respiratory distress syndrome

- Anxiety
- Bathing or hygiene self-care deficit
- Deficient fluid volume
- Denial
- Dysfunctional ventilatory weaning response
- Fear
- Impaired comfort
- Imbalanced nutrition: Less than body requirements
- Impaired gas exchange
- Impaired skin integrity
- Impaired spontaneous ventilation
- Impaired verbal communication
- Ineffective airway clearance
- Ineffective breathing pattern
- Ineffective coping
- Ineffective tissue perfusion (cardiopulmonary)
- Insomnia
- Risk for acute confusion
- Risk for electrolyte imbalance
- Risk for ineffective cardiac tissue perfusion
- Risk for ineffective cerebral tissue perfusion
- Risk for infection
- Risk for shock
- Risk for vascular trauma
- Sleep deprivation

Acute respiratory failure

- Activity intolerance
- Death anxiety
- Decreased cardiac output
- Denial
- Disturbed sensory perception
- Disturbed thought processes
- Fear
- Impaired gas exchange
- Impaired resilience
- Impaired verbal communication
- Ineffective breathing pattern
- Ineffective tissue perfusion (cardiopulmonary)
- Insomnia
- Powerlessness
- Readiness for enhanced spiritual well-being
- Risk for ineffective activity planning
- Risk for acute confusion
- Risk for aspiration
- Risk for electrolyte imbalance
- Risk for ineffective cardiac tissue perfusion
- Risk for ineffective renal tissue perfusion
- Risk for infection
- Risk for shock
- Risk for suffocation
- Spiritual distress

Adrenal insufficiency

- Acute pain
- Chronic low self-esteem
- Compromised family coping
- Disturbed body image

- Disturbed personality identity
- Readiness for enhanced resilience
- Readiness for enhanced self-care
- Risk for electrolyte imbalance
- Risk for imbalanced body temperature
- Risk for impaired skin integrity
- Risk for infection
- Risk-prone health behavior
- Sexual dysfunction
- Sleep deprivation

Adrenocortical insufficiency

- Risk for disproportionate growth
- Risk for infection

Affective disorders

- Anxiety
- Disturbed personality identity
- Disturbed sensory perception (specify)
- Disturbed thought processes
- Hopelessness
- Impaired mood regulation
- Impaired religiosity
- Ineffective coping
- Ineffective impulse control
- Ineffective relationship
- Ineffective role performance
- Insomnia
- Labile emotional control
- Readiness for enhanced coping
- Readiness for enhanced emancipated decision making
- Risk for loneliness
- Risk for other-directed violence
- Risk-prone health behavior
- Risk for self-directed violence
- Sexual dysfunction
- Disturbed sleep pattern
- Stress overload

Alcohol addiction and abuse

- Acute confusion
- Bathing or hygiene self-care deficit
- Defensive coping
- Deficient knowledge (specify)
- Disturbed personality identity
- Dysfunctional family processes: Alcoholism
- Functional urinary incontinence
- Imbalanced nutrition: Less than body requirements
- Impaired emancipated decision making
- Impaired resilience
- Impaired physical mobility
- Ineffective activity planning
- Ineffective community therapeutic regimen management
- Ineffective coping
- Ineffective denial
- Ineffective family health management
- Ineffective impulse response
- Insomnia
- Labile emotional control
- Powerlessness
- Readiness for enhanced emancipated decision making
- Readiness for enhanced family processes
- Readiness for enhanced family coping
- Readiness for enhanced self-concept
- Risk for acute confusion
- Risk for compromised human dignity
- Risk for electrolyte imbalance
- Risk for imbalanced fluid volume
- Risk for impaired emancipated decision making
- Risk for impaired liver function
- Risk for poisoning
- Risk for self-directed violence
- Risk-prone health behavior
- Self-neglect
- Sexual dysfunction
- Sleep deprivation
- Spiritual distress
- Social isolation
- Stress overload

Alzheimer's disease

- Anxiety
- Bathing or hygiene self-care deficit
- Bowel incontinence
- Caregiver role strain
- Chronic confusion
- Chronic functional constipation
- Chronic low self-esteem
- Complicated grieving
- Compromised family coping
- Deficient knowledge (specify)
- Disturbed sensory perception
- Disturbed thought processes
- Frail elderly syndrome
- Functional urinary incontinence
- Grieving
- Hopelessness
- Imbalanced nutrition: Less than body requirements
- Impaired comfort

- Impaired emancipated decision making
- Impaired home maintenance
- Impaired memory
- Impaired verbal communication
- Ineffective coping
- Ineffective health maintenance
- Ineffective role performance
- Ineffective sexuality patterns
- Interrupted family processes
- Moral distress
- Readiness for enhanced knowledge
- Readiness for enhanced self-care
- Relocation stress syndrome
- Risk for caregiver role strain
- Risk for chronic functional constipation
- Risk for compromised human dignity
- Risk for frail elderly syndrome
- Risk for impaired emancipated decision making
- Risk for injury
- Risk for poisoning
- Risk for trauma
- Social isolation
- Stress urinary incontinence
- Wandering

Amniotic fluid embolism
- Ineffective tissue perfusion (cardiopulmonary)
- Risk for electrolyte imbalance
- Risk for ineffective cardiac tissue perfusion
- Risk for ineffective peripheral tissue perfusion
- Risk for injury
- Risk for shock

Amputation
- Acute pain
- Anxiety
- Chronic low self-esteem
- Chronic pain
- Decisional conflict
- Deficient knowledge (specify)
- Delayed surgical recovery
- Denial
- Disturbed body image
- Disturbed personality identity
- Grieving
- Impaired resilience
- Impaired wheelchair mobility
- Impaired walking
- Ineffective activity planning
- Impaired transfer ability
- Readiness for enhanced self-care
- Readiness for enhanced hope
- Readiness for enhanced knowledge
- Risk for impaired resilience
- Risk for compromised human dignity
- Risk for impaired tissue integrity
- Risk for injury
- Risk for pressure ulcer
- Risk-prone health behavior

Amyotrophic lateral sclerosis
- Bowel incontinence
- Caregiver role strain
- Chronic low self-esteem
- Complicated grieving
- Compromised family coping
- Constipation
- Death anxiety
- Disturbed personality identity
- Dressing or grooming self-care deficit
- Dysfunctional ventilatory weaning response
- Grieving
- Hopelessness
- Impaired physical mobility
- Impaired sitting
- Impaired skin integrity
- Impaired spontaneous ventilation
- Impaired standing
- Impaired verbal communication
- Impaired walking
- Impaired wheelchair ability
- Ineffective airway clearance
- Ineffective breathing pattern
- Ineffective coping
- Ineffective health maintenance
- Ineffective sexuality patterns
- Readiness for enhanced knowledge
- Risk for aspiration
- Risk for caregiver role strain
- Risk for constipation
- Risk for dysfunctional gastrointestinal motility
- Risk for electrolyte imbalance
- Risk for falls
- Risk for imbalanced fluid volume
- Risk for impaired skin integrity
- Risk for ineffective peripheral tissue perfusion
- Risk for infection
- Risk for pressure ulcer
- Social isolation

Anaphylactic shock
- Decreased cardiac output
- Impaired gas exchange
- Ineffective tissue perfusion (cardiopulmonary)

- Ineffective tissue perfusion (renal)
- Ineffective tissue perfusion (cerebral)

Anemias

- Activity intolerance
- Decreased cardiac output
- Fatigue
- Impaired gas exchange
- Impaired skin integrity
- Ineffective breathing patterns
- Ineffective protection
- Ineffective tissue perfusion (cardiopulmonary)
- Readiness for enhanced resilience
- Risk for infection

Angina pectoris

- Activity intolerance
- Acute pain
- Anxiety
- Deficient knowledge (specify)
- Impaired comfort
- Ineffective denial
- Ineffective role performance
- Ineffective sexuality patterns
- Readiness for enhanced knowledge
- Risk for ineffective activity planning
- Risk for ineffective cardiac tissue perfusion
- Risk for ineffective cerebral tissue perfusion
- Risk for ineffective renal tissue perfusion
- Sedentary lifestyle
- Stress overload

Anorexia nervosa

- Anxiety
- Constipation
- Deficient fluid volume
- Disturbed body image
- Disturbed personality image
- Hyperthermia
- Imbalanced nutrition: Less than body requirements
- Impaired resilience
- Ineffective denial
- Ineffective impulse control
- Ineffective relationships
- Interrupted family processes
- Readiness for enhanced emancipated decision making
- Readiness for enhanced nutrition
- Readiness for enhanced relationship
- Readiness for enhanced sleep
- Risk for chronic low self-esteem
- Risk for constipation
- Risk for dysfunctional gastrointestinal motility
- Risk-prone health behavior
- Sleep deprivation
- Social isolation
- Spiritual distress
- Stress overload

Antisocial personality disorder

- Chronic low self-esteem
- Defensive coping
- Disturbed personal identity
- Disturbed sensory perception
- Dysfunctional family processes: Alcoholism
- Impaired home maintenance
- Impaired resilience
- Ineffective coping
- Ineffective role performance
- Interrupted family processes
- Readiness for enhanced relationships
- Readiness for enhanced family coping
- Risk for other-directed violence
- Risk for self-mutilation
- Risk for suicide
- Sexual dysfunction
- Social isolation

Anxiety disorder

- Anxiety
- Caregiver role strain
- Chronic low self-esteem
- Constipation
- Defensive coping
- Diarrhea
- Disturbed sensory perception
- Disturbed thought processes
- Hopelessness
- Impaired emancipated decision making
- Impaired home maintenance
- Impaired mood regulation
- Ineffective denial
- Interrupted family processes
- Posttrauma syndrome
- Powerlessness
- Readiness for enhanced communication
- Readiness for enhanced coping
- Readiness for enhanced emancipated decision making
- Readiness for enhanced nutrition
- Readiness for enhanced self-concept
- Readiness for enhanced sleep
- Readiness for enhanced spiritual well-being

- Risk for imbalanced nutrition: Less than required
- Risk for impaired religiosity
- Risk for loneliness
- Risk for posttrauma syndrome
- Social isolation
- Sleep deprivation
- Stress overload

Aortic aneurysm
- Acute pain
- Excess fluid volume
- Impaired gas exchange
- Ineffective tissue perfusion (cardiopulmonary)
- Ineffective tissue perfusion (peripheral)
- Ineffective tissue perfusion (renal)
- Risk for bleeding
- Risk for electrolyte imbalance
- Risk for imbalanced fluid volume
- Risk for ineffective cerebral tissue perfusion
- Risk for shock

Aortic insufficiency
- Activity intolerance
- Decreased cardiac output
- Deficient knowledge (specify)
- Impaired gas exchange
- Ineffective tissue perfusion (cardiopulmonary)
- Risk for decreased cardiac output
- Risk for impaired cardiovascular function
- Risk for ineffective renal tissue perfusion

Aortic stenosis
- Activity intolerance
- Decreased cardiac output
- Deficient knowledge (specify)
- Impaired gas exchange
- Ineffective tissue perfusion (cardiopulmonary)
- Risk for decreased cardiac output

Appendicitis
- Acute pain
- Delayed surgical recovery
- Imbalanced nutrition: Less than body requirements
- Impaired comfort
- Risk for imbalanced fluid volume
- Risk for infection
- Arterial insufficiency
- Chronic pain
- Impaired tissue integrity
- Readiness for enhanced knowledge
- Risk for ineffective peripheral tissue perfusion

Arterial occlusion
- Acute pain
- Deficient knowledge (specify)
- Disturbed sensory perception (tactile)
- Impaired comfort
- Impaired skin integrity
- Ineffective tissue perfusion (cerebral)
- Ineffective tissue perfusion (peripheral)
- Risk for ineffective peripheral tissue perfusion
- Risk-prone health behavior

Asphyxia
- Hypothermia
- Ineffective breathing pattern
- Ineffective gas exchange
- Risk for aspiration
- Risk for injury
- Risk for hypothermia
- Risk for suffocation

Asthma
- Activity intolerance
- Anxiety
- Deficient knowledge (specify)
- Dressing or grooming self-care deficit
- Dry eye
- Impaired gas exchange
- Impaired oral mucous membrane
- Ineffective airway clearance
- Ineffective breathing pattern
- Ineffective coping
- Latex allergy response
- Readiness for enhanced comfort
- Readiness for enhanced family coping
- Readiness for enhanced knowledge
- Risk for impaired resilience
- Risk for infection
- Risk for latex allergy response
- Risk-prone health behavior
- Sleep deprivation
- Stress overload

Atelectasis
- Anxiety
- Bathing or hygiene self-care deficit
- Impaired gas exchange
- Impaired physical mobility
- Ineffective airway clearance
- Ineffective breathing pattern
- Impaired gas exchange
- Readiness for enhanced self-care

Attention deficit hyperactivity disorder
- Denial
- Disturbed sleep pattern
- Family therapeutic regimen management
- Ineffective activity planning
- Interrupted family processes
- Readiness for enhanced family processes
- Readiness for enhanced relationships
- Risk for delayed development
- Stress overload

Autism
- Compromised family coping
- Disabled family coping
- Impaired emancipated decision making
- Ineffective denial
- Interrupted family processes
- Labile emotional control
- Risk for delayed development
- Risk for impaired emancipated decision making
- Risk for self-mutilation

Bell's palsy
- Acute pain
- Anxiety
- Chronic low self-esteem
- Disturbed body image
- Disturbed sleep pattern
- Disturbed sensory perception (gustatory)
- Impaired comfort
- Impaired swallowing
- Impaired verbal communication
- Ineffective sexuality patterns
- Powerlessness
- Risk for compromised human dignity
- Social isolation
- Stress overload
- Unilateral neglect

Benign prostatic hypertrophy
- Deficient knowledge (specify)
- Impaired comfort
- Impaired urinary elimination
- Ineffective sexuality patterns
- Sexual dysfunction
- Urinary retention

Bipolar disorder: Depressive phase
- Chronic low self-esteem
- Constipation
- Disturbed personality identity
- Disturbed sensory perception
- Disturbed thought processes
- Feeding self-care deficit
- Hopelessness
- Imbalanced nutrition: Less than body requirements
- Impaired emancipated decision making
- Impaired mood regulation
- Ineffective coping
- Ineffective denial
- Ineffective relationships
- Ineffective health maintenance
- Insomnia
- Readiness for enhanced communication
- Readiness for enhanced coping
- Readiness for enhanced self-concept
- Risk for compromised human dignity
- Risk for ineffective activity planning
- Risk for injury
- Risk for self-directed violence
- Self-neglect
- Sexual dysfunction
- Sleep deprivation
- Social isolation
- Spiritual distress
- Stress overload

Bipolar disorder: Manic phase
- Chronic low self-esteem
- Disabled family coping
- Disturbed personality identity
- Disturbed sensory perception
- Disturbed thought processes
- Feeding self-care deficit
- Impaired home maintenance
- Impaired physical mobility
- Impaired verbal communication
- Ineffective coping
- Ineffective denial
- Ineffective impulse control
- Ineffective sexuality pattern
- Insomnia
- Risk for impaired resilience
- Readiness for enhanced family coping
- Interrupted family processes
- Risk for falls
- Risk for impaired religiosity
- Risk for injury
- Risk for other-directed violence
- Risk-prone health behavior
- Sexual dysfunction
- Spiritual distress

Bladder cancer
- Acute pain
- Fear
- Impaired tissue integrity
- Impaired urinary elimination
- Readiness for enhanced self-care
- Risk for compromised human dignity
- Risk for latex allergy response
- Overflow urinary incontinence
- Urge urinary incontinence

Blindness
- Deficient diversional activity
- Deficient knowledge (specify)
- Disturbed body image
- Disturbed sensory perception (visual)
- Fear
- Hopelessness
- Impaired physical mobility
- Ineffective health management
- Powerlessness
- Risk for falls
- Risk for injury
- Risk for loneliness
- Social isolation

Bone marrow transplantation
- Activity intolerance
- Complicated grieving
- Contamination
- Decreased cardiac output
- Deficient diversional activity
- Diarrhea
- Disturbed body image
- Excess fluid volume
- Grieving
- Imbalanced nutrition: Less than body requirements
- Impaired oral mucous membrane
- Impaired skin integrity
- Ineffective activity planning
- Ineffective protection
- Ineffective therapeutic management
- Risk for contamination
- Risk for electrolyte imbalance
- Risk for imbalanced fluid balance
- Risk for infection

Bone sarcomas
- Activity intolerance
- Acute pain
- Deficient knowledge
- Impaired comfort
- Impaired physical mobility
- Impaired tissue integrity
- Readiness for enhanced knowledge
- Risk for falls
- Risk for injury
- Risk for infection

Borderline personality disorder
- Chronic low self-esteem
- Disturbed personality identity
- Fear
- Impaired religiosity
- Ineffective coping
- Ineffective impulse control
- Ineffective relationships
- Risk for impaired resilience
- Risk for self-directed violence
- Risk for self-mutilation
- Social isolation

Bowel fistula
- Chronic functional constipation
- Risk for chronic functional constipation
- Risk for deficient fluid volume
- Risk for infection

Bowel resection
- Anxiety
- Delayed surgical recovery
- Dysfunctional gastrointestinal motility
- Deficient knowledge
- Diarrhea
- Imbalanced nutrition: Less than required
- Impaired skin integrity
- Risk for delayed surgical recovery
- Risk for disturbed personal identity
- Risk for infection

Brain abscess
- Acute pain
- Decreased intracranial adaptive capacity
- Disturbed body image
- Impaired physical mobility
- Impaired skin integrity
- Ineffective sexuality patterns
- Ineffective tissue perfusion (cerebral)
- Risk for aspiration
- Risk for infection
- Risk for injury
- Risk for urge urinary incontinence

Brain tumors
- Acute confusion
- Bowel incontinence
- Constipation

- Decreased intracranial adaptive capacity
- Disturbed personality identity
- Disabled family processes
- Disturbed sensory perception
- Disturbed thought processes
- Fear
- Grieving
- Impaired memory
- Impaired physical mobility
- Impaired tissue integrity
- Impaired urinary elimination
- Impaired verbal communication
- Ineffective coping
- Ineffective thermoregulation
- Risk for falls
- Risk for injury
- Total urinary incontinence

Breast cancer
- Acute pain
- Anxiety
- Complicated grieving
- Death anxiety
- Decisional conflict (specify)
- Deficient knowledge (specify)
- Disturbed body image
- Fear
- Grieving
- Impaired skin integrity
- Ineffective coping
- Moral distress
- Powerlessness
- Readiness for enhanced hope
- Readiness for enhanced spiritual well-being
- Readiness for enhanced resilience
- Risk for compromised human dignity
- Spiritual distress

Breast engorgement
- Acute pain
- Impaired comfort
- Impaired skin integrity
- Ineffective breast-feeding
- Readiness for enhanced breast-feeding
- Risk for infection

Bronchiectasis
- Compromised family coping
- Deficient knowledge
- Imbalanced nutrition: Less than body requirements
- Impaired gas exchange
- Ineffective airway clearance
- Ineffective breathing pattern
- Risk for electrolyte imbalance
- Risk for imbalance in fluid volume
- Risk for infection

Bulimia nervosa
- Anxiety
- Constipation
- Deficient fluid volume
- Disabled family coping
- Disturbed body image
- Hyperthermia
- Imbalanced nutrition: Less than body requirements
- Impaired dentition
- Ineffective denial
- Interrupted family processes
- Powerlessness
- Risk for constipation
- Risk for electrolyte imbalance
- Risk for self-mutation
- Risk for self-directed violence
- Sleep deprivation
- Social isolation

Burns
- Acute pain
- Chronic functional constipation
- Constipation
- Deficient diversional activity
- Deficient fluid volume
- Disabled family coping
- Disturbed body image
- Disturbed personal identity
- Dysfunctional ventilatory weaning response
- Electrolyte imbalance
- Grieving
- Hyperthermia
- Hypothermia
- Imbalanced nutrition: Less than body requirements
- Impaired comfort
- Impaired physical mobility
- Impaired skin integrity
- Impaired spontaneous ventilation
- Ineffective breathing pattern
- Ineffective tissue perfusion (renal)
- Powerlessness
- Readiness for enhanced hope
- Readiness for enhanced self-care

- Risk for chronic functional constipation
- Risk for deficient fluid volume
- Risk for electrolyte imbalance
- Risk for falls
- Risk for imbalanced body temperature
- Risk for impaired tissue integrity
- Risk for infection
- Risk for injury
- Risk for hypothermia
- Risk for shock

Cancer
- Chronic functional constipation
- Chronic pain syndrome
- Chronic sorrow
- Death anxiety
- Deficient knowledge
- Disabled family coping
- Grieving
- Ineffective health maintenance
- Nausea
- Readiness for enhanced emancipated decision making
- Readiness for enhanced knowledge
- Readiness for enhanced religiosity
- Readiness for enhanced self-concept
- Readiness for enhanced spiritual well-being
- Risk for chronic functional constipation
- Risk for impaired tissue integrity
- Risk for infection
- Risk for spiritual distress

Cardiac arrhythmias
- Anxiety
- Decreased cardiac output
- Excess fluid volume
- Fear
- Ineffective sexuality patterns
- Ineffective tissue perfusion (cardiopulmonary)
- Risk for decreased cardiac output
- Risk for electrolyte imbalance
- Risk for imbalanced fluid volume
- Risk for impaired cardiovascular function
- Stress overload

Cardiac disease: End-stage
- Activity intolerance
- Caregiver role strain
- Death anxiety
- Decisional conflict
- Decreased cardiac output
- Defensive coping
- Excess fluid volume
- Grieving
- Hopelessness
- Ineffective breathing pattern
- Ineffective coping
- Impaired physical mobility
- Risk for aspiration
- Risk for caregiver role strain
- Risk for decreased cardiac output
- Risk for electrolyte imbalance
- Risk for falls
- Risk for impaired cardiovascular function
- Risk for infection
- Risk for injury
- Risk for perioperative hypothermia
- Sedentary lifestyle
- Self-care bathing, feeding, dressing, toileting deficit
- Situational low self-esteem

Cardiogenic shock
- Death anxiety
- Decreased cardiac output
- Excess fluid volume
- Fear
- Impaired gas exchange
- Ineffective breathing pattern
- Ineffective tissue perfusion (cardiac)
- Risk for decreased cardiac output
- Risk for impaired cardiovascular function

Carpal tunnel syndrome
- Acute pain
- Impaired physical mobility
- Ineffective tissue perfusion (peripheral)
- Risk for peripheral neurovascular dysfunction
- Sleep deprivation
- Readiness for enhanced comfort

Cataracts
- Disturbed body image
- Disturbed sensory perception (visual)
- Impaired physical mobility
- Ineffective coping
- Ineffective health maintenance
- Risk for falls
- Risk for injury

Cellulitis
- Acute pain
- Anxiety
- Deficient knowledge (specify)
- Impaired physical mobility
- Impaired skin integrity
- Risk for ineffective activity planning

Cerebral aneurysm
- Decreased intracranial adaptive capacity
- Fear
- Impaired physical mobility
- Impaired skin integrity
- Ineffective airway clearance
- Ineffective breathing pattern
- Ineffective tissue perfusion
- Risk for bleeding
- Risk for falls
- Risk for ineffective cerebral tissue perfusion
- Risk for injury
- Risk for shock

Cerebral edema
- Decreased intracranial adaptive capacity
- Impaired gas exchange
- Ineffective thermoregulation
- Risk for electrolyte imbalance
- Risk for ineffective cerebral tissue perfusion

Cerebral palsy
- Impaired physical mobility
- Impaired sitting
- Impaired standing
- Impaired walking
- Impaired verbal communication
- Powerlessness
- Readiness for enhanced self-care
- Risk for caregiver role strain
- Risk for compromised human dignity
- Social isolation
- Toileting self-care deficit
- Total urinary incontinence

Cervical cancer
- Acute pain
- Disturbed body image
- Disturbed personal identity
- Fatigue
- Fear
- Impaired skin integrity
- Ineffective protection
- Deficient knowledge
- Risk-prone health behavior

Chemotherapy
- Constipation
- Deficient diversional activity
- Deficient fluid volume
- Diarrhea
- Disturbed sensory perception (auditory)
- Imbalanced nutrition: Less than body requirements
- Impaired gas exchange
- Impaired oral mucous membrane
- Impaired physical mobility
- Ineffective protection
- Ineffective tissue perfusion
- Nausea
- Readiness for enhanced hope
- Risk for compromised human dignity
- Risk for impaired oral mucous membrane
- Risk for impaired skin integrity
- Risk for impaired tissue integrity
- Risk for infection
- Sexual dysfunction

Chest trauma
- Dysfunctional ventilatory weaning response
- Impaired comfort
- Impaired gas exchange
- Impaired spontaneous ventilation
- Ineffective airway clearance
- Ineffective breathing pattern
- Risk for aspiration
- Risk for ineffective cardiac tissue perfusion
- Risk for shock

Child abuse
- Fear
- Impaired parenting
- Deficient knowledge
- Imbalanced nutrition: Less than body requirements
- Parental role conflict
- Readiness for enhanced parenting
- Risk for impaired parenting
- Risk for other directed violence
- Disturbed sleep pattern

Childbirth
- Deficient knowledge (specify)
- Ineffective childbearing process
- Interrupted family processes
- Readiness for enhanced childbearing process
- Readiness for enhanced knowledge
- Readiness for enhanced parenting
- Risk for ineffective childbearing process
- Risk for disturbed maternal–fetal dyad

Chlamydia
- Ineffective health management
- Ineffective sexuality patterns
- Risk for infection
- Risk-prone health behavior

Chloride imbalance
- Imbalanced nutrition: Less than body requirements
- Impaired breathing pattern
- Nausea
- Risk for electrolyte imbalance

Cholecystitis
- Acute pain
- Deficient fluid volume
- Imbalanced nutrition: Less than body requirements
- Risk for impaired liver function
- Risk for infection

Chronic bronchitis
- Activity intolerance
- Deficient knowledge (specify)
- Fatigue
- Fear
- Hopelessness
- Impaired comfort
- Impaired gas exchange
- Impaired spontaneous ventilation
- Ineffective airway clearance
- Ineffective breathing pattern
- Risk for ineffective cardiac tissue perfusion
- Risk for infection

Chronic fatigue syndrome
- Acute pain
- Disturbed sleep pattern
- Fatigue
- Hopelessness
- Powerlessness
- Readiness for enhanced therapeutic regimen management
- Social isolation
- Risk for spiritual distress

Chronic obstructive pulmonary disease
- Activity intolerance
- Anxiety
- Caregiver role strain
- Compromised family coping
- Defensive coping
- Deficient fluid volume
- Deficient knowledge (specify)
- Dysfunctional ventilatory weaning response
- Fatigue
- Fear
- Hopelessness
- Imbalanced nutrition: Less than body requirements
- Impaired gas exchange
- Impaired home maintenance
- Impaired oral mucous membrane
- Impaired spontaneous ventilation
- Impaired verbal communication
- Ineffective airway clearance
- Ineffective breathing pattern
- Ineffective denial
- Ineffective health maintenance
- Ineffective health management
- Ineffective tissue perfusion (cardiopulmonary)
- Insomnia
- Noncompliance
- Powerlessness
- Readiness for enhanced coping
- Readiness for enhanced health management
- Readiness for enhanced religiosity
- Risk for falls
- Risk for infection
- Risk for injury
- Risk for suffocation
- Sleep deprivation

Chronic pain
- Anxiety
- Chronic functional constipation
- Chronic low self-esteem
- Chronic pain
- Chronic pain syndrome
- Defensive coping
- Disturbed sleep pattern
- Hopelessness
- Risk for chronic functional constipation
- Risk-prone health behavior
- Situational low self-esteem
- Sleep deprivation

Chronic renal failure
- Caregiver role strain
- Compromised family coping
- Death anxiety
- Deficient knowledge (specify)
- Disturbed body image
- Excess fluid volume
- Ineffective denial
- Ineffective therapeutic management
- Ineffective tissue perfusion (renal)
- Interrupted family processes
- Powerlessness
- Risk for ineffective renal perfusion
- Risk for impaired liver function
- Risk for impaired skin integrity
- Risk for infection

- Risk for vascular trauma
- Sexual dysfunction

Cirrhosis

- Compromised family coping
- Bowel incontinence
- Deficient fluid volume
- Diarrhea
- Disturbed thought processes
- Imbalanced nutrition: Less than body requirements
- Ineffective breathing pattern
- Interrupted family processes: Alcoholism
- Ineffective health management
- Moral distress
- Nausea
- Risk for bleeding
- Readiness for enhanced religiosity
- Risk for electrolyte imbalances
- Risk for falls
- Risk for impaired liver function
- Risk for impaired skin integrity
- Risk for ineffective gastrointestinal tissue perfusion
- Risk for injury
- Risk-prone health behavior
- Self-neglect
- Stress urinary incontinence
- Total urinary incontinence

Cleft lip or palate

- Compromised family coping
- Imbalanced nutrition: Less than body requirements
- Impaired verbal communication
- Ineffective breast-feeding
- Ineffective infant feeding pattern
- Risk for aspiration
- Risk for compromised human dignity

Colic

- Disorganized infant behavior
- Impaired comfort
- Interrupted breast-feeding

Colitis

- Acute pain
- Deficient knowledge
- Deficient fluid volume
- Diarrhea
- Dysfunctional gastrointestinal motility
- Disturbed body image
- Imbalanced nutrition: Less than body requirements
- Ineffective tissue perfusion (GI)
- Risk for imbalanced body temperature
- Risk-prone health behavior

Colon and rectal cancer

- Acute pain
- Anxiety
- Chronic functional constipation
- Constipation
- Deficient fluid volume
- Deficient knowledge (specify)
- Diarrhea
- Fear
- Impaired comfort
- Deficient knowledge
- Risk for chronic functional constipation
- Risk for dysfunctional gastrointestinal motility
- Risk for urinary tract injury

Colostomy

- Complicated grieving
- Deficient fluid volume
- Delayed surgical recovery
- Disturbed body image
- Dysfunctional gastrointestinal motility
- Imbalanced nutrition: Less than body requirements
- Impaired skin integrity
- Ineffective sexuality patterns
- Ineffective tissue perfusion (GI)
- Readiness for enhanced hope
- Readiness for enhanced knowledge
- Readiness for enhanced self-care
- Risk for compromised human dignity
- Situational low self-esteem
- Spiritual distress

Conduct disorder

- Chronic low self-esteem
- Disturbed personal identity
- Hopelessness
- Impaired resilience
- Ineffective impulse control
- Interrupted family processes
- Risk for other-directed violence
- Risk for self-directed violence
- Risk for suicide

Congenital anomalies

- Disabled family coping
- Interrupted family coping
- Risk for falls
- Risk for injury
- Total urinary incontinence

Congenital heart disease
- Activity intolerance
- Decreased cardiac output
- Disturbed body image
- Ineffective breathing pattern
- Interrupted family processes
- Risk for decreased cardiac output
- Risk for impaired cardiovascular function
- Risk for ineffective activity planning
- Risk for disproportionate growth
- Risk for infection
- Risk for injury

Coronary artery disease
- Activity intolerance
- Acute pain
- Anxiety
- Decreased cardiac output
- Deficient knowledge (specify)
- Health-seeking behaviors
- Impaired gas exchange
- Impaired home maintenance
- Ineffective sexuality patterns
- Ineffective therapeutic regimen management
- Ineffective tissue perfusion (cardiopulmonary)
- Readiness for enhanced knowledge
- Readiness for enhanced health management
- Risk for decreased cardiac output
- Risk for impaired cardiovascular function
- Risk for injury
- Risk for overweight
- Risk for perioperative hypothermia
- Risk-prone health behavior
- Sedentary lifestyle
- Stress overload

Cor pulmonale
- Activity intolerance
- Decreased cardiac output
- Excess fluid volume
- Fatigue
- Grieving
- Hopelessness
- Impaired gas exchange
- Ineffective airway clearance
- Ineffective breathing pattern
- Ineffective coping
- Risk for decreased cardiac output
- Risk for impaired cardiovascular function
- Risk for infection

Craniotomy
- Acute pain
- Bathing, feeding, toileting self-care deficit
- Decreased intracranial adaptive capacity
- Delayed surgical recovery
- Disturbed body image
- Disturbed sensory perception
- Disturbed sleep pattern
- Hyperthermia
- Imbalanced nutrition: Less then body requirements
- Impaired physical mobility
- Impaired skin integrity
- Ineffective airway clearance
- Ineffective breathing pattern
- Ineffective tissue perfusion (cerebral)
- Risk for falls
- Risk for infection
- Risk for injury
- Spiritual distress
- Sleep deprivation

Crohn's disease
- Acute pain
- Anxiety
- Compromised family coping
- Deficient fluid volume
- Deficient knowledge (specify)
- Diarrhea
- Disturbed body image
- Dysfunctional gastrointestinal motility
- Fear
- Imbalanced nutrition: Less than body requirements
- Impaired skin integrity
- Insomnia
- Nausea
- Noncompliance
- Readiness for enhanced hope
- Readiness for enhanced self-care
- Risk for imbalanced fluid volume
- Risk for infection
- Stress overload

Cushing's syndrome
- Activity intolerance
- Complicated grieving
- Disturbed body image
- Disturbed thought processes
- Excess fluid volume
- Hopelessness
- Impaired skin integrity

- Ineffective coping
- Risk for acute confusion
- Risk for imbalanced body temperature
- Risk for imbalanced fluid volume
- Risk for overweight

Cystic fibrosis
- Activity intolerance
- Caregiver role strain
- Compromised family coping
- Deficient diversional activity
- Deficient fluid volume
- Imbalanced nutrition: Less than body requirements
- Impaired gas exchange
- Ineffective activity planning
- Ineffective airway clearance
- Ineffective breathing pattern
- Parental role conflict
- Risk for delayed development
- Risk for deficient fluid volume
- Risk for imbalanced body temperature
- Risk for imbalanced fluid volume
- Risk for ineffective activity planning
- Risk for infection

Cystitis
- Acute pain
- Impaired urinary elimination
- Noncompliance
- Overflow urinary incontinence
- Risk for urge urinary incontinence
- Sleep deprivation
- Urge urinary incontinence

Deafness
- Chronic low self-esteem
- Defensive coping
- Disturbed sensory perception (auditory)
- Fear
- Impaired verbal communication
- Ineffective coping
- Readiness for enhanced coping
- Risk for falls
- Risk for injury
- Risk for trauma

Delusional disorder
- Disturbed personality identity
- Impaired home maintenance
- Risk for self-directed violence
- Risk for other directed violence
- Risk for self-mutilation

Dementia
- Activity intolerance
- Acute confusion
- Caregiver role strain
- Chronic confusion
- Disturbed sensory perception
- Disturbed thought processes
- Frail elderly syndrome
- Functional urinary incontinence
- Impaired emancipated decision making
- Impaired memory
- Impaired verbal communication
- Interrupted family processes
- Risk for frail elderly syndrome
- Risk for loneliness
- Powerlessness
- Risk for impaired emancipated decision making
- Risk for injury
- Risk for self-directed violence
- Risk for suicide
- Self-neglect
- Social isolation
- Wandering

Depression
- Caregiver role strain
- Chronic functional constipation
- Chronic low self-esteem
- Constipation
- Deficient diversional activity
- Disturbed body image
- Disturbed personality identity
- Fatigue
- Functional urinary incontinence
- Hopelessness
- Imbalanced nutrition: Less than body requirements
- Impaired home maintenance
- Impaired mood regulation
- Ineffective coping
- Ineffective denial
- Posttrauma syndrome
- Powerlessness
- Rape-trauma syndrome
- Readiness for enhanced nutrition
- Readiness for enhanced resilience
- Readiness for enhanced hope
- Risk for chronic functional constipation
- Risk for impaired resilience
- Risk for constipation
- Risk for injury

- Risk for loneliness
- Risk for poisoning
- Risk for posttrauma syndrome
- Risk for self-directed violence
- Sexual dysfunction
- Sleep deprivation
- Social isolation
- Spiritual distress

Detached retina
- Acute pain
- Anxiety
- Disturbed sensory perception (visual)
- Risk for falls
- Risk for injury

Developmental disorder
- Disabled family coping
- Impaired sitting
- Impaired standing
- Risk for impaired parent–infant–child attachment
- Risk for injury
- Risk for self-mutilation

Diabetes insipidus
- Deficient fluid volume
- Impaired oral mucous membrane
- Risk for deficient fluid volume
- Risk for imbalanced body temperature
- Risk for unstable glucose level

Diabetes mellitus
- Chronic low self-esteem
- Compromised family coping
- Constipation
- Decreased cardiac output
- Deficient knowledge (specify)
- Disturbed body image
- Disturbed sensory perception
- Grieving
- Hopelessness
- Hyperthermia
- Impaired oral mucous membrane
- Impaired skin integrity
- Impaired urinary elimination
- Ineffective coping
- Ineffective health maintenance
- Ineffective sexuality patterns
- Ineffective therapeutic regimen management
- Ineffective tissue perfusion (peripheral)
- Ineffective tissue perfusion (renal)
- Interrupted family coping
- Noncompliance
- Obesity
- Overweight
- Powerlessness
- Readiness for enhanced fluid balance
- Readiness for enhanced nutrition
- Readiness for enhanced resilience
- Readiness for enhanced therapeutic regimen management
- Readiness for enhanced urinary elimination
- Risk for delayed surgical recovery
- Risk for imbalanced fluid volume
- Risk for imbalanced body temperature
- Risk for impaired skin integrity
- Risk for infection
- Risk for injury
- Risk for overweight
- Risk for unstable glucose level
- Risk for vascular trauma
- Risk-prone health behavior
- Self-neglect
- Social isolation

Diabetic ketoacidosis
- Deficient fluid volume
- Deficient knowledge
- Noncompliance
- Risk for acute confusion
- Risk for imbalanced body temperature
- Risk for unstable glucose level
- Risk-prone health behavior

Diarrhea
- Deficient fluid volume
- Diarrhea
- Disturbed body image
- Dysfunctional gastrointestinal motility
- Readiness for enhanced fluid balance
- Risk for electrolyte imbalance
- Risk for imbalanced fluid volume

Digoxin toxicity
- Decreased cardiac output
- Deficient knowledge (specify)
- Risk for decreased cardiac output
- Risk for impaired cardiovascular function
- Risk for ineffective cardiac tissue perfusion
- Risk for poisoning

Disseminated intravascular coagulation
- Decreased cardiac output
- Death anxiety
- Deficient fluid volume
- Fear

- Impaired gas exchange
- Risk for bleeding
- Risk for decreased cardiac output
- Risk for impaired cardiovascular function
- Risk for ineffective cardiac tissue perfusion
- Risk for shock

Dissociative disorder
- Disturbed personality identity
- Disturbed thought processes
- Impaired home maintenance
- Interrupted family processes
- Risk for self-directed violence
- Risk for other-directed violence

Diverticulitis
- Acute pain
- Chronic functional constipation
- Constipation
- Deficient fluid volume
- Diarrhea
- Dysfunctional gastrointestinal motility
- Hyperthermia
- Imbalanced nutrition: Less than body requirements
- Risk for chronic functional constipation
- Risk for electrolyte imbalance

Down syndrome
- Compromised family coping
- Deficient knowledge (specify)
- Defensive coping
- Interrupted family processes
- Readiness for enhanced knowledge
- Readiness for enhanced self-care
- Risk for aspiration
- Risk for delayed development
- Risk for infection
- Risk for injury
- Situational low self-esteem
- Toileting self-care deficit

Drug addiction
- Acute confusion
- Decisional conflict
- Defensive coping
- Deficient community health
- Disturbed personality identity
- Dysfunctional family processes: Alcoholism
- Impaired resilience
- Ineffective community therapeutic regimen management
- Ineffective coping
- Ineffective denial
- Ineffective family health management
- Ineffective health maintenance
- Moral distress
- Risk for compromised human dignity
- Risk for falls
- Risk for injury
- Risk for impaired liver function
- Risk for poisoning
- Risk for self-directed violence
- Risk for sudden infant death syndrome
- Sexual dysfunction
- Sleep deprivation

Drug overdose
- Disturbed thought processes
- Functional urinary incontinence
- Hyperthermia
- Hypothermia
- Impaired comfort
- Impaired gas exchange
- Impaired resilience
- Ineffective coping
- Ineffective thermoregulation
- Risk for compromised human dignity
- Risk for hypothermia
- Risk for poisoning
- Risk for suffocation
- Risk for self-directed violence
- Risk for suicide
- Risk for trauma

Drug toxicity
- Functional urinary incontinence
- Hyperthermia
- Hypothermia
- Impaired resilience
- Impaired gas exchange
- Ineffective protection
- Risk for hypothermia
- Risk for impaired cardiovascular function
- Risk for poisoning

Duodenal ulcer
- Acute pain
- Anxiety
- Imbalanced nutrition: Less than body requirements
- Ineffective tissue perfusion (GI)
- Dysfunctional gastrointestinal motility
- Risk for shock
- Risk for ineffective gastrointestinal tissue perfusion

Ectopic pregnancy
- Acute pain
- Anxiety
- Deficient fluid volume
- Disturbed personal identity
- Fear
- Ineffective tissue perfusion (cardiopulmonary)
- Risk for electrolyte imbalance
- Risk for infection
- Risk for shock
- Situational low self-esteem

Emphysema
- Activity intolerance
- Deficient knowledge (specify)
- Fatigue
- Fear
- Hopelessness
- Imbalanced nutrition: Less than body requirements
- Impaired gas exchange
- Impaired spontaneous ventilation
- Ineffective airway clearance
- Ineffective breathing pattern
- Noncompliance
- Readiness for enhanced coping
- Readiness for enhanced decision making
- Readiness for enhanced knowledge
- Readiness for enhanced resilience
- Readiness for enhanced sleep
- Risk for infection

Empyema
- Deficient fluid volume
- Impaired gas exchange
- Ineffective breathing pattern
- Risk for infection

Encephalitis
- Activity intolerance
- Acute pain
- Anxiety
- Constipation
- Deficient fluid volume
- Hyperthermia
- Impaired physical mobility
- Ineffective coping
- Ineffective thermoregulation
- Risk for infection

Endocarditis
- Activity intolerance
- Acute pain
- Anxiety
- Decreased cardiac output
- Deficient knowledge (specify)
- Excess fluid volume
- Hyperthermia
- Imbalanced nutrition: Less than body requirements
- Readiness for enhanced knowledge
- Risk for decreased cardiac output
- Risk for impaired cardiovascular function
- Risk for infection
- Risk for ineffective cardiac tissue perfusion

Endometrial cancer
- Acute pain
- Chronic sorrow
- Fear
- Grieving
- Impaired tissue integrity
- Ineffective protection

Endometriosis
- Anxiety
- Decisional conflict
- Deficient fluid volume
- Deficient knowledge (specify)
- Grieving
- Moral distress
- Risk for infection
- Sexual dysfunction
- Spiritual distress

Esophageal cancer
- Acute pain
- Dysfunctional intestinal motility
- Fatigue
- Fear
- Imbalanced nutrition: Less than body requirements
- Impaired resilience
- Impaired swallowing
- Ineffective coping
- Ineffective health management
- Risk for aspiration
- Risk for deficient fluid volume
- Risk for infection

Esophageal fistula
- Imbalanced nutrition: Less than body requirements
- Risk for aspiration
- Risk for deficient fluid volume

Esophageal varices
- Deficient fluid volume
- Disturbed personal identity
- Dysfunctional family processes: Alcoholism
- Imbalanced nutrition: Less than body requirements
- Moral distress
- Readiness for enhanced hope
- Risk for bleeding
- Risk for imbalanced fluid volume
- Risk for impaired skin integrity
- Risk for shock

Failure to thrive
- Deficient fluid volume
- Disorganized infant behavior
- Frail elderly syndrome
- Imbalanced nutrition: Less than body requirements
- Impaired parenting
- Ineffective community coping
- Risk for deficient fluid volume
- Risk for disorganized infant behavior
- Risk for frail elderly syndrome
- Risk for impaired parenting

Fetal alcohol syndrome
- Compromised family coping
- Dysfunctional family processes: Alcoholism
- Ineffective community coping
- Moral distress
- Risk for delayed development
- Risk for disproportionate growth
- Disturbed sleep pattern
- Food poisoning
- Acute pain
- Contamination
- Diarrhea
- Disturbed sensory perception (visual)
- Dysfunctional gastrointestinal motility
- Hyperthermia
- Impaired physical mobility
- Impaired verbal communication
- Ineffective breathing pattern
- Nausea
- Risk for contamination
- Risk for electrolyte imbalance
- Risk for imbalance of fluid volume

Fractures
- Activity intolerance
- Acute pain
- Bathing or hygiene self-care deficit
- Compromised family coping
- Deficient diversional activity
- Deficient fluid volume
- Disturbed sensory perception
- Hopelessness
- Impaired parenting
- Impaired physical mobility
- Impaired wheelchair mobility
- Impaired skin integrity
- Impaired transfer ability
- Ineffective breathing pattern
- Ineffective denial
- Risk for constipation
- Risk for disuse syndrome
- Risk for falls
- Risk for infection
- Risk for injury
- Risk for perioperative positioning injury
- Risk for peripheral neurovascular dysfunction
- Risk for trauma
- Risk-prone health behavior

Gallbladder disease
- Acute pain
- Anxiety
- Decisional conflict
- Deficient knowledge
- Delayed surgical recovery
- Fear
- Risk for infection

Gastric cancer
- Imbalanced nutrition: Less than body requirements
- Ineffective tissue perfusion (GI)
- Risk for adverse reaction to iodinated contrast media

Gastric ulcer
- Acute pain
- Anxiety
- Deficient knowledge
- Imbalanced nutrition: Less than body requirements
- Ineffective tissue perfusion (GI)
- Risk for bleeding
- Risk-prone health behavior
- Stress overload

Gastroenteritis
- Deficient fluid volume
- Diarrhea
- Dysfunctional gastrointestinal motility

- Risk for bleeding
- Risk for imbalanced fluid volume
- Risk for imbalanced body temperature

Genital herpes
- Chronic low self-esteem
- Deficient knowledge (specify)
- Hopelessness
- Ineffective community coping
- Ineffective sexuality patterns
- Impaired social interaction
- Powerlessness
- Risk for chronic low self-esteem
- Risk for infection
- Risk for loneliness
- Risk-prone health behavior
- Risk for impaired skin integrity
- Social isolation

Gestational diabetes
- Risk for infection
- Risk for imbalanced fluid level
- Risk for unstable glucose level
- Urge urinary incontinence

Gestational hypertension
- Activity intolerance
- Acute pain
- Deficient fluid volume
- Deficient knowledge (specify)
- Disturbed sensory perception (visual)
- Excess fluid volume
- Fear
- Ineffective tissue perfusion (cerebral)
- Urinary retention

Glaucoma
- Anxiety
- Deficient knowledge (specify)
- Disturbed sensory perception (visual)
- Grieving
- Hopelessness
- Risk for dry eye
- Risk for falls
- Risk for injury
- Social isolation

Glomerulonephritis
- Compromised family coping
- Excess fluid volume
- Imbalanced nutrition: Less than body requirements
- Ineffective tissue perfusion (renal)
- Risk for electrolyte imbalance
- Risk for ineffective renal perfusion
- Risk for infection

Gonorrhea
- Deficient community health
- Deficient knowledge (specify)
- Ineffective community coping
- Ineffective sexuality patterns
- Moral distress
- Noncompliance
- Risk for infection
- Risk-prone health behavior

Gout
- Activity intolerance
- Acute pain
- Deficient knowledge (specify)
- Disturbed body image
- Impaired physical mobility
- Ineffective health management
- Noncompliance
- Risk-prone behavior

Guillain–Barré syndrome
- Activity intolerance
- Acute pain
- Anxiety
- Bathing or hygiene self-care deficit
- Bowel incontinence
- Fatigue
- Impaired gas exchange
- Impaired physical mobility
- Impaired spontaneous ventilation
- Ineffective airway clearance
- Ineffective breathing pattern
- Ineffective coping
- Powerlessness
- Risk for urge urinary incontinence

Headaches
- Acute pain
- Ineffective coping
- Insomnia
- Spiritual distress

Head injury
- Activity intolerance
- Acute confusion
- Bowel incontinence
- Chronic confusion
- Chronic sorrow
- Decreased intracranial adaptive capacity
- Deficient knowledge (specify)

- Disturbed sensory perception
- Disturbed thought processes
- Dressing or grooming self-care deficit
- Fear
- Impaired emancipated decision making
- Impaired gas exchange
- Impaired memory
- Impaired physical mobility
- Impaired social interaction
- Impaired swallowing
- Impaired verbal communication
- Ineffective thermoregulation
- Ineffective tissue perfusion
- Posttrauma syndrome
- Powerlessness
- Risk for activity intolerance
- Risk for aspiration
- Risk for constipation
- Risk for delayed development
- Risk for disuse syndrome
- Risk for falls
- Risk for imbalanced body temperature
- Risk for imbalanced fluid volume
- Risk for impaired parenting
- Risk for injury
- Risk for trauma
- Risk for urge urinary incontinence
- Sleep deprivation
- Total urinary incontinence
- Unilateral neglect

Head or neck cancer
- Acute pain
- Anxiety
- Disturbed body image
- Disturbed sensory perception
- Impaired oral mucous membrane
- Impaired swallowing
- Impaired tissue integrity
- Impaired verbal communication
- Ineffective airway clearance
- Situational low self-esteem
- Risk for aspiration
- Risk for imbalanced fluid volume

Heart failure
- Activity intolerance
- Acute pain
- Caregiver role strain
- Death anxiety
- Decreased cardiac output
- Deficient knowledge (specify)
- Excess fluid volume
- Fatigue
- Hopelessness
- Impaired gas exchange
- Impaired home maintenance
- Ineffective airway clearance
- Ineffective breathing pattern
- Ineffective tissue perfusion
- Powerlessness
- Risk for activity intolerance
- Risk for caregiver role strain
- Risk for decreased cardiac output
- Risk for deficient fluid volume
- Risk for imbalanced fluid volume
- Risk for impaired cardiovascular function
- Risk for ineffective cardiac tissue perfusion
- Risk for ineffective renal tissue perfusion
- Risk for injury
- Risk for falls

Hemodialysis
- Complicated grieving
- Deficient fluid volume
- Deficient knowledge (specify)
- Disturbed body image
- Excess fluid volume
- Interrupted family processes
- Readiness for enhanced hope
- Risk for falls
- Risk for deficient fluid volume
- Risk for electrolyte imbalance
- Risk for imbalanced fluid volume
- Risk for ineffective renal tissue perfusion
- Risk for ineffective cardiac tissue perfusion
- Risk for infection
- Spiritual distress

Hemophilia
- Acute pain
- Chronic low self-esteem
- Impaired gas exchange
- Ineffective protection
- Parental role conflict
- Readiness for enhanced family coping
- Risk for bleeding
- Risk for falls
- Risk for imbalanced body temperature
- Risk for injury
- Risk for trauma
- Risk-prone health behavior

Hemorrhage
- Deficient fluid volume
- Impaired oral mucous membrane
- Ineffective thermoregulation
- Ineffective tissue perfusion (renal)
- Risk for aspiration
- Risk for bleeding
- Risk for ineffective cardiac tissue perfusion
- Risk for electrolyte imbalance
- Risk for shock

Hemorrhoids
- Acute pain
- Constipation
- Deficient knowledge (specify)
- Impaired comfort
- Impaired skin integrity

Hemothorax
- Acute pain
- Anxiety
- Deficient fluid volume
- Fear
- Impaired gas exchange
- Impaired spontaneous ventilation
- Ineffective breathing pattern
- Ineffective tissue perfusion
- Risk for bleeding
- Risk for shock

Hepatic coma
- Acute confusion
- Deficient fluid volume
- Disturbed sensory perception
- Excess fluid volume
- Imbalanced nutrition: Less than body requirements
- Impaired skin integrity
- Ineffective health management
- Moral distress
- Risk for acute confusion
- Risk for falls
- Risk for infection
- Risk for injury
- Risk for dysfunctional gastrointestinal motility
- Risk for electrolyte imbalance
- Risk for ineffective cerebral tissue perfusion

Hepatitis
- Deficient knowledge (specify)
- Ineffective community coping
- Ineffective community therapeutic regimen management
- Nausea
- Readiness for enhanced community coping
- Risk for electrolyte imbalance
- Risk for imbalanced fluid volume

Hip fracture
- Compromised family coping
- Deficient knowledge (specify)
- Ineffective denial
- Ineffective sexuality patterns
- Powerlessness
- Risk for activity intolerance
- Risk for falls
- Risk for impaired skin integrity
- Risk for infection
- Risk for injury
- Risk for pressure ulcer
- Spiritual distress

Hodgkin's disease
- Deficient knowledge
- Grieving
- Imbalanced nutrition: Less than body requirements
- Impaired physical mobility
- Impaired skin integrity
- Impaired tissue integrity
- Ineffective breathing pattern
- Ineffective oral mucous membrane
- Ineffective protection
- Risk for complicated grieving
- Risk for infection

Huntington's disease
- Bathing or hygiene self-care deficit
- Bowel incontinence
- Caregiver role strain
- Compromised family coping
- Deficient knowledge (specify)
- Hopelessness
- Impaired physical mobility
- Impaired verbal communication
- Ineffective health maintenance
- Risk for loneliness
- Moral distress
- Risk for injury
- Social isolation

Hydatidiform mole
- Acute pain
- Deficient fluid volume
- Grieving
- Risk for situational low self-esteem

Hydrocephalus
- Acute pain

- Anxiety
- Chronic low self-esteem
- Compromised family coping
- Disturbed body image
- Ineffective coping
- Imbalanced nutrition: Less than body requirements
- Interrupted family processes
- Readiness for enhanced family processes
- Risk for impaired skin integrity
- Risk for infection
- Risk for falls

Hyperbilirubinemia
- Interrupted breast-feeding
- Neonatal jaundice
- Risk for injury
- Risk for neonatal jaundice

Hyperemesis gravidarum
- Deficient fluid volume
- Excess fluid volume
- Imbalanced nutrition: Less than body requirements
- Risk for electrolyte imbalance
- Risk for imbalanced fluid volume
- Situational low self-esteem

Hyperosmolar hyperglycemic nonketotic syndrome
- Deficient fluid volume
- Impaired skin integrity
- Ineffective tissue perfusion
- Risk for infection
- Risk for unstable glucose level

Hyperparathyroidism
- Acute pain
- Anxiety
- Deficient knowledge
- Delayed surgical recovery
- Hopelessness
- Imbalanced nutrition: Less than body requirements
- Ineffective breathing pattern
- Ineffective coping
- Risk for imbalanced body temperature
- Risk for impaired skin integrity

Hyperpituitarism
- Acute pain
- Disturbed body image
- Ineffective coping
- Risk for compromised human dignity
- Sexual dysfunction

Hypertension
- Decreased cardiac output
- Deficient knowledge (specify)
- Excess fluid volume
- Health-seeking behaviors
- Impaired resilience
- Ineffective denial
- Ineffective sexuality patterns
- Noncompliance (specify)
- Powerlessness
- Readiness for enhanced urinary elimination
- Risk for decreased cardiac output
- Risk for impaired cardiovascular function
- Risk for situational low self-esteem
- Risk-prone health behavior

Hyperthermia
- Deficient knowledge (specify)
- Hyperthermia
- Impaired oral mucous membrane
- Impaired comfort
- Ineffective thermoregulation

Hyperthyroidism
- Activity intolerance
- Decreased cardiac output
- Disturbed body image
- Disturbed thought processes
- Ineffective thermoregulation
- Insomnia
- Risk for decreased cardiac output
- Risk for imbalanced body temperature
- Risk for impaired cardiovascular function
- Sleep deprivation

Hypoparathyroidism
- Anxiety
- Compromised family coping
- Decreased cardiac output
- Imbalanced nutrition: Less than body requirements
- Ineffective coping
- Ineffective thermoregulation
- Risk for decreased cardiac output
- Risk for impaired cardiovascular function
- Risk for trauma

Hypopituitarism
- Risk for delayed development
- Risk for disproportionate growth

Hypothermia
- Deficient knowledge (specify)
- Hypothermia

- Impaired comfort
- Ineffective thermoregulation

Hypothyroidism
- Activity intolerance
- Chronic functional constipation
- Compromised family coping
- Constipation
- Decreased cardiac output
- Disturbed body image
- Functional urinary incontinence
- Ineffective coping
- Ineffective sexuality patterns
- Ineffective thermoregulation
- Risk for chronic functional constipation
- Risk for decreased cardiac output
- Risk for delayed development
- Risk for disproportionate growth
- Risk for hypothermia
- Risk for imbalanced body temperature
- Risk for impaired cardiovascular function
- Risk for overweight
- Disturbed sleep pattern

Ileostomy
- Anxiety
- Deficient fluid volume
- Deficient knowledge
- Diarrhea
- Disturbed body image
- Fear
- Imbalanced nutrition: Less than body requirements
- Impaired skin integrity
- Ineffective sexuality patterns
- Ineffective tissue perfusion (GI)
- Risk for infection
- Risk for dysfunctional gastrointestinal motility
- Risk for situational low self-esteem

Impotence
- Deficient knowledge (specify)
- Disturbed body image
- Risk for compromised human dignity
- Sexual dysfunction
- Situational low self-esteem
- Urinary retention

Incest
- Ineffective coping
- Interrupted family processes
- Moral distress
- Posttrauma syndrome

Infertility
- Chronic sorrow
- Complicated grieving
- Deficient knowledge (specify)
- Ineffective coping
- Risk for situational low self-esteem
- Stress overload

Inhalation injuries
- Ineffective thermoregulation
- Risk for injury
- Risk for suffocation

Interstitial pulmonary fibrosis
- Activity intolerance
- Anxiety
- Deficient knowledge (specify)
- Grieving
- Impaired gas exchange
- Impaired resilience
- Ineffective airway clearance
- Ineffective breathing pattern
- Ineffective coping
- Insomnia
- Spiritual distress

Intestinal obstruction
- Acute pain
- Chronic functional constipation
- Constipation
- Imbalanced nutrition: Less than body requirements
- Ineffective tissue perfusion (GI)
- Risk for aspiration
- Risk for chronic functional constipation
- Risk for deficient fluid volume
- Risk for dysfunctional gastrointestinal motility
- Risk for electrolyte imbalance
- Risk for imbalanced fluid volume
- Urinary retention

Intoxication
- Disturbed sensory perception
- Hypothermia
- Impaired verbal communication
- Ineffective community therapeutic regimen management
- Moral distress
- Risk for aspiration
- Risk for compromised human dignity
- Risk for falls
- Risk for hypothermia
- Risk for injury

Joint replacement
- Acute pain
- Compromised family coping
- Deficient knowledge (specify)
- Delayed surgical recovery
- Disturbed sensory perception (kinesthetic)
- Impaired physical mobility
- Ineffective peripheral tissue perfusion
- Risk for contamination
- Risk for falls
- Risk for infection
- Risk for injury

Juvenile rheumatoid arthritis
- Acute pain
- Caregiver role strain
- Compromised family coping
- Defensive coping
- Disturbed body image
- Disturbed sensory perception (tactile)
- Grieving
- Impaired resilience
- Impaired physical mobility
- Ineffective health maintenance
- Ineffective role performance
- Interrupted family processes
- Risk for unstable glucose level

Kidney transplantation
- Deficient fluid volume
- Deficient knowledge (specify)
- Delayed surgical recovery
- Disturbed body image
- Ineffective protection
- Interrupted family processes
- Risk for bleeding
- Readiness for enhanced hope
- Readiness for enhanced decision making
- Readiness for enhanced hope
- Readiness for enhanced resilience
- Risk for complicated grieving
- Risk for electrolyte imbalance
- Risk for infection

Labor and delivery
- Acute pain
- Anxiety
- Deficient knowledge (specify)
- Effective breast-feeding
- Impaired skin integrity
- Ineffective breast-feeding
- Ineffective coping
- Insufficient breast milk
- Labor pain
- Readiness for enhanced childbearing
- Risk for bleeding
- Risk for disturbed maternal–fetal dyad
- Risk for injury
- Urinary retention

Leukemia
- Acute pain
- Grieving
- Hopelessness
- Imbalanced nutrition: Less than body requirements
- Impaired gas exchange
- Impaired oral mucous membrane
- Impaired tissue integrity
- Ineffective protection
- Ineffective tissue perfusion (cardiopulmonary)
- Ineffective tissue perfusion (renal)
- Risk for bleeding
- Risk for contamination
- Risk for falls
- Risk for imbalanced body temperature
- Risk for infection
- Risk for injury

Liver transplantation
- Anxiety
- Compromised family coping
- Defensive coping
- Deficient knowledge (specify)
- Delayed surgical recovery
- Fear
- Ineffective coping
- Ineffective protection
- Ineffective tissue perfusion (cardiopulmonary)
- Ineffective tissue perfusion (GI)
- Ineffective tissue perfusion (renal)
- Moral distress
- Risk for impaired liver function
- Risk for electrolyte imbalance
- Risk for imbalanced fluid volume
- Risk for infection
- Risk for injury

Lung abscess
- Acute pain
- Anxiety
- Impaired gas exchange
- Ineffective airway clearance
- Ineffective breathing pattern
- Ineffective coping
- Ineffective tissue perfusion (cardiopulmonary)

- Risk for imbalanced body temperature

Lung cancer
- Activity intolerance
- Death anxiety
- Fear
- Grieving
- Hopelessness
- Imbalanced nutrition: Less than body requirements
- Impaired gas exchange
- Impaired tissue integrity
- Impaired verbal communication
- Ineffective airway clearance
- Ineffective breathing pattern
- Powerlessness
- Risk for infection

Lupus erythematosus
- Acute pain
- Decreased cardiac output
- Deficient knowledge
- Fatigue
- Hyperthermia
- Imbalanced nutrition: Less than body requirements
- Impaired oral mucous membrane
- Impaired physical mobility
- Impaired skin integrity
- Ineffective coping
- Ineffective tissue perfusion
- Risk for infection
- Risk-prone health behavior

Lyme disease
- Activity intolerance
- Acute pain
- Fatigue
- Hyperthermia
- Impaired skin integrity

Lymphomas
- Death anxiety
- Disturbed sleep pattern
- Grieving
- Hopelessness
- Impaired tissue integrity
- Ineffective protection
- Readiness for enhanced decision making
- Risk for impaired religiosity
- Risk for infection
- Macular degeneration
- Activity intolerance
- Deficient knowledge
- Disturbed sensory perception (visual)
- Ineffective denial
- Powerlessness
- Readiness for enhanced hope
- Risk for caregiver role strain
- Risk for low situational self-esteem
- Risk for falls
- Risk for trauma

Malnutrition
- Imbalanced nutrition: Less than body requirements
- Ineffective community coping
- Risk for electrolyte imbalance
- Risk for impaired oral mucous membrane
- Risk for injury

Maternal psychological stress
- Anxiety
- Deficient knowledge
- Ineffective breast-feeding
- Ineffective infant feeding pattern
- Ineffective role performance
- Interrupted breast-feeding
- Parental role conflict
- Risk for impaired attachment
- Risk for disturbed maternal–fetal dyad
- Risk for ineffective childbearing process
- Risk for sudden infant death syndrome
- Powerlessness

Meconium aspiration syndrome
- Ineffective breathing pattern
- Impaired gas exchange
- Impaired spontaneous ventilation
- Risk for aspiration
- Risk for injury

Melanoma
- Death anxiety
- Decisional conflict
- Defensive coping
- Disturbed body image
- Fatigue
- Hopelessness
- Impaired resilience
- Impaired oral mucous membrane
- Impaired skin integrity
- Powerlessness
- Spiritual distress

Ménière's disease
- Disturbed sensory perception (auditory)
- Impaired physical mobility

- Insomnia
- Nausea
- Risk for falls
- Risk for injury
- Risk for trauma

Meningitis
- Acute pain
- Bowel incontinence
- Deficient fluid volume
- Disturbed sensory perception
- Excess fluid volume
- Fatigue
- Fear
- Hyperthermia
- Ineffective airway clearance
- Ineffective breathing pattern
- Risk for imbalanced fluid volume
- Risk for infection
- Risk for injury

Menopause
- Ineffective sexuality patterns
- Insomnia
- Sexual dysfunction
- Situational low self-esteem
- Stress overload
- Risk for imbalanced body temperature

Metabolic acidosis
- Deficient knowledge (specify)
- Impaired airway clearance
- Impaired gas exchange
- Impaired oral mucous membrane
- Ineffective breathing pattern
- Risk for acute confusion
- Risk for electrolyte imbalance
- Risk for injury
- Risk for poisoning
- Risk for shock
- Metabolic alkalosis
- Deficient fluid volume
- Disturbed thought processes
- Impaired oral mucous membrane
- Ineffective breathing pattern
- Risk for electrolyte imbalance
- Risk for injury

Mitral insufficiency
- Activity intolerance
- Decreased cardiac output
- Deficient knowledge (specify)
- Fatigue
- Ineffective tissue perfusion (cardiopulmonary)
- Mitral stenosis
- Activity intolerance
- Decreased cardiac output
- Deficient knowledge (specify)
- Fatigue
- Ineffective tissue perfusion (cardiopulmonary)
- Risk for infection

Mood disorders
- Impaired religiosity
- Ineffective health management
- Ineffective community therapeutic regimen management
- Labile emotional control
- Powerlessness
- Readiness for enhanced health management
- Risk for impaired resilience
- Risk for suicide
- Self-mutilation
- Social isolation
- Spiritual distress

Multiple births
- Anxiety
- Deficient knowledge (specify)
- Impaired parenting
- Ineffective coping
- Interrupted family processes
- Risk for injury
- Risk for impaired parenting
- Risk for urinary tract injury
- Stress urinary incontinence

Multiple myeloma
- Activity intolerance
- Acute pain
- Excess fluid volume
- Fatigue
- Grieving
- Imbalanced nutrition: Less than body requirements
- Ineffective tissue perfusion (cerebral)
- Risk for infection

Multiple sclerosis
- Acute pain
- Bowel incontinence
- Caregiver role strain
- Chronic low self-esteem
- Death anxiety
- Deficient knowledge (specify)
- Disturbed sensory perception
- Dressing or grooming self-care deficit
- Fatigue

- Grieving
- Imbalanced nutrition: Less than body requirements
- Impaired bed mobility
- Impaired comfort
- Impaired memory
- Impaired physical mobility
- Impaired sitting
- Impaired spontaneous ventilation
- Impaired standing
- Impaired urinary elimination
- Impaired wheelchair mobility
- Ineffective airway clearance
- Ineffective health maintenance
- Ineffective sexuality patterns
- Ineffective therapeutic regimen management
- Readiness for enhanced family coping
- Readiness for enhanced spiritual well-being
- Risk for activity intolerance
- Risk for caregiver role strain
- Risk for infection
- Risk for spiritual distress
- Risk for urge urinary incontinence
- Risk-prone health behavior

Multisystem trauma
- Anxiety
- Bathing or hygiene self-care deficit
- Deficient fluid volume
- Dysfunctional ventilatory weaning response
- Ineffective tissue perfusion
- Impaired spontaneous ventilation
- Powerlessness
- Risk for electrolyte imbalance
- Risk for ineffective cardiac tissue perfusion
- Risk for ineffective cerebral tissue perfusion
- Risk for infection
- Risk for suffocation
- Risk for trauma

Muscular dystrophy
- Caregiver role strain
- Deficient knowledge (specify)
- Disturbed sensory perception (kinesthetic)
- Feeding self-care deficit
- Hopelessness
- Impaired physical mobility
- Impaired sitting
- Impaired standing
- Impaired swallowing
- Impaired transfer ability
- Ineffective health maintenance
- Readiness for enhanced family coping
- Risk for caregiver role strain
- Risk for pressure ulcer
- Risk for urge urinary incontinence
- Risk-prone health behavior

Myasthenia gravis
- Bowel incontinence
- Chronic low self-esteem
- Dressing or grooming self-care deficit
- Dysfunctional ventilatory weaning response
- Fatigue
- Fear
- Impaired gas exchange
- Impaired physical mobility
- Impaired verbal communication
- Ineffective airway clearance
- Readiness for enhanced self-care
- Risk for urge urinary incontinence

Myocardial infarction
- Activity intolerance
- Acute pain
- Anxiety
- Compromised family coping
- Death anxiety
- Decreased cardiac output
- Health-seeking behaviors
- Ineffective coping
- Ineffective denial
- Ineffective role performance
- Ineffective sexuality patterns
- Ineffective tissue perfusion
- Readiness for enhanced spiritual well-being
- Readiness for enhanced relationships
- Risk for decreased cardiac function
- Risk for impaired cardiovascular function
- Risk for ineffective cardiac tissue perfusion
- Risk for spiritual distress
- Risk-prone health behavior
- Sedentary lifestyle
- Sexual dysfunction
- Situational low self-esteem
- Sleep deprivation
- Spiritual distress

Neonatal asphyxia
- Compromised family coping
- Hypothermia
- Ineffective breathing pattern
- Risk for aspiration
- Risk for hypothermia

- Risk for injury
- Risk for sudden infant death syndrome
- Risk for suffocation
- Risk for sudden infant death syndrome

Neonatal hyperbilirubinemia
- Interrupted breast-feeding
- Neonatal jaundice
- Risk for neonatal jaundice

Neurologic impairment (neonatal)
- Compromised family coping
- Ineffective infant feeding pattern
- Disorganized infant behavior
- Readiness for enhanced organized infant behavior
- Risk for disorganized infant behavior

Neuromuscular trauma
- Impaired skin integrity
- Impaired swallowing
- Overflow urinary incontinence
- Posttrauma syndrome
- Risk for aspiration
- Risk for constipation
- Risk for disuse syndrome
- Unilateral neglect

Nutritional deficiencies
- Imbalanced nutrition: Less than body requirements
- Impaired skin integrity
- Risk for impaired parenting
- Risk for infection

Obesity
- Obesity
- Readiness for enhanced nutrition
- Readiness for enhanced self-concept
- Risk for constipation
- Risk for impaired skin integrity
- Risk for impaired tissue integrity
- Situational low self-esteem
- Stress urinary incontinence

Obsessive-compulsive disorder
- Anxiety
- Compromised family coping
- Decisional conflict
- Disturbed personal identity
- Impaired home maintenance
- Ineffective coping
- Ineffective denial
- Insomnia
- Risk for impaired religiosity
- Risk for injury
- Risk for spiritual distress
- Risk for self-directed violence
- Risk for other-directed violence
- Risk for suicide
- Self-mutilation
- Sleep deprivation
- Social isolation

Organic brain syndrome
- Frail elderly syndrome
- Impaired verbal communication
- Risk for deficient fluid volume
- Risk for frail elderly syndrome
- Wandering

Osteoarthritis
- Activity intolerance
- Acute pain
- Compromised family coping
- Deficient knowledge (specify)
- Disturbed body image
- Dressing or grooming self-care deficit
- Impaired home maintenance
- Impaired physical mobility
- Impaired wheelchair ability
- Ineffective health maintenance
- Ineffective health management
- Risk for injury
- Risk for falls
- Risk for injury
- Osteomyelitis
- Acute pain
- Disturbed body image
- Impaired coping
- Impaired physical mobility
- Impaired skin integrity
- Impaired tissue integrity
- Ineffective coping
- Ineffective tissue perfusion (specify)
- Risk for infection
- Risk for injury
- Risk for falls

Osteoporosis
- Deficient knowledge (specify)
- Disturbed body image
- Fear
- Ineffective denial
- Ineffective health management
- Ineffective sexuality patterns
- Loneliness
- Nutrition imbalanced: Less than body requirements

- Powerlessness
- Risk for falls
- Risk for injury
- Risk for trauma
- Risk-prone health behaviors
- Self-neglect
- Social isolation

Ovarian cancer
- Constipation
- Death anxiety
- Fear
- Grieving
- Imbalanced nutrition: Less than body requirements
- Impaired tissue integrity
- Ineffective coping
- Ineffective protection
- Nausea
- Powerlessness
- Readiness for enhanced hope
- Readiness for enhanced resilience
- Readiness for enhanced spiritual well-being
- Risk for falls
- Spiritual distress
- Urinary retention

Panic disorder
- Anxiety
- Chronic low self-esteem
- Deficient knowledge (specify)
- Fear
- Impaired emancipated decision making
- Impaired resilience
- Impaired mood regulation
- Ineffective coping
- Insomnia
- Powerlessness
- Risk for impaired emancipated decision making
- Risk for posttrauma syndrome
- Sleep deprivation
- Risk for spiritual distress

Paralysis
- Autonomic dysreflexia
- Bowel incontinence
- Caregiver role strain
- Complicated grieving
- Compromised family coping
- Disuse syndrome
- Hopelessness
- Impaired bed mobility
- Impaired physical mobility
- Impaired sitting
- Impaired skin integrity
- Impaired standing
- Impaired walking
- Ineffective coping
- Ineffective health maintenance
- Ineffective role performance
- Ineffective sexuality patterns
- Powerlessness
- Reflex urinary incontinence
- Risk for caregiver role strain
- Risk for impaired skin integrity
- Risk for impaired tissue integrity
- Risk for pressure ulcer

Parkinson's disease
- Activity intolerance
- Bowel incontinence
- Caregiver role strain
- Chronic low self-esteem
- Compromised family coping
- Death anxiety
- Deficient knowledge (specify)
- Disturbed body image
- Disturbed sensory perception (tactile)
- Feeding self-care deficit
- Grieving
- Hopelessness
- Imbalanced nutrition: Less than body requirements
- Impaired home maintenance
- Impaired resilience
- Impaired physical mobility
- Impaired transfer ability
- Ineffective breathing pattern
- Ineffective coping
- Ineffective health maintenance
- Ineffective role performance
- Ineffective sexuality patterns
- Loneliness
- Powerlessness
- Readiness for enhanced therapeutic regimen management
- Risk for aspiration
- Risk for caregiver role strain
- Risk for compromised human dignity
- Risk for injury
- Risk for falls
- Risk for loneliness
- Risk for urge urinary incontinence
- Social isolation

Pelvic inflammatory disease
- Acute pain
- Deficient fluid volume
- Ineffective sexuality pattern
- Risk for infection
- Risk-prone health behavior
- Sexual dysfunction

Pericarditis
- Activity intolerance
- Acute pain
- Anxiety
- Decreased cardiac output
- Deficient knowledge
- Ineffective tissue perfusion (cardiopulmonary)
- Risk for decreased cardiac output
- Risk for impaired cardiovascular function
- Risk for ineffective cardiac tissue perfusion
- Risk for infection
- Risk for shock

Perinatal trauma
- Decisional conflict
- Hypothermia
- Impaired gas exchange
- Impaired spontaneous ventilation
- Risk for hypothermia
- Risk for injury
- Risk for ineffective cardiac tissue perfusion
- Risk for ineffective cerebral tissue perfusion
- Risk for ineffective renal tissue perfusion
- Risk for shock
- Risk for vascular trauma

Peripheral vascular disease
- Activity intolerance
- Acute pain
- Deficient diversional activity
- Deficient knowledge (specify)
- Impaired physical mobility
- Impaired skin integrity
- Impaired tissue integrity
- Ineffective health management
- Risk for falls
- Risk for impaired skin integrity
- Risk for ineffective peripheral tissue perfusion
- Risk for vascular trauma
- Risk for impaired tissue integrity
- Risk for infection
- Risk for injury
- Risk for peripheral neurovascular dysfunction
- Risk-prone health behavior

Peritoneal dialysis
- Caregiver role strain
- Defensive coping
- Deficient fluid volume
- Deficient knowledge (specify)
- Disabled family coping
- Disturbed body image
- Excess fluid volume
- Imbalanced nutrition: Less than body requirements
- Impaired resilience
- Interrupted family processes
- Risk for electrolyte imbalance
- Risk for infection
- Risk for injury

Peritonitis
- Acute pain
- Anxiety
- Decreased cardiac output
- Deficient fluid volume
- Nausea
- Risk for decreased cardiac output
- Risk for electrolyte imbalance
- Risk for ineffective gastrointestinal tissue perfusion
- Risk for ineffective cardiac tissue perfusion
- Risk for ineffective renal tissue perfusion
- Risk for imbalanced fluid volume
- Risk for impaired cardiovascular function
- Risk for infection
- Risk for shock

Personality disorders
- Decisional conflict
- Deficient knowledge
- Disturbed personal identity
- Impaired resilience
- Interrupted family processes
- Loneliness
- Risk for loneliness
- Risk for self-directed violence
- Risk for suicide
- Sexual dysfunction
- Social isolation

Phobic disorder
- Anxiety
- Disturbed personal identity
- Fear
- Hopelessness

- Ineffective coping
- Powerlessness
- Risk for impaired resilience
- Risk for loneliness
- Social isolation

Placenta previa
- Anxiety
- Fear
- Ineffective denial
- Risk for disturbed maternal–fetal dyad
- Risk for situational low self-esteem

Pleural effusion
- Acute pain
- Dysfunctional ventilatory weaning response
- Hyperthermia
- Impaired gas exchange
- Ineffective breathing pattern
- Risk for infection

Pleurisy
- Acute pain
- Fatigue
- Impaired gas exchange
- Ineffective breathing pattern

Pneumonia
- Bathing or hygiene self-care deficit
- Feeding and toileting self-care deficit
- Deficient fluid volume
- Imbalanced nutrition: Less than body requirements
- Impaired gas exchange
- Impaired physical mobility
- Impaired spontaneous ventilation
- Impaired verbal communication
- Ineffective airway clearance
- Ineffective breathing pattern
- Ineffective tissue perfusion (cardiopulmonary)
- Readiness for enhanced sleep
- Risk for aspiration
- Risk for electrolyte imbalance
- Risk for imbalanced fluid volume
- Risk for infection

Pneumothorax
- Anxiety
- Ineffective breathing pattern
- Fear
- Impaired gas exchange
- Acute pain
- Ineffective tissue perfusion (cardiopulmonary)
- Impaired spontaneous ventilation

Poisoning
- Contamination
- Disturbed sensory perception
- Ineffective tissue perfusion (renal)
- Nausea
- Risk for aspiration
- Risk for bleeding
- Risk for injury
- Risk for poisoning
- Risk for shock

Polycystic kidney disease
- Acute pain
- Anxiety
- Defensive coping
- Deficient knowledge (specify)
- Fear
- Ineffective tissue perfusion (renal)
- Interrupted family processes
- Moral distress
- Risk for infection
- Risk for urinary tract injury

Polycythemia vera
- Acute pain
- Disturbed sensory perception (visual) Fatigue
- Impaired gas exchange
- Impaired skin integrity
- Ineffective breathing pattern
- Risk for bleeding
- Risk for injury

Postpartum hemorrhage
- Anxiety
- Deficient fluid volume
- Ineffective tissue perfusion
- Risk for bleeding
- Risk for ineffective renal tissue perfusion
- Risk for shock

Posttraumatic stress disorder
- Ineffective impulse control
- Ineffective relationships
- Defensive coping
- Disabled family coping
- Disturbed personal identity
- Disturbed sensory perception
- Hopelessness
- Ineffective activity planning
- Interrupted family processes

Posttrauma syndrome
- Powerlessness
- Risk for loneliness

- Risk for posttrauma syndrome
- Risk for other-directed violence
- Risk for self-directed violence
- Risk for self-mutilation
- Risk for suicide
- Situational low self-esteem
- Sleep deprivation

Pregnancy
- Anxiety
- Deficient knowledge (specify)
- Impaired tissue integrity
- Ineffective coping
- Ineffective tissue perfusion (peripheral)
- Interrupted family processes
- Readiness for enhanced childbearing
- Readiness for enhanced fluid balance
- Readiness for enhanced relationships
- Risk for constipation

Premature labor
- Anxiety
- Deficient knowledge (specify)
- Effective breast-feeding
- Impaired parenting
- Ineffective coping
- Risk for disturbed maternal–fetal dyad
- Risk for infection
- Situational low self-esteem

Premature rupture of membranes
- Risk for infection

Prematurity
- Compromised family coping
- Disorganized infant behavior
- Hypothermia
- Imbalanced nutrition: Less than body requirements
- Impaired verbal communication
- Ineffective breast-feeding
- Ineffective breathing pattern
- Ineffective infant feeding pattern
- Ineffective thermoregulation
- Interrupted breast-feeding
- Readiness for enhanced parenting
- Risk for aspiration
- Risk for delayed development
- Risk for disorganized infant behavior
- Risk for disturbed maternal–fetal dyad
- Risk for hypothermia
- Risk for impaired parent–infant–child attachment
- Risk for sudden infant death syndrome

Pressure ulcers
- Imbalanced nutrition: Less than body requirements
- Impaired physical mobility
- Impaired skin integrity
- Impaired tissue integrity
- Ineffective protection
- Risk for deficient fluid volume
- Risk for infection

Prolapsed intervertebral disc
- Acute pain
- Impaired physical mobility
- Powerlessness
- Reflex urinary incontinence
- Urinary retention

Prostate cancer
- Acute pain
- Chronic sorrow
- Deficient knowledge
- Impaired skin integrity
- Impaired tissue integrity
- Risk for situational low self-esteem
- Risk for urinary tract injury
- Sexual dysfunction
- Urinary retention

Prostatectomy
- Acute pain
- Disturbed body image
- Ineffective protection
- Ineffective role performance
- Impaired skin integrity
- Risk for infection
- Urinary retention

Pseudomembranous colitis
- Deficient fluid volume
- Diarrhea
- Impaired skin integrity
- Ineffective tissue perfusion (cardiopulmonary)
- Ineffective tissue perfusion (GI)
- Ineffective tissue perfusion (renal)
- Risk for bleeding
- Risk for electrolyte imbalance

Psoriasis
- Deficient knowledge
- Disturbed body image
- Impaired skin integrity
- Powerlessness

- Risk for imbalanced body temperature
- Social isolation
- Risk for infection

Pulmonary edema
- Activity intolerance
- Bathing or hygiene self-care deficit
- Decreased cardiac output
- Dysfunctional ventilatory weaning response
- Excess fluid volume
- Fear
- Impaired gas exchange
- Impaired verbal communication
- Ineffective airway clearance
- Ineffective breathing pattern
- Ineffective tissue perfusion (cardiopulmonary)
- Risk for decreased cardiac output
- Risk for impaired cardiovascular function
- Risk for ineffective cardiac tissue perfusion
- Risk for ineffective cerebral tissue perfusion
- Risk for ineffective renal tissue perfusion

Pulmonary embolus
- Acute pain
- Anxiety
- Activity intolerance
- Decreased cardiac output
- Deficient fluid volume
- Impaired gas exchange
- Impaired verbal communication
- Ineffective breathing pattern
- Ineffective tissue perfusion (cardiopulmonary)
- Risk for decreased cardiac output
- Risk for impaired cardiovascular function
- Risk for ineffective cardiac tissue perfusion

Pyelonephritis
- Acute pain
- Excess fluid volume
- Impaired physical mobility
- Risk for infection
- Risk for electrolyte balance
- Risk for imbalanced fluid volume

Pyloric stenosis
- Acute pain
- Imbalanced nutrition: Less than body requirements
- Risk for aspiration
- Risk for imbalanced body temperature

Radiation therapy
- Acute pain
- Deficient fluid volume
- Diarrhea
- Imbalanced nutrition: Less than body requirements
- Impaired oral mucous membrane
- Impaired physical mobility
- Impaired tissue integrity
- Ineffective protection
- Nausea
- Risk for impaired oral mucous membrane
- Risk for impaired tissue integrity
- Sexual dysfunction

Rape
- Anxiety
- Complicated grieving
- Fear
- Posttrauma syndrome
- Rape-trauma syndrome
- Risk for compromised human dignity
- Risk for thermal injury
- Situational low self-esteem
- Social isolation

Raynaud's disease
- Deficient knowledge (specify)
- Disturbed sensory perception (tactile)
- Impaired tissue integrity
- Ineffective tissue perfusion (peripheral)
- Risk for impaired skin integrity
- Risk for ineffective peripheral tissue perfusion

Renal calculi
- Acute pain
- Ineffective denial
- Risk for infection
- Risk for urinary tract injury
- Urinary retention

Renal cancer
- Acute pain
- Deficient fluid volume
- Risk for electrolyte balance
- Risk for imbalanced fluid volume

Renal disease: End-stage
- Caregiver role strain
- Chronic low self-esteem
- Decisional conflict
- Defensive coping
- Excess fluid volume
- Grieving
- Hopelessness
- Ineffective coping

- Ineffective denial
- Ineffective role performance
- Ineffective sexuality patterns
- Risk for caregiver role strain
- Risk for disuse syndrome
- Risk for infection
- Risk for poisoning
- Risk for spiritual distress
- Spiritual distress

Respiratory distress syndrome
- Dysfunctional weaning response
- Impaired gas exchange
- Impaired spontaneous ventilation
- Ineffective airway clearance
- Ineffective breathing pattern
- Ineffective thermoregulation
- Risk for infection

Reye's syndrome
- Decreased intracranial adaptive capacity
- Hyperthermia
- Impaired physical mobility
- Ineffective thermoregulation

Rheumatoid arthritis
- Activity intolerance
- Acute pain
- Deficient knowledge (specify)
- Disturbed body image
- Dressing or grooming self-care deficit
- Impaired physical mobility
- Impaired skin integrity
- Impaired transfer ability
- Ineffective coping
- Ineffective denial
- Ineffective health maintenance
- Ineffective protection
- Ineffective therapeutic regimen management
- Insomnia
- Risk for disuse syndrome
- Risk for falls
- Risk for ineffective activity planning
- Risk for injury
- Risk-prone health management
- Sexual dysfunction

Salmonella
- Constipation
- Diarrhea
- Hyperthermia
- Nausea
- Risk for imbalanced fluid volume
- Risk for dysfunctional gastrointestinal motility
- Risk for electrolyte imbalance
- Risk for imbalanced fluid volume
- Risk for infection
- Urinary retention

Sarcoidosis
- Activity intolerance
- Acute pain
- Decreased cardiac output
- Disturbed body image
- Impaired gas exchange
- Ineffective breathing pattern

Schizophrenia
- Anxiety
- Bathing or hygiene self-care deficit
- Caregiver role strain
- Disturbed personal identity
- Disturbed sensory perception
- Dysfunctional family processes
- Functional urinary incontinence
- Hopelessness
- Impaired emancipated decision making
- Impaired home maintenance
- Impaired mood regulation
- Impaired social interaction
- Interrupted family processes
- Ineffective coping
- Ineffective therapeutic family regimen management
- Ineffective health maintenance
- Ineffective relationships
- Ineffective role performance
- Interrupted family processes
- Insomnia
- Labile emotional control
- Risk for caregiver role strain
- Risk for impaired emancipated decision making
- Risk for injury
- Risk for poisoning
- Risk for self-directed violence
- Risk for suicide
- Sexual dysfunction
- Social isolation

Seizure disorders
- Anxiety
- Chronic low self-esteem
- Disturbed sensory perception (tactile)
- Impaired memory
- Ineffective airway clearance

- Ineffective breathing pattern
- Ineffective coping
- Ineffective therapeutic management
- Risk for delayed development
- Risk for falls
- Risk for impaired oral mucous membrane
- Risk for injury
- Risk for spiritual distress
- Risk for trauma
- Risk-prone health behavior
- Social isolation
- Self-neglect

Self-destructive behavior
- Anxiety
- Chronic low self-esteem
- Ineffective denial
- Risk for poisoning
- Risk for self-directed violence
- Risk for self-mutilation

Sepsis
- Acute confusion
- Acute pain
- Diarrhea
- Dysfunctional ventilatory weaning response
- Hyperthermia
- Hypothermia
- Nausea
- Imbalanced nutrition: Less than body requirements
- Impaired spontaneous ventilation
- Ineffective thermoregulation
- Risk for hypothermia
- Risk for ineffective cardiac tissue perfusion
- Risk for ineffective renal perfusion
- Risk for shock

Sexual assault
- Posttrauma syndrome
- Rape-trauma syndrome
- Risk for self-directed violence
- Risk for suicide

Shaken baby syndrome
- Disabled family coping
- Impaired parenting
- Interrupted family processes
- Risk for impaired parenting
- Risk for ineffective cerebral tissue perfusion
- Risk for impaired attachment
- Risk for injury
- Risk for other-directed violence

Shock
- Decreased cardiac output
- Deficient fluid volume
- Impaired gas exchange
- Impaired oral mucous membrane
- Impaired spontaneous ventilation
- Ineffective airway clearance
- Ineffective tissue perfusion (cardiopulmonary)
- Ineffective tissue perfusion (cerebral)
- Ineffective tissue perfusion (renal)
- Risk for decreased cardiac output
- Risk for electrolyte imbalance
- Risk for impaired cardiovascular function
- Risk for infection

Sickle cell anemia
- Acute pain
- Impaired gas exchange
- Impaired physical mobility
- Ineffective protection
- Ineffective tissue perfusion (peripheral)
- Ineffective tissue perfusion (renal)

Sjögren's syndrome
- Acute pain
- Disturbed sensory perception (gustatory)
- Risk for corneal injury
- Risk for dry eye
- Impaired oral mucous membrane

Spina bifida
- Bowel incontinence
- Impaired skin integrity
- Latex allergy response
- Risk for physical immobility
- Risk for latex allergy response
- Urinary incontinence

Spinal cord defects
- Chronic low self-esteem
- Impaired urinary elimination
- Overflow urinary incontinence
- Readiness for enhanced family coping
- Risk-prone health behavior
- Total urinary incontinence

Spinal cord injury
- Activity intolerance
- Autonomic dysreflexia
- Bathing or hygiene self-care deficit
- Bowel incontinence
- Chronic functional constipation
- Chronic pain
- Chronic sorrow
- Complicated grieving

- Constipation
- Deficient diversional activity
- Deficient knowledge (specify)
- Disturbed body image
- Disturbed sensory perception
- Fear
- Hopelessness
- Impaired physical mobility
- Impaired sitting
- Impaired spontaneous ventilation
- Impaired standing
- Impaired transfer ability
- Impaired urinary elimination
- Ineffective airway clearance
- Ineffective health maintenance
- Ineffective sexuality patterns
- Ineffective therapeutic regimen management
- Moral distress
- Posttrauma syndrome
- Powerlessness
- Readiness for enhanced communication
- Readiness for enhanced therapeutic regimen management
- Reflex urinary incontinence
- Risk for autonomic dysreflexia
- Risk for chronic functional constipation
- Risk for constipation
- Risk for delayed development
- Risk for disuse syndrome
- Risk for impaired skin integrity
- Risk for impaired tissue integrity
- Risk for infection
- Risk for pressure ulcer
- Risk for trauma
- Risk for urge urinary incontinence
- Risk-prone health behavior
- Sleep deprivation
- Social isolation
- Total urinary incontinence
- Urinary retention

Spinal tumor
- Autonomic dysreflexia
- Bowel incontinence
- Chronic low self-esteem
- Disturbed sensory perception (kinesthetic)
- Dressing or grooming self-care deficit
- Impaired physical mobility
- Impaired urinary elimination
- Ineffective breathing pattern
- Reflex urinary incontinence
- Risk for autonomic dysreflexia
- Risk for impaired skin integrity
- Risk for injury
- Risk for urge urinary incontinence
- Sexual dysfunction
- Situational low self-esteem
- Total urinary incontinence

Spouse abuse
- Anxiety
- Defensive coping
- Deficient knowledge (specify)
- Fear
- Hopelessness
- Impaired emancipated decision making
- Posttrauma syndrome
- Powerlessness
- Rape-trauma syndrome
- Readiness for enhanced hope
- Readiness for enhanced knowledge
- Readiness for enhanced parenting
- Readiness for enhanced power
- Readiness for enhanced self-concept
- Readiness for enhanced health management
- Risk for impaired emancipated decision making
- Risk for other-directed violence
- Risk for suicide
- Stress overload

Streptococcal throat
- Acute pain
- Hyperthermia
- Impaired oral mucous membrane
- Risk for infection

Stroke
- Acute confusion
- Bathing or hygiene self-care deficit
- Bowel incontinence
- Caregiver role strain
- Chronic confusion
- Chronic functional constipation
- Chronic sorrow
- Compromised family coping
- Constipation
- Death anxiety
- Decreased intracranial adaptive capacity
- Deficient knowledge (specify)
- Disturbed body image
- Disturbed sensory perception (tactile)
- Fatigue
- Frail elderly syndrome

- Functional urinary incontinence
- Hopelessness
- Imbalanced nutrition: Less than body requirements
- Impaired bed mobility
- Impaired gas exchange
- Impaired home maintenance
- Impaired memory
- Impaired physical mobility
- Impaired sitting
- Impaired social interaction
- Impaired standing
- Impaired swallowing
- Impaired urinary elimination
- Impaired verbal communication
- Impaired walking
- Ineffective airway clearance
- Ineffective breathing pattern
- Ineffective health maintenance
- Ineffective sexuality patterns
- Ineffective thermoregulation
- Ineffective tissue perfusion (cerebral)
- Interrupted family processes
- Powerlessness
- Readiness for enhanced family processes
- Risk for activity intolerance
- Risk for aspiration
- Risk for caregiver role strain
- Risk for chronic functional constipation
- Risk for compromised human dignity
- Risk for disuse syndrome
- Risk for frail elderly syndrome
- Risk for impaired skin integrity
- Risk for injury
- Risk for poisoning
- Risk for pressure ulcer
- Situational low self-esteem
- Sleep deprivation
- Social isolation
- Stress urinary incontinence
- Total urinary incontinence
- Unilateral neglect

Suicidal behavior
- Anxiety
- Chronic low self-esteem
- Disturbed personal identity
- Ineffective denial
- Readiness for enhanced spiritual well-being
- Risk for poisoning
- Risk for self-directed violence
- Risk for self-mutilation

Tendinitis
- Acute pain
- Activity intolerance
- Impaired physical mobility
- Ineffective role performance

Testicular cancer
- Acute pain
- Death anxiety
- Disturbed body image
- Fear
- Hopelessness
- Powerlessness
- Sexual dysfunction
- Risk for situational low self-esteem

Thoracic surgery
- Acute pain
- Deficient fluid volume
- Fatigue
- Fear
- Impaired gas exchange
- Ineffective airway clearance
- Ineffective breathing pattern
- Risk for bleeding
- Risk for delayed surgical recovery
- Risk for infection
- Risk for perioperative position injury

Thrombophlebitis
- Acute pain
- Impaired gas exchange
- Impaired skin integrity
- Ineffective tissue perfusion (peripheral)
- Risk for impaired skin integrity
- Risk for infection
- Risk for injury
- Risk for vascular trauma

Tracheoesophageal fistula
- Imbalanced nutrition: Less than body requirements
- Risk for aspiration

Tracheostomy
- Imbalanced nutrition: Less than body requirements
- Impaired skin integrity
- Impaired verbal communication

Transient ischemic attacks
- Acute confusion
- Disturbed sensory perception (tactile)
- Impaired memory
- Ineffective tissue perfusion (cerebral)

- Risk for bleeding
- Risk for ineffective cerebral tissue perfusion

Trauma
- Death anxiety
- Disabled family coping
- Disturbed sensory perception (auditory)
- Risk for bleeding
- Risk for corneal injury
- Risk for self-directed violence
- Risk for shock
- Risk for urinary tract injury

Trigeminal neuralgia
- Acute pain
- Anxiety
- Deficient knowledge (specify)
- Imbalanced nutrition: Less than body requirements

Tuberculosis
- Deficient community health
- Deficient knowledge
- Fatigue
- Fear
- Impaired dentition
- Impaired gas exchange
- Ineffective airway clearance
- Ineffective breathing pattern
- Ineffective community coping
- Risk for infection
- Risk for loneliness
- Social isolation

Urinary calculi
- Acute pain
- Anxiety
- Impaired urinary elimination
- Ineffective tissue perfusion (renal)
- Readiness for enhanced urinary elimination
- Risk for infection
- Risk for urinary tract injury

Urinary diversion
- Acute pain
- Constipation
- Disturbed personal identity
- Grieving
- Impaired skin integrity
- Ineffective breathing pattern
- Ineffective sexuality patterns
- Risk for infection
- Sexual dysfunction

Urinary incontinence
- Anxiety
- Functional urinary incontinence
- Impaired skin integrity
- Overflow urinary incontinence
- Reflex urinary incontinence
- Social isolation
- Stress urinary incontinence
- Total urinary incontinence

Urinary tract infection
- Acute pain
- Impaired urinary elimination
- Readiness for enhanced urinary elimination
- Risk for infection
- Risk for urge urinary incontinence
- Stress urinary incontinence
- Urge urinary incontinence

Uterine prolapse
- Disturbed body image
- Stress urinary incontinence
- Risk for situational low self-esteem

Uterine rupture
- Acute pain
- Deficient fluid volume
- Ineffective tissue perfusion (cardiopulmonary)
- Ineffective tissue perfusion (cerebral)
- Ineffective tissue perfusion (renal)
- Risk for bleeding
- Risk for electrolyte imbalance
- Risk for shock

Vascular insufficiency
- Impaired tissue integrity
- Risk for peripheral neurovascular dysfunction

Viral hepatitis
- Deficient fluid volume
- Imbalanced nutrition: Less than body requirements
- Impaired skin integrity
- Risk for impaired skin integrity
- Risk for infection
- Social isolation

Index

A

B

C

D

E

F

G

H

I

J

K

L

M

N

O

P

R

S

T

U

V

W

NANDA International Nursing Diagnoses 2015–2017

Chapter 1 Adult Health Diagnoses

A
Activity Intolerance
Risk for Activity Intolerance
Ineffective Activity Planning
Risk for Ineffective Activity Planning
Decreased Intracranial Adaptive Capacity
Ineffective Airway Clearance
Risk for Allergy Response
Anxiety
Risk for Aspiration
Autonomic Dysreflexia
Risk for Autonomic Dysreflexia

B
Risk for Bleeding
Risk for Unstable Blood Glucose Level
Disturbed Body Image
Ineffective Breathing Pattern

C
Decreased Cardiac Output
Risk for Decreased Cardiac Output
Impaired Comfort
Acute Confusion
Risk for Acute Confusion
Chronic Confusion
Constipation
Risk for Constipation
Perceived Constipation
Defensive Coping
Ineffective Coping
Compromised Family Coping
Disabled Family Coping

D
Death Anxiety
Decisional Conflict
Ineffective Denial
Diarrhea
Risk for Disuse Syndrome
Deficient Diversional Activity
Risk for Dry Eye
Risk for Peripheral Neurovascular Dysfunction

E
Risk for Electrolyte Imbalance

F
Interrupted Family Processes
Fatigue
Fear
Deficient Fluid Volume
Risk for Deficient Fluid Volume
Excess Fluid Volume
Risk for Imbalanced Fluid Volume

G
Impaired Gas Exchange
Dysfunctional Gastrointestinal Motility
Risk For Dysfunctional Gastrointestinal Motility
Risk for Ineffective Gastrointestinal Perfusion
Grieving
Complicated Grieving
Risk for Complicated Grieving

H
Risk-Prone Health Behavior
Ineffective Health Management
Ineffective Family Health Management
Impaired Home Maintenance
Hopelessness
Risk for Compromised Human Dignity
Hyperthermia
Hypothermia

I
Bowel Incontinence
Functional Urinary Incontinence
Overflow Urinary Incontinence
Reflex Urinary Incontinence
Stress Urinary Incontinence
Urge Urinary Incontinence
Risk for Infection
Risk for Injury
Risk for Urinary Tract Injury
Insomnia

K
Deficient Knowledge

L
Latex Allergy Response
Risk for Latex Allergy Response
Sedentary Lifestyle
Risk for Impaired Liver Function
Risk for Loneliness

M
Impaired Memory
Impaired Physical Mobility
Moral Distress
Impaired Oral Mucous Membrane

N
Nausea
Noncompliance
Imbalanced Nutrition: Less Than Body Requirements

O
Obesity

P
Acute Pain
Chronic Pain
Chronic Pain Syndrome
Risk for Poisoning
Risk for Perioperative-Positioning Injury
Post-Trauma Syndrome
Risk for Post-Trauma Syndrome
Powerlessness
Risk for Powerlessness
Risk for Pressure Ulcer
Ineffective Protection

R
Risk for Adverse Reaction to Iodinated Contrast Media
Impaired Religiosity
Readiness for Enhanced Religiosity
Risk for Impaired Religiosity
Relocation Stress Syndrome
Risk for Ineffective Renal Perfusion
Ineffective Role Performance
Caregiver Role Strain
Risk for Caregiver Role Strain

S

Bathing Self-Care Deficit
Dressing Self-Care Deficit
Feeding Self-Care Deficit
Toileting Self-Care Deficit
Readiness for Enhanced Self-Care
Chronic Low Self-Esteem
Situational Low Self-Esteem
Risk for Situational Low Self-Esteem
Self-Neglect
Sexual Dysfunction
Ineffective Sexuality Pattern
Risk for Shock
Impaired Sitting
Impaired Skin Integrity
Risk for Impaired Skin Integrity
Sleep Deprivation
Disturbed Sleep Pattern
Impaired Social Interaction
Spiritual Distress
Risk for Spiritual Distress
Impaired Spontaneous Ventilation
Impaired Standing
Stress Overload
Risk for Suffocation
Delayed Surgical Recovery
Impaired Swallowing

T

Risk for Thermal Injury
Ineffective Thermoregulation
Impaired Tissue Integrity
Risk for Impaired Tissue Integrity
Risk for Decreased Cardiac Tissue Perfusion
Risk for Ineffective Cerebral Tissue Perfusion
Risk for Ineffective Peripheral Tissue Perfusion
Impaired Transfer Ability
Risk for Trauma
Risk for Vascular Trauma

U

Unilateral Neglect
Impaired Urinary Elimination
Readiness for Enhanced Urinary Elimination
Urinary Retention

V

Dysfunctional Ventilatory Weaning Response
Impaired Verbal Communication

W

Impaired Walking
Wandering

Chapter 2 Adolescent Health Diagnoses

B

Disturbed Body Image

D

Decisional Conflict

H

Ineffective Health Maintenance

P

Risk for Poisoning

R

Risk for Caregiver Role Strain

S

Risk for Self-Directed Violence
Situational Low Self-Esteem
Social Isolation

T

Risk for Trauma

Chapter 3 Child Health Diagnoses

A

Risk for Aspiration
Risk for Impaired Attachment

B

Disturbed Body Image
Risk for Imbalanced Body Temperature
Ineffective Breathing Pattern

C

Chronic Functional Constipation
Disabled Family Coping

D

Impaired Dentition
Risk for Delayed Development
Diarrhea
Deficient Diversional Activity

F

Fear
Deficient Fluid Volume
Risk for Deficient Fluid Volume

G

Grieving
Risk for Disproportionate Growth

H

Hyperthermia

I

Risk for Injury
Risk for Corneal Injury

K

Deficient Knowledge

N

Imbalanced Nutrition: Less Than Body Requirements

O

Overweight
Risk for Overweight

P

Acute Pain
Impaired Parenting
Risk for Impaired Parenting

R

Parental Role Conflict

S

Bathing Self-Care Deficit
Dressing Self-Care Deficit
Feeding Self-Care Deficit
Toileting Self-Care Deficit

T

Ineffective Thermoregulation

V

Impaired Verbal Communication

Chapter 4 Maternal-Neonatal Health Diagnoses

A

Anxiety
Risk for Aspiration

B

Disorganized Infant Behavior
Readiness for Enhanced Organized Infant Behavior
Risk for Disorganized Infant Behavior
Insufficient Breast Milk
Ineffective Breast-feeding
Interrupted Breast-feeding

Readiness for Enhanced Breast-feeding
Ineffective Breathing Pattern

C
Ineffective Childbearing Process
Risk for Ineffective Childbearing Process
Ineffective Coping
Compromised Family Coping

F
Interrupted Family Processes
Readiness for Enhanced Family Processes
Ineffective Infant Feeding Pattern
Deficient Fluid Volume

H
Hypothermia
Risk for Hypothermia

I
Risk for Infection
Risk for Injury

J
Neonatal Jaundice
Risk for Neonatal Jaundice

K
Deficient Knowledge

M
Risk for Disturbed Maternal–Fetal Dyad

N
Imbalanced Nutrition: Less Than Body Requirements

P
Acute Pain
Labor Pain
Impaired Parenting
Readiness for Enhanced Parenting

S
Risk for Situational Low Self-Esteem
Impaired Skin Integrity
Risk for Sudden Infant Death Syndrome

T
Ineffective Thermoregulation

U
Impaired Urinary Elimination

Chapter 5 Geriatric Health Diagnoses

A
Risk for Activity Intolerance

B
Disturbed Body Image
Risk for Imbalanced Body Temperature

C
Decreased Cardiac Output
Risk for Impaired Cardiovascular Function
Constipation
Ineffective Coping
Compromised Family Coping

D
Ineffective Denial

F
Risk for Falls
Frail Elderly Syndrome
Risk for Frail Elderly Syndrome

G
Impaired Gas Exchange
Grieving

H
Impaired Home Maintenance
Risk for Perioperative Hypothermia

I
Stress Urinary Incontinence
Risk for Urge Urinary Incontinence
Risk for Injury

K
Deficient Knowledge (Specify)

M
Impaired Bed Mobility
Impaired Wheelchair Mobility
Risk for Impaired Oral Mucous Membrane

N
Readiness for Enhanced Nutrition

P
Risk for Poisoning
Powerlessness

R
Risk for Relocation Stress Syndrome
Ineffective Role Performance

S
Risk for Self-Directed Violence
Situational Low Self-Esteem
Ineffective Sexuality Pattern
Risk for Impaired Skin Integrity
Social Isolation
Readiness for Enhanced Spiritual Well-Being

V
Impaired Verbal Communication

Chapter 6 Psychiatric and Mental Health Diagnoses

A
Anxiety

C
Ineffective Coping

E
Impaired Emancipated Decision Making
Readiness for Enhanced Emancipated Decision Making
Risk for Impaired Emancipated Decision Making
Labile Emotional Control

F
Dysfunctional Family Processes
Interrupted Family Processes

H
Hopelessness

I
Ineffective Impulse Control
Risk for Injury

K
Deficient Knowledge

M
Impaired Mood Regulation

O
Risk for Other-Directed Violence

P
Disturbed Personal Identity
Risk for Disturbed Personal Identity
Posttrauma Syndrome
Powerlessness

R
Rape-Trauma Syndrome
Ineffective Relationship
Risk for Ineffective Relationship
Impaired Resilience
Risk for Impaired Resilience
Caregiver Role Strain

S
Risk for Chronic Low Self-Esteem
Self-Mutilation
Risk for Self-Mutilation
Sexual Dysfunction
Social Isolation
Chronic Sorrow
Risk for Suicide

V
Impaired Verbal Communication

Chapter 7 Community-Based Health Diagnoses

C
Contamination
Risk for Contamination
Ineffective Community Coping

F
Fear

G
Grieving

H
Deficient Community Health
Ineffective Health Maintenance

I
Risk for Infection

K
Deficient Knowledge

N
Imbalanced Nutrition: Less Than Body Requirements

P
Risk for Poisoning

R
Risk for Caregiver Role Strain

S
Readiness for Enhanced Spiritual Well-Being
Impaired Spontaneous Ventilation

Chapter 8 Wellness Diagnoses

C
Readiness for Enhanced Childbearing Process
Readiness for Enhanced Comfort
Readiness for Enhanced Communication
Readiness for Enhanced Coping
Readiness for Enhanced Community Coping
Readiness for Enhanced Family Coping

D
Readiness for Enhanced Decision Making

F
Readiness for Enhanced Fluid Balance

H
Readiness for Enhanced Hope

K
Readiness for Enhanced Knowledge

P
Readiness for Enhanced Power

R
Readiness for Enhanced Relationship
Readiness for Enhanced Resilience

S
Readiness for Enhanced Self-Care
Readiness for Enhanced Self-Concept
Readiness for Enhanced Sleep
Readiness for Enhanced Spiritual Well-Being
